THE VEIN BOOK

THE VEIN BOOK

SECOND EDITION

EDITED BY

John J. Bergan

Nisha Bunke-Paquette

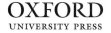

OXFORD
UNIVERSITY PRESS

OXFORD
UNIVERSITY PRESS

Oxford University Press is a department of the University of
Oxford. It furthers the University's objective of excellence in research,
scholarship, and education by publishing worldwide.

Oxford   New York

Auckland   Cape Town   Dar es Salaam   Hong Kong   Karachi
Kuala Lumpur   Madrid   Melbourne   Mexico City   Nairobi
New Delhi   Shanghai   Taipei   Toronto

With offices in

Argentina   Austria   Brazil   Chile   Czech Republic   France   Greece
Guatemala   Hungary   Italy   Japan   Poland   Portugal   Singapore
South Korea   Switzerland   Thailand   Turkey   Ukraine   Vietnam

Oxford is a registered trademark of Oxford University Press
in the UK and certain other countries.

Published in the United States of America by
Oxford University Press
198 Madison Avenue, New York, NY 10016

Library of Congress Cataloging-in-Publication Data
The vein book / edited by John J. Bergan, Nisha Bunke-Paquette.—2nd ed.
p. ; cm.
Includes bibliographical references and index.
ISBN 978–0–19–539963–9
I. Bergan, John J., 1927–   II. Bunke-Paquette, Nisha.
[DNLM: 1. Venous Insufficiency.   2. Veins—physiopathology.   3. Venous Thromboembolism. WG 600]
RC695
616.1′4—dc23
2013016280

3 5 7 9 8 6 4
Printed in China on acid-free paper

CONTENTS

PART V
CONGENITAL VENOUS ABNORMALITIES

CONTRIBUTING AUTHOR LIST

Ali F. AbuRahma
Robert C. Byrd Health Sciences Center
West Virginia University
Charleston, WV

Claudio Allegra
University La Sapienza
Rome, Italy

Jose I. Almeida
Miami Vein Center
Miami, FL

Niren Angle
University of California, San Diego Health System
San Diego, CA

J. I. Arcelus
Hospital Virgen de las Nieves
University of Granada
Granada, Spain

John J. Bergan
University of California, San Diego
La Jolla, CA

David Bergqvist
Uppsala University Hospital
Uppsala, Sweden

Kevin Broder
University of California, San Diego Health Systems
VA San Diego Healthcare System
La Jolla, CA

Warner P. Bundens
VA San Diego Healthcare System
La Jolla, CA

Nisha Bunke-Paquette
La Jolla Vein Care
VA San Diego Healthcare System
La Jolla, CA

Juan Cabrera
Instituto Internacional de Flebologia
Barcelona, Spain

Juan Cabrera Jr.
University Clinic of Navarra
Granada, Spain

Alberto Caggiati
University La Sapienza
Rome, Italy

Joseph A. Caprini
Evanston Northwestern Healthcare
Evanston, IL

Teresa L. Carman
University Hospitals Case Medical Center
Case Western Reserve University School of Medicine
Cleveland, OH

Attilio Cavezzi
Clinic Stella Maris
Tronto, Italy

Santiago Chahwan
Jobst Vascular Center
The Toledo Hospital
Toledo, OH

S. Chastanet
Riviera Vein Institute
Nice, France

Amy Clough
Melbourne Vascular Ultrasound
Melbourne, Australia

Anthony J. Comerota
Jobst Vascular Center
The Toledo Hospital
Toledo, OH

Michael H. Criqui
University of California, San Diego
La Jolla, CA

Michael C. Dalsing
Indiana University School of Medicine
Indianapolis, IN

Alun H. Davies
Charing Cross Hospital
London, United Kingdom

Meryl Davis
Charing Cross Hospital
London, United Kingdom

Marianne De Maeseneer
University Hospital of Antwerp
Edegem, Belgium

Julie O. Denenberg
University of California, San Diego
La Jolla, CA

Jose A. Diaz
School of Medicine, University of Michigan
Ann Arbor, MI

Walter N. Duran
New Jersey Medical School
Newark, NJ

Bo Eklöf
Doctors Office Center
Helsingborg, Sweden

David A. Frankel
Scripps Healthcare System
La Jolla, CA

Arnost Fronek
University of California, San Diego
La Jolla, CA

Steven S. Gale
Jobst Vascular Center
The Toledo Hospital
Toledo, OH

Peter Gloviczki
Mayo Clinic
Rochester, MN

Linda M. Graham
Cleveland Clinic Lerner Research Institute
Cleveland, OH

Jean-Jérôme Guex
Phlebology Clinic
Nice, France

John A. Heit
Mayo Clinic
Rochester, MN

Russell D. Hull
Foothills Hospital
Calgary, Alberta, Canada

Marcello Izzo
University of Ferrara
Ferrara, Italy

Colleen M. Johnson
Division of Vascular Surgery
Southern Illinois University School of Medicine
Springfield, IL

Damien Jolley
Monash University
Victoria, Australia

Manju Kalra
Mayo Clinic
Rochester, MN

Nikhil Kansal
Steward Health Care System
Brighton, MA

Robert M. Kaplan
UCLA School of Public Health
Los Angeles, CA

Robert L. Kistner
Kistner Vein Clinic
Honolulu, HI

Brajesh K. Lal
University of Maryland Medical Center (UMMC)
Baltimore, MD

Robert D. Langer
Jackson Hole Center for Preventive Medicine
Jackson, WY

James Laredo
George Washington University School of Medicine
Washington, D.C.

Byung-Boong (B.B.) Lee
George Washington University School of Medicine
Washington, DC

Andrew Li
University of California, San Diego School of Medicine
San Diego, CA

Timothy K. Liem
Oregon Health & Science University
Portland, OR

T. Locret
Riviera Vein Institute
Nice, France

Nicole Loerzel
La Jolla Vein Care
La Jolla, CA

Joann M. Lohr
Lohr Surgical Specialists
Cincinnati, OH

Fedor Lurie
Kistner Vein Clinic
Honolulu, HI

Oscar Maleti
Hesperia Hospital Modena
Modena, Italy

William Marston
University of North Carolina, Chapel Hill
Chapel Hill, NC

Elna Masuda
Straub Clinic & Hospital
Honolulu, HI

John C. McCallum
University of California, San Diego Health System
San Diego, CA

Robert B. McLafferty
Southern Illinois University School of Medicine
Springfield, IL

Nick Morrison
Morrison Vein Institute
Scottsdale, AZ

Geza Mozes
Mayo Clinic
Rochester, MN

Daniel D. Myers Jr.
University of Michigan School of Medicine
Ann Arbor, MI

Kenneth Myers
Epworth Hospital
Richmond, Australia

Francisco J. Osse
Vein Center of Sao Paulo
Sao Paulo, Brazil

Frank T. Padberg Jr.
New Jersey Medical School
Newark, NJ

Peter J. Pappas
New Jersey Medical School
Newark, NJ

Hugo Partsch
University of Vienna
Vienna, Austria

Luigi Pascarella
Duke University Medical Center
Durham, NC

Michel Perrin
Clinique du Grande Large
Chassieu, France

Graham F. Pineo
Foothills Hospital
Calgary, Alberta, Canada

Paul Pittaluga
Riviera Vein Institute
Nice, France

Alessandra Puggioni
Scottsdale Vascular Services
Scottsdale, AZ

Joseph D. Raffetto
VA Boston Healthcare System
Boston, MA

Jeffrey K. Raines
Miami Vein Center
Miami, FL

Seshadri Raju
The RANE Center for Venous and Lymphatic Diseases
River Oaks Hospital
Jackson, MS

Albert-Adrien Ramelet
Lausanne, Switzerland

Virginia Ratcliff
La Jolla Vein Care
La Jolla, CA

Pritham P. Reddy
Southern Illinois University School of Medicine
Springfield, IL

Graeme D. Richardson
Rural Clinical School
Wagga Wagga, Australia

Stefania Roberts
Victoria Vein Clinic
East Melbourne, Australia

Maria V. Rubia
Instituto Internacional de Flebologia
Barcelona, Spain

Teresa Russell
VA San Diego Healthcare System
La Jolla, CA

Robert B. Rutherford
The University of Colorado Medical Center
Corpus Christi, TX

Neil Sadick
Sadick Dermatology
New York, NY

Richard J. Sanders
Denver Vascular Surgical Associates
Denver, CO

Jocelyn A. Segall
Oregon Health & Science University
Portland, OR

A. C. Shepherd
Charing Cross Hospital
London, United Kingdom

Philip Coleridge Smith
British Vein Institute
London, United Kingdom

Lian Sorhaindo
Weill Cornell Medical College of Cornell University
New York, NY

Patrick A. Stone
CAMC Health Systems
Charleston, WV

Paul K. Thibault
Central Vein & Cosmetic Medical Centre
Broadmeadow, Australia

Patricia E. Thorpe
University of Arizona Medical Center
Arizona Heart Hospital
Phoenix, AZ

Thomas W. Wakefield
University of Michigan School of Medicine
Ann Arbor, MI

Theodore E. Warkentin
McMaster University
Hamilton General Hospital
Hamilton, Ontario, Canada

Margaret A. Weiss
Johns Hopkins School of Medicine
Baltimore, MD

Robert A. Weiss
Johns Hopkins School of Medicine
Baltimore, MD

Robert W. Zickler
New Jersey Medical School
Newark, NJ

Steven E. Zimmet
Zimmet Vein and Dermatology Clinic
Austin, TX

PART I

BASIC CONSIDERATIONS

1.

HISTORICAL INTRODUCTION

Alberto Caggiati and Claudio Allegra

In 1628, William Harvey explained in his *De Motu Cordis* the theory of the blood circulation (see Figure 1.1). However, the discovery of the circulation was not complete until 1661, when Marcello Malpighi in his *De Pulmonibus* demonstrated by microscopy the existence of the capillaries (see Figure 1.2).

The heart has been regarded as the center of the vascular system (Empedocles of Agrigentum; 500–430 BC) since the fifth century BC. The great epic of India, *Mahabharata*, stated that "all veins proceed from the heart, upwards, downwards and sideways and convey the essences of food to all parts of the body." The Chinese Wang Shu Ho reported in his *Mei ching* that "the heart regulates all the blood in the body… The blood current flows continuously in a circle and never stops." Herasistratus (310–250 BC) was so close to the discovery of the circulation as to guess the existence of capillaries: "the blood passes from the veins into arteries thorough 'anastomoses,' small inter-communicating vessels."

These correct theories were darkened by Hippocratic dogma for centuries. Hippocrates of Cos, the "father of Medicine" (460–377 BC) affirmed in *De Nutritione* that the liver is the "root" of all veins, that the veins alone contain blood destined for the body's nourishment, and that arteries contain an elastic ethereal fluid, the "spirit of life." This incorrect theory, based on the Pythagorean doctrine of the four humors (blood, phlegm, yellow bile, and black bile), remained the basis for medical practice for more than 2000 years.

Beginning in the fourteenth century, many authors confuted the Hippocratic theory, allowing, and sometimes anticipating, Harvey's discovery; but more than three centuries (1316–1661) passed before it was abolished. In 1316, Mondino de Luzzi furnished a rudimental but exact description of the circulatory system that was omitted by all subsequent authors:

Postea vero versus pulmonem est aliud orificium venae arterialis, quae portat sanguinem ad pulmonem a corde; quia cum pulmo deserviat cordi secundum modum dictum, ut ei recompenset, cor ei transmittit sanguinem per hanc venam, quae vocatur vena arterialis; est vena, quia portat sanguinem, et arterialis, quia habet duas tunicas; et habet duas tunicas, primo quia vadit ad membrum quod existit in continuo motu, et secundo quia portat sanguinem valde subtilem et cholericum.

The same occurred to the Spanish Ludovicus Vassaeus and Michael Servetus. The anatomy of the cardiovascular system was so well depicted by Vassaeus (*De Anatomen Corporis Humani Tabulae Quator*, 1544) that Marie Jean Pierre Florens affirmed that he "described the blood circulation a century before William Harvey." In 1546, the anti-Arabist theologician and physician Servetus exactly described the pulmonary circulation: "the blood enters the lungs by the way of the pulmonary artery in greater quantities than necessary for their nutrition, mixes with the pneuma and returns by way the pulmonary veins." Servetus's discovery did not diffuse among contemporary physicians, probably because it was reported in a theological book. Servetus's theories were so innovative that he was accused of heresy by Calvinists and burned. Andrea Cesalpino, professor of medicine at Rome, first identified the function of the valves ("certain membranes placed at the openings of the vessels prevent the blood from returning") and the centripetal direction of the flow in the veins (1571). He also supposed the existence of "*vasa in capillamenta resoluta*" (capillaries) and affirmed that in the lung the blood "is distributed into fine branches and comes in contact with the air" (1583). Finally, he coined the term "circulation." According to important historians like Florens, Richet, and Castiglioni, Cesalpino did the groundwork for Harvey's revelation.

VENOUS ANATOMY

The first systematic description of the venous system was given by André Vesale (alias Vesalius) in *De Humanis Corporis Fabrica* (1543). Vesalius's venous anatomy was almost complete (see Figure 1.3) though it contained some

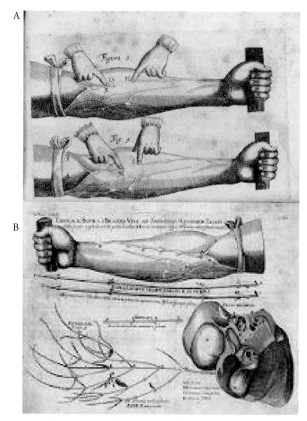

Figure 1.1 (A) The famous illustration used by Harvey in his *De Motu Cordis* (1661) showing the direction of flow into the veins and (B) the plate published sixty years before by Hyeronimus Fabricius of Acquapendente (1603).

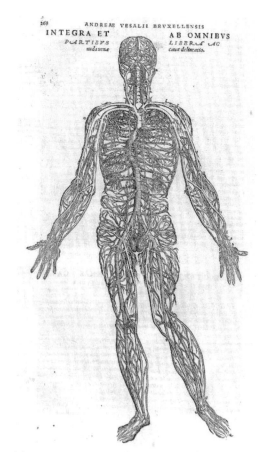

Figure 1.3 The venous system according to Vesalius (1545).

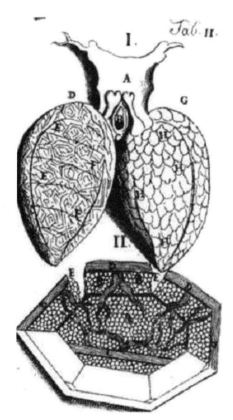

Figure 1.2 The original Malpighi's representation of the lung capillary bed (*De Pulmonibus*, 1661).

omissions, such as venous valves and perforating veins. Vesalius furnished a good description of the structure of the venous wall. He differentiated the internal coat of the veins in two layers. The internal one contained contractile fibers, though "dissimilar from those of skeletal muscles, arranged, from within outwards, circularly, obliquely and longitudinally." The outer coat was formed by a loose network borrowed from surrounding structures.

VESALIUS'S OMISSION I: VENOUS VALVES

Giovanni Battista Canano from Ferrara, was the first to describe venous valves in 1540 ("*ostiola sive opercula*"), in the renal, azygos, and external iliac veins. According to Franck Cockett, "he identified correctly the function of the valves, i.e., to avoid blood reflux." Further sporadic descriptions of venous valves were given by the Spanish anatomist Vassaeus (1544) and, one year later, by Charles Estienne ("*apophyses membranarum*"). Valves in the veins of the lower limbs first were reported by Sylvius Ambianus in 1555, and their first illustrations appeared in the Salomon Alberti's *De valvulis membraneis vasorum* (1585). Finally, Hyeronimus Fabricius of Acquapendente published in 1603 an exhaustive description of the valves of the veins with magnificent figures (see Figure 1.4) that were used by his pupil Harvey to demonstrate the direction of flow (see Figure 1.1). Four centuries

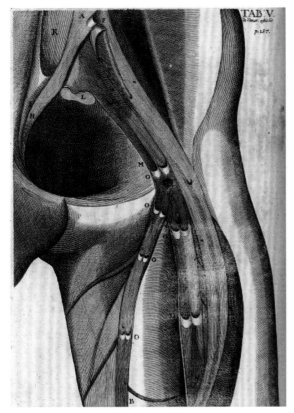

Figure 1.4 The saphenofemoral junction according to Fabricius (1603).

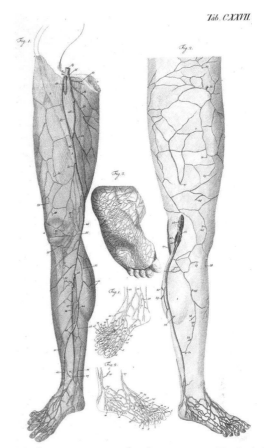

Figure 1.5 The first representation of perforating veins in Von Loder's *Anatomische Tafeln* (1803).

passed before it was demonstrated that venous valves not only steer blood return and prevent reflux but also, according to Lurie et al, modulate venous flow.[1]

VESALIUS'S OMISSION II: PERFORATING VEINS

The second gap in Vesalius's venous anatomy was filled at the beginning of the nineteenth century (1803), when the anatomist Justus Christian Von Loder represented exactly the more important perforating veins of the human body (see Figure 1.5). Von Loder omitted a description of their function; that was clarified only in 1855, when Aristide August Verneuil described the presence of valves within perforating veins and the direction of blood flow in them.

THE RETURN OF THE VENOUS BLOOD

The mechanisms allowing blood to flow centripetally along the veins were described more than two hundreds years ago (see Table 1.1). The "*vis a tergo*" was described in 1670 by Richard Lower: "the return of the venous blood is the result of the impulse given to the arterial blood." Furthermore, Lower acknowledged an important role to the "*venarum tono*" in venous return, and described the effects of the muscular pumping. Antonio Valsalva, pupil of Malpighi, described in 1710 the aspiratory forces that enhance venous return to the heart: the "*vis a fronte*" due to the rhythmic respiratory changes of thoracoabdominal pressure. In 1728, Giovanni Lancisi demonstrated experimentally the spontaneous rhythmical contraction of larger veins. Finally, John Hunter suggested in 1793 that the pulsation of arteries assists the blood return in certain veins. J. F. Palmer, the editor of the posthumous Hunterian *Of the Vascular System* (1837), added a footnote: "especially when a common sheath exists."

ETIOLOGY AND PATHOGENESIS OF VARICOSE VEINS

Hippocrates was the first to deal with the pathogenesis and epidemiology of varicose disease when he affirmed that

Table 1.1 MECHANISMS OF VENOUS PROPULSION

1670	Richard Lower	*Propulsive vis a tergo*
1670	Richard Lower	Muscle pump
1670	Richard Lower	Tone of the venous wall
1710	Antonio Valsalva	*Aspirative vis a fronte*
1728	Giovanni Lancisi	Contraction of the venous wall
1793	John Hunter	Pulsation of neighboring arteries

varicose veins were more frequent in Scythians because of the prolonged time spent on the horseback with the legs hanging down. In 1514, Marianus Sanctus noted that varicose veins were more frequent after pregnancy and in people who stood for long periods of time ("standing too much before kings"). In 1545, Ambroise Paré related varicose veins to pregnancy and long traveling and affirmed that they are more frequent in melancholic subjects. Ten years later, Jean Fernel (1554), professor of medicine at Paris, stated that varicose veins can develop after an effort or a trauma: "the varix comes also from a blow, from a contusion, from an effort." Rudolf Virchow (1846) was the first to point out the hereditary tendency to varicose veins. Finally, the rare syndrome due to congenital absence of venous valves was first reported by Josephus Luke in 1941.

The first to attribute the onset of varicose veins to valvular incompetence was Hyeronimus Fabricius (1603). The parietal theory first was promulgated by Richard Lower, who in 1670 affirmed that a *"relaxatio venarum tono"* (wall muscular looseness) is the cause of venous stasis and dilation. Pierre Dionis credited in 1707 an important role to mechanical compression of large trunks in the development of varicose veins, whereas Jean Louis Petit (1774), the eminent French surgeon, reported their possible occurrence during obstruction of proximal veins. According to these two authors, the clinical syndromes due to compression of the left common iliac vein were described by the Canadian James McMurrich in 1906, and of the popliteal vein by Norman Rich and Carl Hughes in 1967. Al Sadr described in 1950 the compression of the left renal vein by the aorta and the superior mesenteric artery. Paul Briquet was the first to affirm in 1824 that varicose veins are due to abnormal flow coming from deep veins via the perforators. In 1944, E Malan described the occurrence of varicose veins in limbs with abnormal arteriovenous connections. The theory of a subclinical parietal phlogosis inducing venous valve disruption has been proposed only recently by Takashi Ono, John J. Bergan, Geert Schmid-Schonbein.[2]

VENOUS THROMBOSIS

In 1544, the Spanish anatomist Vassaeus first identified the "vascular dessication" described by Hippocratic medicine with the phenomena of "coagulation," that is, loss of the liquid state of the blood. One year later, Paré first described superficial phlebitis ("a swollen vein, with jelly blood, spontaneously painful"). In 1793, John Hunter introduced the term "phlebothrombosis" and affirmed that inflammation of the venous wall is always accompanied by the formation of a clot. Matthew Baillie (1793), in contrast to Hunter, considered flow deceleration the cause of thrombosis. Virchow, the greatest pathologist of all time, defined in 1846 the famous triad of conditions essential for development of thrombosis: slowing of flow or its cessation, excess of circulating thrombogenic factors, and disruption

of the endothelial lining. Only one century later (1946), MacFarlane and Biggs described the "cascade" mechanism for coagulation.

The "white swelling" of the lower limb or *phlegmasia alba dolens* was accounted for by Charles White in 1784. In 1857, Jean Baptiste Cruveilhier described the *"phlébite bleue"* (*phlegmasia coerulea dolens*) and affirmed it is due to the thrombosis of all the veins with patency of the arteries (see Figures 1.6 and 1.7). Sir James Paget investigated the pathogenesis of phlebitis and described in 1866 a great number of possible causes: traumatic phlebitis; distension phlebitis; phlebitis occurring in exhaustion or during either acute or chronic disease; phlebitis due to extension of inflammation from an ulcer; idiopathic, puerperal, and pyemial phlebitis; and finally, phlebitis occurring in varicose limbs. A clear nosologic discrimination between phlebothrombosis and thrombophlebitis was finally indicated by Ochsner and De Bakey in 1939. The possible occurrence of venous thrombosis of the leg due to prolonged sitting was first described by John Homans (1954). Incorrectly, the association of prolonged sitting and venous thrombosis was then limited to air travel and assumed the name "Economy Class Syndrome."

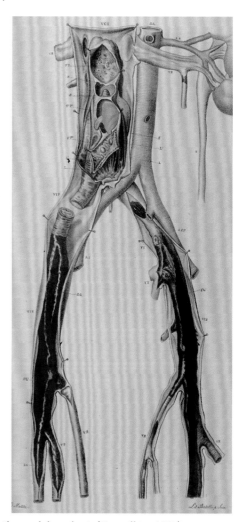

Figure 1.6   Ileocaval thrombosis (Cruveilhier, 1857).

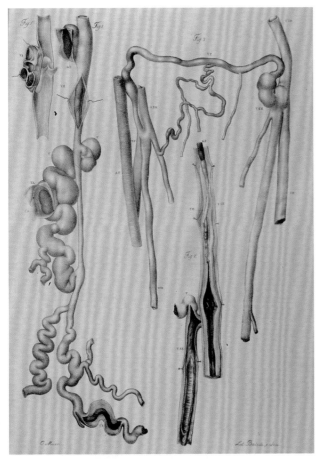

Figure 1.7   Postthrombotic varicose veins (Cruveilhier, 1857).

Lipiodol. In 1929, McPheeters and Rice performed the first dynamic varicography and described the movement of blood in the varicose veins. Further developments were due to Ratschow (who in 1930 introduced water soluble contrast media for angiography), Dos Santos (who demonstrated in 1938 the utility of direct ascending contrast venography to detect deep venous thrombosis, or DVT), and Farinas (who performed the first pelvic venography in 1947). Intraosseus phlebography was then proposed by Schobinger in 1960 and refined by Lea Thomas in 1970. Finally, Dow described in 1973 the technique to perform retrograde phlebography.

Traditional venography is even less used in daily practice due to the achievement of duplex sonography. However, radiologic venous imaging recently improved due to the introduction of computed tomography (CT) and magnetic resonance (MR) techniques. CT was introduced in 1980 to demonstrate venous thrombosis by Zerhouni. Multislice CT, proposed first in 1994 by Stehling to evaluate the venous bed of the lower limb, also is indicated for the contemporary evaluation of the pulmonary vessels. More recently, multislice CT has been proposed to obtain 3D images (see Figure 1.8) of superficial veins[3] with special reference to the preoperative evaluation of varicose limbs.[4] MR was introduced in the field of the diagnosis of DVT in 1986 by Erdman. MR venous imaging improved after 2001, when the group of Jorge Debatin proposed the technique called "low-dose, direct-contrast-injection 3D MR venography."[5]

DIAGNOSIS OF VENOUS DISORDERS

CLINICAL SEMIOTICS

Clinical semiotics started in 1806, when the Swiss surgeon Tommaso Rima described a simple test for the diagnosis of saphenous reflux. In 1846, Sir Benjamin Brodie described a method of testing for incompetent valves by constriction of the limb and palpation. These two tests were reproposed by Friedrich Trendelenburg in 1890. In 1896, Georg Perthes of Bonn described the famous test to verify the patency of the deep veins. Finally, in 1938, John Homans described a test for detection of deep venous obstruction based on foot dorsiflexion. Surprisingly, these tests and maneuvers still appear in modern texts of vascular medicine and venous surgery.

PHLEBOGRAPHY

The history of phlebography started in 1923, when Berberich and Hirsch described the technique to demonstrate the venous system in living humans by infusion of strontium bromide. One year later, Sicard and Forestier performed the first phlebography in humans using

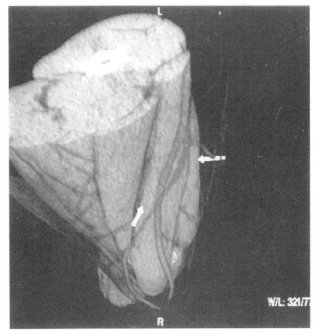

Figure 1.8   The first contrastless 3D venography by multislice CT (Caggiati, 1999).

ULTRASONIC VENOUS FLOW EVALUATION AND IMAGING

The history of ultrasound in venous medicine started in 1961, when Stegall and Rushmer described the first Doppler instrument and the basis for its practical use. A refinement of the Doppler techniques for venous investigations was made in 1967 by Sigel and coworkers. One year later, fundamentals of Doppler investigation of deep venous thrombosis were furnished separately by Evans and Cockett, and Sumner and Strandness. The technique to evaluate valvular competence was deeply investigated in 1970 by Folse and Alexander.

The history of venous echotomography started in 1976, when Day focused the possible role of B-mode imaging of venous thrombi. Duplex scanning was proposed for the diagnosis of venous disorders in 1986 by the group of Szendro, Nicolaides, Myers, Malouf et al[6] and by that of Luizy, Franceschi, and Franco.[7]

OTHER DIAGNOSTIC TECHNIQUES

Other techniques have been proposed in the daily clinical evaluation of venous disorders (see Table 1.2).

COMPRESSION THERAPY

It has been well known since ancient civilizations that compression is the main therapeutic option for the conservative management of limbs afflicted with chronic venous insufficiency. Henry de Mondeville (1260–1320) affirmed that "compression expels bad humors that infiltrate legs and ulcers." The effectiveness of compression was explained in 1824 by Sir Astley Paston Cooper, who affirmed that it allows the venous valves to regain their competence. Clinical and hemodynamic effects of compression and bandages in

Table 1.2 **PROPOSALS FOR EVALUATION OF VENOUS DISORDERS**

1948	Pollack and Wood	Dynamic measurement of venous pressure
1953	Whitney	Impedance plethysmography
1960	Hobbs and Davies	Detection of thrombi by radioactive iodium
1968	Dahn	Strain gauge plethysmography
1969	Webber	Detection of thrombi by radioactive technetium
1971	Rosenthal	Radionuclide venography
1973	Norgren and Thulesius	Foot volumetry
1973	Cranley	Phleborheography
1979	Abramovitz	Photoplethysmography
1987	Van Rijn	Air plethysmography

the field of treatment of any form of venous insufficiency and of phlebitis are still deeply investigated.[8]

Techniques of bandaging changed minimally over the course of the centuries. In the fifth century BC, Hippocrates meticulously described how to apply leg bandages and how to obtain an eccentric compression by placing a sponge under the bandage. Giovanni Michele Savonarola (grandfather of the theologian Girolamo Savonarola) in 1440 recommended extending the application of bandages to the thigh. Bell (1778) proposed associating bandaging with bed rest, and Underwood (1787) with deambulation. In 1849, Thomas Hunt warned that bandages must be applied only by surgeons.

The use of compressive bandaging was extended to treatment of acute phlebitis in 1826 by Alfred Armand Louis Marie Velpeau, and associated with immediate mobilization by Einrich Fisher in 1910 in order to enhance its beneficial effects. Intermittent compression for the prevention of DVT and of its sequelae was proposed in 1971 by Sabri.

Materials for bandages varied greatly over the centuries. Celsus used linen rollers, Galen preferred wool, as well as split and sewn bandages. Aetius put bandages in an ear-of-corn shaped fashion. Fabricius introduced laced stockings made from dog's skin. At the end of the eighteenth century, dog skin was abandoned and laced stockings were made with linen. In 1783, Underwood first used an elastic bandage obtained with a Welsh flannel. At the same time (1797) Baynton introduced the eponymous bandage done with small plasters of pitch, resin, and lithargyre. Adhesive bandaging was introduced by Dickson Wright in 1830. Five years later, Muray and Claney described the first mechanical device for compression of the limb. Thanks to the introduction of rubber vulcanization in 1839 by Goodyear, elastic stockings were ideated and patented by William Brown in 1848. In 1878, Martin proposed obtaining elastic compression with rubber bandages. In 1896, Paul Gerson Unna combined local treatment with compression for treatment of venous ulcer by incorporating emollient compounds in a dressing that becomes increasingly rigid. The first seamless compression stocking is dated 1904, the first rubber-free in 1917. Ultrathin rubber strings were introduced in the late 1930s.

In 1902, Hoffmeister described the principles of mercury compression obtained by placing the edematous limb in a reservoir with 50 ml of mercury. Pneumatic devices with laced chambers adaptable to any form of extremities were proposed in 1955 by Brush and, in the same year, Samson and Kirby described the first sequential pressure pneumatic device furnished with fourteen compartments.

SCLEROTHERAPY

The beginning of sclerotherapy is commonly dated back to the invention of the syringe by Pravaz (1831), and of the hypodermic needle by Rynd (1845). However, earlier phlebologists could not wait for Rynd's and Pravaz's discoveries.

In fact, the first endovenous treatment goes back to 1665, when Sigismond Johann Elsholz treated venous ulcers by irrigating them with intravenous injection of distilled water and essences from plants using a chicken bone as a needle and a bladder of pigeon as a syringe. Some authors credit Zolliker as the first to perform sclerotherapy in 1682, by injecting acid into varicose veins. The rationale of sclerotherapy was furnished by Joseph Hodgson (1815) who noted first that "thrombosis extinguished varicose veins." In the second half of the eighteenth century, various substances were used (see Table 1.3), but adverse sequelae (local tissue necrosis, extravasation, pulmonary embolism, and scarring caused by poor technique and causticity of solutions) were so frequent and serious that, in 1894, at the Medical Congress of Lyon, sclerotherapy of varicose veins was firmly stopped. The adoption of safer sclerosants allowed, primarily in Europe, the renaissance of sclerotherapy at the beginning of the twentieth century.

The renaissance of sclerotherapy was also due to safer techniques and to its use in combination with surgery. Tavel (1904) injected varicose veins after high ligation of the saphena. In order to avoid innumerable skin incisions, Benedetto Schiassi, from Bologna (1909), performed multiple injections of a combined iodine and potassium iodide immediately after saphenous interruption (see Figure 1.9). Linser (1916) suggested using compression to reduce complication and to enhance the effects of the therapy. Ungher (1927) used a urethral catheter to perfuse varicose veins with sclerosing agents. Mc Ausland in 1939 recommended emptying the vein to be injected by elevating the leg and bandaging the leg after treatment.

Modern sclerotherapy developed in the 1960s. The tactics and the techniques to obtain even safer and more effective

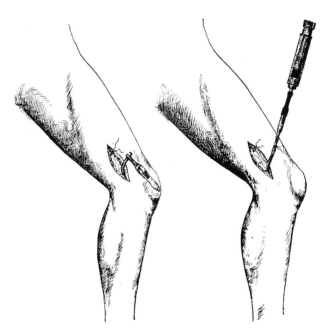

Figure 1.9 Schiassi's method to inject the GSV at the same time of its interruption (1909).

venous obliterations varied greatly between countries: the Swiss technique was proposed by Sigg; the French method by Tournay; Fegan popularized the so-called Irish technique, and Hobbs the English method. These techniques differed with relation to: (1) position of the patient; (2) progression of injections (from larger to smaller veins, or vice versa); (3) sclerosant agents, their concentrations, and quantity; (4) modalities, duration, extension, and strength of compression; and (5) size of the needle and modalities of injection.

In early 1990s, the safety and accuracy of sclerotherapy were greatly enhanced by the introduction of real-time control of needle position and wall reaction by echotomography ("echosclerosis," according to Schadeck). In the late 1990s to early 200s, the effectiveness of sclerotherapy was further improved thanks to the use of sclerosing foams, obtained by mixing slerosants with air (Tessari, Monfreux) or inert gas (Cabrera). However, the use of gas-sclerosant mixtures dates back to 1939 (Stuard Mc Ausland) and to 1944 (the "air-block technique" of Egmont James Orbach).

SURGERY OF SUPERFICIAL VEINS: THE DETRACTORS

In ancient civilizations, surgery of "serpent-shaped dilatations of lower limb veins" was advised to avoid dangerous hemorrhages and death (Papyrus of Ebers, 1550 BC). Only minimally invasive procedures were performed: "the varix itself is to be punctured in many places, as circumstances may indicate" in order to avoid that "large ulcers be the consequence of the incisions" (Hippocrates). This detracting theory persisted through the centuries. As an example, Wiseman (1676) discouraged surgery of varicose veins

Table 1.3 SOME OF THE SCLEROSANT AGENTS USED

1840	Monteggio	Absolute alcohol
1853	Pravaz	Iron perchloride
1855	Desgranges	Iodotannin
1880	Negretti	Iron chloride
1894	Medical Congress of Lyon: to stop sclerotherapy!	
1904	Tavel	Phenol + surgery
1909	Schiassi	Iodine and potassium iodide + surgery
1917	Kaush	Inverted sugar
1919	Sicard	Sodium saliciate
1926	Linser	Hypertonic saline
1930	Higgins and Kittel	Sodium morruate
1933	Jausion	Chromated glycerine
1946	Reiner	Sodium tetradecyl sulphate
1959	Imhoff and Sigg	Stabilized polyiodated ions
1966	Henschel and Eichenberg	Polidocanol

"unless they were painful, formed a large tumour, ulcerated, or bled" or when "purging and bleeding, not once or twice, but often repeated, fail."

SURGERY OF SUPERFICIAL VEINS: FORERUNNERS

First described by the Roman Celsus, hook extraction of the varicose vein, double ligation, and venectomy (or cautery) is the rough operation performed for centuries. Galenum used the hook to perform multiple ultrashort stripping of varicose veins. A great boost to varicose vein surgery come from the Byzantine physician Oribasius of Pergamum (325–405 AD), who devoted three chapters of his book to the treatment of varicose veins, an operation using a special hook called a *cirsulce*. Many of his recommendations are still valid:

1. Remove the veins, because if only ligated, they can form new varices.

2. Shave and bathe the leg to be operated.

3. When the leg is still warm, the surgeon has to mark varicose veins with the patient standing.

4. Extirpate varicose veins of the leg first, then at the thigh.

5. Remove clots by external compression of the limb.

Further important contributions were from Paulus of Aegina (seventh century), who described the main anatomy of varicose veins and identified the great saphenous vein (GSV) as their source. He isolated the varicose veins at the thigh by a longitudinal incision, and, after bloodletting, ligated them at both ends. The tied-off portion was excised or allowed to slough off later with the ligatures.

In Arab medicine, treatment of varicose veins was dominated by cautery. However, the Spanish El Zahrawi (Albucasis of Cordova) (936–1013) is credited by Anning as the first to use an external stripper. William of Saliceto advocated in his *Cyrurgia* (1476) the reintroduction of the knife into surgery and, a few decades later, Amboise Paré (1545) abandoned definitively external cauterization of varicose veins to reintroduce their ligation: "the incision must be placed a little above the knee, where a varicose vein is usually found to develop.…Ligature was needed for the purpose of cutting the channel and making a barrier against the blood and the humors contained within it which flow to varicose veins and fill any ulcer." A similar technique was used by Sir Benjamin Collins Brodie (1816): "after the skin over a varix was incised, the varix was divided with a curved bistoury and pressure was applied to prevent haemorrhage." Lorenz Heister (1718) placed a wax thread transcutaneously around the distal end of a varicose vein. Eight to ten ounces of the grumous and viscid blood was allowed to escape as the varix was laid open longitudinally. The wound was then bandaged and compressed. This technique was reproposed one century later by Alfred Armand Louis Marie Velpeau (1826) who "introduced a pin or needle through the skin, which is passed underneath the vein, and at right angles to it. A twisted suture is then applied round the two ends of the pin, so as to compress the vein sufficiently

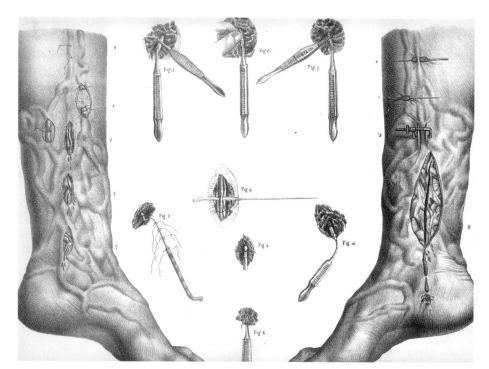

Figure 1.10 Techniques for venous obliteration from Davat (1), Velpeau (2), Sanson (3), Beclard (4), Wise (5), Fricke (6), and Richerand (7). Courtesy of Doctor Michel Georgiev. AU: Okay?

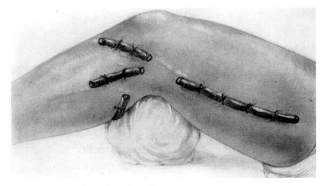

Figure 1.11 Velpeau's method (1826).

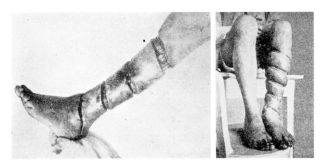

Figure 1.13 Rindfleish intervention (left) and its sequelae (1908) (right).

to produce its obliteration." (see Figures 1.10 and 1.11). Max Schede in 1877 operated on varicose limbs by multiple ligature or venesections and percutaneous ligations. Delbet described in 1884 the reimplantation of the terminal portion of the GSV just below a healthy femoral valve. In the same year, Madelung proposed a complete excision of the GSV (see Figure 1.12) through a long incision much like those used today in vein harvest for coronary bypass. On the contrary, in the operation proposed by Rindfleish and Friedel in 1908, the incision was spiral (see Figure 1.13) and the lancet plunged deep to the fascia. Saphenous ligation followed by sclerotherapy (see Figure 1.14) was proposed by Tavel (1904), whereas Schiassi (1905) injected varicose veins at the time of surgery (see Figure 1.9).

MODERN SURGERY OF SUPERFICIAL VEINS

Modern surgery of varicose veins started in 1806, when Tommaso Rima proposed a hemodynamic treatment with ligation of the upper GSV. This operation was reproposed in 1890 by Friedrich Trendelenburg: "the saphenous reflux must be the first step in control distal varicosities." It consisted of a double ligation of the GSV just inferior to the saphenofemoral junction, thanks to a 3-cm incision. He boasted that he could do "the operation so fast that no anaesthesia was required." Trendelenburg made it clear that this technique had to be applied only to those limbs in which the

compression tests, described by Brodie in 1846, revealed the incompetency of the saphenofemoral valve. In 1896, Moore of Melbourne refined the Trendelenburg operation, with the skin incision performed parallel and close to the inguinal fold, almost exactly as it is today. In the same year, Thelwall Thomas emphasized the importance of ligation and division of all branches at the saphenofemoral junction.

SAPHENOUS STRIPPING

The stripping technique was introduced by Charles Mayo (1904), who used an extraluminal device. In 1905, Keller described an intraluminal stripper to extirpate the GSV (see Figure 1.15). A twisted and rigid wire was passed into the

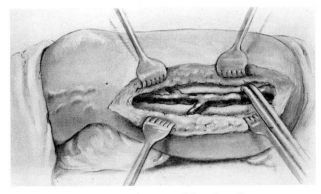

Figure 1.12 GSV excision according to Madelung (1884).

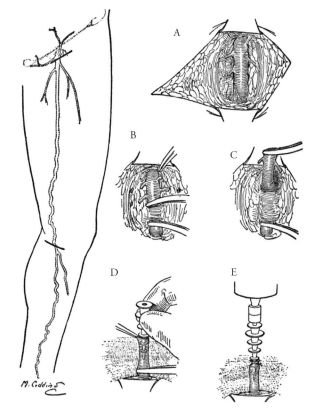

Figure 1.14 Saphenous interruption and its incannulation with the instrument called a *pagoda*.

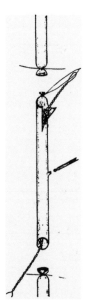

Figure 1.15 Keller's operation for saphenous extraction (1905).

vein lumen. The wire was brought throughout its lumen at a site distal to the divided end of the vein. Its end was tied to the ligated and divided end of the varicose vein. Extracting the wire distally inverted the end of the vein into itself as the vein was extracted. This technique was then refined by van der Stricht in 1963. In 1907, Babcock modified Keller's technique and proposed using an acorn tip and a flexible rod, which was more sophisticated than a twisted wire. His operation avoided tearing of the vein at the tributary junction, which occurs in the inversion technique. In 1920, Cole suggested limiting saphenectomy to the tract located between the groin and the knee. In 1930, De Takats refined the technique of Schiassi by proposing the ambulatory treatment of saphenous vein insufficiency followed by sclerotherapy. In 1947, Myers and Smith further refined the endoluminal flexible stripper.

BEYOND STRIPPING

Many effective techniques alternative to stripping were proposed in the second half of the twentieth century. First of all, the ancient art of hook phlebectomy was so improved by Robert Muller (1956) that it became possible to operate, with local anesthesia and small incisions, on both saphenae for their entire length. Muller's stab avulsion technique was further refined and diffused worldwide in 1995 by Ricci, Georgiev, and Goldman.[9] In 1988, Claude Franceschi proposed a minimally invasive surgical approach (conservatrice et hemodynamique de l'insuffisance veineuse en ambulatoire [CHIVA]) aimed to a hemodynamic correction, more than to a radical avulsion of the varicose bed, based on a meticulous preoperative Duplex examination. External banding of the terminal saphena has been largely adopted by many centers, but its results are good only if performed in limbs with

early disease, as demonstrated by Corcos et al in 1997.[10] This procedure was refined in 2002 by Yamaki,[11] who associated valvuloplasty of the subterminal valve combined to the axial transposition of a competent tributary vein.

ENDOVASCULAR TECHNIQUES

The first to use endovascular techniques for treatment of the varicose saphena was Gaetano Conti from Naples, who in 1854 proposed a complex method based on "electropuncture and cauterizations of varicose veins" (see Figure 1.16). Modern endovascular techniques developed beginning in 1964 with Werner and McPheeters ("electrofulguration") and Politowski ("endovenous electrosurgical dessication"). A similar technique was proposed by Watts (1972) to treat saphenous varicosities by endovenous diathermy. In 1981, a freezing technique was proposed by Milleret and Le-Pivert to treat saphenous trunk insufficiency. This technique was refined in 1997 by Constantin, who combined ligation and division of the saphenous junction with saphenous trunk removal by a cryoprobe. The field of *physical sclerotherapy* was drastically revolutionized by two innovative techniques

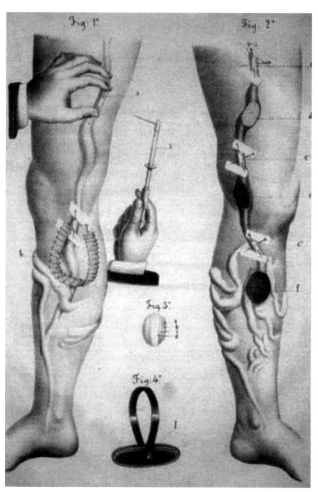

Figure 1.16 Gaetano Conti's method for endovascular fulguration of the GSV (1854). Courtesy of Doctor Michel Georgiev.

that obtained the obliteration of the varicose trunks by endovascular radiofrequency and laser. Endovascular radiofrequency diffused in the late 1990s, and the first positive results were reported by Mitchell Goldman in 2000. The use of endovenous laser in the treatment of the varicose saphena was proposed first by Puglisi at the IUP World Congress of 1989 held in Strasbourg. Endovenous laser technique was deeply refined and diffused worldwide in 1999 by Bone. Many centers are still at work to evaluate exact indications and results of these techniques.

Historically, removal of the GSV from superficial circulation has been considered the first essential step in treating primary varicose veins. While the newer endovenous thermal and chemical ablation procedures also accomplish this, the need to ablate the saphenous vein is increasingly being questioned, as discussed in more detail in Chapter 25.

PERFORATING VEIN SURGERY

The first to suggest selective interruption of perforators to treat varicose veins was probably Remy in 1901. In 1938, Linton proposed a medial subfascial approach to treat incompetent perforators. In 1953, Cockett and Jones proposed the epifascial ligature of medial ankle perforators. Two years later, Felder recommended that the fascial incision for perforating vein ligature should be placed in the posterior midline of the calf in order to avoid placing the lower end of the incision over the ulcer itself or in the compromised skin of the medial leg: the so-called posterior stocking seam approach. Glauco Bassi and Robert Muller used a hook for transcutaneous stripping of perforators through small incisions. Special instruments have been proposed to facilitate subfascial perforator interruption, like those of Albanese (1965) and Edwards (1976). The use of endoscopy to interrupt perforators in the subfascial space goes back to 1985 by Hauer, but only extensive technical improvements allowed its even wider and safer use.[12] Despite new techniques and instrumentations, the problem still remains open: Which perforators must be treated? And when?[13,14]

SURGERY OF THE DEEP VEINS

Ochsner and De Bakey publicized in 1943 the interruption of the inferior vena cava to prevent embolic migration from the leg. John Hunter is credited as the first to ligate it in 1739. Bottini (1893) and Trendelenburg (1910) also are credited with performing this intervention. A temporary caval ligation was proposed by Dale in 1958. In the same year, De Weese and Hunter partially interrupted the inferior vena cava by an intraluminal "hard grip." Spencer obtained caval interruption by suture plication (1965), Ravitch by stapler plication (1966), and finally, Pate by a detachable clip (1969). Mobin-Huddin described in 1967 an umbrella

filter for the prevention of pulmonary embolism. This instrument was then refined by Greenfield, who introduced a steel filter. One year later, Eichelter and Schenk proposed a temporary caval filtration with a removable balloon.

In order to control symptoms of venous insufficiency, Parona in 1894 suggested ligating the popliteal vein, whereas Linton in 1948 suggested interrupting the femoral vein.

Fundamentals of reconstructive venous surgery were developed during the nineteenth century, and in 1912, Carrel and Guthrie received the Nobel Prize for their improvements to vascular surgery techniques. However, safe and effective venous interventions for venous obstructions of the trunk and limbs developed only after World War II (see Table 1.4).

THROMBECTOMY

Paré was probably the first to perform a superficial vein thrombectomy, in 1545: He suggested performing an incision along the vein and squeezing it to expel the thrombus. The first thrombectomy of deep veins was performed by

Table 1.4 VENOUS RECONSTRUCTIVE SURGERY

	The Pioneers of Venous Reconstructive Surgery	
1816	Travers	Sutured a traumatic lesion of the femoral vein
1830	Guthrie	Sutured a traumatic lesion of the jugular vein
1872	Eck	Portacaval anastomosis
1878	Agnew	Lateral suture of traumatized veins
1889	Kummel	First termino-terminal anastomosis of the femoral vein
1901	Clermont	First termino-terminal anastomosis of the inferior vena cava
1912	Carrel & Guthrie	Nobel prize for improvements of vascular surgery techniques
	Main Steps in Venous Reconstructive Surgery	
1950	Wanke	Surgical decompression of the left common iliac vein
1953	Kunlin	Venovenous grafting
1954	Warren & Thayer	GSV bypass of obstructed femoral veins
1958	Palma & Esperón	Cross-pubic bypass for iliac vein occlusion
1964	Stansel	Synthetic graft for caval reconstruction
1970	Husni	Saphenopopliteal bypass for femoral venous obstruction
1982	Fiore	Reconstruction with prosthetic grafts of superior vena cava
1984	Gloviczki; Dale	Reconstruction with prosthetic grafts of inferior vena cava
1988	Zolliker	Endovascular disobliteration and stenting

Lawen in 1937. In 1939, Leriche and Geisendorf associated a periarterial sympathectomy of the nonpulsatile but unoccluded femoral artery to a successful thrombectomy of the femoral vein in a patient with phlegmasia coerulea dolens. In 1966, Fogarthy described how to remove vascular obstruction by a catheter and affirmed this is the "most rationale, most effective and safest way of dealing with iliofemoral thrombosis."

SURGERY OF VALVES

The first attempt to restore valvular function was performed in 1953 by Eisemann and Malette, who proposed producing valve-like structures by gathering folds at two sites of the venous wall opposite each other. In 1963, Psathakis proposed entwining the tendon of the gracilis muscle between the popliteal artery and vein in order to obtain the compression of the vein during contraction of the muscle. A few years later, Ferris and Kistner proposed a transvalvular approach for internal repair of venous valve (1968). In 1984, Raju modified this technique by using a supravalvular approach. Finally, Sottiurai (1988) proposed an internal approach, modifying the original technique of Raju for supravalvular repair of the incompetent venous valves. In 1972, Hallberg proposed the external banding of the incompetent valves of deep veins by sheathing the region with a plastic tube. An extravenous valve substitute in the popliteal space was described by Psathakis in 1984. In 1982, Taheri proposed transferring a valvulated segment of the axillary vein into the lower femoral vein to treat chronic venous insufficiency. In 1986, Jessup and Lane developed an external technique of banding incompetent valves with a silastic cuff. One year later, Kistner developed an external suture technique to "band" incompetent valves.

Reparative or substitutive surgery of venous valves continued to improve greatly. In 1999, Dalsing introduced the use of cryopreserved venous valve allografts for the treatment of chronic deep venous insufficiency.[15] One year later, Raju, Berry, and Neglen[16] described a variation of closed external venous valve repair (transcommissural valvuloplasty). In 2001, Tripathy and Ktenidis reported a new technique of exposure of the valve commissure, called the "trapdoor" internal valvuloplasty.[17] In 2003, Pavcnik experimented with small-intestinal submucosa square-stent bicuspid venous valve in sheep jugular veins and in three patients. In the same year, Corcos[18] proposed a monocuspid valve reconstruction obtained with an intimal flap.

VENOUS ULCERS—WHY TO TREAT THEM

Spender (1866) categorized ulcers of venous origins as "varicose ulcers" and "venous ulcers" ("ulcers of the varicose type without varicose veins"), attributing the latter to failure of deep veins. One year later, John Gay first identified induration and bronzing of the skin as circulatory complications of venous disorders, and, having noted that varicose veins can be present for many years without any ulcer or bronzing of the skin, affirmed that "ulceration is not a direct consequence of varicosity, but all of other conditions of the venous system with which varicosity is not infrequently a complication." Gay's intuitions had already been explained by Fabricius (1603), who affirmed that varicose veins carry "fecaloid humours" that cause skin damage. The "bad humours" could be the hemosiderin that spreads from the capillary bed into the interstitium,[19] or other substances that produce a pericapillary fibrin cuff, poorly permeable to gases,[20] or that induce leukocyte trapping, migration, and release of cytotoxic substances.[21]

AND WHY NOT TO HEAL THEM

A few authors devoted to the Pythagorean theory of the four humours argued against healing ulcers, because they are considered as beneficial in expelling dangerous substances. Galen of Pergamum (130–200 AD) believed that black bile would be trapped by a healing ulcer. Thus, black bile could leak outside while the ulcer remains unhealed. If the ulcer heals, madness and other disasters would follow. Avicenna even proposed reopening varicose ulcers if these spontaneously closed. In modern times, among those reluctant to treat ulcers were Lorenz Heister (1718) and Henry Françoise Le Dran (1731). Both of them considered the ulcer to be a drain for humors that caused severe illness if not expelled. Laufman stated: "A number of British surgeons took up the same cry in the eighteenth century and even into the nineteenth century."

ULCER THERAPY

Modern ulcer therapy is based on (1) topical medications, (2) compressive bandaging, and (3) surgery of related veins. The same was true more than two thousand years ago.

In fact, for many centuries, venous ulcers have been treated by topical applications of substances (like the fig poultice used by the Prophet Isaiah) and combined with bandages (Celsus) and local hygienic treatments (Hippocrates). Principles of local treatments were meticulously described in 1446 by an anonymous surgical textbook (quoted by Partsch, 2002), which treated extensively (9,000 words) the treatment of leg ulcers. Four steps are reported: (1) enlargement of the ulcer mouth, to obtain drainage; (2) *mortification* (debridement); (3) *mundification* (cleansing); (4) *fleshing* (production of granulation tissue).

Ulcer therapies based only on topical remedies were strongly criticized in 1797 by Everard Home: "It must appear obvious, that there is no probability that any one medicine can ever be discovered which, whether internally administered or locally applied, shall have powers adapted to the cure of all ulcer on the legs; and it would appear, the idea that such a medicine may exist, has retarded very considerably, the advancement of our knowledge in the treatment of ulcers." In addition, Brodie (1846) warned against the frequent occurrence of cutaneous sensitization due to drugs and other remedies used topically to treat ulcers.

The importance of using bandages along with local treatment of ulcers was well known since Hippocrates, and in 1676, the Englishman Richard Wiseman warned that venous ulcers healed by compression usually recur once the compression is discontinued. In 1771 Else tried to determine what compression therapy would do in old ulcers of the leg, without administering any internal medicine, and found it so exceedingly efficacious that he believed it will seldom fail where there is no carious bone. It has been discussed at length, whether bandaged patients must walk or if it is better that they rest in bed (see Table 1.5). Besides clinical argumentations, ambulatory treatment of venous ulcers was justified by the analysis of the costs of hospitalization reported by Underwood in 1783 and by Philip Boyers in 1831.

Besides topical treatments, surgery of the varicose veins, when present, has been recommended since old times. Hyeronimus Fabricius of Acquapendente (1603) suggested combining compression with double ligation and division of the varix above the ulcer. In turn, John Gay (1867) randomly divided all the veins around the ulcers by several incisions. It was only one century later that selective interruption of perforating veins below the ulcer was emphasized by Franck Cockett. Currently, sclerotherapy is used to obliterate periulcerative varicose veins. Nevertheless, the first to perform an endovenous treatment of ulcers was Sigismond Johann Elsholz in 1665, using a chicken bone as a needle and a bladder of pigeon as a syringe.

Other suggestions included using a "divine factor" to heal ulcers (Fabricius, 1603) or the "delicate massages from sweet maiden or boy, according with own preferences," proposed by the Roman physician Asclepiade.

Table 1.5 **WALKING OR BED REST TO HEAL ULCERS?**

1778	Benjamin Bell	Absolute bed rest
1783	Michel Underwood	Immediate mobilization
1793	John Hunter	Bed rest
1797	Thomas Baynton	Walking
1799	Whately	"to walk with no scruples"
1861	Hilton	Bed rest
1886	Dechambre	Walking

ADDENDUM: THE INTERNATIONAL UNION OF PHLEBOLOGY (IUP)

It was on March 24, 1959, at the Château de Meyrargues in France near Aix-en-Provence, at the close of a joint meeting of the responsible representatives of the four existing Societies of Phlebology (the French Society of Phlebology created in 1947, the Benelux Society of Phlebology created in 1957, the German Society of Phlebology created in 1958, and the Italian Society of Phlebology, which came into being at the same time) that the foundations of an International Union of Phlebology were laid. Those responsible were Tournay and Wallois (France), van der Molen (Benelux), Krieg (Germany), and Bassi and Comel (Italy). Currently, the IUP includes the phlebological societies of more than forty countries

REFERENCES[1]

1. Lurie F, Kistner RL, Eklof B, Kessler D. Mechanism of venous valve closure and role of the valve in circulation: A new concept, *J Vasc Surg.* 2003. *38*: 955–961.
2. Ono T, Bergan JJ, Schmid-Schonbein GW, Takase S. Monocyte infiltration into venous valves, *J Vasc Surg.* 1998. *27*: 158–166.
3. Caggiati A, Luccichenti G, Pavone P. Three-dimensional phlebography of the saphenous venous system, *Circulation.* 2000. *102*: E33–E35.
4. Uhl JF, Verdeille S, Martin-Bouyer Y. Three-dimensional spiral CT venography for the pre-operative assessment of varicose patients, *Vasa.* 2003. *32*: 91–94.
5. Ruehm SG, Zimny K, Debatin JF. Direct contrast-enhanced 3D MR venography, *Eur Radiol.* 2001. *11*: 102–112.
6. Szendro G, Nicolaides AN, Zukowski AJ, et al. Duplex scanning in the assessment of deep venous incompetence, *J Vasc Surg.* 1986. *4*: 237–242.
7. Luizy F, Franceschi C, Franco G. A method of venous study by real time ultrasonography associated with directional and continuous Doppler ultrasonography, *Ann Med Interne (Paris).* 1986. *137*: 484–487.
8. Partsch H, Rabe E, Stemmer R. *Compression therapy of the extremities.* Paris: Editions Phlebologiques Francais. 2002.
9. Ricci S, Georgiev M, Goldman MP. *Ambulatory phlebectomy.* St Louis: Mosby. 1995.
10. Corcos L, De Anna D, Zamboni P, et al. Reparative surgery of valves in the treatment of superficial venous insufficiency: External banding valvuloplasty versus high ligation or disconnection: A prospective multicentric trial, *J Mal Vasc.* 1997. *22*: 128–136.
11. Yamaki T, Nozaki M, Sasaki K. Alternative greater saphenous vein-sparing surgery: Valvuloplasty combined with axial transposition of a competent tributary vein for the treatment of primary valvular incompetence, 18-month follow-up, *Dermatol Surg.* 2002. *28*: 162–167.
12. Mozes G, Gloviczki P, Menawar SS, Fisher DR, Carmichael SW, Kadar A. Surgical anatomy for endoscopic subfascial division of perforating veins, *J Vasc Surg.* 1996. *24*: 800–808.
13. Labropoulos N, Mansour MA, Kang SS, Gloviczki P, Baker WH. New insights into perforator vein incompetence, *Eur J Vasc Endovasc Surg.* 1999. *18*: 228–234.

[1.] The chronology of the main innovations in the field of venous medicine and surgery that occurred during the last decades was derived mainly by a PubMed investigation.

14. van Neer PA, Veraart JC, Neumann HA. Venae perforantes: A clinical review, *Dermatol Surg.* 2003. *29:* 931–942.

15. Dalsing MC, Raju S, Wakefield TW, Taheri S. A multicenter, phase I evaluation of cryopreserved venous valve allografts for the treatment of chronic deep venous insufficiency, *J Vasc Surg.* 1999. *30:* 854–864.

16. Raju S, Berry MA, Neglen P. Transcommissural valvuloplasty: Technique and results, *J Vasc Surg.* 2000. *32:* 969–976.

17. Tripathi R, Ktenedis KD. Trapdoor internal valvuloplasty: A new technique for primary deep vein valvular incompetence, *Eur J Vasc Endovasc Surg.* 2001. *22:* 86–89.

18. Corcos L, Peruzzi G, Procacci T, Spina T, Cavina C, De Anna D. A new autologous venous valve by intimal flap: One case report. *Minerva Cardioangiol.* 2003. *51:* 395–404.

19. Zamboni P, Izzo M, Fogato L, Carandina S, Zanzara V. Urine hemosiderin: A novel marker to assess the severity of chronic venous disease, *J Vasc Surg.* 2003. *37:* 132–136.

20. Browse NL, Burnand KG. The cause of venous ulceration, *Lancet.* 1982. *2*(8292): 243–245.

21. Coleridge Smith PD, Thomas P, Scurr JH, Dormandy JA. Causes of venous ulceration: A new hypothesis, *Br Med J (Clin Res Ed).* 1988. *296:* 1726–1727.

2.

VENOUS EMBRYOLOGY AND ANATOMY

Geza Mozes and Peter Gloviczki

INTRODUCTION

Substantial knowledge has accumulated in recent years on development and anatomy of the venous system. Progress in medical genetics resulted in identification of genes linked to development of circulation and in recognition of growth factors affecting normal and abnormal development of blood vessels. Perfection of ultrasound technology combined with an increasing clinical interest in venous disease resulted in identification of new compartments and clinically important anatomic structures.[1] Finally, a new, clinically relevant anatomic terminology of the veins of the leg and pelvis was introduced.[2] In this chapter we discuss the embryology of the venous system and present the most frequent venous anomalies. We describe the histology of large veins and present a detailed anatomy of the veins of the trunk and the upper and lower limbs. Discussion of the anatomy of the visceral and cervical veins is beyond the scope of this review. The new terminology of veins will be used in this chapter (see Table 2.1).

EMBRYOLOGY

During embryogenesis the earliest veins develop from capillary plexuses; these carry blood into the sinus venosus, the inflow end of the forming heart. The right and left common cardinal veins drain directly into the sinus venosus (see Figure 2.1). The common cardinal veins form at the junction of the anterior and posterior cardinal veins on both sides. Between this junction and the heart the common cardinal veins receive the vitelline and umbilical veins. The vitelline veins initially drain the yolk sac and later the intestines. The right umbilical vein regresses completely, the left drains the placenta.[3,4]

The anterior cardinal veins drain the cranial part of the embryo and are connected to each other by a large central anastomosing channel. The segment of the left anterior cardinal vein located proximal to the anastomosis will regress. The oblique vein of the left atrium and the coronary

sinus develop from the regressed proximal segment of the left anterior cardinal vein. The remaining distal segment becomes the left internal jugular vein, and the anastomosis between the anterior cardinal veins forms the left brachiocephalic vein. The right internal jugular and brachiocephalic veins develop from the proximal segment of the right anterior cardinal vein. The external jugular veins develop secondarily. Failure of the regression of the proximal left anterior cardinal vein results in double superior vena cava (SVC), whereas erroneous regression on the right side results in left-sided SVC (see Figure 2.2A and B).

The posterior cardinal veins run caudal to the heart and distally develop an interconnecting iliac anastomosis. Contrary to their anterior counterparts, the posterior cardinal veins regress almost completely. Only a small proximal segment remains on the right side to form the azygos arch and the iliac anastomosis to transform into the common, external, and internal iliac and median sacral veins.

Most veins, caudal to the heart, develop from the sub- and supracardinal veins, which arise dorsal and ventral to the regressed posterior cardinal veins, respectively. The subcardinal veins anastomose with each other (subcardinal anastomosis) and with the supracardinal veins (subsupracardinal anastomosis). The majority of the left-sided cardinal veins regress. The right subcardinal vein develops to drain most of the upper, the right supracardinal vein most of the lower part of the abdomen.

The majority of the azygos system develops from the cranial part of the supracardinal veins. The infrarenal segment of the inferior vena cava (IVC) develops from the caudal right supracardinal vein. The renal segment of the IVC arises from the subsupracardinal anastomosis, a venous network located circumferentially around the aorta (renal collar). Eventually, the posterior segment of the collar regresses and the anterior part gives the left renal vein. Most of the suprarenal segment of the IVC develops from the right subcardinal vein, except for the short hepatic segment, which originates directly from hepatic sinusoids.[5] Variation in the complex development of IVC and left renal vein is not uncommon. If the right subcardinal vein fails to connect to

Table 2.1 HISTORIC AND NEW ANATOMIC TERMS OF LOWER EXTREMITY VEINS

HISTORIC TERM	NEW TERM
Greater or long saphenous vein	Great saphenous vein (GSV)
Smaller or short saphenous vein	Small saphenous vein (SSV)
Saphenofemoral junction	Confluence of the superficial inguinal veins
Giacomini's vein	Intersaphenous vein
Posterior arch vein or Leonardo's vein	Posterior accessory great saphenous vein of the leg
Superficial femoral vein	Femoral vein
Cockett perforators (1,11,11)	Posterior tibial perforators (lower, middle, upper)
Boyd's perforator	Paratibial perforator (proximal)
Sherman's perforators	Paratibial perforators
24-cm perforators	Paratibial perforators
Hunter's and Dodd's perforators	Perforators of the femoral canal
May's or Kuster's perforators	Ankle perforators

supracardinal vein is associated with regression of the right supracardinal vein (see Figure 2.2D).[7] Developmental variations of the left renal vein include persistent (circumaortic) renal collar (1–9%) and retroaortic left renal vein (1–2%) (see Figure 2.3).[8]

Capillaries of the primitive limb buds initially drain into the marginal sinuses. In the arm the ulnar portion of the marginal sinuses dominate over the radial ones, and eventually form the basilic, axillary, and subclavian veins. The subclavian vein drains into the proximal anterior cardinal vein. The cephalic vein develops secondarily from segments of the radial marginal sinuses and attaches to the axillary vein later. In the leg, segments of the primitive marginal sinuses persist only distally and develop into the peroneal, anterior tibial, and small saphenous veins (SSV). The great saphenous vein (GSV) originates from the posterior cardinal vein and later gives off the femoral, popliteal, and posterior tibial veins.

the liver sinusoids, the suprarenal segment of the IVC will not develop, consequently the lower part of the body will be drained through the azygos system and the liver will drain directly into the heart. Double IVC (0.2–3%) occurs due to the persistence of the left supracardinal vein, therefore it usually involves only the infrarenal segment (see Figure 2.2C).[6] Left-sided IVC (<0.5%) develops if persistence of the left

HISTOLOGY

The venous wall has three layers: intima, media, and adventitia. The intima is made up by endothelial cells and an underlying thin connective tissue layer. Valves are formed by infolding of the intima, therefore they are covered with endothelium on both sides and have a very thin connective tissue skeleton. Venous valves are bicuspid. The veins are distended at the base of the valves, probably secondary to

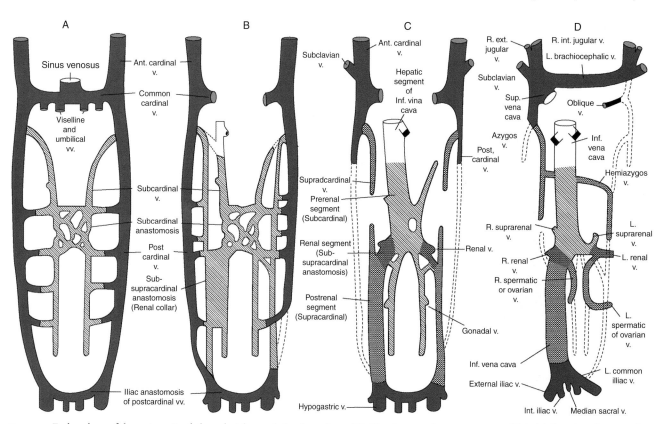

Figure 2.1 Embryology of the major veins (adapted with permission from Avery LB. *Developmental anatomy*, rev. 7e. Philadelphia: Saunders, 1974).

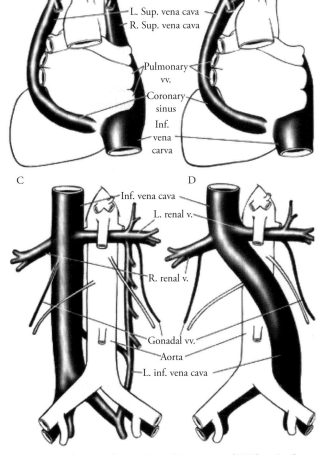

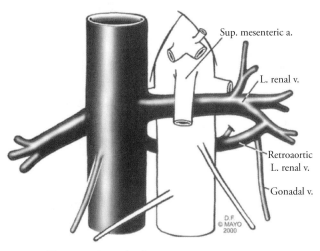

Figure 2.2 Developmental anomalies of the superior (SVC) and inferior vena cava (IVC). A) Double SVC (posterior view); B) Left SVC (posterior view); C) Double IVC; D) Left IVC.

the effects of local flow reversal. The border of the intima is marked by the internal elastic lamina: a layer of thick elastic fibers. The internal elastic lamina is well developed only in large veins; it is incomplete in medium-sized and absent

Figure 2.3 Circumaortic renal collar.

in small ones. The media is composed of smooth muscle cells and connective tissue fibers, most of which is collagen. Larger superficial veins, such as the GSV, have thick muscular media with the ability of significant contraction. Smaller tributaries of the GSV have thinner media, and therefore are more prone to varicosity. Media of the deep calf veins contain plenty of collagen, providing better wall strength. More central deep veins, such as femoral, iliac, axillary, and subclavian veins, contain less and less smooth muscle cell. The media of the superior and inferior vena cava is built up almost exclusively from connective tissue. The adventitia is poorly differentiated from the media, in particular in larger veins. It consists of some loose connective tissue with vasa vasorum and nerve fibers.[9,10]

ANATOMY OF THE THORACIC VEINS

The superior vena cava (SVC) starts at the confluence of the brachiocephalic veins behind the first right costal cartilage, and ends at the level of the third right costal cartilage, where it drains into the right atrium. The SVC is about 7 cm long and 2 cm wide. Halfway along its course, before it enters the pericardium, the SVC receives the azygos arch. The brachiocephalic veins are formed at the confluence of the subclavian and internal jugular veins behind the sternoclavicular joints (see Figure 2.4). The right brachiocephalic vein is short, about 2–3 cm, and lies anterior to the innominate artery.[7] The left one is about 6 cm long and courses obliquely behind the manubrium from left to right, anterior to the left subclavian, common carotid arteries, and superior to the aortic arch. Major tributaries of the brachiocephalic veins are the vertebral, internal thoracic, and inferior thyroid veins. The first intercostal vein drains into the brachiocephalic veins on both sides. The left superior intercostal vein is connected to the left brachiocephalic vein, whereas on the right it joins the azygos vein. There are no valves in either the SVC or the brachiocephalic veins.

The azygos-hemiazygos system forms an H-shaped network in the posterior mediastinum, anterior to the body of the thoracic vertebrae (see Figure 2.4). The azygos vein gives the entire right arm of the H, the hemiazygos gives the left lower and the accessory hemiazygos vein the left upper segment. The azygos vein starts at T12 to L2 with the confluence of the right ascending lumbar and subcostal veins. The azygos vein ascends on the right side up to the level of T4, then passes anterior to form an arch joining the SVC. Major tributaries of the azygos vein are the right posterior fifth to eleventh intercostal veins and the right superior intercostal vein draining the second to fourth intercostal veins. The hemiazygos vein starts similar to the azygos vein but on the left side of the vertebral column at T12 to L2. It courses cranial and at the level of T8 it crosses over to join the azygos vein. Major tributaries of the hemiazygos vein are the left azygos-hemiazygos system provides an important collateral pathway in case of IVC or SVC obstruction.[7]

ANATOMY OF THE UPPER EXTREMITY VEINS

The dorsal and palmar digital veins join to form the metacarpal veins, which drain into the superficially located dorsal venous network of the hand. The cephalic and basilic veins arise from this network on the radial and ulnar side of the wrist, respectively. The superficial veins on the palmar side of the hand are richly anastomosed to the deep veins. A superficial and a more proximal deep venous arch is formed from the interconnection of the palmar veins and parallel the corresponding arterial arches.

The cephalic vein originates at the anatomical snuff box from the dorsal venous network. It courses over the distal radius to the ventral aspect of the forearm and ascends on the lateral side of the arm. The cephalic vein runs in the deltopectoral groove, it enters the infraclavicular fossa behind the pectoralis major muscle and pierces the clavipectoral fascia before empting into the axillary vein (see Figure 2.5). The basilic vein begins on the ulnar side of the wrist, passes along the ulnar aspect of the forearm, and courses more ventrally at the level of the elbow. Above the elbow the basilic vein runs medial to the biceps and at about midway in the upper arm it perforates the deep fascia and joins the brachial vein. After receiving the brachial vein, the basilic vein continues in the axillary vein. The median cubital vein connects the cephalic and basilic veins in the antecubital fossa. The medial antebrachial vein originates from the superficial palmar venous plexus and runs on the ventral side of the forearm. It joins either the cephalic or basilic vein or both in the proximal forearm. The accessory cephalic vein originates from the dorsal venous plexus on the ulnar side and crosses over dorsally to join the cephalic vein in the forearm. Variations in the anatomy of superficial arm veins are countless.

Deep veins of the hand join to form the paired radial, ulnar, and interosseus veins, which accompany the corresponding arteries. The three pairs of deep veins of the forearm form the brachial veins at the level of the elbow. The paired brachial veins join the basilic vein to form the axillary vein at the lower border of the teres major muscle (at the lateral border of the scapula on an anteroposterior chest X-ray). The axillary vein is located medial and inferior to the axillary artery and the medial cord of the brachial plexus lies between the two vessels. The axillary vein ends at the outer border of the first rib, where it becomes the subclavian vein. The subclavian vein runs posterior and superior to the subclavian artery and receives its only major tributary, the external jugular vein. The subclavian vein ends at the medial border of the scalenus anterior muscle, where it joins the internal jugular vein to form the brachiocephalic vein.

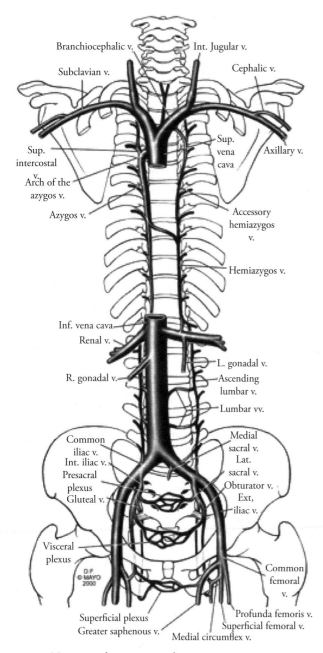

Figure 2.4 Thoracic and retroperitoneal veins.

posterior eighth to eleventh intercostal veins. The accessory hemiazygos vein has more variation than the azygos and hemiazygos veins. Usually it drains the left superior intercostal vein (which in turn drains the left second to fourth intercostal veins) and the left posterior fifth to seventh intercostal veins. At the level of T7 it either crosses over to the right and joins the azygos or stays on the left and joins the hemiazygos vein. If the connection between the accessory hemiazygos and the rest of the azygos-hemiazygos system is not developed, the accessory hemiazygos vein will drain through the left superior intercostal vein into the left brachiocephalic vein. The azygos-hemiazygos system receives several small veins from the viscera of the chest and freely anastomoses with the vertebral venous plexuses as well. The

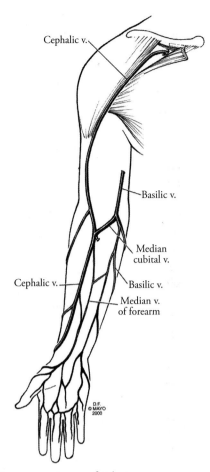

Figure 2.5 Upper extremity superficial veins.

There are valves in the superficial and deep veins of the arm, although they are not so numerous as in the leg. Valves in the axillary vein usually are located proximal to the junction with the brachial and cephalic veins. The subclavian vein has a valve just proximal to the confluence of the external jugular vein. Upper extremity venous return is maintained mainly by the work of the heart without significant contribution of a muscle pump. Therefore the valves are less important from a functional standpoint. Perforators between the deep and superficial veins are scarce.

ANATOMY OF THE ABDOMINAL AND PELVIC VEINS

The inferior vena cava (IVC) begins at the confluence of the common iliac veins and ascends on the right side of the vertebral column, passes through the tendinous portion of the diaphragm, and after a short course (approximately 2.5 cm) in the chest it terminates in the right atrium at the level of T9. In the upper abdomen the IVC is located posterior to the duodenum, the head and neck of the pancreas, the lesser sac, and the liver. The intrahepatic portion of the IVC lies in a groove along the posterior aspect of the caudate lobe. Tributaries of the IVC are the paired lumbar and renal veins

and the hepatic veins, additionally on the right side the right gonadal, suprarenal, and inferior phrenic veins also drain into the IVC (see Figure 2.4). The left gonadal and suprarenal veins join the left renal vein; the left inferior phrenic vein drains into the left suprarenal vein. In case of IVC obstruction, communication between the veins of the thoracic and abdominal wall (thoracoepigastric, internal thoracic, and epigastric veins), the lumbar-azygos anastomosis, and the vertebral plexuses provide important collateral pathways.

The common iliac veins begin at the sacroiliac joint on both sides and end at L5, where they form the IVC. The only tributary of the right common iliac vein is the right ascending lumbar vein; the left common iliac vein drains the left ascending lumbar and median sacral veins (see Figure 2.4). The right common iliac vein lies posterolateral to the right common iliac artery. The distal segment of the left common iliac vein is medial and posterior to the left common iliac artery, the proximal segment is posterior to the right iliac artery and distal aorta. Compression of the proximal left common iliac vein may occur due to the overlying arterial structures. The external iliac vein starts at the level of the inguinal ligament, it courses along the pelvic brim and ends anterior to the sacroiliac joint where the external and internal iliac veins form the common iliac vein. On the right the distal external iliac vein is medial to the artery; however, as it ascends, more proximally, it courses posterior to it. The left external iliac vein remains medial to the artery along its entire course. Tributaries of the external iliac vein are the inferior epigastric, deep circumflex iliac, and pubic veins. The internal iliac vein runs posteromedial to the internal iliac artery on both sides. The short trunk of internal iliac vein is formed by the confluence of extra and intrapelvic venous tributaries. The extrapelvic tributaries include the gluteal (superior and inferior), internal pudendal, and obturator veins, which drain the pelvic wall and the perineum. Intrapelvic tributaries of the internal iliac vein are the lateral sacral and visceral (middle rectal, vesical, uterine, and vaginal) veins, which drain the presacral and pelvic visceral venous plexuses (rectal, vesical, prostatic, uterine, and vaginal).

Both the IVC and the common iliac veins are valveless. There is usually one valve in the external iliac vein, but often it is without any valves.

ANATOMY OF THE LOWER EXTREMITY VEINS

Thorough knowledge of the fascial compartments of the leg is a prerequisite of understanding the relationship between superficial and deep veins. The fascia surrounding the calf and thigh muscles separates two compartments: the superficial compartment, consisting of all tissues between the skin and the fascia, and the deep compartment, which includes all tissues between the fascia and the bones (see Figure 2.6).[11]

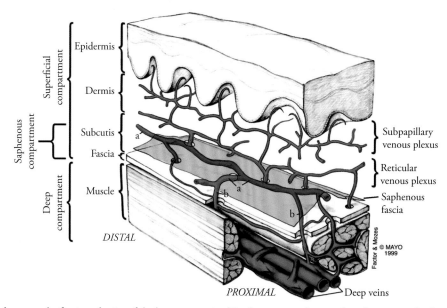

Figure 2.6   Relationship between the fascia and veins of the lower extremity. The fascia covers the muscle and separates the deep from the superficial compartment. Superficial veins (a) drain the subpapillary and reticular venous plexuses, and are connected to deep veins through perforating veins (b). The saphenous fascia invests the saphenous vein. The saphenous compartment is a subcompartment of the superficial compartment.

Superficial veins run in the superficial, deep veins in the deep compartments. Perforating veins pierce through the fascia and connect the superficial to deep veins.[12] Communicating veins connect veins within the same compartment: superficial to superficial or deep to deep veins. The saphenous veins are covered by a fibrous sheath, the saphenous fascia. The saphenous fascia is thinner than the deep fascia and it is more pronounced in the upper-mid thigh, than more distally.[1,13] The space between the saphenous and muscular deep fascia is the saphenous compartment. The saphenous compartment is a subcompartment of the superficial compartment.

The superficial venous system of the foot is divided into the dorsal and plantar subcutaneous venous network (see Figure 2.7). Superficial vein tributaries drain blood into the dorsal venous arch on the dorsum of the foot at the level of the proximal head of the metatarsal bones. The medial and lateral end of this arch continues through the medial and lateral marginal vein into the GSV and SSV, respectively.

Small superficial veins drain the subpapillary and reticular plexuses of the skin and subcutaneous tissues to form bigger tributaries, which eventually all connect to the saphenous veins.[14,15] The GSV begins just anterior to the medial ankle, crosses in front of the tibia, and ascends medial to the knee (see Figure 2.8).[16–18] Proximal to the knee, the GSV ascends on the medial side of the thigh and enters the fossa ovalis 3 cm inferior and 3 cm lateral to the pubic tubercle.[19] The GSV is doubled in the calf in 25% of the population, in the thigh in 8%.[20] The saphenous nerve runs in close proximity to the GSV in the distal two-thirds of the calf. Accessory GSVs are frequently present, and they run parallel to the GSV both in the thigh and in the leg; they lie either anterior, posterior, or superficial to the main trunk.

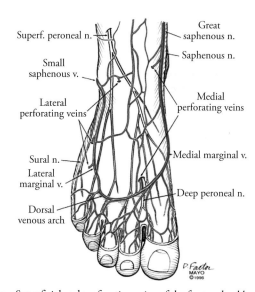

Figure 2.7   Superficial and perforating veins of the foot and ankle.

The posterior accessory GSV of the leg (Leonardo's vein or posterior arch vein) is a common tributary, it begins posterior to the medial malleolus, ascends on the posteromedial aspect of the calf, and joins the GSV distal to the knee (see Figure 2.8). The anterior accessory GSV of the leg drains the anterior aspect of the leg below the knee. The posterior accessory GCV of the thigh, if present, drains the medial and posterior thigh.[11] The anterior accessory GSV of the thigh collects blood from the anterior and lateral side of the thigh (see Figure 2.8). The anterior and posterior accessory GSVs join the GSV just before it ends at the confluence of superficial inguinal veins (saphenofemoral junction). The superficial circumflex iliac, superficial epigastric, and external pudendal veins join each other and the distal GSV to

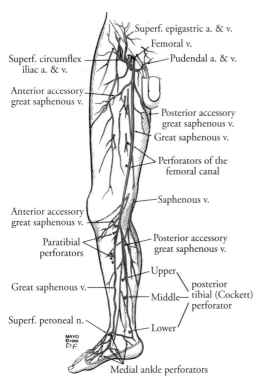

Figure 2.8   Superficial and perforating veins of the leg.

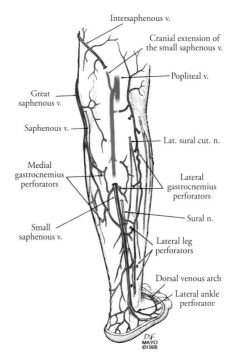

Figure 2.10   The SSV and lateral venous system of the calf.

form the confluence of superficial inguinal veins (sapheno-femoral junction) (see Figure 2.9).[21] Rarely, the GSV terminates high on the lower abdomen or joins the femoral vein very low and the superficial inguinal veins empty individually into the femoral vein.[22] Other occasional tributaries of the GSV in the groin include the posterior and anterior thigh circumflex veins.

The SSV lies lateral to the Achilles tendon in the distal calf (see Figure 2.10).[23] In the lower two-thirds of the calf the SSV runs in the subcutaneous fat, then it pierces the fascia and runs between the two heads of the gastrocnemius

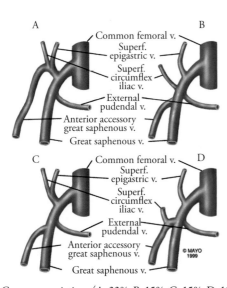

Figure 2.9   Common variations (A. 33%, B. 15%, C. 15%, D. 13%) in the anatomy of the confluence of inguinal veins (saphenofemoral junction).

muscle. In the popliteal fossa at about 5 cm proximal to the knee crease, the main trunk of the SSV drains into the popliteal vein. A smaller vein, the cranial extension of the SSV, frequently continues in cephalad direction (see Figure 2.10).[24] Uncommonly the main trunk of the SSV continues without draining into the popliteal vein and eventually empties into the femoral vein or GSV.[11] The intersaphenous vein (vein of Giacomini) is a communicating vein connecting the SSV to the GSV in the posteromedial thigh. The sural nerve courses along the SSV in the distal calf. Superficial veins of the lateral leg and thigh form the lateral venous system. The lateral venous system is drained through multiple small tributaries into the GSV and SSV.

Deep veins of the foot form two divisions: the plantar and the dorsal veins. The richly anastomosing deep plantar venous arch drains the plantar digital veins through the plantar metatarsal veins. The deep plantar venous arch drains into the medial and lateral plantar veins, which in turn continue in the posterior tibial veins behind the medial ankle (see Figure 2.11).[25] On the dorsum of the foot the pedal vein drains the deep dorsal digital veins through the dorsal metatarsal veins. The pedal vein continues in the anterior tibial veins. Pairs of the posterior and anterior tibial and peroneal veins accompany the corresponding arteries, and all drain into the popliteal vein (see Figure 2.11). Large soleal and gastrocnemius (medial, lateral, and intergemellar) veins drain venous sinuses of calf muscles and join the popliteal vein (Figure 2.12). Venous sinuses are closely related to deep veins. They are embedded in the belly of calf muscles, such as the soleus and gastrocnemius, and are able to dilate and hold a large amount of blood. With the contraction of calf muscles at walking the blood is pumped to

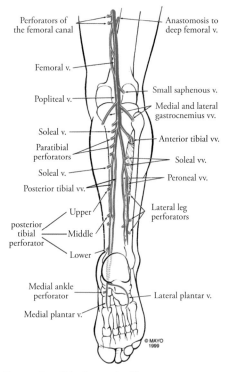

Figure 2.11   Deep veins of the foot and calf.

more proximal deep veins (calf muscle pump). The popliteal vein continues into the femoral vein as it passes through the adductor canal. The popliteal and femoral veins are frequently duplicated.[26] Distally the femoral vein runs lateral to the femoral artery; however, more proximally it runs

medial to it. The deep femoral (profunda femoris) vein joins the femoral vein to form the common femoral vein at about 9 cm below the inguinal ligament.[27] The common femoral vein is medial to the common femoral artery and it becomes the external iliac vein at the level of the inguinal ligament. The GSV joins the common femoral vein at the confluence of the superficial inguinal veins. Other tributaries of the common femoral vein are the circumflex femoral veins (lateral and medial). In the distal thigh the femoropopliteal segment frequently communicates through a large collateral with the deep femoral vein providing an important alternative avenue for venous drainage in case of femoral vein occlusion. The sciatic vein, the main trunk of the primordial deep venous system, runs along the sciatic nerve.

There are as much as 150 perforating veins (PVs) in the lower extremity; however, only a few of these are clinically important. Significant variation exists in the location of individual PVs; however, distribution of clusters of PVs follows a predictable pattern. Dorsal, plantar, medial, and lateral foot perforators are the main groups of PVs in the foot.[28] A large PV runs between the first and second metatarsal bones and connects the superficial dorsal venous arch to the pedal vein.[29] Clusters of PVs at the ankle are the anterior, medial, and lateral ankle perforators (see Figure 2.13).[30] The medial calf perforators have two groups: posterior tibial and paratibial PVs. Three groups (lower, middle, upper) of posterior tibial PVs (Cockett I–III perforators) connect the posterior accessory GSV to the posterior tibial veins (see Figures 2.8, 2.11, 2.12, and 2.13).[31,32] The paratibial perforators drain the GSV into the posterior tibial veins.[33,34] Other perforators of the leg below the knee are the anterior, lateral, medial, and lateral gastrocnemius; intergemellar; and Achillean PVs (see Figure 2.11). Infra- and suprapatellar and popliteal fossa PVs are located around the knee. Perforators of the femoral canal connect tributaries of the GSV to the femoral vein (see Figure 2.8). Inguinal perforators drain into the femoral vein in the proximal thigh.

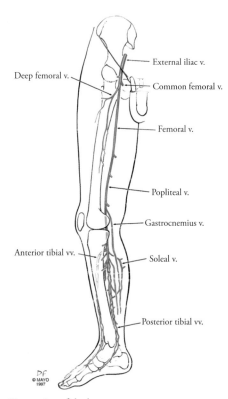

Figure 2.12   Deep veins of the leg.

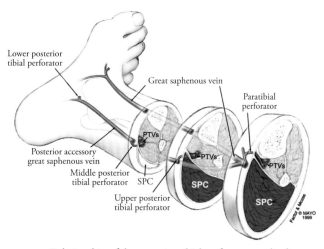

Figure 2.13   Relationship of the posterior tibial perforators to the deep and superficial posterior compartments (SPC) of the calf (PTVs, posterior tibial veins).

Valves in superficial veins of the lower extremity usually are located near the termination of major tributaries. Some valves are well developed with marked sinusoid dilation at their base, others are more delicate in their structure. In the GSV there are about six valves, with more valves located below than above the knee. A nearly constant valve of GSV is at 2–3 cm distal to its confluence with the femoral vein. Valves in the SSV are closer to each other than in the GSV. Valves in communicating branches between the SSV and GSV are oriented to direct blood from the SSV to the GSV. Like superficial veins, deep veins have more valves in the calf than in the thigh. Tibial veins are densely packed with valves, whereas there are only one or two valves in the popliteal vein. In the femoral vein there are three to five valves, with one of them located just distal to the junction of the deep femoral vein. There is usually one valve in the common femoral vein. Major PVs have one to three valves, all located below the level of the fascia, that direct flow toward the deep veins. Small PVs are usually valveless. PVs of the foot are without any valves or with valves that direct flow toward the superficial veins.

CUTANEOUS NERVES OF THE LOWER EXTREMITIES

Nerve injury is a potential complication of varicose vein procedures and is the most frequent cause for litigation following varicose vein surgery.[35] Knowledge of lower extremity nerve anatomy can minimize adverse outcomes. The most common nerve injury is to the common peroneal nerve where it crosses the neck of the fibula.[36] Other nerves of importance during varicose vein procedures include the saphenous, tibial, and sural nerves. Their anatomical locations have been previously described and illustrated in Figures 2.8 and 2.10.

REFERENCES

1. Caggiati A. Fascial relationships of the long saphenous vein, *Circulation*. 1999. *100*(25): 2547–2549.
2. Caggiati A, Bergan JJ, Gloviczki P, Jantet G, Wendell-Smith CP, Partsch H; International Interdisciplinary Consensus Committee on Venous Anatomical Terminology. Nomenclature of the veins of the lower limbs: An international interdisciplinary consensus statement, *J Vasc Surg*. 2002. *36*(2): 416–422.
3. Carlson BM. The development of the circulatory system. In: Carlson B, ed. *Patten's Foundation of embryology*, 5e. New York: McGraw-Hill. 1988. 586–627.
4. Nicholson CP, Gloviczki P. Embryology and development of the vascular system. In: White RA, Hollier LH, eds. *Vascular surgery: Basic science and clinical correlations*. Philadelphia: JB Lippincott. 1994. 3–20.
5. Lundell C, Kadir S. Inferior vena cava and spinal veins. In: Kadir S, ed. *Atlas of normal and variant angiographic anatomy*. Philadelphia: Saunders. 1991. 187–202.
6. Hirsch DM, Chan K. Bilateral inferior vena cava, *JAMA*. 1963. *18S*: 729–732.
7. Lundell C, Kadir S. Superior vena cava and thoracic veins. In: Kadir S, ed. *Atlas of normal and variant angiographic anatomy*. Philadelphia: Saunders. 1991. 163–175.
8. Mozes G, Carmichael SW, Gloviczki P. Development and anatomy of the venous system. In: Gloviczki P, Yao ST, eds. *Handbook of venous disorders*. London: Arnold. 2001. 11–24.
9. Parum DV. Histochemistry and immunochemistry of vascular disease. In: Stehbens WE, Lie JT, eds. *Vascular pathology*. London: Chapman & Hall. 1995. 313–327.
10. Patrick JG. Blood vessels. In: Sternberg SS, ed. *Histology for pathologists*. New York: Raven Press. 1992. 195–213.
11. Hollinshead WH. The back and limbs. In: Hollinshead WH, ed. *Anatomy for surgeons*. New York: Harper & Row. 1969. 617–631, 754–758, 803–807.
12. May R. Nomenclature of the surgically most important connecting veins. In: May R, Partsch H, Staubesand J, eds. *Perforating veins*. Baltimore: Urban & Schwarzenberg. 1981. 13–18.
13. Caggiati A. Fascial relationships of the short saphenous vein. *J Vasc Surg*. 2001. *34*(2): 241–246.
14. Negus D, Coleridge Smith P. The blood vessels of the lower limb: Applied anatomy. In: Negus D, Coleridge Smith P, Bergan J, eds. *Leg ulcers: Diagnosis and management*, 3e. CRC Press. 2005. 15–24.
15. Braverman IM. The cutaneous microcirculation: Ultrastructure and microanatomical organization, *Microcirculation*. 1997. *4*(3): 329–340.
16. Scultetus AH, Villavicencio JL, Rich NM. Facts and fiction surrounding the discovery of the venous valves [comment], *J Vasc Surg*. 2001. *33*(2): 435–441.
17. Caggiati A, Bergan JJ. The saphenous vein: Derivation of its name and its relevant anatomy, *J Vasc Surg*. 2002. *35*(1): 172–175.
18. Caggiati A, Bertocchi P. Regarding "fact and fiction surrounding the discovery of the venous valves" [comment], *J Vasc Surg*. 2001. *33*(6): 1317.
19. Gardner E, O'Rahilly R. Vessels and lymphatic drainage of the lower limb. In: Gardner E, O'Rahilly R, eds. *Anatomy: A regional study of human structure*, 5e. Philadelphia: W.B. Saunders. 1986. 190–196.
20. Thomson H. The surgical anatomy of the superficial and perforating veins of the lower limb, *Ann R Coll Surg Engl*. 1979. *61*(3): 198–205.
21. Daseler EH, Anson BJ, Reimann AF, Beaton LE. The saphenous venous tributaries and related structures in relation to the technique of high ligation: Based chiefly upon a study of 550 anatomical dissections, *Surg Gynecol Obstet*. 1946. *82*: 53–63.
22. Browse NL Burnand K, Irvine AT, Wilson NM. Embryology and radiographic anatomy. In: Browse NL, Burnand K, Irvine AT, Wilson NM, eds. *Diseases of the veins*, 2e. London: Arnold. 1999. 23–48.
23. Kosinski C. Observations on the superficial venous system of the lower extremity, *J Anat*. 1926. *60*: 131–142.
24. Bergan JJ. Surgical management of primary and recurrent varicose veins. In: Gloviczki P, Yao J, eds. *Handbook of venous disorders: Guidelines of the American Venous Forum*. London: Chapman & Hall Medical. 1996. 394–415.
25. White JV, Katz ML, Cisek P, Kreithen J. Venous outflow of the leg: Anatomy and physiologic mechanism of the plantar venous plexus, *J Vasc Surg*. 1996. *24*(5): 819–824.
26. Zbrodowski A, Gumener R, Gajisin S, Montandon D, Bednarkiewicz M. Blood supply of subcutaneous tissue in the leg and its clinical application, *Clin Anat*. 1995. *8*(3): 202–207.
27. Dodd H, Cockett F. Surgical anatomy of the veins of the lower limb. In: Dodd H, Cockett F, ed. *The pathology and surgery of the veins of the lower limb*. London: Livingstone. 1956. 28–64.
28. Kuster G, Lofgren EP, Hollinshead WH. Anatomy of the veins of the foot, *Surg Gynecol Obstet*. 1968. *127*(4): 817–823.
29. Stolic E. Terminology, division and systematic anatomy of the communicating veins of the lower limb. In: May R, Staubesand J, eds. *Perforating veins*. Baltimore: Urban & Schwarzenberg. 1981. 19–34.
30. May R. Nomenclature of the surgically most important connecting veins. In: May R, Staubesand J, eds. *Perforating veins*. Baltimore: Urban & Schwarzenberg. 1981. 13–18.
31. Mozes G, Gloviczki P, Menawat SS, Fisher DR, Carmichael SW, Kadar A. Surgical anatomy for endoscopic subfascial division of perforating veins, *J Vasc Surg*. 1996. *24*(5): 800–808.

32. Mozes G, Gloviczki P, Kadar A, Carmichael SW. Surgical anatomy of perforating veins. In: Gloviczki P, Bergan J, eds. *Atlas of endoscopic perforator vein surgery*. London: Springer-Verlag. 1998. 17–28.

33. Boyd AM. Discussion on primary treatment of varicose veins, *Proc R Soc Med*. 1948. *61*: 633–639.

34. Sherman RS. Varicose veins: Anatomic findings and an operative procedure based upon them, *Ann Surg*. 1944. *120*: 772–232.

35. Campbell WB, France F, Goodwin HM. Medicolegal claims in vascular surgery. *Ann R Coll Surg Engl*. 2002. 84181–84184.

36. Tennant WG, Ruckley CV, Medicolegal action following treatment for varicose veins, *Br J Surg*. 1996. *83*: 291–292.

3.

EPIDEMIOLOGY OF CHRONIC PERIPHERAL VENOUS DISEASE

Michael H. Criqui, Julie O. Denenberg, Robert D. Langer, Robert M. Kaplan, and Arnost Fronek

INTRODUCTION

The term "chronic venous disease," or more specifically of interest here, "chronic peripheral venous disease" (CPVD) has been used more generally to refer to either visible and/or functional abnormalities in the peripheral venous system. The most widely used classification of such abnormalities is the CEAP (clinical, etiological, anatomic, pathophysiologic), which employs both anatomic (superficial, deep, or perforating veins) and pathophysiologic (reflux, obstruction, or both) categories.[1] The CEAP classification is further described in Chapter 10.

The CEAP classification reflects the clinical situation in which patients are typically referred to a vascular specialist for clinically significant venous disease. In contrast to the clinical situation, population studies of CPVD have typically focused on broader categories determined by visual inspection only. The three major categories of interest have been varicose veins (VV), chronic venous insufficiency (CVI), and venous ulcers. However, there has not been a standard definition of these categories. VV has been defined at differing levels of visible disease severity. CVI has typically been defined by skin changes and/or edema in the distal leg. Venous ulcers, both active and healed, have been defined by visible inspection and subjective inference as to etiologic origin.

Two studies have now reported results on defined free-living populations with simultaneous assessment of both visible abnormalities and functional impairment by Duplex ultrasound.[2,3] The Duplex examination for the San Diego Population Study (SDPS) determined both obstruction and reflux, while the Edinburgh study determined only the latter. The results were revealing in that to some degree the validity of both the assumptions of earlier population studies and of the CEAP classification, at least as applied to population samples, were brought into question. Specifically, the general concept that visible disease necessarily implied underlying functional disease, and vice versa, was true in the large majority of affected limbs, but not universally so.

Although these discrepancies occurred in a minority of cases, they were frequent enough to lead us to separately classify visible and functional CPVD in each limb evaluated in the SDPS. Specifically, we classified each limb into four visible categories: normal, telangiectasias/spider veins (TSV), VV, and trophic changes (TCS); the latter category being one or more of hyperpigmentation, lipodermatosclerosis, or active or healed ulcer. The presence or absence of edema was not by itself a criterion for TCS. For functional disease, we determined the presence of obstruction and reflux separately for the superficial, perforating, and deep systems. The presence of either reflux or obstruction in superficial or deep veins was categorized as functional disease, and because of small numbers, abnormalities of the perforating veins were considered as deep disease. Three functional categories were defined: normal, superficial functional disease (SFD), and deep functional disease (DFD). Here, the term "functional" is essentially interchangeable with "anatomic." Also, in this population study, obstruction was uncommon and virtually all legs with obstruction also had reflux, such that SFD and DFD essentially refer to reflux.

In addition to separately assessing edema, we asked about a history of superficial venous thrombosis (SVT) and deep venous thrombosis (DVT), with or without pulmonary embolism.

Table 3.1 shows the prevalence of various manifestations of CPVD in the SDPS by age, gender, and ethnicity. Specifically, prevalence rates are given for TSV, VV, TCS, SFD, DFD, edema on physical examination, and SVT and DVT by history.

AGE AND CVPD

Using mutually exclusive categories for both visible and functional CVPD, we found a graded relationship with increasing age for VV, with those aged 70–79 years having nearly twice the prevalence of those aged 40–49 years. TSV also increased with age, but this difference was obscured by the mutually exclusive categories, with increasing numbers

Table 3.1 VISIBLE AND FUNCTIONAL CHRONIC VENOUS DISEASE, EDEMA AND THROMBOTIC EVENTS BY STRATA OF SEX, AGE, AND ETHNICITY, SAN DIEGO, CALIFORNIA, 1994–1998

STUDY GROUP	N	%	VISIBLE DISEASE, %				FUNCTIONAL DISEASE, %			EDEMA AND THROMBOTIC EVENTS, %		
			NL	TSV	VV	TCS	NL	SFD	DFD	EDEMA	SVT	DVT
All subjects	2211	100	19.0	51.6	23.3	6.2	72.1	19.0	9.0	5.8	2.4	3.2
Men	780	35.3	33.6	43.6	15.0	7.8	75.6	13.1	11.3	7.4	1.5	4.0
Women	1431	64.7	11.0	55.9	27.7	5.3	70.1	22.2	7.8	4.9	2.8	2.7
Age, yrs <50	534	24.2	33.0	47.9	16.9	2.3	81.8	11.2	6.9	2.6	2.1	2.4
50–59	608	27.5	22.5	52.8	20.7	4.0	78.0	14.5	7.6	4.1	2.5	2.5
60–69	557	25.2	12.4	52.8	26.0	8.8	66.1	23.5	10.4	6.1	2.2	3.8
70+	512	23.2	7.4	52.5	29.9	10.2	61.3	27.3	11.3	10.7	2.7	4.1
Ethnicity												
NHW	1282	58.0	14.3	54.8	24.0	6.9	69.7	20.0	10.3	7.8	2.6	4.4
Hispanic	338	15.3	18.9	50.0	26.3	4.7	71.0	22.8	6.2	1.8	3.6	1.5
Afr. Am.	318	14.4	27.7	45.3	20.8	6.3	76.7	16.4	6.9	4.1	0.9	1.9
Asian	273	12.4	31.1	45.4	18.7	4.8	78.8	12.5	8.8	3.3	1.5	1.1

ABBREVIATIONS: NL = normal, TSV = spider veins, VV = varicose veins, TCS = trophic changes, SFD = superficial functional disease, DFD = deep functional disease
NHW = Non-Hispanic white, Afr. Am.= African American
STE = superficial thrombotic event, DTE = deep thrombotic event

of participants with TSV also having VV or TCS at older ages. TCS showed the most dramatic age-related increase, with the oldest age group having more than four times the prevalence of the youngest.[3] These findings for visible disease are consistent with most previous population studies, which generally have found a linear increase in TSV and or VV with age (reviewed in References 4, 5). Earlier studies typically defined CVI only by venous (assumed) ulcers, and reported exponential increases in CVI with age, findings similar to the dramatic age increase we reported for the broader TCS category.

For functional CVPD, SFD was more than twice as common and DFD 64% more common in the oldest age group. SFD showed both a higher prevalence and a steeper age gradient than did DFD.[3] The only other population data on functional disease were from the Edinburgh study; these were limited to reflux and showed similar gradients with age.[2]

Edema was strongly age-related as expected, but a history of SVT and DVT somewhat less so, perhaps reflecting selective recall bias in older participants.[3] Nonetheless, our data for DVT overall are quite similar to the lifetime prevalence in a large population-based study.[6]

GENDER AND CPVD

For visible disease, we found nearly twice as much VV in women as in men, but TCS were 50% more common in men.[3] These findings for VV are consistent with earlier studies, but earlier studies have also suggested a small excess of CVI in women, in contrast to our findings for the broader category of TCS. However, more concordant with our findings, the Edinburgh study reported that CVI was twice as common in men as women. For functional CPVD, only the Edinburgh study has comparable data, and only for reflux, and found a gender ratio for functional disease similar to the SDPS.

Edema was about 50% more common in men than women, consistent with a 50% greater history of DVT in men.[3] The Edinburgh group reported more edema in women, but a discordance with CVI being more common in men.[2] In contrast, in our study a history of SVT was more than twice as common in women, which has been linked to hormonal factors and pregnancy.[7,8]

ETHNICITY AND CPVD

The SDPS reported data for four ethnicities, non-Hispanic White, Hispanic, African American, and Asian. Non-Hispanic Whites showed the highest prevalence of CPVD, with only 14.3% with a normal visual examination. Non-Hispanic Whites had the highest rates of TSV, TCS, and DFD, and the second highest rates (after Hispanics) of VV and SFD. African Americans and Asians had a somewhat lower prevalence of CPVD. Consistent with the visible and functional findings, non-Hispanic Whites also had the highest rates of edema and of DVT by history, and Hispanics the highest rate of SVT by history.[3]

Several previous studies have suggested a higher prevalence in developed than developing countries, although these studies are not entirely consistent (reviewed in Reference 4). The SDPS is the first population study to evaluate multiple ethnic groups who were residents of the same geographical area.

CONCORDANCE OF VISIBLE AND FUNCTIONAL DISEASE

Figure 3.1 shows the concordance of visible and functional disease in the individual 4,422 legs of the 2,211 participants for this analysis. The majority of legs showed TSV, but the majority of legs were also functionally normal. If we consider TSV as a "normal" visible finding, visible disease would be defined as VV or TCS, and functional disease as SFD or DFD. The concordance between visible and functional disease was 92%, 17.4% concordant for disease presence and 74.6% concordant for disease absence. Discordance was thus 8%, 4.9% of the legs with visible but not functional disease and 3.1% with functional but not visible disease. Surprisingly, 21% of all legs with VV were normal functionally (3.7%/17.7%), as were 26% of all legs with TCS (1.2%/4.6%). Thus, although the concordance was strong, visible disease did not invariably mark underlying functional disease, and functional disease was sometimes present in the absence of any visible venous disease.[3] In contrast with our findings, Engelhorn, mapped the venous flow of 269 limbs in women with telangiectasias as the only visible sign of disease and found that 46% had reflux in the saphenous vein.[9]

CONCORDANCE OF CPVD WITH EDEMA, SVT, AND DVT

Table 3.2 shows edema on examination and SVT and DVT by history, cross-classified by visible and functional disease. Significant differences from the normal/normal reference group are noted. Edema was closely associated with TCS. For limbs with TSV or VV, the presence of SFD or DFD greatly increased the probability of edema, as did DFD in legs visibly normal. Of legs with edema, 26% were normal functionally and had either normal or TSV visible findings, providing an estimate of the minimum number of legs on a population basis with edema of nonvenous etiology. SVT was not related to visible disease in legs with normal function, but was increased similarly by both SFD and DFD. This finding is consistent with the large proportion of DFD legs that also had SFD (48%). DVT was related to both TCS and DFD, but not to VV or SFD. By far the highest prevalence of reported DVT, 25%, was in legs with both TCS and DFD. Thus although edema, SVT, and DVT were much more common in the presence of visible and/or functional disease, they also sometimes occurred in normal legs.[3]

RISK FACTORS FOR CPVD

In evaluating risk factors for CPVD in the SDPS, for simplicity we defined as "normal" legs as visibly normal or with TSV and normal functionally; moderate CPVD as VV or

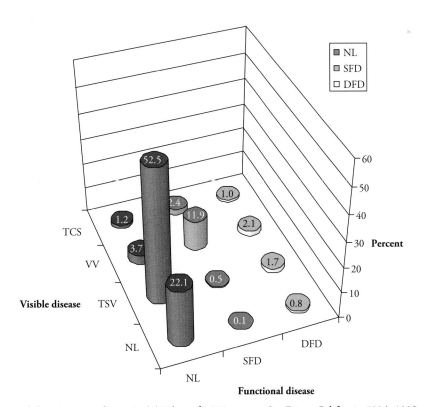

Figure 3.1   Visible and functional chronic venous disease in 4,422 legs of 2,211 persons, San Diego, California, 1994–1998.

Table 3.2 PREVALENCE OF EDEMA, HISTORY OF SUPERFICIAL THROMBOTIC EVENTS, AND HISTORY OF DEEP THROMBOTIC EVENTS BY VISIBLE AND FUNCTIONAL DISEASE, SAN DIEGO, CALIFORNIA, 1994–1998

	NL	SFD	DFD
Edema			
NL	1.7*	0.6	6.6
TSV	1.8	14.9+	10.5+
VV	3.9	7.4+	15.6+
TCS	40.8+	30.0+	48.2+
Superficial Events			
NL	0.6*	0.0	5.3+
TSV	0.4	10.0+	0.0
VV	1.2	4.1+	1.2
TCS	0.2	4.9+	11.3+
Deep Events			
NL	1.3*	0.0	5.4
TSV	1.7	0.0	5.4+
VV	3.0	2.4	6.6+
TCS	7.7+	7.6+	26.6+

Abbreviations: NL = normal, TSV = spider veins, VV = varicose veins, TCS = trophic changes
SFD = superficial functional disease, DFD = deep functional disease
* = reference group
+ = p < 0.005

Table 3.3 RISK FACTORS FOR MODERATE AND SEVERE VENOUS DISEASE

	MODERATE DISEASE		SEVERE DISEASE	
	MEN	WOMEN	MEN	WOMEN
Variable	Point estimate	Point estimate	Point estimate	Point estimate
Age (10 years)	1.59	1.43	1.41	1.43
African American	0.64	0.84	0.63	0.44
Asian	0.55	0.90	1.50	0.99
Hispanic	1.48	1.21	0.63	0.71
Family Hx of Ven. Dis.	2.87	2.34	2.13	1.92
Flat Feet	—	1.39	1.63	—
Hernia Surgery	1.85	1.81		
Flat Arch (vs. normal)			—	3.28
Small Arch (vs. normal)			—	1.84
Leg Injury			—	1.67
CVD History	0.22	—	—	2.02
Hypertension	0.58	0.64		
Dias. BP (10 mm/Hg)			0.80	—
Current Walking (per hr)	1.14	—		
Adult Sitting (per hour)	—	0.92		
Curr. Move after Sitting	0.31	—		
Current Stand. (per hr)			—	1.14
Laborer			3.24	—
Weight (10 kilograms)	—	1.32		
Waist Circumf. (10 cm)	—	0.83	1.37	1.24
Current Cigs. (20/day)			2.24	—
Oophorectomy	na	1.37		
Number of Births	na	1.14	na	1.14

Abbreviations: Hx of Ven. Dis. = history of venous disease, CVD = cardiovascular disease, Dias. BP = diastolic blood pressure, Curr = currently, Stand. = standing, Circumf. = circumference, Cigs. = cigarettes, na = not applicable

SVD; and severe CPVD as TCS or DVD.[10] Each participant was classified by their worst leg. Table 3.3 summarizes this work and shows odds ratios for significant predictors of visible and functional venous disease in our population.

Age was positively consistently related to moderate and severe disease in both sexes. African Americans had less CVPD than non-Hispanic Whites, a finding that was significant for severe disease in women.

Family history of venous disease based on subject recall was a risk factor for both moderate and severe disease in both sexes, with a somewhat stronger association for moderate than severe disease. Although this finding could be biased by selective recall; it is consistent with many other studies,[5,11,12,13] although not all.[14]

Connective tissue laxity, as manifested by previous hernia surgery or findings of flat feet, was a consistent risk factor for both moderate and severe disease. The association of increasing laxity in connective tissue with venous disease corroborated previous research (reviewed in Reference 10).

Lower limb injury was a risk factor in women for severe disease. Coughlin et al., in a case-control study, found serious lower limb trauma to be a risk factor for CVI.[14]

Cardiovascular disease-related factors, such as a cardiovascular disease history, hypertension, and diastolic pressure were associated with less moderate disease for men

and women and less severe disease in men. Although some studies have found a relationship between atherosclerosis and venous disease (reviewed in Reference 10), others have not.[11] The reason for any protective effect of cardiovascular disease and hypertension on CPVD is not readily apparent, although venous vasoconstriction and microthrombosis could conceivably be involved.

The number of hours spent walking or standing was positively associated with moderate disease in men and severe disease in women, respectively. Working as a laborer was strongly associated with severe disease in men. Hours spent sitting was inversely related to moderate disease in women, as was moving about when sitting for long periods of time in men. Fowkes et al.[15] found that walking was a risk factor for women with venous insufficiency when age-adjusted, but less so when multiply adjusted. They found walking to be related to lessened risk of venous insufficiency in men.[15] Both Carpentier et al. and Tuchsen et al. found that men performing unskilled work were at risk for varicose veins.[13,16] Our data indicate that standing was a strong risk factor for venous disease in women. This is concordant with a number of studies,[11,12,16] and contrasts with some other studies.[15]

Weight and waist circumference were risk factors for moderate and severe disease in women and severe disease in men. A number of studies have found an association of obesity with venous disease. Gourgou et al.[12] found a relationship in both men and women with VV. Our finding of increased waist circumference with severe disease was consistent with previous reports reviewed in Reference 10. In contrast, Coughlin et al. and Fowkes et al. both found that obesity was not a factor in venous insufficiency among women.[14,15] Fowkes et al. extended this finding to men as well.[15] Other studies have also found no association between obesity and venous disease.[11] However, the Edinburgh group also found that for men and women combined, persons with greater severity of varices (i.e., more segments with reflux) had higher body mass indices than those with fewer segments involved. Additionally, Fowkes et al. found that varicosities in the superficial system, but not in the deep system, were related to body mass index (BMI) in women.[15]

Current cigarette smoking was associated with severe disease in men. Gourgou et al. found a similar relationship with VV.[12]

Oophorectomy and parity were both positively associated with moderate disease in women, and parity with severe disease as well. Gourgou et al. and Traber et al. each found increasing VV prevalence with increasing numbers of births.[5,12] Coughlin et al. found that multiparity was associated with varicose veins in pregnant women.[14] Changes can reportedly occur with only one pregnancy.[11]

Our data indicate that age and family history were the strongest risk factors for CPVD, and neither is subject to intervention. Other significant findings on inherent factors included associations with connective tissue laxity and inversely with African American ethnicity. Cardiovascular disease-related factors were associated with lower rates of venous disease. Among volitional factors important findings were a relationship of CPVD with central adiposity, positional factors such as hours spent standing or sitting, exercise, smoking, and selected hormonal factors in women. In contrast with prior studies, we found no relationship with dietary fiber intake. In women but not men we confirmed the importance of a previous lower limb injury for DFD.

SYMPTOMS AND CPVD

The SDPS reported data for ever having any of seven symptoms of venous disease: aching, cramping, tired legs, swelling, heaviness, restless legs, and itching.[17] Aching legs was the most commonly reported venous symptom, with an overall prevalence of 17.7%. Cramping was present in 14.3% of legs, tired legs in 12.8%, and swelling in 12.2%. Heaviness and restless legs had similar prevalence at 7.5 and 7.4%. Itching was the least commonly reported symptom, affecting 5.4 % of legs. With the exception of restless legs, all these symptoms increased in prevalence with increasing severity of venous functional disease (see Figure 3.2). The rate was lowest in normal legs, increased in legs with SFD, and highest in legs with DFD. These differences were statistically significant (p < 0.01) for all symptoms except for restless legs (p = 0.56). Although each symptom was more common in women than men, trends were similar in both sexes.

Escalating rates of symptoms were also found across categories of visible venous disease.[17] Figure 3.3 shows the prevalence rates by symptom and visible category for each sex. Symptom prevalence in subjects with TSV, the most common category of visible disease, was only marginally greater than in normal participants. Symptoms were generally about twice as common when VV was present. Rates were further increased in the presence of TCS. Again, with the exception of restless legs (p = 0.06), these differences were highly statistically significant (p < 0.01). Similar to functional disease, symptom prevalence was uniformly greater in women although trends were similar in both sexes.

SYMPTOMS BY VISIBLE AND FUNCTIONAL DISEASE

To estimate the relative importance of each symptom to the clinical picture of venous disease we evaluated the odds ratios (OR) for each symptom in each of the twelve categories of venous status formed by crossing the three categories of functional disease with the four categories of visible disease using logistic regression adjusted for age, sex, BMI, education, and racial/ethnic group (Table 3.4). Aching (OR 2.20) and swelling (OR 2.99) were significantly associated with DFD even in subjects without visible disease. These two symptoms were significantly associated with DFD across all categories of visible disease with the strongest association in subjects with TCS. Aching was significantly associated with VV regardless of venous functional status and was associated with TCS except in those with normal functional examinations. Itching followed a similar pattern being significantly associated with VV regardless of visible status, and with TCS except in those with normal functional exams. However, the OR for itching with VV and DFD was twice the level of the parallel ratio for aching (5.31 and 2.82,

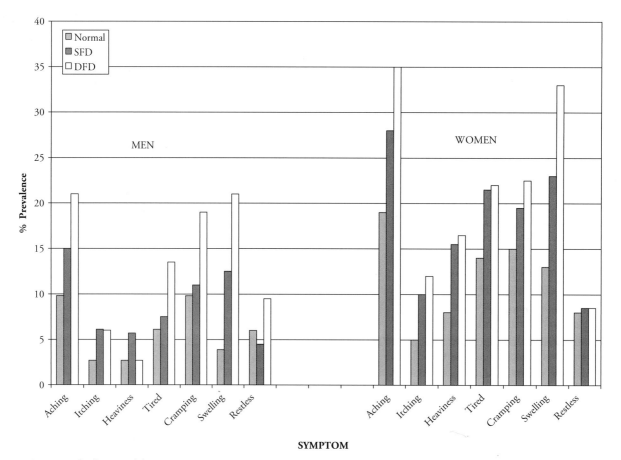

Figure 3.2   Symptoms by functional disease status.

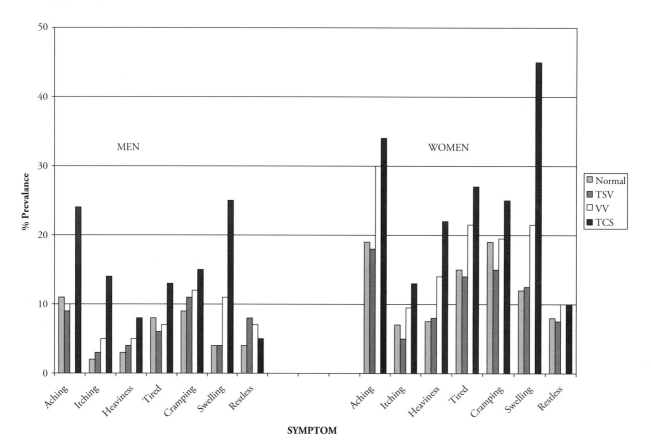

Figure 3.3   Symptoms by visible disease status.

	NORMAL	TSV	VV	TCS
N				
Normal	1024	2519	184	58
SFD	5	22	591	117
DFD	39	87	107	55
Aching				
Normal	ref	1.11	2.05*	0.85
SFD	0.03	1.56	2.29*	3.90*
DFD	2.20*	1.93*	2.82*	6.17*
Itching				
Normal	ref	1.11	1.98*	2.63
SFD	0.04	5.88*	2.33*	4.81*
DFD	1.10	0.32	5.31*	6.94*
Heaviness				
Normal	ref	1.33	1.60	0.02
SFD	0.01	1.44	2.69*	5.68*
DFD	0.59	1.65	2.82*	5.27*
Tired				
Normal	ref	1.09	1.63*	0.42
SFD	0.01	0.30	2.07*	3.80*
DFD	1.52	1.04	2.95*	4.79*
Cramping				
Normal	ref	0.95	1.45	0.46
SFD	0.03	1.36	1.41*	1.82*
DFD	1.53	1.57	1.44	3.82*
Swelling				
Normal	ref	1.15	1.91*	5.41*
SFD	0.02	4.13*	2.31*	6.73*
DFD	2.99*	2.57*	5.82*	11.61*
Restless				
Normal	ref	1.44*	2.36*	1.13
SFD	0.03	1.50	1.64*	0.95
DFD	2.32	0.82	1.18	3.78*

* p<0.05.

TSV = Telangiectasias and Spider Veins, VV = Varicose Veins, TCS = Trophic Changes, SFD = Superficial Functional Disease, DFD = Deep Functional Disease

legs was associated with disease for subjects with both DFD and TCS, it did not consistently distinguish disease as rates were elevated in subjects with normal functional examinations who had either TSV or VV. In general, a combination of visible and functional findings tended to increase ORs compared with only a visible or functional finding.[17]

SYMPTOM SPECIFICITY AND CPVD

In this population-based study, aching was the most commonly reported symptom related to venous disease. However, it was relatively nonspecific as about 15% of normal subjects (assessed by either functional or visible status) reported it. Swelling was a more specific marker for prevalent disease with less than 10% of normal subjects reporting this symptom and at least a two-fold higher rate associated with functional disease or any visible disease besides TSV. Likewise, heaviness and itching were reported in legs with functional or visible findings at more than twice the rate reported in normal legs. Tired legs and cramping were also increased in legs with functional or visible findings, but the contrasts with normal legs were not as strong. The joint occurrence of aching and swelling, or aching and tired legs was useful in distinguishing diseased legs.[17]

Our finding that swelling correlates strongly with symptoms is concordant with several other reports. A study of patients attending a vascular clinic found an association between vascular endothelial growth factor (VEGF) and CEAP classification, and between VEGF and swelling.[18] The Edinburgh study, conducted in patients from clinical practices, evaluated associations by leg as in the present report. Disease was defined by the presence of superficial and deep reflux. For isolated superficial reflux, associations were found for heaviness and itching in women; there were no significant associations in men. For venous disease defined as combined superficial and deep reflux, associations were found between swelling, cramps, and itching for men, and between aching and cramps in women.[19] A study of a large employed population found swelling and nocturnal cramps to be the most common symptoms.[20] Surprisingly, in that population the strongest association was found for people with small cutaneous veins, the equivalent of TSV in our study. In a clinical population evaluated by color-flow duplex, the strongest associations were found for aching and swelling that were associated with below-knee reflux.[21]

Women were more likely to report symptoms than men. Similar results have been reported by other investigators.[20,22] This is not simply an artifact of the greater prevalence of visible disease and superficial functional disease in women[(3)] since it was evident on a percentage basis for each category and was also found for deep functional disease, which was more prevalent in men.

respectively). Swelling had associations very similar to itching for VV, but was associated with much higher rates when TCS was present (ORs 11.61, 6.94, and 6.17 for swelling, itching, and aching, respectively, in subjects with DFD and TCS). Heaviness, tired legs, and cramping each had modest associations with disease in the presence of both functional and visible abnormalities. Although the symptom of restless

QOL AND CPVD

Despite the high prevalence of venous disease, the impact on daily functioning and quality of life is still poorly documented. Venous disease has been considered as a cosmetic problem that might affect emotional well-being. Several studies have shown that venous disease affects selected aspects of daily functioning (reviewed in Reference 23). An ad hoc committee of the Society of Vascular Surgery (SVS)/International Society of Cardiovascular Surgery (ISCVS) recommended the expansion of outcome measures in studies of venous disease to include patient-reported functioning and quality-of-life measures.[24] In their review, the ad hoc committee noted that comprehensive evaluation of venous disease must include assessment of clinical outcomes and quality of life.[24] However, only a limited number of studies have measured quality of life in patients with venous disease. At least six previous studies have used the Medical Outcomes Study 36 Item Short Form (SF-36) for patients with varicose veins. With some exceptions[25,26] patients in these studies were not well described in terms of disease status.

SF-36 AND CPVD

The SF-36 includes eight subscales. These subscales have been factor analyzed and clustered into two groups: physical and mental health.[27] Physical health components are regarded as measures of functioning, whereas mental health components are thought of as indicators of well-being. Functioning describes what people are able to do, while well-being characterizes how people feel, particularly on mental health or emotional dimensions.

Scores for the four physical health components of SF-36, broken down by visible disease categories in the SDPS, are summarized in the top portion of Figure 3.4.[23] The mental health components of the SF-36 are shown in the bottom portion of the figure. The differences between visual categories of disease were highly significant with a strong linear component for the physical health subscales of the SF-36. In particular, there were strong linear effects for the Physical Functioning $p < 0.0001$, Role-Physical ($p < 0.0001$), Pain ($p < 0.0001$), and General Health Perception scales ($p < 0.001$). The only significant effect for the mental health or well-being scales was for Vitality, and this effect was relatively weak in relation to the SF-36 functional scales ($p < 0.03$).[23]

Similar trends were observed for the functional categories based on the duplex ultrasound evaluations. However, these trends were not as strong as for the visual categories (Figure 3.5). There were strong linear trends for all four SF-36 physical health scales (Physical Functioning, $p < 0.01$; Role-Physical, $p < 0.001$; Pain, $p < 0.01$; General Health Perceptions, $p < 0.001$). Similar trends were not observed for any of the mental health scores and all tests of differences between groups and linear trends were nonsignificant.[23]

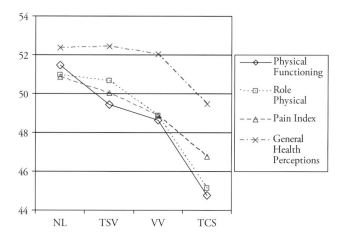

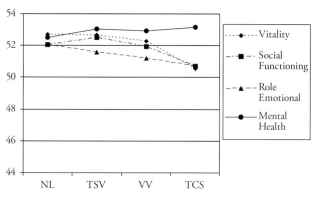

Figure 3.4 SF-36 scores by visual disease status for physical (top) and mental (bottom) health scores.

After adjustment for sex and ethnicity, age was significantly inversely correlated with the physical but positively correlated with the mental summary component scores (PCS, $r = -0.26$; MCS, $r = 0.18$). This suggests that older participants had lower physical health scores but slightly higher mental health scores. Men scored significantly higher on the PCS summary score than women ($p < 0.01$) and marginally higher on the MCS summary score ($p < 0.10$). There were also significant differences in SF-36 summary scores by ethnicity, with the Asian group scoring highest on both the PCS and MCS components. For the MCS component, the non-Hispanic White group obtained the lowest mean score. Despite the univariate effects of age, gender, and ethnicity, adjustments for these variables did not affect the results for either visible category or functional category. This suggests that differences in quality of life are explained primarily by disease category. Ethnicity, age, and gender contribute to the prediction of quality of life, but do so independently of disease category.[23]

A final set of analyses examined the effect of visible category adjusting for functional category and the effect of functional category adjusting for visible category. These analyses focused on the PCS and MCS summary scores. Using a general linear model, we observed very strong differences in PCS by visible category ($p < 0.001$). However,

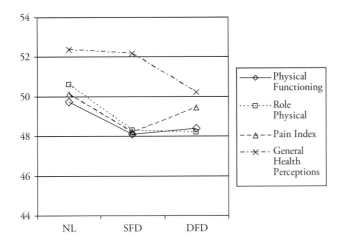

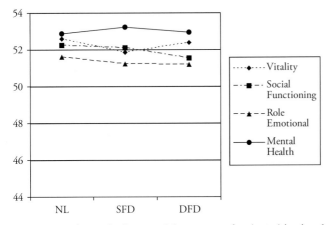

Figure 3.5 SF-36 scores by functional disease status for physical (top) and mental (bottom) health scores.

once visible category was entered, functional category did not explain additional variance (p = 0.74). The model entering the functional categories with the visible category as a covariate still favored the visible category. These findings suggest that the visible categories explain most of the variance in the SF-36 PCS. In the MCS model, differences between both the visible and functional categories were nonsignificant, and adjustments did not have significant effects.[23]

Evidence from this study suggests that venous disease affects the functional scales (what people can do) but does not appear to affect the well-being aspects (how people feel). Very similar results were reported in a recent European study. Kurz et al. also found significant gradations in SF-36 PCS scores by disease severity, but found few differences for the MCS components.[26] In addition to evidence suggesting that quality-of-life measures are associated with disease severity, some evidence suggests that the measures are also responsive to changes following therapeutic intervention.[28]

In summary, even modest venous disease is associated with significant limitations on the physical functioning scales of the SF-36. Venous disease did not appear to affect emotional aspects of health-related quality of life.

CONCLUSIONS

CPVD PREVALENCE

CPVD increased with age and was most common in NHW. Women had more superficial and men more deep venous disease. Visible and functional disease were highly concordant, but in 8% of legs they were discordant. Although edema and venous thrombotic events were increased dramatically with TCS and DFD, they also occurred in their absence as well as in the absence of milder forms of CPVD.

RISK FACTORS FOR CVPD

Family history was the strongest risk factor. Although some risk factors were immutable, such as family history, age, and ligamentous laxity, other risk factors are amenable to intervention, including weight, physical activity, and cigarette smoking. These latter findings allow for the potential of CPVD prevention.

SYMPTOMS IN CPVD

Venous symptoms were more common in the presence of either visible or functional disease, and increased with the severity of venous disease. Women reported more symptoms than men. Swelling was the most specific predictor; heaviness, itching, and aching also helped to distinguish CPVD.

QOL IN CPVD

CPVD had a substantial effect on the physical health aspects of quality of life. These findings were stronger for visible than for functional categories of disease. CVPD showed only weak associations with mental health components of quality of life.

REFERENCES

1. Eklof B, Rutherford RB, Bergan JJ, et al. Revision of the CEAP classification for chronic venous disorders: Consensus statement, *J Vasc Surg*. 2004. *40*: 1248–1252.
2. Evans CJ, Allan PL, Lee AJ, Bradbury AW, Ruckley CV, Fowkes FG. Prevalence of venous reflux in the general population on duplex scanning: The Edinburgh vein study, *J Vasc Surg*. 1998. *28*: 767–776.
3. Criqui MH, Jamosmos M, Fronek A, et al. Chronic venous disease in an ethnically diverse population: The San Diego Population Study, *Am J Epidemiol*. 2003. *158*: 448–456.
4. Adhikari A, Criqui MH, Wooll V, et al. The epidemiology of chronic venous diseases, *Phlebology*. 2000. *15*: 2–18.
5. Traber J, Mazzolai L, Lauchli S. Epidemiology of chronic venous insufficiency: Swiss survey with surprising results, *Praxis*. 2009. *98*: 749–755.
6. Saarinen J, Laurikka J, Sisto T, Tarkka M, Hakama M. The incidence and cardiovascular risk indicators of deep venous thrombosis, *Vasa*. 1999. *28*: 195–198.

7. McColl MD, Ramsay JE, Tait RC, et al. Superficial vein thrombosis: Incidence in association with pregnancy and prevalence of thrombophilic defects, *Thromb Haemost*. 1998. *79*: 741–742.

8. Helmerhorst FM, Bloemenkamp KW, Rosendaal FR, Vandenbroucke JP. Oral contraceptives and thrombotic disease: Risk of venous thromboembolism, *Thromb Haemost*. 1997. *78*: 327–333.

9. Engelhorn CA, Engelhorn AL, Cassou MF, Salles-Cunha S. Patterns of saphenous venous reflux in women presenting with lower extremity telangiectasias, *Dermatol Surg*. 2007. *33*: 288.

10. Criqui MH, Denenberg JO, Bergan J, Langer RD, Fronek A. Risk factors for chronic venous disease: The San Diego Population Study, *J Vasc Surg*. 2007. *46*: 331–337.

11. Komsuoglu B, Goldeli O, Kulan K, Cetinarslan B, Komsuoglu SS. Prevalence and risk factors of varicose veins in an elderly population, *Gerontology*. 1994. *40*: 25–31.

12. Gourgou S, Dedieu F, Sancho-Carnier H. Lower limb venous insufficiency and tobacco smoking: A case-control study, *Am J Epidemiol*. 2002. *155*: 1007–1015.

13. Carpentier PH, Maricq HR, Biro C, Poncot-Makinen CO, Franco A. Prevalence, risk factors, and clinical patterns of chronic venous disorders of lower limbs: A population-based study in France, *J Vasc Surg*. 2004. *40*: 650–659.

14. Coughlin LB, Gandy R, Rosser S, de Cossart L. Factors associated with varicose veins in pregnant women, *Phlebology*. 2001. *16*: 41–50.

15. Fowkes FG, Lee AJ, Evans CJ, Allan PL, Bradbury AW, Ruckley CV. Lifestyle risk factors for lower limb venous reflux in the general population: Edinburgh Vein Study, *Int J Epidemiol*. 2001. *30*: 846–852.

16. Tuchsen F, Hannerz H, Burr H, Krause N. Prolonged standing at work and hospitalisation due to varicose veins: A 12 year prospective study of the Danish population, *Occup Environ Med*. 2005. *62*: 847–850.

17. Langer RD, Ho E, Denenberg JO, Fronek A, Allison M, Criqui MH. Relationships between symptoms and venous disease: The San Diego population study, *Arch Intern Med*. 2005. *165*: 1420–1424.

18. Howlader MH, Smith PD. Symptoms of chronic venous disease and association with systemic inflammatory markers, *J Vasc Surg*. 2003. *38*: 950–954.

19. Bradbury A, Evans CJ, Allan P, Lee AJ, Ruckley CV, Fowkes FG. The relationship between lower limb symptoms and superficial and deep venous reflux on duplex ultrasonography: The Edinburgh Vein Study, *J Vasc Surg*. 2000. *32*: 921–931.

20. Kroger K, Ose C, Rudofsky G, Roesener J, Hirche H. Symptoms in individuals with small cutaneous veins, *Vasc Med*. 2002. *7*: 13–17.

21. Labropoulos N, Leon M, Nicolaides AN, Giannoukas AD, Volteas N, Chan P. Superficial venous insufficiency: Correlation of anatomic extent of reflux with clinical symptoms and signs, *J Vasc Surg*. 1994. *20*: 953–958.

22. Bradbury A, Evans C, Allan P, Lee A, Ruckley CV, Fowkes FG. What are the symptoms of varicose veins? Edinburgh vein study cross sectional population survey, *Br Med J*. 1999. *318*: 353–356.

23. Kaplan RM, Criqui MH, Denenberg JO, Bergan J, Fronek A. Quality of life in patients with chronic venous disease: San Diego population study, *J Vasc Surg*. 2003. *37*: 1047–1053.

24. McDaniel MD, Nehler MR, Santilli SM, et al. Extended outcome assessment in the care of vascular diseases: Revising the paradigm for the 21st century, *J Vasc Surg*. 2000. *32*: 1239–1250.

25. Smith JJ, Guest MG, Greenhalgh RM, Davies AH. Measuring the quality of life in patients with venous ulcers, *J Vasc Surg*. 2000. *31*: 642–649.

26. Kurz X, Lamping DL, Kahn SR, et al. Do varicose veins affect quality of life? Results of an international population-based study, *J Vasc Surg*. 2001. *34*: 641–648.

27. Ware JE, Jr., Gandek B. Overview of the SF-36 Health Survey and the International Quality of Life Assessment (IQOLA) Project, *J Clin Epidemiol*. 1998. *51*: 903–912.

28. Baker DM, Turnbull NB, Pearson JCG, Makin GS. How successful is varicose vein surgery: A patient outcome study following varicose vein surgery using the SF-36 health assessment questionnaire, *Eur J Vasc Endovasc Surg*. 1995. *9*: 299–304.

4.

VENOUS ANATOMY, PHYSIOLOGY, AND PATHOPHYSIOLOGY

John J. Bergan and Luigi Pascarella

In order to understand treatment of various venous disorders, it is necessary to know the normal anatomy of the venous system of the lower extremities as well as the normal functioning of its elements and the mechanisms that cause derangements in its normal functioning.

In 2001, an International Interdisciplinary Committee was designated by the presidents of the International Union of Phlebology (IUP) and the International Federation of Anatomical Associations to update the official Terminologia Anatomica regarding the veins of the lower limbs. The relative deficiency of the official Terminologia Anatomica[1] with regard to the veins of the lower limbs was responsible for a nonuniform anatomical nomenclature in clinical literature, which caused both difficulty in international exchange of information and inappropriate treatment of venous disease.[2] The Committee, with the participation of members of the Federative International Committee for Anatomical Nomenclature (FICAT), outlined a consensus document at a meeting held in Rome on the occasion of the 14th World Congress of the IUP. Terminological recommendations of the Committee were published,[3] and these terms are used in the following exposition.

ANATOMY

For purposes of understanding, the venous system in the lower extremities can be divided into three systems: the deep venous system, which parallels the tibia and femur; the superficial venous system, which resides in the superficial tissue compartment between the deep muscular fascia and the skin; and the perforating or connecting veins, which join the superficial to the deep systems. It is because these latter veins penetrate anatomic barriers that they are called perforating veins.

Although the superficial veins are the targets of most therapy, the principal return of blood flow from the lower extremities is through the deep veins. In the calf, these deep veins are paired and named for their accompanying arteries. Therefore, the anterior tibial, posterior tibial, and peroneal arteries are accompanied by their paired veins, which are interconnected. These crural veins join and form the popliteal vein. Occasionally the popliteal veins as well as more proximal deep veins are also paired like the calf veins.

As the popliteal vein ascends, it becomes the femoral vein. Formerly, this was called the superficial femoral vein, but that term has been abandoned.[3] Near the groin the femoral vein is joined by the deep femoral vein, and the two become the common femoral vein, which ascends to become the external iliac vein proximal to the inguinal ligament.

Ultrasound imaging has shown that the superficial compartment of the lower extremities consists of two compartments, one enclosing all the structures between the muscular fascia and the skin, and the other, within the superficial compartment enclosing the saphenous vein and bounded by the muscular fascia inferiorly and the superficial fascia superiorly, is termed the "saphenous compartment" (see Figure 4.1). The importance of this anatomic structure is underscored by its being targeted during percutaneous placement of endovenous catheters and the instillation of tumescent anesthesia.[4,5]

The main superficial veins are the great saphenous vein and the small saphenous vein. These receive many interconnecting tributaries, and these tributaries may be referred to as communicating veins. They are correctly called tributaries rather than branches of the main superficial veins. The great saphenous vein has its origin on the dorsum of the foot. It ascends anterior to the medial malleolus of the ankle and further on the anteromedial aspect of the tibia. At the knee, the great saphenous vein is found in the medial aspect of the popliteal space. It then ascends through the anteromedial thigh to join the common femoral vein, just below the inguinal ligament. Throughout its course, it lies within the saphenous compartment. The small saphenous vein originates laterally from the dorsal venous arch of the foot and travels subcutaneously behind the lateral malleolus at the ankle. As it ascends in the calf, it enters the deep fascia and ascends between the heads of the gastrocnemius muscle to join the popliteal vein behind the knee (see Figure 4.2).

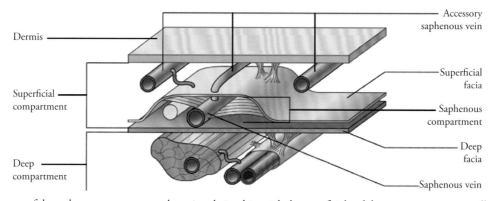

Figure 4.1   This diagram of the saphenous compartment shows its relationships with the superficial and deep compartments as well as the saphenous vein and nerve and their relationships to the medial, anterior, and lateral accessory saphenous veins. (Redrawn with permission from Caggiati A, Bergan JJ, Gloviczki P, et al. Nomenclature of the veins of the lower limbs: An international interdisciplinary consensus statement, *J Vasc Surg*. 2002. *36*: 416–422.)

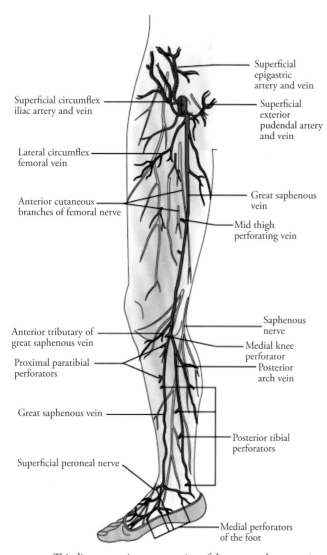

Figure 4.2   This diagrammatic representation of the great saphenous vein emphasizes it relationship to perforating veins and the posterior arch vein. (Redrawn with permission from Mózes G, Gloviczki P, Kádár A, Carmichael SW. Anatomy of the perforating veins. In Gloviczki P, and Bergan JJ, eds. *Atlas of endoscopic perforating vein surgery*. London: Springer. 1998.)

In fact, there are many variations of the small saphenous vein as it connects both to the popliteal vein and to cranial extensions of the saphenous vein, as well as connections to the posteromedial circumflex vein (vein of Giacomini).

The third system of veins is called the perforating vein system. As indicated earlier, they connect the superficial and deep systems of veins. There is a fundamental fact that confuses understanding of perforating veins. This relates to flow direction. Some perforating veins produce normal flow from the superficial to the deep circulation, others conduct abnormal outflow from the deep circulation to the superficial circulation. This is termed perforating vein reflux. Any of these perforating veins may demonstrate bidirectional flow (see Table 4.1).

In the leg, the principal clinically important perforating veins are on the medial aspect of the ankle and leg, and are found anatomically at approximately 6-cm intervals from the base of the heel through the upper portion of the leg. They are therefore at roughly 6, 12, 18, and 24 cm from the

Table 4.1 **SUMMARY OF IMPORTANT CHANGES IN NOMENCLATURE OF LOWER EXTREMITY VEINS**

OLD TERMINOLOGY	NEW TERMINOLOGY
Femoral Vein	Common Femoral Vein
Superficial Femoral Vein	Femoral Vein
Sural Veins	Sural Veins
	Soleal Veins
	Gastrocnemius Veins (Medial and Lateral)
Huntarian Perforator	Mid Thigh Perforator
Cockett's Perforators	Paratibial Perforator
	Posterior Tibial Perforators
May's Perforator	
Gastrocnemius Point	Intergemellar Perforator

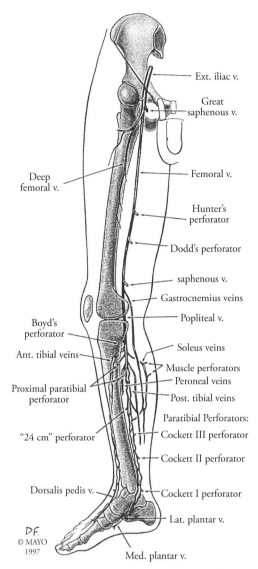

Ext. iliac v.

Great
saphenous v.

Deep
femoral v.

Femoral v.

Hunter's
perforator

Dodd's perforator

saphenous v.

Gastrocnemius veins

Popliteal v.

Boyd's
perforator

Soleus veins

Ant. tibial veins

Muscle perforators

Peroneal veins

Proximal paratibial
perforator

Post. tibial veins

Paratibial Perforators:

Cockett III perforator

"24 cm" perforator

Cockett II perforator

Dorsalis pedis v.

Cockett I perforator

Lat. plantar v.

DF.
© MAYO
1997

Med. plantar v.

Figure 4.3 Deep connections of the main thigh and leg perforating veins are shown in this diagram of the deep veins of the lower extremity. (Redrawn with permission from Mózes G, Gloviczki P, Kádár A, Carmichael SW. Anatomy of the perforating veins. In Gloviczki P, and Bergan JJ, eds. *Atlas of endoscopic perforating vein surgery.* London: Springer. 1998.)

floor (see Figure 4.3). These medial perforating veins may become targets for treatment of severe chronic venous insufficiency (CVI). Smaller perforating veins can be found along intermuscular septa and these allow direct drainage of blood from surface veins into the deep venous system.[6] Conversely, when they are dysfunctional, they allow muscular compartment pressure to be transmitted directly to unsupported cutaneous and subcutaneous veins and venules.

VENOUS PHYSIOLOGY

It is estimated that 60 to 75% of the blood in the body is to be found in the veins. Of this total volume, about 80% is contained in the veins that are less than 200 μm in diameter. It is important to understand this reservoir function as it

is related to the major components. The splanchnic venous circulation and the veins of the skin are richly supplied by the sympathetic nervous system fibers, but muscular veins have little or none of these. The veins in skeletal muscle, on the other hand, are responsive to catecholamines.

Although arterial pressures are generated by muscular contractions of the heart, pressures in the venous system largely are determined by gravity. In the horizontal position, pressures in the veins of the lower extremity are similar to the pressures in the abdomen, chest, and extended arm. However, with the assumption of the upright position, there are dramatic changes in venous pressure. The only point in which the pressure remains constant is the hydrostatic indifferent point just below the diaphragm. All pressures distal to this point are increased due to the weight of the blood column from the right atrium. When assuming the upright position, there is an accumulation of approximately 500 ml of blood in the lower extremities, largely due to reflux through the valveless vena cava and iliac veins. There is some loss of fluid into the tissues, and this is collected by the lymphatic system and returned to the venous system.

Venous valves play an important role in transporting blood from the lower extremities to the heart. In order for valve closure to occur, there must be a reversal of the normal transvalvular pressure gradient. A pressure and generated velocity flow exceeding 30 cm/sec leads to valve closure. Direct observation of human venous valves has been made possible by specialized ultrasound techniques.[7] Venous flow is not in a steady state but is normally pulsatile, and venous valves undergo regular opening and closing cycles. Even when fully opened, the cross-sectional area between the leaflets is 35% smaller than that of the vein distal to the valve. Flow through the valve separates into a proximally directed jet and vortical flow into the sinus pocket proximal to the valve cusp. The vortical flow prevents stasis and ensures that all surfaces of the valve are exposed to shear stress. Valve closure develops when the vortical flow pressure exceeds the proximally directed jet flow.

The role of venous valves in an individual quietly standing is not well understood. Pressures in the superficial and deep veins are essentially the same during quiet standing, but, as Arnoldi has found, the pressure in the deep veins is 1 mm higher, which would tend to keep the valves in the perforating veins closed.[8] Normally functioning perforating vein valves protect the skin and subcutaneous tissues from the effects of muscular contraction pressure. This muscular contraction pressure may exceed 100 to 130 mmHg.

Intuitively, the role of venous valves during muscular exercise is obvious, since their major purpose is to promote antegrade flow from superficial to deep. Volume and pressure changes in veins within the calf occur with muscular activity. In the resting position, with the foot flat on the floor, there is no flow. However, in the heel strike position, the venous plexus under the heel and plantar surface of the foot (Bejar's plexus) is emptied proximally. Blood flows from the foot and ankle into the deep veins of the calf. Then, calf contraction transports this blood into the deep veins of the thigh, and henceforth, blood flow proceeds to the pelvic veins, vena cava, and ultimately to the heart all due to the influence of lower extremity muscular contraction.[9]

PATHOPHYSIOLOGY

Abnormal functioning of the veins of the lower extremities is recognized clinically as venous dysfunction or, more commonly, venous insufficiency. Cutaneous telangiectases and subcutaneous varicose veins usually are grouped together under the title "primary venous insufficiency," and limbs with skin changes of hyperpigmentation, edema, and healed or open venous ulceration are categorized as CVI.

PRIMARY VENOUS INSUFFICIENCY

A dysfunctional venous system follows injury to vein walls and venous valves. This injury is largely due to inflammation, an acquired phenomenon.[10] Factors that are not acquired also enter into such injury. These include heredity, obesity, female gender, pregnancy, and a standing occupation in women. Vein wall injury allows the vein to elongate and dilate thus producing the visual manifestations of varicose veins. An increase in vein diameter is one cause of valve dysfunction that results in reflux. The effect of persistent reflux through axial veins is a chronic increase in distal venous pressure. This venous pressure increases as one proceeds from the inguinal ligament past the knee to the ankle. Prolonged venous hypertension initiates a cascade of pathologic events. These manifest themselves clinically as lower extremity edema, pain, itching, skin discoloration, and ulceration.[11]

The earliest signs of venous insufficiency often are elongated and dilated veins in the epidermis and dermis, called *telangiectasias*. Slightly deeper and under the skin are flat, blue-green veins of the reticular (network) system. These may become dilated and elongated as well (see Figure 4.4). And finally, still deeper but still superficial to the superficial fascia are the varicose veins themselves. All of these abnormal veins and venules have one thing in common: they are elongated, tortuous, and have dysfunctional venous valves. This implies a common cause, which is inflammation.

CVI

Skin changes of hyperpigmentation, scarring from previous ulceration, and active ulcerations are grouped together under the term CVI. Numerous theories have been postulated regarding the cause of CVI and the cause of venous ulceration.[12,13] All the theories proposed in the twentieth century have been disproved. An example is the theory of venous stasis, first proposed in a manuscript by John Homans of Harvard in 1916.[14] In this treatise on diagnosis and management of patients with CVI, Dr. Homans coined the term "post-phlebitic syndrome" to describe the skin changes of CVI. He stated that, "Overstretching of the vein walls and destruction of the valves…interferes with the nutrition of the skin…therefore, skin which is bathed under pressure with stagnant venous blood will form

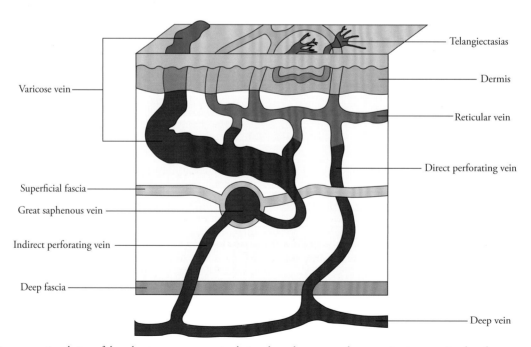

Figure 4.4   This cross-sectional view of the subcutaneous venous circulation shows how venous hypertension is transmitted to the unsupported veins of the dermis and subcutaneous tissues from axial veins and the deep veins of the muscular compartments. (Redrawn with permission from Somjen GM. Anatomy of the superficial venous system, *Dermatol Surg*. 1995. *21*: 35–45.)

permanent open sores or ulcers." That statement, like many others that describe venous conditions and their treatments, is steeped in dogma and is short of observational fact. The erroneous term "stasis ulcer" honors that misconception, as do the terms "venous stasis disease" and "stasis dermatitis."

Alfred Blalock, who later initiated cardiac surgery, disproved the stasis theory by studying oxygen content from varicose veins and normal veins.[15] He pointed out that the oxygen content of the femoral vein in patients with severe CVI was greater than the oxygen content of the contralateral nonaffected limb. Because oxygen content was higher, some investigators felt that arteriovenous fistulas caused venous stasis and varicose veins.[16,17] Though disproved, that explanation has some basis in fact, since the entire thermal regulatory apparatus in limbs depends on the opening and closing of arteriovenous shunts. These shunts are important as they explain some terrible accidents that happen during sclerotherapy when sclerosant entering a vein is shunted into the arterial system and distributed in its normal territory.[18] Microsphere investigations have failed to show any shunting, and the theory of arteriovenous communications has died despite the fact that these shunts actually exist and do open under the influence of venous hypertension.

Hypoxia and its part in causation of CVI was investigated throughout the last 25 years of the twentieth century. English investigators thought that a fibrin cuff, observed histologically, blocked transport of oxygen and was responsible for skin changes of CVI at the ankles and distally.[19] That theory has been abandoned even though a true periarteriolar cuff is easily identified histologically.

The two elements that make up all the manifestations of lower extremity venous insufficiency are failure of the vein valves and vein walls and skin changes at the ankles, both of which are related to venous hypertension.[20]

FAILURE OF VEIN WALLS AND VALVES

Our work suggests that venous hypertension causes a shear stress–dependent leukocyte-endothelial interaction, which has all the manifestations of chronic inflammation.[21] These are leukocyte rolling, firm adhesion to endothelium, and subsequent migration of the cells through the endothelial barrier into parenchyma of valves and vein walls.[22] There, macrophages elaborate matrix metalloproteases, which destroy elastin and possibly collagen as well. Vein walls become stretched and elongated. Vein valves become perforated, torn, and even scarred to the point of near total absence. These changes are seen both macroscopically and angioscopically.[23] Similar changes have been produced in the experimental animal by constructing an arteriovenous fistula to mimic the venous hypertension of venous dysfunction in humans.[24]

The second manifestation of CVI is expressed in the skin, where leukocytes also are implicated in the observed changes. There is evidence that leukocyte activation in the skin, perhaps related to venous hypertension, plays a major role in the pathophysiology of CVI. Thomas, working with Dormandy, reported that 25% fewer white cells and platelets left the dependent foot of the patients with venous hypertension. When the foot was elevated there was a significant washout of white cells but not platelets, suggesting platelet consumption within the microcirculation of the dependent foot.[25] They concluded that the decrease in white cell exodus was due to leukocyte trapping in the venous microcirculation secondary to venous hypertension. They further speculated that trapped leukocytes may become activated, resulting in release of toxic metabolites causing damage to the microcirculation and overlying skin. Apparently, the primary injury in the skin is extravasation of macromolecules and red blood cells into the dermal interstitium. Red blood cell degradation products and interstitial protein extravasations are potent chemoattractants and represent the initial chronic inflammatory signal responsible for leukocyte recruitment.

The important observations of Dormandy's group were historically the first to implicate abnormal leukocyte activity in the pathophysiology of CVI.

The importance of leukocytes in the development of dermal skin alterations was further emphasized by Coleridge Smith and his team.[26] They obtained punch biopsies from patients with primary varicose veins, lipodermatosclerosis, and patients with lipodermatosclerosis and healed ulcers. They counted the median number of white blood cells per high power field in each group but there was no attempt to identify the types of leukocytes. In patients with primary varicose veins, lipodermatosclerosis, and healed ulceration there was a median of 6, 45, and 217 WBCs per mm^2, respectively. This demonstrated a correlation between clinical disease severity and the number of leukocytes in the dermis of patients with CVI.

The types of leukocytes involved in dermal venous stasis skin changes remain controversial. T-lymphocytes, macrophages, and mast cells have been observed on immunohistochemical and electron microscopic examinations.[27,28] The variation in types of leukocytes observed may reflect the types of patients investigated. The London group biopsied patients with erythematous and eczematous skin changes, whereas Pappas has evaluated predominantly older patients with dermal fibrosis. Patients with eczematous skin changes may have an autoimmune component to their CVI, whereas patients with dermal fibrosis may have experienced pathologic alterations consistent with chronic inflammation and altered tissue remodeling. Skin biopsies have shown that in liposclerotic, eczematous skin macrophages and lymphocytes were predominant in such diseased skin. Infiltration of leukocytes into the extracellular space has been documented by observing the localization of these leukocytes around capillaries and postcapillary venules. Accompanying the leukocytes is a disorganized collagen deposition. Clearly, CVI of the skin and its subcutaneous tissues is a disease of chronic inflammation, again dependent on venous hypertension.

SUMMARY AND CONCLUSIONS

Knowing the normal anatomy of the venous system of the lower extremities and the normal functioning of its elements is essential to understanding the pathologic processes of venous dysfunction. Both processes, valve and vein wall damage, and the advanced skin changes of CVI are the result of sterile inflammatory reactions. Both appear to be triggered by venous hypertension and, therefore, therapy must be directed at correcting such venous hypertension.

REFERENCES

1. Federative International Committee for Anatomical Terminology. *Terminologia Anatomica.* Stuttgart: George Thieme Verlag. 1998.
2. Bundens WP, Bergan JJ, Halasz NA, Murray J, Drehobl M. The superficial femoral vein: A potentially lethal misnomer, *JAMA.* 1995. *274*: 1296–1298.
3. Caggiati A, Bergan JJ, Gloviczki P, et al. Nomenclature of the veins of the lower limbs: An international interdisciplinary consensus statement, *J Vasc Surg.* 2002. *36*: 416–422.
4. Weiss RA, Weiss MA. Controlled radiofrequency endovenous occlusion using a unique radiofrequency catheter under duplex guidance to eliminate saphenous varicose vein reflux: A 2-year follow-up, *Dermatol Surg.* 2002. *28*: 38–42.
5. Bush RG, Hammond KA. Tumescent anesthetic technique for long saphenous stripping, *J Am Coll Surg.* 1999. *189*: 626–628.
6. Somjen GM. Anatomy of the superficial venous system, *Dermatol Surg.* 1995. *21*: 35–45.
7. Lurie F, Kistner RL, Eklof B, Kessler D. Mechanism of venous valve closure and role of the valve in circulation: A new concept, *J Vasc Surg.* 2003. *38*: 955–961.
8. Arnoldi CC. Venous pressures in the leg of healthy human subjects at rest and during muscular exercise in the nearly erect position, *Acta Chir Scand.* 1965. *130*: 520–534.
9. Gardner AMN, Fox RH. *The return of blood to the heart*, 2e. London: John Libbey. 1993. 81.
10. Schmid-Schönbein GW, Takase S, Bergan JJ. New advances in the understanding of the pathophysiology of chronic venous insufficiency, *Angiology.* 2001. *52*(Suppl *1*): S27–S34.
11. Ballard JL, Bergan JJ, eds. *Chronic venous insufficiency: Diagnosis and treatment.* London: Springer-Verlag. 2000.
12. Homans J. The etiology and treatment of varicose ulcer of the leg, *Surg Gynecol Obstet.* 1917. *24*: 300–311.
13. Browse NL, Burnand KG. The cause of venous ulceration, *Lancet.* 1982. *320*(8292): 243–245.
14. Homans J. The operative treatment of varicose veins and ulcers based on a classification of these lesions, *Surg Gynec Obst.* 1916. *22*: 143–158.
15. Blalock A. Oxygen content of blood in patients with varicose veins, *Arch Surg.* 1929. *19*: 898–904.
16. Piulachs P, Vidal Baraquer F. Pathogenic study of varicose veins, *Angiology.* 1953. *4*: 59–100.
17. Brewer AC. Arteriovenous shunts, *Br Med J.* 1950. *2*: 270.
18. Bergan JJ, Weiss RA, Goldman MP. Extensive tissue necrosis following high-concentration sclerotherapy for varicose veins, *Derm Surg.* 2000. *26*: 535–542.
19. Coleridge Smith PD. Microcirculation disorders in venous leg ulcer: Microcirculation in CVI, *Microcirculation.* 2001. *8*: 1–10.
20. Takase S, Lerond L, Bergan JJ, Schmid-Schonbein GW. The inflammatory reaction during venous hypertension in the rat, *Microcirculation.* 2000. *7*: 41–52.
21. Takase S, Schmid-Schonbein G, Bergan JJ. Leukocyte activation in patients with venous insufficiency, *J Vasc Surg.* 1999. *30*: 148–156.
22. Takase S, Pascarella L, Lerond L, Bergan JJ, Schmid-Schonbein GW. Venous hypertension, inflammation, and valve remodeling, *Eur J Vasc Endovasc Surg.* 2004. *28*: 484–493.
23. Hoshino S, Satokawa H, Ono T, Igari T. Surgical treatment for varicose veins of the legs using intraoperative angioscopy. In: Raymond-Martimbeau P, Prescott R, Zummo M, eds. *Phlebologie 92.* Paris: John Libbey Eurotext. 1992. 1083–1085.
24. Takase S, Pascarella L, Lerond L, Bergan JJ, Schmid-Schonbein GW. Venous hypertension, inflammation, and valve remodeling, *Eur J Vasc Endovasc Surg.* 2004. *28*: 484–493.
25. Thomas PR, Nash GB, Dormandy JA. White cell accumulation independent legs of patients with venous hypertension: A possible mechanism for trophic changes in the skin, *Br Med J (Clin Res Ed).* 1988. *296*(6638): 1693–1695.
26. Scott HJ, Smith PDC, Scurr JH. Histological study of white blood cells and their association with lipodermatosclerosis and venous ulceration, *Br J Surg.* 1991. *78*: 210–211.
27. Wilkerson LS, Bunker C, Edward JCW, Scurr JH, Coleridge Smith PD. Leukocytes, their role in the etiopathogenesis of skin damage in venous disease, *J Vasc Surg.* 1993. *27*: 669–675.
28. Pappas PJ, DeFouw DO, Venezio LM, et al. Morphometric assessment of the dermal microcirculation in patients with chronic venous insufficiency, *J Vasc Surg.* 1997. *26*: 784–795.

5.

ROLE OF PHYSIOLOGIC TESTING IN VENOUS DISORDERS

Jeffrey K. Raines and Jose I. Almeida

Of the 25 million Americans with venous insufficiency, approximately 7 million exhibit serious symptoms such as edema, skin changes, and venous ulcers.[1] About 1 million seek formal medical advice annually and do so for symptoms of venous insufficiency. Approximately 80% of venous patients are managed conservatively with observation, leg elevation, and support stockings; while the remainder are treated surgically with vein stripping or endovenous ablation. Most investigators acknowledge with the development of safe, less traumatic, and effective endovenous techniques for venous insufficiency, more individuals in the population will seek treatment, and physicians will be more inclined to move from conservative therapy to surgical therapy.

Physiologic testing is used to define deep venous thrombosis and identify, grade, and follow venous insufficiency. Since more patients will be presenting for therapy because of improved outcomes with endovenous techniques over traditional surgery, physiologic testing will take on increasing importance. For purposes of this chapter, physiologic testing includes the various devices based on plethysmographic concepts, and color flow duplex imaging. The goal of these studies is to provide accurate information describing the hemodynamic or anatomic characteristics of the patient with chronic venous insufficiency, precluding the need for invasive studies.[2]

BACKGROUND

Venous insufficiency of the lower extremity is far more frequent than venous insufficiency in any other part of the human circulation. This chapter will therefore be limited to the lower extremity. The venous system in the lower extremities is composed of three interconnected parts: the deep system, perforating (i.e., communicating) system, and superficial system. By virtue of the venous muscular pump and bicuspid/unidirectional valves, in healthy veins, blood flows toward the right side of the heart (i.e., upward) and from the superficial system to the deep system (i.e., inward).

Lower extremity muscle compartments contract during ambulation. This contraction compresses the deep veins, producing a pumping action, which propels blood upward toward the right side of the heart. This pumping action is significant; transient pressures in the deep system have been recorded as high as 5 atmospheres during strenuous lower extremity exertion. This pumping action secondary to ambulation has the effect of reducing pressure within the superficial system. With this in mind, it is instructive to comment on the hydrostatic pressure under which all three venous systems of the lower extremity are subjected. A fluid column has weight and can produce a pressure gradient. In an individual 6 feet in height, the distance from the level of the right atrium to the ankle is 120 cm and produces a hydrostatic pressure of approximately 90 mmHg.

Deep veins can withstand elevated pressure because the fascia in which they exist limits dilation. In contrast, the superficial system, surrounded by elastic skin, is constructed for low pressure; therefore, elevated pressure in the superficial system can produce dilation, elongation, and valve failure. Dilation increases the diameter of the veins and elongation causes them to be more tortuous.

Consider the following cascade of events. Because of valve failure, above-physiologic pressure develops in the superficial system. With time, nearby superficial valves begin to fail (i.e., lose their ability to direct flow in one direction). With dilation and multiple valve failure, venous blood will flow in the direction of the pressure gradient, which is downward and outward. This flow direction is directly opposite physiologic flow (i.e., upward and inward). The early result is varicose veins and telangiectasia, which are visible on the skin surface.

Early or mild venous insufficiency produces low-level pain, edema, burning, throbbing, and leg cramping. As the disease progresses patients can develop venous stasis changes that can lead to debilitating severe soft tissue ulceration. We know from hemodynamics and clinical experience, on eliminating high pressure or flow in diseased superficial venous channels, symptoms can improve dramatically.

In understanding lower extremity venous hemodynamics, the following experiment is instructive (see Figure 5.1). First, a superficial vein in the foot of a normal subject is cannulated and connected to a fluid column (sterile saline with Vitamin A to add color to the column). With the subject standing erect, the fluid column will rise to the level of the right atrium. This is due to the fact that the pressure at the right atrium is near zero and therefore, the venous pressure at the cannulation site is almost entirely based on the subject's hydrostatic blood column (the subject's blood and the fluid in the column have nearly the same specific weight). When the subject is asked to perform sustained ankle flexion, the fluid column drops to between 50–60% of its resting height. This simulates walking and the reduction in superficial venous pressure secondary to the ambulatory venous pump. In subjects with venous insufficiency, the fluid column will not drop to normal levels. If a subject's fluid column falls to normal levels while occluding the superficial system, the observer knows the deep system is intact and the superficial system is incompetent. If the fluid column remains elevated with exclusion of the superficial system, the observer knows the deep system is incompetent. As will be illustrated, physiologic venous testing is based on the principles outlined in this experiment.

While the morbidity secondary to venous insufficiency and varicose veins is significant,[3] the most devastating consequence is due to life threatening venous thromboembolism to the lungs. In a study from the Mayo Clinic, during 14,629 person-years of follow-up, 1,333 patients died.

Seven-day, 30-day, and 1-year venous thromboembolism survival rates were 75%, 72%, and 64%, respectively.[4]

Two statements may summarize this section. First, the culprit in venous insufficiency syndrome is elevated pressure when limbs are dependent or ambulating. Measuring and understanding venous hemodynamics is the cornerstone of this diagnosis. Second, deep venous thromboembolism may result in venous insufficiency and may develop independently. This diagnosis is less hemodynamically oriented and more focused on sonographic visualization of thrombi.

PLETHYSMOGRAPHY

Plethysmographs are devices that measure volume change. Over the last 50 years plethysmographs that employ completely different principles have been developed and used clinically. The impedance plethysmograph (IPG), based on a fundamental principle of electronics, is not widely used.[5,6] The strain-gauge plethysmograph (SGP) measures circumference of a selected limb segment and estimates volume.[7,8] Like IPG, this technique is not in widespread use and will not be more completely defined.

PHOTOPLETHYSMOGRAPH (PPG)

Photoplethysmographs are not true plethysmographs because the measure they provide is qualitative and cannot be used to determine volume. Despite this limitation, PPG is used in many clinics to assess venous insufficiency.[9,10] The device measures phenomena limited to the microvasculature of the cutaneous skin. PPG instrumentation includes a surface transducer, which is taped to the lower leg just above the medial malleolus and connected to an electrical circuit. The electrical circuit excites the transducer and records and interprets the returning signal.

The PPG transducer is designed with an infrared light–emitting diode and a photosensor. The transducer transmits light to the skin, which is both scattered and absorbed by the tissue in the illuminated field. Blood is more opaque than surrounding tissue and therefore attenuates the reflected signal more than other tissue in the field. The intensity of reflected light is reduced with more blood in the field. If the electrical circuit filters the higher frequency arterial pulsations it is possible to register a signal, which qualitatively corresponds to venous volume in the segment of interest. PPG is therefore able to detect changes in venous filling secondary to various patient maneuvers, which will be described below. PPG has found a role in the clinical assessment of venous insufficiency.

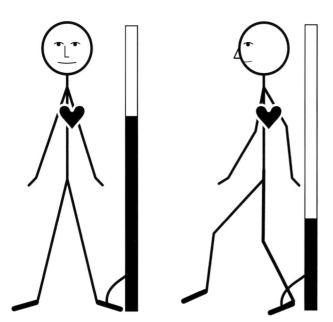

Figure 5.1 The stick figure on the left illustrates a normal subject erect and motionless with a venous cannulation in the left foot. Venous pressures rises to the level of the right atrium. The stick figure on the right illustrates the effect of the normal lower extremity venous pump and the unidirectional valves activated by walking or ankle flexion. The fluid column is reduced to between 50–60% of its resting value. Failure to reduce the height of the fluid column results in ambulatory venous hypertension (i.e., venous insufficiency).

AIR PLETHYSMOGRAPH (APG)

Properly designed air plethysmographs more accurately measure true volume than IPG, SGP, or PPG and are easier to use in the clinical setting.[11–14] The instrumentation is characterized by three major components. The first component is the transducer, which is a form of closed air bladder used to surround the limb segment of interest. The second component is a pressure sensor, which can accurately measure the pressure in the air bladder as a function of time. The third component is the electrical circuit necessary to control the pressure sensor and display the measured results.

As mentioned above, use of the APG is relatively simple. The air bladders are generally self-contained units similar to standard blood pressure cuffs and are designed for specific limb segments. The connection to the console is generally limited to a single rubber tube with connector. With the air bladder surrounding the limb segment of interest, any change in volume in the limb segment will cause the pressure within the bladder to change. For example if limb volume increases the bladder volume with decrease. Since the bladder is a closed system, this will cause the bladder pressure to increase. Accurate APG carefully correlate bladder state (i.e., mean bladder pressure and volume), instantaneous change in bladder pressure, and limb volume change. APG is able to detect changes in venous limb volume secondary to various patient maneuvers. The maneuvers and outputs are similar for all plethysmographs described in this chapter and are given below. APG is used in the clinical assessment of venous insufficiency and deep venous thrombosis.

DEFINITION OF PARAMETERS AND MANEUVERS USED IN GENERIC PLETHYSMOGRAPHY FOR VENOUS INSUFFICIENCY

Venous insufficiency causes the three venous systems in the lower extremity to misdirect venous blood volume. Therefore, the goal of this testing is to characterize misdirection of venous blood volume, if present.

Our test subject is placed in the supine position. This will lower venous pressure in the lower extremities to a value only slightly above right atrial pressure ($\sim$ 0 mmHg). Using a plethysmograph an operator can obtain a baseline volume in the segment of interest. When the subject is placed in the erect position lower extremity venous pressure increases due to the hydrostatic column of blood extending from the right atrium to the segment of interest. Since veins are compliant (i.e., increase volume with increased internal pressure), vein blood volume in the segment of interest increases. This volume increase is displayed on a graph from which measurements may be taken. The Y-axis is volume and the X-axis is time. Since all measurements are either times or ratios, the Y-axis is not required to be strictly calibrated as volume. However, its display on the graph must correlate with volume change (see Figure 5.2).

The measurement between the supine baseline volume and the erect volume plateau is known as the *venous volume* (VV). From this same curve the operator can determine

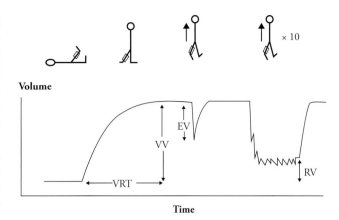

Figure 5.2 This figure illustrates parameter definitions and maneuvers used generically in plethysmographic studies for venous insufficiency.

the *venous refilling time* (VRT). This is the time measured from when the baseline volume begins to increase to its plateau. With the subject in the erect position, the operator instructs the subject to perform a single brisk ankle flexion. This will produce a momentary reduction in Y-axis volume. This change in volume is called the *ejection volume* (EV). To calculate the *ejection fraction* (EF), the operator divides EV by VV. The subject is then instructed to perform 10 brisk ankle flexions. This will produce a reduction in Y-axis volume, which will be larger than the volume reduction experienced with one flexion. This allows the operator to measure *residual volume* (RV). This is defined as the difference between the volume after 10 flexions and the baseline volume. Finally, the operator can calculate the *residual volume fraction* (RVF) by dividing RV by VV.[15–17]

SIMPLIFIED DIAGNOSTIC CRITERIA FOR VENOUS INSUFFICIENCY

These criteria may be applied to any plethysmograph. The only restriction is that the volume measurements be taken accurately. In order to simplify the diagnostic criteria for venous plethysmographic studies we have focused on three parameters. The first is VRT. In patients with significant venous insufficiency, venous refilling develops secondary to venous reflux and clearly reduces the time necessary to complete the process. If VRT is >20 seconds, the limb is not demonstrating significant reflux. If VRT is <20 seconds, the diagnosis of venous reflux should be considered.[17] The second parameter is EF. In patients with deep or superficial venous insufficiency or deep venous thrombosis, EF is reduced. If EF is >60% the limb is presenting with normal venous hemodynamics. For superficial venous insufficiency the average EF is 50%. Average EF is reduced to 40% in subjects with deep venous insufficiency and 35% in deep venous obstruction. The third measurement is RVF. If RVF is elevated, the limb is demonstrating venous ambulatory hypertension. A normal value for RVF is <35%. Subjects with RVF > 35% should be evaluated further for venous disease.[17]

DEEP VENOUS THROMBOSIS (DVT)—EXAMINATION BY PLETHYSMOGRAPHY

The four plethysmographs described above have been used for the identification and monitoring of DVT. For purposes of this text a generic procedure for DVT will be described.

DVT is a life-threatening disease; for that reason alone accurate diagnosis and therapy is essential. The deep venous system is not only a conduit for returning blood to the right side of the heart; it is also a storage or capacitant system. This means its volume changes rapidly as pressure within the deep system changes. If one examines a vein at low pressure the walls are nearly fully collapsed and only a small flow channel is present. It takes very little increase in internal fluid pressure to expand the flow channel of a vein. Finally, if there is obstruction in a segment of deep vein, despite rich venous collateral channels, venous pressure distal to the obstruction will increase. Examination by plethysmograph makes use of these two principles (i.e., volume change with increased pressure and resistance).

Typically a plethysmograph transducer is placed at the calf or distal thigh with the patient lying supine on a table. In the case of APG the transducer is an air bladder inflated to 5 mmHg; in the case of PPG the transducer is a light emitting diode. Proximal to the transducer a method of rapidly occluding the deep system must be used. For all transducers this can be a thigh cuff inflated rapidly by hand bulb or automatic inflator.

With the transducer recording a stable venous signal at 5 mm/sec chart speed, the pressure in the proximal occluding cuff is rapidly elevated to 50 mmHg. The transducer is measuring absolute levels of volume.

With the increased pressure in the proximal cuff, venous blood in the deep system cannot pass under the cuff until the venous pressure reaches approximately occluding cuff pressure. This increase in venous pressure (i.e., pooling) develops because the proximal cuff does not obstruct the arterial inflow. After about 20 to 40 seconds, pressure in the distal venous system reaches the pressure in the occluding cuff and venous volume reaches a plateau. Once the plateau has been reached, the operator rapidly releases the pressure in the occluding cuff. The pooled venous blood can then return to the right side of the heart via the larger veins upstream. Two measures of venous hemodynamics are taken during this test. First, there is the volume increase from the baseline to the plateau. This is known as *segmental venous capacitance* (SVC) and represents the blood storage capacity of the segment vein. This is generally quoted in millimeters of deflection, or milliliters if the system is calibrated to volume. The second measurement is the slope of the volume-time curve immediately after the pressure in the occluding cuff is released. This is known as *maximum venous outflow* (MVO) and represents resistance to blood flow in the deep system. This may be quoted in millimeters of deflection per second or milliliters per second if the system is calibrated to volume. The next two sections define the diagnostic use of these parameters.

Segmental Venous Capacitance (SVC)

With experience, vascular technologists and physicians are able to identify a normal range of SVC with their specific plethysmographic equipment. With the subject supine, normal veins have significant capacitance. If proximal deep venous obstruction is present, pressure distal to the obstruction increases and SVC is markedly reduced. Therefore, if SVC reduces more than 25% when compared with normal levels, venous abnormality is suggested.[11] It is recommended that SVC always be measured bilaterally. In the case of unilateral disease, the normal limb can serve as a control, which increases both sensitivity and specificity.

Maximum Venous Outflow (MVO)

As in the case of SVC, vascular technologists and physicians are able to identify a normal range of MVO with their specific plethysmographic equipment. Normal veins exhibit a very rapid decrease in volume on deflation of the occluding cuff. When deep system resistance is increased due to deep venous obstruction the reduction in MVO is dramatic. Again, in the case of unilateral disease, the normal limb can serve as a control. A difference in MVO between limbs of 25% is abnormal.[11]

When continuous-wave venous Doppler measurements, SVC, and MVO are performed as a diagnostic package, sensitivity and specificity of the combined testing reaches 85% respectively.[11] It should be acknowledged duplex venous Doppler ultrasonic imaging, which requires more expensive equipment, clearly demonstrates a higher sensitivity and specificity. Further, ultrasound is able to more accurately localize obstruction and age thrombus. For this reason, plethysmographic methods have limited diagnostic use. There is one area in venous disease where SVC and MVO provide unique and important information. This is in the determination of venous collaterization following a DVT. Patients that normalize SVC and MVO rapidly have an improved prognosis when compared with subjects in which normalization is prolonged.

CONTINUOUS-WAVE VENOUS DOPPLER (CW DOPPLER)

CW Doppler instruments are widely available, relatively inexpensive, and used extensively to rapidly investigate the peripheral vascular system. CW Doppler measurements can be used independently or, as mentioned above, combined with measurements from a plethysmograph. The purpose of this section is to outline how CW Doppler is used to facilitate the diagnosis of venous insufficiency of the deep system, specifically deep vein reflux and DVT.

Strandness and Baker introduced CW Doppler in the 1960s.[18] Its initial application was peripheral arterial assessment. With the development of additional maneuvers the instrumentation was applied first to the diagnosis of DVT and later to deep vein insufficiency.

We recommend that the subject be studied on a flat examining table in which the lower extremities may be placed in the dependent position at approximately 15 degrees. This slight angle dilates the deep system, which makes the identification of veins easier and improves the velocity signals. We recommend that target veins include the common femoral vein at the inguinal ligament, popliteal vein at the popliteal fossa, and the posterior tibial vein just behind the medial malleolus.

With the pencil-like probe positioned toward the venous flow and at 60 degrees to the flow streamline, the target velocity is optimized. The fact that a velocity is identified means the vein is patent at the target level, and this is the first of three major diagnostic criteria. The second diagnostic criterion is associated with the spontaneous and phasic nature of the signal. When veins are not obstructed proximal to the target vein, the local pressure is low and local velocity changes as a function of respiration. Low-pressure veins collapse and local velocity is often reduced to zero shortly after inspiration. This is due to the fact that when the diaphragm moves down on inspiration, pressure in the closed abdominal cavity increases and collapses veins at low pressure. With proximal obstruction this phasic velocity is disturbed in the sense that velocity is no longer phasic with respiration and in fact may be continuous. The third criterion is associated with velocity response secondary to distal compression. When veins are unobstructed proximal to the target and compression is performed distally, the local velocity will increase in response to compression. In a high resistance proximal venous system, distal compression will not evoke increased velocity.

If a subject demonstrates at the femoral, popliteal, and posterior tibial veins good velocity signals that are phasic with respiration and augment with distal compression, the chance of DVT involving the iliac, common femoral, femoral, or popliteal veins is very low. DVT limited to the calf veins is more problematic due to vein duplication at this level. As mentioned above, when CW Doppler is combined with venous plethysmography (SVC and MVO) the sensitivity and specificity of the combined package is 85% respectively.[11]

VENOUS INSUFFICIENCY

The main use of CW Doppler in venous insufficiency is in assessing reflux in the major deep veins of the lower extremity (common femoral, femoral, and popliteal veins). This procedure is most effectively performed with the subject standing. To the extent possible, weight should be shifted to the contralateral leg. A bidirectional CW Doppler with a stereo audio signal and printout is recommended. For venous work an ultrasound frequency range of 5 to 7 MHz is suggested. As a quick review, the pencil-like probe of the CW Doppler should be aligned toward the flow and at an angle of approximately 60 degrees to the anticipated flow streamline. Unlike duplex ultrasound, with CW Doppler the exact path of the target vein is not well defined. Therefore, in practice the operator will have to manually adjust the probe angle to obtain the maximum signal (audio level and velocity level). The concept is quite simple; target veins are assessed for reversal of flow velocity after rapid manual limb compression and release. The more reversal, the more reflux. In terms of diagnostic criteria, a normal vein demonstrates no evidence of reflux using this technique. Flow reversal can be assessed both by audio signal and by examination of velocity versus time printouts.[17]

ASSESSMENT OF THE DEEP AND SUPERFICIAL VENOUS SYSTEMS USING DUPLEX ULTRASOUND

The two sections preceding this text described pure physiologic measures. This section will focus on the combination of physiologic and imaging measures. Further, duplex ultrasound has become the "gold standard" in the diagnosis of both deep venous thrombosis and venous insufficiency. The method is so pervasive that it has replaced in most venous centers the use of venous plethysmographs and CW Dopplers. It should also be stated that the accuracy, speed, and cost of this procedure to diagnose deep venous thrombosis has been so attractive that venography is rarely indicated or necessary.

Power Color Pulsed-Wave Doppler and High-Resolution B-mode Imaging characterize state-of-the-art duplex ultrasound. Descriptions of these devices are found elsewhere in this book and are commonplace in medical literature. The remaining sections describe our approach to the assessment of the deep and superficial systems using duplex ultrasound.

RISK FACTORS, VASCULAR HISTORY, PRESENTING SIGNS AND SYMPTOMS, AND CEAP CLASSIFICATION

In addition to demographic data we suggest risk factors and associated history be recorded. This includes parameters like obesity, pregnancy, hormone use, and hypercoagulability. Also recorded for each leg are presenting signs and symptoms like edema, pain/tenderness, skin changes, varicose veins, and previous DVT. We have found the CEAP classification to be helpful in describing degree of disease and in developing management plans.[19]

DEEP VENOUS SYSTEM ASSESSMENT

We recommend that the subject be studied on a flat examining table in which the lower extremities may be placed in the dependent position at approximately 15 degrees. This slight angle dilates the deep system, which makes the identification of veins easier and improves the velocity signals. We recommend deep vein interrogation from the level of the inguinal ligament to the distal calf. This includes the common femoral, femoral, popliteal, and tibial veins. In special cases the deep femoral vein may be added to this list. Effective imaging requires that the technologist have a comprehensive understanding of venous and arterial anatomy.

The evaluation begins by obtaining a B-mode image of the structures at the level of the inguinal ligament. In a single transverse view it is generally possible to see the common femoral vein, common femoral artery, and great saphenous vein (GSV). In Florida, we refer to this image as the "Mickey Mouse Image" because of the similarity to the Disney character. We have found keeping the lateral (arterial) structures on the left side of the screen for both the right and left leg to be helpful. This requires that the technologist rotate the linear array probe 180 degrees when moving from the right to the left leg. The marker on the probe should be oriented to the lateral aspect of the leg. With this orientation, Mickey's face is the common femoral vein and is the larger and lower of the three structures. The common femoral artery is Mickey's right ear and the GSV is Mickey's left ear. As the probe is moved distally, the GSV will disappear, and the common femoral artery will divide into the superficial femoral artery and the deep femoral artery. As the probe continues distally the technologist should focus on keeping the superficial femoral artery and the femoral vein in clear view. The popliteal artery and the popliteal vein are difficult to visualize in the adductor canal, therefore, these structures are identified by placing the probe in the popliteal crease. Below the knee, the duplicated posterior tibial and peroneal veins with their associated single arteries can be viewed with the probe at a medial location. In general, the anterior tibial veins can be ignored because they are rarely pathologic.

During this examination a number of maneuvers are necessary. First, the technologist may change from transverse to longitudinal views. When longitudinal views are used the vein walls (proximal and distal) should be seen across the entire screen, left to right. The technologist may use the Doppler portion of the duplex system to verify artery versus vein and determine flow direction.

With the probe, the technologist can compress the vein. The ability to fully compress the vein walls confirms vein patency and absence of thrombus formation. The technologist also looks for visible thrombus formation in the vein structures. Acute thrombi are characterized by vein dilatation and noncompressible echo lucent intraluminal material. Chronic thrombi take on a speckled ultrasonic appearance.

If the evaluated system from the common femoral vein through the tibial veins is compressible and no evidence of thrombus formation is seen, the study is considered negative for DVT. Color Doppler, Power Doppler, compression maneuvers, and respiratory maneuvers can be used to supplement this procedure, if necessary.

SUPERFICIAL VENOUS SYSTEM ASSESSMENT

Most investigators agree assessment of the superficial venous system is more challenging for the technologist and interpreting physician than the deep system.[20,21] We agree with this contention. In our facility we always perform deep system assessment in advance of superficial venous system assessment.

In contrast to the deep system, for superficial assessment we always evaluate subjects in the erect position. We have our subjects stand on a standard medical step, which is approximately 8 inches high. The patient is asked to rotate the leg of interest to expose the medial surface of the lower extremity from the groin to the ankle. To the extent possible, weight should be shifted from the leg of interest in order to relax the musculature. A degree of arm support may be needed.

With the subject properly positioned, the technician moves the probe to the inguinal ligament and produces the Mickey Mouse image described above. The Mickey Mouse image is the most important landmark of the venous examination. At this point the focus is on the GSV. Starting from the three-vessel image in the transverse view the probe is slowly moved down the leg following the course of the GSV. The GSV is kept near midscreen. The normal GSV extends from the saphenofemoral junction to the distal calf and is surrounded by superficial fascia above and muscular fascia below. As a minimum we record diameter measurements in millimeters and the presence of reflux (positive or negative) at three locations in the GSV (saphenofemoral junction, mid thigh, and below knee).

Reflux is determined at locations of interest using the following technique. The technologist adjusts the color box of the duplex system in the measurement location. The velocity scale is adjusted (maximum 25 cm/sec). While a signal is being obtained the technologist compresses the calf (below the probe) in a brisk manner. The vein highlighted in the color box should demonstrate an increase in velocity toward the heart with compression. On release the vein should demonstrate no velocity or minimal velocity away from the heart. We have found that reflux (venous flow away from the heart after release) lasting between 0.5 to 2.0 seconds is mild. Reflux is severe if present > 2.0 seconds.

The same evaluation is repeated for the small saphenous vein (SSV). This vein originates in the distal calf and can terminate in the upper thigh. We access this vessel with ultrasound by rotating the subject to expose the back of the legs.

We identify the SSV at the distal calf, and advance over the course of the SSV. Multiple levels may be assessed; however, we generally record a characteristic SSV diameter (mm) and assess reflux in the most diseased location.

At this point it is important to note that there are variations in superficial venous anatomy. For example, the GSV may be quite small and complemented by an anterior accessory saphenous vein (AASV), which may be competent or incompetent. Further, the GSV may be duplicated in portions of its course. It is worth repeating that these variations are common and must be known and anticipated by the technologist, if a comprehensive report is to be generated.

The lower extremity has some common perforators that play significant roles in venous insufficiency. Huntarian perforating veins are located in the mid thigh. The Dodd's perforator is located in the distal thigh. The Boyd perforating vein is located below the level of the popliteal fossa. Finally, we have Cockett #1, #2, and #3 perforating veins located respectively between the ankle and the lower calf. Newer terminology of perforating veins that describe their anatomical location, is discussed in Chapter 2. This assessment must also be part of this work-up. If present, perforators should be assessed regarding diameter, degree of reflux, and extension to other superficial structures.

Finally, there are tributaries of the GSV and SSV that deserve attention. We look for seven tributaries in the GSV and three in the SSV. If present, we record diameter, degree of reflux, and connection to other superficial structures.

In closing, we emphasize that duplex ultrasound is not only diagnostic, but also plays crucial roles in endovenous ablation, ultrasound-guided sclerotherapy, and monitoring the success of vein closure procedures.

REFERENCES

1. Barron HC, Ross BA. *Varicose veins: A guide to prevention and treatment.* New York: Facts on File. 1995. vii.
2. Marston WA. PPG, APG, or Duplex: Which noninvasive tests are most appropriate for the management of patients with chronic venous insufficiency?, *Semin Vasc Surg.* 2002. *15*(1): 13–20.
3. Prandoni P, Villalta S, Bagatelle P, et al. The clinical course of deep vein thrombosis: Prospective long-term follow-up of 528 symptomatic patients, *Haematologica.* 1997. *82*(4): 423–428.
4. Heit JA, Silverstein MD, Mohr DN, et al. Predictors of survival after deep vein thrombosis and pulmonary embolism: A population-based, cohort study, *Arch Intern Med.* 1999. *159*(5): 445–453.
5. Wheeler HB. Diagnostic tests for deep vein thrombosis: Clinical usefulness depends on probability of disease, *Arch Intern Med.* 1994. *154*: 1921–1928.
6. Huisman MV, Buller HR, ten Cate JW, Vreeken J. Serial impedance plethysmography for suspected deep venous thrombosis in outpatients: The Amsterdam General Practitioner Study, *N Engl J Med.* 1986. *314*: 823–828.
7. Croal S, Birkmyre J, McNally M, Hamilton C, Mollan R. Straingauge plethysmography for the detection of deep venous thrombosis, *J Biomed Eng.* 1993. *15*: 135–139.
8. Maskell NA, Cooke S, Meecham Jones DJ, Prior JG, Butland RJA. The use of automated strain gauge plethysmography in the diagnosis of deep vein thrombosis, *Br J Radiology.* 2002. *75*: 648–651.
9. Fronek A. Photoplethysmography in the diagnosis of venous disease, *Dermatol Surg.* 1995. *21*(1): 64–66.
10. Schultz-Ehrenburg U, Blazek V. Value of quantitative photoplethysmography for functional vascular diagnostics: Current status and prospects, *Skin Pharmacol Appl Skin Physiol.* 2001. *14*(5): 316–323.
11. Raines, J, Traad, E. Noninvasive evaluation of peripheral vascular disease, *Med Clin N Am.* 1980. *64*: 283–304.
12. Owens LV, Farber MA, Young ML, et al. The value of air plethysmography in predicting clinical outcome after surgical treatment of chronic venous insufficiency, *J Vasc Surg.* 2000. *32*(5): 961–968.
13. Asbeutah AM, Riha AZ, Cameron JD, McGrath BP. Reproducibility of duplex ultrasonography and air plethysmography used for the evaluation of chronic venous insufficiency, *J Ultrasound Med.* 2005. *24*(4): 475–482.
14. Fukuoka M, Sugimoto T, Okita Y. Prospective evaluation of chronic venous insufficiency based on foot venous pressure measurements and air plethysmography findings, *J Vasc Surg.* 2003. *38*(4): 891–895.
15. Nicolaides AN, Christopoulos D, Vasdekis S. Progress in the evaluation of chronic venous insufficiency, *Ann Vasc Surg.* 1989. *3*: 278–292.
16. Abramowitz HB, Queral LA, Flinn WR, et al. The use of photoplethysmography in the assessment of venous insufficiency: A comparison to venous pressure measurements, *Surgery.* 1979. *86*: 434–441.
17. Needham T. Assessment of lower extremity venous valvular insufficiency examinations, *J Vasc Ultrasound.* 2005. *29*(3): 123–129.
18. Strandness DE. History of ultrasonic duplex scanning, *Cardiovasc Surg.* 1996. *4*(3): 273–280.
19. Porter JM, Moneta GL. Reporting standards in venous disease: An update: International Consensus Committee on Chronic Venous Disease, *J Vasc Surg.* 1995. *21*(4): 635–645.
20. Labropoulos N, Touloupakis E, Giannoukas AD, et al. Recurrent varicose veins: Investigation of the pattern and extent of reflux with color flow duplex imaging, *Surgery.* 1996. *119*: 406–409.
21. Valentin LI, Valentin WH, Mercado S, et al. Venous reflux localization: Comparative study of venography and DU, *Phlebology.* 1993. *8*: 124–127.

6.

INAPPROPRIATE LEUKOCYTE ACTIVATION IN VENOUS DISEASE

Philip Coleridge Smith

INTRODUCTION

Venous ulceration remains a common problem in medical practice. A great deal has been learned about the causes of this problem, but a simple solution for all patients remains elusive. Although the presence of a leg ulcer is easy to establish, it may be the result of a number of diseases, not just venous disease. In a recent study patients with leg ulcers had venous disease, arterial disease, diabetes, lymphedema, and rheumatoid disease.[1] In this study patients had combined pathologies in 35% of cases. The overall prevalence of open venous ulceration in published epidemiological studies in adults over the age of 18 years is about 0.3%.[2–5] For every patient with an open ulcer there are probably three or four with healed venous ulcers. This means that approximately 1% of the adult population are affected by ulceration, either open or healed. Since these ulcers require regular management by health care services, the cost of this disease remains high.

Venous ulceration occurs when valves fail in the deep, superficial, or perforating veins. This results in impairment of the venous muscle pumps in the lower limb.[6] Superficial venous reflux accounts for 20 to 50% of venous leg ulcers,[7,8] with deep vein and perforating vein reflux involved in many. The consequence of incompetent lower limb vein valves is that the pumping mechanism no longer reduces the pressure in the superficial veins to low levels during walking. This is reflected in the microcirculation of the skin leading, in some patients, to lipodermatosclerosis and leg ulceration.

MECHANISMS OF ULCERATION

FIBRIN CUFFS

In 1982 Browse and Burnand proposed that oxygen diffusion into the tissues of the skin was restricted by a pericapillary fibrin cuff that they had observed histologically.[9] They suggested that increased capillary pressure as a consequence of venous hypertension results in an increased loss of plasma proteins through the capillary wall. This includes fibrinogen, which polymerizes to provide the fibrin cuff that may be seen around capillaries in the skin, using both histochemical and immunohistochemical methods. Subsequent measurements of fibrinolysis have shown that patients with venous disease have reduced fibrinolytic activity in the blood and veins, which might explain why the fibrin cuff persists.[10]

The clearance of [133]xenon from the skin as an assessment of the efficiency of the microcirculation in handling a molecule of similar size to oxygen had been measured. This gas has a molecular weight four times that of oxygen, so its diffusion rate would be half that of oxygen, assuming similar solubility for oxygen and xenon in body fluids (water). Measurements were made in the liposclerotic skin of patients with venous disease, and compared with control subjects under conditions of reactive hyperemia after five minutes of cuff occlusion of the arterial supply to the leg. No difference in xenon clearance was found between patients with venous disease and control subjects.[11] These findings lead to the conclusion that in patients with chronic venous insufficiency, skin changes are not principally attributable to failure of skin oxygenation.

THE WHITE CELL TRAPPING HYPOTHESIS

The search for alternative mechanisms of skin damage in venous disease has resulted in investigation of the blood itself. Thomas investigated a series of patients and control subjects who were subjected to experimental venous hypertension by sitting with the legs dependent for a period of 60 minutes.[12] Blood samples were taken from the great saphenous vein at the ankle. After 60 minutes patients with venous disease were trapping 30% of the white cells and control subjects were trapping 7%.

White cell margination is a normal event in the arterioles, capillaries, and venules. This phenomenon is thought to be important in the mechanism that results in tissue injury following ischemia. White blood cells are substantially larger than red cells and are responsible for many of the rheological properties of blood. White cells take 1,000 times longer than red cells to deform on entering a capillary bed, and are responsible for about half the peripheral vascular resistance despite their small numbers in the circulation compared with red cells.[13] In myocardial infarction they cause capillary occlusion, which can be prevented in experimental animals by first rendering the animal leukopenic.[14,15] White blood cells have been implicated as the mediators of ischemia in many tissues including myocardium, brain, lung, and kidneys.[16–19] Polymorphonuclear leukocytes, particularly those attached to capillary endothelium, may become activated, in which cytoplasmic granules containing proteolytic enzymes are released.[20] In addition, a nonmitochondrial respiratory burst permits these cells to release free radicals, including the superoxide radical, which have nonspecific destructive effects on lipid membranes, proteins, and many connective tissue compounds.[21] Leukotactic factors also are released, attracting more polymorphonuclear cells.

In conjunction with other authors I published a hypothesis suggesting that white cell trapping resulted in neutrophil activation, causing damage to the tissues (see Figure 6.1).[22]

Based on the literature on myocardial ischemia, we proposed that white cells might cause occlusion of capillaries. If some of the capillaries were occluded this might result in heterogeneous perfusion and therefore tissue hypoxia and ischemia. This seemed a reasonable suggestion at the time, since it predated our attempts to measure the severity of the diffusion block, and we included this to explain the hypoxia observed by transcutaneous oximetry. I subsequently have concluded that this part of the original hypothesis is not of major importance in producing skin damage in patients with venous disease.

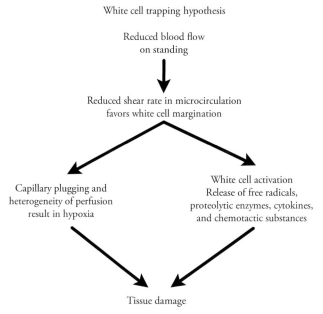

White cell trapping hypothesis

Reduced blood flow
on standing

Reduced shear rate in microcirculation
favors white cell margination

Capillary plugging and
heterogeneity of perfusion
result in hypoxia

White cell activation
Release of free radicals,
proteolytic enzymes, cytokines,
and chemotactic substances

Tissue damage

Figure 6.1   White cell trapping hypothesis as originally published in Coleridge Smith PD, Thomas P, Scurr JH, Dormandy JA. Causes of venous ulceration: A new hypothesis, *Br Med J.* 1988. *296*: 1726–1727.

LEUKOCYTE ACTIVATION

The effect of venous hypertension on leukocyte activation subsequently has been studied in human volunteers using a series of plasma and cellular markers. Control subjects exposed to lower limb venous hypertension produced by standing were studied by taking blood samples from the hand and the leg veins. Degranulation of neutrophils was studied by measuring plasma levels of neutrophil elastase (a primary neutrophil granule enzyme) and lactoferrin (a secondary neutrophil granule enzyme). After a 30-minute period of experimental venous hypertension, a rise in plasma lactoferrin concentration was observed in the blood taken from both the foot and the arm.[23] When venous hypertension was produced by inflation of a cuff around one lower limb, a rise in lactoferrin was observed only in that limb. Subsequently expression of the surface neutrophil ligand, CD11b, has been investigated as a marker of neutrophil activation. The experiment was repeated as before on control subjects. Blood was taken from a dorsal foot vein. CD11b expression was assessed by fluorescent labeled monoclonal antibody used to label neutrophils in whole blood, which were counted using flow cytometry. During the period of venous hypertension in control subjects no rise in CD11b expression was seen in the lower limb blood.[24] Following return to the supine position, when neutrophils might be expected to leave the lower limb, according to the studies of Thomas,[12] increased levels of CD11b were observed. This indicates that neutrophils were upregulated by their period of adhesion to normal endothelium. An increased white cell: red cell ratio also was observed during this phase, confirming white cell egress from the lower limb.

A similar study also has been conducted in patients with venous disease, including only subjects with unulcerated skin to avoid the possibility that the inflammatory processes involved in the ulcer may result in upregulation of inflammatory mediators in a way unrelated to the development of the ulcer. Two groups of patients were studied: one group with uncomplicated varicose veins and one with skin changes (lipodermatosclerosis) attributable to venous disease. The adhesion of neutrophils and monocytes to endothelium was investigated. This is a two-stage process. Initially these cells roll along the endothelium, binding in a loose manner using a ligand on the leukocytes known as CD62L or L-selectin. When binding occurs a fragment of L-selectin is released into the plasma (soluble L-selectin) and can be detected by an ELISA. It was found that the concentration of soluble L-selectin rose during venous hypertension, confirming that endothelial-leukocyte binding had occurred. There was no major difference in magnitude between the two groups of patients.[25]

Subsequently, firm binding of neutrophils and monocytes occurs using CD11b/CD18 ligands, which link to endothelial ICAM. This is reflected in the peripheral blood by a fall in the cells expressing most CD11b. Just such a fall was seen in the blood taken from the leg in both groups of patients. On returning patients to the supine position I had expected to see an egress of leukocytes expressing more CD11b in these patients, but this was not observed, in contrast to the studies on control subjects. In the time scale of this experiment (up to 10 minutes following venous hypertension), the more activated neutrophils and monocytes remained bound to the endothelium of the lower limb.[26]

Plasma lactoferrin and elastase have been assessed in groups of patients with active venous disease. Blood was taken from the arm veins (not the lower limb veins) of patients with varicose veins, liposclerotic skin change, and active venous ulceration.[27,28] In all samples, the levels of lactoferrin and elastase were higher in the patients than the age and sex-matched control groups (see Figures 6.2 and 6.3).

However, it was found that the highest levels of plasma lactoferrin were present in patients with active varicose veins. Subsequently blood was taken from the arms of patients for measurement of neutrophil CD11b expression. This was elevated in patients with varicose veins, but depressed in patients with lipodermatosclerosis.[29] The explanation may be that the more active leukocytes are attracted to the

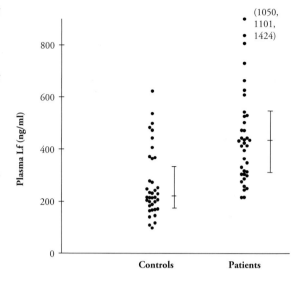

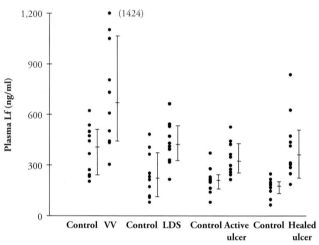

Figure 6.3   Results of plasma neutrophil lactoferrin measurements in patients and control subjects. Error bars show the median and interquartile range of data.

region of the inflammatory process and do not circulate in the peripheral blood. Alternatively, such patients may have high circulating levels of neutrophil inhibitors.

HISTOLOGY

Histological studies have been used to investigate the biological processes at work in the skin in chronic venous disease. A quantitative histological study has been reported in which three groups of patients were studied.[30] The first was a group of patients with no evidence of skin changes as a consequence of their venous disease. The next group exhibited lipodermatosclerosis without a history of ulceration. The third group had healed ulcers with residual lipodermatosclerosis. Patients with normal skin had a low number of white blood cells visible (4 per mm^2) in the upper 0.5 mm of the skin. There were eight times as many in patients with liposclerotic skin, and 40 times as many in patients with healed venous ulcers. Subsequently an immunohistological

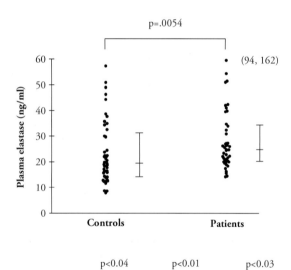

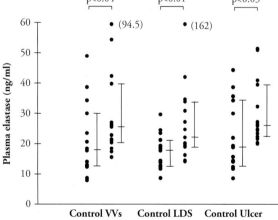

Figure 6.2   Results of plasma neutrophil elastase measurements in patients and control subjects. Error bars show the median and interquartile range of data. Statistical significance was tested by the Mann-Whitney U test.

study was undertaken to determine the types of white cell present in this infiltrate.[31] The majority of cells are macrophages with a T-lymphocyte component, but no excess of neutrophils compared with control sections taken from normal limbs. So this infiltrate is a reflection of a chronic inflammatory process.

THE ENDOTHELIUM

The microcirculation of the skin has been investigated by histology[32] and by capillary microscopy.[33] Both methods demonstrate capillary proliferation in patients with chronic venous insufficiency—vastly more capillaries are visible by both techniques (see Figure 6.4). However, capillary microscopy shows that these probably arise from a single capillary loop and appear like a glomerulus, rather than an increase in the numbers of capillaries. Quantitative measurement of the capillary convolution in patients from each of the CEAP (clinical, etiological, anatomic, pathophysiologic) clinical classes has been published (see Figure 6.5).[34] Immunohistochemical investigations have shown that the pericapillary cuff contains far more than fibrin. The capillary endothelium is perturbed, expressing increased amounts of

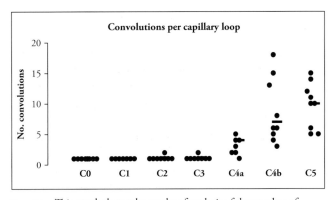

Figure 6.5   This graph shows the results of analysis of the number of convolutions per capillary loop in images such as those shown in Figure 6.4. The vertical axis shows the number of convolutions per capillary in CEAP stages C0–C5. Capillary abnormalities are mainly present in C4a, C4b, and C5 limbs.

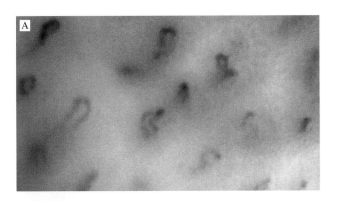

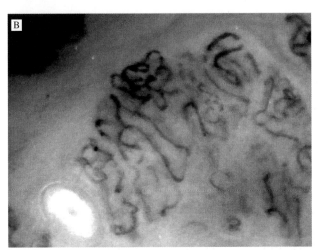

Figure 6.4   Images from the capillary microscope. Normal capillary loops in the skin of the lower limb show one reversal of direction as the vessel rises to the top of the papillary dermis and then descends (A). In a patient with lipodermatosclerosis, numerous convolutions are seen in each capillary (B).

factor VIII–related antigen[31,35] and adhesion molecules, especially ICAM-1. ELAM-1 may be slightly upregulated, but VCAM appears to be normal in patients without venous ulceration. Perturbed endothelium is more likely to attract the adhesion of leukocytes. The presence of the pericapillary fibrin cuff has been confirmed, but it also contains collagen IV, laminin, fibronectin, and tenascin.[36] A strong leukocyte infiltration has been measured in patients with venous disease.[37] These cells are macrophages and T-lymphocytes. The cytokines involved include IL-1α and IL-1β. TNFα has not been detected in these histological sections. The presence of the perivascular fibrin cuff (with other components) is a reflection of the inflammatory process and is seen in other chronic inflammatory conditions. In patients with venous disease, increased plasma D-dimer levels have been observed, suggesting enhanced deposition of fibrin.[38] The perturbed state of the endothelium allows the passage of large molecules though the endothelium permitting their perivascular accumulation, and explains the presence of the fibrin cuff.

A search for systemic markers of endothelial activation has been performed by undertaking measurements of plasma levels of soluble endothelial adhesion molecules and von Willebrand factor.[39] Patients with chronic venous disease (a group with uncomplicated varicose veins and a group with skin changes) again were studied and compared with normal controls. The concentration of soluble VCAM (vascular endothelial adhesion molecule) was elevated in both patient groups compared with control subjects, and was highest in the group with skin changes (see Figure 6.6).

HISTOLOGICAL SEARCH FOR ANGIOGENIC FACTORS

The vascular proliferation seen in the skin of patients with venous disease has been known for many years, but has not been explained. In recent years many angiogenic factors that stimulate the growth of blood vessels have been recognized.

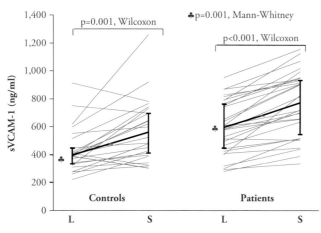

Figure 6.6 Plasma VCAM-1 levels in normal controls and patients with chronic venous disease (with and without skin changes), before and after venous hypertension produced by sitting with the lower limbs dependent for 30 min. Descriptors: medians and inter-quartile ranges; statistics; Wilcoxon and Mann-Whitney U tests for unpaired data. L = lying, S = standing.

Immunohistochemistry was used to evaluate the presence of a number of such factors in the skin of patients with venous disease.[40] Skin biopsies were taken at the time of surgery for varicose veins from the legs of patients with and without skin changes as well as of breast skin in patients without clinical evidence of venous disease, for use as a control. There was an increase in platelet-derived growth factor, subtype BB (PDGF-BB) in patients with venous disease. This was found in the capillary wall in vessels of the dermal papillae. There was also considerable upregulation of the production of vascular endothelial growth factor (VEGF) in the epidermis of patients with venous disease, most marked in those with skin changes. It seems likely that VEGF may account for at least some of the vascular proliferation seen in the skin of patients with venous disease. This growth factor is also responsible for increased vascular permeability to large molecules, a feature of the skin microangiopathy that has been reported from capillary microscopy studies.[33] The mechanism of stimulation of epidermal VEGF production is unclear at present.

SKIN FIBROSIS IN VENOUS DISEASE

The role of transforming growth factor beta 1 (TGF-β_1) in the skin damage of chronic venous insufficiency has been studied in considerable detail by Pappas et al using immunohistochemical examination, electron microscopy, and examination of TGF-β_1 gene expression.[41] This investigation indicated that activated leukocytes traverse perivascular cuffs and release active TGF-β_1. Positive TGF-β_1 staining of dermal fibroblasts was observed and suggests that fibroblasts are the targets of activated interstitial leukocytes. A potential mechanism for quick access and release is storage of TGF-β_1 in the extracellular matrix. TGF-β_1 was elevated exclusively in areas of clinically active disease,

indicating a localized response to injury. These data suggest that alterations in tissue remodeling occurs in patients with chronic venous insufficiency and that dermal tissue fibrosis in chronic venous insufficiency is regulated by TGF-β_1.

The fibrosis seen in the skin of patients with lipodermatosclerosis also has been investigated by other authors.[42] This study shows that enhanced cell proliferation and an increase in the number of procollagen mRNA-expressing fibroblasts contribute to the development of lipodermatosclerosis (see Figure 6.7). The fibrotic changes that result may not only be mediated by inflammatory cell-derived factors but by additional profibrotic agents released in the skin as a consequence of chronic venous hypertension.

Some authors have studied the distribution of growth substances and connective tissue proteins in skin biopsies using immunohistochemical staining.[43] In particular they studied the pericapillary cuffs, which were once thought to inhibit oxygen transfer to the tissues. The cuffs were positive for actin, type IV collagen, factor XIIIa, and alpha 2-macroglobulin, and there was increased TGF-β_1. They observed that TGF-β_1 immunoreactivity was present within the fibrin cuffs, but not in the provisional matrix in the ulcer bed around the cuffs. These observations suggest that growth factors critical in wound healing, such as TGF-β_1, are present within venous ulcers, but are abnormally distributed. Their distribution within fibrin cuffs and

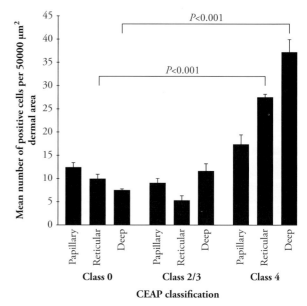

Figure 6.7 Increased procollagen type I–expressing cells in lipodermatosclerotic skin. The number of positive dermal cells, as demonstrated by in situ hybridization, was assessed in skin sections from the control patients (CEAP Class 0, n = 12), from patients with chronic venous insufficiency but no clinical evidence of lipodermatosclerosis (CEAP Class 2/3, n = 10), and from patients with lipodermatosclerosis (CEAP Class 4, n = 12). Data represent mean and SEM. (From Degiorgio-Miller AM, Treharne LJ, McAnulty RJ, Coleridge Smith PD, Laurent GJ, Herrick SE. Procollagen type I gene expression and cell proliferation are increased lipodermatosclerosis, *Br J Dermatol*. 2005. 152: 242–249.)

colocalization with extravasated plasma proteins, particularly alpha 2-macroglobulin, which is a recognized scavenger molecule for TGF-β and other growth factors, provides evidence for a possible trapping of growth factors in venous ulcers. This proposal has been advanced as a cause for failure of venous leg ulcers to heal.[44]

INTERPRETATION OF DATA FROM EXISTING STUDIES

Endothelial adhesion is a normal physiological activity of neutrophils and monocytes. During venous hypertension the fall in blood flow to the lower limb and increase in diameter of capillaries result in a fall in the shear rate in cutaneous capillaries. This favors leukocyte adhesion, which may be observed even in control subjects but is of greater magnitude in patients with venous disease, presumably due to the modifications that take place in the endothelium in chronic venous disease.

It has been found that leukocyte-endothelial interaction occurs during short-term venous hypertension (within 30 minutes) and that during this period neutrophil degranulation may be detected, releasing primary and secondary granule enzymes into the region of the endothelium. At the same time an increase in von Willebrand factor and soluble endothelial adhesion molecules can be found in the leg blood. These arguments apply to control subjects as well as to patients, although the magnitude of change is always greater in the patients rather than the control subjects.

The research shows that when the venous system becomes deranged, endothelial injury may be the result. Activated leukocytes leave the lower limbs of control subjects following venous hypertension. In patients with venous disease, these cells appear to remain in the lower limb, perhaps attached to the abnormal endothelium.

The chronic changes seen in lipodermatosclerotic skin may be the response to sustained, low-grade injury to the endothelium by neutrophils and monocytes over many months or years. The perivascular infiltration of vessels in the papillary dermis by macrophages and T-lymphocytes may simply be a tissue response to the chronic inflammatory processes referred to earlier (see Figure 6.8). Endothelial activation is seen during this phase with increased expression of endothelial adhesion molecules. This would favor the adhesion of further leukocytes encouraging this process to continue.

The chronic inflammatory process results in the release of cytokines, which encourage vascular proliferation. VEGF has been shown to be involved in this process. Whether this is simply an associated phenomenon or crucial to subsequent ulceration remains unclear at present. Extensive skin fibrosis, which is part of the clinical syndrome of lipodermatosclerosis, is a feature of chronic venous disease. The macrophages present in the perivascular inflammatory process release TGF-β, and this in turn stimulates fibroblasts to synthesize more collagen and connective tissue proteins.

The progression from the chronic skin damage to actual ulceration remains difficult to understand. A possible explanation is that an initiating stimulus causes massive activation

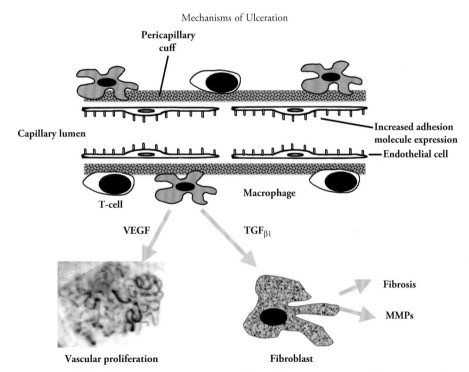

Mechanisms of Ulceration

Figure 6.8   Diagrammatic summary of findings from many investigations in skin capillaries in patients with chronic venous disease. The capillaries comprise endothelial cells showing activation. The vessels are surrounded by an inflammatory cuff with a cellular infiltrate, which includes macrophages. These and other cell types release a range of cytokines that, among other things, produce vascular proliferation and skin fibrosis.

of the perivascular macrophages, resulting in extensive tissue and blood vessel destruction. This might occur spontaneously, or minor trauma to the region may set in motion the series of events that lead to ulcer formation.

The data collected in the studies of neutrophil, monocyte, and endothelial cell activity have so far failed to identify major differences between those patients who develop skin changes and are at risk of ulcerasion and those who do not. Inflammatory mechanisms are very complex, and identifying those which predispose to the development of skin changes and ulceration will be a complex task.

IMPLICATIONS FOR PHARMACOLOGICAL TREATMENT IN VENOUS DISEASE

Although bandaging and stockings have been used effectively in the treatment of chronic venous insufficiency for many years, modern pharmacological science may provide assistance in healing venous ulcers and perhaps some insight into the mechanisms of the disease.

Pentoxifylline has been used for the treatment of claudication for a number of years, with moderate success. Its mechanism of action is probably through an effect on inhibition of cytokine-mediated neutrophil activation.[45] Its efficacy in healing venous leg ulcers has been reported in a recent meta-analysis.[46] Nine trials involving 572 adults were included. Pentoxifylline plus compression is more effective than placebo plus compression (relative risk of healing with pentoxifylline 1.30, 95% confidence interval 1.10–1.54). This drug could be considered for use in patients with venous leg ulceration when used in combination with compression.

Prostaglandin E_1 (PGE_1) has a number of profound effects on the microcirculation, including reduction of white cell activation, platelet aggregation inhibition, small vessel vasodilatation, and reduction of vessel wall cholesterol levels. Recently the results of a randomized, placebo-controlled, single-blind study in which 87 patients who had venous leg ulcers has been reported.[47] Patients were treated with compression bandaging and conventional wound management. They also received treatment for 20 days with an infusion of prostaglandin E_1 analogue (Prostavasin, Schwarz Pharma) or placebo. After four months, all ulcers were healed in the active treatment group but only 32 of 38 in the placebo group. This is a potentially useful drug, but the limitation of giving intravenous infusions restricts it applicability.

Laurent et al investigated micronized purified flavonoid fraction (MPFF)[48] and showed that this drug reduced the symptoms of venous disease (aching, itching, feeling of swelling) and also reduced ankle edema. More recently MPFF has been studied for its effects on venous leg ulcer healing. A meta-analysis has been published in which five prospective, randomized, controlled studies involving 723 patients with venous ulcers were included.[49] Patients were treated with compression bandaging and local wound care

in all cases. In two studies MPFF was compared with placebo, and in three studies MPFF was compared with standard treatment alone. At six months, the chance of healing ulcer was 32% better in patients treated with adjunctive MPFF than in those managed by conventional therapy alone. The main benefit of MPFF was present in the subgroup of ulcers between 5 and 10 cm^2 in area and those present for 6 to 12 months duration. MPFF therefore may be a useful drug to combine with compression management in countries where it is licensed.

CONCLUSIONS

The precise mechanisms through which venous hypertension causes ulceration remain to be discovered. There is clear evidence of leukocyte activation in venous disease, and many inflammatory mechanisms are upregulated in the skin. So far it has been impossible to say which of these is the main cause of the problem and which are simply a response to the inflammatory process. Drugs that mitigate leukocyte activation appear to benefit ulcer healing. A better understanding of the initiating processes may lead to improvements in the management of patients with venous ulceration.

REFERENCES

1. Moffatt CJ, Franks PJ, Doherty DC, Martin R, Blewett R, Ross F. Prevalence of leg ulceration in a London population, *QJM*. 2004. *97*: 431–437.
2. Evans CJ, Fowkes FG, Ruckley CV, Lee AJ. Prevalence of varicose veins and chronic venous insufficiency in men and women in the general population: Edinburgh Vein Study, *J Epidemiol Community Health*. 1999. *53*: 149–153.
3. Callam MJ, Ruckley CV, Harper DR, Dale JJ. Chronic ulceration of the leg: Extent of the problem and provision of care, *Br Med J*. 1985. *290*: 1855–1856.
4. Baker SR, Stacey MC, Singh G, et al. Aetiology of chronic leg ulcers, *Eur J Vasc Surg*. 1992. *6*: 245–251.
5. Nelzen O, Bergqvist D, Lindhagen A, Hallbook T. Chronic leg ulcers: An underestimated problem in primary health care among elderly patients, *J Epidemiol Community Health*. 1991. *45*: 184–187.
6. Nicolaides AN, Zukowski A, Lewis R, Kyprianou P, Malouf GM. Venous pressure measurements in venous problems. In: Bergan JJ, Yao JST, eds. *Surgery of the Veins*. Orlando: Grune and Stratton. 1985. 111–118.
7. Dodd H, Cockett FB. *The pathology and surgery of the veins of the lower limb*. Edinburgh: Churchill Livingstone. 1976.
8. Hoare MC, Nicolaides AN, Miles CR, et al. The role of primary varicose veins in venous ulceration, *Surgery*. 1982. *92*: 450–453.
9. Browse NL, Burnand KG. The cause of venous ulceration, *Lancet*. 1982. *320*(8292): 243–245.
10. Browse NL, Gray L, Jarrett PEM, Morland M. Blood and vein-wall fibrinolytic activity in health and vascular disease, *Br Med J*. 1977. *1*(6059): 478–481.
11. Cheatle TR, McMullin GM, Farrah J, Coleridge Smith PD, Scurr JH. Three tests of microcirculatory function in the evaluation of treatment for chronic venous insufficiency, *Phlebology*. 1990. *5*: 165–172.
12. Thomas PRS, Nash GB, Dormandy JA. White cell accumulation in the dependent legs of patients with venous

hypertension: A possible mechanism for trophic changes in the skin, *Br Med J.* 1988. *296*: 1693–1695.

13. Braide M, Amundson B, Chien S, Bagge U. Quantitative studies of leucocytes on the vascular resistance in a skeletal muscle preparation, *Microvasc Res.* 1984. *27*: 331–352.

14. Engler RL, Dahlgren MD, Peterson MA, Dobbs A, Schmid-Schoenbein GW. Accumulation of polymorphonuclear leucocytes during three hour myocardial ischemia, *Am J Physiol.* 1986. *251*: H93–100.

15. Romson JL, Hook BG, Kunkel SL, Abrams GD, Schork MA, Lucchesi BR. Reduction of the extent of ischemic myocardial injury by neutrophil depletion in the dog, *Circulation.* 1983. *67*: 1016–1023.

16. Wilson JW. Leucocyte sequestration and morphologic augmentation in the pulmonary network following haemorrhagic shock and related forms of stress, *Adv Microcirc.* 1972. *4*: 197–232.

17. Linas SL, Shanley PF, Whittenburg D, Berger E, Repine JE. Neutrophils accentuate ischemia-reperfusion injury in isolated perfused rat kidneys, *Am J Physiol.* 1988. *255*: F728–F735.

18. Yamakawa T, Suguyama I, Niimi H. Behaviour of white blood cells in microcirculation of the cat brain cortex during hemorrhagic shock: Intravital microscopic study, *Int J Microcirc: Clin Exp.* 1984. *3*: 554.

19. Braide M, Blixt A, Bagge U. Leukocyte effects on the vascular resistance and glomerular filtration of the isolated rat kidney at normal and low flow rates, *Circulatory Shock.* 1986. *20*: 71–80.

20. Weissman G, Smolen JE, Korchak HM. Release of inflammatory mediators from stimulated neutrophils, *N Engl J Med.* 1980. *303*: 27–34.

21. Babior BM. Oxidants from phagocytes: Agents of defense and destruction, *Blood.* 1984. *64*: 959–966.

22. Coleridge Smith PD, Thomas P, Scurr JH, Dormandy JA. Causes of venous ulceration: A new hypothesis, *Br Med J.* 1988. *296*: 1726–1727.

23. Shields DA, Andaz S, Abeysinghe RD, Porter JB, Scurr JH, Coleridge Smith PD. Neutrophil activation in experimental ambulatory venous hypertension, *Phlebology.* 1994. *9*: 119–124.

24. Shields D, Andaz SK, Timothy-Antoine CA, Scurr JH, Porter JB. CD11b/CD18 as a marker of neutrophil adhesion in experimental ambulatory venous hypertension, *Phlebology.* 1995. *1995* (Suppl 1): 108–109.

25. Saharay M, Shields DA, Porter JB, Scurr JH, Coleridge Smith PD. Leukocyte activity in the microcirculation of the leg in patients with chronic venous disease, *J Vasc Surg.* 1997. *26*: 265–273.

26. Shields DA, Andaz S, Sarin S, Scurr JH, Coleridge Smith PD. Neutrophil activation in experimental venous hypertension, *Phlebologie.* 1993. *46*: 687–689.

27. Shields DA, Andaz S, Abeysinghe RD, Porter JB, Scurr JH, Coleridge Smith PD. Plasma lactoferrin as a marker of white cell degranulation in venous disease, *Phlebology.* 1994. *9*: 55–58.

28. Shields DA, Andaz SK, Sarin S, Scurr JH, Coleridge Smith PD. Plasma elastase in venous disease, *Br J Surg.* 1994. *81*: 1496–1499.

29. Shields D, Saharay M, Timothy-Antoine CA, Porter JB, Scurr JH. Neutrophil CD11b expression in patients with venous disease, *Phlebology.* 1995. *1995*(Suppl 1): 108–109.

30. Scott HJ, McMullin GM, Coleridge Smith PD, Scurr JH. A histological study into white blood cells and their association with lipodermatosclerosis and ulceration, *Br J Surg.* 1990. *78*: 210–211.

31. Wilkinson LS, Bunker C, Edwards JC, Scurr JH, Coleridge Smith PD. Leukocytes: Their role in the etiopathogenesis of skin damage in venous disease, *J Vasc Surg.* 1993. *17*: 669–675.

32. Burnand KG, Whimster I, Naidoo A, Browse NL. Pericapillary fibrin in the ulcer-bearing skin of the leg: The cause of lipodermatosclerosis and venous ulceration, *Br Med J.* 1982. *285*: 1071–1072.

33. Haselbach P, Vollenweider U, Moneta G, Bollinger A. Microangiopathy in severe chronic venous insufficiency evaluated by fluorescence video-microscopy, *Phlebology.* 1986. *1*: 159–169.

34. Howlader MH, Coleridge Smith PD. Microangiopathy in chronic venous insufficiency: Quantitative assessment by capillary microscopy, *Eur J Vasc Endovasc Surg.* 2003. *26*: 325–331.

35. Veraart JC, Verhaegh ME, Neumann HA, Hulsmans RF, Arends JW. Adhesion molecule expression in venous leg ulcers, *Vasa.* 1993. *22*: 213–218.

36. Herrick SE, Sloan P, McGurk M, Freak L, McCollum CN, Ferguson MW. Sequential changes in histologic pattern and extracellular matrix deposition during the healing of chronic venous ulcers, *Am J Pathol.* 1992. *141*: 1085–1095.

37. Scott HJ, McMullin GM, Coleridge Smith PD, Scurr JH. A histological study into white blood cells and their association with lipodermatosclerosis and ulceration, *Br J Surg.* 1990. *78*: 210–211.

38. Falanga V, Kruskal J, Franks JJ. Fibrin and fibrinogen-related antigens in patients with venous disease and venous ulceration, *Arch Dermatol.* 1991. *127*: 75–78.

39. Saharay M, Shields DA, Georgiannos SN, Porter JB, Scurr JH, Coleridge Smith PD. Endothelial activation in patients with chronic venous disease, *Eur J Vasc Endovasc Surg.* 1998. *15*: 342–349.

40. Pardoe HD. *The expression of angiogenic growth factors in the skin of patients with chronic venous disease of the lower limb.* MSc Thesis, University College London. September 1996. 1–61.

41. Pappas PJ, You R, Rameshwar P, et al. Dermal tissue fibrosis in patients with chronic venous insufficiency is associated with increased transforming growth factor-beta1 gene expression and protein production, *J Vasc Surg.* 1999. *30*: 1129–1145.

42. Degiorgio-Miller AM, Treharne LJ, McAnulty RJ, Coleridge Smith PD, Laurent GJ, Herrick SE. Procollagen type I gene expression and cell proliferation are increased lipodermatosclerosis, *Br J Dermatol.* 2005. *152*: 242–249.

43. Higley HR, Ksander GA, Gerhardt CO, Falanga V. Extravasation of macromolecules and possible trapping of transforming growth factor-beta in venous ulceration, *Br J Dermatol.* 1995. *132*: 79–85.

44. Falanga V, Eaglstein WH. The "trap" hypothesis of venous ulceration, *Lancet.* 1993. *341*: 1006–1008.

45. Sullivan GW, Carper HT, Novick WJ, Mandell GL. Inhibition of the inflammatory action of interleukin-1 and tumour necrosis factor (alpha) on neutrophil function by pentoxifylline, *Infect Immunol.* 1988. *56*: 1722–1729.

46. Jull AB, Waters J, Arroll B. Pentoxifylline for treating venous leg ulcers, *Cochrane Database Syst Rev.* 2002. *1*: CD001733.

47. Milio G, Mina C, Cospite V, Almasio PL, Novo S. Efficacy of the treatment with prostaglandin E-1 in venous ulcers of the lower limbs, *J Vasc Surg.* 2005. *42*: 304–308.

48. Laurent R, Gilly R, Frileux C. Clinical evaluation of a venotropic drug in man: Example of Daflon 500 mg. *Int Angiol.* 1988. *7*(Suppl 2): 39–43.

49. Coleridge-Smith P, Lok C, Ramelet AA. Venous leg ulcer: A meta-analysis of adjunctive therapy with micronized purified flavonoid fraction, *Eur J Vasc Endovasc Surg.* 2005. *30*: 198–208.

7.

CHRONIC VENOUS INSUFFICIENCY

MOLECULAR ABNORMALITIES AND ULCER FORMATION

Joseph D. Raffetto

INTRODUCTION

Chronic venous insufficiency (CVI) is a condition that affects the venous system of the lower extremities rendering the superficial, perforating, and deep veins incompetent. This results from venous hypertension and causes various pathologies including pain, swelling, edema, skin changes, and ulcerations. The underlying pathology leading to CVI is a consequence of venous hypertension from valve incompetence causing venous reflux and/or obstructive disease.[1] Varicose veins by definition have incompetent valves with increased venous pressure leading to progressive dilation and tortuosity. The formation of primary varicose veins is unknown, but is likely a multifactorial process related to heredity, female sex hormones, hydrostatic force, and hydrodynamic muscular compartments.[2] The significance of protracted venous hypertension from abnormal venous hemodynamics is the formation of dermal skin changes called *lipodermatosclerosis*, which leads to dermal and subcutaneous tissue fibrosis and eventual ulceration.[3] This chapter will review the recent literature supporting the formation of varicose veins, with specific interest in the molecular changes in the vein wall of varicosities, and basic scientific studies that have investigated the molecular alterations that are present in advanced CVI disease, namely dermal tissue fibrosis and venous ulcer formation.

VARICOSE VEINS

ABNORMALITIES WITH MATRIX METALLOPROTEINASE METABOLISM

Varicose veins have characteristically tortuous and dilated venous walls. A possible explanation for these findings may be the influences of proteolytic enzymes known as matrix metalloproteinases (MMPs) and their inhibitors known as tissue inhibitors of metalloproteinases (TIMPs), which lead to venous wall remodeling and subsequent dilatation and valvular incompetence. MMPs are highly homologous zinc-dependent endopeptidases that cleave most of the constituents of the extracellular matrix. To date there are 26 human MMPs, which are classified according to their substrate specificity and structural similarities. The four major subgroups of MMPs are gelatinases, interstitial collagenases, stromelysins, and membrane-type MMPs (MT-MMPs). MMPs are important enzymes in embryogenesis, acute tissue healing, remodeling, neoplastic invasion and metastasis, skin and granulomatous diseases, aging, and chronic wounds. MMPs are regulated by cytokines, growth factors, and activation of TIMPs, which specifically degrade and inactivate MMPs.

In the recent decade there has been a significant interest in the role of MMPs in the pathophysiology of varicose vein formation. An early report evaluating the collagen and elastin content of nonthrombophlebitic varicose veins compared with normal saphenous veins found that there was increased collagen and a significant decrease in elastin in both varicose veins and in the vein segment not affected by valvular incompetence but with varicosities at other sites. In this study gelatin zymography and elastase activity failed to demonstrate any differences, indicating the presence of an imbalance in tissue matrix but not attributable to proteolytic activity.[4] In support of this prior study, evaluation of the vein segment at the saphenofemoral junction in patients with varicose veins demonstrated that MMPs' activity was unchanged with that of control and with most of the MMPs located in the adventitia, and the content of MMP-2 was decreased but TIMP-1 content was increased.[5] Neither of these studies supported the role of MMPs in extracellular matrix degradation in the formation of varicose veins; however, both of these studies examined normal vein tissue in patients with varicose veins. An additional study investigated the TIMP-1/MMP-2 in varicose veins. A three-fold ratio increase was found in varicose veins compared with normal veins, and the authors concluded that, due to the favored proteolytic inhibition, extracellular matrix accumulation could account for the pathogenesis observed in varicose veins.[6]

To demonstrate that MMPs were induced by postural changes in patients with varicose veins, a study sampled blood from the brachial vein and lower extremity varicose vein in erect patients following 30 minutes of stasis. The investigators found that there was an abundant increase of pro-MMP-9 in the plasma of sampled blood from the varicose vein compared with arm vein. In addition, the proteolytic activity was associated with increased levels of endothelial membrane intercellular adhesion molecule-1, vascular cell adhesion molecule-1, angiotensin converting enzyme, and L-selectins indicating endothelial cell and polymorphonuclear cell activation and enzymatic granule release in varicose veins during periods of stasis.[7] This study provided evidence that MMPs are important proteolytic enzymes in patients with CVI that affect the interface of the leukocytes and endothelium in varicose veins. A number of investigators have specifically examined various MMPs in varicose veins. A current study examining MMP-1, MMP-3, and MMP-13 in the proximal and distal vein segments in patients with CVI versus normal control demonstrated that transcriptional products (mRNA) were not different for MMP-1 or MMP-13 in varicose veins versus control nor in proximal versus distal varicose segments. However, the protein expression of MMP-1 was elevated in varicose veins compared with controls. In addition, regional variation of MMP-1 and MMP-13 expression were increased significantly in proximal versus distal varicose segments.[8] Other investigators have found that the morphologic variations of MMPs differ in localization by immunohistochemical technique within the endothelium, media, and adventitia, with elevated amounts of MMP-1 in smooth muscle and adventitia of varicose veins, but without any differences in TIMPs. In another study, MMP-9 was found to have increased immunopositive staining in smooth muscle cells. These findings, although not causative, suggest that MMPs may lead to venous wall degradation and affect the extracellular matrix of the normal venous wall structure.

Of interest is whether varicose veins with concomitant thrombophlebitis have variations in MMPs' expression compared with varicose veins. In a recent study evaluating MMP-1, MMP-2, MMP-3, and MMP-9 activity, it was found that thrombophlebitic varicose veins had elevated content of MMPs in the vein wall, with increased gelatinase activity and MMP-1 activity. Varicose veins had increased activity of MMP-2. It was concluded that the wall of varicose veins, especially those affected with thrombophlebitis, have extensive alterations in content and activity of MMPs that may lead to remodeling and influence venous wall mechanical properties.[9]

ALTERATIONS IN SMOOTH MUSCLE CELLS, DERMAL FIBROBLASTS, AND COLLAGEN

Several studies have investigated cultured smooth muscle cells derived from varicose veins to determine whether the extracellular matrix modifications seen in varicose vein tissue are related to smooth muscle cells. Smooth muscle cells cultured from varicose veins were found to have decreased number of cells staining for collagen type III and fibronectin, although the transcriptional products of these two proteins were not dissimilar. The synthesis and deposition of collagen type III but not type I was significantly lower in varicose veins. When MMPs and TIMPs were analyzed from the supernatant of confluent cells no differences were observed. These findings suggested that the regulation was altered during posttranscriptional events for both collagen type III and fibronectin in smooth muscle cells.[10] Further work in this area demonstrated that varicose great saphenous vein has a smaller spiraled collagen distribution specifically in the intima and media.

In an interesting study, investigators evaluated abnormal collagen in cultured dermal fibroblasts, to determine whether the phenotypic changes observed in venous smooth muscle cells of patients with varicose veins are also present in their dermal fibroblasts. The findings from this study demonstrated that the synthesis of collagen type I and the transcript mRNA product were increased in dermal fibroblasts, but as in smooth muscle cells, dermal fibroblasts also had decreased synthesis of collagen type III despite normal transcript. Among the various MMPs evaluated, pro-MMP-2 was increased in dermal fibroblasts cultured from patients with venous disease. The authors concluded that the synthesis of collagen type III is dysregulated in dermal fibroblasts and is comparable to the observations of smooth muscle cells derived from patients with varicose veins, suggesting a systemic alteration in tissue remodeling.[11] The same investigators demonstrated that with inhibition of MMP with Marimastat, the production of collagen type III in smooth muscle cells from varicose veins was partially restored. In addition, MMP-3, which degrades fibronectin, was elevated in both transcription product and protein expression. The authors concluded that the mechanism involved in collagen type III and fibronectin degradation in the smooth muscle cells cultured from varicose veins likely is linked to the expression of MMP-3.

ALTERATIONS WITH PROGRAMMED CELL DEATH (APOPTOSIS)

Apoptosis involves cell suicide in response to intrinsic signals (mitochondrial pathway) or extrinsic stimuli (death receptor pathway) in order to maintain homeostasis of the organism. The intrinsic mechanism of apoptosis involves the mitochondrial pathway. In normal cells the mitochondria express the bcl-2 (b-cell lymphoma 2) protein on their surface that is bound to Apaf-1 (apoptotic protease activating factor 1). Internal damage of a cell by oxygen reactive species, drugs, toxins, and radiation leads to Apaf-1 dissociation with concomitant Bax protein to enter the mitochondria with resultant cytochrome c egression in the cytosol. Cytochrome c and Apaf-1 bind to caspase 9 (cysteinyl aspartate-specific protease), cleave at specific aspartic acid residues, forming an apoptosome that activates other caspases that digest structural proteins and cleave chromosomal DNA, causing DNA fragmentation. In the extrinsic pathway, the events that commit a cell to either a path of apoptosis or necrotic cell death after a specific stimulus is dictated in the former and not the latter by the activation of the central cell death signal via a specific set of surface death receptors that form a specific death domain effector and activate caspase 8. The specific inducers of apoptosis include tumor necrosis factor, neurotransmitters, growth factor withdrawal, IL-2 withdrawal, Fas ligands (expressed on cytotoxic T lymphocytes), whereas oxygen reactive metabolites, viral infection, chemotherapeutic drugs, radiation (UV and gamma), and toxins can affect both the intrinsic and extrinsic pathways.[12]

Alteration in apoptosis is responsible for many intractable human diseases including neurodegenerative disorders (Alzheimer's, Parkinson's), autoimmune diseases (lupus, rheumatoid arthritis), and cancer. In the past five years investigators have examined the role of apoptosis in varicose vein formation. In an earlier report the apoptotic index was 48% in control veins and only 15% in varicose veins. Apoptosis was observed only in the adventitia, and immunoreactivity was similar for bcl-2 protein, but cyclin D1 was increased significantly in varicose veins, indicating inhibition of apoptosis in varicose veins may be related to changes in expression of cell cycle events.[13] In further exploring the observed reduced apoptosis in varicose veins, the same authors examined the expression of Bax protein and of poly ADP-ribose polymerase (PARP, involved in repair of DNA damage), which is inhibited by caspases 3 and 6 activation. In twenty patients with varicose veins, the immunoreactivity expression of Bax and PARP was decreased in the distal portion of the varicose veins compared with distal control vein specimens. Both of these studies imply that reduced apoptosis may lead to functional abnormalities required in maintaining the integrity and homeostasis of the vein wall. Other studies support the role of changes in apoptosis regulatory proteins in varicose vein pathophysiology. A recent study evaluating the distal segment of varicose veins and controls demonstrated disorganized architecture with increased collagen fibers and a decrease in the density and size of elastic fibers. In addition, varicose veins exhibited fewer immunoreactive cells in the media for Bax and caspase 9, suggesting that the dysregulation of the intrinsic pathway of apoptosis disrupts normal tissue integrity leading to varicose vein formation.[14]

ANIMAL MODELS OF VENOUS HYPERTENSION

The underlying disturbance leading to varicose vein formation is venous hypertension and valvular incompetence. There are a few animal models that have investigated the effect of acute and chronic venous hypertension on molecular changes of the vein wall and valvular function. By creating a femoral artery and vein arteriovenous fistula an acute rat model of venous hypertension evaluated valvular changes and vein wall biochemical characteristics. At three weeks, three of four rats had demonstrable venous reflux and increased venous pressure (94 ± 9 mmHg, control 11 ± 2 mmHg) compared with the contralateral control femoral vein. The pressurized veins were dilated with valve leaflets, and length and width were reduced. There was a significant inflammatory response represented by leukocytes infiltrating the entire vein wall, and upregulation of P-selectin and intercellular adhesion molecules. In this study there were no differences in MMP-2 or MMP-9 at three weeks, and interestingly the number of apoptotic cells in the vein wall was increased.[15] In a subsequent study, these investigators evaluated both acute and chronic venous hypertension in the femoral vein of 60 rats by the same methodology. The findings were an increased pressure in the femoral vein (96 ± 9 mmHg) with progressive reflux at 42 days post arteriovenous fistula formation. As previously determined, the valves distal to the fistula demonstrated increased diameter, decreased height, and fibrosis of the valve in the media and adventitia. Of interest, valve obliteration was observed and MMP-2 and MMP-9 were elevated significantly after 21 and 42 days of venous hypertension.[16] Based on these studies, a model of venous hypertension is feasible, and significant endothelial, biochemical, and valve structure changes of inflammation and fibrosis are present. However, only proximal segments of veins were analyzed, and whether the venous changes are a result from venous hypertension, venous arterialization, or a combination will require further work to evaluate if these venous abnormalities are transmitted to distal segments of the axial veins as observed in human CVI pathology.

ADVANCED CVI: LIPODERMATOSCLEROSIS AND VENOUS ULCERS

THEORETICAL PERSPECTIVES IN CVI DERMAL FIBROSIS AND ULCER FORMATION

The formation of venous ulcer and the mechanisms for dermal fibrosis are not known. In the early 1980s and through the 1990s various investigators proposed possible explanations for the underlying cause of advanced forms of dermal pathology in CVI patients. In 41 patients with venous ulcers, tissue biopsies were stained for fibrin. The tissues were found to have layers of fibrin around dermal capillaries of lipodermatosclerotic skin, but no fibrin was found in control normal skin. The pericapillary fibrin cuff observed in skin with lipodermatosclerosis was proposed to cause tissue fibrosis and hypoxia, causing ulcer formation.[17] A series of investigations on CVI patients determined that there were 24% fewer leukocytes leaving the dependent lower limb, which was reversed upon elevation of the limb.[18] This led to the hypothesis that leukocytes trapped in the microcirculation (dermal capillaries) resulted in tissue ischemia and venous ulceration.[19] Growth factors are considered important mediators toward wound healing. A possible mechanism for venous ulcer formation proposed that growth factors became bound or "trapped" by macromolecules such as α-2 macroglobulin and fibrinogen.[20] These proposed theories were important because they led to further investigation to define the role of pericapillary changes, leukocyte function, and the effect of cytokines and growth factors on the pathogenesis of tissue fibrosis and venous ulcer formation.

THE ROLE OF LEUKOCYTES

The role of leukocytes in CVI was demonstrated by the increased number of cells in the dermis of patients with lipodermatosclerosis and healed ulceration.[18] Further work in this area aimed to define cell type and function responsible for the formation of the dermal skin fibrosis and ulceration. In a study evaluating the number of white blood cells in tissue biopsies of patients with CVI, it was determined that the number of leukocytes was highest in the dermis of patients with a history of ulceration followed by tissue with lipodermatosclerosis and lowest in patients with uncomplicated skin and CVI.[21] A careful histological study using immunohistochemistry in patients with severe lipodermatosclerotic skin changes determined that the predominant cell types were T lymphocytes and macrophages, expression of intercellular adhesion molecule-1 was elevated but not endothelial leukocyte adhesion molecule-1 or vascular cell adhesion molecule, and neutrophils were rarely observed, concluding that the accumulation of macrophages and T lymphocytes are associated with CVI skin changes and ulceration.[22] To further evaluate the activity of circulating markers on leukocytes in patients with CVI and confirm prior findings of dermal tissue histological findings, a study determined that compared with normal control patients, patients with CVI had decreased CD3+/CD38+ markers on T lymphocytes and increased expression of CD14+/CD38+ markers on monocytes, and no neutrophil activation was present.[23] Function of mononuclear cells was evaluated by proliferation response assays in the presence of staphylococcal enterotoxin antigen challenge. The study concluded that mononuclear cell function deteriorated with CVI, and that diminished proliferative response was

observed with greater severity of CVI disease (venous ulcers and lipodermatosclerosis), indicating that decrease mononuclear cell proliferation may be involved in poor wound healing.[24] In a quantitative study using electron microscopy to evaluate differences in endothelial cell structure, leukocyte cell type and their relationship to the microcirculation in dermal biopsies of patients with advanced CVI were investigated. The authors determined that patients with severe lipodermatosclerosis and healed ulcers contained a significant number of mast cells around arterioles and postcapillary venules, and in active ulcers macrophages were predominant in the postcapillary venule. Fibroblasts were the most abundant cell type in all biopsies evaluated without regard to severity of disease, and no differences in interendothelial junction widths were observed.[25]

The involvement of leukocytes in CVI pathology requires leukocyte/endothelial signaling for the cells to extravasate and enter the dermal tissue. A study evaluating changes in adhesion molecules in patients with severe lipodermatosclerosis and active ulceration by immunohistochemistry of biopsies adjacent to ulcerated skin demonstrated that increased expression of intracellular adhesion molecule-1 and vascular cell adhesion molecule-1 was present. In addition, the expression of leukocyte function-associated antigen-1 and very late activated antigen-4 was increased dramatically on perivascular leukocytes compared with healthy skin, indicating that the upregulation of adhesion molecules in CVI patients are important mediators toward facilitating leukocyte endothelial adhesion, activation, and transendothelial migration.[26]

Although the evidence suggests that neutrophils are rarely found in the dermis of patients with severe CVI and that activation has not been detected, several studies have identified a role for neutrophils in CVI. Investigators evaluating patients with varicose veins with and without skin changes took blood samples from dependent legs in the foot in the supine position. Leukocyte surface marker CD11b and L-selectin expression were analyzed by flow cytometry, and plasma soluble L-selectin was measured by ELISA. In dependent legs with skin changes, both the median neutrophil and monocyte CD11b and L-selectin levels decreased and remained low after venous hypertension was reversed (supine position). This also was seen in patients with uncomplicated varicose veins. The soluble L-selectin increased in the plasma in both patient groups with varicose veins during venous hypertension, indicating leukocyte adhesion to the endothelium. The authors concluded that venous hypertension resulted in sequestration of activated neutrophils and monocytes in the microcirculation, which persisted despite removal of venous hypertension.[27] Systemic activation of leukocytes was studied in patients with lipodermatosclerosis and venous ulcers, using blood samples and looking at granulocyte activation with nitroblue tetrazolium reduction. There was increased neutrophil activation from patients' plasma, but not patients' whole blood, which was greater for lipodermatosclerosis and ulcer patients than those with varicose veins and edema. Their results suggested that patients' plasma may contain activating factors for granulocytes that also activated neutrophils, which were fewer in patients' whole blood than control healthy blood, which suggests that activated neutrophils in CVI patients become trapped in the peripheral circulation and may be important in the development of CVI and dermal skin changes.[28]

ALTERATIONS IN CELLULAR PROLIFERATION, MOTILITY, AND REGULATION

Fibroblasts are important in healing in acute and chronic wounds and, in microscopic analysis, have been determined to be a major cell type in dermal biopsies from venous ulcer and lipodermatosclerotic skin.[25] Interest in alterations in fibroblast growth and growth factor response from patients with venous ulcers was evaluated by biopsies taken from the ulcer margin and compared with normal ipsilateral thigh fibroblasts of the same patients. The authors found a significant reduction in proliferation and the fibroblasts were morphologically larger and polygonal with less uniform nuclear features. However, response to growth factors (basic fibroblast growth factor [bFGF], epidermal growth factor [EGF]) was maintained in venous ulcer fibroblasts, albeit not to the same degree as control fibroblasts. These results indicated a functional abnormality with dermal fibroblasts in venous ulcers and suggested that cellular senescence may contribute to the pathophysiology of venous ulcer formation.[29] Other investigators also have determined that venous ulcer fibroblasts have a diminished proliferative rate and an attenuated response to growth factors including platelet-derived growth factor (PDGF). In addition, the fibroblasts from patients with ulcers older than three years grew significantly slower than those from patients with ulcers less than three years.[30] Certain characteristics of cellular senescence were elucidated in subsequent experiments. Venous ulcer fibroblasts contained more cells that stained positive for senescent associated-α galactosidase (specific marker for senescent state) and had increased expression of protein and mRNA product for cellular fibronectin. The authors speculated that increased accumulation of senescent cells in venous ulcers may lead to the observed impaired healing.[31] Of interest, taking ulcer fibroblasts and subjecting them to progressive passage had a significant effect on the expression of senescent associated-α galactosidase compared with normal fibroblast or fibroblasts cultured from patients with varicose veins only. Not only did the ulcer fibroblasts have an increased mean number of senescent associated-α galactosidase expressing cells (63.8 ± 8.9% vs. 11.2 ± 3.1%), but after six passages nearly all the ulcer fibroblasts were senescent (>95%). These data indicated that venous ulcer fibroblasts were significantly advanced in cellular age and

closer to replicative exhaustion, suggesting that the accumulation of senescent cells in venous ulcer wounds may lead to recalcitrant healing.[32] In experiments evaluating the effect of bFGF on fibronectin and MMP-2 expression, fibroblasts from venous ulcer and CVI patients and in normal controls were found to increase the expression of these proteins. The implications were that bFGF mediated its effects by increasing both extracellular matrix protein and matrix proteinase, indicating that the upregulation of fibronectin and MMP-2 may be a normal, transient, and inducible response of these cells to bFGF. Furthermore, that ulcer fibroblasts at baseline have higher levels of fibronectin may not signify that they possess more of a senescent-like phenotype, but rather that they have been subjected to more mitogenic stimuli as a result of their slow growth or location in the ulcer environment.[33]

Functional studies evaluating fibroblast motility by time lapse digital photoimaging were performed in both venous ulcer fibroblasts and fibroblasts cultured from the medial malleolar skin of patients with varicose veins. The findings demonstrated a significant reduction in venous ulcer fibroblast motility compared with ipsilateral normal thigh fibroblasts and in fibroblasts from patients without any CVI, and interestingly fibroblasts from varicose vein patients also had significant lower motility. The decreased fibroblast motility was associated with the expression of α-sma, a marker for myofibroblast differentiation. These data supported that altered motility in CVI fibroblasts and myofibroblast differentiation are important functional characteristics and provide further explanation in altered wound healing.[34]

The response to PDGF by venous ulcer fibroblast previously has been demonstrated to be attenuated.[30] Although these authors were unable to demonstrate any differences in PDGF receptors, a recent report demonstrated that venous ulcer fibroblasts had no growth response to PDGF αβ, and the basal levels of PDGF α and PDGF β receptors were decreased.[35] A possible explanation for these differences is that in the latter, fibroblasts were cultured from biopsies taken from the ulcer margin,[35] and in the former, biopsies were from the central portion of granulation tissue and from lipodermatosclerotic skin.[30]

The regulatory mechanisms for fibroblast-reduced growth and attenuated response to growth factors remain unknown. In a recent report the mitogen-activated protein kinase (MAPK) pathways ERK1 and ERK2 were studied in venous ulcer fibroblasts treated with PDGF AB. The ulcer fibroblasts were found to activate MAPK, and inhibition of the upstream kinase MEK1 significantly reduced fibroblast proliferation, which was reversible with the addition of PDGF. In addition venous ulcer wound fluid inhibited MAPK directly. These data suggest the importance of the MAPK ERK pathway in regulating venous ulcer fibroblasts proliferation.[36]

Key cell-cycle regulatory proteins for proliferation and apoptosis specifically involved with epithelialization have been investigated. In biopsies of venous ulcers, diabetic ulcers, and control subjects no major differences in keratinocyte immunohistochemical staining was observed for cell-cycle regulatory proteins or apoptosis-related proteins.[37] In a follow-up study these investigators compared the edge of venous ulcer with that of the central granulation tissue for growth factors and cytokines in keratinocytes and endothelial cells by immunohistochemistry and phenotype characterization. Significant findings were that on the ulcer margin, keratinocytes and endothelial cells retained their secretory potential for growth factors and cytokines, whereas the ulcer bed was significant for very few fibroblasts and mainly scavenging cells (macrophages) being present.[38] From these data the authors speculated that the wound bed organization was altered by chronic infections, and impaired nutrition inhibited keratinocyte migration. It is well known that fibronectin is an important protein of the extracellular matrix and involved in keratinocyte reepithelialization. A study evaluating biopsies from venous ulcer wound margin, acute wounds, and normal skin determined that the transcription product for fibronectin was increased significantly in venous ulcer. However, immunostaining for alpha5beta1 integrin, the cell surface receptor for fibronectin, was undetectable in venous ulcer biopsies. The authors concluded that although fibronectin mRNA was expressed, the lack of integrin receptor may prevent keratinocyte migration and wound closure.[39]

ALTERATIONS IN TRANSFORMING GROWTH FACTOR FUNCTION

Transforming growth factor beta1 (TGF-β1) is an important growth factor with functional properties in regulating cell proliferation, extracellular matrix production, and immunosuppressive effects. A number of investigators have studied the role of TGF in patients with venous ulcer and lipodermatosclerotic skin changes. In an immunohistochemical study of venous ulcer and normal skin graft donor sites, in the venous ulcer biopsies there was increased α-2 macroglobulin, increased number of type I procollagen fibroblasts, and elevated immunoreactivity of TGF-β1 within fibrin cuffs but not in the provisional matrix of the ulcer bed around the cuffs. In comparison, normal skin had restriction of α-1 macroglobulin to the vessel lumen, and procollagen and TGF-β1 were present within the granulating matrix and adjacent to the wound margin. These data suggested that although TGF is present in venous ulcers it is distributed in the fibrin cuff and not available in the wound matrix due to binding by α-2 macroglobulin.[40] The responsiveness of venous ulcer fibroblasts to TGF was tested. Investigation determined that ulcer fibroblasts compared with normal fibroblasts at baseline had the same capacity for procollagen synthesis by tritiated proline incorporation assay, and no difference was detected in total TGF-β1 synthesis. As well, similar mRNA levels of α-1 procollagen and

TGF-β1 were present. In exogenously TGF-β1-stimulated fibroblasts, venous ulcer fibroblasts failed to increase collagen production and were associated with a four-fold decrease in TGF-β type II receptors.[41] Another investigation with CVI patients evaluated lipodermatosclerotic skin, healed ulcers, and active ulcers. Compared with control skin, the transcriptional product for TGF-β1 was elevated only in lipodermatosclerotic biopsies, and total TGF-β1 protein was increased in all CVI specimens and significantly higher in biopsies closer to the diseased skin than the thigh. Immunohistochemical examination of TGF-β1 localized the protein to the epidermis, fibroblasts, and leukocytes, which appeared to be mast cells; in contrast, normal skin had TGF-β1 present only in the epidermis. The authors concluded that fibroblasts are target cells that are activated by leukocytes, and that alterations in tissue remodeling leads to fibrosis in patients with advanced CVI.[42] Evaluation of fibroblast response to TGF-β1 was performed in early (C2 and C3) and late stages (C4–6) of CVI, and the composition of the extracellular matrix tissue cultures was tested for proliferative effect of TGF-β1 treated fibroblasts. Response to TGF-β1 was normal in C2 and C3 CVI fibroblast, with diminished proliferation of C4 that was reversible in TGF-β1–treated cells. In C5 and C6 fibroblasts TGF-β1 was unable to cause any increase in proliferation. Changing the composition of the extracellular matrix from polystyrene, collagen, or fibronectin had no effect in increasing TGF-β1 treated advanced CVI fibroblasts.[43]

Recent investigations on the mechanisms of fibroblasts unresponsive to TGF-β1 from venous ulcer and lipodermatosclerotic skin have been evaluated. A previous study demonstrated that the TGF-β type II receptors were lower.[41] A recent study of venous ulcer fibroblasts determined that the transcript for TGF-β type II receptors and number of receptors was decreased. Decreased receptor expression was associated with inhibited phosphorylation of S-mad 2 and S-mad 3 proteins and MAPK ERK1 and ERK2, which are important downstream cell regulatory kinases that are phosphorylated in response to TGF-β type II receptor activation by ligand. These findings indicate abnormal signaling pathways that may be responsible for altered fibroblast proliferation in venous ulcers.[44]

ALTERATIONS IN EXTRACELLULAR REMODELING AND THE WOUND FLUID ENVIRONMENT

The extracellular matrix (ECM) is an important structural and functional scaffolding made up of proteins that are necessary for cell function, wound repair, epithelialization, blood vessel support, cell differentiation and signaling, and cellular migration. The ECM is particularly important in providing a substrate for keratinocytes to migrate and establish coverage in both acute and chronic wounds.[39] Alterations in protease activity and the relation to abnormalities in ECM metabolism in wounds have been areas of active investigation in the past decade. In an early report evaluating wound fluid collected from patients with venous ulcers, the investigators determined that compared with acute wound fluid, the chronic wound fluid contained up to ten-fold increased levels of MMP-2 and MMP-9 as well as increased activity of the enzymes, suggesting high tissue turnover.[45] Increased MMP-1 and gelatinase activity from the exudates of chronic venous leg ulcers also has been confirmed by other investigators, and the doxycycline inhibition studies suggested that the protease activity was that of fibroblasts, mononuclear cells, keratinocytes, or endothelial cells and not neutrophils.[46] It is important to note that MMP's levels and activity, although abnormal in venous ulcers, is not specific to just venous disease, and alterations are found in other inflammatory wounds including burn and pressure ulcers.[47] The excess proteolytic activity in venous leg ulcers has been found to degrade essential plasminogen, which is important in activating pro-MMP to MMP necessary for fibrinolysis and cell migration, and MMPs inhibit plasmin production by keratinocytes, which may lead to reduced cell migration.[48] Of interest, a study evaluating fibroblasts cultured from venous ulcers determined that there was a marked reduction in MMP-1 and MMP-2 level and activity, and a significant increase in TIMP-1 and TIMP-2 production. The authors concluded that the inhibition of proteinase activity by TIMP in fibroblasts causes impaired function to reorganize the ECM in chronic wounds, leading to delayed healing.[49]

The abnormalities in structure and healing process seen in lipodermatosclerotic skin have also been attributed to MMP pathophysiology. A study where dermal biopsies were obtained from liposclerotic skin and compared with healthy skin and analyzed by immunohistochemistry, reverse transcriptase polymerase chain reaction, immunoblot, and zymography found that lipodermatosclerotic skin had increased expression of mRNA and protein for MMP-1, MMP-2, and TIMP-1, and increased levels of active MMP-2. The MMP-2 was localized predominantly in the basal and suprabasal layers of the epidermis, perivascular region, and reticular dermis, and had less TIMP-2 in the basement membrane of the diseased skin. The relevance of this study was that lipodermatosclerotic skin is characterized by elevated ECM turnover.[50] The regulation of MMP production is complex. Posttranslational modifications of MMPs appear to be essential, and dermal fibroblasts and leukocytes are sources for MMPs, especially MMP-2, and likely regulated by TGF-β1.[51] The interplay of MAPK with MMP activation has also been investigated in fibroblasts. The cytokine tumor necrosis factor alpha has been demonstrated to induce MMP-19 expression, which is inhibited by blocking MAPK pathways ERK1 and ERK2 with PD98059 and p38 with SB203580. In addition, adenovirus-mediated induction of ERK 1 and ERK 2 in combination with p38 resulted in potent MMP-19 expression in fibroblasts and the

activation of c-JNK also produced abundant pro-MMP-19. These data indicated the important regulatory functions of MAPK and proteolytic activity in dermal fibroblasts.[52]

The venous ulcer microenvironment consists of dermal fibroblasts, keratinocytes, inflammatory cells, ECM, bacteria, and microcirculation. An interesting aspect of the venous ulcer milieu is the presence of the chronic wound fluid. The wound fluid is known to have properties of excess protease activity, as stated earlier. In addition, the venous ulcer wound fluid has been demonstrated to cause inhibition of fibroblast proliferation and induce changes of cellular senescence.[34,53] The venous ulcer wound fluid has been demonstrated to inhibit the growth of fibroblasts with the majority of cells with a G1 and G2 DNA content in the cell cycle (quiescent state, unable to enter S phase). Proliferation of fibroblasts treated with chronic venous ulcer wound fluid could be reestablished by heat inactivation or reversed by removal and placement of cells in 10% serum.[54] In addition to fibroblasts, wound fluid from venous ulcers also inhibits the proliferation of endothelial cells and keratinocytes. Although the inhibitory component(s) and the responsible source(s) for production of wound fluid are not known, the active inhibitory substance can be fractionated and consists of a molecular weight of less than 30 kd.[55] In neonatal fibroblasts, venous ulcer wound fluid was demonstrated to inhibit the expression of MAPK, specifically ERK1 and ERK2, with simultaneous decrease in proliferation.[36] In addition, the mechanism of cell inhibition by wound fluid, in part, involves downregulation of phosphorylated retinoblastoma tumor suppression gene and cyclin D1, via inhibition of the Ras-dependent MAPK pathway.[56]

REFERENCES

1. Flanigan DP, Goodreau JJ, Burnham SJ, Bergan JJ, Yao JST. Vascular laboratory diagnosis of clinically suspected acute deep vein thrombosis, *Lancet.* 1978. *2:* 331–334.
2. Bergan JJ. Surgical management of primary and recurrent varicose veins. In: Gloviczki P, Yao JST, eds. *Handbook of venous disorders: Guidelines of the American venous forum,* 1e. New York: Chapman and Hall. 1996. 394–415.
3. Burnand KG, Whimster I, Naidoo A, Browse NL. Pericapillary fibrin in the ulcer-bearing skin of the leg: The cause of lipodermatosclerosis and venous ulceration, *Br Med J.* 1988. *285:* 1071–1072.
4. Gandhi RH, Irizarry E, Neckman GB, Halpern VJ, Mulcare RJ, Tilson MD. Analysis of the connective tissue matrix and proteolytic activity of primary varicose veins, *J Vasc Surg.* 1994. *20:* 814–820.
5. Parra JR, Cambria RA, Hower CD, et al. Tissue inhibitor of metalloproteinase-1 is increased in the saphenophemoral junction of patients with varices in the leg, *J Vasc Surg.* 1998. *28:* 669–675.
6. Badier-Commander C, Verbeuren T, Lebard C, Michel JB, Jacob MP. Increased TIMP/MMP ratio in varicose veins: A possible explanation for extracellular matrix accumulation, *J Pathol.* 2000. *192:* 105–112.
7. Jacob MP, Cazaubon M, Scemama A, et al. Plasma matrix metalloproteinase-9 as a marker of blood stasis in varicose veins, *Circulation.* 2002. *106:* 535–538.
8. Gillespie DL, Patel A, Fileta B, et al. Varicose veins possess greater quantities of MMP-1 than normal veins and demonstrate regional variation in MMP-1 and MMP-13, *J Surg Res.* 2002. *106:* 233–238.

9. Kowalewski R, Sobolewski K, Wolanska M, Gacko M. Matrix metalloproteinases in the vein wall, *Int Angiol*. 2004. *23*: 164–169.

10. Sansilvestri-Morel P, Nonotte I, Fournet-Bourguignon MP, et al. *J Vasc Res*. 1998. *35*: 115–123.

11. Sansilvestri-Morel P, Rupin A, Jaisson S, Fabiani JN, Verbeuren TJ, Vanhoutte PM. Synthesis of collagen is dysregulated in cultured fibroblasts derived from skin of subjects with varicose veins as it is in venous smooth muscle cells, *Circulation*. 2002. *106*: 479–483.

12. Green DR, Reed JC. Mitochondria and apoptosis, *Science*. 1998. *281*: 1309–1312.

13. Ascher E, Jacob T, Hingorani A, Gunduz Y, Mazzariol F, Kallakuri S. Programmed cell death (apoptosis) and its role in the pathogenesis of lower extremity varicose veins, *Ann Vasc Surg*. 2000. *14*: 24–30.

14. Ducasse E, Giannakakis K, Chevalier J, et al. Dysregulated apoptosis in primary varicose veins. *Eur J Vasc Endovasc Surg*. 2005. *29*: 316–323.

15. Takase S, Pascarella L, Bergan JJ, Schmid-Schonbein GW. Hypertension-induced venous valve remodeling, *J Vasc Surg*. 2004. *39*: 1329–1334.

16. Pascarella L, Schmid-Schonbein GW, Bergan JJ. An animal model of venous hypertension: The role of inflammation in venous valve failure, *J Vasc Surg*. 2005. *41*: 303–311.

17. Burnand KG, Whimster I, Naidoo A, Browse NL. Pericapillary fibrin in the ulcer-bearing skin of the leg: The cause of lipodermatosclerosis and venous ulceration, *Br Med J*. 1982. *285*: 1071–1072.

18. Thomas PR, Nash GB, Dormandy JA. White cell accumulation in dependent legs of patients with venous hypertension: A possible mechanism for trophic changes in the skin, *Br Med J*. 1988. *296*: 1693–1695.

19. Coleridge Smith PD, Thomas P, Scurr JH, Dormandy JA. Causes of venous ulceration: A new hypothesis, *Br Med J*. 1988. *296*: 1726–1727.

20. Falanga V, Eaglstein WH. The "trap" hypothesis of venous ulceration, *Lancet*. 1993. *341*: 1006–1008.

21. Scott HJ, Coleridge Smith PD, Scurr JH. Histological study of white blood cells and their association with lipodermatosclerosis and venous ulceration, *Br J Surg*. 1991. *78*: 210–211.

22. Wilkinson LS, Bunker C, Edwards JC, Scurr JH, Coleridge Smith PD. Leukocytes: Their role in the etiopathogensis of skin damage in venous disease, *J Vasc Surg*. 1993. *17*: 669–675.

23. Pappas PJ, Fallek SR, Garcia A, et al. Role of leukocyte activation in patients with venous stasis ulcers, *J Surg Res*. 1995. *59*: 553–559.

24. Pappas PJ, Teehan EP, Fallek SR, et al. Diminished mononuclear cell function is associated with chronic venous insufficiency, *J Vasc Surg*. 1995. *22*: 580–586.

25. Pappas PJ, DeFouw DO, Venezio LM, et al. Morphometric assessment of the dermal microcirculation in patients with chronic venous insufficiency, *J Vasc Surg*. 1997. *26*: 784–795.

26. Weyl A, Vanscheidt W, Weiss JM, Pesschen M, Schopf E, Simon J. Expression of the adhesion molecules ICAM-1, VCAM-1, and E-selectins and their ligands VLA-4 and LFA-1 in chronic venous leg ulcers, *J Am Acad Dermatol*. 1996. *34*: 418–423.

27. Saharay M, Shields DA, Porter JB, Scurr JH, Coleridge Smith PD. Leukocyte activity in the microcirculation of the led in patients with chronic venous disease, *J Vasc Surg*. 1997. *26*: 265–273.

28. Takase S, Schmid-Schonbein G, Bergan JJ. Leukocyte activation in patients with venous insufficiency, *J Vasc Surg*. 1999. *30*: 148–156.

29. Stanley AC, Park HY, Phillips TJ, Russakovsky V, Menzoian JO. Reduced growth of dermal fibroblasts from chronic venous ulcers can be stimulated with growth factors, *J Vasc Surg*. 1997. *26*: 994–1001.

30. Agren MS, Steenfos HH, Dabelsteen S, Hansen JB, Dabelsteen E. Proliferation and mitogenic response to PDGF-BB of fibroblasts isolated from chronic venous leg ulcers is ulcer-age dependent, *J Invest Dermatol*. 1999. *112*: 463–469.

31. Mendez MV, Stanley AC, Park HY, Shon K, Phillips TJ, Menzoian JO. Fibroblasts cultured from venous ulcers display cellular characteristics of senescence, *J Vasc Surg*. 1998. *28*: 876–883.

32. Raffetto JD, Mendez MV, Phillips TJ, Park HY, Menzoian JO. The effect of passage number on fibroblast cellular senescence in patients with chronic venous insufficiency with and without ulcer, *Am J Surg*. 1999. *178*: 107–112.

33. Seidman CS, Raffetto JD, Marien BJ, Kroon CS, Seah CC, Menzoian JO. bFGF induced alterations in cellular markers of senescence in growth rescued fibroblasts from chronic venous ulcer and venous reflux patients, *Ann Vasc Surg*. 2003. *17*: 239–244.

34. Raffetto JD, Mendez VM, Marien BJ, et al. Changes in cellular motility and cytoskeletal actin in fibroblasts from patients with chronic venous disease and in newborn fibroblasts in the presence of chronic wound fluid, *J Vasc Surg*. 2001. *33*: 1233–1241.

35. Vasquez R, Marien BJ, Gram C, Goodwin DG, Menzoian JO, Raffetto JD. Proliferative capacity of venous ulcer fibroblasts in the presence of platelet-derived growth factor, *Vasc Endovascular Surg*. 2004. *38*: 355–360.

36. Raffetto JD, Vasquez R, Goodwin DG, Menzoian JO. Mitogen activated protein kinase pathway regulates cell proliferation in venous ulcer fibroblasts, *Vasc Endovasc Surg*. 2006. *40*: 59–66.

37. Galkowska H, Olszewsk WL, Wojewodzka U, Mijal J, Filipiuk E. Expression of apoptosis- and cell cycle-related proteins in epidermis of venous leg and diabetic foot ulcers, *Surgery*. 2003. *134*: 213–220.

38. Galkowska H, Olszewsk WL, Wojewodzka U. Keratinocyte and dermal vascular endothelial cell capacities remain unimpaired in the margin of chronic venous ulcer, *Arch Dermatol Res*. 2005. *296*: 286–295.

39. Ongenae KC, Phillips TJ, Park HY. Level of fibronectin mRNA is markedly increased in human chronic wounds, *Dermatol Surg*. 2000. *26*: 447–451.

40. Higley HR, Ksander GA, Gerhardt CO, Falanga V. Extravasation of macromolecules and possible trapping of transforming growth factor-beta in venous ulceration, *Br J Dermatol*. 1995. *132*: 79–85.

41. Hasan A, Murata H, Falabella A, et al. Dermal fibroblasts from venous ulcers are unresponsive to the action of transforming growth factor-beta 1, *J Derm Sci*. 1997. *16*: 59–66.

42. Pappas PJ, You R, Rameshwar P, et al. Dermal tissue fibrosis in patients with chronic venous insufficiency is associated with increased transforming growth factor-beta1 gene expression and protein production, *J Vasc Surg*. 1999. *30*: 1129–1145.

43. Lal BK, Saito S, Pappas PJ, et al. Altered proliferative responses of dermal fibroblasts to TGF-beta1 may contribute to chronic venous stasis ulcer, *J Vasc Surg*. 2003. *37*: 1285–1293.

44. Kim BC, Kim HT, Park SH, et al. Fibroblasts from chronic wounds show altered TGF-beta-signaling and decreased TGF-beta type II receptor expression, *J Cell Physiol*. 2003. *195*: 331–336.

45. Wysocki AB, Staiano-Coico L, Grinnell F. Wound fluid from chronic leg ulcers contains elevated levels of metalloproteinases MMP-2 and MMP-9, *J Invest Dermatol*. 1993. *101*: 64–68.

46. Weckroth M, Vaheri A, Lauharanta J, Sorsa T, Konttinen TY. Matrix metalloproteinases, gelatinase, and collagenase, in chronic leg ulcers, *J Invest Dermatol*. 1996. *106*: 1119–1124.

47. Yager DR, Zhang LY, Liang HX, Diegelmann RF, Cohen IK. Wound fluid from human pressure ulcers contain elevated matrix metalloproteinase levels and activity to surgical wound fluids, *J Invest Dermatol*. 1996. *107*: 743–748.

48. Hoffman R, Starkey S, Coad J. Wound fluid from venous leg ulcers degrades plasminogen and reduces plasmin generation by keratinocytes, *J Invest Dermatol*. 1998. *111*: 1140–1144.

49. Cook H, Stephens P, Davies KJ, Harding KG, Thomas DW. Defective extracellular matrix reorganization by chronic wound fibroblasts is associated with alterations in TIMP-1, TIMP-2, and MMP-2 activity, *J Invest Dermatol*. 2000. *115*: 225–233.

50. Herouy Y, May AE, Pornschlegel G, et al. Lipodermatosclerosis is characterized by elevated expression and activation of matrix metalloproteinases: Implications for venous ulcer formation, *J Invest Dermatol*. 1998. *111*: 822–827.

51. Saito S, Trovato MJ, You R, et al. Role of matrix metalloproteinases 1, 2, and 9 and tissue inhibitor of matrix metalloproteinase-1 in chronic venous insufficiency, *J Vasc Surg*. 2001. *34*: 930–938.

52. Hieta N, Impola U, Lopez-Otin C, Saarialho-Kere U, Kahari VM. Matrix metalloproteinase-19 expression in dermal wounds and by fibroblasts in culture, *J Vasc Surg*. 2003. *121*: 997–1004.

53. Mendez MV, Raffetto JD, Phillips TJ, Menzoian JO, Park HY. The proliferative capacity of neonatal skin fibroblasts is reduced after exposure to venous ulcer fluid: A potential mechanism for senescence in venous ulcers, *J Vasc Surg*. 1999. *30*: 734–743.

54. Phillips TJ, Al-Amoudi HO, Leverkus M, Park HY. Effect of chronic wound fluid on fibroblasts, *J Wound Care*. 1998. *7*: 527–532.

55. Bucalo B, Eaglstein WH, Falanga V. Inhibition of cell proliferation by chronic wound fluid, *Wound Rep Reg*. 1993. *1*: 181–186.

56. Seah CC, Phillips TJ, Howard CE, et al. Chronic wound fluid suppresses proliferation of dermal fibroblasts through a Ras-mediated signaling pathway, *J Invest Dermatol*. 2005. *124*: 466–474.

8.

PATHOPHYSIOLOGY OF CHRONIC VENOUS INSUFFICIENCY

Peter J. Pappas, Brajesh K. Lal, Frank T. Padberg Jr., Robert W. Zickler, and Walter N. Duran

INTRODUCTION

Ten to 35% of adults in the United States have some form of chronic venous insufficiency (CVI), with venous ulcers affecting 4% of people over the age of 65.[1,2] Because of the high prevalence of the disease, the population-based costs to the U.S. government for CVI treatment and venous ulcer care has been estimated at over one billion dollars a year. In addition, 4.6 million work days per year are lost to vein-related illnesses.[3,4] The recurrent nature of the disease, the high cost to the health care system, and the ineffectiveness of current treatment modalities underscore the need for CVI-related research. Research has further defined the role of leukocyte-mediated injury and elucidated the role of inflammatory cytokines in lower extremity dermal pathology. In addition, several laboratories have performed investigations on pathologic alterations in cellular function and the molecular regulation of these processes observed in patients with CVI. This chapter will discuss the pathophysiology of varicose vein formation and the molecular regulation of inflammatory damage to the lower extremity dermis caused by persistent ambulatory venous hypertension.

VARICOSE VEIN FORMATION (MACROSCOPIC ALTERATIONS)

GENETICS AND THE ROLE OF DEEP VENOUS THROMBOSIS (DVT)

Unlike arteries, veins are thin-walled, low-pressure conduits whose function is to return blood from the periphery to the heart. Muscular contractions in the upper and lower extremities propel blood forward, and a series of intraluminal valves prevent retrograde flow, or reflux. Venous reflux is observed when valvular destruction or dysfunction occurs in association with varicose vein formation. Valvular reflux causes an increase in ambulatory venous pressure and a cascade of pathologic events that manifest themselves clinically as lower extremity edema, pain, itching, skin discoloration,

varicose veins, venous ulceration, and, in its severest form, limb loss. These clinical symptoms collectively refer to the disorder known as CVI.[5] Age, gender, pregnancy, weight, height, race, diet, bowel habits, occupation, posture, previous deep venous thrombosis, and genetics all have been proposed as predisposing factors associated with varicose vein formation. Except for previous deep vein thrombosis and genetics, there is poor evidence that indicates a causative relationship between these predisposing factors and the formation of varicose veins. Refer to Kevin Burnand's textbook *Diseases of the Vein* for further discussion on these predisposing factors.[6]

There are few reported epidemiologic investigations that suggest a relationship between varicose vein formation and a genetic predisposition.[7,8] It was previously thought that axial destruction of venous valves led to transmission of ambulatory venous hypertension causing reflux and varix formation.[6] However, a publication by Labropoulos et al. indicated that the most frequent location for initial varicose vein formation was in the below-knee great saphenous vein (GSV) and its tributaries, followed by the above-knee GSV and the saphenofemoral junction.[9] This study clearly indicates that vein wall degeneration with subsequent varix formation can occur in any segment of the superficial and deep systems at any time and suggests a genetic component to the disease. In 1969, Gunderson and Hauge reported on the epidemiology of varicose veins observed in the vein clinic in Malmo, Sweden, over a 2-month period.[7] Of 250 patients, 154 female and 24 male patients provided complete survey information on their parents and siblings. Although biased by the predominance of women and dependence on survey data, this report suggested that patients with varicose veins had a higher likelihood of developing varicosities if their fathers had varicose veins. Furthermore, the risk of developing varicose veins increases if both parents had varicosities. Cornu-Thenard et al. prospectively examined 67 patients and their parents. Patients' nonaffected spouses and parents were used as controls for a total of 402 subjects.[8] These investigators reported that the risk of developing varicose veins was 90% when both parents were affected, 25% for males and 62% for females if one parent is affected, and 20% when neither parent is affected. These data suggest an autosomal dominant with variable penetrance mode of genetic transmission. The decreased incidence in males with an affected parent and the spontaneous development in patients without affected parents suggests that males are more resistant to varix formation and that other multifactorial etiologies in patients with predispositions to the disease must exist. To further elucidate the genetic component of the disease, molecular analyses with gene chip technologies is required. The chromosome responsible for the disease and its protein byproducts are currently unknown.

An injury to the venous endothelium or local procoagulant environmental factors leads to thrombus formation in the venous system. It is currently well accepted that a venous thrombus initiates a cascade of inflammatory events that contributes to or causes vein wall fibrosis.[10] Thrombus formation at venous confluences and valve pockets leads to activation of neutrophils and platelets. Activation of these cells leads to formation of inflammatory cytokines, procoagulants, and chemokines leading to thrombin activation and further clot formation. Production of inflammatory mediators creates a cytokine/chemokine gradient leading to leukocyte invasion of the vein wall at the thrombus wall interface and from the surrounding adventitia. Upregulation of adhesion molecules perpetuates this process, eventually leading to vein wall fibrosis, valvular destruction, and alteration of vein wall architecture.[10,11] Although the mechanisms associated with vein wall damage secondary to venous thrombosis are beginning to be unraveled, the majority of varicose veins occur in patients with no prior history of deep venous thrombosis. The etiology of primary varicose veins continues to be a mystery.

VEIN WALL ANATOMY, HISTOPATHOLOGY, AND FUNCTIONAL ALTERATIONS

Whatever the initiating event, several unique anatomic and biochemical abnormalities have been observed in patients with varicose veins. Normal and varicose GSVs are characterized by three distinct muscle layers within their walls. The media contains an inner longitudinal and an outer circular layer, and the adventitia contains a loosely organized outer longitudinal layer.[12–14] In normal GSVs, these muscle layers are composed of smooth muscle cells (SMCs), which appear spindle-shaped (contractile phenotype) when examined with electron microscopy (see Figure 8.1).[15] These cells lie in close proximity to each other, are in parallel arrays, and are surrounded by bundles of regularly arranged collagen fibers. In varicose veins, the orderly appearance of the muscle layers of the media is replaced by an intense and disorganized deposition of collagen.[15–17] Collagen deposits separate the normally closely opposed SMCs and are particularly striking in the media. SMCs appear elliptical

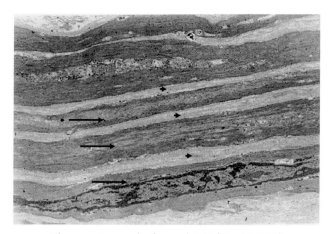

Figure 8.1 Electron micrograph of normal GSV (Mag 11,830×). Note organized structure of alternating smooth muscle cells (long arrows) with spindle-shaped contractile phenotype, interspersed by longitudinally arranged collagen bundles (short arrows).

rather than spindle-shaped, and demonstrate numerous collagen-containing vacuoles imparting a secretory phenotype (see Figure 8.2).[15] What causes SMCs to dedifferentiate from a contractile to a secretory phenotype is currently unknown. Ascher et al. theorized that SMC dedifferentiation may be related to dysregulation of apoptosis.[18,19] These investigators reported a decrease in the proapoptotic mediators Bax and PARP (poly ADP-ribose polymerase) in the adventitia of varicose veins compared with normal veins. Although no difference in these mediators was observed in the media or intima of varicose veins, a decrease in SMC turnover was postulated as a possible cause for the increase in secretory phenotype. Increased phosphorylation of the retinoblastoma protein, an intracellular regulator of cellular proliferation and differentiation, has been observed in varicose veins, and may similarly contribute to this process.[13]

Vein wall remodeling has been observed consistently in histologic varicose vein specimens.[12,14-17,20] Gandhi et al.

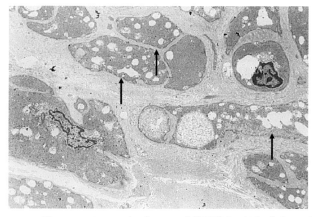

Figure 8.2 Electron micrograph of varicosed GSV (Mag 4240×). Smooth muscle cells exhibit prominent vacuoles (arrows) and an elliptical appearance consistent with a secretory phenotype. Smooth muscle cells are separated by diffusely deposited collagen bundles, which impart a disorganized architectural appearance to the vein wall.

quantitatively demonstrated an increase in collagen content and a decrease in elastin content compared with normal GSVs.[20] The net increase in the collagen/elastin ratio suggested an imbalance in connective tissue matrix regulation. As a result, several investigators have observed alterations in matrix metalloproteinase and fibrinolytic activity in varicose veins. TIMP-1 and MMP-1 protein levels are increased at the saphenofemoral junction compared with normal controls, whereas MMP-2 levels are decreased.[21] No overall differences in MMP-9 protein or activity levels have been identified, however, the number of cells expressing MMP-9 by immunohistochemistry has been reported to be elevated in varicose veins compared with normal veins.[22,23] There are conflicting reports regarding the role of plasmin activators and their inhibitors. Shireman et al. reported that uPA (urokinase plasminogen activator) levels are increased three to five times compared with normal controls in the media of vein specimens cultured in an organ bath system.[24] No differences were noted in tPA (tissue plasminogen activator) or PAI-1 (plasmin activator inhibitor-1) levels. However, other investigations have reported a decrease in uPA and tPA activity by enzyme zymography in varicose veins.[22,25] These data suggest that the plasminogen activators may play a role in matrix metalloproteinase activation leading to vein wall fibrosis and varix formation; however, further research into the mechanisms regulating vein wall fibrosis clearly are needed.

What effect vein wall fibrosis has on venous function needs further elucidation. The contractile responses of varicose and normal GSV rings to noradrenaline, potassium chloride, endothelin, calcium ionophore A23187, angiotensin II, and nitric oxide have been evaluated by several investigators.[26,27] These studies have demonstrated decreased contractility of varicose veins when stimulated by noradrenaline, endothelin, and potassium chloride. Similarly, endothelium-dependent and - independent relaxations after A23187 or nitric oxide administration were diminished compared with normal GSVs, respectively. The mechanisms responsible for decreased varicose vein contractility appear to be receptor mediated.[27,28] Utilizing Sarafotoxin S6c (selective pharmacologic inhibitor of endothelin B) and competitive inhibition receptor assays with ^{131}I-endothelin-1, a decrease in endothelin B receptors have been observed in varicose veins compared with normal GSVs.[28] Feedback inhibition of receptor production secondary to increased endothelin-1 is postulated to mediate the decreased receptor content in varicose vein walls. Other possible mechanisms for decreased contractility appear related to cAMP levels and the ratio of prostacyclin to thromboxane-A2.[29] Cyclic-AMP is increased in varicose vein specimens compared with normal GSVs. In addition, the ratio of prostacyclin to thromboxane-A2 is increased even though absolute protein levels do not differ between normal veins and varicosities. Whether venodilation of varicosities is caused by diminished endothelin receptor levels and responsiveness to cAMP or by a secondary effect of

varix formation is not known. However, it is clear that with the development of vein wall fibrosis, varicose veins demonstrate decreased contractile properties that probably exacerbate the development of ambulatory venous hypertension.

HISTORICAL THEORIES

In the twentieth century numerous theories were postulated regarding the etiology of CVI and the cause of venous ulceration. The venous stasis, arteriovenous fistula, and diffusion block theories have been disproven over time and are discussed here for historical interest only. The etiology for dermal skin pathology is primarily a chronic inflammatory process, and the events regulating these events are discussed later.

VENOUS STASIS THEORY

In 1917, John Homans published a manuscript titled "The Etiology and Treatment of Varicose Ulcer of the Leg," in *Surgery, Gynecology, and Obstetrics*.[30] This manuscript was a clinical treatise on the diagnosis and management of patients with CVI. In this manuscript Dr. Homans coined the term "post-phlebitic syndrome" and speculated on the cause of venous ulceration. He stated that "Overstretching of the vein walls and destruction of the valves upon which the mechanism principally depends bring about a degree of surface stasis which obviously interferes with the nutrition of the skin and subcutaneous tissues.... It is to be expected, therefore that skin which is bathed under pressure in stagnant venous blood will readily form permanent, open sores or ulcers."[30] This statement resulted in a generation of investigators trying to seek a causal relationship between hypoxia, stagnant blood flow, and the development of CVI.

The first investigator to address the question of hypoxia and CVI scientifically was Alfred Blalock.[31] He obtained venous samples from the femoral, great saphenous, and varicose veins in ten patients with CVI isolated to one limb and compared their oxygen content with samples taken from corresponding veins in the opposite limb. Seven of the patients had active ulcers at the time. All samples were collected in the recumbent and standing positions. He reported that in patients with unilateral CVI the oxygen content was higher in the femoral vein of the affected limb. He speculated that this observation may be reflective of increased venous flow rather than stagnation.

ARTERIOVENOUS FISTULA THEORY

The concept of increased venous flow in the dermal venous plexus was expanded upon by Pratt, who reported that increased venous flow in patients with CVI could be clinically observed.[32] He attributed the development of venous ulceration to the presence of arteriovenous connections and coined the term "arterial varices." He reported that in a series of 272 patients with varicose veins who underwent vein ligation, 24% had arteriovenous connections. Of the 61 patients who developed recurrences, 50% had arteriovenous communications identified clinically by the presence of arterial pulsations in venous conduits. Pratt hypothesized that increased venous flow shunted nutrient- and oxygen-rich blood away from the dermal plexus, leading to areas of ischemia and hypoxia and resulting in venous ulceration. Pratt's clinical observations however, have never been confirmed with objective scientific evidence. Experiments with radioactively labeled microspheres have never demonstrated shunting and have therefore cast serious doubts on the validity of this theory.

DIFFUSION BLOCK THEORY

Hypoxia and alterations in nutrient blood flow again were proposed as the underlying etiology of CVI in 1982 by Burnand et al.[33] These authors performed a study in which skin biopsies were obtained from 109 limbs of patients with CVI and 30 limbs from patients without CVI. Foot vein pressures were measured in the CVI patients at rest and after 5, 10, 15, and 20 heel raises. Vein pressure measurements were then correlated with the number of capillaries observed on histologic section. The authors reported that venous hypertension was associated with increased numbers of capillaries in the dermis of patients with CVI. Whether the histologic sections represented true increases in capillary quantity or an elongation and distension of existing capillaries was not answered by this study. However, in a canine hind-limb model, the authors were able to induce enlargement in the number of capillaries with experimentally induced hypertension.[34] This important investigation was one of the first studies to demonstrate a direct effect of venous hypertension on the venous microcirculation. In a later study, Browse and Burnand noted that the enlarged capillaries observed on histologic examination exhibited pericapillary fibrin deposition and coined the term "fibrin cuff."[35] They speculated that venous hypertension led to widening of endothelial gap junctions with subsequent extravasation of fibrinogen leading to the development of fibrin cuffs. These authors theorized that the cuffs acted as a barrier to oxygen diffusion and nutrient blood flow, resulting in epidermal cell death. Although pericapillary cuffs do exist, it has never been demonstrated that they act as a barrier to nutrient flow or oxygen diffusion.

LEUKOCYTE ACTIVATION

Dissatisfaction with the fibrin cuff theory and subsequent observations of decreased circulating leukocytes in blood samples obtained from the GSVs in patients with CVI led Coleridge Smith and colleagues to propose the leukocyte trapping theory.[36] This theory proposes that circulating neutrophils are trapped in the venous microcirculation secondary to venous hypertension. The subsequent sluggish capillary blood flow leads to hypoxia and neutrophil activation. Neutrophil activation leads to degranulation of toxic metabolites with subsequent endothelial cell damage. The ensuing heterogeneous capillary perfusion causes alterations in skin blood flow and eventual skin damage. The problem with the leukocyte trapping theory is that neutrophils have never been directly observed to obstruct capillary flow, therefore casting doubt on its validity. However, there is significant evidence that leukocyte activation plays a major role in the pathophysiology of CVI.

ROLE OF LEUKOCYTE ACTIVATION AND FUNCTIONAL STATUS IN CVI

In 1988, Thomas et al. reported that 24% fewer white cells left the venous circulation after a period of recumbency in patients with CVI as compared with normal patients.[37] They studied three groups of ten patients each. Group 1 consisted of patients with no signs of venous disease. Group 2 were patients with uncomplicated primary varicose veins, and Group 3 were patients with long-standing CVI as determined by Doppler ultrasonography, strain-gauge plethysmography, and foot volumetry. Patients had the GSV cannulated just above the medial malleolus. Venous samples were obtained at various time points with patients in the sitting and supine position. Samples were then placed in an automated cell counter, and the number of leukocytes and erythrocytes determined. The ratios of white cells to red cells at the various time points were then compared. The authors reported that with leg dependency, packed cell volume significantly increased in patients with CVI as compared with normal controls, whereas patients with primary varicose veins showed no difference from controls. They also noted that the relative number of white cells were significantly decreased compared to control and primary varicose vein patients (28% vs. 5%, p < 0.01). The authors concluded that the decrease in white cell number was due to leukocyte trapping in the venous microcirculation secondary to venous hypertension. They further speculated that while trapped, leukocytes may be activated and release toxic metabolites, causing damage to the microcirculation and the overlying skin. These important observations were the first to implicate abnormal leukocyte activity in the pathophysiology of CVI.

The importance of leukocytes in the development of dermal skin alterations was emphasized by Scott et al.[38] These authors obtained punch biopsies from patients with primary varicose veins, patients with lipodermatosclerosis, and patients with lipodermatosclerosis and healed ulcers, and determined median number of white blood cells (WBCs) per high power field (40× magnification) in each group. No patients with active ulcers were included, and no attempt to identify the type of leukocytes was made. The authors reported that in patients with primary varicose veins, lipodermatosclerosis, and healed ulceration there was a median of 6, 45, and 217 WBCs per mm², respectively. This study demonstrated that with clinical disease progression and increasing severity of CVI, there was a progressive increase in the number of leukocytes in the dermis of CVI patients.

The types of leukocytes involved in dermal venous stasis skin changes are controversial. In a study performed by Wilkerson et al., skin biopsies were obtained from twenty-three patients who required surgical ligation, stripping, and/or avulsion for their varicose veins.[39] The condition of the skin was recorded as liposclerotic, eczematous, or normal. Lipodermatosclerosis was defined clinically as palpable induration of the skin, and subcutaneous tissues and eczema as visible erythema with scaling of the skin. Using immunohistochemical techniques, the authors stained for leukocyte-specific cell surface markers and reported that macrophages and lymphocytes were the predominant leukocytes observed in this patient population. Neutrophils and B lymphocytes rarely were observed. T lymphocytes and macrophages were predominantly observed perivascularly and in the epidermis. However, Pappas et al. performed a quantitative morphometric assessment of the dermal microcirculation using electron microscopy and reported that macrophages and mast cells were the predominant cells observed in patients with CVI dermal skin changes.[40] Furthermore, lymphocytes were never observed. This discrepancy may reflect the types of patients that were studied. Wilkerson et al. biopsied patients with erythematous and eczematous skin changes, whereas Pappas predominantly evaluated older patients with dermal fibrosis. Patients with eczematous skin changes may have an autoimmune component to their CVI, whereas patients with dermal fibrosis may reflect changes consistent with chronic inflammation and altered tissue remodeling.

Given the predominant role of leukocytes in CVI pathology, there has been great interest in the activation state and functional status of leukocytes in CVI patients. Pappas et al. explored the hypothesis that circulating leukocytes in CVI patients were in an altered state of activation and therefore may be involved in leukocyte-mediated injury. They measured the expression of cell surface activation markers of circulating leukocytes using fluorescence flow cytometry.[41] Relative to normal individuals, patients with chronic venous stasis ulcers had a decreased expression of the CD3+/DR+ and CD3+/CD38+ markers on T lymphocytes and an increased expression of CD14+/CD38+ markers on monocytes. Circulating neutrophils demonstrated no evidence of activation.

Although Pappas et al. identified a population of circulating cells demonstrating altered activation markers, their results did not test the functional status of these cells. In a follow-up study, Pappas et al. tested the hypothesis that circulating mononuclear cells in CVI patients were dysfunctional by challenging monocytes with test mitogens.[42] Lymphocyte and monocyte cell function was measured as the degree of proliferation in response to a mitogenic challenge. Fifty patients were separated into four groups: Group 1, fourteen patients with normal limbs; Group 2, ten patients with class 2 CVI (stasis dermatitis only); Group 3, fifteen patients with active venous ulcers; Group 4, eleven patients with healed venous ulcers and current evidence of lipodermatosclerosis. Systemically circulating lymphocytes and monocytes were obtained by antecubital venipuncture from Groups 1–4. Cells were cultured in the presence of staphylococcal enterotoxins (SEs) A, B, C_1, D, and E (mitogens) and PHA (phytohemagglutinin), a control mitogen. Proliferative responses to PHA indicated that lymphocytes and monocytes from CVI patients were not globally depressed. However, patients in Group 2 did not exhibit the same degree of proliferation to PHA as did Groups 1, 3, and 4. Differences in proliferative responses between Groups 2 and 1 (44.38 ± 43.9 vs. 118.87 ± 27.1, $p < 0.05$) and Groups 2 and 3 (44.38 ± 43.9 vs. 105.95 ± 60.99, $p < 0.05$) were significant. Challenges with staphylococcal enterotoxin A and B revealed significant diminution of proliferative responses in Groups 2 (42.73 ± 11.55, $p < 0.05$) and 3 (45.57 ± 9.1, $p < 0.05$) and Groups 3 (36.81 ± 6.9, $p < 0.05$) and 4 (35.04 ± 7.5, $p < 0.05$), compared with SEA controls (68.68 ± 9.9) and SEB controls (66.25 ± 13.56), respectively. A trend toward diminished cellular function with progression of CVI was observed with staphylococcal enterotoxins B, C_1, D, and E, strongly suggesting biologic significance. Furthermore, patients with lipodermatosclerosis and a history of healed ulcers uniformly exhibited the poorest proliferative responses. This study indicated that deterioration of mononuclear cell function was associated with CVI and suggested that lymphocyte and monocyte function diminished with clinical disease progression. The authors speculated that the decreased capacity for mononuclear cell proliferation in response to various challenges may manifest itself clinically as poor and prolonged wound healing.

THE VENOUS MICROCIRCULATION

Numerous investigations have attempted to evaluate the microcirculation of patients with CVI.[40,43–46] The majority of these investigations were qualitative descriptions of vascular abnormalities, which lacked uniformity of biopsy sites and patient stratification. Prior to 1997 it was widely accepted that endothelial cells from the dermal microcirculation appeared abnormal, contained Weibel-Palade bodies, were edematous, and demonstrated widened interendothelial gap junctions.[45] Based on these descriptive observations it was assumed that the dermal microcirculation of CVI patients have functional derangements related to permeability and ulcer formation. It was not until 1997 that a quantitative morphometric analysis of the dermal microcirculation was reported.[40] The objectives of this investigation were to quantify differences in endothelial cell structure and local cell type with emphasis on leukocyte cell type and their relationship to arterioles, capillaries, and postcapillary venules (PCVs). Variables assessed were number and types of leukocytes, endothelial cell thickness, endothelial vesicle density, interendothelial junctional width, cuff thickness, and ribosome density. Thirty-five patients had two 4-mm punch biopsies obtained from the lower calf (gaiter region) and lower thigh. Patients were separated into one of four groups according to the 1995 ISCVS/SVS (International Society for Cardiovascular Surgery/Society for Vascular Surgery) CEAP classification.[5] Group 1 consisted of five patients with no evidence of venous disease. Skin biopsies from these patients served as normal controls. Groups 2 through 4 consisted of patients with CEAP Class 4 (n = 11), Class 5 (n = 9), and Class 6 (n = 10) CVI.

ENDOTHELIAL CELL CHARACTERISTICS

No significant differences were observed in endothelial cell thickness of arterioles, capillaries, and PCVs from either gaiter or thigh biopsies.[40] Qualitatively, endothelial cells appeared metabolically active. Many nuclei exhibited a euchromatic appearance, implying active mRNA transcription. In most instances ribosome numbers were so abundant that they exceeded the resolution capacity of the image analysis system and could not be quantified. The prominence in ribosome content and the euchromatic appearance of the endothelial cell nucleus strongly suggested active protein production. No significant differences in vesicle density were observed in gaiter biopsies between groups. Class 6 patients exhibited an increased number of vesicles in arterioles and PCV endothelia from thigh biopsies but did not differ compared with gaiter biopsies. Mean interendothelial junctional width varied within a normal range of 20–50 nm. Significantly widened interendothelial gap junctions were not observed and thus conflicted with the reports of Wenner et al.[45] Mean basal lamina thickness differed significantly at the capillary level in both gaiter and thigh biopsies. Differences were most pronounced in patients with Class 4 disease. These data indicated that endothelial cells from the dermal microcirculation of CVI patients were far from normal. They demonstrated increased metabolic activity suggestive of active cellular transcription and protein production. Most surprising was the observation of uniformly tight gap junctions. Previously these gap junctions were reported to be as wide as 180 nm, and it was assumed that these widened junctions were responsible for

macromolecule extravasation and edema formation.[33,45] Pappas et al. suggested that alternate methods for tissue edema such as increased transendothelial vesicle transport, formation of transendothelial channels, and alterations in the glycocalyx lining the junctional cleft may be involved in CVI edema and macromolecule transport.[40]

TYPES AND DISTRIBUTION OF LEUKOCYTES

The most striking differences in cell type and distribution were observed with mast cells and macrophages (see Figure 8.3). In both gaiter and thigh biopsies, mast cell numbers were two to four times greater than control in Class 4 and 5 patients around arterioles and PCVs (p < 0.05). Class 6 patients demonstrated no difference in mast cell number compared to controls. Mast cell numbers around capillaries did not differ across groups in either gaiter or thigh biopsies. Macrophages demonstrated increased numbers in Class 5 and 6 patients around arterioles and PCVs, respectively (p < 0.05). Differences in macrophage numbers around capillaries were observed primarily in Class 4 patients in both gaiter and thigh biopsies. Surprisingly, lymphocytes, plasma cells, and neutrophils were not present in the immediate perivascular space. Fibroblasts were the most common cells observed in both gaiter and thigh biopsies. It was speculated that mast cells and macrophages may function to regulate tissue remodeling resulting in dermal

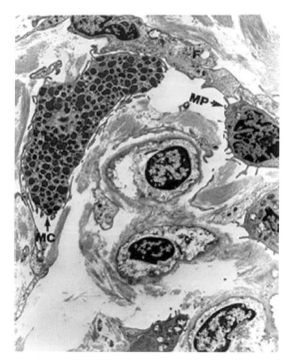

Figure 8.3 Electron micrograph (Mag 4300×) of mast cells (MC), macrophages (MP) and fibroblast (F) surrounding a central capillary from dermal biopsy of a patient with CEAP class 4 chronic venous insufficiency.

fibrosis.[40] The mast cell enzyme chymase is a potent activator of matrix metalloproteinase-1 and -3 (collagenase and stromelysin).[47–49] In an in vitro model using the human mast cell line HMC-1, these cells were reported to spontaneously adhere to fibronectin, laminin, and collagen types I and III, all components of the perivascular cuff (see later).[49] Chymase also causes release of latent transforming growth factor-beta 1 (TGF-β_1) secreted by activated endothelial cells, fibroblasts, and platelets from extracellular matrices.[50] Release and activation of TGF-,β_1 initiate a cascade of events in which macrophages and fibroblasts are recruited to wound healing sites and stimulated to produce fibroblast mitogens and connective tissue proteins, respectively.[51] Mast cell degranulation leading to TGF-β_1 activation and macrophage recruitment may explain why decreased mast cell and increased macrophage numbers were observed in Class 6 patients. Macrophage migration, as evidenced by the frequent appearance of cytoplasmic tails in perivascular macrophages, further substantiates the concept of inflammatory cytokine recruitment (see Figure 8.4).

EXTRACELLULAR MATRIX ALTERATIONS

Once leukocytes have migrated to the extracellular space they localize around capillaries and postcapillary venules. The perivascular space is surrounded by extracellular matrix (ECM) proteins and forms a perivascular cuff. Adjacent to these perivascular cuffs and throughout the dermal interstitium is an intense and disorganized collagen deposition.[33,40] Perivascular cuffs and the accompanying collagen deposition are the sine qua non of the dermal microcirculation in CVI patients (see Figure 8.4). The perivascular cuff originally was thought to be the result of fibrinogen extravasation

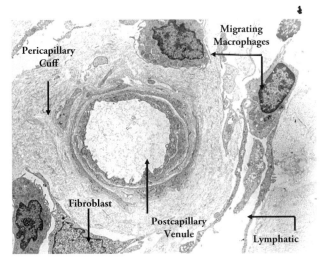

Figure 8.4   Electron micrograph (Mag 4300×) of a well-developed perivascular cuff in close proximity to a fibroblast in a patient with CEAP class 6 chronic venous insufficiency. Long arrow points to macrophages that appear to be entering a lymphatic lumen.

and erroneously referred to as a fibrin cuff.[5] It is now known that the cuff is a ring of ECM proteins consisting of collagen types I and III, fibronectin, vitronectin, laminin, tenascin, and fibrin.[52] The role of the cuff and its cell of origin is not completely understood. The investigation by Pappas et al. suggested that the endothelial cells of the dermal microcirculation were responsible for cuff formation.[40] The cuff was once thought to be a barrier to oxygen and nutrient diffusion; however, recent evidence suggests that cuff formation is an attempt to maintain vascular architecture in response to increased mechanical load.[53] Although perivascular cuffs may function to preserve microcirculatory architecture, several pathologic processes may be related to cuff formation. Immunohistochemical analyses have demonstrated TGF-β_1 and α_2-macroglobulin in the interstices of perivascular cuffs.[54] It has been suggested that these "trapped" molecules are distributed abnormally in the dermis, leading to altered tissue remodeling and fibrosis. Cuffs may also serve as a lattice for capillary angiogenesis, explaining the capillary tortuosity and increased capillary density observed in the dermis of CVI patients.

PATHOPHYSIOLOGY OF STASIS DERMATITIS AND DERMAL FIBROSIS

The mechanisms modulating leukocyte activation, fibroblast function, and dermal extracellular matrix alterations have been the focus of investigation in the 1990s. CVI is a disease of chronic inflammation due to a persistent and sustained injury secondary to venous hypertension. It is hypothesized that the primary injury is extravasation of macromolecules (i.e., fibrinogen and α_2-macroglobulin) and red blood cells (RBCs) into the dermal interstitium.[33,34,44,45,54] RBC degradation products and interstitial protein extravasation are potent chemoattractants and presumably represent the initial underlying chronic inflammatory signal responsible for leukocyte recruitment. It has been assumed that these cytochemical events are responsible for the increased expression of ICAM-1 (intercellular adhesion molecule-1) on endothelial cells of microcirculatory exchange vessels observed in CVI dermal biopsies.[39,55] ICAM-1 is the activation-dependent adhesion molecule utilized by macrophages, lymphocytes, and mast cells for diapedesis. As stated earlier, all these cells have been observed by immunohistochemistry and electron microscopy in the interstitium of dermal biopsies.[39,40]

CYTOKINE REGULATION AND TISSUE FIBROSIS

Leukocyte recruitment, ECM alterations, and tissue fibrosis are characteristic of chronic inflammatory diseases caused by alterations in TGF-β₁ gene expression and protein production. To determine the role of TGF-β₁ in CVI, dermal biopsies from normal patients and CEAP Class 4, 5, and 6 CVI patients were analyzed for TGF-β₁ gene expression, protein production, and cellular location.[56] Quantitative RT-PCR for TGF-β₁ gene expression was performed on twenty-four skin biopsies obtained from twenty-four patients. Patients were separated into four groups according to the ISCVS/SVS classification for CVI: normal skin (n = 6), CEAP Class 4 (n = 6), CEAP Class 5 (n = 5), and CEAP class 6 (n = 7). TGF-β₁ gene transcripts for controls, Class 4, 5, and 6 patients were 7.02 ± 7.33, 43.33 ± 9.0, 16.13 ± 7.67, and 7.22 ± 0.56 x 10^{-14} moles/g total RNA, respectively. The differences in TGF-β₁ gene expression in Class 4 patients was significantly elevated compared with control and Class 5 and 6 patients ($p < 0.05$).[56] An additional 38 patients had 54 biopsies from the lower calf (LC) and lower thigh (LT) analyzed for TGF-β₁ protein concentration. The amounts of active TGF-β₁ in picograms/gram (pg/g) of tissue from LC and LT biopsies compared to normal skin biopsies were as follows: Normal skin (<1.0 pc/g), Class 4 (LC, 5061 ± 1827; LT 317.3 ± 277), Class 5 (LC, 8327 ± 3690; LT 193 ± 164), and Class 6 (LC, 5392 ± 1800; LT, 117 ± 61; see Figure 8.5). Differences between normal skin and Class 4 and 6 patients were significant ($p < 0.05$ and $p < 0.01$, respectively). No differences between Class 4, 5, and 6 patients were observed. Differences between LC and LT within each CVI group were significant (Class 4, $p < 0.003$, Class 5, $p < 0.008$, Class 6, $p < 0.02$). These data demonstrate that in areas of clinically active CVI, increased amounts of active TGF-β₁ are present compared with normal skin. Furthermore, active TGF β₁ protein concentrations of

biopsies from the LT did not differ from normal skin demonstrating a regionalized response to injury.[56]

Immunohistochemistry and immunogold labeling experiments were performed to identify the sources of active TGF-β₁ protein production. Immunohistochemistry of normal skin and ipsilateral thigh biopsies of CVI patient demonstrated mild TGF-β₁ in the basal layer of the epidermis. The dermis demonstrated few capillaries, ordered collagen architecture, and no interstitial leukocytes. CVI dermal biopsies from areas of clinically active disease demonstrated staining of the basal layer of the epidermis, interstitial leukocytes, and fibroblasts. Many perivascular leukocytes demonstrated positive staining of intracellular granules and appeared morphologically similar to previously reported mast cells (see Figures 8.3 and 8.6).[56] Numerous capillaries with perivascular cuffs were observed; however, cuffs did not stain positively for TGF-β₁.[56] This study conflicts with the observations reported by Higley et al. in which they reported positive TGF-β₁ staining in perivascular cuffs and an absence of TGF-β₁ in the provisional matrix of the venous ulcer compared to healing donor skin graft sites.[54] They concluded that TGF-β₁ was therefore abnormally "trapped" in the perivascular cuff and therefore unavailable for normal granulation tissue development. Differences between the two studies may relate to biopsy site selection. Higley et al. biopsied chronic, nonhealing venous ulcer edges and ulcer bases, whereas patients with active ulcers in the study by Pappas et al. were biopsied 5 to 10 cm away from an active ulcer. Therefore, the former study reflects the biology of chronic wound healing, and our data suggest active tissue remodeling in response to a chronic injury stimulus.

Immunogold labeling confirmed the presence of TGF-β₁ in dermal leukocytes. Positive labeling of gold particles similarly were observed in collagen fibrils of the ECM. This observation may explain why the molecular regulation of TGF-β₁ in CVI patients demonstrates differential gene and protein production according to disease classification. As

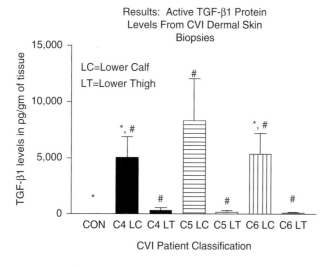

Results: Active TGF-β1 Protein Levels From CVI Dermal Skin Biopsies

LC=Lower Calf
LT=Lower Thigh

* Control vs Class 4 and 6 (p≤0.05)
# LC vs LT biopsies within each class (p≤0.02)

Figure 8.5   Active TGF-β₁ levels indicating increased levels in class 4, 5, and 6 patients compared with controls and ipsilateral thigh biopsies. Con-Control patients without venous disease, LT-Ipsilateral thigh, LC-Ipsilateral diseased skin.

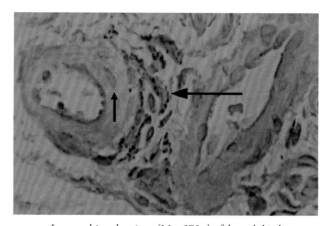

Figure 8.6   Immunohistochemistry (Mag 575×) of dermal skin biopsy demonstrating transforming growth factor-β₁ positive granules (long arrow) in leukocytes surrounding a perivascular cuff and leukocytes migrating through a perivascular cuff (short arrow).

stated earlier, the gene expression of TGF-β_1 was increased in Class 4 patients only, and the protein production essentially was increased in Class 4, 5, and 6 patients. These differences may be related to disease severity and the pluripotential responses of TGF-β_1. TGF-β_1 can have inhibitory and stimulatory effects that are primarily dependent on local concentration, cell source, and surrounding ECM. In the study by Pappas et al., Class 4 patients were younger than the other study groups, never experienced an episode of venous stasis ulceration, and clinically demonstrated less dermal tissue fibrosis. TGF-β_1 in these patients therefore may be involved in limiting the response to injury. Indeed, one could speculate that early on in the disease process, a low-grade production of TGF-β_1 is a normal wound-healing response and may serve to prevent the onset and development of tissue fibrosis. With continued and prolonged exposure, an imbalance in tissue remodeling in patients with Class 5 and 6 disease clinically manifests itself as dermatofibrosis. A pathologic effect of increased ECM deposition is an alteration in the storage and release of growth factors.[57] The latent form of TGF-β_1 is secreted from cells bound to one of three latent TGF-β_1 binding proteins (LTBPs). Once secreted, LTBPs mediate binding of latent TGF-β_1 to matrix proteins. Matrix release of TGF-β_1 is mediated by multiple serine proteinases including plasmin, mast cell chymase, and leukocyte elastase.[50,58–60] An increase in the number of mast cells and circulating leukocyte elastase have been reported previously in CVI patients.[40,61] The increase in active TGF-β_1 observed in Class 5 and 6 patients therefore may result from ECM release of latent TGF-β_1, resulting in tissue fibrosis. This hypothesis is consistent with the demonstration of immunogold labeling to collagen fibrils in the ECM of CVI patients. The modulation of TGF-β_1 release from the ECM may therefore provide a faster means of signal transduction than simple control of gene expression, and therefore may explain the sustained increase of TGF-β_1 in Class 5 and 6 patients in the absence of increased gene expression. This study did not demonstrate increased TGF-β_1 staining in the ECM by ICC because the primary antibody used was specific only for active TGF-β_1 and therefore may have missed latency associated peptide (LAP) and LTBP associated TGF-β_1.

The distribution and location of several other growth factors in the skin of CVI patients have also been investigated. Peschen et al. reported on the role of platelet-derived growth factor receptor alpha and beta (PDGFR-α and -β) and vascular endothelial growth factor (VEGF).[62] Skin biopsies from 30 patients were separated into five groups: Group 1, patients with reticular veins; Group 2, venous eczema; Group 3, skin pigmentation; Group 4, lipodermatosclerosis; and Group 5, patients with active leg ulcers; with a total of six patients in each group. Biopsies were studied with immunohistochemistry and the degree of immunoreactivity assessed with a scoring system by two blinded reviewers. Peschen et al. reported that PDGFR-α and -β and vascular endothelial growth factor (VEGF) expression was strongly increased in the stroma of CVI patients with eczema and active ulcers compared with patients with reticular veins and pigmentation changes only.[62] To a lesser degree, patients with lipodermatosclerosis demonstrated immunoreactivity to PDGFR-α and -β and VEGF as well. PDGFR-α and -β expression was elevated considerably in the capillaries and surrounding fibroblasts and inflammatory cells of venous eczema patients. In addition, immunoreactivity was increased in dermal fibroblasts, smooth muscle cells, and vascular cells of lipodermatosclerosis patients compared with patients with reticular veins only. The greatest expression of PDGFR-α and -β was observed in mesenchymal cells and vascular endothelial cells of patients with active venous ulcers. VEGF immunoreactivity correlated with disease severity. VEGF positive capillary endothelial cells and pericapillary cells increased in patients with venous eczema, lipodermatosclerosis, and active venous ulceration, respectively. In a subsequent investigation, these authors reported that with progression of CVI dermal pathology the endothelial cell adhesion molecules intercellular and vascular adhesion molecules (ICAM-1, VCAM-1) and their corresponding leukocyte ligands LFA-1 and VLA-4 were upregulated on leukocytes and endothelial cells.[55] Based on these observations, the authors speculated that leukocyte recruitment, capillary proliferation, and interstitial edema in CVI patients may be regulated through PDGF and VEGF by upregulation of adhesion molecules leading to leukocyte recruitment, diapedesis, and release of chemical mediators.[55]

In summary, these investigations indicate that progression of CVI dermal pathology is mediated by a cascade of inflammatory events. Venous hypertension causes extravasation of macromolecules like fibrinogen and red blood cells that act as potent inflammatory mediators. These mediators cause an upregulation of adhesion molecules and the expression of growth factors like PDGF and VEGF, which result in leukocyte recruitment. Monocytes and mast cells travel to the site of injury, which activate or release TGF-β_1 and probably other undiscovered chemicals as well. What effect growth factor binding has on fibroblast and endothelial cell function has been the focus of numerous investigations in the 1990s.

DERMAL FIBROBLAST FUNCTION

Several studies have reported aberrant phenotypic behavior of fibroblasts isolated from venous ulcer edges when compared to fibroblasts obtained from ipsilateral thigh biopsies of normal skin in the same patients. Hasan et al. compared the ability of venous ulcer fibroblasts to produce αI procollagen mRNA and collagen after stimulation with TGF-β_1.[63] These authors were not able to demonstrate differences in αI procollagen mRNA levels after stimulation with TGF-β_1 between venous ulcer fibroblasts and normal fibroblasts (control) from ipsilateral thigh biopsies. However, collagen production was increased by 60% in a dose-dependent manner in controls, whereas venous ulcer fibroblasts were unresponsive. This unresponsiveness was associated with a four-fold decrease in TGF-β_1 type II receptors. In a follow-up report, Kim et al. indicated that the decrease in TGF-β_1 type II receptors was associated with a decrease in phosphorylation of the TGF-β_1 receptor substrates SMAD 2 and 3 as well as p42/44 mitogen activated protein kinases.[64] A similar investigation reported a decrease in collagen production from venous ulcer fibroblasts and similar amounts of fibronectin production when compared to normal controls.[65]

Fibroblast responsiveness to growth factors was further delineated by Stanley et al.[66] These investigators characterized the proliferative responses of venous ulcer fibroblasts when stimulated with basic fibroblastic growth factor (bFGF), epidermal growth factor (EGF), and interleukin 1-β (IL-1β). In their initial study, they reported that venous ulcer fibroblast growth rates were markedly suppressed when stimulated with bFGF, EGF, and IL-1β. In a follow-up investigation these authors noted that the previously observed growth inhibition could be reversed with bFGF.[67] Lal et al. reported that the proliferative responses of CVI fibroblasts to TGF-β_1 correlated with disease severity.[68] Fibroblasts from patients with CEAP Class 2 and 3 disease retain their agonist-induced proliferative capacity. Class 4 and 5 fibroblasts demonstrated diminished agonist-induced proliferation, whereas Class 6 (venous ulcer fibroblasts) did not proliferate after TGF-β_1 stimulation, confirming the observations made by the previous investigators. Phenotypically, venous ulcer fibroblasts appeared large and polygonal with varied nuclear morphologic features, whereas normal fibroblasts appeared compact and tapered with well-defined nuclear morphologic features. Venous ulcer fibroblasts appeared morphologically similar to fibroblasts undergoing cellular senescence. Therefore, the blunted growth response of CVI venous ulcer fibroblasts appears related to development of cellular senescence.[66,69]

Other characteristics of senescent cells are an overexpression of matrix proteins such as fibronectin (cFN) and enhanced activity of β-galactosidase (SA-β-Gal). In an evaluation of seven patients with venous stasis ulcers, it was noted that a higher percentage of SA-β-Gal positive cells in venous ulcers compared to normal controls (6.3% vs. 0.21%, $p < 0.0.6$).[67] It was also reported that venous ulcer fibroblasts produced one to four times more cFN by Western blot analysis compared to controls.[69] These data support the hypothesis that venous ulcer fibroblasts phenotypically behave like senescent cells. However, senescence is probably the end manifestation of a wide spectrum of events that lead to proliferative resistance and cellular dysfunction. Telomeres and telomerase activity are the sine qua non of truly senescent cells. To date, there are no reported studies indicating an abnormality in CVI fibroblast telomere or telomerase activity. Absent these investigations, the true role of senescence in CVI remains ill-defined.

ROLE OF MATRIX METALLOPROTEINASES AND THEIR INHIBITORS IN CVI

The signaling event responsible for the development of a venous ulcer and the mechanisms responsible for prolonged wound healing are poorly understood. Wound healing is an orderly process that involves inflammation, re-epithelialization, matrix deposition, and tissue remodeling. Tissue remodeling and matrix deposition are processes controlled by matrix metalloproteinases (MMPs) and tissue inhibitors of matrix metalloproteinases (TIMPs). In general, MMPs and TIMPs are not constitutively expressed. They are induced temporarily in response to exogenous signals such as various proteases, cytokines or growth factors, cell-matrix interactions, and altered cell-cell contacts. TGF-β_1 is a potent inducer of TIMP-1 and collagen production and inhibitor of MMP-1 through regulation of gene expression and protein synthesis. Several studies have demonstrated that prolonged and continuous TGF-β_1 production causes tissue fibrosis by stimulating ECM production and inhibiting degradation by affecting MMP and TIMP production. Alterations in MMP and TIMP production may similarly modulate the tissue fibrosis of the lower extremity in CVI patients. Several investigators have reported that the gelatinases MMP-2 and -9 as well as TIMP-1 are increased in the exudates of patients with venous ulcers compared to acute wounds.[70-72] However, analyses of biopsy specimens have demonstrated variable results. Herouy et al. reported that MMP-1 and -2 and TIMP-1 are increased in patients with lipodermatosclerosis compared with normal skin.[73] In a subsequent investigation, biopsies from venous ulcer patients were found to have increased levels of the active form of MMP-2 compared with normal skin[74] as well as increased immunoreactivity to EMMPRIN (extracellular inducer of MMP), MT1-MMP (membrane type 1), and MT2-MMP in the dermis and perivascular regions of venous ulcers.[75] Saito et al. were unable to identify differences in overall MMP-1, -2, and -9 and TIMP-1 protein levels or activity in CVI patients with CEAP Class 2 through 6 disease compared with normal controls or CVI groups.[76] However, within a clinical class, MMP-2 levels were elevated compared with MMP-1, and -9 and TIMP-1 in patients with Class 4 and Class 5 disease. These data indicate that active tissue remodeling is occurring in patients with CVI. Which matrix metalloproteinases are involved and how they're activated and regulated are currently unclear. It appears that MMP-2 may be activated by urokinase plasminogen activator (uPA). Herouy et al. observed increased uPA and urokinase-type plasminogen activator receptor (uPAR) mRNA and protein levels in patients with venous ulcers compared to normal skin.[77] The elevated levels of active TGF-β_1 in the dermis of CVI patients suggests a regulatory role for TGF-β_1 in MMP and TIMP synthesis and activity. However, there is currently no direct evidence indicating such a relationship.

CONCLUSION

The mechanisms regulating varicose vein development and the subsequent dermal skin sequelae caused by chronic ambulatory venous hypertension only recently have been investigated. It is clear that varicose vein formation has a genetic component that is linked to environmental stimuli. Susceptible patients develop vein wall fibrosis and loss of valvular competence that leads to venous hypertension. The transmission of high venous pressures to the dermal microcirculation causes extravasation of macromolecules and red blood cells that serve as the underlying stimulus for inflammatory injury. Activation of the microcirculation results in cytokine and growth factor release leading to leukocyte migration into the interstitium. At the site of injury, a host of inflammatory events is set into action. TGF-β_1 appears to be a primary regulator of CVI induced injury. TGF-β_1 secretion from leukocytes with subsequent binding to dermal fibroblasts is associated with intense dermal fibrosis and tissue remodeling. In addition, decreased TGF-β_1 type II receptors on venous ulcer fibroblasts are associated with diminished fibroblast proliferation. Fibroblast proliferation diminishes with disease progression, ultimately leading to senescence and poor ulcer healing. In addition, increases in MMP-2 synthesis appear to increase tissue remodeling and further impede ulcer healing. As our understanding of the underlying cellular and molecular mechanisms that regulate CVI and ulcer formation increase, therapeutic interventions for treatment and prevention will ultimately follow.

REFERENCES

1. White GH. Chronic venous insufficiency. In: Veith F, Hobson RW II, Williams RA, Wilson SE, eds. *Vascular surgery*. New York: McGraw-Hill. 1993. 865–888.
2. Callam MJ. Epidemiology of varicose veins, *Br J Surg*. 1994. *81*: 167–173.
3. Hume M. Presidential address: A venous renaissance?, *J Vasc Surg*. 1992. *6*: 947–951.
4. Lawrence PF, Gazak CE. Epidemiology of chronic venous insufficiency. In: Gloviczki P, Bergan JJ, eds. *Atlas of endoscopic perforator vein surgery*. London: Springer-Verlag. 1998. 31–44.
5. Porter JM, International Consensus Committee on Chronic Venous Disease. Reporting Standards in venous disease: An update, *J Vasc Surg*. 1995. *21*: 635–645.
6. Browse NL, Burnand KG, Irvine AT, Wilson NM, eds. Varicose veins: Pathology. In: *Diseases of the veins*. London and New York: Oxford University Press. 1999. 145–162.
7. Gunderson J, Hauge M. Hereditary factors in venous insufficiency, *Angiology*. 1969. *20*(6): 346–355.
8. Cornu-Thenard A, Boivin P, Baud MM, De Vincenzi I, Carpentier PH. Importance of the familial factor in varicose disease: Clinical study of 134 families, *J Derm Surg Onc*. 1994. *20*: 318–326.
9. Labropoulos N, Giannoukas AD, Delis K, et al. Where does the venous reflux start? *J Vasc Surg*. 1997. *26*: 736–742.
10. Wakefield TM, Strietert RM, Prince MR, Downing LJ, Greenfield LJ. Pathogenesis of venous thrombosis: A new insight, *Cardiovasc Surg*. 1997. *5*(1): 6–15.
11. Takase S, Bergan JJ, Schmid-Schonbein G. Expression of adhesion molecules and cytokines on saphenous veins in chronic venous insufficiency, *Ann Vasc Surg*. 2000. *14*: 427–435.
12. Rose A. Some new thoughts on the etiology of varicose veins, *J Cardiovasc Surg*. 1986. *27*: 534–543.
13. Pappas PJ, Gwertzman GA, DeFouw DO, et al. Retinoblastoma protein: A molecular regulator of chronic venous insufficiency, *J Surg Res*. 1998. *76*: 149–153.
14. Travers JP, Brookes CE, Evans J, et al. Assessment of wall structure and composition of varicose veins with reference to collagen, elastin, and smooth muscle content, *Eur J Vasc Endovasc Surg*. 1996. *11*: 230–237.
15. Jurukova Z, Milenkov C. Ultrastructural evidence for collagen degradation in the walls of varicose veins, *Exp and Molec Path*. 1982. *37*: 37–47.
16. Venturi M, Bonavina L, Annoni F, et al. Biochemical assay of collagen and elastin in the normal and varicose vein wall, *J Surg Res*. 1996. *60*: 245–248.
17. Maurel E, Azema C, Deloly J, Bouissou H. Collagen of the normal and the varicose human saphenous vein: A biochemical study, *Clinica Chimica Acta*. 1990. *193*: 27–38.
18. Ascher E, Jacob T, Hingorani A, Gunduz Y, Mazzariol F, Kallakuri S. Programmed cell death (apoptosis) and its role in the pathogenesis of lower extremity varicose veins, *Ann Vasc Surg*. 2000. *14*: 24–30.
19. Ascher E, Jacob T, Hingorani A, Tsemekhin B, Gunduz Y. Expression of molecular mediators of apoptosis and their role in the pathogenesis of lower-extremity varicose veins, *J Vasc Surg*. 2001. *33*: 1080–1086.
20. Gandhi RH, Irizarry E, Nachman GB, Halpern JJ, Mulcare RJ, Tilson MD. Analysis of the connective tissue matrix and proteolytic activity of primary varicose veins, *J Vasc Surg*. 1993. *18*: 814–820.
21. Parra JR, Cambria RA, Hower CD, et al. Tissue inhibitor of metalloproteinase-1 is increased in the saphenofemoral junction of patients with varices in the leg, *J Vasc Surg*. 1998. *28*: 669–675.
22. Kosugi I, Urayama H, Kasashima F, Ohtake H, Watanabe Y. Matrix metalloproteinase-9 and urokinase-type plasminogen activator in varicose veins, *Ann Vasc Surg*. 2003. *17*(3): 234–238.
23. Woodside KJ, Hu M, Burke A, et al. Morphologic characteristics of varicose veins: Possible role of metalloproteinases, *J Vasc Surg*. 2003. *38*: 162–169.
24. Shireman PK, McCarthy WJ, Pearce WH, et al. Plasminogen activator levels are influenced by location and varicosity in greater saphenous vein, *J Vasc Surg*. 1996. *24*(5): 719–724.
25. Badier-Commander C, Verbeuren T, Lebard C, Michel J, Jacob M. Increased TIMP/MMP ratio in varicose veins: A possible explanation for extracellular matrix accumulation, *J Pathol*. 2000. *192*: 105–112.
26. Lowell RC, Gloviczki P, Miller VM. In vitro evaluation of endothelial and smooth muscle function of primary varicose veins, *J Vasc Surg*. 1992. *16*: 679–686.
27. Rizzi A, Quaglio D, Vasquez G, et al. Effects of vasoactive agents in healthy and diseased human saphenous veins, *J Vasc Surg*. 1998. *28*: 855–861.
28. Barber DA, Wang X, Gloviczki P, Miller VM. Characterization of endothelin receptors in human varicose veins, *J Vasc Surg*. 1997. *26*: 61–69.
29. Nemcova S, Gloviczki P, Rud KS, Miller VM. Cyclic nucleotides and production of prostanoids in human varicose veins, *J Vasc Surg*. 1999. *30*: 876–884.
30. Homans J. The etiology and treatment of varicose ulcer of the leg, *Surg Gynecol Obstet*. 1917. *24*: 300–311.
31. Blalock A. Oxygen content of blood in patients with varicose veins, *Arch Surg*. 1929. *19*: 898–905.
32. Pratt GH. Arterial varices: A syndrome, *Am J Surg*. 1949. *77*: 456–460.
33. Burnand KG, Whimster I, Naidoo A, Browse NL. Pericapillary fibrin deposition in the ulcer bearing skin of the lower limb: The cause of lipodermatosclerosis and venous ulceration, *Br Med J*. 1982. *285*: 1071–1072.

34. Burnand KG, Clemenson G, Gaunt J, Browse NL. The effect of sustained venous hypertension in the skin and capillaries of the canine hind limb, *Br J Surg*. 1981. *69*: 41–44.

35. Browse NL, Burnand KG. The cause of venous ulceration, *Lancet*. 1982. *2*: 243–245.

36. Smith PDC, Thomas P, Scurr JH, Dormandy JA. Causes of venous ulceration: A new hypothesis, *Br Med J*. 1988. *296*: 1726–1727.

37. Thomas P, Nash GB, Dormandy JA. White cell accumulation in dependent legs of patients with venous hypertension: A possible mechanism for trophic changes in the skin, *Br Med J*. 1988. *296*: 1693–1695.

38. Scott HJ, Smith PDC, Scurr JH. Histological study of white blood cells and their association with lipodermatosclerosis and venous ulceration, *Br J Surg*. 1991. *78*: 210–211.

39. Wilkinson LS, Bunker C, Edward JCW, Scurr JH, Smith PDC. Leukocytes: Their role in the etiopathogenesis of skin damage in venous disease, *J Vasc Surg*. 1993. *17*: 669–675.

40. Pappas PJ, DeFouw DO, Venezio LM, et al. Morphometric assessment of the dermal microcirculation in patients with chronic venous insufficiency, *J Vasc Surg*. 1997. *26*: 784–795.

41. Pappas PJ, Fallek SR, Garcia A, et al. Role of leukocyte activation in patients with venous stasis ulcers, *J Surg Res*. 1995. *59*: 553–559.

42. Pappas PJ, Teehan EP, Fallek SR, et al. Diminished mononuclear cell function is associated with chronic venous insufficiency, *J Vasc Surg*. 1995. *22*: 580–586.

43. Leu AJ, Leu HJ, Franzeck UK, Bollinger A. Microvascular changes in chronic venous insufficiency: A review, *Cardiovasc Surg*. 1995. *3*: 237–245.

44. Leu HJ. Morphology of chronic venous insufficiency-light and electron microscopic examinations, *Vasa*. 1991. *20*: 330–342.

45. Wenner A, Leu HJ, Spycher M, Brunner U. Ultrastructural changes of capillaries in chronic venous insufficiency, *Expl Cell Biol*. 1980. *48*: 1–14.

46. Scelsi R, Scelsi L, Cortinovis R, Poggi P. Morphological changes of dermal blood and lymphatic vessels in chronic venous insufficiency of the leg, *Int Angiol*. 1994. *13*: 308–311.

47. Saarien J, Lalkkinen N, Welgus HG, Kovannen PT. Activation of human interstitial procollagenase through direct cleavage of the Leu83-Thr84 bond by mast cell chymase, *J Biol Chem*. 1994. *269*: 18134–18140.

48. Lees M, Taylor DJ, Woolley DE. Mast cell proteinases activate precursor forms of collagenase and stromelysin, but not of gelatinases A and B, *Eur J Biochem*. 1994. *223*: 171–177.

49. Kruger-Drasagakes S, Grutzkau A, Baghramian R, Henz BM. Interactions of immature human mast cells with extracellular matrix: Expression of specific adhesion receptors and their role in cell binding to matrix proteins, *J Invest Dermatol*. 1996. *106*: 538–543.

50. Taipale J, Keski-Oja J. Growth factors in the extracellular matrix, *FASEB J*. 1997. *11*: 51–59.

51. Roberts AB, Flanders KC, Kondaiah P, et al. Transforming growth factor β: Biochemistry and roles in embryogenesis, tissue repair, and remodeling, and carcinogenesis, *Recent Prog Horm Res*. 1988. *44*: 157–197.

52. Herrick S, Sloan P, McGurk M, Freak L, McCollum CN, Ferguson WJ. Sequential changes in histologic pattern and extracellular matrix deposition during the healing of chronic venous ulcers, *Am J Pathol*. 1992. *141*: 1085–1095.

53. Bishop JE. Regulation of cardiovascular collagen deposition by mechanical forces, *Molec Med Today*. 1998. *4*: 69–75.

54. Higley HR, Kassander GA, Gerhardt CO, Falanga V. Extravasation of macromolecules and possible trapping of transforming growth factor-β1 in venous ulceration, *Br J Surg*. 1995. *132*: 79–85.

55. Peschen M, Lahaye T, Gennig B, Weyl A, Simon JC, Wolfgang V. Expression of the adhesion molecules ICAM-1, VCAM-1, LFA-1, and VLA-4 in the skin is modulated in progressing stages of chronic venous insufficiency, *Acta Derm Venereol*. 1999. *79*: 27–32.

56. Pappas PJ, You R, Rameshwar P, et al. Dermal tissue fibrosis in patients with chronic venous insufficiency is associated with increased transforming growth factor-β1 gene expression and protein production, *J Vasc Surg*. 1999. *30*: 1129–1145.

57. Taipale J, Saharinen J, Hedman K, Keski-oja J. Latent transforming growth factor-β1 and its binding protein are components of extracellular matrix microfibrils, *J Histochem Cytochem*. 1996. *44*: 875–889.

58. Border WA, Noble NA. Transforming growth factor β in tissue fibrosis, *N Engl J Med*. 1994. *331*: 1286–1292.

59. O'Kane S, Ferguson WJ. Transforming growth factor βs and wound healing, *Int J Biochem Cell Biol*. 1997. *29*: 63–78.

60. Grande JP. Role of transforming growth factor-β in tissue injury and repair, *PSEBM*. 1997. *214*: 27c40.

61. Shields DA, Sarin AS, Scurr JH, Smith PDC. Plasma elastase in venous disease, *Br J Surg*. 1994. *81*: 1496–1499.

62. Peschen M, Grenz H, Brand-Saberi B, et al. Increased expression of platelet-derived growth factor receptor alpha and beta and vascular endothelial growth factor in the skin of patients with chronic venous insufficiency, *Arch Dermatol Res*. 1998. *290*: 291–297.

63. Hasan A, Murata H, Falabella A, et al. Dermal fibroblasts from venous ulcers are unresponsive to the action of transforming growth factor-β1, *J Derm Sci*. 1997. *16*: 59–66.

64. Kim B, Kim HT, Park SH, et al. Fibroblasts from chronic wounds show altered TGF-β signaling and decreased TGF-β type II receptor expression, *J Cell Physiol* 2003. *195*: 331–336.

65. Herrick SE, Ireland GW, Simon D, McCollum CN, Ferguson MW. Venous ulcer fibroblasts compared with normal fibroblasts show differences in collagen but not in fibronectin production under both normal and hypoxic conditions, *J Invest Dermatol*. 1996. *106*: 187–193.

66. Stanley AC, Park H, Phillips TJ, Russakovsky V, Menzoian JO. Reduced growth of dermal fibroblasts from chronic venous ulcers can be stimulated with growth factors, *J Vasc Surg*. 1997. *26*: 994–1001.

67. Mendez MV, Stanley A, Park H, Shon K, Phillips TJ, Menzoian JO. Fibroblasts cultured from venous ulcers display cellular characteristics of senescence, *J Vasc Surg*. 1998. *28*: 876–883.

68. Lal BK, Saito S, Pappas PJ, et al. Altered proliferative responses of dermal fibroblasts to TGF-β1 may contribute to chronic venous stasis ulcers, *J Vasc Surg*. 2003. *37*: 1285–1293.

69. Mendez MV, Stanley A, Phillips TJ, Murphy M, Menzoian JO, Park H. Fibroblasts cultured from distal lower extremities in patients with venous reflux display cellular characteristics of senescence, *J Vasc Surg*. 1998. *28*: 1040–1050.

70. Weckroth M, Vaheri A, Lauharanta J, Sorsa T, Konttinen YT. Matrix metalloproteinases, gelatinase, and collagenase, in chronic leg ulcers, *J Invest Dermatol*. 1996. *106*: 1119–1124.

71. Wysocki AB, Staiano-Coico L, Grinell F. Wound fluid from chronic leg ulcers contains elevated levels of metalloproteinases MMP-2 and MMP-9, *J Invest Dermatol*. 1993. *101*: 64–68.

72. Bullen EC, Longaker MT, Updike DL, et al. Tissue inhibitor of metalloproteinases-1 is decreased and activated gelatinases are increased in chronic wounds, *J Invest Dermatol*. 1995. *104*: 236–240.

73. Herouy Y, May AE, Pornschlegel G, et al. Lipodermatosclerosis is characterized by elevated expression and activation of matrix metalloproteinases: Implications for venous ulcer formation, *J Invest Dermatol*. 1998. *111*: 822–827.

74. Herouy Y, Trefzer D, Zimpfer U, Schopf E, Vanscheidt W, Norgauer J. Matrix metalloproteinases and venous leg ulceration, *Eur J Dermatol*. 2000. *9*: 173–180.

75. Norgauer J, Hildenbrand T, Idzko M, et al. Elevated expression of extracellular matrix metalloproteinase inducer (CD 147) and membrane-type matrix metalloproteinases in venous leg ulcers, *Br J Dermatol*. 2002. *147*: 1180–1186.

76. Saito S, Trovato MJ, You R, et al. Role of matrix metalloproteinases 1, 2, and 9 and tissue inhibitor of matrix metalloproteinase-1 in chronic venous insufficiency, *J Vasc Surg*. 2001. *34*(5): 930–938.

77. Herouy Y, Trefzer D, Hellstern MO, et al. Plasminogen activation in venous leg ulcers, *Br J Dermatol*. 2000. *143*: 930–936.

9.

MECHANISM AND EFFECTS OF COMPRESSION THERAPY

Hugo Partsch

Compression therapy is a very effective treatment modality whose mechanisms are not yet fully understood.

The clinical effects depend mainly on two factors, interface pressure and stiffness.

Interface pressure is the pressure exerted by a compression device on a specific skin area. Stiffness is defined by the increase of the interface pressure induced by the increase of the circumference of a limb segment when muscles are contracting.[1]

INTERFACE PRESSURE

COMPRESSION HOSIERY

The pressure ranges given for compression hosiery are measured in the laboratories of the producers by determining the force that is necessary to stretch the ankle part of the stocking in transverse direction. The pressure values are calculated from the force-extension diagram of the elastic fabric, the so-called hysteresis curve, projected to a leg model with defined circular cross sections using Laplace's law. This formula describes the relationship between the interface pressure (P), which is directly proportional to the tension (T) of the bandage and inversely proportional to the radius (R) of the curvature to which it is applied (P = T/R). The proportion of stretch and force, which corresponds to the steepness of the so-called slope in the hysteresis curve, reflects the elasticity of the material of the stocking.

Several industrial measuring systems for obtaining hysteresis curves are used, such as the Hosy method, the Hatra tester, the Instron method, the French ITF method, and others.[2]

Table 9.1 gives a comparison of compression classes for ready-to-wear and custom stockings used in several countries. The range of compression pressures and the description of these classes vary among different countries. Therefore, it is recommended to use the pressure range in mmHg rather than compression classes for a better universal understanding.

However, comparisons may also be problematic because the given ranges are measured by different methods. These facts underline the necessity of in vivo pressure measurements on the individual leg, at least in future clinical studies.

The unit for pressure is 1 Pascal (Pa), which is 1 Newton (N) per square meter. In the medical field, for example, measuring blood pressure, the usual unit for pressure is the weight of one cubic millimeter of mercury.

The pressure values in Table 9.1 refer to the ankle region, called the level B. Proximal measuring points on the leg are:[1]

- B1, the point at which the Achilles tendon changes into the calf muscle

- C, corresponding to the calf at its maximum girth

- D, just below the tibial tuberosity

- E, over the patella

- F, between K and E

- G, 5 cm below K in the upright position

- H, at the greatest lateral trochanteric projections of the buttock

- K, at the center point of the crotch

As the circumference of the leg progressively increases, a compression gradient is produced, which is defined by the European prestandard as follows: for level B1, 70–100%; for C and D, 50–80%; and for F or G, 20–40% for compression class III and IV, 20–60% for the classes A–I, and 20–50% for class II.

COMPRESSION BANDAGES

The interface pressure of compression bandages depends on the experience and the skill of the bandager and only rarely is declared. For future trials it will be essential to measure the interface pressure as a parameter characterizing the "dosage" and hence the efficacy of the bandage.

Table 9.1 COMPRESSION CLASSES OF COMPRESSION STOCKINGS USED IN SEVERAL COUNTRIES (VALUES ARE MMHG, 1 MMHG = 1333 HPA)

COMPRESSION CLASS	EU (CEN)64	USA	UK (BS 6612)65	FRANCE	GERMANY66
A	10–14 (light)	15–20 (moderate)	14–17 (light)	10–15	18–21 (light)
I	15–21 (mild)	20–30 (firm)	18–24 (medium)	15–20	23–32 (medium)
II	23–32 (moderate)	30–40 (extra firm)	25–35 (strong)	20–36	34–46 (strong)
III	34–46 (strong)	40+		>36	>49 (very strong)
IV	>49 (very strong)				

The values indicate the compression exerted by the hosiery at a hypothetical cylindrical ankle

Several devices for measuring the interface pressure on the individual leg have been described.[2,3] The pressure measured under static (resting) conditions is termed resting pressure; that measured on the moving patient is known as working pressure.

When pressure data are reported it is essential to indicate the type and size of the transducer and the exact localization on the extremity.[4]

The ankle region, which is a reference point for stocking manufacturers (B-segment), is not a suitable location for reliable in vivo measurement because of the radius changes varying widely due to the bony prominences and tendons prevailing in this segment. This is the reason why some reports of stocking pressures have given lower values from B than from the more proximal segment B1.

STIFFNESS

It has been shown that compression devices exerting the same resting pressure have different hemodynamic effects on venous reflux and venous pumping function depending on the elastic property of the material.[5] This can be characterized by the stiffness, which plays an important role concerning the performance of a compression device during standing and walking, and which can be measured in vivo.

Stiffness is defined by the increase of compression per centimeter increase in the circumference of the leg, expressed in hectopascals per centimeter and/or millimeters of mercury per centimeter.[1] A very appropriate method to measure a dynamic stiffness index during walking has been described by a Dutch group.[6] However, this technique requires sophisticated instrumentation and can be performed only in specialized laboratories.

We have proposed a very simple method that is able to differentiate inelastic from elastic material by measuring the difference between the standing pressure and the supine pressure at the B1 region, which is the area where the tendinous part of the medial gastrocnemius muscle changes into the muscular part.[7] The standing position is considered to be a snapshot of the walking cycle. Therefore pressure sensors also may be used that are not able to register continuous pressure changes.

Especially when several textiles are combined in a multilayer bandage, the stiffness of the final bandage will increase because of the friction of the layers.[2] The same is true when two compression stockings are donned over each other.

Compared with in vivo measurements stiffness corresponds to the slope of the hysteresis curve in vitro.[8]

COMPRESSION MATERIAL

Based on the principles mentioned earlier, several textiles used for compression therapy can be differentiated (see Table 9.2).

PERFORMANCE OF COMPRESSION MATERIALS

Elastic textiles exert pressure by being stretched. During walking only small pressure peaks will occur, because the elastic material gives way with every step. The working pressure is therefore not much higher than the resting pressure (see Figure 9.1). Because of the retraction of the elastic fibers there is only a small reduction of interface pressure in the sitting and lying position. A continuous high resting

Table 9.2 COMPRESSION MATERIALS

ELASTIC, LONG-STRETCH MATERIAL	INELASTIC, SHORT-STRETCH MATERIAL	NONSTRETCH MATERIAL
Compression stockings	Short-stretch bandages	Zinc paste bandages, Unna boot
Long-stretch bandages	Multilayer short-stretch bandages*	Velcro band devices (also short stretch)
Extensibilty >100%	Extensibility <100%*	Extensibility 0–10%
Low stiffness	Medium stiffness	High stiffness
Exerts pressure when applied with stretch	Pressure increases when movement causes calf muscle to contract	Pressure increases when movement causes calf muscle to contract

*Bandages consisting of several elastic components with an extensibility of the single layer >100% for example as the "four-layer bandage," will become relatively inelastic when applied in more layers and therefore may also be ranged into this category.

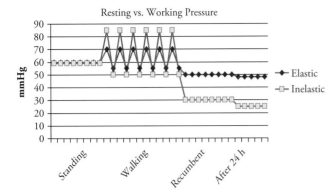

Resting vs. Working Pressure

Figure 9.1   Interface pressure measured on the medial aspect of the leg (B1) of an elastic and an inelastic bandage. Both bandages are firmly applied and exert a pressure of 60 mmHg immediately after application in the standing position. During walking much higher pressure peaks are obtained with inelastic than with elastic material. When the patient lies down and also after 24 hours, elastic bandages show only a mild reduction of pressure. The more intense pressure loss of the inelastic material is the reason why these bandages also are tolerated during nighttime, and why they should be renewed when getting too loose.

pressure may cause unpleasant feelings during rest and is strictly contraindicated in patients with arterial occlusive disease. Therefore elastic bandages and firm medical compression stockings should be removed over nighttime. The main advantage of elastic material is that it can also be handled by nonexperienced staff and even by the patients themselves.

Short-stretch material and completely rigid devices show a high working pressure with high peaks during walking that are able to occlude leg veins intermittently, thereby reducing ambulatory venous hypertension.[9]

During walking, nonyielding material will exert similar effects as intermittent pneumatic compression, especially concerning the release of anti-inflammatory, anticoagulatory, and vasoactive mediators from the endothelial cells.[10] These effects are probably the reason for the fact that the best healing rates of venous ulcers have been described with multilayer high-pressure bandages.[11] A considerable fall of pressure will occur when the patient lies down, so that short-stretch bandages may better be tolerated in the resting position. The pressure loss of up to 40% in the first two hours is caused by an immediate reduction of the limb volume and should be taken into account by applying an inelastic bandage with a much higher strength than an elastic bandage, which needs some experience. Due to the pressure fall, inelastic bandages are well tolerated also during nighttime. In patients with massive edema they should be reapplied after short periods of time in the initial phase when they get loose. Later on they may be worn for one week and longer. In the presence of arterial occlusions inelastic bandages should be applied with a very low resting pressure, which should be adjusted to the systolic ankle pressure in order not to interfere with the reduced arterial inflow. During movement there will be a massage of the limb, which may be compared with intermittent pneumatic compression. Bandages

applied with several elastic layers get similar elastic properties as short-stretch bandages.

Intermittent pneumatic compression offers adjunctive beneficial effects, especially in patients with a restricted walking ability. In addition to the decongestive effect, an increase of arterial flow and a release of vasoactive and anticoagulatory mediators from the endothelial cells have been documented during the last few years.[10,12]

THERAPY PHASE AND MAINTENANCE PHASE OF COMPRESSION THERAPY

In general, we prefer multilayer short-stretch or completely nonelastic material for the therapy phase of severe stages of chronic venous insufficiency like venous ulcers, for lymphedema, and also for acute phlebitis and deep vein thrombosis.[13] When the leg ulcers are healed and when the extremity is fairly free from edema, elastic material (preferably compression stockings) is used in order to maintain this condition (maintenance phase).

PHYSIOLOGICAL EFFECTS OF COMPRESSION THERAPY

Some physiological effects of compression therapy as documented in several studies are summarized in Table 9.3.[1,14]

The application of continuous compression is contraindicated in patients with advanced peripheral arterial disease or severe sensory impairment.

Several effects of compression therapy have been demonstrated in the acute experiment using intermittent pneumatic compression. It may be assumed that similar effects will also occur during walking with inelastic bandages.

TISSUE PRESSURE AND EDEMA

By increasing the tissue pressure, compression works against filtration, which is the most important mechanism to

Table 9.3 EFFECTS OF COMPRESSION THERAPY STOCKINGS AND BANDAGES

PARAMETERS	EFFECT
Tissue pressure	Increase
Edema	Decrease
Venous volume	Decrease
Venous velocity	Increase
Blood shift into central compartments	Increase
Venous refluxes	Decrease
Venous pump	Improvement
Arterial flow	Increase (intermittent compression)
Microcirculation	Improvement
Lymph drainage	Improvement

prevent or to remove edema. Occupational leg swelling in sitting and standing professions can be prevented by light compression stockings, which are also able to reduce mild edema.[15] Reduction in intradermal edema can be measured with ultrasonography in patients with CVI and lipodermatosclerosis. Severe stages of limb swelling benefit more from inelastic compression devices exerting higher pressure.

Compression may reveal beneficial effects also in non-phlebological causes of edema like inflammatory edema (arthritis, cellulitis), cardiac, dysproteinemic, renal edema, lymphedema, and cyclic idiopathic edema.[2]

VENOUS VOLUME AND VENOUS BLOOD FLOW VELOCITY

Depending on the exerted pressure and the body position, external compression is able to narrow or to occlude superficial and deep leg veins.[16]

In the supine position an external pressure of 10–15 mmHg is enough to decrease the venous diameter. The resulting increase of blood flow velocity as clearly shown by measuring the circulation time with isotopes[17] is the rationale for recommending light compression stockings for thromboprophylaxis in bedridden patients.

Venous volume can be assessed using air-plethysmography (APG), which shows a significantly more pronounced reduction by inelastic than by elastic compression, even when the resting pressure is the same.[5]

In the upright position elastic stockings will have only a minor effect on decreasing the diameter of the leg veins.[18] However, a very small decrease of venous diameter will result in an overproportional decrease of the local blood volume as demonstrated by several plethysmographic studies[5,14]

BLOOD SHIFT INTO CENTRAL COMPARTMENTS

Firm compression bandages applied on both lower extremities may redistribute blood toward the central parts of the body. This can lead to an increase of the preload of the heart by about 5% and should be avoided in patients with borderline cardiac function.[19]

DECREASE OF VENOUS REFLUXES AND IMPROVEMENT OF THE VENOUS PUMP

Using APG in patients with deep venous incompetence, it could be shown that compression with increasing interface pressure was associated with a decreasing amount of total reflux measured by venous filling index.

A statistically significant reduction of refluxes was achieved with pressures over 30 mmHg for inelastic and over 40 mmHg for elastic material.[5]

The reduction of venous refluxes in patients with chronic venous insufficiency by external compression explains the improvement of the venous pumping function. Plethysmographic studies have shown an increasing improvement of the venous pump with increasing stocking pressures, starting with an ankle pressure of around 20 mmHg.[9,20–23]

Higher compression pressure using stiff material leads to short phases of intermittent occlusion of the deep veins with every step during muscle contraction. Such intermittent occlusions of deep veins on the leg can be visualized by Duplex.[16] By encasing the veins in a rigid envelope ambulatory venous hypertension may thereby be reduced in patients with deep venous incompetence.[9] Similarly, a progressively increasing pressure on the thigh by using a blood pressure cuff blown up to 40–80 mmHg led to a progressively decreasing vein diameter and to an abolishment of reflux when the femoral vein segment contained incompetent valves.[20] Reduction of venous refluxes and improvement of ambulatory venous hypertension by external cuff compression could be demonstrated even in patients without any valves (avalvulia). This effect therefore cannot be explained by the common explanation of a coaptation of distended valve leaflets, but seems rather to be due to the intermittent occlusion of the incompetent vein during walking.[21]

Conflicting results have been reported concerning an improvement of ambulatory venous hypertension by compression stockings.[2,9] This may be explained by the fact that the pressure exerted by stockings is too low in order to sufficiently compress the veins in the leg in the upright position. In addition, the elastic material gives way with every step, whereas inelastic, short-stretch bandages with a double as high resting pressure are able to achieve intermittently short venous occlusions during muscle systole while walking. In patients with severe stages of chronic venous insufficiency a higher compression pressure is needed to improve the disturbed venous pumping function, whereas lower pressure is sufficient in simple varicose veins.[22]

The key mechanism of compression therapy to reduce ambulatory venous hypertension in patients with severe chronic venous insufficiency is an intermittent occlusion of the veins during walking.

In contrast, continuous obliteration of veins by external compression may be desirable after varicose vein surgery in order to stop bleeding and after sclerotherapy to prevent refilling of blood.

To achieve complete venous occlusion the external pressure has to be higher than the intravenous pressure, depending on the body position. By Duplex ultrasonography and by MRI it could be demonstrated that an occlusion of superficial leg veins can be obtained with an external pressure in the range of 20 mmHg in the supine position, but that in the sitting and standing positions the pressure has to be between 50 and 70 mmHg.[16,24] With compression stockings such pressure ranges can be achieved only when rolls or pads are applied over the vein. According to the law of Laplace this will increase the local pressure due to the reduction of the local radius.[25]

ARTERIAL FLOW AND MICROCIRCULATION

A reduction of arterial flow will occur when the external compression pressure exceeds the intra-arterial pressure. This may happen in patients with arterial occlusive disease with a reduced peripheral arterial pressure. In order to avoid ischemic skin lesions from external compression it is therefore essential to measure the peripheral arterial pressure by a Doppler probe before strong compression bandages or stockings are applied. It is generally accepted that a Doppler ankle-brachial index (ABI) of less than 0.5 is a contraindication for compression therapy. However, external compression does not invariably mean reduction of arterial flow. H. N. Mayrovitz reported on several experiments concerning arterial blood flow and compression and was able to demonstrate an increase of the pulsatile flow below the knee in healthy volunteers using nuclear magnetic resonance flowmetry.[26] An increase of arterial flow under the bandages could also be shown in patients with mixed, arteriovenous ulcers and an ABPI of >0.6 when inelastic material was applied up to a pressure of 40 mmHg.[27]

Patients with edematous legs and with an ABI between 0.5 and 0.8 may benefit from inelastic or short-stretch bandages applied with a mild resting pressure due to the edema-removing massage effect that will occur with every ankle movement. In patients with mixed ulceration it could be demonstrated that inelastic bandages applied with a pressure up to 40 mmHg were able to increase arterial flow and to improve the venous pumping function.[27] Completely inelastic bandages together with walking have a similar effect as intermittent pneumatic compression. The rhythmic pressure peaks of an inelastic bandage during walking can be compared with those exerted by an intermittent pneumatic pressure pump. Several experiments with intermittent pneumatic compression have demonstrated an increase of arterial flow in patients with arterial occlusive disease.[28,29] The deciding mechanisms of action are the reduction of edema, an increase of the arteriovenous pressure gradient, myogenic mechanisms, and the release of vasoactive substances from the endothelial cells[30]

Compression accelerates blood flow in the enlarged capillary loops and reduces capillary filtration due to enhanced tissue pressure. Blood flow and partial oxygen tension in the skin increase and the endothelial adhesion of leukocytes is normalized. Different studies using electron microscopy were able to show a restoration of the structural changes in the media myocytes in stripped veins and a tightening of intercellular junctions. Increasing flow velocity

demonstrated by laser Doppler fluxmetry may reduce the likelihood of white blood cells interacting or sticking to endothelium with release of various factors.[31] Effects on mediators involved in the local inflammatory response may explain both the immediate pain relief that occurs with good compression, and ulcer healing.

Model experiments with intermittent pneumatic compression were able to demonstrate that there is an increased release of fibrinolytic mediators and of the endothelial relaxing factor (EDRF) nitrogen oxide from the endothelial cells depending on the amount of shear stress produced by the compression waves.[10,30]

LYMPH DRAINAGE

Several beneficial mechanisms of compression therapy on the swollen extremity may be explained by its effects on the lymphatic system:[32]

- Reduction of capillary filtration
- Shift of fluid into noncompressed parts of the body
- Increase of lymphatic reabsorption and lymphatic transport
- Breakdown of fibrosclerotic tissue
- Downregulation of proinflammatory cytokines and receptors for growth factors.

External compression increases the interstitial pressure and prevents fluid from filtering out of the capillary network. The amount of the lymphatic load is thereby decreased.

Compression removes more water than protein from the tissue, thereby increasing oncotic tissue pressure and reinforcing the need for sustained compression. Therefore in chronic edema, success is dependent on continued compression.

Compression together with movement enhances the contraction of the lymphangion.

It has been demonstrated that both compression bandaging and exercise stimulate the movement of stagnating lymph through the lymph collector in lymphedema patients, in which the lymphatic trunks are filled. This is probably one explanation for the reduction of intralymphatic hypertension by complex decongestive therapy.

Intermittent pneumatic compression enhances prefascial lymph drainage. Unna boots are able to increase subfascial lymph transport, which is reduced in postthrombotic syndrome.

Consequent compression leads to a morphological improvement of pathological initial lymphatics in patients with lipodermatosclerosis, which can be demonstrated by indirect x-ray lymphography.

CLINICAL EFFECTS OF COMPRESSION THERAPY

The use of compression therapy in various clinical indications is based mainly on experience.

Only a few randomized controlled trials (RCTs) are available that prove the efficacy of compression treatment on the level of evidence-based medicine.[33]

Table 9.4 summarizes the outcome of an international consensus meeting in which all RCTs and systematic reviews have been scored.

There are only three areas for which evidence-based medicine data show clear clinical benefits of compression therapy: active venous ulceration, prevention of postthrombotic syndrome after deep vein thrombosis, and prevention of thromboembolic events after surgery when combined with anticoagulatory prophylaxis.

In venous ulcers several RCTs have shown that compression is better than no compression and that high pressure is more effective than low pressure. Conflicting results are coming from studies comparing different compression materials, mainly due to the fact that frequently, good bandages have been compared with poor bandages applied by inadequately trained staff. This underlines the need to measure pressure and stiffness of the compression products in future trials.

Compression stockings after proximal deep vein thrombosis are able to reduce the incidence of a postthrombotic syndrome some years after the acute event to one half. Immediate mobilization of mobile patients with deep vein thrombosis using compression has been shown not only to reduce pain and swelling in the acute stage but also to achieve less postthrombotic changes after some years.

The overview given in Table 9.4 does not mean that compression is less or not effective in areas with recommendation levels B and C, but that we need more trials in order to improve the scientific evidence for compression devices in the future.

REFERENCES

1. CEN European Prestandard. *Medical compression hosiery*. Brussels: European Committee for Standardization. 2001. 1–40.
2. Partsch H, Rabe E, Stemmer R. *Compression therapy of the extremities*. Paris: Editions Phlébologiques Francaises. 1999.
3. Partsch H, Mosti G. Comparison of three portable instruments to measure compression pressure, *Int Angiol*. 2010. *29*(5): 426–430.
4. Partsch H, Clark M, Bassez S, et al. Measurement of lower leg compression in vivo: Recommendations for the performance of measurements of interface pressure and stiffness: A consensus statement, *Dermatol Surg*. 2006. *32*: 229–238.
5. Partsch H, Menzinger G, Mostbeck A. Inelastic leg compression is more effective to reduce deep venous refluxes than elastic bandages, *Dermatol Surg*. 1999. *25*: 695–700.
6. Stolk R, Wegen van der-Franken CPM, Neumann, HAM. A method for measuring the dynamic behavior of medical compression hosiery during walking, *Dermatol Surg*. 2004. *30*: 729–736.
7. Partsch H. The static stiffness index: A simple method to assess the elastic property of compression material in vivo, *Dermatol Surg*. 2005. *31*: 625–630.
8. Partsch H, Partsch B, Braun W. Interface pressure and stiffness of ready made compression stockings: Comparison of in vivo and in vitro measurements. *J Vasc Surg*. 2006. *44*(4): 809–814.

Table 9.4 RCTS AND SYSTEMATIC REVIEWS ON COMPRESSION THERAPY

FIRST COLUMN: INDICATIONS, FOLLOWING THE CEAP CLASSIFICATION; SECOND COLUMN: NUMBER OF RCTS IDENTIFIED; COLUMNS 3–7: LEVELS OF RECOMMENDATION A, B, C (SEE LATER) FOR BANDAGES (COLUMN 3) OR DIFFERENT STOCKINGS WITH THEIR PRESSURE RANGES (COLUMNS 4–7)

INDICATION	REF #	BANDAGE	STOCKING 10–14	STOCKING 15–21	STOCKING 23–32	STOCKING 34–46
C0S, C1S	3		B	B		
C1 Sclerother	2				B	B
C2A	1				C	
C2S	1					C
C2 Pregnancy	1			B	B	
C2 Surgery	7	C	C		C	C
C2 Sclerother	3	C		C		C
C3	1				B	
C4b (LDS)	1				B	
C5	Multiple			B	B	B
C6	Multiple	A			B	
DVT	Multiple		A–B	A–B		
Prevention	2					
Flight	3		B	B		
DVT Therapy	3	B		B		
PTS					A	A
Prevention						
Lymphedema	5	B			C	C

Levels of Recommendation:
A: Large RCTs, meta-analysis of homogeneous results
B: Only one or smaller RCTs
C: Observational studies, consensus among participants of the consensus meeting

9. Partsch H. Improvement of venous pumping function in chronic venous insufficiency by compression depending on pressure and material, *VASA*. 1984. *13*: 58–64.

10. Dai G, Tsukurov O, Orkin RW, Abbott WM, Kamm RD, Gertler JP. An in vitro cell culture system to study the influence of external pneumatic compression on endothelial function, *J Vasc Surg*. 2000. *32*: 977–987.

11. O'Meara S, Cullum NA, Nelson EA. Compression for venous leg ulcers, *Cochrane Database Syst Rev*. 2009. *1*: CD000265.

12. Kessler CM, Hirsch DR, Jacobs H, et al. Intermittent pneumatic compression in chronic venous insufficiency favorably affects fibrinolytic potential and platelet activation, *Blood Coagul Fibrinolysis*. 1996. *7*: 437–446.

13. Blättler W, Partsch H. Leg compression and ambulation is better than bed rest for the treatment of acute deep vein thrombosis, *Int Angiol*. 2003. *22*: 393–400.

14. Vin F, Benigni JP. Compression therapy: International Consensus Document Guidelines according to scientific evidence, *Int Angiol*. 2004. *23*: 317–345.

15. Partsch H, Winiger J, Lun B. Compression stockings reduce occupational swelling, *J Derm Surg*. 2004. *30*: 737–743.

16. Partsch B, Partsch H. Pressure dose for leg vein compression therapy?, *J Vasc Surg*. 2005. *42*: 734–738.

17. Partsch H, Kahn P. Venöse Strömungsbeschleunigung in Bein und Becken durch "Anti-Thrombosestrümpfe," *Klinikarzt*. 1982. *11*: 609–615.

18. Lord RS, Hamilton D. Graduated compression stockings (20–30 mm Hg) do not compress leg veins in the standing position, *ANZ J Surg*. 2004. *74*: 581–583.

19. Mostbeck A, Partsch H, Peschl L. Änderungen der Blutvolumenverteilung im Ganzkörper unter physikalischen und pharmakologischen Maßnahmen, *VASA*. 1977. *6*: 137–141.

20. Partsch H, Menzinger G, Borst-Krafek B, Groiss E. Does thigh compression improve venous hemodynamics in chronic venous insufficiency?, *J Vasc Surg*. 2002. *36*: 948–952.

21. Partsch B, Mayer W, Partsch H. Improvement of ambulatory venous hypertension by narrowing of the femoral vein in congenital absence of venous valves, *Phlebology*. 1992. *7*: 101–104.

22. Stöberl C, Gabler S, Partsch H. Indikationsgerechte Bestrumpfung: Messung der venösen Pumpfunktion, *VASA*. 1989. *18*: 35–39.

23. Mosti G, Partsch H. Measuring venous pumping function by strain-gauge plethysmography, *Int Angiol*. 2010. *29*(5): 421–425.

24. Partsch H, Mosti G, Mosti F. Narrowing of leg veins under compression demonstrated by magnetic resonance imaging (MRI), *Int Angiol*. 2010. *29*(5): 408–410.

25. Partsch B, Partsch H. Which pressure do we need to compress the great saphenous vein on the thigh?, *Dermatol Surg*. 2008. *34*(12): 1726–1728.

26. Mayrovitz HN. Compression-induced pulsatile blood flow changes in human legs, *Clin Physiol*. 1998. *18*: 117–124.

27. Mosti G, Iabichella ML, Partsch H. Compression therapy in mixed ulcers increases venous output and arterial perfusion, *J Vasc Surg*. 2012. *55*(1): 122–128.

28. Delis KT, Nicolaides AN. Effect of intermittent pneumatic compression of foot and calf on walking distance, hemodynamics, and quality of life in patients with arterial claudication: A prospective randomized controlled study with 1-year follow-up, *Ann Surg*. 2005. *241*(3): 431–441.

29 Labropoulos N, Wierks C, Suffoletto B. Intermittent pneumatic compression for the treatment of lower extremity arterial disease: A systematic review, *Vasc Med*. 2002. *7*(2): 141–148.

30 Chen AH, Frangos SG, Kilaru S, Sumpio BE. Intermittent pneumatic compression devices: Physiological mechanisms of action, *Eur J Vasc Endovasc Surg*. 2001. *21*(5): 383–392.

31. Abu-Own A, Shami SK, Chittenden SJ, Farrah J, Scurr JH, Smith PD. Microangiopathy of the skin and the effect of leg compression in patients with chronic venous insufficiency, *J Vasc Surg*. 1994. *19*: 1074–1083.

32. Földi E, Jünger M, Partsch H. *The science of lymphoedema bandaging, EWMA Focus Document: Lymphoedema bandaging in practice*. London: MEP. 2005. 2–4.

33. Partsch H, Flour M, Smith PC, International Compression Club. Indications for compression therapy in venous and lymphatic disease consensus based on experimental data and scientific evidence, *Int Angiol*. 2008. *27*(3): 193–219.

10.

CLASSIFYING VENOUS DISEASE

Bo Eklöf

The Swedish physician and scientist Carl von Linné published a classification of plants based on the number of stamina and pistils in 1735 in *Systema Naturae*. Today, classification of diseases is a basic instrument for uniform diagnosis and meaningful communication about disease. In chronic venous disorders (CVD), reliance for too long has been placed on the clinical appearance of the superficial effects of CVD, such as spider veins, varicose veins, swelling, skin changes, and ulcerations, without requiring accurate objective testing of the venous system to substantiate the diagnosis. This practice has caused errors of diagnosis and has been largely responsible for the poor correlation of results between treatment methods. There have been several classifications in the past that have added to our understanding of CVD, but all lack the completeness and objectivity needed for scientific accuracy.

PREVIOUS CLASSIFICATIONS OF CVD

The most commonly used classification, particularly in Europe, was Widmer's 1978[1] classification of chronic venous insufficiency:

Stage I: Edema and dilated subcutaneous veins with corona phlebectatica

Stage II: Trophic lesions of the skin with hyper- or depigmented areas

Stage III: Healed or active ulcer

This clinical classification was criticized for the nonspecificity of Stage I and the absence of differentiation between trophic changes in Stage II.

In 1979[2] Hach suggested a grading of great saphenous vein (GSV) incompetence:

Grade I: Reflux in the groin

Grade II: Reflux to above the knee

Grade III: Reflux to just below the knee

Grade IV: Total reflux to the ankle

Hach's thesis was that in severe reflux of the GSV, a vicious internal circle developed because of the large venous blood volume with dilatation of the popliteal and femoral veins leading to deep venous incompetence if the GSV incompetence was not treated.

In 1980,[3] Partsch asked whether in patients with CVD one could achieve further improvement from other means after compression therapy. Could surgery or sclerotherapy be helpful? He recommended a classification based on involvement of superficial, perforator, and deep veins using objective measures such as foot volumetry and ambulatory venous pressure to discriminate between "betterable" (*bess-erbare*) and "not betterable" (*nicht besserbare*) patients.

In 1985,[4] Sytchev published a classification very similar to the present CEAP (clinical, etiological, anatomic, pathophysiologic) classification, as follows.

CLINICAL CLASSES

Stages of regional circulatory-trophic disorders:

• Compensation

• Decompensation (cyanosis, edema, cruralgia, or leg pain)

Degrees:

• By the end of the day

• By midday

• At the beginning of the day

Phases:

• Functional trophic disorders (hyper-, hypo-, and anhidrosis of the skin)

- Preulcer condition of tissues
- Trophic ulcers

Etiology:

- Primary venous dilatation
- Secondary (postthrombotic) occlusion and recanalization
- Congenital dysplasias

Central hemodynamics

- Compensation
- Decompensation
  — Underloaded
  — Overloaded

The same year,[5] Pierchalla and Tronnier suggested differentiation between primary and secondary (postthrombotic) disease, and between superficial, perforator, and deep venous disease using objective measures.

In 1988,[6] Porter et al. published reporting standards for venous disease developed by an ad hoc committee for the Society for Vascular Surgery (SVS) and the North American chapter of the International Society for Cardiovascular Surgery (ISCVS). This was similar to and based on the Widmer classification with the addition of etiology and anatomic distribution. This was the stimulus for the CEAP classification that followed later.

In 1991,[7] Cornu-Thénard et al. published a clinical classification of the severity of varicose veins by inspection and palpation and calculated the sum of maximum diameter at seven sites of the leg.

In 1992,[8] Enrici and Caldevilla published a clinical classification on the evolution of the postthrombotic syndrome:

Stage 1: Early postthrombotic syndrome with painful swelling of the leg with distal venous hypertension and venographically demonstrating residual obstruction of the deep veins with competent perforators

Stage 2: Compensatory hypertrophy of the musculovenous calf muscle pump

Stage 3: Stage 2 plus appearance of secondary varicose veins. Venography shows recanalization with varying reflux with incompetent perforators;

Stage 4: Advanced chronic venous insufficiency with development of a vicious venous recirculation with lipodermatosclerosis and ulceration due to venous hypertension

Stage 5: Phleboarthrotic syndrome with immobilization of the ankle.

Stage 6: Secondary, postthrombotic lymphedema

In 1993,[9] Miranda et al. published a clinical classification:

Stage I: Dilatation of GSV 7 mm by duplex scanning

Stage II: Dilatation of GSV > 7 mm without skin changes

Stage III: Stage II plus skin changes

Stage IV: Stage III plus active or healed ulcer

THE CREATION OF THE CEAP CLASSIFICATION

At the fifth annual meeting of the American Venous Forum (AVF) in 1993, John Porter suggested using the TNM classification for cancer as a model to develop a classification system for venous diseases. Following a year of intense discussions a consensus conference was held at the sixth annual meeting of AVF in February 1994 on the island of Maui, Hawaii, at which an international ad hoc committee, chaired by Andrew Nicolaides, and with representatives from Australia, Europe, and the United States, developed the first CEAP consensus document.[10] It contained two parts, a classification of CVD and a scoring system of the severity of CVD. The classification was based on clinical manifestations (C), etiologic factors (E), anatomic distribution of disease (A), and the underlying pathophysiologic findings (P), thus the name CEAP. The severity scoring system was based on three elements: the number of anatomic segments affected, grading of symptoms and signs, and disability. The CEAP consensus statement was published in 26 journals and books in nine languages, truly a universal document for CVD. It was endorsed by the Joint Councils of the SVS and the North American Chapter of the ISCVS, and its basic elements were incorporated into venous reporting standards.[11] Today most published clinical papers on CVD use all or portions of the CEAP classification.

REVISION OF CEAP

Diagnosis and treatment of CVD were developed rapidly in the 1990s, and the need for an update of the classification logically followed. Now, it is important to stress that CEAP is a descriptive classification. Venous Severity Scoring (VSS)[12] was developed to allow longitudinal outcomes assessment, but it became apparent that CEAP itself required updating and modification. In April 2002, the AVF appointed an ad hoc committee on CEAP to review the classification and make recommendations for change by 2004, 10 years after its introduction (see Table 10.1). An International ad hoc committee was also established to assure continued universal utilization (see Table 10.2).

The two committees held four joint meetings in Hawaii, November 2002; Cancun, Mexico, February 2003; San Diego, August 2003; and Orlando, February 2004.

The following passages summarize the results of these deliberations, by describing the new aspects of the revised CEAP.[13]

The recommended changes, detailed next, include additions to or refinements of several definitions used in describing CVD, refinement of the C-classes of CEAP, addition of the descriptor *n* (no venous abnormality identified), incorporation of the date of classification and level of clinical investigation, and the description of basic CEAP, introduced as a simpler alternative to the full (advanced) CEAP classification.

TERMINOLOGY AND NEW DEFINITIONS

The CEAP classification deals with all forms of chronic venous disorders. The term "chronic venous disorder" (CVD) includes the full spectrum of morphological and functional abnormalities of the venous system from telangiectasias to venous ulcers. Some of these, like telangiectasias, are highly prevalent in the normal adult population, and in many cases the use of the term "disease" is not appropriate. The term "chronic venous insufficiency" (CVI) implies a functional abnormality of the venous system and usually is reserved for patients with more advanced disease including those with edema (C3), skin changes (C4), or venous ulcers (C5–C6).

It was agreed to maintain the overall structure of the CEAP classification, but to add more precise definitions. The following recommended definitions apply to the clinical C classes in CEAP:

Telangiectasia: A confluence of dilated intradermal venules of less than 1 mm in caliber. Synonyms include "spider veins," "hyphen webs," and "thread veins."

Reticular veins: Dilated bluish subdermal veins usually from 1 mm in diameter to less than 3 mm in diameter. They usually are tortuous. This excludes normal visible veins in people with thin, transparent skin. Synonyms include "blue veins," "subdermal varices," and "venulectasies."

Varicose veins: Subcutaneous dilated veins equal to or more than 3 mm in diameter measured in the upright position. These may involve saphenous veins, saphenous tributaries, or nonsaphenous superficial leg veins. Varicose veins usually are tortuous, but tubular saphenous veins with demonstrated reflux may be classified as varicose veins. Synonyms include "varix," "varices," and "varicosities."

Corona phlebectatica: A fan-shaped pattern of numerous small intradermal veins on the medial or lateral aspects of the ankle and foot. This commonly is thought to be an early sign of advanced venous disease. Synonyms include "malleolar flare" and "ankle flare."

Edema: A perceptible increase in volume of fluid in the skin and subcutaneous tissue characteristically indenting with pressure. Venous edema usually occurs in the ankle region, but it may extend to the leg and foot.

Pigmentation: A brownish darkening of the skin resulting from extravasated blood, which usually occurs in the ankle region but may extend to the leg and foot.

Eczema: An erythematous dermatitis, which may progress to a blistering, weeping, or scaling eruption of the skin of the leg. It is most often located near varicose veins but may be located anywhere in the leg. Eczema usually is seen in uncontrolled CVD but may reflect sensitization to local therapy.

Lipodermatosclerosis (LDS): Localized chronic inflammation and fibrosis of the skin and subcutaneous tissues of the lower leg, sometimes associated with scarring or contracture of the Achilles tendon. LDS is sometimes preceded by diffuse inflammatory edema of the skin, which may be painful and which is often referred to as *hypodermitis*. This condition must be distinguished from lymphangitis, erysipelas, or cellulitis by their characteristically different local signs and systemic features. LDS is a sign of severe chronic venous disease.

Atrophie blanche or white atrophy: Localized, often circular whitish and atrophic skin areas surrounded by dilated capillaries and sometimes hyperpigmentation. This finding is a sign of severe chronic venous disease and not to be confused with healed ulcer scars. Scars of healed ulceration also may have atrophic skin with pigmentary changes but are distinguishable by history of ulceration and appearance from atrophie blanche and are excluded from this definition.

Venous ulcer: Full thickness defect of the skin most frequently in the ankle region that fails to heal spontaneously and is sustained by CVD.

REFINEMENT OF C-CLASSES IN CEAP

The essential change here is the division of class C4 into two subgroups that reflect different severity of disease, and carry a different prognosis in terms of risk of ulceration:

C0: No visible or palpable signs of venous disease
C1: Telangiectasies or reticular veins
C2: Varicose veins—distinguished from reticular veins by a diameter of 3 mm or more
C3: Edema
C4: Changes in the skin and subcutaneous tissue secondary to CVD (now divided into two subclasses to better define the differing severity of venous disease):
C4a: Pigmentation and/or eczema
C4b: Lipodermatosclerosis and/or atrophie blanche
C5: Healed venous ulcer
C6: Active venous ulcer

Each clinical class is further characterized by a subscript for the presence of symptoms (S, symptomatic) or absence of symptoms (A, asymptomatic), for example, $C2_A$ or $C5_S$. Symptoms include aching, pain, tightness, skin irritation, heaviness, and muscle cramps, as well as other complaints attributable to venous dysfunction.

REFINEMENT OF E, A, AND P IN CEAP

To improve the assignment of designations under E, A, and P, a new descriptor *n* is now recommended for use where no venous abnormality is identified. This *n* could be added to E (E*n*: no venous etiology identified), A (A*n*: no venous location identified), and P (P*n*: no venous pathophysiology identified). In the past, the lack of a "normal" option may have contributed to observer variability in assigning designations. Further definition of the A and P has also been afforded by the new venous severity scoring system,[12] which was developed by the ad hoc Committee on Outcomes of the AVF to complement CEAP. It includes not only a Clinical Severity Score but a Venous Segmental Score. The latter is based on imaging studies of the leg veins, for example, duplex scan, and the degree of obstruction or reflux (P) in each major segment (A) and forms the basis for the overall score.

This same committee also is pursuing a prospective multicenter investigation of variability in vascular diagnostic laboratory assessment of venous hemodynamics in patients with CVD. The last revision of the venous reporting standards[11] still cites changes in ambulatory venous pressure or plethysmographically measured venous return time (VRT) as objective measures of change. The current multicenter study aims to establish the variability of, and thus limits of, "normal" for the VRT and the newer noninvasive venous tests as an objective basis for claiming significant improvement as a result of therapy, and will hopefully provide improved reporting standards for definitive diagnosis and results of competitive treatments in patients with CVD.

DATE OF CLASSIFICATION

CEAP is not a static classification; the patient can be reclassified at any point in time. Classification starts with the initial visit, but can be better defined after further investigations. A final classification may not be complete until after surgery and histopathologic assessment. We therefore recommend that any CEAP classification be followed by the date; for example, C4b,S, Ep, As,p, Pr (August 21, 2003).

LEVEL OF INVESTIGATION

A precise diagnosis is the basis for correct classification of the venous problem. The diagnostic evaluation of the patient with CVD can be logically organized into one or more of three levels of testing, depending on the severity of the disease:

Level I: The office visit with history and clinical examination, which may include use of a hand-held Doppler

Level II: The noninvasive vascular laboratory, which now routinely includes duplex color scanning, with some plethysmographic method added as desired

Level III: Invasive investigations or more complex imaging studies including varicography, ascending and descending venography, venous pressure measurements, spiral CT scan, or MRV

We recommend that the level of investigation (L) should also be added to the classification, for example, C2,4b,S, Ep, As,p, Pr (2003-08-21,L II).

BASIC CEAP

A new basic CEAP is offered here. Use of all components of CEAP is still encouraged, but unfortunately many physicians merely use only the C-classification, which is just a modest advance beyond the previous classifications and is based solely on the clinical appearance. Venous disease is complex, but can be described by use of well-defined categorical descriptions. For the practicing physician, CEAP can be a valuable instrument for correct diagnosis to guide treatment and assess prognosis. In modern phlebological practice the vast majority of patients will have a duplex scan of the venous system of the leg, which largely will define the E, A, and P categories.

Nevertheless, it is recognized that the merits of using the *full* (advanced) CEAP classification system hold primarily for the researcher and for standardized reporting in scientific journals. It allows grouping of patients so that the same types of patients can be analyzed together, and such subgroup analysis allows their treatments to be more accurately assessed. Furthermore, reports using CEAP can be compared with one another with much greater certainty. This more complex classification, for example, also allows any of the eighteen named venous segments to be identified as the location of venous pathology. Take a patient with pain, varicose veins, and lipodermatosclerosis where duplex scan confirms primary reflux of the GSV and incompetent perforators in the calf. The classification here would be C2,4b,S, Ep, As,p, Pr2,3,18.

Although the detailed elaboration of venous disease in this form may seem unnecessarily complex, even intimidating, to some clinicians, it provides universal understandable descriptions that may be essential to

investigators in the field. To serve the needs of both, the full CEAP classification, as modified earlier, is retained as advanced CEAP, and the following simplified form is offered as basic CEAP.

In essence, Basic CEAP applies two simplifications: (1) In basic CEAP, *the single highest descriptor can be used for clinical classification.* For example, a patient with varicose veins, swelling, and lipodermatosclerosis would be C4b. The more comprehensive clinical description, in advanced CEAP, would be C2,3,4b. (2) In basic CEAP, where duplex scan is performed, E, A, and P should also be classified using the multiple descriptors recommended, but the complexity of applying these to the eighteen possible anatomic segments is avoided in favor of applying the simple *s*, *p*, and *d* descriptors to denote the superficial, perforator, and deep systems. Thus, using basic CEAP, the same patient cited in a previous example (painful varicosities plus lipodermatosclerosis and duplex scan–determined reflux involving the superficial and perforator systems) would be classified as C4b,S, Ep, As,p Pr (rather than C2,4b,S, Ep, As,p, Pr2,3,18).

REVISION OF CEAP: SUMMARY

CLINICAL CLASSIFICATION

C0: No visible or palpable signs of venous disease
C1: Telangiectasias or reticular veins
C2: Varicose veins
C3: Edema
C4a: Pigmentation and/or eczema
C4b: Lipodermatosclerosis and/or atrophie blanche
C5: Healed venous ulcer
C6: Active venous ulcer
S: Symptoms including ache, pain, tightness, skin irritation, heaviness, muscle cramps, as well as other complaints attributable to venous dysfunction
A: Asymptomatic

ETIOLOGIC CLASSIFICATION

Ec: Congenital
Ep: Primary
Es: Secondary (postthrombotic)
En: No venous etiology identified

ANATOMIC CLASSIFICATION

As: Superficial veins
Ap: Perforator veins
Ad: Deep veins
An: No venous location identified

PATHOPHYSIOLOGIC CLASSIFICATION

Basic CEAP:

Pr: Reflux

Po: Obstruction

Pr,o: Reflux and obstruction

Pn: No venous pathophysiology identifiable

ADVANCED CEAP

Same as basic, with the addition that any of eighteen named venous segments can be utilized as locators for venous pathology:

Superficial veins:

1. Telangiectasias/reticular veins
2. GSV above knee
3. GSV below knee
4. Small saphenous vein
5. Nonsaphenous veins

Deep veins:

6. Inferior vena cava
7. Common iliac vein
8. Internal iliac vein
9. External iliac vein
10. Pelvic: gonadal, broad ligament veins, other
11. Common femoral vein
12. Deep femoral vein
13. Femoral vein
14. Popliteal vein
15. Crural: anterior tibial, posterior tibial, peroneal veins (all paired)
16. Muscular: gastrocnemial, soleal veins, other

Perforating veins:

17. Thigh
18. Calf

Example: A patient presents with painful swelling of the leg and varicose veins, lipodermatosclerosis, and active ulceration. Duplex scanning on May 17, 2004, showed axial reflux of GSV above and below the knee, incompetent calf perforators, and axial reflux in the femoral and popliteal veins. No signs of postthrombotic obstruction.

- Classification according to basic CEAP: C6,S, Ep, As,p,d, Pr

- Classification according to advanced CEAP: C2,3,4b,6,S, Ep, As,p,d, Pr2,3,18,13,14 (2004-05-17, L II)

REVISION OF CEAP—AN ONGOING PROCESS

With improvement in diagnostics and treatment there will be continued demands to adapt the CEAP classification to better serve future developments. There are several conditions that arc not included in the CEAP classification but that can influence the management of the patients:

- Combined arterial/venous etiology
- Postthrombotic lymphedema
- Ankle ankylosis with atrophy of the calf
- Venous aneurysms
- Venous neuropathy
- Corona phlebectatica
- Pelvic congestion syndrome
- Morbid obesity

The role of corona phlebectatica (CP) was discussed during the meetings, and the Atlantic Ocean was a clear divider. In parts of Europe CP has been used as an early indicator of advanced CVD. Its scientific significance is now under investigation, particularly in France. There is a need to incorporate appropriate new features without too frequent disturbances of the stability of the classification. As one of the committee members (F. Padberg) stated in our deliberations, "It is critically important that recommendations for change in the CEAP standard be supported by solid research. While there is precious little that we are recommending which meets this standard, we can certainly emphasize it for the future. If we are to progress we should focus on levels of evidence for changes rather than levels of investigation. While a substantial portion of our effort will be developed from consensus opinion, we should still strive to achieve an evidence-based format."

ACKNOWLEDGMENT

Part of this article was previously published in Eklof B, Rutherford RB, Bergan JJ, et al.; for the American Venous Forum International Ad Hoc Committee for Revision of the CEAP classification. Revision of the CEAP classification for chronic venous disorders: Consensus statement, *J Vasc Surg.* 2004. 40:1248–1252.

The author wishes to thank the Society for Vascular Surgery for permission to reproduce the relevant section.

REFERENCES

1. Widmer LK. *Peripheral venous disorders: Prevalence and socio-medical importance: Observations in 4529 apparently healthy persons: Basle III study.* Bern, Switzerland: Hans Huber. 1978.
2. Hach W, Schirmers U, Becker L. Veränderungen der tiefen Leitvenen bei inner Stammvaricose der V. saphena magna. In: Muller-Wiefel H, ed. *Microzirkulation und Blutrheologie.* Baden, Germany: Witzstrock. 1980. 468–470.
3. Partsch H. "Betterable" and "nonbetterable" chronic venous insufficiency: A proposal for a practice oriented classification, *Vasa.* 1980. *9*: 165–167.
4. Sytchev GG. Classification of chronic venous disorders of lower extremities and pelvis, *Int Angiol.* 1985. *4*: 203–206.
5. Pierchalla P, Tronnier H. Diagnosis and classification of venous insufficiency of the leg, *Dtsch Med Wschr.* 1985. *110*: 1700–1702.
6. Porter JM, Rutherford RB, Clagett GP, et al. Reporting standards in venous disease, *J Vasc Surg.* 1988. *8*: 172–181.
7. Cornu-Thénard A, DeVincenzi G, Maraval M. Evaluation of different systems for clinical quantification of varicose veins, *J Derm Surg Onc.* 1991. *17*: 345–348.
8. Enrici EA, Caldevilla HS. Classification de la insuficiencia venosa chronica. In: Enrici EA, Caldevilla HS, eds. *Insuficiencia venosa cronica de los miembros inferiores.* Buenos Aires, Argentina: Editorial Celcius. 1992. 107–114.
9. Miranda C, Fabre M, Meyer P, Marescaux J. Evaluation of a reference anatomo-clinical classification of varices of the lower limbs, *Phlebologie.* 1993. *46*: 235–239.
10. Bergan JJ, Eklof B, Kistner RL, Moneta GL, Nicolaides AN; and the International Ad Hoc Committee of the American Venous Forum. Classification and grading of chronic venous disease in the lower limbs: A consensus statement, *Vasc. Surg.* 1996. *30*: 511.
11. Porter JM, Moneta GL; International Consensus Committee on Chronic Venous Disease. Reporting standards in venous disease: An update, *J. Vasc. Surg.* 1995. *21*: 635–645.
12. Rutherford RB, Padberg FT, Comerota AJ, et al. Venous severity scoring: An adjunct to venous outcome assessment, *J. Vasc. Surg.* 2000. *31*: 1307–1312.
13. Eklöf B, Rutherford RB, Bergan JJ, et al.; for the American Venous Forum International Ad Hoc Committee for Revision of the CEAP classification. Revision of the CEAP classification for chronic venous disorders: Consensus statement, *J. Vasc. Surg.* 2004. *40*: 1248–1252.

PART II

PRIMARY SUPERFICIAL VENOUS INSUFFICIENCY

11.

RISK FACTORS, MANIFESTATIONS, AND CLINICAL EXAMINATION OF THE PATIENT WITH PRIMARY VENOUS INSUFFICIENCY

John J. Bergan

Knowledge of the risk factors that enter into causation of primary venous insufficiency provides an understanding that aids in care of the patient. Some risk factors, such as heredity, female gender, and aging, cannot be altered (see Table 11.1). Others, such as pregnancy, are acquired but cannot be modified. And there are those with little or no influence, such as smoking, hypercholesterolemia, vitamin intake, and leg crossing. These and the historical and largely abandoned physical tests of the patient with venous insufficiency are the subject of this chapter.

HEREDITY

Although development of varicose veins usually can be ascribed to many conditions, conventional examinations may not disclose the apparent source of the high-pressure leak from the deep to the superficial system.[1] Therefore other inherent factors such as vein wall weakness, increased primary valvular dysfunction or agenesis, and other genetic factors may enhance the development of varicose veins.

In an extensive study in France, 134 families were examined. Of these, 67 were families with patients with varicose veins, and 67 were control families without familial varicose veins. A total of 402 subjects were examined and the results demonstrated a prominent role of hereditary in the development of varicose veins (p < 0.001). For the children, the risk of developing varicose veins was 90% when both parents were afflicted. When only one parent was affected, the risk of developing varicose veins was 25% for men and 62% for women. The overall risk of varicose vein development is 20% when neither parent is affected by varicosities.[2]

A familial tendency toward the development of varicose veins has been described in many population groups.[3,4] This may also be demonstrated by the development over time of varicose veins bilaterally when patients with unilateral varicose and telangiectatic veins are followed for 10 years.[5] A limited study of fifty patients with varicose veins in Great Britain disclosed a simple dominant type of inheritance.[6] Only 28% of patients had no family history of varicose veins. In Scandinavia, questionnaires completed by 124 women with varicose veins disclosed a 72% prevalence of varicose veins of an autosomal type in the women's siblings.[7] Of these cases, 28% were of a recessive pattern. Troisier and Le Bayon examined 154 families with 514 descendants. They found that if both parents had varicose veins, 85% of children had evidence of varicose veins, whereas 27% of the children were affected if neither parent had varicose veins, and 41% of the children were affected if one parent had varicosities. These authors conclude that the inheritance of varicose disease is recessive. However, some studies have not found a significant familial tendency.[8,9]

A single study on unselected twins found that 75% of twelve monozygotic pairs were concordant with regard to varicose veins. Of 25 dizygotic, same-sexed pairs, 52% had varicose veins.[10]

Other studies have found more of a multifactorial inheritance. In a detailed study from Sweden of 250 probands of patients with varicose veins requiring treatment, the overall frequency of varicose veins in female relatives was 43%, compared with 19% in male relatives.[11]

The absence of venous valves in the external iliac and femoral veins has been shown to be a marker of varicose veins in a limited radiographic study of twelve male volunteers, some with and some without varicose veins,[12] and in a venous Doppler study of fifty-four patients with varicose veins.[12] In addition, a simple dominant mode of inheritance has been reported in fourteen patients with congenital partial or total absence of venous valves of the leg.[13] Thus this genetic predisposition may be the result of multiple factors, and the subsequent development of varicose veins may depend on one or more occupational or hormonal factors.

Recent studies on varicose and normal veins using gene expression profiling based on cDNA microarray analysis suggest that pathways associated with fibrosis and wound healing may be altered in varicose veins.[14] Whether the upregulated varicose vein genes are a sequel to the changes in the varicose vein wall rather than a primary contributing factor to varicose pathogenesis awaits additional study.

Table 11.1 RISK FACTORS FOR VARICOSE VEINS AND TELANGIECTASIAS

Certain
  Heredity
  Female Gender
  Pregnancy
  Aging

Conjectural
  Diet
  Abdominal Straining
  Tight Clothing
  Leg Crossing

PREGNANCY

Pregnancy typically is associated with secondary valvular incompetence. Many epidemiologic studies have found a significantly increased incidence of varicose veins in women who have been pregnant.[15] However, some epidemiologic studies have failed to confirm this association when the effect of age is controlled.[16] Varices are often first noted during pregnancy and are exceedingly rare before puberty. Indeed, population studies have found that only 12% of women with varicose veins have never been pregnant.[17]

In pregnancy, hormonal factors are primarily responsible for venous dilation. As many as 70 to 80% of patients develop varicose veins during the first trimester, when the uterus is only slightly enlarged. In the second trimester, 20 to 25% of patients develop varicose veins, and 1 to 5% of patients develop them in the third trimester.[18,19]

Varicose veins of the legs are first apparent as early as six weeks into gestation, a time when the uterus is not yet large enough to significantly impede venous return from the leg veins. Mullane[20] notes that symptoms of varicose veins can be the first sign of pregnancy and can occur even before the first missed menstrual period. This confirms observations of many multiparous women and argues for a profound influence of progesterone on venous dilation and valvular insufficiency.

AGING

The incidence of varicose veins increases with age, therefore vein wall damage should be more pronounced in the veins of older patients. An autopsy study of the popliteal vein in 127 persons demonstrated diffuse changes, with an increase in connective tissue in the media that become most pronounced in the fifth decade and are progressive thereafter. This is associated with the loss of muscle cells in the media.[21] The finding correlated with an abnormality in the physical property of axial tension testing in ninety-three specimens of saphenous veins from twenty-two patients harvested during coronary bypass surgery.[22] However, one study of thirty-one normal veins and forty-one varicose

veins in patients and autopsy samples ranging in age from twenty-five to ninety-two failed to disclose an age-related difference.[23] The latter study concluded that varicose veins were a predetermined disease unrelated to aging effects.

THEORETICAL RISK FACTORS

One popular hypothesis for the development of varicose veins is Western dietary and defecation habits, which cause an increase in intra-abdominal pressure. Population studies have demonstrated that a high-fiber diet is evacuated within an average of 35 hours.[24] In contrast, a low-fiber diet has an average transit time of 77 hours. An intermediate diet has a stool transit time of 47 hours.

Defecatory straining induced by Western-style toilet seats has also been cited as a cause of varicose veins, in contrast to the African custom of squatting during defecation.[25,26]

An association between prostatic hypertrophy, inguinal hernia, and varicose veins may be caused by straining at micturition with a resultant increase in intra-abdominal pressure.

Another mechanism for increasing distal venous pressure by proximal obstruction is the practice of wearing girdles or tight-fitting clothing. A statistically significant excess of varicose veins is noted in women who wear corsets compared with women who wear less constrictive garments.

Leg crossing and sitting on chairs are two other potential mechanisms for producing a relative impedance in venous return. Habitual leg crossing is commonly thought to result in extravenous compression, but this has never been scientifically verified.

Most,[27] but not all,[28] studies have found that obesity is associated with the development of varicose veins. Careful examination of some of these epidemiologic studies shows that when the patient's age is correlated with obesity, the statistical significance is eliminated. Varices may be secondary to decreased exercise and associated medical problems specific to obesity such as hypertension, diabetes, hypercholesterolemia, and sensory impairment.

Finally, it commonly is noted that occupations that require standing for prolonged periods have an increased incidence of varicose veins. This may be exacerbated by tall height, although this factor has not been supported by other studies.

VALVE REMODELING

Our interest and focus on the venous valve dysfunction as a fundamental cause of distal venous hypertension began with unpublished observations using angioscopy. The angioscope provided a direct view of the internal architecture of saphenous veins. Patients taken to surgery who demonstrated preoperative reflux verified by duplex ultrasonography showed a variety of pathologic lesions in the valves themselves. The first indication was a relative paucity of valves. The observation of decrease in number of great saphenous vein (GSV) valves was reported by Cotton in 1961.[29] Next, we encountered actual valve lesions. These observations were an extension of those reported by Hoshino et al.,[30] who classified valve damage in the saphenous vein into three categories ranging from stretched commissures to perforations and valve splitting.

From the preceding observations we suggest that the earliest valve defects are an increase in the commissural space, which allows reflux on the border of the vein. This may be one of the earliest causes of reflux in varicose veins. Later, thinning, elongation, stretching, splitting, and tearing of the valves develop. The latest stages are thickening, contraction, and possibly even adhesion between valves. These observations have been confirmed by Van Cleef et al.[31] Although we have proposed that this valve damage is acquired and causes axial reflux as well as outflow through check valves in perforating veins, others have proposed that the cause of primary venous insufficiency is an actual reduced number of valves in the saphenous system.[32]

The angioscopic observations could be confirmed by gross morphologic studies that, when extended to microscopic observations using monoclonal antibody labeling, have demonstrated monocytic infiltration into damaged venous valves.[33] Others have found leukocytic infiltration into varicose veins and have called attention to the fact that the cells observed release vasoactive substances, including histamine, tryptase, prostaglandins, leukotrienes, and cytokines. Observations in patients led to the conclusions that venous hypertension was related to leukocytic infiltration on the cranial surfaces of the venous valve and venous wall and that leukocytes there were greater in quantity than on the caudal portion of valve leaflets and venous wall.[34]

Therefore a model of venous hypertension was developed in which microvessels in rat mesentery were examined microscopically. Venous occlusion and subsequent venous hypertension were produced by pipette blockade of venules about 40 μm in diameter. Videomicroscopy revealed early signs of inflammation, such as progressive leukocyte rolling, adhesion, and subsequent migration as well as parenchymal cell death.

This inflammatory sequence occurred early during the phase of venous hypertension and progressed further after release of the occlusion. The model showed that venous occlusion with elevation of the hydrostatic pressure caused a highly injurious process for the surrounding tissues. It was accompanied by formation of microhemorrhages on the high-pressure side of the postcapillary venule and rolling and adhesion of leukocytes on the venular endothelium.

van Bemmelen et al.[35] created a model of venous hypertension by performing arteriovenous fistulas in Wistar rats using microsurgical techniques. Valvular incompetence was seen as early as one day after creation of the arteriovenous fistula, and valvular structural changes were noticeable within two months of production of venous hypertension. Elongation of the cusps was observed. Separation and leakage of the cusps were encountered along the entire valvular free border, and, in later stages beyond four months, valve areas became difficult to recognize because commissures were lost and bulging of the valve sinus disappeared.

We have pursued this line of investigation and have reproduced the human observations in the animal model.[36,37]

Another model of venous hypertension has been produced by Lalka. This model creates venous hypertension by ligation of the inferior vena cava, the common iliac veins, and the common femoral veins. This preparation elevates rat hind limb venous pressures compared with forelimb pressures. Myeloperoxidase assay indicates leukocyte trapping in hind leg tissues just as it occurs in humans.

The observations just mentioned suggest that valve damage in venous insufficiency is an acquired phenomenon related to leukocyte and endothelial interactions and an inflammatory reaction. This observation is not universally accepted. A study on thirteen valve structures from varicose GSV showed an absence of lymphomonocyte infiltration in 85%, and rare isolated "nonsignificant" inflammatory cells in 15%. However, if this hypothesis is correct, pharmacologic intervention to block leukocyte adhesion, activation, and subsequent valve damage may be a possibility.

SYMPTOMS OF PRIMARY VENOUS INSUFFICIENCY

It is well known that the presence and severity of symptoms do not correlate with the size or severity of the varicose veins present. Symptoms usually attributable to varicose veins include feelings of heaviness, tiredness, aching, burning, throbbing, itching, and cramping in the legs (see Table 11.2). These symptoms are generally worse with prolonged sitting or standing and are improved with leg elevation or walking. A premenstrual exacerbation of symptoms is also common. Generally, patients find relief with the use of compression in the form of either support hose or an elastic bandage. Weight loss or the commencement of a regular program of lower extremity exercise may also lead to a diminution in the severity of varicose vein symptoms. Clearly, these symptoms are not specific, as they may also be indicative of a variety of rheumatologic or orthopedic problems. However, their relationship to lower extremity movement and compression is usually helpful in establishing a venous origin for the symptoms. Significant symptoms suggestive of venous disease should prompt further evaluation for valvular insufficiency and calf muscle pump dysfunction. If a venous etiology is suspected but all examinations are negative, repeat examination during a symptomatic period is warranted and often fruitful.

Table 11.2 SYMPTOMS OF VARICOSE VEINS AND TELANGIECTASIAS

Aching Heaviness (on standing, prolonged sitting)
Aching Pain (on standing, prolonged sitting)
Burning (venous neuropathy)
Itching (cutaneous inflammation)
Nocturnal Cramps (recumbent edema reduction)

Table 11.3 TESTS OF HISTORIC INTEREST

Trendelenburg Test
Cough Test
Schwartz Test
Perthes' Test

The recent development of an extremely painful area on the lower leg at the ankle associated with an overlying area of erythema and warmth may be indicative of lipodermatosclerosis, which may be associated with insufficiency of an underlying perforator vein, and examination for this lesion should be performed. Lipodermatosclerosis may precede ulceration and has been shown to be improved by stiff compression and certain pharmacologic interventions.

Patients with a history of iliofemoral thrombophlebitis who describe "bursting" pain with walking may be suffering from venous claudication. In these patients an evaluation for persistent hemodynamically significant obstruction, possibly treatable with angioplasty and stenting, may be in order.

PHYSICAL EXAMINATION

Using no special equipment, the practitioner can obtain a degree of information regarding overall venous outflow from the leg, the sites of valvular insufficiency, the presence of primary versus secondary varicose veins, and the presence of deep venous thrombosis (DVT). The screening physical examination consists of careful observation of the legs. Any patient with the following conditions should be examined more fully: large varicose veins; bulges in the thigh, calf, or the inguinal region representative of incompetent perforating veins (IPVs) or a saphena varix; signs of superficial venous hypertension such as an accumulation of telangiectasias in the ankle region (corona phlebectatica); or any of the findings suggestive of venous dermatitis (pigmentation, induration, eczema). This includes patients with obvious cutaneous signs of venous disease such as venous ulceration, atrophie blanche, or lipodermatosclerosis. An obvious but often forgotten point is the necessity of observing the entire leg and not confining the examination simply to the area that the patient feels is abnormal.

Finally, because the veins of the leg empty into the pelvic and abdominal veins, inspection of the abdomen is very important, since dilation of veins on the abdominal wall or across the pubic region suggests an old iliofemoral thrombus. Dilated veins along the medial or posterior aspect of the proximal thigh or buttocks most often arise from varicosities involving the pudendal or other pelvic vessels, and these can be of ovarian reflux origin.

CLINICAL TESTING

Historically important tests of venous function have been part of the physical examination of venous insufficiency (see Table 11.3). These tests have been laid aside largely because of their lack of specificity and sensitivity. The continuous-wave Doppler examination has replaced most of these tests, and confirmatory duplex testing has relegated them to an inferior role. However, the educated physician who treats venous insufficiency must have knowledge of these tests and their physiologic background, such as the Trendelenburg test or Brodie-Trendelenburg test.

TRENDELENBURG TEST

A tourniquet may be placed around the patient's proximal thigh while the patient is standing. The patient then assumes the supine position with the affected leg elevated 45 degrees. The tourniquet is removed, and the time required for the leg veins to empty, which is indicative of the adequacy of venous drainage, is recorded.

When compared with the contralateral leg, the method just described may demonstrate a degree of venous obstructive disease. Another approach is to elevate the leg while the patient is supine and to observe the height of the heel in relation to the level of the heart that is required for the prominent veins to collapse. Unfortunately, these procedures are neither sufficiently sensitive nor accurate and do not differentiate acute from chronic obstruction; thus they are of minimal assistance in current medical practice.

COUGH TEST

One hand is placed gently over the GSV or saphenofemoral junction (SFJ), and the patient is asked to cough or perform a Valsalva maneuver. Simply palpating an impulse over the vein being examined may be indicative of insufficiency of the valve at the SFJ and below to the level of the palpating hand.

PERCUSSION/SCHWARTZ TEST

One hand is placed over the SFJ or saphenopopliteal junction (SPJ), and the other hand is used to tap very lightly on a distal segment of the GSV or small saphenous vein (SSV). The production of an impulse in this manner implies insufficiency of the valves in the segment between the two hands. Confirmation of the valvular insufficiency can be achieved by tapping proximally while palpating distally. This test can also be used to detect whether an enlarged tributary is in direct connection with the GSV or SSV by palpating over the main trunk and tapping lightly on the dilated tributary, or vice versa. The presence of a direct connection results in a palpable impulse being transmitted from the percussing to the palpating hand. As might be expected, these tests are far from infallible.

PERTHES' TEST

The Perthes' test has several uses, including distinguishing between venous valvular insufficiency in the deep, perforator, and superficial systems and screening for DVT. To localize the site of valvular disease, the physician places a tourniquet around the proximal thigh with the patient standing. When the patient walks, a decrease in the distension of varicose veins suggests a primary process without underlying deep venous disease because the calf muscle pump effectively removes blood from the leg and empties the varicose veins. Secondary varicose veins do not change caliber (if there is patency of the deep venous system) because of the inability to empty blood out of the veins as a result of impairment of the calf muscle pump. In the setting of a current DVT, they may increase in size. If there is significant chronic or acute obstructive disease in the iliofemoral segment, the patient may note pain (venous claudication) as a result of the obstruction to outflow through both the deep and superficial systems. The Perthes' test is now of more historical than actual clinical importance.

ACKNOWLEDGMENT

Much of the material in this manuscript was derived and modified from the scholarly research of Mitchel Goldman, MD, and was published in his volume on sclerotherapy.

REFERENCES

1. Thompson H. The surgical anatomy of the superficial and perforating veins of the lower limb, *AM R Coll Surg Engl*. 1979. *61*: 198.
2. Cornu-Thenard A, Boivin P, Baud JM, et al. Importance of the familial factor in varicose disease, *J Derm Surg Onc*. 1994. *20*: 318.
3. Arnoldi C. The heredity of venous insufficiency, *Dan Med Bull*. 1958. *5*: 169.
4. Carpentier PH, Maricq HR, Biro C, et al. Prevalence, risk factors, and clinical patterns of chronic venous disorders of lower limbs: A population-based study in France, *J Vasc Surg*. 2004. *40*: 650–659.
5. Arenander E, Lindhagen A. The evolution of varicose veins studied in a material of initially unilateral varices, *Vasa*. 1978. *7*: 180.
6. Ottley C. Heredity and varicose veins, *Br Med J*. 1934. *1*: 528.
7. Alxlolt EC. The heredity of venous insufficiency, *Dan Med Bull*. 1958. *5*: 169.
8. King ESJ. The genesis of varicose veins, *ANZ J Surg*. 1950. *20*: 126.
9. Weddell IM. Varicose veins pilot survey, 1966, *Br J Prev Soc Med*. 1969. *23*: 179.
10. Niermann H. *Zwillingsdermatologie*. Berlin: Springer-Verlag. 1964.
11. Gundersen J, Hauge M. Hereditary factors in venous insufficiency, *Angiology*. 1969. *20*: 346.
12. Folse R. The influence of femoral vein dynamics on the development of varicose veins, *Surgery*. 1970. *68*: 974.
13. Almgren B. Non-thrombotic deep venous incompetence with special reference to anatomic, haemodynamic, and therapeutic aspects, *Phlebology*. 1990. *5*: 255.
14. Lee S, Lee W, Choe Y, et al. Gene expression profiles in varicose veins using complementary DNA microarray, *Dermatol Surg*. 2005. *31*: 391–395.
15. Coughlin LB, Gandy R, Rosser S, de Cossart L. Factors associated with varicose veins in pregnant women, *Phlebology*. 2002. *16*: 167–169.
16. Abramson JH, Hopp C, Epstein LM. The epidemiology of varicose veins: A survey in western Jerusalem, *J Epidemiol Community Health*. 1981. *35*: 213.
17. Henry M, Corless C. The incidence of varicose veins in Ireland, *Phlebology*. 1989. *4*: 133.
18. Tournay R, Wallois P. *Les varices de la grossesse et leur traitement principalement par les injections sclerosantes, expansion*. Paris: Scient Franc. 1948.
19. McCausland AM. Varicose veins in pregnancy, *Cal West Med*. 1939. *50*: 258.
20. Mullane DJ. Varicose veins in pregnancy, *Am J Obstet Gynecol*. 1952. *63*: 620.
21. Lev M, Saphir O. Endophlebohypertrophy and phlebosclerosis, *Arch Pathol Lab Med*. 1951. *51*(2): 154.
22. Donovan DL, Schmidt SP, Townshend SP, et al. Material and structural characterization of human saphenous veins, *J Vasc Surg*. 1990. *12*: 531.
23. Bouissou H, Julian M, Pieraggi M-Th, et al. Structure of healthy and varicose veins. In: Vanhoutte PM, ed. *Return circulation and norepinephrine: An update*. Paris: John Libbey Eurotext. 1991.
24. Cambell GD, Cleave TL. Diverticular disease of the colon, *Br Med J*. 1968. *3*(5620): 741.
25. Burkitt DP. Varicose veins, deep vein thrombosis, and haemorrhoids: Epidemiology and suggested etiology, *Br Med J*. 1972. *2*:556.
26. Myers TT. Varicose veins. In: Barker and Hines, eds. *Barker and Hines's peripheral vascular diseases*, 3e. 1962. Philadelphia: Saunders. 1962.
27. Fowkes FGR. Prevalence and risk factors for chronic venous insufficiency, *Acta Phlebol*. 2000. *1*: 69–78.
28. Widmer LK. *Peripheral venous disorders: Prevalence and socio-medical importance: Observations in 4529 apparently healthy persons, Basle Study III*. Berne, Switzerland: Huber. 1978.
29. Cotton LT. Varicose veins: Gross anatomy and development, *Br J Surg*. 1961. *48*: 589.
30. Hoshino S, Satakawa H, Iwaya F, et al. External valvuloplasty under preoperative angioscopic control, *Phlebologie*. 1993. *46*: 521.
31. Van Cleef JF, Desvaux P, Hugentobler JP, et al. Etude endoscopique des reflux valvulaires sapheniens, *J Maladies Vasculaires*. 1992. *17*: 113.
32. Sales CM, Rosenthal D, Petrillo ICA, et al. The valvular apparatus in venous insufficiency: A problem of quantity?, *Ann Vasc Surg*. 1998. *12*: 153.
33. Takase S, Lerond L, Bergan JJ, Schmid-Schonbein GW. The inflammatory reaction during venous hypertension in the rat, *Microcirculation*. 2000. *7*: 41.
34. Takase S, Pascarella L, Bergan JJ, Schmid-Schonbein GW. Hypertension-induced venous valve remodeling, *J Vasc Surg*. 2004. *39*: 1329–1334.
35. van Bemmelen SP, Hoynck van Papendrecht AA, Hodde KC, Klopper PJ. A study of valve incompetence that developed in an experimental model of venous hypertension, *Arch Surg*. 1986. *121*: 1048.
36. Takase S, Pascarella L, Lerond L, Bergan JJ, Schmid-Schonbein GW. Venous hypertension, inflammation, and valve remodeling, *Eur J Vasc Endovasc Surg*. 2004. *28*(5): 484–493.
37. Takase S, Lerond L, Bergan JJ, Schmid-Schonbein GW. Enhancement of reperfusion injury by elevation of microvascular pressures, *Am J Physiol Heart Circ Physiol*. 2002. *282*: H1387–H1394.

12.

SCLEROSANT AGENTS

MECHANISMS OF ACTION, CLASSIFICATION, AND PHARMACOLOGY

Attilio Cavezzi and Marcello Izzo

MECHANISM OF ACTION

To sclerose a vein means to induce endothelial damage and subsequent thrombus formation (sclerothrombus) by the injection of a chemical into the vein lumen. The result of this process is occlusion and fibrosis of the diseased vein. Modern sclerosing substances act directly on the vein endothelium. Three hours after the injection, endothelial swelling with desquamation is detected. After 15 hours, a deposition of a mixed thrombus takes place and after about 24 hours it fixes to the vessel wall until its final connective organization. Finally fibrosis of the vein may occur between 60 and 90 days after the injection.

Perivenous inflammatory reactions can appear when adventitia is involved (which is usually caused by excessive doses of the sclerosant drug), with or without intima and media lesions.

In 1989 Mancini et al. investigated histology of proximal segments of great saphenous vein (GSV), which were submitted to liquid sclerotherapy followed by surgical excision (at different time intervals) and investigated by optical and electronic microscopy. The main findings of this study were the following: (1) an endothelial lesion develops immediately; (2) 15 minutes after the injection the first fibrin content deposits; (3) after two and a half hours, the formation of a lamellar platelet microthrombus occurs; (4) between the second and third day massive (sclero) thrombosis develops; (5) at two months, the complete occlusion of vein lumen with connective and fibrous organization usually occurs.

Sclerosing substances have been experimentally studied on animals since 1920. The outcomes of animal studies are summarized here:

1. Endothelial damage is low in vessels injected with chromated glycerin (CG), polidocanol (POL) 0.25%, dextrose-sodium chloride (DSC), and ethanolamine oleate (EO) 0.5%; an early recanalization takes place;

2. POL 0.5%, sodium morrhuate (SM) 0.5–1%, EO 1%, and hypertonic saline solution 11.7% do not cause endothelial necrosis but only partial damage, and, although an

organized thrombus appears, vessel recanalization invariably occurs;

3. Vessels injected with sodium tetradecylsulfate (STS) at 0.5% concentration, or with SM 2.5%, present endothelial necrosis and an incomplete recanalization by numerous newly formed microchannels with clinical disappearance of treated venules.

More specifically the study of Goldman et al. on rabbit ear veins shows that increasing concentrations of POL and STS (from 0.25 to 1%) result in sclerofibrosis of the vessel but with recanalization within 14 days, and in some cases the reappearance of the vein takes place. Endothelial damage may be caused by the sum of a number of different mechanisms depending on the action of the substance used. Changes in surface tension of plasma membranes can be produced; physical, chemical changes in endothelial cells matrix through pH variations or changes of osmolarity may occur; also direct cellular destruction may occur due to caustic chemical actions or other physical factors like cold and heat.

Classification of sclerosing solutions:

1. Detergent solutions with decreasing sclerosant power: STS, SM, POL, EO

2. Osmotic solutions: Sodium salicylate (SS; or potassium salicylate [PS]), saline hypertonic solutions with very high osmolality (about 7533.8 mOsm/kg), DSC

3. Chemical solutions with a caustic-like effect on the endothelium: Iodine solutions.

Currently used sclerosing substances have different mechanisms of action and aggression on vein walls, but basically they are all osmotically active and in general, their action on the endothelium may be just irritative, necrotizing, or colliquative.

Factors that influence the sclerosing power are: (1) dose and concentration of medication, (2) physical-chemical variables (pH, liquid or foam) of the agents and of the blood, (3) physical-hemodynamic reasons inherent to local

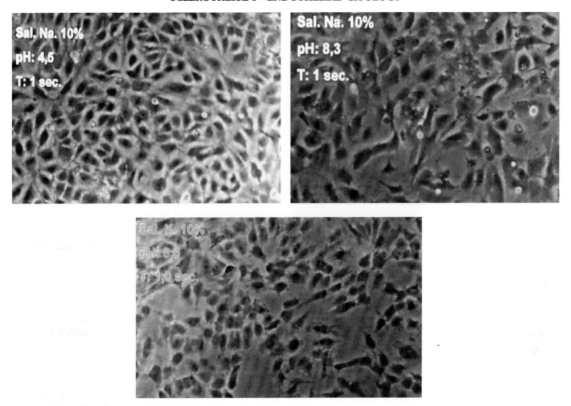

Figure 12.1   Endothelial cytology findings after injection of: traditional (top left) sodium salicylate, alkalinized (top right) sodium salicylate, potassium salicylate (bottom).

flow conditions, (4) injection technique, and (5) variability of the factors related to thrombosis and fibrosis of the treated vessels.

All sclerosant drugs have a different mechanism of action, but changing (usually increasing) the pH of a drug renders it a more powerful sclerosant. Dietrich and Sinapsius already demonstrated an increased colliquative action of a higher ph sclerosant drug. More recently Izzo et al. showed a remarkably higher colliquation and aniso-poikilocytosis in cytohistology samples of human umbilical veins treated with 8.4 pH sclerosant drug, when compared to the samples treated with the same sclerosant at an acidic pH (see Figure 12.1). Similarly modifying the physical form of detergents (e.g., POL, STS) from liquid to foam increases the sclerosing power.

The introduction of the foamy sclerosing form of the drug (foam sclerotherapy or endovenous chemical ablation) has led to a kind of mass effect (sclerosant foam [SF] is a "viscoelastic body"), for which it is possible to inject a nearly empty vein, at least in close proximity of the injected point.

Sclerosing substances are grouped, depending on the power, in three main groups: (1) major sclerosants: iodine solutions and STS; (2) medium sclerosants: POL, SS, and SM; and (3) minor sclerosants: CG, DCS, hypertonic saline solution 23.4%, and EO.

PHYSICS OF THE SCLEROSING AGENTS

Experimental studies carried out by Stemmer show that blood and sclerosant liquid always move toward the area of lowest pressure according to a pressure gradient. Compression can facilitate movement of the liquid toward a vein segment (e.g., perforator) or increase the contact time with the endothelium; It was also demonstrated that the vessel size of the treated vein influences the distribution of the sclerosant substance.

In small veins (4 mm or less) the injected liquid determines a contact zone with the wall around the injection point and a central streak to the vessel of a few inches; the streak touches the wall only when it encounters an obstacle (e.g., the tortuosity of the varicose veins); medium size varicose veins (approximately 6 mm) exhibit a laminar flow of the injected drug, and a central turbulence zone is produced around the needle tip with two streaks of laminar flow to the extremities; finally in larger veins (8 mm or more) there is a turbulence zone that fades more slowly than the smaller caliber tubes and completely occupies the lumen. The so-called air block technique (which has been proposed for small varices) involves an injection of a quantity of air before the liquid sclerosant, to displace some blood from the injected segment, obtaining a better contact between the substance and the endothelium, as shown in Stemmer's studies.

Orbach also proposed the creation of a froth (large bubble foam dispersion) by means of an agitation of STS in a vial, thus obtaining a froth that was aspirated into the syringe with the aim of depositing the drug along the vein in a uniform way and acting longer at the injection site.

In Stemmer's and our own experimental studies, the caliber of the needle affects the dynamics of the injection: at the same injection speed rate and with the same amount of time, the quantity of substance that touches the wall increases or decreases according to the dimensions of the needle.

While Stemmer's experience demonstrates that the injection rate does not affect the sclerosis effect, Zelikovski demonstrated that the rapid injection of labeled iodine solution 4% results in a longer contact time with the vein wall compared to a slow technique. It is agreed that the bending of the needle is completely irrelevant as to liquid injection dynamics.

Chemical and physical constants of blood and of sclerosant agents interact and are detailed in Table 12.1.

An endothelial injury may be caused by alteration of the electrical charge, of blood pH, of osmolality, and of the surface tension. The injection of an alkaline substance modifies the blood/tissue pH and causes endothelial damage, while a solution with acidic pH causes fewer lesions. This histochemical finding may represent a basic knowledge in the management and exploitation of the sclerosant drugs, with the aim of possibly potentiating their action on the venous wall. In fact, the pH of any single sclerosant drug is different, and any possible change of this chemical variable may interfere with the final outcome as well. The lowering of surface tension induced by detergent agents and the osmotic variations of hypertonic solutions determine significant changes in the endothelium. The viscosity of the sclerosant agent does not influence the effect, but a strong viscosity slows the progression of the product along the venous route (which is the case, for example for CG).

Density is important in the distribution of the liquid in the vessel: if the specific weight of a sclerosant agent considerably differs from that of blood (mean 1.050) it will tend to float or sediment (depending on whether it is lighter or heavier, respectively), which affects the necrotizing effect on the endothelium.

Table 12.1 **CHEMICAL AND PHYSICAL CONSTANTS OF BLOOD AND SCLEROSANT AGENTS**

The circulating blood and the venous endothelium present chemical and physical constants that can be considered stable:
the pH of venous blood varies between 7.27 and 7.43;
the specific weight is between 1.050 and 1.060;
the osmolality is between 275 and 295 milliosmoles;
the surface tension of the serum at 37 ° C is 47 dyn/cm;
the endothelium's electrical charge is negative (glycocalyx)
(Glycosaminoglycans of normal veins and their alterations in varicose veins and varicose veins complicated by thrombophlebitis.)

Factors related to thrombosis and fibrosis of venous vessels may be different from those in Virchow's triad: the thrombus composition is poor of fibrin, and there is a reduced participation of coagulation mechanisms. The slowdown of blood flow and hypercoagulability do not play an important role in the formation of postsclerotherapy fibrosis and for example, no decrease of the sclerosing POL activity has been reported in anticoagulated patients, as the endothelial injury is the key mechanism that provokes the localized sclerothrombosis.

Wuppermann in 1991 studied the sclerotherapy-coagulation interactions before and after sclerotherapy, and he concluded that hyperfibrinolysis occurs immediately after endothelial destruction (release of tissue activators), together with a denaturation of coagulation proteins; similarly this author showed fibrinogen infiltration into the wall and coagulation related to fibrinopeptide release (usually between the 5th and 7th day after treatment) until the fibrin degradation products and fibrinogen peptides attract chemotaxis cellular infiltration from the supporting tissue and the consequent organization of the sclerothrombus and vein wall altogether.

More recently Parsi accurately investigated several changes in coagulation factors/mechanisms that occur in sclerotherapy. His several in vitro studies and publications highlighted the following interactions between sclerosant agents (namely STS and POL) and the blood components:

1. Higher STS (especially) and POL concentrations (>0.6%) have anticoagulant properties, and STS, not POL, may enhance heparin activity.

2. Lower concentrations of STS and POL (e.g., 0.1–0.3%) have procoagulant properties (POL > STS).

3. High concentrations (STS > 0.3%, POL > 0.45%) produce hemolysis, platelet lysis, and endothelial cell lysis.

4. Plasma proteins, especially albumin, neutralize sclerosants.

To summarize the results of all these heterogeneous tests, STS at high concentration has an antithrombotic effect, while POL at high concentration is probably neutral. Conversely, both STS and POL at low concentrations have a net prothrombotic effect. Through these studies Parsi concluded that the effective sclerosant concentration can be reduced if a lower content of blood/albumin/plasma is obtained in the target vein (which confirms Fegan's old studies on the "empty vein technique"), but more generally higher concentrations and lower volumes are preferable to lower concentrations and higher volumes. Similarly, Parsi speculated on the low incidence of postsclerotherapy deep venous thrombosis (DVT), which could be possibly explained through the neutralization of sclerosants by blood proteins in deep veins; finally, due to the chemical phenomena reported above, the possible distal neurological/pulmonary effects of the foamed sclerosants should be unlikely related to the presence of the drug on the circulating bubbles.

In another recent publication, furthermore, Watkins showed how approximately 2 ml of a 4% blood protein solution deactivates 1 ml of 3% STS; hence, from his experimental studies it is possible to extrapolate the concept that about 0.5 ml of whole blood should deactivate 1 ml of 3% STS.

Recent in vivo studies from Tessari et al. also pointed out how the chemical activity of STS sclerosing foam is nearly zero after less than 1 minute (no active STS in the common femoral vein after STS foam injection in a leg varicose vein; 13th Annual European Venous Forum, 2012, Florence, Italy).

Several physical variables may positively or negatively interfere with the sclerosis process, and the volume of the target vein is one of the most important. When injecting a sclerosant agent into the vein, the blood dilution plays a major role because of the interaction of blood components (primarily proteins) with the sclerosant drugs. Intuitively, the larger the vein, the higher the blood/protein content, the higher the negative interference with the sclerosant drug action on the blood content itself and finally on the vein walls.

Vein caliber reduction, prior to any injection is hence suggested in liquid or foam sclerotherapy, to maximize the sclerosant effect on the vein walls. This simple statement brings most sclerotherapists to inject patients only in supine position; in this position vein size decreases by about 50% from standing position and according to Feied's reports, the

dilution of the sclerosant drug at 5 cm from the injected site is about three times lower. The possibility of raising the limb before any sclerosing treatment commences, may lead to a further reduction of the dilution of the sclerosant drug 5 cm away from the injected site (eight times higher concentration in comparison with a standing position); similarly, with a limb elevated at 30°–50°, a 60–80% caliber reduction is expected in the saphenous and tributary veins (personal unpublished data; Figure 12.2). To overcome the possible difficulty of cannulating a vein in a raised limb, many physicians prefer to raise the limb after entering the vein in supine position and after fixing the needle/catheter to the skin. Limb elevation does not necessarily pertain to sclerotherapy of minor varicosities, as the latter reduce in size much less (or not at all) because of their location in the dermal space and the minor changes in inner pressure with postural changes. For reticular varices and telangiectasias a possible option to improve the blood reduction/clearing effect in the treated segment could be to inject and retrieve the sclerosant drug within the vessel a few times. In our empirical experience this procedure seems to reduce clot retention while increasing the sclerosing power even of low concentration drugs (e.g., POL 0,25%, STS 0,1%, SS 8 %).

As vein caliber and blood content are strictly regulated by the transmural pressure (external pressure versus inner vein pressure), it is possible to increase external pressure through stockings or bandages (with or without pads to increase local pressure according to Laplace's law), which is more easily achievable for varicose tributaries or for subcutaneous veins in general. In the case of major veins

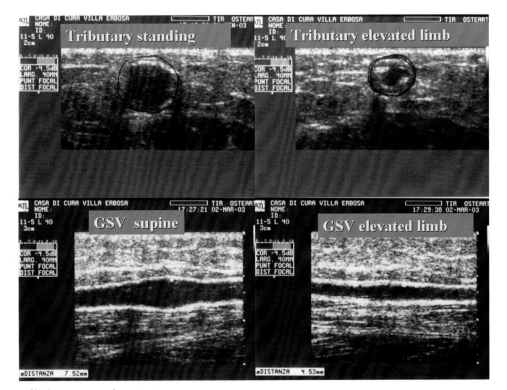

Figure 12.2   Influence of limb position on the vein sizes.

(e.g., GSV, small saphenous vein [SSV], anterior accessory saphenous vein, Giacomini vein, thigh extension of SSV, groin or popliteal fossa recurrence, etc.), which are deeper, Partsch's studies showed high pressure is needed to occlude a saphenous vein, or to significantly reduce its caliber (i.e., 70–80 mm Hg for GSV at mid thigh in standing position).

Thibault proposed another mechanical method to minimize blood content and vein size. Through the infiltration of saline solution in the subcutaneous space or in the saphenous compartment after a sclerosant foam injection, he got a prolonged decrease of vein size (decrease of blood reappearance in the treated area). Fewer side effects and ultimately better results have been shown by the author through this adjuvant procedure.

A further reappraisal of this proposal led Parsi and Cavezzi to inject tumescent saline solution (with or without anaesthetics, with or without adrenaline inclusion, the latter drug having the ability to minimize vein diameter) immediately prior to the sclerotherapy session. In fact if a long catheter is inserted in the target vein (GSV, SSV, etc.), the tumescence infiltration is performed before sclerosant foam (or liquid) is delivered into the vein through the catheter retrieval; similarly tumescence is possibly applicable to previously cannulated varicose tributaries. In a preliminary study Ramelet proposed the tumescence infiltration also in sclerotherapy of resistant reticular varices/telangiectasias, with some contrasting evidence.

These procedures, though not scientifically validated so far, may increase the obliteration rate also in larger veins, while decreasing the necessary dose of SF or liquid and possibly decreasing the side effects. In our experience, additional tumescence has resulted in improved outcomes in patients treated with long catheter foam sclerotherapy of GSV or SSV or AASV + phlebectomy of the varicose vein tributaries.

Diffusion of the sclerosant drug from the injection site and blood (re-)entrance in the treated vein/s is another major factor that may influence the extension of the sclerothrombus.

After Stemmer's experiments and Feied's published data, the movement of the sclerosant liquid drug (and of SF, though in a lesser extent) from the injected site has been elucidated as another factor that may jeopardize the sclerosant drug effect. Passariello and Schadeck in the early nineties highlighted the "erasure" effect from the local tributaries/veins on the sclerosis process of the saphenous stem; when injecting a vein, the washing effect of the local tributaries will interfere with the extension of the sclerothrombus, for mechanical and chemical reasons: open veins flush and limit the proximal segment of the sclerothrombus where these enter the sclerosed vein (and provide fresh lytic factors). This is the case, for example with thrombosis of the GSV and common femoral vein or just with epigastric/abdominal veins and endovenous procedures on GSV.

Since the introduction of foam sclerotherapy and its worldwide diffusion thanks to Tessari's method, a significant reappraisal of sclerosant drug chemical and physical activities has been proposed. Some of the considerations and data that have been mentioned above for liquid drugs, may not necessarily be pertinent to the injections of sclerosant foam. In fact foam dynamics significantly differ from liquid dynamics, both in supine and raised limbs. A potentiated action of SF over a liquid drug has been proven in different studies, which can be referred to the prolonged contact between drug and vein wall, to the great multiplication of the active surface of the drug over the microbubble surface, to the reduced blood content in the injected segment and to many other factors that intervene in foam activity and that are still under investigation.

The role of air as the gas component of the sclerosant foam has been questioned, as to the possible nitrogen-based distant side effects of the microbubbles. More biocompatible gases, such as CO_2 and O_2, preferably in a 70% to 30% combination, have been proposed in place of air to form sclerosant foam. Morrison's studies showed an overall improved safety for CO_2, alone or in combination with O_2, over room air, as to a few side effects.

PHARMACOLOGY OF SCLEROSANT AGENTS: AN OVERVIEW

CHROMATED GLYCERIN (CG)

Glycerin or glycerol is a glycol (bivalent alcohol) used as an osmotic diuretic and it is a sclerosant liquid, when combined with chrome alum, with strong coagulating properties. Today a bluish-colored and oily sterile solution of chromated glycerin is commonly used, composed of 72% glycerin and 1.11% chrome alum; alternatively, in a few countries the single glycerin or glycerol is used as a compound drug. Thanks to Kern's studies CG has regained some popularity in the scientific community, as it proved to achieve good results in the treatment of telangiectasias over the use of POL, STS, or sclerosant foam. CG has an irritating chemical action on the endothelium, and it is a weak, viscous sclerosant that may result in some minor local side effects such as pigmentation, perivenous inflammation (rarely necrosis), skin redness, and/or short-lasting pain in the surrounding area. Systemic reactions are those common to all sclerosant agents plus a dark colored urine emission in rare cases. Generally, CG dose per session and per injection never surpasses 10 ml and 3 ml respectively (usually a few drops per injection in telangiectasias), and this "weak" drug is used for telangiectasias and reticular varices only.

SALICYLATES (SS AND PS)

The salicylates, an ancient remedy known to Hippocrates and Galen and also in the Middle Ages, exist in nature (e.g., salicylic and methyl salicylate). Used in 1876 in rheumatic fever, and as the basic components of acetylsalicylic acid (ASA) 20 years later, salicylates were introduced by Jean Sicard in 1919 in France (SS) in sclerotherapy of varicose veins. SS has been used worldwide (mainly in France, Italy, Canada, and Argentina) in the last 60 years, basically for minor varicosities only, more frequently under the form of a compound drug.

SS is usually used at 10–20% concentration, with xylocaine included to compensate the hyperalgesia that SS may generate in the first seconds after the injection. Mariani and Izzo introduced PS to potentiate salicylate ion activity on endothelial cells, using an alkaline pH formulation (Figure 12.1); this also resulted in a lower pigmentation rate in the authors' experience. SS and PS have also shown a beneficial effect on venous symptoms such as cramps and heaviness, though a short-lasting painful injection is associated with higher concentrations. Side effects include skin necrosis (if injected extravenously) and rarely pigmentation. Allergy to ASA and deafness are common contraindications to usage of SS or PS. Ten ml of SS 20% is the recommended maximum dose per session, while 0.1–0.5 ml of SS or SP are commonly used per injection.

The combination of glycerin and SS has been proposed by Capurro in treatment of minor varicosities to exploit the mildness of the first drug and the low-pigmentation property of SS.

HYPERTONIC SALINE SOLUTION (HSS) 23.4%

HSS damages endothelial wall and induces a thrombus within 1 hour after injection, while the sclerosis is completed in 2–4 weeks. Addition of heparin to HSS resulted in more "matting," probably due to the angiogenesis action of heparin, without any improvement of the outcomes.

Local side effects are similar to those of salicylates, while the lack of selectivity of action of HSS on the diseased vessel walls may explain the higher incidence of DVT and pulmonary embolism (PE) in literature. Finally caution is recommended if large amounts are injected in hypertensive patients. Generally, 15 ml is the suggested highest dose per session, and 1 to 3 ml of HSS is the dose per injection, while few drops are used in telangiectasias.

DSC

DSC is a mixture of dextrose 250 mg/ml, NaCl 100 mg/ml, phenethylic alcohol 8 mg/ml, propylene glycol 100 mg/ml, and water up to 10 ml. This hypertonic solution with 5.9 pH value causes dehydration and necrosis of endothelial cells, 3 minutes post injection. The deposition of fibrin and thrombus formation occurs because of a change of electrostatic charges in the endothelium. Local side effects of DSC may include pigmentation and rare skin necrosis, while, like HSS, a lack of the selectivity of action may raise the risk of DVT/PE if large amounts are injected (total volume of 10 ml per session is recommended). The dose per injection is up to 3 ml, and DSC is usually recommended in telangiectasias and reticular varices only.

POL OR LAUROMACROGOL 400

POL is an alcohol that was introduced in 1936 as a surface anaesthetic. The basic molecule (hydroxypoliethoxy-dodecane) is formed by a lipophilic and by a hydrophilic part, and the amphipathic properties of POL explain the interaction with veins and skin. In 1960 Henschel used POL in varicose vein treatment; since 1967 this usage has spread worldwide, and several clinical trials have been performed to test this molecule in small and large varices. Different concentrations of POL (0.25–3%) are available on the market, to treat from telangiectasias to larger saphenous veins. POL is an alcohol with the characteristics of a nonionic surfactant or detergent substance, which makes POL well transformable in foam; furthermore POL reversibly inhibits the sensory receptors and the conductivity of the sensory nerve fibers (anaesthetic proprieties). POL dilution with distilled water is possible thanks to its long carbon chain; and Lauromacrogol 400 is the stabilized POL preparation at neutral pH. Experimental and in vivo studies demonstrated that placenta is an effective barrier for POL and 64% protein binding of POL molecules has been calculated in humans; similarly no teratogenicity, mutagenicity, or carcinogenicity have been shown. Local reactions commonly include urticaria-like reactions, pigmentation due to clot retention, perivenous inflammation, and skin necrosis. Systemic reactions are those common to all sclerosant agents (allergies, nausea, etc.), while major neurologic, cardiac, and thromboembolic complications have been rarely reported for POL both in liquid and foamy form.

STS

STS is an anionic "surfactant" with corrected pH that was discovered by Reiner in 1946 and since then diffused in several countries worldwide. This detergent drug can be easily transformed in foam form and has been extensively used in foam sclerotherapy since 1997. With reference to sclerosant foam, STS microbubbles basically have smaller size than POL bubbles, whereas their half-liquid time is shorter compared with POL foam. Its 7–8.1 pH helps to cause endothelial maceration within 1 hour after injection, and STS quickly combines with serum and endothelial proteins. The possible local side reactions are rare: pain, urticaria-like skin reactions, pigmentation, perivenous inflammation, and necrosis. Hemolysis, transient fever, nausea, and vomiting are possible systemic reactions when large doses are employed. Cerebral and thromboembolic complications have been reported in literature for STS as liquid or sclerosant foam. The drug is available in different concentrations (0.2%, 0.5%, 1%, 3%) and it is mostly used for medium-large size veins, though 0.1% STS is proposed in sclerotherapy of telangiectasias too.

POLYIODIDE SOLUTIONS

Iodated solution (IS) was of major importance for large-vessel sclerotherapy in the last decades (especially in Sigg's technique), being gradually replaced by detergent agents, both liquid and foam. IS is a dark brown stabilized aqueous solution of monoiodic and polyiodic ions, sodium ions in various concentrations with the addition, in some preparations, of benzyl alcohol. IS has always been recommended for medium-large varices only. IS has a cell-damaging action on the venous endothelium, a marked and time-lasting toxic effect because it acts as a sort of vital dye stuck to the wall. Lindemayr and Santler indicate that IS does not likely produce activation of blood coagulation, resulting in low risk of thrombosis propagation induced on the damaged venous segments. IS necrotic and algesic power is extremely high if injected into the extravascular space, but high concentrations often result in painful intravenous injections. IS shares similar local and general complications with POL and STS, while visual disorders, dizziness, and iodine taste sensation are more typical for IS. A typical general contraindication to IS usage is hyperthyroidism, and the total dose of 2–8% IS per session should never exceed 3–4 ml.

SM

SM is a mixture of saturated and unsaturated fatty acids of sodium salts of soap-like cod liver oil, synthesized for intravenous use by Ghosh and Cutting (1926) with surfactant (detergent) characteristics and a 6.9–9.6 pH; SM causes endothelium maceration through an action on membrane lipids, with subsequent thrombosis between the 2nd and 10th day. Typical local reactions are: cramp-like pain, burning sensation in the injection area, remarkable perivenous inflammation, and necrosis, whereas systemic reactions are those of the other sclerosants. The usual dose in adults to sclerose small-to-large varicose veins is 50 to 250 mg (1–5 ml 5%). SM is not generally recommended for sclerotherapy of spider veins.

EO

EO is a viscous detergent aqueous solution containing ethanolamine oleate at 5%, with a 8–9 pH. EO causes endothelium maceration, intense extravascular inflammatory reactions, hemolytic reactions, and the activation in vitro of coagulation (which accounts for the risk of disseminated intravascular coagulation, occasionally associated to EO). Beside the typical local and systemic complications, an acute renal failure was reported in treating an obese patient with high doses. The injected dose should not exceed 10 ml per session, and normally no more than 2 ml per injection site is used. EO is mostly used for esophageal varices, but lower-limb medium-large varicose veins are also an indication for the use of liquid (or foamed) EO sclerotherapy.

ACKNOWLEDGMENTS

Thanks to Fabrizio Mariani and to Lorenzo Tessari for their invaluable scientific inputs and thanks to Elio Concettina for her help in the literature review.

REFERENCES

1. Schneider W. In: Tournay R et al., eds. *Terapia sclerosante delle varici*. Milan, Italy: Cortina. 1984. 79–90.
2. Mancini S, Mariani F, De Sando D, et al. La sclérose de la grande saphéne: Histologie et microscopie électronique des altérations chez l'homme. In: Davy A, Stemmer R, eds. *Phlebologie '89*. 10éme Congres Mondial Union Internationale des Phlebologie; Strasbourg, Sep 25–29, 1989. London: John Libbey Eurotext. 1989. 769–771.
3. Mancini S, Lassueur F, Mariani F. La sclérose de la veine grande saphéne: Étude expérimentale chez l'homme sur l'action sclérosante de la solution iodo-iodurée et le polidodécane (histologie et microscopie électronique), *Phlebologie*. 1991. *44*(2): 461–468.
4. Wolf E. Die histologischen Veranderungen der venen nach intravenosen sub limatein Spritzungen, *Med Klin*. 1920. *16*: 806.
5. Dietrich VHP, Sinapsius D. Experimental endothelial damage by varicosclerosation drugs, *Arznittel Forsh*. 1968. *18*: 116.
6. Imhoff E, Stemmer R. Classification and mechanism of action of sclerosing agents, *Soc Fr Phlebol*. 1969. *22*: 143–148.
7. Goldman MP, Kaplan RP, Oki LN, et al. Sclerosing agents in the treatment of telangiectasia: Comparison of the clinical and histological effects of intravascular polidocanol, sodium tetradecyl sulfate, and hypertonic saline in the dorsal rabbit ear vein model, *Arch Dermatol*. 1987. *123*: 1196–1201.
8. Martin DE, Goldman MP. A comparison of sclerosing agents: Clinical and histological effects of intravascular sodium tetradecyl sulfate and chromated glycerine in the dorsal rabbit ear vein, *J Derm Surg Onc*. 1990. *16*: 18–22.
9. Goldman MP. Mechanism of action of sclerotherapy. In: Goldman MP, ed. *Sclerotherapy: Treatment of varicose and teleangiectatic leg veins*. St. Louis, MO: Mosby Year Book. 1991. 183–218.
10. Hanschell HM. Treatment of varicose veins, *Br Med J*. 1947. *2*: 630–631.
11. Oscher A, Garside E. Intravenous injection of sclerosing substances: Experimental comparative studies of changes in vessels, *Ann Surg*. 1932. *96*(4): 691–718.
12. Merlen JF, Curri SB, Saout J, Coget J. Histological changes in a sclerosed vein, *Phlebologie*. 1978. *31*: 17–34.
13. Stemmer R. In: Tournay R, ed. *Terapia sclerosante delle varici*. Milan, Italy: Cortina. 1984. 65–77.
14. Stemmer R, Kopp C, Voglet P. Etude physique de l'injection sclerosante, *Phlebologie*. 1969. *22*: 149–172.
15. Steinacher J, Kammerhuber F. Weg und Verweildauer eines Kontrastmittels im oberflachlichen Venesystem unter Bedingung

der Varicenverodung: Eine Studie zur Technik der Varicenverodung [Passage and duration of stay of contrast media in the superficial venous system under conditions of varicose sclerozation: A study of the technique of varicose sclerozation], *Z Haut- und Geschlechtskrankheiten.* 1968. *43*: 369–376.

16. Orbach EJ. Has injection treatment of varicose veins become obsolete?, *J Am Med Assoc.* 1958. *166*(16): 1964–1966.

17. Zelikovski A, et al. Compression sclerotherapy of varicose veins: A few observations and some practical suggestions, *Folia Angiologica.* 1978. *26*: 61–64.

18. Dastain, JY. Sclerotherapy of varices when the patient is on anticoagulants, with reference to 2 patients on anticoagulants, *Phlebologie.* 1981. *34*: 73–76.

19. Wuppermann Th. Mécanisme de la sclérose des varices: Explorations hémostatiques, isotopiques, et histologiques, *Phlebologie.* 1991. *44*(1): 23–29.

20. Goldman MP, Bergan JJ, Guex JJ. *Sclerotherapy: Treatment of varicose and telangiectatic leg veins,* 4e. London: Mosby. 2007.

21. Cutting RA. The preparation of sodium morrhuate, *J Lab Clin Med.* 1926. *11*: 842–845.

22. Dick ET. The treatment of varicose veins, *NZ Med J.* 1966. *65*: 310–313.

23. Reiner L. The activity of anionic surface active compounds in producing vascular obliteration, *Proc Soc Exp Biol Med.* 1946. *62*: 49–54.

24. Schneider W, Fischer H. Fixierung und bindegewebige organization artefizieller Thromben bei der Varizenuerodung, *Dtsch Med Wschr.* 1964. *89*: 2410.

25. Fegan G. *Varicose veins: Compression sclerotherapy.* London: Heinemann Medical. 1967. Reprint, Hereford, UK: Berrington Press. 1990.

26. Tournay PR. Sclerosing treatment of very fine intra or subdermal varicosities, *Soc Fr Phlebol.* 1966. *19*: 235–241.

27. Olesch B. Recent investigations on pharmacokinetics of Polidocanol (Aethoxysklerol) in animals and men. In: Kreussler, ed. *Phlebol.* Bonn: Vasomed. 1992.

28. Goor W. Phlebologie in der Schwangerschaft, *Swiss Med.* 1982. *4*: 49–50; 1983. *4a*: 86–88.

29. Bodian EL. Sclerotherapy, *Semin Dermatol.* 1987. *6*: 238–248.

30. Martindale W. *The extra pharmacopoeia,* 28e. London: Pharmaceutical Press. 1982.

31. Ouvry P, Arlaud R. Le traitement sclérosant des télangiectasies des membres inférieurs, *Phlebologie.* 1979. *32*: 365–370.

32. Ouvry P, Davy A. Le traitement sclérosant des télangiectasies des membres inférieurs, *Phlebologie.* 1982. *35*: 349–359

33. Wallois P. Incidents et accidents del la sclérose. In Tournay R, ed. *La sclérose des varices,* 4e. Paris: Expansion Scientifique Française. 1985. 297–319.

34. Reid RG Rothine NG. Treatment of varicose veins by compression sclerotherapy, *Br J Surg.* 1968. *55*: 889–895.

35. Kang JH, et al. Mechanism of the haemostatic effect of ethanolamine oleate in the injection sclerotherapy for oesophageal varices, *Br J Surg.* 1987. *74*: 50–53.

36. Yamaga H, et al. Platelet aggregability after endoscopic intravariceal injection of 5 per cent ethanolamine oleate into oesophageal varice, *Br J Surg.* 1989. *76*: 939–942.

37. Meyer NE. Monoethanolamine oleate: A new chemical for obliteration of varicose veins, *Am J Surg.* 1938. *40*: 628–629.

38. Maling TJB, Cretney MJ. Ethanolamine oleate and acute renal failure. *NZ Med J.* 1975. *82*: 269–270.

39. Lindemayr H, Santler R. The fibrinolytic activity of the vein wall, *Phlebologie.* 1977. *30*(2): 151–160.

40. Kern HM, Angle LW. The chemical obliteration of varicose veins: A clinical and experimental study, *JAMA.* 1929. *93*: 595–601.

41. McPheeters HO, Anderson JK. *Injection treatment of varicose veins and hemorrhoids,* 2e. Philadelphia: F.A. Davis. 1939.

42. Bodian EL. Techniques of sclerotherapy for sunburst venous blemishes, *J Derm Surg Onc.* 1985. *11*: 696–704.

43. Sadick N. Treatment of varicose and telangiectatic leg veins with hypertonic saline: A comparative study of heparin and saline, *J Derm Surg Onc.* 1990. *16*: 24–28.

44. Foley WT. The eradication of venous blemishes, *Cutis.* 1975. *15*: 665–668.

45. Thornton SC, Mueller SN, Levine EM. Human endothelial cells: Use of heparin in cloning and long-term serial cultivation, *Science.* 1983. *222*: 623–625.

46. Mantse LA. Mild sclerosing agent for telangiectasias, *J Derm Surg Onc.* 1985. *11*: 855.

47. Gallagher PG. Varicose veins-primary treatment with sclerotherapy, *J Derm Surg Onc.* 1992. *18*: 39–42.

48. Morrison RT, Boyd RN. *Chimica organica.* Milan: Ambrosiana. 1970. 539–604, 937–969.

49. Mariani F, Izzo M, Di Stefano R. I farmaci sclerosanti: Proprietà chimiche e effetto lesivo. *Flebologia.* 1998. *9*(1–3): 29–30.

50. Carcassi U. *Trattato di reumatologia.* Rome: Società Editrice Universo. 1993. Vol. 1, 673–674.

51. Tessari L, Cavezzi A, Frullini A. Preliminary experience with a new sclerosing foam in the treatment of varicose veins, *Dermatol Surg.* 2001. *27*(1): 58–60.

52. Wright DD. What is the current role of foam sclerotherapy in treating reflux and varicosities?, *Semin Vasc Surg.* 2010. *23*(2): 123–126.

53. Goldman MP. My sclerotherapy technique for telangiectasia and reticular veins, *Dermatol Surg.* 2010. *36*(Suppl 2): 1040–1045.

54. Palm MD, Guiha IC, Goldman MP. Foam sclerotherapy for reticular veins and nontruncal varicose veins of the legs: A retrospective review of outcomes and adverse effects, *Dermatol Surg.* 2010. *36*(Suppl 2): 1026–1033.

55. Duffy DM. Sclerosants: A comparative review, *Dermatol Surg.* 2010. *36*(Suppl 2): 1010–1025.

56. Palm MD. Commentary: Choosing the appropriate sclerosing concentration for vessel diameter, *Dermatol Surg.* 2010. *36* (Suppl 2): 982.

57. Rabe E, Pannier F. Sclerotherapy of varicose veins with polidocanol based on the guidelines of the German Society of Phlebology, *Dermatol Surg.* 2010. *36*(Suppl 2): 968–975.

58. Rabe E, Schliephake D, Otto J, Breu FX, Pannier F. Sclerotherapy of telangiectases and reticular veins: A double-blind, randomized, comparative clinical trial of polidocanol, sodium tetradecyl sulphate, and isotonic saline (EASI study), *Phlebology.* 2010. *25*(3): 124–131.

59. Blaise S, Bosson JL, Diamand JM. Ultrasound-guided sclerotherapy of the great saphenous vein with 1% vs. 3% polidocanol foam: A multicentre double-blind randomised trial with 3-year follow-up, *Eur J Vasc Endovasc Surg.* 2010. *39*(6): 779–786.

60. Guex JJ. Complications and side-effects of foam sclerotherapy, *Phlebology.* 2009. *24*(6): 270–274.

61. Cavezzi A, Tessari L. Foam sclerotherapy techniques: Different gases and methods of preparation, catheter versus direct injection, *Phlebology.* 2009. *24*(6): 247–251.

62. Hamel-Desnos C, Allaert FA. Liquid versus foam sclerotherapy, *Phlebology.* 2009. *24*(6): 240–246.

63. Rao J, Wildemore JK, Goldman MP. Double-blind prospective comparative trial between foamed and liquid polidocanol and sodium tetradecyl sulfate in the treatment of varicose and telangiectatic leg veins, *Dermatol Surg.* 2005. *31*(6): 631–635; discussion 635.

64. Passariello F, Carbone R. Chirurgia dell' Arco della Safena Esterna, *Min Angiol.* 1992. *17*(Suppl. 3 al n. 2): 149–156.

65. Parsi K, Exner T, Ma DDF, Joseph JE. In vitro effects of detergent sclerosant on fibrinolytic enzymes and inhibitors, *Thromb Res.* 2010. *126*: 328–336.

66. Wollman JC. Sclerosant foams: Stabilities, physical properties, and rheological behaviour, *Phlebologie.* 2010. *39*(4): 208–217.

67. Parsi K, Exner T, Connor DE, Ma DDF, Joseph JE. *In vitro* effects of detergent sclerosants on coagulation, platelets and microparticles, *Eur J Vasc Endovasc Surg.* 2007. *34*: 731–740.

68. Parsi K, Exner T, Connor DE, Herbert A, Ma DDF, Joseph JE. The lytic effects of detergent sclerosants on erythrocytes, platelets, endothelial cells, and microparticles are attenuated by albumin and

other plasma components *in vitro*, *Eur J Vasc Endovasc Surg*. 2008. *36*: 216–223.

69. Cavezzi A, Carigi V, Buresta P, Di Paolo S, Sigismondi G. Flebectomía de las várices + espuma esclerosante del tronco safénico: Una propuesta terapéutica innovadora, *Flebologia y Linfologia*. 2008. *8*: 426–427.

70. Partsch B, Partsch H. Which pressure do we need to compress the great saphenous vein on the thigh?, *Dermatol Surg*. 2008. *34*(12): 1726–1728.

71. Feied C. Sclerosing solutions. In: Bergan J, ed. *The vein book*. Boston: Elsevier.2007. 125–131.

72. Thibault P. Sclerotherapy and ultrasound-guided sclerotherapy. In: Bergan J, ed. *The vein book*. Boston: Elsevier.2007. 189–199.

73. Cavezzi A, Carigi V, Collura M, et al. Phlebectomy of varicose tributaries combined with transcatheter foam sclerotherapy of the saphenous vein, *Int Angiol*. 2009. *28*(Suppl 1): 78.

74. Hamel-Desnos C, Desnos P, Wollmann JC, et al. Evaluation of the efficacy of Polidocanol in the form of foam compared with liquid form in sclerotherapy of the long saphenous vein: Initial results. *Dermatol Surg*. 2003. *29*: 1170–1175.

75. Kern P, Ramelet AA, Wutschert R, Bounameaux H, Hayoz D. Single-blind, randomized study comparing chromated glycerin, polidocanol solution, and polidocanol foam for treatment of telangiectatic leg veins, *Dermatol Surg*. 2004. *30*(3): 367–372; discussion 372; comment *Dermatol Surg*. 2004. *30*(9): 1272; author reply, 1272–1273.

76. Capurro S. La phlébothérapie régénératrice tridimensionnelle ambulatoire (TRAP): Concept innovant de traitement de la varicose, *Phlebologie*. 2010. *63*: 1–5.

77. Mariani F, Izzo M, Trapassi S, Mancini S. Sclerotherapy of reticular varices and teleangiectasias: Therapeutic strategy and result, *Acta Phlebol*. 2001. *2*: 71–76.

78. Izzo M, Amitrano M, Bacci PA, Mancini S, Mariani F. Pigmentation post-sclérothérapie: Physiopathologie et traitement, *Phlebologie*. 2001. *54*: 273–277.

79. Izzo M, Mariani F, Bianchi V, Bacci PA, Di Stefano R. A new sclerosing agent: Potassium salicylate, *Int Angiol*. 2001. *20*(Suppl 1): 2.

80. Parsi K. Catheter-directed sclerotherapy, *Phlebology*. 2009. *24*: 98–107.

81. Cavezzi A, Parsi K. Complications of foam sclerotherapy, *Phlebology*. 2012. *27*(Suppl 1): 46–51.

82. Morrison N, Neuhardt DL, Rogers CR, et al. Incidence of side effects using carbon dioxide oxygen foam for chemical ablation of superficial veins of the lower extremity, *Eur J Vasc Endovasc Surg*. 2010. *40*: 407–413.

83. Watkins MR. Deactivation of sodium tetradecyl sulphate injection by blood proteins, *Eur J Vasc Endovasc Surg*. 2011. *41*(4): 521–525.

84. Peterson JD, Goldman MP, Weiss RA, et al. Treatment of reticular and telangiectatic leg veins: Double-blind, prospective comparative trial of polidocanol and hypertonic saline, *Dermatol Surg*. 2012. *38*: 1–9.

85. Schuller-Petrović S, Brunner F, Neuhold N, Pavlović MD, Wölkart G. Subcutaneous injection of liquid and foamed polidocanol: Extravasation is not responsible for skin necrosis during reticular and spider vein sclerotherapy, *JEADV*. 2011. *25*: 983–986.

86. Ramelet AA. Sclerotherapy in tumescent anesthesia of reticular veins and telangiectasias, *Dermatol Surg*. 2012. *38*(5): 748–751.

13.

SCLEOTHERAPY TREATMENT OF TELANGIECTASIAS

Robert A. Weiss and Margaret A. Weiss

INTRODUCTION

Isolated small reticular veins and telangiectasias often cause severe symptoms that are worsened by prolonged standing or sitting and may be relieved by wearing support hose or by elevation of the legs.[1] Vein size alone does not predict the presence of symptoms. Vessels causing symptoms may be as small as 1 mm in diameter or less.[2] Besides symptoms of pain, burning, and fatigue, women typically curtail their activities and modify their lifestyles to avoid situations in which their legs are easily seen. Sclerotherapy not only offers the possibility of remarkably good cosmetic results, but also has been reported to yield an 85% reduction in symptoms.[1] Prior experience with venipuncture helps very little with treatment of larger veins and is completely irrelevant in the treatment of the smallest veins. Successful treatment requires the correct technique, the correct diagnosis, and the correct treatment plan for the type and size of vein to be treated.

TELANGIECTASIA FROM RETICULAR VEINS

Telangiectasia can develop as a result of reflux from reticular veins, thin-walled blue superficial venules that are part of an extensive network of the lateral subdermic venous system; a system that is separate from the saphenous system. A typical network is shown in Figure 13.1. Reticular veins associated with telangiectasia are commonly called "feeder" veins. Both handheld Doppler and duplex ultrasound have been used to map the path of transmission of venous hypertension from small reticular veins into telangiectasia.[3,4]

ISOLATED ARBORIZING WEBS

High-pressure reflux through failed valves is at the root of nearly all telangiectatic webs, although there are some exceptions due to arteriovenous malformations or shunts. This has been estimated to occur approximately one in twenty times, although this may be a high estimate.[5] Typically, localized valve failure will produce arborizing networks of dilated cutaneous venules that are direct tributaries of underlying larger veins. Arborization occurs through a recruitment phenomenon in which high pressure causes dilatation of a venule, failure of its valves, and transmission of the high pressure across the failed valves into an adjacent vein. Treatment of an arborizing system must be directed at the entire system, because if the point source of reflux is not ablated, the web will rapidly recur.

PRETREATMENT INSTRUCTIONS

Patients are told to wear shorts and not to use moisturizers or shave their legs on the day of treatment. Shaving the leg may cause erythematous streaks, making it difficult to visualize patterns of reticular and telangiectatic veins. Use of moisturizers causes poor adhesion of tape used to secure compression following injections and causes slower evaporation of alcohol used to prep the leg. Patients are encouraged to eat at least a small meal beforehand in order to minimize vasovagal reactions.

FIRST TREATMENT TEST

The first treatment session usually is limited to a small number of sites in order to observe the patient for any allergic reactions and the ability to tolerate the burning or cramping of a hypertonic solution, to judge the effectiveness of a particular concentration and class of sclerosing agent, and to observe the ability to comply with compression. It also serves to familiarize the patient with the treatment, treating physician, clinic surroundings, and the sensation of the fine needle. This allows more extensive treatment on the second visit with the patient being familiar with the technique and surroundings. The test site also complies with the suggestion in the package insert of sodium tetradecyl sulfate (STS; Sotradecol, Bioniche Pharma, Belleville, Ontario).

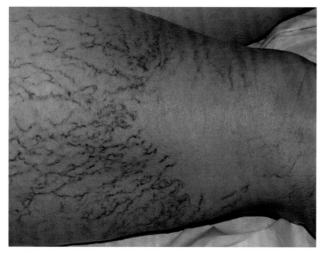

Figure 13.1 Typical telangiectatic web–reticular vein complex of the lateral subdermic venous system.

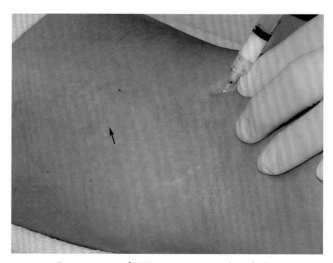

Figure 13.2 Foam mixture of STS 0.1% comprising liquid sclerosant agitated with air at a ratio of one part liquid to four parts air. Here the foam is seen injected into a reticular vein. Foam is visualized in the vein up to arrow.

When the patient returns in 4 to 8 weeks, the test site or limited treatment area is compared with pretreatment photographs. Any side effects such as matting and pigmentation can be explained to the patient. Reasonable time intervals for clearance of treated vessels can be reinforced. At each session, all sites treated are noted in anatomic diagrams in the chart.

TREATMENT PLAN

With increasing experience and recognition of common patterns, injection sites are based on known patterns of reflux. For example, reticular veins usually feed a group of telangiectasias on the lateral thigh from a varicose lateral subdermic venous system. During the treatment session, treatment would begin with reticular veins from which reflux is suspected to arise and would proceed along the course of the reticular vein, with injections every 3–4 cm along the feeder.

Our typical treatment regimen is to foam or agitate STS at 0.1 to 0.2% using a ratio of one part sclerosant to four parts air. This foam mixture is injected into reticular veins that are directly connected to visible telangiectasias (see Figure 13.2). It is not advisable to treat every reticular vein of the thigh; only those reticular veins visibly connected to a telangiectatic web should be targeted.

As sclerosing solution/foam flows away from the point of injection, it is clearly seen for a distance of several centimeters before it is diluted by blood and becomes less potent.

When injecting a reticular vein, the sclerosing foam is sometimes seen flowing into the telangiectasia. When this is observed, the telangiectasias do not need to be injected directly. Similarly, sclerosing solution injected into a telangiectasia may be seen flowing into the feeder vein, but reticular veins usually still need to be injected directly, because it

is difficult to deliver an effective volume and concentration of sclerosant foam to the reticular vein indirectly.

TECHNIQUE

The technique used for injection of small reticular feeder veins is the direct cannulation technique used for the injection of larger, deeper reticular veins and varicose veins.

The patient is recumbent in a position that allows convenient access to the reticular veins to be treated. A 3-cc syringe with a 27 or 30 gauge is used, and the needle is bent to an angle of 10 to 30 degrees to facilitate cannulation of the vein (see Figure 13.3). The syringe is held in the dominant hand, which rests on the patient's leg, and the needle is advanced at a shallow angle through the skin and into the reticular vein. When the physician feels the typical "pop-through" sensation of piercing the vein, the plunger is pulled back gently until blood return is seen in the transparent plastic hub. Typically one injects up to 2 cc of foamed sclerosant and then massages the solution toward any associated telangiectasias. Injection must stop immediately if any signs of leakage occur or if a bleb or bruising is noted. As the needle is withdrawn, pressure is applied immediately either with cotton ball then tape, or compression bandaging.

The cannulation of a reticular vein can be quite difficult at times, because reticular veins can go into spasm, and may virtually disappear during an attempt at cannulation. It is best to avoid applying alcohol to the skin just prior to treatment as the evaporative cooling may cause venospasm of the reticular vein. Any resistance to injection means the needle tip is not inside the vein. When this happens, the injection should be terminated immediately and the needle withdrawn. Failed cannulation will rapidly produce a bruise at the site of injection.

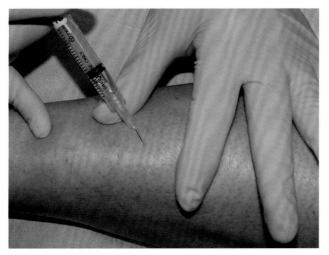

Figure 13.3 The position of the syringe with needle bend in the hands of the injecting physician for injecting reticular and telangiectatic veins. This shows the injection of 72% glycerine into telangiectasias. Some blanching is seen.

syringes. We have not yet seen allergic reactions to STS in over 500,000 injections since switching to latex-free syringes in 1994.

PATIENT PREPARATION

The patient is recumbent in a position that allows convenient access to the telangiectasias to be treated. If available, a motorized table with height adjustment will facilitate easy access to all regions of the leg. Use of double polarized lighting (InVu Vantage, Syris Scientific, Grey, ME) has also proven to be helpful (see Figure 13.4). The neck and back position of the treating physician must be optimal to avoid injury over the long term to the physician. Indirect lighting is best, as harsh halogen surgical lights bleach out reticular veins and some telangiectasias.

EQUIPMENT

- Cotton balls soaked with 70% isopropyl alcohol
- Protective gloves
- 1-cc or 3-cc disposable syringes
- 3-way intravenous stopcock for agitation/foaming
- 30-gauge 1/2-inch disposable transparent hub needles
- Cotton balls or foam pads for compression
- Hypoallergenic tape (synthetic silk or paper)
- Topical nitroglycerine ointment (2%)
- Sclerosing solutions (stored separately from other injectables in the clinic)
- Magnifying loupes or lenses (2–3×)

The choice of syringe is a personal one. Some phlebologists believe that a 3-cc syringe allows optimal control. Others hold that a 1-cc syringe is preferable because the smaller plunger offers reduced plunger friction and allows smoother control with less jerkiness, but higher pressures may induce quicker vessel rupture. It is worth the effort to try a variety of syringes, as there is a marked difference in plunger friction among different types of syringes and among syringes from different manufacturers.

With use of STS, it is recommended to use latex-free syringes. In high enough concentration, STS (0.5% and greater) will dissolve the rubber from the plunger, thereby releasing rubber and rubber products into solution. There is a relatively high and increasing incidence of latex allergy in the general population.[6] Theoretically the risk of a severe allergic reaction may be increased with latex-containing

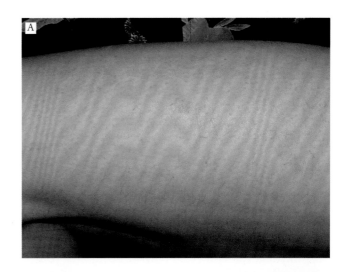

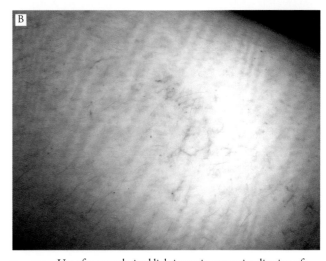

Figure 13.4 Use of cross-polarized lighting to increase visualization of telangiectasias. A) Thigh telangiectasias as seen with conventional light. B) Group of telangiectasias in center of thigh as visualized using cross-polarized light (InVu Vantage, Syris Scientific, Grey, ME).

A syringe of sclerosant is prepared with a 30-gauge needle that has been bent to an angle of 10 to 30 degrees with the bevel up. The needle is placed flat on the skin so that the needle is parallel to the skin surface. The nondominant hand plays an important role in stabilization of the syringe. The injecting hand rests on the patient's leg with the fourth and fifth finger providing stabilization in a fixed position to facilitate controlled penetration of the vessel. The non-dominant hand is used to stretch the skin around the needle and may offer additional support for the syringe. The firmly supported needle is then moved slowly 1 to 2 mm forward, piercing the top of the tiny vein just sufficiently to allow infusion of solution with the most minimal pressure on the plunger.

CANNULATION OF THE VESSEL

The technique requires a gentle, precise touch, but with practice the beveled tip of the 30-gauge (0.3-mm diameter) needle may be used to cannulate vessels as small as 0.1 mm. The bevel of the needle usually can be seen within the lumen of the telangiectasias with use of 1.75 to 2× magnification. Needles smaller than 30 gauge or longer than ½ inch are difficult to use because they tend to veer off course when advanced through the skin. Depending on the patient's skin type, needles can become dull rather quickly, and should be replaced whenever resistance to skin puncture is noted. This typically occurs within three to 10 punctures. In the United States, one must follow OSHA blood-borne pathogen guidelines when changing needles.

Once the needle tip is seen in the lumen of the vessel, a tiny bolus of air (<0.05 cc) may be injected to help demonstrate that the needle is within the vein. With the use of glycerine as a sclerosant we often utilize an air block technique, in which a small bolus of air (0.1 cc) is used to clear the arborizing vessels of blood before the sclerosing solution is infused. This is much smaller than previously described.[7]

Concentrations of sclerosants used for telangiectasias are less than those used for reticular veins. Typically the solutions are not foamed. We now prefer to use 72% glycerine for the telangiectasias of a telangiectatic web–reticular vein complex (see Table 13.1). When sclerosing solutions are injected into telangiectasia, blood usually is flushed out of the vessel ahead of the solution, thus the sclerosant usually is not diluted at all. For this reason, the initial treatment of telangiectatic webs begins with the minimal effective concentration of sclerosant.[8] At the next visit, the same concentration is used if sclerosis was effective, and a higher concentration is used if sclerosis was ineffective.

The injection of telangiectasias is performed very slowly, with minimal pressure on the syringe. A few drops of sclerosant are sufficient to fill the vein and maintain contact with the vessel wall for 10 to 15 seconds. The amount infused is approximately 0.1 cc to 0.2 cc per site, and this often is sufficient to produce blanching in a radius of 2 cm from the site of injection. Rapid flushing of the vessels with larger volumes of sclerosant or with higher pressures leads to problems with extravasation, tissue necrosis, and ulceration, as well as an increased incidence of telangiectatic matting and of hyperpigmentation.[9,10]

For glycerine injection, the telangiectasias are filled with solution and the injection is stopped. Glycerine has the least risk of causing subsequent matting or pigmentation.[11] When detergent sclerosants are used, small volumes and small areas of short-duration blanching are still important to minimize side effects such as telangiectatic matting. Sometimes there is no blanching at the site of injection, but the sclerosing solution flows easily through the telangiectasia or can even be seen flowing through adjacent telangiectasias or reticular veins several centimeters away from the injection site. In this case the injection is stopped after no more than 0.5 cc of sclerosant has been injected. Immediately after injection, the treated area is gently massaged in the desired direction of further spread of sclerosant. We strongly recommend against the use of hypertonic saline as it is painful and highly ulcerogenic.

Table 13.1 SCLEROSANT CONCENTRATIONS FOR TELANGIECTASIA AND RETICULAR VEINS

SIZE OF VESSEL	MINIMUM EFFECTIVE CONCENTRATION	MAX CONCENTRATION	FOAMED	SCLEROSANT
Reticular 1–3 mm	0.1%	0.25%	Yes	Sodium tetradecyl sulfate (STS)
Reticular 1–3 mm	0.25%	0.5%	Yes	Polidocanol (Laureth-9)
Telangiectasias 0.2–1 mm	0.2%	0.5%	No	Polidocanol (Laureth-9)
Telangiectasias 0.2–1 mm	0.1%	0.2%	No	STS
Telangiectasias 0.2–1 mm	72% in water	Same	No	Glycerine 72%
Telangiectasias 0.2–1 mm	10% hypertonic saline and 25% dextrose	Same	No	SclerodexTM

To minimize skin necrosis, extravasation must be avoided, although the risks are minimized with glycerine or very low doses of liquid 0.1% STS.[12] If there is resistance to the flow of sclerosant, or if a bleb begins to form at the injection site, the injection must be stopped immediately. Extravasation of low concentrations of polidocanol does not cause tissue necrosis, but significant extravasation of higher concentration (>0.1%) STS or of hypertonic saline will cause necrosis and ulceration.[13] A randomized study in animals found the incidence of ulceration to be greater when attempts were made to dilute the extravasated sclerosant by the injection of normal saline into the area.[14] Vigorous massage of any blebs is recommended to minimize the chance of necrosis. Application of 2% nitroglycerine paste if bone white blanching is observed is used to cause immediate vasodilatation and minimize risks of small areas of necrosis.

COMPRESSION

Compression will speed vessel clearance and reduce staining from any vessel that protrudes above the surface of the skin. After treatment of telangiectasias, compression is provided by ready-to-wear gradient compression hose (15–20 mm Hg) placed over cotton balls secured with tape at the sites of injection. If larger reticular veins (>3 mm) are treated at the same session, then compression consists of Class I 20–30 mm Hg compression. Some authorities recommend that continuous compression be applied for as long as the patient will tolerate it (usually 1–3 days). Then the stockings are removed and the cotton balls discarded; the patient bathes and reapplies his or her stockings, wearing them for the next two weeks except when bathing and sleeping. We have the patient remove both stockings and cotton balls at bedtime of the day of treatment. Compression hose are then worn daily for 2 weeks except when bathing and sleeping. Patients are encouraged to walk, and the only restrictions on activity are those such as heavy weightlifting that result in sustained forceful muscular contraction and venous pressure elevation.

TREATMENT INTERVALS

Physician and patient preferences play a large role in determining treatment intervals. New areas may be treated at any time, but retreatment of the same areas should be deferred for several weeks, because the immediate post-treatment appearance of telangiectasias is either bruising, matting, or pigmentation; this will ultimately clear after 2 to 4 weeks. Patients often are anxious to speed their course of treatment, but allowing a longer time between treatment sessions may minimize the number of sessions needed. We strongly recommend waiting as long as 4 to 8 weeks between treatments.

The number of treatments needed depends on the extent of the problem and the extent of areas treated at each session. Some patients are highly responsive to treatment and can be treated with weak sclerosants in only a few sessions. Others are highly resistant and may require more sessions and stronger sclerosants. The younger the patient the better and faster the response.

After the initial series of treatments, a rest period of 4 to 6 months will allow time for pigmentation and matting to clear, and for any remaining reticular veins to establish new routes of reflux or drainage. Approximately 80% of patients will clear to their satisfaction during the first course of treatment. Any remaining telangiectatic webs or new telangiectasias are then reassessed to determine the best approach for another round of treatment.

POOR RESPONSE TO TREATMENT

When patients have had a poor response to the initial series of treatments, the original diagnosis must always be called into question. Unsuspected sources of reflux can include truncal varices, incompetent perforating veins, and unrecognized reticular vessels. If no untreated source of reflux can be identified, the patient must be carefully questioned about proper compliance with compression. Many patients abandon compression immediately after sclerotherapy, and this can lead to treatment failures. The concentration and volume of sclerosant used should also be reexamined. It is not uncommon to find that the concentrations selected were ineffective for the size and type of vessel being treated.

SUMMARY

When based on a correct diagnosis and an appropriate treatment plan, sclerotherapy is a highly effective method of treatment for telangiectasias. Formulating an effective treatment plan requires a detailed knowledge of venous anatomy, a thorough understanding of the principles and patterns of reflux, and intimate familiarity with a range of volumes and concentrations of sclerosing solutions. The results obtained depend greatly on the experience of the clinician, but with care and with attention to detail, clearing rates of 90% can be achieved in most patients. Sufficient time must be allowed between treatments.

Patient satisfaction is enhanced through education and informed consent, photographic documentation, and a measured approach to treatment. When the basic principles of diagnosis and treatment are followed meticulously, a successful outcome is highly likely. It is important to educate the patient that telangiectasias may be a lifelong problem. Development of new veins within a few years after successful treatment does not constitute treatment failure; rather, it demonstrates the chronicity of venous insufficiency.

REFERENCES

1. Weiss RA, Weiss MA. Resolution of pain associated with varicose and telangiectatic leg veins after compression sclerotherapy, *J Dermatol Surg Onc.* 1990. *16*: 333–336.
2. Weiss RA, Heagle CR, Raymond-Martimbeau P. The Bulletin of the North American Society of Phlebology: Insurance Advisory Committee Report, *J Dermatol Surg Onc.* 1992. *18*: 609–616.
3. Weiss RA, Weiss MA. Doppler ultrasound findings in reticular veins of the thigh subdermic lateral venous system and implications for sclerotherapy, *J Dermatol Surg Onc.* 1993. *19*(10): 947–951.
4. Somjen GM, Ziegenbein R, Johnston AH, Royle JP. Anatomical examination of leg telangiectases with duplex scanning [see comments], *J Dermatol Surg Onc.* 1993. *19*(10): 940–945.
5. Bihari I, Muranyi A, Bihari P. Laser-doppler examination shows high flow in some common telangiectasias of the lower limb, *Dermatol Surg.* 2005. *31*(4): 388–390.
6. Cheng L, Lee D. Review of latex allergy, *J Am Board Fam Pract.* 1999. *12*(4): 285–292.
7. Bodian EL. Sclerotherapy: A personal appraisal, *J Derm Surg Onc.* 1989. *15*: 156–161.
8. Sadick NS. Sclerotherapy of varicose and telangiectatic leg veins: Minimal sclerosant concentration of hypertonic saline and its relationship to vessel diameter [see comments], *J Derm Surg Onc.* 1991. *17*(1): 65–70.
9. Weiss MA, Weiss RA. Efficacy and side effects of 0.1% sodium tetradecyl sulfate in compression sclerotherapy of telangiectasias: Comparison to 1% polidocanol and hypertonic saline, *J Derm Surg Onc.* 1991. *17*: 90–91.
10. Weiss RA, Weiss MA. Incidence of side effects in the treatment of telangiectasias by compression sclerotherapy: Hypertonic saline vs. polidocanol, *J Derm Surg Onc.* 1990. *16*: 800–804.
11. Georgiev M. Postsclerotherapy hyperpigmentations: Chromated glycerin as a screen for patients at risk (a retrospective study), *J Derm Surg Onc.* 1993. *19*: 649–652.
12. Martin DE, Goldman MP. A comparison of sclerosing agents: Clinical and histologic effects of intravascular sodium tetradecyl sulfate and chromated glycerine in the dorsal rabbit ear vein, *J Derm Surg Onc.* 1990. *16*: 18–22.
13. Duffy DM. Small vessel sclerotherapy: An overview, *Adv Dermatol.* 1988. *3*: 221–242.
14. Zimmet SE. The prevention of cutaneous necrosis following extravasation of hypertonic saline and sodium tetradecyl sulfate, *J Derm Surg Onc.* 1993. *19*: 641–646.

14.

COMPLICATIONS OF LIQUID SCLEROTHERAPY

Nisha Bunke-Paquette

INTRODUCTION

Sclerotherapy remains the gold standard of treatment for lower limb telangiectasia and reticular veins. Sclerotherapy, by definition, is the injection of a chemical irritant into a vein to produce inflammation, eventual fibrosis, and obliteration of the lumen. The cellular mechanisms that occur in vein sclerosis involve endothelial swelling with desquamation, deposition of a mixed thrombus, connective organization, and fibrosis.[1] While endothelial cell injury and inflammation are necessary to effectuate sclerosis, these responses can also be causation for undesirable side effects. Most adverse events are minor and inconsequential, such as local injection site pain, urticaria, itching, erythema, and bruising.[2,3] Other common but usually self-limiting responses include cutaneous hyperpigmentation (HP) and telangiectatic matting (TM). Cutaneous necrosis is infrequent but can be severe and extensive. Systemic life-threatening reactions and fatal anaphylaxis have been reported. As with the use of any medication, other complications such as cardiotoxicity have been attributed to the use of sclerosants but are rare and unlikely.[4] Thrombotic complications are more common with foam sclerotherapy. The use of a sclerosant in foam form, where the sclerosing power is increased and there is the added ability to migrate, carries its own set of unique complications, which are described elsewhere in this text. This chapter describes the common and significant adverse events pertaining to liquid sclerotherapy.

GENERAL CONSIDERATIONS

There are two basic principles that the phlebologist should consider in the approach to sclerotherapy of leg veins. These were described by Ouvry in 1982 and continue to be affirmed by various authors: (1) treat the most proximal source of venous reflux first, and (2) use the lowest effective concentration of the sclerosant.[5] The use of higher sclerosant concentrations is associated with more side effects.[6] Additionally, failure to recognize and treat underlying venous insufficiency can result in suboptimal results.

As a result, sclerotherapy should be performed by trained clinicians who have a knowledge of the pharmacology and side effects of sclerosing medications and the ability to recognize the presence of underlying venous insufficiency and the need for further ultrasound evaluation.

PRETREATMENT ASSESSMENT

PATIENT HISTORY

A thorough medical history and clinical examination will help to identify patients who require further evaluation with ultrasonography, and risk stratification for adverse events.

A detailed history should be obtained from each patient with particular attention to potential risk factors for adverse events such as their vascular history, allergy profile, medication list, history of prior vein treatment, and treatment failures. A personal and/or family history of deep venous thrombosis and spontaneous thrombophlebitis may indicate a hypercoagulable predisposition. A history of poor response to prior treatment, or varicose vein surgery may suggest the need for ultrasonographic evaluation. Atopic individuals may be identified by a history of multiple allergies, asthma, allergies to detergents (if a detergent sclerosant is being considered) or iodine (if polyiodides are used), and repeated exposure to sclerosants.[7] Risks for complications such as pigmentation may be greater in those taking tetracycline or minocycline.[8] With sclerotherapy, aspirin, nonsteroidal anti-inflammatory drugs, and other blood-thinning medications can cause increased capillary leakage and subsequent pigmentation.[9] Hormonal medications that increase the risk of thrombotic events such as ovulatory agents, oral contraceptives, estrogens, and selective estrogen receptor modulators (SERMs) should be addressed.

Clinical Examination

The clinical assessment should be done with the patient standing so as to maximally dilate leg veins. Documentation should be made of the type and location of telangiectatic and reticular veins. Since sclerosant selection and concentration is dependent on vessel size, the type of abnormal veins should be noted: (1) telangiectatic matting or telangiectasias up to 1 mm, (2) venulectasias (1–2 mm), (3) reticular veins (2–4 mm) and (4) presence of varicose veins (greater than 3 mm).[10] The use of vein-imaging devices such as a fiber optic vein transilluminator or near-infrared imaging device may help identify reticular or "feeder veins" that are not readily visible with the naked eye (see Figure 14.1). Particular note should be made of the anatomical location and distribution of telangiectasias and reticular veins, because anatomical location may be suggestive of underlying venous insufficiency. Telangiectasias in the lateral thighs are often accompanied by reticular veins from the lateral plexus. Fan-shaped intradermal telangiectases on the medial or lateral malleoli, known as corona phlebectasia, can be associated with underlying saphenous or perforator insufficiency.[11] Other identifiers to indicate saphenous vein insufficiency may be lacking. Engelhorn reported that 46% of women (125 out of 269) with spider veins had underlying venous insufficiency of either the great or small saphenous veins.[12]

INJECTION SITE REACTIONS

Local injection site reactions are common to all sclerosants and tend to be mild, transient, and somewhat expected. They include localized injection site pain, hematoma, urticaria, pruritis, erythema, and warmth (see Figure 14.2).[3] Polidocanol (POL), which has an anesthetic property, is generally described as well tolerated.[13–15] However, urticaria

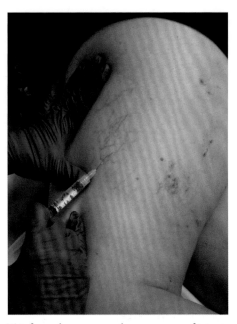

Figure 14.2 This figure demonstrates the appearance of injection-site urticaria immediately following intravenous injection of 0.5% POL. It was associated with localized pruritis.

may be more prevalent with POL. Urticaria is a result of local histamine release occurring with vascular injury. This is transient, and associated itching is usually relieved within 30 minutes. POL analogues have been studied for effects on skin irritation and sensitization and found to produce only negligible skin irritation.[16–18]

TELANGIECTATIC MATTING

Telangiectatic matting (TM) refers to the appearance of new clusters of fine vessels within superficial layers of the dermis that typically appear 4 to 6 weeks after sclerotherapy treatment (see Figure 14.3). They appear as blanching small blood vessels with a blemish-like appearance measuring less than 0.2 mm in diameter. The most common location for TM to appear is on the inner and outer thighs, near the knees and calves.[19] TM may affect up to one-third of

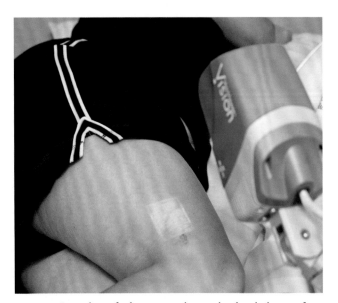

Figure 14.1 Reticular or feeder veins can be visualized with the use of a light source such as near-infrared imaging as demonstrated in this figure.

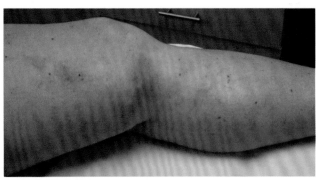

Figure 14.3 Blemish-like appearance of fine vessels attributed to TM following treatment of reticular veins. Duplex ultrasound evaluation revealed underlying insufficiency of the GSV.

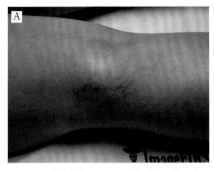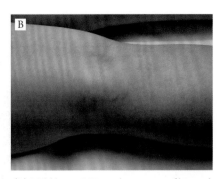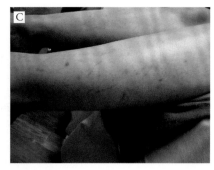

Figure 14.4 (A) Telangiectasias before sclerotherapy. (B) Mild linear HP overlying veins of larger diameter, 6 weeks following sclerotherapy with 0.5% POL. It resolved after 3 months. (C) Macular HP persisting for several months after sclerotherapy with 0.5% POL.

patients undergoing sclerotherapy,[20–22] and usually resolves spontaneously in 3 to 12 months.[21]

The development of TM is attributed to reactive inflammatory or angiogenic mechanisms and is more prevalent with high concentrations of sclerosing solution.[22] Other risk factors that have been associated with the development of TM include being overweight, female, or of a high estrogen state during treatment, and a longer duration of spider veins.[20] Weiss and Weiss found a relative risk of 3.17 (p > 0.003) for development of TM while patients were receiving exogenous estrogen.[20]

In the authors' experience, TM can be observed when underlying venous insufficiency is present; for example, TM on the inner knees can indicate underlying saphenous vein incompetence. Therefore, further investigation with duplex evaluation may be indicated in TM. Often self-resolving, TM can also be treated with lower concentration sclerotherapy or certain lasers.

SKIN HYPERPIGMENTATION

Skin hyperpigmentation (HP) refers to the brown staining of the skin following sclerotherapy that can occur as linear or macular pigmentation (see Figure 14.4, A–C). The general incidence of hyperpigmentation ranges from 10% to 30%, although persistent pigmentation lasting greater than 1 year occurs in approximately 1% of patients. The incidence of hyperpigmentation is related to both vessel size and to the sclerosing agent.[22–24] For example, hypertonic saline has higher rates of HP than POL.

Two explanations permeate medical literature regarding the pathological mechanisms of HP. HP is attributed to either direct hemosiderin deposition or post-inflammatory processes or a combination of the two. Hemosiderin deposits from hemoglobin degradation of red blood cells, enter the dermis by extravasation after rupture of treated vessels[2] or perivenulitis.[9] Histologic evidence of hemosiderin deposition, presented by Goldman et al., supports the theory of extravasation of red blood cells into the dermis following rupture of fragile vessels.[9] Therefore, vessel fragility, increased concentrations, type of solution (the pH levels of sclerosants cause varying degrees of endothelial damage), vessel size, and injection

pressure have been implicated as factors for HP, which thus may be initiated by high sclerosant concentrations in superficial and dermal veins as well as sclerosant-dependent.

Postsclerotherapy HP tends to be more common when greater amounts of intravascular coagula are present. Persistent thrombi are thought to produce a subacute "perivenulitis," which favors extravasation of red blood cells. The presence of intravascular coagulum that is persistent can cause tenderness to the patient. In our experience, extraction almost immediately relieves discomfort and expedites the resolution of hyperpigmentation. Compression stockings minimize the amount of intravascular coagulum and therefore are an important part of posttreatment care.

Additionally, untreated refluxing veins that connect to the affected area should be sought and treated. Gravitational pressure is a generally accepted risk for increased HP. Therefore, veins should be treated in a proximal to distal direction and, in cases of persistent HP, a proximal source of venous insufficiency should be investigated with duplex ultrasonography.

There is no general agreement on whether certain skin types are prone to HP. Munavalli and Weiss report more frequent HP in patients with dark skin and dark hair.[2] Figure 14.5 represents a patient who demonstrated extensive

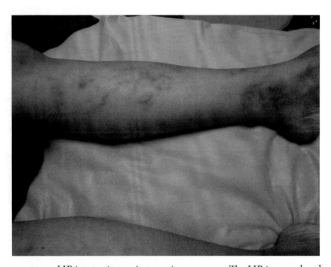

Figure 14.5 HP in a patient prior to vein treatment. The HP is not related to sclerotherapy treatment, but is likely a result of chronic inflammation from venous insufficiency.

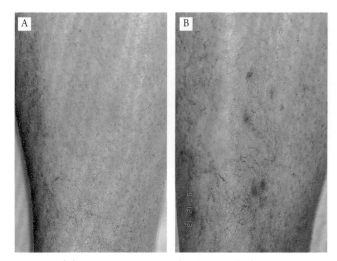

Figure 14.6 (A) Resolution 2 months after the second of two treatments with the Q-switched ruby laser at 8.0 J/cm². (B) Pigmentation from sclerotherapy lasting over 1 year. (Courtesy David Duffy, MD; from Goldman MP, Weiss RA, Bergan JJ, eds. *Varicose veins and telangiectasias: Diagnosis and treatment.* St Louis. MO: Quality Medical Publishing. 1999.)

linear HP along reticular veins in the absence of any type of vein treatment.

The majority of HP will resolve spontaneously in 1 year. Exfoliation by trichloroacetic acid, phenolic peeling agents, and pumice stone have been described with variable results. Treatment with intense pulsed light (IPL) has shown good results (Figure 14.6).[24]

CUTANEOUS NECROSIS

Cutaneous necrosis most commonly presents as an ulceration but can result in extensive loss of tissue (Figures 14.7). It can occur as far out as weeks after the initial insult, and may be associated with pain, localized inflammation, and edema. Etiologic explanations include (1) extravasation of the sclerosant into perivascular tissue, (2) injection into a dermal arteriole or an arteriole feeding into a telangiectatic or varicose veins, or (3) reactive vasospasm of the vessel.[25]

Evidence tends to favor theories of nonextravasation, because in many cases intravenous injection was verified. Miyake et al. showed that vessel size, sclerosant viscosity and strength not extravasation, play a role in cutaneous ulceration.[26]

Bergan et al. proposed a theory of distribution of the sclerosant into the arterial arborization.[27] Based on this theory, the distribution of sclerosant into the arterial tree could result in extensive tissue necrosis (Figure 14.8).

Additionally, Duffy intentionally extravasated 3% POL into a human volunteer's arm, which did not cause ulceration.[18] Schuller-Petrovic demonstrated that subcutaneous injections of POL strengths 0.5%–3% into a rabbit ear did not result in extravasation necrosis.[28]

MICROTHROMBI

"Microthrombi" refers to the common occurrence of palpable intravascular coagulum in a treated vessel appearing

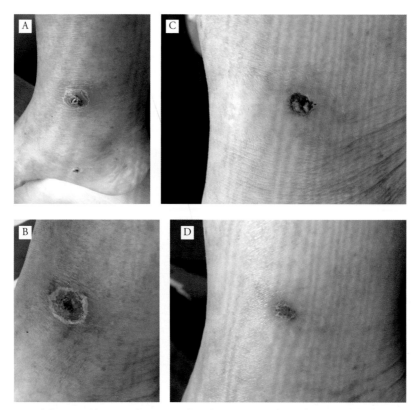

Figure 14.7 This patient documented the natural history of a necrotic skin ulcer over several months, as a result of 1% POL liquid injections on her medial malleolus. (A) 3 weeks after sclerotherapy, (B) 6 weeks, (C) 12 weeks, (D) 16 weeks.

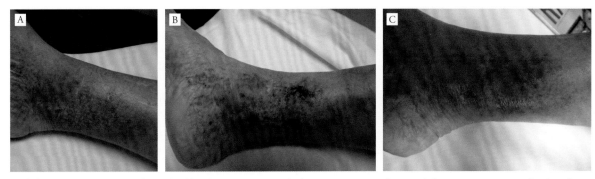

Figure 14.8 (A) Skin pigmentation and atrophie blanche in a patient with chronic venous insufficiency. (B) Cutaneous necrosis developed 3 weeks after treatment of a varicose vein with intravenous injection of 0.5% POL sclerofoam. The feeding varix was located several centimeters proximal to the affected area. The sclerofoam traveled into distal veins and filled small capillary vessels of this already compromised skin. (C) At 3 months.

1 to 6 weeks after sclerotherapy (Figure 14.9). The larger the vessel size, the more frequently intravascular coagulum occurs. The intravascular thrombus tends to remain liquefied. Persistent microthrombi can be a source of tenderness for the patient and result in SH. Persistent microthrombi should prompt evaluation for a proximal source of reflux. Evacuation of microthrombi is indicated to reduce tenderness and decrease risk of residual HP.

Microthrombi and larger volumes of intravascular coagulum can be evacuated by puncture with a 16- or 18-gauge needle (depending on the vessel size) and manually expressed. The coagulum remains highly viscous liquid and can be extracted by applying manual pressure and "milking" the vein (Figure 14.10).

In the author's experience, evacuation of intravascular coagula almost immediately reduces tenderness and inflammation. Continued use of compression is recommended, and evaluation for an underlying source of venous insufficiency may be indicated for persistent or recurrent intravascular coagulum. Microthrombi can be minimized with external compression following sclerotherapy. In the author's experience and others, microthrombi are less prevalent when patients are compliant with the use of posttreatment compression stockings.[29]

HYPERSENSITIVITY REACTIONS

ANAPHYLAXIS AND ANAPHYLACTOID RESPONSES

Most reported allergic reactions after sodium tetradecyl sulfate (STS) administration showed mild intensity.[30,31] The incidence of nonfatal allergic reactions such as hives, asthma, and anaphylactic shock are estimated at 0.3% with STS.[32] Both anaphylaxis and anaphylactoid reactions have been reported following injection of a sclerosant. They can occur at the first exposure to the sclerosant or after several innocuous treatments. As a result, the utility of a test site as the sclerosant package inserts suggest, is not practical nor will it necessarily predict an allergic reaction. In one case, a nonfatal anaphylactic reaction occurred on the second sclerotherapy treatment with STS 6 months following the initial uneventful session. The patient showed initial signs of reaction, such as tongue and lip swelling, within 20 minutes of the injection.[33] Since the risk of anaphylaxis increases with repeated exposures to the antigen, one should always be prepared for this reaction in every patient.

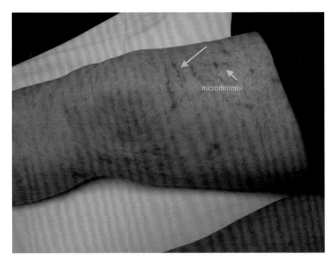

Figure 14.9 Microthrombi in treated venules and reticular veins.

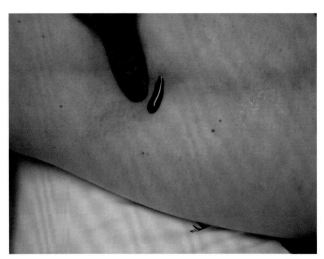

Figure 14.10 Manual evacuation of intravascular coagulum following puncture with a 16-gauge needle. The intravascular coagulum has a highly viscous, "molasses-like" appearance.

Anaphylaxis is an immunoglobulin E (IgE)-mediated mast cell–activated reaction that usually occurs within minutes of antigen exposure. A systemic reaction is caused by antigen-specific cross-linking of IgE molecules on the surface of tissue mast cells and peripheral blood basophils, which results in immediate release of potent mediators.

On occasion, this complication may occur hours to weeks after treatment.

ANAPHYLACTOID REACTION

The same chemical mediators that cause the physical manifestations of anaphylaxis produce anaphylactoid reactions. Anaphylactoid reactions are not IgE mediated and do not require previous exposure to an antigen. In one case, a 49-year-old woman developed anaphylactoid reaction after the administration of STS for varicose veins.[34] In this case report, the patient developed a generalized itch with rash and nausea prior to cardiovascular symptoms. She was promptly treated and had a full recovery.

Benzoyl alcohol[35] and carbitol[36] have been implicated as allergens in sclerosant medications. Benzoyl alcohol is a bacteriostatic agent used in many injectable pharmaceutical agents. It is found in some injectable sclerosants and in bacteriostatic water, which is often used to dilute a sclerosant to a lesser concentration. Benzoyl alcohol has been associated with toxic effects such as respiratory failure, hypotension, vasodilation, hemolysis, convulsions, hypersensitivity reactions, and death.

Carbitol is a contaminant that can be found in impure compounded sclerosants. Impurities have been found in samples of compounded POL, and Goldman has reported significant concentrations of the contaminant carbitol in samples of compounded STS.[37–39]

The following text is reprinted from *The Vein Book*, first edition by Mitchel P. Goldman.

MANIFESTATIONS OF HYPERSENSITIVITY REACTIONS

Systemic reactions caused by sclerotherapy treatment occur very rarely. Anaphylaxis is a systemic hypersensitivity response caused by exposure or, more commonly, reexposure to a sensitizing substance. Anaphylaxis is usually an IgE-mediated, mast cell–activated reaction that occurs most often within minutes of antigen exposure. Other classes of immunoglobulin such as IgG also may produce anaphylaxis. Since the risk of anaphylaxis increases with repeated exposures to the antigen, one should always be prepared for this reaction in every patient.

The principal manifestations of anaphylaxis occur in areas where mast cell concentrations are highest: skin, lungs, and gastrointestinal (GI) tract. Histamine release is responsible for the clinical manifestations of this reaction. Although urticaria and abdominal pain are common, the three principal manifestations of anaphylaxis are airway edema, bronchospasm, and vascular collapse. Urticaria alone does not constitute anaphylaxis and should not be treated as such because of the potential side effects of treatment with epinephrine, especially in older patients.

The signs and symptoms of anaphylaxis initially may be subtle and often include anxiety, itching, sneezing, coughing, urticaria, and angioedema. Wheezing may be accompanied by hoarseness of the voice and vomiting. Shortly after these presenting signs, breathing becomes more difficult, and the patient usually collapses from cardiovascular failure resulting from systemic vasodilation. One helpful clue in distinguishing between anaphylaxis and vasovagal reactions is heart rate. Sinus tachycardia is almost always present in a patient with anaphylaxis, whereas bradycardia or cardiac rhythm disturbances are commonplace in vasovagal reactions.

The recommended treatment is epinephrine, 0.2 to 0.5 ml 1:1000 subcutaneously. This can be repeated three or four times at 5- to 15-minute intervals to maintain a systolic blood pressure above 90 to 100 mm Hg. This should be followed with establishment of an intravenous (IV) line of 0.9% sodium chloride solution. Diphenhydramine hydrochloride, 50 mg, is given next along with cimetidine, 300 mg; both the IV solution and oxygen are given at 4 to 6 L/min. An endotracheal tube or tracheotomy is necessary for laryngeal obstruction. For asthma or wheezing, IV theophylline, 4 to 6 mg/kg, is infused over 15 minutes. At this point it is appropriate to transfer the patient to the hospital. Methylprednisolone sodium succinate, 60 mg, is given intravenously and repeated every 6 hours for four doses. Corticosteroids are not an emergency medication because their effect appears only after 1 to 3 hours. They are given to prevent the recurrence of symptoms 3 to 8 hours after the initial event. The patient should be hospitalized overnight for observation.

SODIUM MORRHUATE

Although touted by the manufacturer as "the natural sclerosing agent," sodium morrhuate causes a variety of allergic reactions, ranging from mild erythema with pruritus to generalized urticaria to GI disturbances with abdominal pain and diarrhea to anaphylaxis. It has been estimated that "unfavorable reactions" from the treatment of varicose leg veins occur in 3% of patients.[40] The reason for the high number of allergic reactions with this product may be related to the inability to remove all the fish proteins present in sodium morrhuate. In fact, 20.8% of the fatty acid composition of the solution is unknown.

Many cases of anaphylaxis have occurred within a few minutes after injection or more commonly when therapy is reinstituted after a few weeks. Most of these cases occurred before 1950. Rarely, anaphylaxis has resulted in fatalities, many of which have not been reported in the medical literature. Bronchospasm developed in one patient being treated with the twelfth injection under anesthesia. This responded readily to antihistamine and epinephrine. The patient was subsequently treated with STS without an adverse reaction.[41]

Prolonged dysrhythmia requiring placement of a permanent pacemaker has been reported in two cases.[42] This complication has been attributed to a direct cardiotoxic effect of sodium morrhuate.

ETHANOLAMINE OLEATE

Ethanolamine oleate (Ethamolin) is a synthetic mixture of ethanolamine and oleic acid with an empirical formula of $C_{20}H_{41}NO_3$. The minimal lethal IV dose in rabbits is 130 mg/kg. The oleic acid component is responsible for the inflammatory action. Oleic acid also may activate coagulation in vitro by release of tissue factor and Hageman factor. Ethanolamine oleate is thought to have a lesser risk of causing allergic reactions compared with sodium morrhuate or STS. However, pulmonary toxicity and allergic reactions have been associated with this sclerosing agent.

The product manufacturer has reported anaphylactic shock after injection in three cases (product information [1989] from Glaxo Pharmaceuticals, Research Triangle Park, NC). Another case of a nearly fatal anaphylactic reaction during the fourth treatment of varicose leg veins with 1 ml of solution also has been reported.[43] In one additional case a fatal reaction occurred in a man with a known allergic disposition (product information [1989] from Glaxo Pharmaceuticals, Research Triangle Park, NC). Another episode of a fatal anaphylactic reaction occurred in a woman having her third series of injections. This represented one reaction in 200 patients from that author's practice. Generalized urticaria occurred in approximately one in 400 patients; this symptom responded rapidly to an antihistamine.[44]

SODIUM TETRADECYL SULFATE

A synthetic detergent developed in the 1940s, STS has been used throughout the world as a sclerosing solution. A comprehensive review of the medical literature (in multiple specialties and languages) until 1987 disclosed a total of forty-seven cases of nonfatal allergic reactions in a review of 14,404 treated patients; this included six case reports.[45] A separate review of treatment in 187 patients with 2,249 injections disclosed no evidence of allergic or systemic reactions.[46] An additional report of 5,341 injections given to an unknown number of patients found "no unfavorable reaction."[47] Fegan[48] has reviewed his experience with STS in 16,000 patients. He reported fifteen cases of "serum sickness, with hot, stinging pain in the skin, and an erythematous rash developing 30 to 90 minutes after injection." These patients subsequently underwent additional

uneventful treatment with STS after premedication with antihistamines. In ten additional patients, "mild anaphylaxis" developed that required treatment with an injection of epinephrine. If one were to combine only those reviews of over 1,000 patients, the incidence of nonfatal allergic reactions would be approximately 0.3%.

The product manufacturer notes two fatalities associated with the use of STS, both from the sclerotherapy procedure itself and not specifically related to STS. One fatality occurred in a patient who was receiving an antiovulatory agent. Another death (fatal pulmonary embolism) was reported in a 36-year-old woman who was not taking oral contraceptives. Wyeth-Ayerst also was required to include in its product insert the deaths of two additional patients who were suspected of dying of anaphylactic shock after sclerotherapy treatment with STS (Mark Coyne, R.Ph., personal communication, Wyeth-Ayerst Pharmaceuticals, August 19, 1998). The company did not have details of the two cases except that one patient had a medical history of asthma. Four deaths attributed to anaphylactoid reactions were reported to the Committee on Safety of Medicines for the United Kingdom between 1963 and 1988, with twenty-two nonfatal allergic reactions such as urticaria noted over the same period.[49]

A fatality has been reported after a test dose of 0.5 ml of STS 0.5% was given to a 64-year-old woman.[50] An autopsy performed by the Hennipin County, Minnesota, coroner's office revealed no obvious cause of death. Subsequently, mast cell tryptase studies were performed on blood collected approximately 1 hour after the reaction while the patient was receiving life support. A normal tryptase level is less than 5 ng/ml; in experimental anaphylactic reactions induced in the laboratory, levels up to 80 ng/ml have been observed. In this patient the levels were extremely high at 6,000 ng/ml, suggesting that an anaphylactoid reaction had caused her death. Unfortunately, tryptase levels are experimental at this time, and it is unclear how such a high level could be obtained. Therefore it is also unclear whether fatal anaphylaxis is a significant possibility with STS.

Since all reported cases of allergic reactions are of the IgE-mediated immediate hypersensitivity type, it is recommended that patients remain in or near the office for 30 minutes after sclerotherapy when STS is used. However, allergic reactions also may develop hours or days after the procedure. Therefore patients should be warned about the possibility of allergic reactions and how to obtain care should a reaction occur. In a review of 2,300 patients treated over 16 years, four cases of allergic reactions were reported (0.17% incidence).[51] Reactions in this study were described as periorbital swelling in one patient and urticaria in three. All reactions were easily treated with oral antihistamines. It is of interest that French phlebologists have advocated a 3-days-before and 3-days-after treatment course with an antihistamine. P. Flurie noted no episodes of allergic reactions in 500 patients treated in this manner.[51]

In a 2-year prospective study of 2,665 patients treated with STS by Paul Thibault,[52] there were four cases of anaphylactoid reactions (0.15%). These occurred 10 to 30 minutes after injection of 3% solution, with patients having facial flushing, urticaria, dizziness, tachycardia, shortness of breath, and finally GI symptoms of nausea, vomiting, and abdominal pain. All four patients responded well to a subcutaneous injection of 0.5 ml of 1:1000 epinephrine followed by promethazine HCL 25 to 50 mg intramuscularly. Urticaria occurred in an additional two patients (0.07%).

Between August 1985 and January 1990, thirty-seven reports of adverse reactions to STS, of which five cases of suspected anaphylaxis and two cases of asthma induced by injection, were reported to the Drug Experience Monitoring Program of the Food and Drug Administration (FDA). One of the cases of anaphylaxis resulted in the death previously discussed. After a detailed review it is unclear to us whether anaphylaxis indeed occurred in every reported case.

The reports of the Clinical Drug Safety Surveillance Group of Wyeth-Ayerst Laboratories are compiled from voluntary reporting to the manufacturer or the FDA, or both. The following are summaries of those reports: January to July 1991 disclosed one episode of erythema multiforme; one episode of acute respiratory distress syndrome (ARDS); one episode of fever, lymphadenopathy, and rash; and three episodes of abdominal pain, nausea, vomiting, and diarrhea. The case report of erythema multiforme was reported in a woman after her thirteenth sclerotherapy treatment. Pruritus developed the morning after the last injection, with a generalized eruption beginning on the legs 4 days later. This was followed by fever the following day. A rapid tapering course of oral prednisone was given, with complete resolution of the rash in 2 weeks.

From September 1991 to November 1992 there were five reports of urticaria and one episode of ARDS. From December 1992 to September 1993 there was only one case of a maculopapular rash. In short, anaphylaxis has been reported, with rare fatal reactions. From September 1993 through October 1994 there was one case of angioedema, and generalized weakness was reported in one patient after receiving 10 ml of 3% STS. From November 1994 through January 1996 there was one case of anaphylaxis. From January 1996 through December 1996, there was one case of allergic vasculitis. From November 1997 through October 1999 there were three cases of urticaria and four cases of nonspecific hypersensitivity reactions. These reactions voluntarily reported to Wyeth-Ayerst occurred with approximately 500,000 2-ml ampoules of 1% and 3% being sold yearly within the United States. Thus the incidence of adverse reactions is rare. (All information regarding adverse reactions from Sotradecol was provided by Paul Minicozzi, Ph.D., Wyeth-Ayerst Laboratories, through yearly correspondence.)

A similar low experience with adverse reactions was reported by STD Pharmaceuticals, the manufacturers of STS (correspondence from Robert Gardiner, Hereford, UK, March 15, 1995, and the Adverse Drug Reaction Information Tracking Product Analysis from the Medicines Control Agency of Great Britain). The adverse drug reaction reported in the United Kingdom between 1963 and 1993 was one nonspecific allergic reaction, two cases of anaphylactic shock, six cases of gastrointestinal disorder, two cases of bronchospasm, four patients with a nonspecific cutaneous eruption, and two patients with urticaria. This summary comprised 30 years, during which time an estimated 7,200,000 ml of STD 1% and 3% was sold within the United Kingdom.

The most common systemic reaction consists of transient low-grade fever and chills lasting up to 24 hours after treatment. This has also been noted in one of our patients. Of note is that three patients with allergic systemic reactions to monoethanolamine oleate had no evidence of allergy to STS.

With any sclerosing solution, reactions can occur that are not allergic in nature but represent the effect of the sclerosing solution on the vascular system. One such reaction is hemolysis, which occurs through lysis of red blood cells that are present in the treated vein. A hemolytic reaction occurred in five patients in a series of more than 900 patients with injection of more than 8 ml of STS 3%. Like a similar reaction that occurred with ethanolamine oleate, patients were described as "feeling generally unwell and shivery, with aching in the loins and passage of red-brown urine. All rapidly recovered with bed rest and were perfectly normal the next day." Injections of less than 8 ml per treatment session did not result in this reaction.

Although the lethal dose in humans has never been reported, the IV median lethal dose (LD_{50}) in mice is 90 mg/kg.[53] In our practice, it is not uncommon for patients to be treated with up to 30 ml of 0.5% STS. We have not observed an adverse reaction from this dose of STS.

My experience in over 20 years in an estimated 20,000 patients is that no patient has developed a serious allergic reaction from the use of STS. Because STS from various sources may have a variable purity, it appears possible that allergic reactions may occur from the impurities such as carbitol and not STS itself.[54] This may explain the decreased reported incidence of allergic reactions with the use of Fibrovein (STD Pharmaceuticals) as compared with Sotradecol (Wyeth-Ayerst) and/or Trombovar (Omega Laboratories, Montreal, Canada). Recently, Sotradecol has been approved for manufacture and sale by Bioniche Life Sciences (Inverin Co. Galway, Ireland). Bioniche claims to have a different method for producing STS that does not involve distillation and thus contains no carbitol. The benefits of this "new" Sotradecol are unknown at the time of this writing.

POLIDOCANOL

Allergic reactions to POL also are quite rare and have been reported in only four patients in a review of the world's literature up to 1987, with an estimated incidence of 0.01%.[45] However, since 1987 rare allergic reactions have been reported, including a case of nonfatal anaphylactic shock to 1 ml of POL 2% injected into a varicose vein during the fourth treatment session.

Guex[55] reported seven cases of minor general urticaria in nearly 11,000 patients treated over 12 years. These patients cleared completely in 1 to 2 days with antihistamine and topical corticosteroid therapy, with one patient requiring systemic corticosteroids. Kreussler GmbH, the product manufacturer in Germany, has documented thirty-five cases of suspected sensitivity from 1987 to 1993 (personal correspondence, January 1994). Of these reports, most were either vasovagal events or unproved allergic reactions. Nine patients were given repeat challenges with POL, with only three demonstrating an allergic reaction (urticaria or erythematous dermatitis). One patient died of anaphylactic shock 5 minutes after injection with 1 ml despite maximal intervention. In 1994, Kreussler reported two patients with urticaria. In 1995, two additional patients were reported with urticaria, two with bronchospasm, and one with angioedema. In 1996, there were four reports of urticaria, two of anaphylactoid reactions, one with angioedema, one with pruritus, and one with contact allergy. Therefore POL is *not* free from allergy, and, as with all sclerosing solutions, physicians must be prepared to evaluate and treat patients who have an allergic reaction to the sclerosing solution.

A detailed account of three serious cases of anaphylaxis was reported from the Netherlands.[56] These patients were anaphylactic within 15 minutes after injection of POL. Two of them received the drug for the first time. One patient, a 70-year-old woman with a complicated medical history of two heart operations, two cerebrovascular accidents, and hyperthyroidism, was successfully resuscitated after cardiac arrest. She was receiving multiple medications, including digoxin, carbimazole, captopril, furosemide, mebeverine, and acenocoumarol. She was treated without complications four previous times with POL. The second patient showed signs of ARDS after being treated with epinephrine and systemic methylprednisolone for shock. The third patient developed urticaria, dyspnea, paresthesia, headache, and chest pain with electrocardiographic (ECG) findings of cardiac ischemia. No further studies were performed on these patients.

The Australian Polidocanol Open Clinical Trial at 2 years, with over 8,000 treated patients, reported nine local urticarial reactions and three generalized reactions, with two patients developing a rash, for a frequency of approximately 0.2%. There were no cases of anaphylaxis.[30] After an additional 8,804 patients were evaluated, an additional three patients developed urticaria, again without any additional significant adverse sequelae.[57] A 5-year experience in 500 patients treated with POL 3% reported five cases of allergic reaction (1% incidence); one patient had nonfatal anaphylactic shock, with the other patients experiencing urticaria.[58]

Two of 689 sequential patients were reported who developed an immediate-type hypersensitivity reaction with systemic pruritus and urticaria.[59] This represented an incidence of 0.3% in their patient population and 0.91%

for the "true" population. These two reactions occurred without prior exposure to POL as a sclerosing agent. Since POL is used as an emulsifying agent in preprocessed foods, patients may have been exposed previously through ingestion. Both patients responded easily to either a single dose of oral diphenhydramine, 50 mg, or 0.3 ml of subcutaneous epinephrine plus 50 mg intramuscular diphenhydramine.

One specific case report describes a 30-year-old woman who underwent four separate sclerotherapy sessions with POL. On the fourth session, 3 ml of POL 1.5% and 12 ml of POL 0.5% were administered. The patient complained of chest heaviness and constriction, which also appeared after two of her other sessions but was not brought to the attention of the medical staff. During the fourth episode she lost consciousness and was found without a pulse or blood pressure with dilated pupils. Spontaneous respiration occurred after 2 to 3 minutes, she began to vomit and complained of headache and earache. She recovered and was discharged after 10 hours well but returned the next day with dysosmia, which lasted 6 weeks. Although a brain CT scan was normal the presumed cause was cerebral.[60]

The median lethal dose (LD_{50}) in rabbits at two hours is 0.2 g/kg, which is three to six times greater than the LD_{50} for procaine hydrochloride. The LD_{50} in mice is 110 mg/kg. The systemic toxicity level is similar to that of lidocaine and procaine.[61]

CHROMATED GLYCERIN

CG 72% (Scleremo) is a sclerosing solution with a very low incidence of side effects (Scleremo product information, 1987). Hypersensitivity is a very rare complication.[62] Contact sensitivity to chromium occurs in approximately 5% of the population.[63] IV potassium dichromate leads to complete desensitization in chromium-sensitized guinea pigs. This effect occurs because chromium needs to bind to skin proteins to become an effective antigen. This may be related to the necessity for epidermal Langerhans' cells to produce an allergic response, whereas T-lymphocyte accessory cooperation is not optimal with IV injection and its resulting endothelial necrosis. Thus it is more common for a sclerotherapist to develop an allergic contact dermatitis to CG than it is for a patient to have an allergic reaction to IV use of CG. Indeed, Ouvry (personal communication, 1995) has developed an allergic contact dermatitis from CG injected without the use of protective gloves.

Ramalet[64] has reported seven patients who developed an allergic reaction to CG. One patient had a vasculitis, and six patients had an eczematous reaction. All allergic patients demonstrated a sensitivity to topically applied chrome.

Hematuria accompanied by urethral colic has been reported to occur transiently after injection of large doses of CG. Ocular manifestations, including blurred vision and a partial visual field loss, have been reported by a single author, with resolution in less than 2 hours.[65] Glycerin-induced (or any sclerotherapy-induced) hemolysis may not be a benign event. Hemoglobin can exert direct cytotoxic, inflammatory, and pro-oxidant effects that adversely affect endothelial function.[66] Hemoglobin from destroyed red blood cells dimerizes and is rapidly bound by the serum protein haptoglobin. The haptoglobin-hemoglobin complex causes endocytosis and degradation, which can lead to a variety of adverse effects.[67]

An additional case was reported of transient hypertension and visual disturbance after the injection of 12 ml of 50% chromated glycerin into spider and "feeder" leg veins in a fourth treatment session.[68] These symptoms occurred 2 ½ hours after treatment and lasted more than 3 hours without treatment. This may have represented a retinal spasm or an ophthalmic migraine.

Although transient hemoglobinuria is common in athletes and without known long-term adverse effects, hemoglobulinemia can cause renal failure.[69] More commonly, hemoglobulinemia can cause a dose-related gastrointestinal dystonia and pain, including esophageal spasm and dysphagia. Refer to an excellent recent review that details more clinical manifestations of hemoglobinemia.[70]

Since we have been using glycerin alone without chromium but mixed 2:1 with 1% lidocaine with or without 1:100,000 epinephrine, we have yet to see an allergic reaction. We have also yet to see hemoglobinuria or adverse effects with the use of up to 12 ml of this glycerin mixture except for a minute or two of epinephrine-induced "rush" that can occur in rare patients who have a sensitivity to epinephrine.

POLYIODIDE IODINE

Polyiodide iodine (Varigloban; Sclerodine 6) is a stabilized water solution of iodide ions, sodium iodine, and benzyl alcohol. Sigg et al.[71,72] reported on their experience with over 400,000 injections with Variglobin reported an incidence of 0.13 allergic cutaneous reactions per 1,000. No systemic allergic reactions were observed. Obvious contraindications to the use of Variglobin are hyperthyroidism and allergies to iodine and benzyl alcohol.

SODIUM SALICYLATE

Saliject (Omega Laboratories, Montreal) has not been reported in a literature review to cause allergic reactions. Dr. Beverly Kemsley has reported one of 6,000 patients who developed an anaphylactic reaction after the use of Saliject. Thirty patients developed localized erythema and urticaria that responded to the oral antihistamine terfenadine 120 mg (personal communication, 1996).

HYPERTONIC SALINE

Alone, hypertonic saline (HS) solution shows no evidence of allergenicity or toxicity. Complications that may arise from its specific use include hypertension that may be exacerbated in predisposed patients when an excessive sodium load is given, sudden hypernatremia, central nervous system disorders, extensive hemolysis, and cortical necrosis of the kidneys (Mary Helenek, written correspondence, American Regent Laboratories, Inc., May 1990). These complications among others have led one manufacturer (American Regent Laboratories) to add to its label the warning "For IV or SC use after dilution" in bold red ink.

As discussed previously, hematuria can occur with any sclerosing agent. Sometimes blood appears in the urine after one or two acts of micturition and occasionally at other times throughout the day. Usually there are no other ill effects, and the hematuria resolves spontaneously. Hematuria probably occurs because of hemolysis of red blood cells during sclerotherapy.

In summary, sclerotherapy with a wide variety of sclerosing solutions is a safe and effective procedure for the treatment of varicose and telangiectatic leg veins. Space does not permit a more complete discussion of other possible adverse effects. Table 14.1 summarizes the different adverse effects

Table 14.1 **SUMMARY OF COMPLICATIONS OF SCLEROSING AGENTS**

AGENTS SOLUTION	PIGMENTATION	ALLERGIC REACTION	NECROSIS	PAIN
Sodium morrhuate	++	++	+++*	+++
Sodium tetradecyl sulfate	++	+	++*	+
Ethanolamine oleate	+	++	++*	++
Polidocanol	+	+	+*	0
Hypertonic saline	+	0	+++*	+++
Sclerodex (+0% saline 5% dextrose)	+	0	+	++
Chromated glycerin	0	+	0	++
Glycerin	0	0	0	+
Polyiodinated iodine	++	+	+++*	+++

+, Minimal; ++, moderate; +++, significant.
*Concentration dependent.

from a variety of available sclerosing solutions. The interested reader is referred elsewhere for a complete review of adverse effects from sclerotherapy treatment.[13]

REFERENCES

1. Cavezzi A, Izzo, M. Sclerosing agents. In: Bergan J, Bunke, N, eds. *The vein book*, 2e. New York: Oxford University Press. Forthcoming.
2. Munavalli GS, Weiss RA. Complications of sclerotherapy, *Semin Cutan Med Surg.* 2007. *26*: 22–8.
3. Rabe E, Pannier F. Sclerotherapy of varicose veins with polidocanol based on the guidelines of the German Society of Phlebology, *Dermatol Surg.* 2010.; *36*(Suppl 2): 968–975.
4. Sylvoz N, Villier C, Blaise S, Seinturier C, Mallaret M. Polidocanol induced cardiotoxicity: A case report and review of the literature, *J Mal Vasc.* 2008. *33*(4–5): 234–238.
5. Ouvry PA. Telangiectasia and sclerotherapy, *J Dermatol Surg Oncol.* 1989. *15*(2): 177–181.
6. Schwartz L, Maxwell H. Sclerotherapy for lower limb telangiectasias, *Cochrane Database Syst Rev.* 2011. *12*: CD008826.
7. Duffy DM. Sclerosants: A comparative review, *Dermatol Surg.* 2010. *36*(Suppl 2): 1010–1025.
8. Green D. Persistent post-sclerotherapy pigmentation due to minocycline: Three cases and a review of post-sclerotherapy pigmentation, *J Cosmet Dermatol.* 2002. *1*(4): 173–182.
9. Goldman MP, Kaplan RP, Duffy DM. Postsclerotherapy hyperpigmentation: A histologic evaluation, *J Dermatol Surg Oncol.* 1987. *13*(5): 547–550.
10. Saddick N, Li C. Small-vessel sclerotherapy, *Dermatol Clin.* 2001. *19*(3): 475–481.
11. Uhl JF, Cornu-Thénard A, Carpentier PH, Widmer MT, Partsch H, Antignani PL. Clinical and hemodynamic significance of corona phlebectatica in chronic venous disorders, *J Vasc Surg.* 2005. *42*(6): 1163–1168.
12. Engelhorn CA, Engelhorn AL, Cassou MF, Salles-Cunha S. Patterns of saphenous venous reflux in women presenting with lower extremity telangiectasias, *Dermatol Surg.* 2007. *33*(3): 282–288.
13. Carlin MC, Ratz JL. Treatment of telangiectasia: Comparison of sclerosing agents, *J Dermatol Surg Oncol.* 1987. *13*(11): 1181–1184.
14. McCoy S, Evans A, Spurrier N. Sclerotherapy for leg telangiectasia: A blinded comparative trial of polidocanol and hypertonic saline, *Dermatol Surg.* 1999. *25*(5): 381–385; discussion 385–386.
15. Peterson JD, Goldman MP, Weiss RA, et al. Treatment of reticular and telangiectatic leg veins: Double-blind, prospective comparative trial of polidocanol and hypertonic saline, *Dermatol Surg.* 2012. *38*(8): 1322–1330.
16. Little AD. *Human safety and environmental aspects of major surfactants.* Report to the Soap and Detergent Association. 1977.
17. Talmadge SS. *Environmental and human safety of major surfactants: Alcohol ethoxylates and alkylphenol ethoxylates.* Boca Raton: Lewis Publishers. 1994.
18. Duffy D. Sclerotherapy. In: Alam M, Silapunt S, eds. *Treatment of leg veins*, 2e. Philadelphia: Elsevier. 2011.
19. Davis LT, Duffy DM. Determination of incidence and risk factors for postsclerotherapy telangiectatic matting of the lower extremity: A retrospective analysis, *J Dermatol Surg Oncol.* 1990. *16*(4): 327–330.
20. Goldman MP, Sadick NS, Weiss RA. Cutaneous necrosis, telangiectatic matting, and hyperpigmentation following sclerotherapy: Etiology, prevention, and treatment, *Dermatol Surg.* 1995. *21*(1): 19–29.
21. Weiss RA, Weiss MA. Incidence of side effects in the treatment of telangiectasias by compression sclerotherapy: Hypertonic saline vs. polidocanol, *J Dermatol Surg Oncol.* 1990. *16*(9): 800–804.
22. Guex JJ, Allaert FA, Gillet JL, Chlier F. Immediate and midterm complications of sclerotherapy report of a prospective multi-center registry of 12,173 sclerotherapy sessions, *Dermatol Surg.* 2005. *31*: 123–128.
23. Norris MJ, Carlin MC, Ratz JL. Treatment of essential telangiectasia: Effects of increasing concentrations of polidocanol, *J Am Acad Dermatol.* 1989. *20*(4): 643–649.
24. Mlosek RK, Wozniak W, Malinowska S, Migda B, Serafin-Kroi M, Milek T. The removal of post-sclerotherapy pigmentation following sclerotherapy alone or in combination with crossectomy, *Eur J Vasc Endovasc Surg.* 2012. *43*(1): 100–105.
25. Goldman, M. Complications and adverse sequelae of sclerotherapy. In: Bergan J, ed. *The Vein Book*, Massachusetts: Elsevier Academic Press. 2007. 139–155.
26. Miyake RK, King JT, Kikuchi R, Duarte FH, Davidson JR, Oba C. Role of injection pressure, flow and sclerosant viscosity in causing cutaneous ulceration during sclerotherapy, *Phlebology.* 2012. *27*(8): 383–389.
27. Bergan JJ, Weiss RA, Goldman MP. Extensive tissue necrosis following high-concentration sclerotherapy for varicose veins. *Dermatol Surg.* 2000. *26*(6): 535–541.
28. Schuller-Petrovic S, Pavlovic MD, Neuhold N, Brunner F, Wolkart G. Subcutaneous injection of liquid and foamed polidocanol: Extravasation is not responsible for skin necrosis during reticular and spider vein sclerotherapy, *J Eur Acad Dermatol Venereol.* 2011. *25*(8): 983–986.
29. Kern P, Ramelet AA, Wutschert R, Hayoz D. Compression after sclerotherapy for telangiectasias and reticular leg veins: a randomized controlled study, *J Vasc Surg.* 2007. *45*(6): 1212–1216.
30. Fronek H, Fronek A, Saltzberg G. Allergic reactions to sotradecol, *J Dermatol Surg Oncol.* 1989. *15*: 684.
31. Nouri K. *Complications in dermatologic surgery.* St. Louis, MO: Mosby/Elsevier. 2008.
32. Scurr JRH, Fisher, RK, Wallace SB, Gilling-Smith GL. Anaphylaxis following foam sclerotherapy: A life threatening complication of non-invasive treatement for varicose veins. *EJVES Extra.* 2007. *13*: 87–89.
33. Brzoza Z, Kasperska-Zajac A, Rogala E, Rogala B. Anaphylactoid reaction after the use of sodium tetradecyl sulfate: A case report, *Angiology.* 2007. *58*(5): 644–646.
34. Shmunes E. Allergic dermatitis to benzyl alcohol in an injectable solution, *Arch Dermatol.* 1984. *120*: 1200–1201.
35. Turvey SE, Cronin B, Arnold AD, et al. Adverse reactions to vitamin B12 injections due to benzyl alcohol sensitivity: Successful treatment with intranasal cyanocobalamin, *Allergy,* 2004. *59*: 1023–1024.
36. Goldman MP, Bergan JJ, Guex JJ. *Sclerotherapy treatments of varicose and telangiectatic leg veins*, 4e. St. Louis, MO: Mosby Elsevier. 2007.
37. Weiss RA, Voigts R, Howell DJ. Absence of concentration congruity in six compounded polidocanol samples obtained for leg sclerotherapy, *Dermatol Surg.* 2011. *37*(6): 812–815.
38. Almeida JI, Raines JK. FDA-approved sodium tetradecyl sulfate (STS) versus compounded STS for venous sclerotherapy, *Dermatol Surg.* 2007. *33*(9): 1037.
39. Goldman MP. Sodium tetradecyl sulfate for sclerotherapy treatment of veins: is compounding pharmacy solution safe?, *Dermatol Surg.* 2004. *30*(12 Pt 1): 1454–1456.
40. Dick ET. The treatment of varicose veins, *NZ Med J.* 1966. *65*: 310.
41. de Lorimier AA. Sclerotherapy for venous malformations, *J Pediatr Surg.* 1995. *30*: 188–194.
42. Perakos PG, Cirbus JJ, Camara S. Persistent bradyarrhythmia after sclerotherapy for esophageal varices, *South Med J.* 1984. *77*: 531.
43. Foote RR. Severe reaction to monoethanolamine oleate, *Lancet.* 1942. *1*: 390.
44. Reid RG, Rothine NG. Treatment of varicose veins by compression sclerotherapy, *Br J Surg.* 1968. *55*: 889.
45. Goldman MP, Bennett RG. Treatment of telangiectasia: a review, *J Am Acad Dermatol.* 1987. *17*: 167.
46. Steinberg MH. Evaluation of sotradecol in sclerotherapy of varicose veins, *Angiology.* 1955. *6*: 519.

47. Nabatoff RA. Recent trends in the diagnosis and treatment of varicose veins, *Surg Gynecol Obstet*. 1950. *90*: 521.

48. Fegan G. *Varicose veins: Compression sclerotherapy*. London: Heinemann Medical. 1967.

49. Tibbs DJ. Treatment of superficial vein incompetence: 2. Compression sclerotherapy. In: Tibbs DJ, ed. *Varicose veins and related disorders*. Oxford: Butterworth-Heinemann. 1992.

50. *Clinical Case 1*. Presented at the Third Annual Meeting of the North American Society of Phlebology, Phoenix, AZ, February 21, 1990.

51. Passas H. One case of tetradecyl-sodium sulfate allergy with general symptoms, *Soc Fr Phlebol*. 1972. *25*: 19.

52. Thibault PK. Sclerotherapy of varicose veins and telangiectasias: A 2-year experience with sodium tetradecyl sulphate, *ANZ J Phlebol*. 1999. *3*: 25.

53. Reiner L. The activity of anionic surface active compounds in producing vascular obliteration, *Proc Soc Exp Biol Med*. 1946. *62*: 49.

54. Goldman MP. Sodium tetradecyl sulfate for sclerotherapy treatment of veins: Is compounding pharmacy solution safe?, *Dermatol Surg*. 2004. *30*: 1454–1456.

55. Guex JJ. Indications for the sclerosing agen polidocanol. *J Dermatol Surg Oncol*. 1993. *19*: 959.

56. Stricker BH, van Oijen JA, Kroon C, et al. Anafylaxie na gebruik van polidocanol, *Ned Tijdschr Geneeskd*. 1990. *134*: 240.

57. Conrad P, Malouf GM, Stacey MC. The Australian polidocanol (aethoxysklerol) study: results at 2 years, *Dermatol Surg*. 1995. *21*: 334.

58. Tombari G, et al. Sclerotherapy of varices: Complications and their treatment. In: Raymond-Martimbeau P, Prescott R, Zummo M, eds. *Phlebologie '92*. Paris: John Libbey Eurotext. 1992.

59. Feied CF, Jackson JJ, Bren TS, et al. Allergic reactions to polidocanol for vein sclerosis: Two case reports, *J Derm Surg Onc*. 1994. *20*: 466.

60. Jenkins D. Severe idiosyncratic reaction to polidocanol, *ANZ J Phlebol*. 2002. *6*: 24–25.

61. Soehring K, Frahm M. Studies on the pharmacology of alkylpolyethyleneoxide derivatives, *Arzneimittelforschung*. 1955. *5*: 655.

62. Ouvry P, Davy A. Le traitement sclerosant des telangiectasias des membres inferieurs, *Phlebologie*. 1982. *35*: 349.

63. Jager H, Pelloni E. Tests epicutanes aux bichromates, posotofs dan l'eczema au ciment, *Dermatologica*. 1950. *100*: 207.

64. Ramelet AA, Ruffieux C, Poffet D. Complications après sclerose a la glycerine chromee, *Phlebologie*. 1995. *48*: 377.

65. Wallois P. Incidents et accidents de la sclerose. In: Tournay R, ed. *La sclerose des varices*, 4e. Paris: Expansion Scientifique Francaise. 1985.

66. Wagener F, Eggert A, Boerman OC, et al. Heme is a potent inducer of inflammation in mice and is counteracted by heme oxygenase, *Blood*. 2001. *98*: 1802–1811.

67. Tabbara IA. Hemolytic anemias: Diagnosis and management, *Med Clin N Am*. 1992. *76*: 649–668.

68. Zimmet SE. Letter to the editor, *J Derm Surg Onc*. 1990. *16*: 1063.

69. Clark DA, Butler SA, Baren V, Hartmann RC, Jenkins DE Jr. The kidneys in paroxysmal nocturnal hemoglobinemia, *Blood*. 1981. *57*: 83–89.

70. Rother RP, Bell L, Hillmen P, Gladwin MT. The clinical sequelae of intravascular hemolysis and extracellular plasma hemoglobin: A novel mechanism of human disease, *JAMA*. 2005. *293*: 1653–1662.

71. Sigg K, Horodegen K, Bernbach H. Varizen-Sklerosierung: Welchos ist das wir Usamste Mittel?, *Deutsohes Arzteblatt*. 1986. *34/35*: 2294.

72. Sigg K, Zelikovski A. Kann die Sklerosierungotherapie der Varizenobne Oparation in jedem Fallwirksam sein?, *Phlebol Proktol*. 1975. *4*: 42.

15.

LASER TREATMENT OF TELANGIECTASIAS AND RETICULAR VEINS

Neil Sadick and Lian Sorhaindo

INTRODUCTION

The incidence of prominent venulectasias and/or telangiectasias on the lower extremities occurs in up to 41% of women and 15% of men within the United States.[1] The current literature subdivides vascular pathology into superficial "spider" veins or telangiectasias, deep reticular veins, and protuberant varicosities. Etiologies include heredity, hormonal dysregulation, prolonged periods of standing obesity, pregnancy, and aging. Although patients may present with symptoms of fatigue, aching, swelling, throbbing, and occasionally pain, patients seek treatment primarily for aesthetic concerns. With this rise in consumer demand since early 2000s, there has been a subsequent increase in the utilization of lasers and intense pulsed light (IPL) sources for the treatment of lower extremity veins.

IDENTIFYING THE PROBLEM

The vasculature of the lower extremity consists of a complex, intertwined network of superficial and deep venous plexuses. The superficial veins lie directly underneath the skin surface. The deep veins, in contrast, traverse the muscle of the leg. The individual flow patterns of these two networks intertwine such that superficial spider veins may be the direct result of increased hydrostatic pressure in the deep reticular veins.

The varying sizes, depths, flow patterns, and vessel thickness of leg veins make the treatment of leg veins challenging. Presently, there is no gold standard of treatment for all leg veins, and lasers often are used as adjunctive therapy in patients undergoing phlebectomy, sclerotherapy, or vein stripping. Laser and light source technology has become particularly useful in the treatment of small spider veins or telangiectasias, and also in the setting of vessels that are scleroresistant that may arise from prior surgical treatment as a result of telangiectatic matting or angiogenic flushing (see Box 15.1).[2] It can also be used in the treatment of large spider and reticular veins; however, sclerotherapy remains the gold standard for the treatment of these vessels. This chapter deals specifically with the laser treatment of telangiectasias and reticular veins; other modalities of treatment including sclerotherapy, ambulatory phlebectomy, and endovenous ablation are discussed elsewhere in the book.

PATIENT SELECTION: WHEN AND HOW TO CHOOSE LASER/ IPL VERSUS SCLEROTHERAPY

Laser therapy is most efficacious for treating telangiectasias/venulectasias or reticular veins less than 3 mm in diameter.[3,4] As mentioned earlier, lasers have become indicated in patients with areas of neovascularization with telangiectatic matting or angiogenic flushing, with scleroresistant/ noncannulable vessels, and who are needle-phobic. Relative contraindications to the use of laser surgery include tanned skin, pregnancy, the use of iron supplements or anticoagulation, history of photosensitivity disorder, or hypertrophic and keloidal scarring (see Table 15.1).

FUNDAMENTALS OF LASER TREATMENT OF LEG VEINS

THEORY OF SELECTIVE THERMOLYSIS: MAJOR PRINCIPLES AND DETERMINANTS

The advent of laser technology for treatment of leg veins began with the concept of selective photothermolysis developed in the late 1980s.[5] The theory of selective photothermolysis states that selective damage to a tissue structure is achieved by means of a wavelength of light preferentially absorbed by a chromophore in light-absorbing molecules and laser exposure time less than or equal to the object's thermal relaxation time (i.e., the time required for the object to lose 50% of its thermal energy). The thermal relaxation times of leg veins vary depending on vessel diameter (see Table 15.2).[6]

A physician employing laser therapy should routinely consider the utility of laser and intense pulsed light (IPL) technologies versus that of sclerotherapy for the treatment of lower extremity vessels.[7] The fundamental requirements for a laser or IPL source in the treatment of leg veins are delineated in Box 15.2.

Laser technology and its role in leg vein reduction is rooted in the molecule hemoglobin and its absorption spectrum, which has broad peaks at 410, 540, and 577 nm and smaller peaks at 920 and 940 nm. The spectra of oxyhemoglobin and deoxyhemoglobin differ, with bluer veins responding to wavelengths targeting the deoxyspectrum and red varicosities responding more effectively to wavelengths targeting the oxyhemoglobin spectrum (see Figure 15.1). Generally speaking, any vessel that is less than 3 mm in diameter may be treated by laser and IPL technologies. However, sclerotherapy is a more efficient modality for eradicating cannulable vessels, and when small, difficult-to-cannulate vessels are present microsclerotherapy may be implemented. Microsclerotherapy, however, is plagued by a number of adverse sequelae, increased incidence of bruising and pigment dyschromia, puncture marks from needle use, microulcerations, and inconsistent results (see Table 15.3). Given the adverse aesthetic outcomes of such procedures, the use of lasers has gained momentum in the management of cosmetic veins.

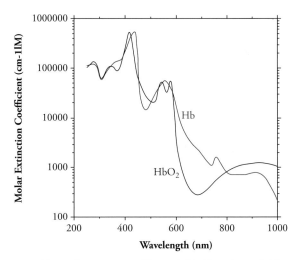

Figure 15.1   Absorption spectrum of hemoglobin/deoxyhemoglobin.

Table 15.1 COMPARISON OF THE 1064 NM ND:YAG,
810 NM DIODE, AND 755 NM ALEXANDRITE LASERS
FOR LEG VEINS 0.3–3 MM IN DIAMETER

LASER	PATIENTS ACHIEVING 75% CLEARANCE AT 3 MONTHS
1064 nm Nd:YAG	88%
810 nm diode	29
755 nm Alexandrite	33

Table 15.2 VESSEL THERMAL RELAXATION TIME

VEIN DIAMETER	TIME (SECONDS)
0.1	0.010
0.2	0.080
0.4	0.16
0.8	0.6
1.0	8.0

Table 15.3 MICROTELANGIECTASIA <0.5 MM:
COMPARISON OF MICROSCLEROTHERAPY AND
LASER TECHNOLOGY

	MICROSCLEROTHERAPY	LASER
Number of treatments	–	–
Bruising	–	+
Discomfort	–	+
Clinical efficiency	–	+
Purpura	–	+
Pigmentation	–	–
Ulceration	–	+
Cost	+	–
Patient satisfaction	–	+
Physician skill	–	–

Table 15.4 OPTIMAL LASER PARAMETERS FOR THE TREATMENT OF LEG VEINS

Wavelength	530–1064 nm
Pulse Duration	2–100 ms
Fluence	30–150 J/cm^2
Spot Size	1.5–10 mm

Adapted from Sadick N. A dual wavelength approach for laser/intense pulsed light source treatment of lower extremity veins, *J Am Acad Dermatol.* 2002. *46:* 66–72.

Table 15.5 MONOMODAL APPROACH TO THE TREATMENT OF LEG VEINS USING THE 1064 NM ND:YAG LASER

VESSEL SIZE	SPOT SIZE	FLUENCE	PULSE DURATION
<1 mm red	Small	High	Short
1–3 mm (blue)	Large	Moderate	Long

Adapted from Sadick N. Laser treatment with a 1064 nm laser for lower extremity class I–III veins employing variable spots and pulse width parameters, *Dermatol Surg.* 2003. *29:* 916–919.

Lasers and intense pulse light (IPL) have not become replacements for sclerotherapy, primarily because hydrostatic pressure considerations are not addressed by light endothelial interactions. It is also more difficult to have sufficient penetration of photons safely through the thick epidermal dermal wall surrounding the lower extremity vessels when utilizing noninvasive treatment modalities like laser technology; direct injection into the target chromophore is intuitively more efficient. Furthermore, an altered pattern of cytokine release may be observed when using laser technology, resulting in injury to the vessel that may lead to increased incidence of postinflammatory hyperpigmentation.

Wavelength, pulse duration, and spot size are the parameters that are most influential during the treatment and management of individual vessels (see Table 15.4). The larger vessels tend to respond to longer wavelengths or the ratio of vessel to epidermal heating increases the probability of achieving complete vessel coagulation.[8] Shorter wavelengths, in contrast, partially coagulate the vessel, ultimately increasing the incidence of treatment failures and subsequent epidermal damage including hyperpigmentation.[9] Maximum efficiency of vessel clearance is achieved when the penetration depth of the beam equals the vessel diameter. The spot size should be as large as possible, at least on the order of four times the optical penetration depth. An adequate spot size minimizes scattering losses in addition to maximizing beam penetration, which increases the probability that panendothelial destruction will be achieved. The disadvantage to this, however, is that the use of larger spot sizes increases the pain and discomfort subjectively reported by the patient.

These parameters have influenced and spurred the development of a bimodal, dual wavelength approach for the treatment of both red and blue lower extremity veins (see Figure 15.2). For the treatment of small, reddish telangiectasias with a high degree of oxyhemoglobin, short wavelengths (500–600 nm) were found to be most effective; longer wavelengths (800–1100 nm) were found to be most effective for the treatment of deeper, blue telangiectasias and reticular veins.

With continuing advances, laser technology can now address both variations in vessel size and depth with a single long wavelength 1064-nm Nd:YAG laser utilizing a varied pulse width as the monomodal approach (see Table 15.5). Delicate, red vessels less than 1 mm in diameter are superficial, having high oxyhemoglobin saturation. Consequently, they can be treated effectively with small spot sizes (<2 mm), higher fluences (350–600 J/cm^2), and short pulse durations (15–30 ms). Larger blue vessels, in contrast, are typically 1–4 mm in diameter, deeper, and possess a lower oxygenated hemoglobin component. As a result, these veins are effectively treated with larger spot sizes (2–8 mm), moderate fluences (100–350 J/cm^2), and long pulse durations (30–50 ms). With the use of the Nd:YAG rapidly gaining momentum, the transition from a bimodal wavelength technique to a monomodal approach has evolved.

TREATMENT APPROACH

CANDIDATES FOR LASER THERAPY

Laser therapy may be considered appropriate in patients who are needle-phobic, cannot tolerate sclerotherapy, are plagued

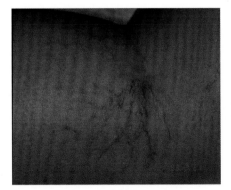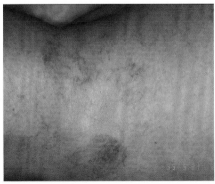

Figure 15.2 Pre- and postclinical pictures of lower extremity veins using biomodal technique.

by legs veins that are scleroresistant, and/or are susceptible to telangiectatic matting (see Box 15.1). Ideal candidates for laser treatment of leg veins previously have undergone appropriate surgery or sclerotherapy for the treatment of varicosities, incompetent perforators, and reticular veins, as well as sclerotherapy to clear the majority of superficial vessels.

PATIENT INTERVIEWS

Diagnosis of spider or varicose veins begins with a thorough medical history detailing potential risk factors or etiologies for vascular pathology such as hormones, prolonged standing associated with occupation, obesity, pregnancy, heredity, or aging.

PHYSICAL EXAMINATION

All potential candidates for laser treatment of leg veins should undergo a thorough physical examination. During the exam, the physician should evaluate the type and size of the leg veins, and the presence/absence of reflux or incompetent valves. The treatment algorithm (see Figure 15.3) suggests that larger varicose veins with reflux should be treated first in an effort to avoid the unsuccessful treatment of smaller telangiectasias and complications such as dyspigmentation and telangiectatic matting.

In keeping with the treatment algorithm in Figure 15.3, initial treatment should include surgical removal, stripping, or ambulatory phlebectomy of varicosities and large feeder vessels. Sclerotherapy should then follow proceeding from large to small vessels. Adhering to this treatment strategy will obliterate, on average, 80 to 90% of vessels in a single session. Laser and light therapy should be utilized in the treatment of any residual vessels including those that are too small in diameter to undergo sclerotherapy with a 30- to 32-gauge needle.

LASER TREATMENT SYSTEMS

A compilation of laser and intense pulsed light sources utilized in the setting of laser treatment of legs veins are presented herein and summarized in Table 15.6. The wavelengths of light range from 515 nm to 1064 nm, depending on the treatment system employed. As mentioned earlier in the chapter, the longer the wavelength, the greater the depth of penetration, as illustrated in Figure 15.4.

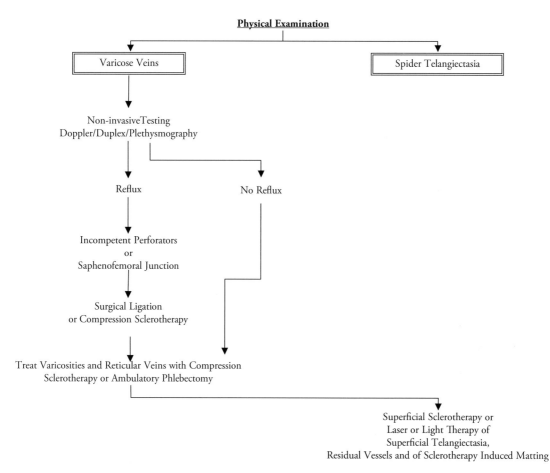

Figure 15.3   Systematic approach to the treatment of leg veins.

Table 15.6 LASERS AND LIGHT SOURCES FOR THE TREATMENT OF LEG VEINS

LASER	WAVELENGTH
Pulsed Dye	585–605 nm
KTP	532 nm
Alexandrite	755 nm
Diode	810 nm
Nd:YAG	1064 nm
Intense Pulsed Light	515–1200 nm

578 NM COPPER BROMIDE (CUBR)

Yellow Light Laser

A new yellow light laser employing a copper bromide medium has demonstrated efficacy in the treatment of red lower extremity telangiectasias that are less than 2 mm in size. An average of 1.7 patient sessions produced significant clearing of 75 to 100% in 71.8% of patients. The positive results have been confined to the treatment of red vessels (1 mm).[10]

PULSED LASERS AND LIGHT SOURCES

POTASSIUM-TITANYL-PHOSPHATE LASER

For small telangiectatic leg veins in fair-skinned patients, the pulsed potassium-titanyl-phosphate (KTP) laser has become the treatment of choice. The Versapulse KTP laser (Lumenis, Santa Clara, California) uses the following parameters: a spot size of 3–5 mm, pulse duration of 10–15 ms, and fluences of 14–20 J/cm², which have proven to be effective. A 4°C chilled tip provides epidermal protection. Side effects include transient erythema crusting superficially, and purpura. When administering the pulsed KTP laser, lower fluences must be employed in the darker skinned or tanned patient because of their increased melanin and

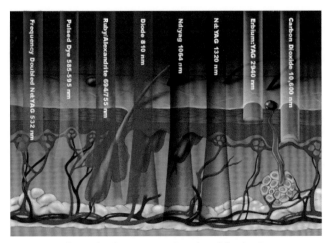

Figure 15.4 Relationship between wavelength and depth of penetration.

its absorption of green light. This increased absorption is more likely to increase the risk of epidermal damage. Treatment failure, consequently, is higher in this subset of patients because the lower fluences are not very effective in coagulating the target vessel. Patient acceptance of this laser treatment system is high with minimal treatment discomfort of the longer penetrating wavelengths and a relatively uncomplicated postoperative course.[11] Other technologies including the Aura (Laserscope, San Jose, California) have produced comparable results.

FLASHLAMP-PUMPED PULSED DYE LASER

The pump pulsed dye laser was the first laser to achieve notable results in the treatment of leg veins in the 1980s. This treatment system utilizes short wavelength technology, at a wavelength of 577 nm. This has become acceptable for treatment of leg vessels <1.0 mm, but cannot be recommended for treatment of blue vessels or red vessels >1.0 mm given its short wavelength, relatively short pulse duration, and moderate energy fluence.[12] This system, in contrast to long wavelength technologies, is less effective and is associated with a number of side effects including bruising and posttherapy hyperpigmentation.

LONGER WAVELENGTH PULSED LASERS

With the advent of longer wavelength technologies, including the long-pulsed alexandrite laser, 1064 nm Nd:YAG, and longer pulse duration lasers and light sources, there has been a great improvement in treatment outcomes. Presently, there are several long-pulse dye lasers available with variable pulse durations capable of deeper penetration into the skin and treatment of larger caliber spider and feeding reticular veins of the lower extremity.

LONG-PULSED ALEXANDRITE LASERS

This system recently has been applied to the treatment of leg telangiectasias and reticular veins, less than 3 mm in diameter, with good results. The longer wavelength (755 nm) provides deeper tissue penetration and an ability to treat larger diameter and more deeply situated vessels. Although hemoglobin absorption of this wavelength is lower than that of 532 and 595 nm wavelengths, it is sufficient to achieve photocoagulation of a wide range of vessel sizes with the use of higher fluences. Optimal treatment parameters for the long-pulsed alexandrite laser include 20 J/cm², double pulsed at a repetition of 1 Hz. To penetrate tissue more deeply and to allow greater thermal diffusion time to treat larger vessels, the alexandrite laser has been modified to provide pulse duration of up to 20 ms. Side effects include purpura, matting, and long-term pigmentary alterations due to melanin absorption.

In a recent study, the alexandrite laser system evoked a significant inflammatory response with concomitant purpura and matting when used at a fluence of 60–70 J/cm^2 and a wavelength of 755 nm, in comparison with other available laser treatment systems. A study conducted by Eremia et al. concluded that the 755-nm wavelength utilized by the alexandrite system is limited to use in nontanned patients with I–III skin types.[13]

DIODE LASERS

The diode lasers utilize a wavelength of 800 nm at 5- to 250-ms duration, and have been indicated in the treatment of superficial leg telangiectasis and reticular veins. This technology system with near infrared wavelengths allows deeper tissue penetration with decreased absorption of melanin. The efficaciousness of the diode was demonstrated in a study conducted by Garden et al. The patients, having a vessel size between 0.2 to 0.5 mm, were treated with an 810-nm quasi-continuous diode laser 20-ms pulse duration. The results of the study showed a 60% mean vessel clearance after a mean of 2.2 treatment sessions.[14] With the recent introduction of higher fluence capability, the diode laser's efficacy continues to increase.[4,15]

LONG-PULSED ND:YAG LASER (1064)

The treatment of choice for spider and feeding reticular veins is the long-pulsed Nd:YAG laser (1064). As discussed earlier in the chapter, spot sizes, energy, and pulse duration can be adjusted to target both small telangiectasias and larger reticular veins with a single device. In addition, this system via its utility of a longer, deeper penetrating wavelength and subsequent epidermal bypass increases the efficacy of this system in treatment of darker skin phenotypes. This system also addresses issues stemming from the hydrostatic pressure of feeder and reticular veins because veins up to 3 mm can be treated, although the patient's tolerance to pain may become an issue as pain increases with treatment of larger vessels. The newer pulsed 1064-nm lasers have pulsed durations between 1 and 200 ms (Vasculight Lumenis [Palo Alto, California], Cool touch Vantage [San Jose, California], Cool Glide Excel [Burlingame, California], Lyra [Laserscope, San Jose, California], Gemini [Laserscope, San Jose, California], and Sciton Profile [Sciton, Palo Alto, California]). For superficial vessels less than 1 mm in diameter, the optimal parameters include small spot sizes of less than 2 mm, short pulse durations of 15–30 ms, and high fluences of 350–600 J/cm^2. For reticular veins, 1 to 4 mm in diameter, larger spot sizes (2–8 mm), longer pulse durations (30–60 ms), and moderate fluences (100–370 J/cm^2) should yield successful results. As a result, the Nd:YAG laser has been embraced by many clinicians worldwide as the state of the art for laser treatment of lower extremity vessels.

The Lyra and Gemini systems use contact cooling and encompass a 1064-nm Nd:YAG technology. Seventy-five

percent improvement of veins of all colors and sizes has been reported with this technology. The Sciton Image has been used predominantly for treatment of the lower extremity telangiectasias and reticular veins up to 3 mm in diameter. Its high energy fluence and large spot size have increased its efficacy in treating both large-diameter vessels (i.e., reticular veins) and small capillary mats less than 1 mm in diameter. A static cooling device also is employed in this treatment system. The Vasculight also has been utilized for treatment of both smaller vessels and larger reticular veins up to 4 mm in diameter. The operator applies a coupling cooling gel in addition to an internal dynamic cooling device (DCD) (1–4°C) and applies the laser tip directly to the treatment vessel under consideration. Superficial red telangiectasias less than 1 mm in diameter may be treated with the hand piece coagulated and defocused off the skin and a lower energy fluence of 90–100 J/cm^2 with a pulse duration of 10 to 12 ms delivered as a single pulse.

Weiss et al. achieved 75% improvement at the 3-month follow-up of 0.3- to 3.0-mm vessels documented by duplex closure. Settings in this study including fluence of 80 to 120 J/cm^2 and single-pulse durations of 10 to 30 ms were utilized.[16] Sadick et al. treated twenty patients with Fitzpatrick skin type II to IV with a similar technology. A mean of 2.5 treatments produced 100% clearance in 88% of patients. Mild purpura was noted in 20% of patients, and postlaser hyperpigmentation was noted in 10% of patients.[17]

IPL

IPL devices have also been indicated in the treatment of leg veins, albeit with variable results. These systems have been shown to have dual success in penetration of both superficial and deep tissues, in addition to absorption by both oxygenated and deoxygenated hemoglobin (Photoderm VL, Vasculight IPL, Lumenis, Palo Alto CA). The main advantage of IPL technology in the treatment of leg veins has been the use of large spot sizes, causing minimal purpura. This technology, in contrast to other treatment modalities, uses a noncoherent pulsed light source with wavelengths between 500–1,200 nm, emitting a spectrum of light rather than a single wavelength in single, double, or triple pulses. The results of this current system are variable. Schroter et al. reported immediate clearing in 73.6% of patients and clearing in 84.3% of patients after 4 weeks. With respect to the immediate response, 82% clearing was seen in the group with veins up to 0–2 mm, 78.9% was seen in the group from 0.2 up to 0.5 mm, and 59.7% was seen in the groups from 0.5 to 1.0 mm.[18]

Other investigators, in contrast, have found lesser success utilizing this technology for management of lower extremity spider veins. Results from a study done by Green showed no improvement in 56% of patients, partial clearing in 25% of patients, and no improvement in 56% of telangiectasias. It is worth mentioning that this particular study was done at the incipient stages of the IPL system's development.[19] Associated side effects include blistering, crusting, and discoloration, especially in darker skinned patients. With growing sophistication and use, however, IPL stands at the forefront of laser vein technology, being the most effective for treating telangiectatic matting associated with diffuse erythema.

COMBINED LASER/ RADIOFREQUENCY TECHNOLOGIES

The most recent development in laser technology in the treatment of leg veins is the combination of bipolar radiofrequency and optical energy, using either the diode laser or an IPL source. The basis of this technology is rooted in the idea that the two forms of energy act synergistically to enhance clearance of the target vessel; with utilization of this system a high energy penetration depth (>2 mm) and a high energy density on the treated vein (>100 J/cm^2) can be achieved. The laser component selectively heats the vessel, allowing the preferential absorption of radiofrequency energy because of the increased temperature and the high electrical conductivity of blood. Moreover, this system has demonstrated 80% clearing of vessels less than 3 mm in diameter after an average of 2.5 treatment sessions by the author.

ADMINISTERING LASER THERAPY

Most laser therapy patients tolerate treatment without difficulty. If a patient exhibits increasing sensitivity to pain or if larger telangiectatic or reticular veins are being treated, a topical anesthetic cream should be applied 1 hour prior to treatment and covered with a plastic dressing. Once the area has been numbed adequately, the area should be cleansed with alcohol. The physician, patient, and any medical assistants present during treatment should wear protective eyewear.

When using the 532-nm KTP laser in the treatment of smaller telangiectasias, a spot size of 3–5 mm, fluence of 12–20 J/cm^2, and a pulse duration of 10–15 ms is recommended. Skin cooling, as discussed earlier in the chapter, should be used before, during, and after treatment to prevent thermal damage to surrounding tissues and decrease patient discomfort. Laser pulses should then be applied individually, separated by at least 1–2 mm. Each laser pulse should be traced along the length of the vein with no overlap or double pulse. A minimal amount of pressure with the application device should be applied to avoid compression of the selected target vessel. The goal of treatment should be

either vessel spasm with immediate clearance or thrombosis with darkening of the vessel. Typically patients require two to three treatment sessions with 6- to 12-week nontreatment intervals because of the intense cytokine release generated by the laser endothelial interaction for maximal results. However, complete clearance may be achieved following one treatment.

For reticular or telangiectasias greater than1 mm, long-pulsed Nd:YAG laser is the treatment of choice. The 1064-nm lasers make it possible to vary spot sizes and pulse width parameters, resulting in a wide treatment range of leg veins including small telangiectasias. For superficial vessels less than 1 mm in diameter, the optimal parameters include small spot sizes of less than 2 mm, short pulse durations of 15–30 ms, and high fluences of 350–600 J/cm^2. For reticular veins 1 to 4 mm in diameter, larger spot sizes (2–8 mm), longer pulse durations (30–60 ms), and moderate fluences (100–370 J/cm^2) yield successful results. As with other laser modalities, cooling before, during, and after the pulse protects the patient's epidermal layer from damage when using higher fluences, and also increases patient comfort. With application of this system, it is often useful to apply mild pressure with the hand piece when treating reticular veins to minimize the diameter and the amount of hemoglobin in the lumen. This allows greater vessel penetration with less total heat and reduced thermal damage to surrounding skin/ tissue. After treatment with the Nd:YAG laser, small vessels experience immediate resolution; larger telangiectasias and reticular veins experience no visual change during the treatment, but demonstrate improvement and ultimately clearance within weeks to months following treatment.

Complications following treatment with any laser system include swelling, urtication, or erythema around the treated vessels. The aforementioned side effects may resolve quickly with the application of ice packs, or a topical steroid. Application of this treatment may also decrease the risk of postinflammatory hyperpigmentation. Although compression stockings are considered unnecessary after the treatment of small telangiectasias, they may improve results, if worn for a week following the treatment of larger telangiectasias and reticular veins, by preventing vessel refilling.

THE BENEFITS OF LASER THERAPY

With its increasing momentum, laser therapy has become one of the most effective treatment options for treating varicosities of the lower extremity. Generally at the time of treatment, both the patient and the physician may observe a disappearance of small telangiectatic vessels giving an immediate visual record of success of treatment. However, the larger telangiectasias and the deeper reticular veins typically do not demonstrate resolution at the time of treatment, often resolving gradually over the course of several months.

A recent study using the monomodal approach with the 1064-nm Nd:YAG and variable spot sizes and pulse width parameters to treat spider telangiectasias and reticular veins produced the following results: Twenty percent of the treated vessels exhibited a 50 to 75% improvement after three treatments administered following 1-month intervals. Gradual improvement was observed at the 6-month follow-up visit, with 80% of the treated vessels exhibiting 75% clearing. Ninety percent of patients were highly satisfied with the treatment.[20]

Another comparative study examined the effectiveness of the 1064-nm Nd:YAG versus the 810 nm diode and the 755 nm alexandrite lasers in the treatment of 0.3–3 mm in diameter. The results summarized in Table 15.1 demonstrated that the Nd:YAG laser was the most effective treatment modality at 3-month follow-up. Purpura and matting were problematic with the alexandrite laser; the results produced by the long-pulsed diode were unpredictable in the subjects enrolled.[13] Presently, no long-term controlled studies have been done regarding the persistence of vessel clearing after laser treatment of leg veins.

ROLE OF COOLING AND OTHER ADVANCES IN LASER TECHNOLOGY

The development of cooling devices (Chess Chamber, VersaPulse, Chill Tip, IPL Chiller, Zimmer Cooler) provides epidermal bypass, which protects the epidermis from damage, allowing delivery of higher fluences of energy. As a result, contact or dynamic cooling devices are presently incorporated into all devices currently manufactured. The increased utilization of extended pulse durations also allows delivery of greater amounts of energy in a more gentle fashion, providing more consistent panendothelial destruction, translating into more consistent results with fewer treatments and lesser side effects. To date, the pulse duration most suited for the thermal destruction of leg telangiectasias appears to be 1–50 ms. Other advances including those made in gentle cavitation, captured pulsing, and the regular use of large diameter beams have all led to improvements in laser/IPL technology.[21]

ADDRESSING THE COMMON PITFALLS IN LASER THERAPY

The laser treatment of leg veins is not free of common pitfalls (see Table 15.3). Retreatment or double pulsing of the target vessels vessel should be avoided to prevent excessive thermal damage that potentially can result in scarring and ulceration. The physician or the medical personnel administering the treatment should be aware that change of the target vessel may take up to several minutes given the time that it takes

for thermocoagulation to occur even when the appropriate parameters are utilized. In the setting of a clearly resistant vessel, it is better to work on a distinctly separate treatment area and return to the resistant vessel in 5 to 10 minutes. It is also important to use the lowest possible fluence that will effectively treat a selected vessel to minimize complications. As a rule a rule of thumb, the physician should always start at the lowest fluence and incrementally increase to higher energy levels as needed depending on the vessel response. Blanching of the skin is a physical manifestation of excessive thermal injury and should be avoided at all costs. Furthermore, the physician should take note of the lateral spread of the thermal energy into surrounding areas, particularly with the longer wavelength 1064-nm laser. Nontreated vessels connected to or adjacent to the desired treatment pulse area may receive enough thermal damage to unintentionally coagulate. All pulses, consequently, ideally should be separated by 1–2 mm. Because of high cytokine, treatment sessions should be spaced at least 6 to 8 weeks apart in order to reduce the risk of postinflammatory hyperpigmentation.

SIDE EFFECTS, COMPLICATIONS, AND ALTERNATIVE APPROACHES

Complications of the laser therapy of leg veins include epidermal damage, thrombosis, hyperpigmentation, matting, and incomplete clearance (see Table 15.4). During the actual procedure patients typically complain of discomfort, but rarely do they feel uncomfortable postoperatively. For those patients who develop telangiectatic matting or incomplete vessel clearance, retreatment should be offered with either laser or microsclerotherapy as deemed appropriate. Localized areas of thrombosis may resolve independently from treatment or easily can be expressed with an 18-gauge needle. Postprocedure hyperpigmentation is usually transient and has become less of an issue with the advent of the longer wavelength technologies and improvement of epidermal cooling devices. Moreover, wound care should follow any procedure that results in epidermal damage, thereby decreasing the incidence of scarring.

THE FUTURE OF LASER THERAPY

The laser treatment of leg veins continues to gain momentum with advances in laser, pulsed light, and combined radiofrequency/IPL technologies. Other advances include enhancement of longer wavelength treatment systems, improved cooling technologies, varied spot size, pulse durations, and fluence-related monomodal approaches and combined lasers/radiofrequency systems. The continued development of laser technologies not only enhances the phlebologist's armamentarium in the treatment and management of telangiectasias and reticular veins, but also provides the patient with an array of safe, noninvasive treatment options with minimal side effects or complications.

REFERENCES

1. Kauvar A. The role of lasers in the treatment of leg veins, *Sem Surg Cutan Med*. 2000. *19*: 245–252.
2. Lupton J, Alster T, Romero P. Clinical comparison of sclerotherapy versus long-pulsed Nd: YAG laser treatment for lower extremity telangiectasias, *Dermatol Surg*. 2002. *28*: 694–697.
3. Fournier N, Brisot P, Murdon S. Treatment of leg telangiectasias with a 532 nm KTP laser in multipulse model, *Dermatol Surg*. 2002. *28*: 564–571.
4. Passeron T, Ollivier V, Duteil L, et al. The new 940 nanometer diode laser: An effective treatment for leg venulectasia, *J Am Acad Dermatol*. 2003. *48*: 768–774.
5. Sonden A, Svensson B, Roman N, Ostmark H, Bismar B. Laser induced shock wave endothelial cell injury, *Lasers Surg Med*. 2002. *6*: 364–375.
6. Dover J, Sadick N, Goldman M. The role of lasers and light sources in the treatment of leg veins, *Dermatol Surg*. 1999. *25*: 328–336.
7. Sadick N. Updated approaches to the management of cosmetic leg veins, *Phlebol*. 2003. *18*: 53–54.
8. Goldman M. Treatment of leg veins with lasers and intense pulse light, *Dermatol Clin*. 2001. *19*: 467–473.
9. Sadick N. A dual wavelength approach for laser/intense pulsed light source treatment of lower extremity veins, *J Am Acad Dermatol*. 2002. *46*: 66–72.
10. Sadick N, Weiss R. The utilization of a new yellow light laser (578 nm) for the treatment of Class I red telangiectasia of the lower extremities, *Dermatol Surg*. 2002. *28*: 21–25.
11. Adrian R. Treatment of leg telangiectasias using a long-pulse frequency-doubled neodymium: YAG laser at 532 nm, *Dermatol Surg*. 1998. *24*: 19–23.
12. Goldman M, Fitzpatrick R. Pulsed dye laser treatment of leg telangiectasia: With and without simultaneous sclerotherapy, *J Dermatol Surg*. 1990. *16*: 338–344.
13. Eremias L, Umars H. A side by side comparative study of 1064 nm Nd: YAG, 310 nm diode and 755 nm alexandrite lasers for treatment of 0.3–3.0 mm leg veins, *Dermatol Surg*. 2002. *28*: 224–230.
14. Garden J, Bakus A, Miller I. Diode laser treatment of leg veins, *Lasers Surg Med*. 1998. *10*(Suppl): 38.
15. Kaudewitz P, Klorekorn W, Rother W. Treatment of leg vein telangiectasias: 1-year result with a new 940 nm diode laser, *Dermatol*. 2002. *28*: 1031–1034.
16. Weiss R, Dover J. Laser surgery of leg veins, *Dermatol Clin*. 2002. *20*: 19–36.
17. Sadick N. Long-term results with a multiple synchronized pulse 1064 nm Nd: YAG laser for the treatment of leg venulectasias and reticular veins, *Dermatol Surg*. 2001. *27*: 365–369.
18. Schroeter C, Wilder D, Reineke T, et al. Clinical significance of an intense, pulsed light source on leg telangiectasias of up to 1 mm diameter, *Eur J Dermatol*. 1997. *7*: 38–42.
19. Green D. Photothermal removal of telangiectases of the lower extremities with the Photoderm VL, *J Am Acad Dermatol*. 1998. *38*: 61–68.
20. Sadick N. Laser treatment with a 1064 nm laser for lower extremity class I–III veins employing variable spots and pulse width parameters, *Dermatol Surg*. 2003. *29*: 916–919.
21. Sadick N, Weiss R, Goldman M. Advances in laser surgery for leg veins: Bimodal wavelength approach to lower extremity vessels, new cooling techniques, and longer pulse durations, *Dermatol Surg*. 2002. *28*: 16–20.

16.

OVERVIEW

TREATMENT OF VENOUS INSUFFICIENCY

John J. Bergan

The term "venous insufficiency" implies that normal functioning is deranged. Terms used to describe the various manifestations of venous insufficiency lend confusion to the general topic. Some of these terms, such as "telangiectasias," "thread veins," and "spider veins," are descriptive but imply different conditions. And it is in the chronic disorders, dominated by venous reflux through failed check valves causing hyperpigmentation, ulceration, and corona phlebectatica, where disorientation reigns. Some order can come from subscribing to a unifying theory of primary venous insufficiency and to a common theory of effects of an inflammatory cascade to clarify both situations.

PRIMARY VENOUS INSUFFICIENCY

The manifestations of simple primary venous insufficiency appear to be different from one another. However, reticular varicosities, telangiectasias, and major varicose veins are all elongated, dilated, and tortuous. Investigations into valve damage and venous wall abnormalities eventually may lead to an understanding of the problem, and therefore, a solution by surgery or pharmacotherapy.[1–4]

Scanning electron microscopy has shown varying degrees of thinning of the varicose venous wall. These areas of thinning coincide with areas of varicose dilation and replacement of smooth muscle by collagen, which is also a characteristic of varicose veins.[5,6] Our approach to this has been to assume that both the venous valve and the venous wall are affected by the elements that cause varicose veins. We and others have observed that in limbs with varicose veins, an absence of the subterminal valve at the saphenofemoral junction is common.[7] Further, perforation, splitting, and atrophy of saphenous venous valves have been seen both by angioscopy[8,9] and by direct examination of surgical specimens.[10]

Supporting the theory of weakness of the venous wall leading to valvular insufficiency is the observation that there is an increase in the vein wall space between the valve leaflets.[10] This is the first and most commonly observed abnormality associated with valve reflux.[11] Realizing these facts, our investigations have led us to explore the possible role of leukocyte infiltration of venous valves and the venous wall as part of the cause of varicose veins. In our investigations of surgical specimens, leukocytes in great number have been observed in the venous valves and wall, and monoclonal antibody staining has revealed their precise identification as monocytes.[10] Similar findings are present in the skin of patients with venous insufficiency.[12]

SURGICAL TREATMENT

Removal of the great saphenous vein (GSV) from the circulation is one of two essential steps in treating lower limb varicose veins. Incompetent valves along the GSV allow blood to reflux down the vein and into its tributaries, transmitting high pressure into smaller tributaries, which become varicose as a result. Much emphasis has been placed on the correct technique of high saphenofemoral ligation, in which meticulous attention is paid to identifying, ligating, and dividing all the tributaries of the GSV as they join the vein in the groin. It has always been a matter of surgical dogma that overlooking any of these allows continued reflux into the residual tributary and subsequent development of recurrent varicose veins.

A number of studies have confirmed that patients in whom the GSV is stripped tend to have fewer recurrences than those undergoing simple high ligation of the saphenofemoral junction (SFJ). Sarin et al. studied eighty-nine limbs in sixty-nine patients with GSV incompetence.[13] Legs were randomized to SFJ ligation with or without stripping, and evaluated by photoplethysmography (PPG), duplex scanning, clinical examination, and patient satisfaction. The follow-up period was 18 months. Significant differences in favor of the stripped group were found in all four parameters at final evaluation.

A similar study of seventy-eight patients (110 limbs) was reported by Dwerryhouse et al. in 1999, with a longer follow-up period of 5 years.[14] This demonstrated a significantly lower reoperation rate among patients undergoing GSV stripping (6%), as opposed to 20% in those undergoing high SFJ ligation alone.

Duplex scanning showed a much lower incidence of residual reflux in the remaining GSV when the proximal vein had been stripped to the knee than when it had not. However, the patient satisfaction rate was not significantly different between the two groups. Ninety percent of the stripped groups were satisfied as opposed to 87% in the nonstripped group (p = ns).

A further study from Jones et al. came to similar conclusions.[15] One hundred patients (133 limbs) were randomized as before. After 2 years, 43% of those who had not had GSV stripping demonstrated recurrent varicose veins as opposed to 25% who had. There was a statistically significant difference.

NEOVASCULARIZATION

Of great importance was the fact that duplex scanning showed that neovascularization in the groin was the most common cause of varicose recurrence. It was often seen in the ligation group that reflux through the neovascularization entered the residual saphenous vein and perpetuated the old varices while new ones developed. The authors concluded that by stripping the GSV, one was removing the runoff into which the new vessels could drain. Again, however, the satisfaction was broadly similar between the two groups: 91% in the stripped group and 87% in the unstripped.

All these authors concluded that stripping the long GSV gave better long-term results than simple high saphenous ligation. This appears to be true in terms of objective assessment of recurrence rates and in objective measurement of postoperative venous function but is not generally reflected in patient satisfaction rates, which tend to be similar whichever procedure is performed. This led Woodyer and Dormandy to reach a contrary conclusion—that stripping the GSV was a procedure based on surgical dogma, and one that did not confer subjective benefit to the patients so treated.[16] This leads one to conclude that a better method of evaluation of treatment results should be developed.

NONSURGICAL TREATMENT

In recent years, endovenous ablation has been found to be safe and effective in eliminating the proximal portion of the GSV from the venous circulation, with even faster

recovery and better cosmetic results than stripping.[17,18] The two currently available methods used to achieve ablation of the GSV are the Closure procedure using a radiofrequency (RF) catheter and generator (VNUS Medical Technologies, Sunnyvale, California), and the endovenous laser ablation (EVLT) procedure using a laser fiber and generator (various manufacturers). Both systems use electromagnetic energy to destroy the GSV in situ.

One of the difficulties in evaluating reports of successful ablation of the GSV lies in the definition of success. Some, especially in the RF ablation reports, define success as "no reflux in any segment longer than 5 cm." Some laser reports refer to success as "stable occlusion" or "reduction in reflux," and Min has applied the much clearer standard of success as "no flow by color flow Doppler."[17] Those who report results have not used the life table method, which takes into consideration dropouts and early and midterm failures. Thus the reported favorable 4- and 5-year rates of elimination of reflux may be exaggerated.

The major difficulty with defining success as reduction or absence of reflux is that attempts to establish whether reflux is present in a portion of a previously closed GSV may be inaccurate. Also, most recurrent patency is seen in the proximal portion of the treated GSV. Therefore, distal compression of the closed portion of the GSV to identify reflux in a proximal segment is futile. Likewise, using the Valsalva maneuver is unreliable and lacks reproducibility. Finally, the importance of distinguishing a partially patent channel with flow, from one with reflux, is academic, since the valves are just as thoroughly destroyed as the rest of the vein wall.[19]

Initially, reports of successful ablation of the GSV using either RF or laser energy without ligation or stripping were treated with great skepticism. However, the absence of neovascularization is striking, and many skeptics have begun to believe that former emphasis on a clean groin dissection may have been in error. Although it is still early, acceptance of endovenous techniques is increasing. Patient acceptance of these minimally invasive procedures is overwhelmingly better than with stripping.

Choosing which procedure to adopt, according to Morrison,[19] is influenced by a variety of factors including reported results (and especially reporting methods); economic factors such as equipment and disposables costs, reimbursement, and procedure time; availability of and experience with ultrasound equipment and trained personnel; individual support by industry before, during, and after acquisition of the generator; and the practitioner's own level of expertise and comfort with ultrasound-guided techniques and minimally invasive surgery.[19]

CHEMICAL VENOUS CLOSURE

Some phlebologists have advocated liquid sclerotherapy of the saphenous vein, but the results of such treatment have been disappointing, and published long-term results are absent. Comparisons between liquid and foam sclerotherapy have been done, and the results strongly favor foam.[20,21] Ultrasound-guided sclerotherapy (USGS) with foam must be considered as a completely new treatment of varicose veins. Although it needs proper training and some skill, it is simple, affordable, and extremely efficient.

Sclerosing agents produce a lesion of the venous wall, predominantly of the endothelium and, to a minor extent, of the media. The reaction that follows depends on the concentration of the agent and on the duration of the contact. If the venous diameter is greater than 3 mm, injections of liquid do not achieve this aim and dilution with blood quickly decreases their efficacy at short distances from the point of injection. Injections of foam have the advantage of a total filling of the vein, at least under 12 mm diameter. A further reduction in venous diameter can be obtained by leg elevation, compression with the hand, duplex probe or bandage, and venous spasm. In very large veins, foam will float over blood and induce a lesion of the upper venous wall despite apparent correct filling of the vein observed on duplex, thus the importance of massaging and compression.

Making the foam is easy and quick. Based on the technique initially described by Tessari, it can be prepared with two 5-cc syringes and a three-way stopcock.[20] Only detergent sclerosing agents can be used: Sotradecol and polidocanol at any desired concentration from 0.25% to 3%. Microbubbles of foam sclerosing agents are hyperechogenic and represent an excellent contrast medium for ultrasound techniques. They appear as a shadow within the lumen early, and like a hyperechogenic mass later with an acoustic shadow. Massaging the sclerosing agent to the desired part of the varicose network with the duplex probe or the hand is also very easily carried out. Progression from the varicose clusters to the GSV and then to the SFJ is always visible, provided a sufficient volume has been injected. Venous spasm usually is observed within minutes. The importance of the initial spasm has been emphasized in several studies and protocols.[22,23]

Postsclerotherapy compression is mandatory: on the varicose clusters for 48 hours, and then whole limb compression with 20- to 30-mm Hg thigh-high medical elastic stockings.[24] They must be worn during the daytime for at least 15 days. Patients must be examined both clinically and with duplex at 7 to 15 days.

The absolute risk of deep venous thrombosis is not confirmed. A few cases have been reported: most of them are gastrocnemius vein thrombosis, typically after telangiectasia and reticular vein sclerotherapy. Most frequent complications are visual disorders. These adverse reactions have been observed also with liquid sclerosing agents, but their incidence is much higher with foam; they can be estimated at 0.5–1 per 100 foam sessions.[25] They are observed more frequently in patients suffering from migraine with visual aura. They usually reproduce this aura. Researchers have questioned the pathophysiology of this phenomenon but have received no answer so far. The existence of a patent foramen ovale is the most likely explanation, as has been the liberation of toxic component associated with endothelial cell destruction (endothelin).

All published results demonstrate an immediate efficacy better than 80% in terms of immediate/primary venous occlusion. Repetition of injections in case of initial failure allows closure to approach 95% of efficacy with two to three sessions. Early and midterm results demonstrate a recurrence rate of about 20%. The redo injections remain as simple as primary injections and at least as efficient.

REFERENCES

1. Takase S, Pascarella L, Bergan J, Schmid-Schönbein, GW. Hypertension-induced venous valve remodeling, *J Vasc Surg*. 2004. *39*: 1329–1334.
2. Takase S, Pascarella L, Lerond L, Bergan JJ, Schmid-Schönbein GW. Venous hypertension, inflammation, and valve remodeling, *Eur J Vasc Endovasc Surg*. 2004. *28*: 484–493.
3. Pascarella L, Schmid-Schönbein GW, Bergan JJ. An animal model of venous hypertension: The role of inflammation in venous valve failure, *J Vasc Surg*. 2005. *41*: 303–311.
4. Pascarella L, Schmid-Schönbein GW, Bergan JJ. Microcirculation and venous ulcers, *Ann Vasc Surg*. 2005. *19*(6): 921–927.
5. Mashiah A, Ross SS, Hod I. The scanning electron microscope in the pathology of varicose veins, *Isr J Med Sci*. 1991. *27*: 202–206.
6. Travers JP, Brookes CE, Evans J, et al. Assessment of wall structure and composition of varicose veins with reference to collagen, elastin, and smooth muscle content, *Eur J Vasc Endovasc Surg*. 1996. *11*: 230–237.
7. Gradman WS, Segalowitz J, Grundfest W. Venoscopy in varicose vein surgery: Initial experience, *Phlebology*. 1993. *8*: 145–150.
8. Van Cleef IF, Desvaux P, Hugentobler JP, et al. Endoscopie veineuse, *J Mal Vasc*. 1991. *16*: 184–187.
9. Van Cleef JF, Desvaux P, Hugentobler JP, et al. Etude endoscopique des reflux valvulaires sapheniens, *J Mal Vasc*. 1992. *17*: 113–116.
10. Ono T, Bergan JJ, Schmid-Schönbein GW, Takase S. Monocyte infiltration into venous valves, *J Vasc Surg*. 1998. *27*: 158–166.
11. Satokawa H, Hoshino S, Igari T. Angioscopic external valvuloplasty in the treatment of varicose veins, *Phlebology*. 1997. *12*: 136–141.
12. Wilkinson LS, Bunker C, Edwards JC, Scurr JH, Coleridge Smith PD. Leukocytes: Their role in the etiopathogenesis of skin damage in venous disease, *J Vasc Surg*. 1993. *17*: 669–675.
13. Sarin S, Scurr JH, Coleridge Smith PD. Stripping of the long saphenous vein in the treatment of primary varicose veins, *Br J Surg*. 1994. *81*: 1455–1458.
14. Dwerryhouse S, Davies B, Harradine K, et al. Stripping of the long saphenous vein reduces the rate of reoperation for recurrent varicose veins: Five year results of a randomized trial, *J Vasc Surg*. 1999. *29*: 589–592.
15. Jones L, Braithwaite BD, Selwyn D, et al. Neovascularisation is the principal cause of varicose vein recurrence: Results of a randomised trial of stripping the long saphenous vein, *Eur J Vasc Endovasc Surg*. 1996. *12*: 442–445.
16. Woodyer AB, Dormandy JA. Is it necessary to strip the long saphenous vein?, *Phlebology*. 1986. 221–224.
17. Min RJ, Zimmet SE, Isaacs MN, Forrestal MD. Endovenous laser treatment of the incompetent greater saphenous vein, *JVIR*. 2001. *12*: 1167–1171.
18. Lurie F, Creton D, Eklof B, et al. Prospective randomized study of endovenous radiofrequency obliteration (Closure Procedure) versus ligation and stripping in a selected patient population (EVOLVeS Study), *J Vasc Surg*. 2003. *38*: 207–214.

19. Morrison NM. Saphenous ablation: What are the choices, laser, or RF energy?, *Semin Vasc Surg*. 2005. *18*(1):15–18.

20. Tessari L, Cavezzi A, Frullini A. Preliminary experience with a new sclerosing foam in the treatment of varicose veins, *Dermatol Surg*. 2001. *27*: 58–60.

20. Yamaki T, Nozaki M, Iwasaka S. Comparative study of duplex-guided foam sclerotherapy and duplex-guided liquid sclerotherapy for the treatment of superficial venous insufficiency, *Dermatol Surg*. 2004. *30*(5): 718–722; discussion 722.

21. Hamel-Desnos C, Desnos P, Wollmann JC, Ouvry P, Mako S, Allaert FA. Evaluation of the efficacy of polidocanol in the form of foam compared with liquid form in sclerotherapy of the greater saphenous vein: Initial results, *Dermatol Surg*. 2003. *29*(12): 1170–1175; discussion 1175.

22. Frullini A, Cavezzi A. Sclerosing foam in the treatment of varicose veins and telangiectases: History and analysis of safety and complications, *Dermatol Surg*. 2002. *28*(1): 11–15.

23. Barrett JM, Allen B, Ockelford A, Goldman MP. Microfoam ultrasound-guided sclerotherapy of varicose veins in 100 legs, *Dermatol Surg*. 2004. *30*(1): 6–12.

24. Barrett JM, Allen B, Ockelford A, Goldman MP. Microfoam ultrasound-guided sclerotherapy treatment for varicose veins in a subgroup with diameters at the junction of 10 mm or greater compared with a subgroup of less than 10 mm, *Dermatol Surg*. 2004. *30*(11): 1386–1390.

25. Guex JJ, Allaert FA, Gillet JL, Chleir F. Immediate and midterm complications of sclerotherapy: Report of a prospective multicenter registry of 12,173 sclerotherapy sessions, *Dermatol Surg*. 2005. *31*(2): 123–128; discussion 128.

17.

ULTRASOUND EXAMINATION OF THE PATIENT WITH PRIMARY VENOUS INSUFFICIENCY

Nicole Loerzel, Virginia Ratcliff, Nisha Bunke-Paquette, and John J. Bergan

INTRODUCTION

Chronic venous insufficiency (CVI) is a common disorder whose manifestations include varicose veins and skin changes such as venous dermatitis, hyperpigmentation, lipodermatosclerosis, and chronic leg ulcers. The signs and symptoms identifying CVI have been clearly demonstrated to be related to venous hypertension.[1,2] Several factors, such as age, gender, hormones, body posture, genetic inheritance, and employment in standing occupations are associated with the development of venous hypertension.[3,4] This, in turn, has been found to trigger vascular remodeling, through a reorganization of extracellular matrix within the venous parenchyma. This leads to the failure of vein valves.[5,6]

Primary valve incompetence is the most important cause of venous hypertension (70–80% of cases). Valve incompetence may be secondary to deep venous thrombosis (DVT) or trauma in 18–25% and due to a congenital anomaly in 1–3% of cases.[7]

The advent of duplex ultrasonography has provided the physician with practical information to assess varicose veins, deep veins, thrombotic states, postthrombotic obstruction, and incompetent perforating veins.[8] Duplex ultrasound examination is an essential diagnostic tool in the evaluation and treatment of venous disorders. Precision anatomical vein mapping and identification of patterns of venous reflux are essential to determine therapeutic options.

EQUIPMENT

The duplex ultrasound system should be able to detect blood flow rates as low as 6 cm/s.[9] This can be done by dedicated high resolution vascular scanners with Color/Power-Doppler functions and pulsed-wave Doppler. Linear transducers in the range of 4–7 MHz are used.[7] The inferior vena cava (IVC), pelvic veins, and deep veins in obese patients may be imaged with 3-MHz transducers.

With advances in technology, duplex systems have become smaller, more transportable, and more operator friendly. Miniaturized devices feature transducers designed with advanced architecture that allow a single probe to image across a greater range of depths within an application and across applications. The transducer for peripheral vascular examinations operates from 5–10 MHz and provides resolution from skin surface to 7 cm in depth. The technology incorporates power Doppler sonography, tissue harmonic imaging, and direct connectivity to a personal computer.

Additional materials needed for a complete examination include a warm room, acoustic gel, towels, handled step stools, and a comprehension worksheet.

CLINICAL EXAMINATION

The clinical examination and complete medical history, will help determine the need for venous duplex ultrasound evaluation. Data concerning family and personal venous history, symptoms, clinical findings, and previous venous treatments should be elicited.

Limbs should be classified into one of seven CEAP classes of increasing severity designated C_0 to C_6 (see Table 17.1) and identified as symptomatic (S) or asymptomatic (A).[10] Common symptoms associated with CVI are leg idling, heaviness, and sensation of itching and swelling; important signs to consider are skin hyperpigmentation, varicose veins, corona phlebectatica, venous dermatitis, lipodermatoclerosis, active ulcers, and/or scars from previous ulceration. The term "chronic venous disease" (CVD) is used for the full spectrum of signs and symptoms associated with classes $C_{0.s}$ to C_6, and the term "CVI" is used for classes C_4 to C_6.[11]

A history of previous DVT or pulmonary embolism provides information regarding etiology. The method of diagnosing DVT always should be recorded. The anatomic distribution and the pathophysiology within the CEAP system are revealed by the ultrasound examination.

Table 17.1 CEAP CLASSIFICATION OF CVD AND CVI[17]

CLASS	SIGNS OF VENOUS DISEASE
Class 0	No visible or palpable signs of venous disease (only symptoms)
Class 1 (A,S)	Telangiectasias or Reticular Veins
Class 2 (A,S)	Varicose Veins
Class 3 (A,S)	Edema
Class 4 (A,S)	Skin changes ascribed to venous disease (e.g., pigmentation, venous eczema, lipodermatosclerosis)
Class 5 (A,S)	Skin changes as defined above with healed ulceration
Class 6 (A,S)	Skin changes as defined above with active ulceration

Table 17.2 SUMMARY OF IMPORTANT CHANGES IN NOMENCLATURE OF LOWER EXTREMITY VEINS[19,25]

OLD TERMINOLOGY	NEW TERMINOLOGY
Femoral Vein	Common Femoral Vein
Superficial Femoral Vein	Femoral Vein
Deep Vein of the thigh	Profunda Femoris Vein
Greater/Long Saphenous Vein	Great Saphenous Vein
Smaller/Short Saphenous Vein	Small Saphenous Vein
Sural Veins	Solcal Veins
Dodd's Perforator	Gastrocnemius Veins
Boyd's Perforator	Medial Gastrocnemius Vein
Sherman's Perforator (24 cm)	Lateral Gastrocnemius Vein
Cockett's Perforators	Intergemellar Vein
	Perforator of the Femoral Canal
	Paratibial Perforator (upper third of the leg)
	Paratibial Perforator (middle third of the leg)
	Posterotibial Perforators

INDICATIONS FOR DUPLEX EVALUATION

Its generally accepted that all patients presenting with varicose veins, skin changes associated with chronic venous insufficiency, edema, leg ulceration (CEAP clinical stages 2–6) should undergo duplex ultrasound evaluation. Duplex scanning is also indicated to further evaluate patients with venous symptoms (CEAP clinical stage 0), venous malformations and for post-treatment surveillance.[12] It is the authors opinion that select patients with telangiectactic or reticular veins (CEAP clinical stage 1) should also be scanned for underlying venous insufficiency. Patients who have extensive reticular veins and/or telangiectasias, especially located in the inner thighs, medial or lateral malleolus or associated with corona phlebectasia are more likely to have underlying venous insufficiency than patients with minimal or isolated spider veins. The Edinborough Vein Study showed there was a significant trend between grade of telangiectasias and reflux in the GSV (upper and lower segments) in the limbs of 1092 subjects. [13,14] Engelhorn demonstrated either greater or small saphenous vein reflux in 46% of patients with CEAP 1 telangiectasias.[15] Other clinical signs such as corona phlebectasia, as defined as fan-shaped intradermal telangiectases in the medial and sometimes lateral portions of the ankle and foot has been associated with an increased prevalence of GSV reflux.[16] Additionally, risk of underlying incompetence in the calf perforators by duplex ultrasound is 4.4 times greater in patients with corona phlebectasia.[16] Patients who have failed spider vein treatment should also be evaluated for an underlying source of venous reflux.

ULTRASOUND EXAMINATION

In 2002, an international interdisciplinary consensus committee on venous anatomical terminology proposed a revision and extension of the Terminologia Anatomica of the lower extremity venous system (see Table 17.2).[17]

The ultrasound examination is carried out with the patient standing in an upright position.[18] This position elicits reflux by challenging venous valves and maximally dilates the leg veins. Sensitivity and specificity in detecting reflux are increased in examinations performed with the patient standing rather than when the patient is supine.[8,18,19] It is further recommended that the patient stand for several minutes prior to a duplex examination, allowing for equilibration of the venous system. The standing examination of the lower extremity venous system has become the standard of care and the supine examination should be considered inadequate. If the patient is physically unable to stand or if the history reveals a tendency to fainting because of vasovagal response, the examination may need to be modified with the patient in the semi-upright position.

VEIN MAPPING.

Transverse rather than longitudinal scans, and continuous scanning are performed in order to provide a clear mapping of the venous system. This can be recorded on a premade data sheet simultaneously with the venous reflux examination (see Figure 17.1). Patency usually is assessed by compression of the vein, and reflux is detected on release. The augmentation of flow, distal compression, and release of thigh and calf [7] should be done sharply and quickly. Automated rapid inflation/deflation cuffs are cumbersome but may be used for this purpose, and offer the advantage of a standardized stimulus.[8,20] The Valsalva maneuver is a reverse flow augmentation stimulus and is best used for the saphenofemoral junction (SFJ) because a competent valve at that level will render the test useless on more distal segments.

REFLUX

The presence of vein reflux through incompetent vein valves is the most important pathologic finding in CVI. Reflux is measured during the release phase of the flow augmentation maneuver and during the closed epiglottis apneic phase of the Valsalva maneuver (see Figure 17.2). It should be noted

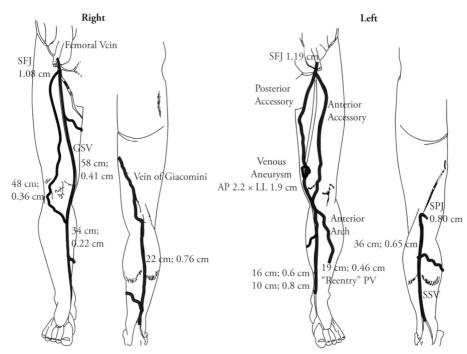

Figure 17.1   This data entry form outlines the saphenous veins and the relevant deep veins. Refluxing veins are added in heavy black lines and selected vein diameters are recorded. Location of PVs and aneurysms can be added and distance from the floor indicated.

that retrograde backflow is present in normal vein valves immediately before their closure, but a cutoff value of 500 ms defines pathologic reflux in the saphenous veins. The value of 350 ms is used in perforator veins (PVs) and 1,000 ms for femoropopliteal veins.[18,21] Time of day is a relative consensus regarding the position for reflux determination.

THE SAPHENOFEMORAL JUNCTION

With the patient standing and the transducer gently applied in the groin, the SFJ, common femoral vein, femoral vein,

and deep femoral veins are identified (see Figure 17.3). The SFJ also known as the confluence of superficial inguinal veins, is complex and highly variable. It includes the great saphenous vein (GSV), pudendal veins, and superficial epigastric and superficial circumflex iliac veins (see Figure 17.4A).[17,22] Imaging of the pudendal veins is particularly important in cases of pelvic congestive syndrome, in which vulvar varicosities and pudendal reflux can be observed.[23] Incompetence of the ovarian veins is the most important cause of this syndrome.[24]

The diameter of the SFJ at the confluence of the GSV and the femoral vein is recorded. The SFJ is usually the location

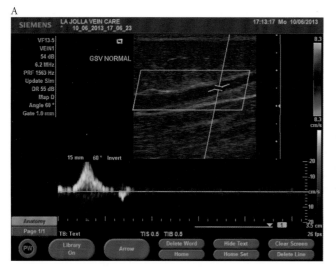

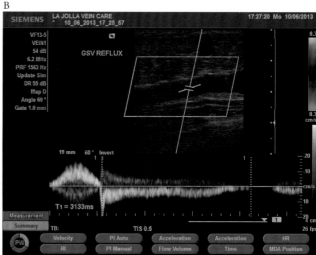

Figure 17.2   Flow augmentation maneuvers elicit reflux in incompetent veins. Reflux is defined as retrograde outflow measured during the release phase of the augmentation maneuver and the Valsava maneuver's closed epiglottis apneic phase for the SFJ only. Figure 17.2 (A) demonstrates examination of a normal GSV. In contrast, Figure 17.3 (B) demonstrates an incompetent GSV with reflux duration greater than 3 seconds.

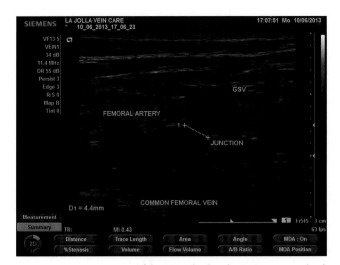

Figure 17.3 A transverse scan of the SFJ is displayed. Major anatomic landmarks to be noted are femoral vein, femoral artery, SFJ diameter, GSVs.

of the terminal valve.[25] More distally another valve, known as subterminal, is also identifiable (see Figure 17.4B).[25]

The Valsalva and thigh/calf compression-release maneuvers define the presence of reflux at the saphenofemoral junction as well as in the femoral vein.

THE GSV

The GSV is scanned from the groin in proximal-to-distal direction.

In the thigh, the GSV lies within the saphenous compartment (see Figure 17.5).[17] The superficial fascia and the muscular fascia define the saphenous compartment and provide the typical ultrasound image of an Egyptian eye (see Figure 17.5C).[25]

Anterior and posterior accessory veins are often identified in the thigh (see Figure 17.6). These veins are often incompetent and receive reflux from the saphenous vein.[17]

Varying patterns of reflux through the different components of the SFJ and GSV system have been documented. Classification of abnormal, refluxing venous patterns has been a difficult task because of the anatomic variability of the vascular structures involved. In 2005 a panel of experts proposed a new classification of GSV reflux describing the different types and extent of GSV insufficiency (Figure 17.7).[26,27] Furthermore, using this classification system, Chastanet and Pittaluga have demonstrated that the more extensive the GSV reflux, the more it was positively correlated with increasing age and advanced clinical stage.[28] Younger patients were more likely to have non-saphenous varicose veins with less advanced clinical signs. Older patients were more likely to have incompetence at the saphenofemoral junction and GSV reflux to the ankle.

Diameters of the GSV, should be measured with B-mode ultrasound in transverse section at several levels. These measurements should be recorded at proximal, middle, and distal regions and especially at diameter variation locations. The term "superficial venous aneurysms" has been proposed for segmental dilations of the GSV and small saphenous vein (SSV).[29] The term "varicosities" refers to more elongated and dilated superficial veins. The level, distance from the heel pad or floor, and anteroposterior and laterolateral diameters of venous aneurysms should be recorded.[29]

Intersaphenous veins are often present as communications between the GSV and SSV.

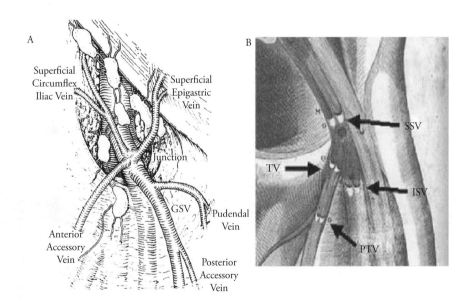

Figure 17.4 (A) The SFJ includes the GSV, the superficial iliac circumflex, the superficial epigastric, and the pudendal veins. (B) Illustration of the SFJ with its valves. Modified from the *De Venarum Ostiolis* of Jeronimus Fabricius ab Aquapendente, Venice, 1603. TV, Terminal valve; PTV, preterminal valve; SSV, suprasaphenic valve; ISV, infrasaphenic valve. (Adapted from Reference 25.)

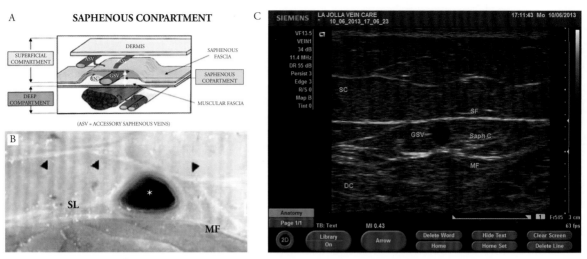

Figure 17.5 (A) The saphenous compartment (SaphC) is bound superficially by the saphenous fascia (SF) and deeply by the muscular fascia (MF). It contains the saphenous veins (SV) and the saphenous nerve (SN). The accessory saphenous veins (ASV) lie external to this compartment, close to the dermis (D). SC, Superficial compartment; DC, deep compartment. (Adapted from Reference 17.) (B) Axial section from a cadaveric limb. The GSV enclosed in the saphenous compartment is clearly visualized. MF, Muscular fascia; SL saphenous ligament. (Adapted from Reference 25.) (C) Sonography of the GSV at mid thigh. The hyperechoic saphenous fascia (SF) and muscular fascia (MF) define the saphenous compartment in which the GSV courses.

THE SSV

The posterior leg should be carefully interrogated prior to venous treatment, due to the variability in its anatomy and proximity to nerves and arteries. The patient should stand and facing opposite the examiner. The knee should be slightly bent, heel on the ground and weight bearing on the opposite limb. The study of the SSV starts at the popliteal fossa by identification of the saphenopopliteal junction (SPJ). Compression-release of the calf provides information concerning junctional reflux. If reflux is present in the SSV, the diameter of the small saphenous vein should be measured 3 cm distal to the SPJ and at mid-calf.[12]

The SSV is an important and often overlooked cause of superficial venous insufficiency. The SSV usually empties in to the popliteal vein directly or via the gastrocnemius vein, but there are many anatomic variations in its points of connection to the popliteal vein.

A thigh extension (TE), also known as the cranial extension of the SSV, is present in the majority of limbs.[30] It can be identified between the biceps femoris and semimembranous muscles.[17] The TE of the SSV may give rise to vein of Giacomini, that connects with the GSV in the posteriomedial aspect of the thigh.[17] In the calf, the SSV courses within a duplication of the superficial fascia similar to the GSV in the saphenous compartment.[19]

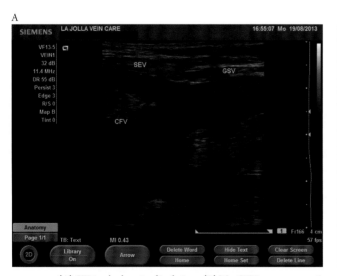

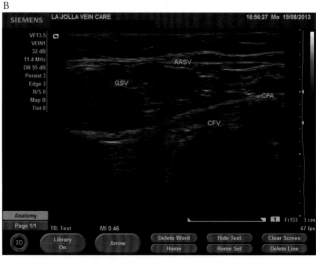

Figure 17.6 (A) SFJ in the longitudinal view. (B) The SFJ in transverse view will demonstrate the presence of accessory saphenous veins.

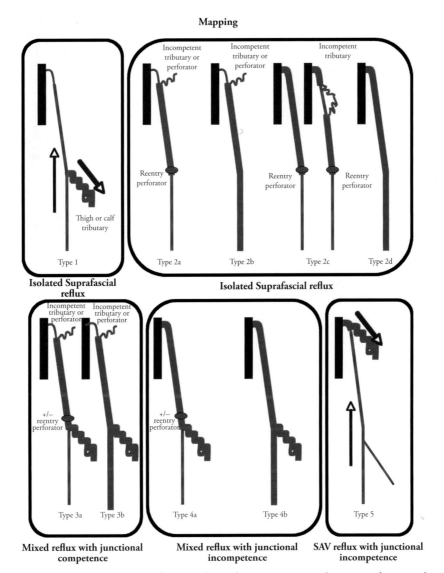

Mapping

Type 1 — Isolated Suprafascial reflux

Type 2a, Type 2b, Type 2c, Type 2d — Isolated Suprafascial reflux

Type 3a, Type 3b — Mixed reflux with junctional competence

Type 4a, Type 4b — Mixed reflux with junctional incompetence

Type 5 — SAV reflux with junctional incompetence

Figure 17.7 In 2005, a panel of experts proposed a new classification to he used in a prospective multicenter study testing the A.S.V.A.L. (selective ablation of varicose veins in local anesthesia) method. The classification reports five major types of saphenofemoral reflux.

Throughout the entire examination, compression-release maneuvers serve to elicit reflux in the various venous segments

PERFORATING VEINS

PVs penetrate anatomic layers (see Figure 17.8). Communicating veins, such as intersaphenous veins, connect veins within the same anatomic layer.[17]

One of the innovations of the new Terminologia Anatomica of the venous system of lower limbs is the complete elimination of eponyms such as the Boyd, Sherman, and Cockett perforators. Descriptive terms designating location have been adopted.[17] A classification of them is shown in Table 17.3. No doubt, all the eponyms will persist.

During the examination, the location of each perforator is recorded by measuring its distance (in centimeters) from the floor. The diameter (in centimeters) of each perforator

should be recorded. Many authors have observed a correlation between an enlarged perforating vein diameter and incompetence. One study reported that perforating diameters of 3.5 mm or larger in the calf and thigh were associated with reflux in more than 90% of cases.[31]

Reflux is assessed by manual compression and release maneuvers. Blood flow direction and duration following the compression must be noted.

It has been suggested that an outward (toward the superficial veins) blood flow of duration greater than 350 ms, following manual distal compression, defines a PV as incompetent.[7]

Perforators can be distinguished as exit and reentry veins. Exit veins are refluxing perforators usually associated with clusters of varicose veins and/or important skin changes, such as hyperpigmentation.[7]

Reentry perforators usually are found distal to major varicose veins and clusters. Their blood flow direction is inward (toward the deep veins) and they are not pathologic

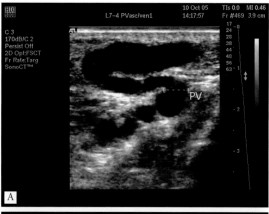

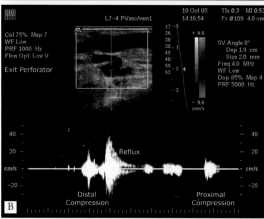

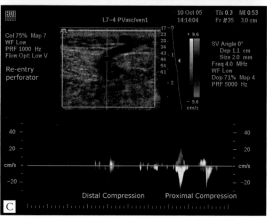

Figure 17.8   PVs penetrate anatomic layers (A). Distal limb compression rather than proximal (B and C) elicits reflux. Reflux is measured on the release phase of the augmentation maneuver and is detected as outward flow (B) whose duration is greater than in incompetent exit perforators. Reentry perforators show little or no outward flow following distal compressions (C).

Table 17.3 PERFORATING VEINS[19]

MAIN GROUPS	SUBGROUPS
Foot perforators	Medial foot PV
	Plantar foot PV
	Dorsal foot PVs or intercapillary veins
	Plantar PV
Ankle Perforators	Anterior Ankle PV
	Medial Ankle PV
	Lateral Ankle PV
Leg Perforators	Medial Leg PV
	Paratibial PV
	Posterior Tibial PV
	Anterior Leg
	Lateral Leg
	Posterior Leg
	Medial Gastrocnemius
	Lateral Gastrocnemius
	Intergemellar PV
	Para-achillean PV
Knee Perforators	Medial Knee PV
	Suprapatellar PV
	Lateral P.V
	Infrapatellar PV
	Popliteal Fossa
Thigh Perforators	Medial Thigh PV
	PV of the femoral canal
	Inguinal PV
	Anterior thigh PV
	Lateral thigh PV
	Posterior Thigh PVs
	Pudendal PV

ULTRASOUND MAPPING OF VENOUS ULCERS

Venous ulcers usually are associated with varicose veins and refluxing perforators located in the immediate vicinity of the ulcerated area. A superficial network of enlarged and dilated veins often can be observed underneath the ulcer (see Figure 17.9).[32] The description and the documentation of reflux in these veins can help to indicate a particular therapeutic approach.[32–34]

DEEP VEINS

The ultrasound examination also must include the deep veins. Femoral and popliteal veins usually are studied with the patient in supine position.[35] Patency is assessed by distal compression. Irregularities of the vascular wall may appear as hyperechoic areas and always should be noted in patients with superficial reflux and a clinical history suggestive of previous DVT or pulmonary embolism. Sural, anterior tibial, posterior tibial, and peroneal veins are imaged while the patient is in the sitting position, usually starting from the ankle and proceeding toward the knee.[35] Compression and flow augmentation maneuvers assess their patency

but merely competent.[7] Skin changes are not seen adjacent to reentry perforating veins.

Incompetent perforators usually are observed at the medial thigh, middle and distal third of the leg, and middle third of the calf.[7,9]

Scanning of the lateral aspect of the lower limb also is recommended. The lateral venous system that is seen on the lateral aspect of the thigh and the leg can show varicosities and important exit and reentry perforators. These are not as well characterized as the medial perforating veins.

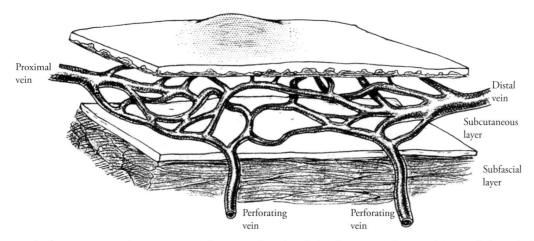

Figure 17.9 A network of varicose veins and incompetent perforators is often identified in the vicinity of venous ulcers usually beneath the ulcer.

and presence of reflux. Deep vein abnormalities must be recorded.

DISCUSSION

Duplex ultrasound sonography represents the best choice in evaluation of venous reflux in lower limbs.[7–9] This test is noninvasive, generally acceptable to the patient, and inexpensive. It provides direct imaging, localization, and extent of venous reflux with a surprisingly high sensitivity (95%) and specificity (100%).[36]

Duplex ultrasound findings correlate with the angioscopic observation of incompetent vein valves in advanced chronic venous insufficiency.[37] As demonstrated by Yamaki et al., high peak reflux velocities (>30 cm/s), reflux duration greater than 3 s, and an enlarged valve annulus measured by duplex ultrasonography at the SFJ are closely related to angioscopically deformed and incompetent terminal valves (Type III and Type IV valves).[37]

In contrast, duplex ultrasound PV identification and characterization have shown to be more difficult and less accurate.[36] Lower sensitivity rates (51%) have been reported when the number of perforators identified by ultrasound, ascending phlebography (AP), and subfascial endoscopic perforator surgery (SEPS) were compared.[36]

CONCLUSION

Duplex ultrasound sonography is the optimal diagnostic modality for assessment of lower extremity reflux. Insights into pathology, proper technique, and uniform testing are essential.[9] A clear graphic notation of significant vein diameters, anomalous anatomy, superficial venous aneurysms, PVs, and presence and extent of reflux should always be recorded during the examination. The most important interrogation points for the venous reflux examination are

Table 17.4 **MAJOR INTERROGATION POINTS FOR VENOUS REFLUX EXAMINATION**

INTERROGATION POINTS
Femoral vein
Saphenofemoral junction
Great saphenous vein
Accessory veins (anterior and posterior)
Popliteal vein-gastrocnemius Veins
Small saphenous vein
Thigh Extension
Vein of Giacomini
Intersaphenous veins
Medial thigh PVs
Leg PVs
Ankle PVs

indicated in Table 17.4. These serve as basic guidelines because the interested vascular ultrasonographer must trace out duplicated veins and note reflux in major tributaries, such as the accessory veins.

REFERENCES

1. Takase S, Bergan J. Molecular mechanisms in chronic venous insufficiency. *Ann Vasc Surg.* 2007. *21*(3): 260–266. Review.
2. Bergan JJ, Pascarella L, Schmid-Schenbein GW. Pathogenesis of primary chronic venous disease: Insights from animal models of venous hypertension. *J Vasc Surg.* 2008. *47*(1): 183–92. Review.
3. Criqui MH, Denenberg JO, Bergan J, Langer RD, Fronek A. Risk factors for chronic venous disease: the San Diego Population Study. *J Vasc Surg.* 2007. *46*(2):331–337.
4. Evans CJ, Fowkes FG, Ruckley CV, Lee AJ. Prevalence of varicose veins and chronic venous insufficiency in men and women in the general population: Edinburgh Vein Study, *J Epidemiol Community Health.* 1999. 53(3): 149–153.
5. Takase S, Pascarella L, Bergan JJ, Schmid-Schonbein GW. Hypertension induced venous valve remodeling, *J Vasc Surg.* 2004. *39*(6): 1329–1334.

6. Pascarella L, Schmid-Schönbein GW, Bergan J. An animal model of venous hypertension: The role of inflammation in venous valve failure, *J Vasc Surg.* 2005. *41*(2): 303–311.

7. Labropoulos N, Leon LR Jr. Duplex evaluation of venous insufficiency, *Semin Vasc Surg.* 2005. *18*(1): 59.

8. Lynch TG, Dalsing MC, Ouriel K, Ricotta JJ, Wakefield TW. Developments in diagnosis and classification of venous disorders: Non-invasive diagnosis, *Cardiovasc Surg.* 1999. *7*(2): 160–178.

9. Ballard JL, Bergan JJ, DeLange MD. Venous imaging for reflux using duplex ultrasonography. In: AbuRahma AF, Bergan JJ, eds. *Noninvasive vascular diagnosis.* London: Springer-Verlag. 2000. 339–334.

10. Kistner RL, Eklof B, Masuda EM. Diagnosis of chronic venous disease of the lower extremities: The "CEAP" classification, *Mayo Clin Proc.* 1996. *71*(4): 338–345.

11. Eklof B, Rutherford RB, Bergan JJ, et al. Revision of the CEAP classification for chronic venous disorders: Consensus statement, *J Vasc Surg.* 2004. *40*(6): 1248–1252.

12. Coleridge-Smith P, Labropoulos N, Partsch H, Myers K, Nicolaides A, Cavezzi A. Duplex ultrasound investigation of the veins in chronic venous disease of the lower limbs—UIP consensus document. Part I. Basic principles, *Eur J Vasc Endovasc Surg.* 2006. *31*(1): 83–92. Review.

13. Ruckley CV, Allan PL, Evans CJ, Lee AJ, Fowkes FG. Telangiectasia and venous reflux in the Edinburgh Vein Study, *Phlebology.* 2012. *27*(6): 297–302.

14. Ruckley CV, Evans CJ, Allan PL, Lee AJ, Fowkes FG. Telangiectasia in the Edinburgh Vein Study: epidemiology and association with trunk varices and symptoms, *Eur J Vasc Endovasc Surg.* 2008. *36*(6): 719–724.

15. Engelhorn CA, Engelhorn ALV, Cassou MF, Salles-Cunha S. Patterns of saphenous venous reflux in women presenting with lower extremity telangiectasias. *Dermatol Surg* 2007. *33*: 282–288.

16. Uhl JF, Cornu-Thenard A, Carpentier PH, Widmer MT, Partsch H, Antignani PL.Clinical and hemodynamic significance of corona phlebectatica in chronic venous disorders. *J Vasc Surg.* 2005. *42*(6):1163–1168.

17. Caggiati A, Bergan JJ, Gloviczki P, Jantet G, Wendell-Smith CP, Partsch H. Nomenclature of the veins of the lower limbs: An international interdisciplinary consensus statement, *J Vasc Surg.* 2002. *36*(2): 416–422.

18. Labropoulos N, Tiongson J, Pryor L, et al. Definition of venous reflux in lower-extremity veins, *J Vasc Surg.* 2003. *38*(4): 793–798.

19. Phillips GW. Review of venous vascular ultrasound, *World J Surg.* 2000. *24*(2): 241–248.

20. Masuda EM, Kistner RL, Eklof B. Prospective study of duplex scanning for venous reflux: Comparison of Valsalva and pneumatic cuff techniques in the reverse Trendelenburg and standing positions, *J Vasc Surg.* 1994. *20*(5): 711–720.

21. Labropoulos N, Giannoukas AD, Delis K, et al. Where does venous reflux start? *J Vasc Surg.* 1997. *26*(5): 736–742.

22. Goldman MP, Fronek A. Anatomy and pathophysiology of varicose veins, *J Derm Surg Onc.* 1989. *15*(2): 138–145.

23. Scultetus AH, Villavicencio JL, Gillespie DL, Kao TC, Rich NM. The pelvic venous syndromes: Analysis of our experience with 57 patients, *J Vasc Surg.* 2002. *36*(5): 881–888.

24. Nascimento AB, Mitchell DG, Holland G. Ovarian veins: Magnetic resonance imaging findings in an asymptomatic population, *J Magn Reson Imaging.* 2002. *15*(5): 551–556.

25. Caggiati A, Bergan JJ, Gloviczki P, Eklof B, Allegra C, Partsch H. Nomenclature of the veins of the lower limb: Extensions, refinements, and clinical application, *J Vasc Surg.* 2005. *41*(4): 719–724.

26. Pittaluga P, Réa B, Barbe R, Guex JJ. Méthode ASVAL (ablation selective des varices sous anesthésie locale): Principes et résultats préliminaires, *Phlebologie.* 2005. *58*(2): 175–181.

27. Pittaluga P, Réa B, Barbe R, Guex. In: Becquemin JP, Alimi YS, Watelet J., eds. *Updates and controversies in vascular surgery, A.S.V.A.L. method: Principles and preliminary results.* Turin, Italy: Minerva Medica. 2005. 182–189.

28. Chastanet S, Pittaluga P. Patterns of reflux in the great saphenous vein system, *Phlebology.* 2013. *28* Suppl 1: 39–46.

29. Pascarella L, Al-Tuwaijri M, Bergan JJ, et al. Lower extremity superficial venous aneurysms, *Ann Vasc Surg.* 2005. *19*(1): 6973.

30. Georgiev M, Myers KA, Belcaro G. The thigh extension of the lesser saphenous vein: from Giacomini's observations to ultrasound scan imaging, *J Vasc Surg.* 2003. *37*: 558–563.

31. Sandri JL, Barros FS, Pontes S, Jacques C, Salles-Cunha SX. Diameter-reflux relationship in perforating veins of patients with varicose veins, *J Vasc Surg.* 30(5): 119–199.

32. Yamaki T, Nozaki M, Sasaki K. Color duplex ultrasound in the assessment of primary venous leg ulceration, *Dermatol Surg.* 1998. *24*(10): 1124–1128.

33. Magnusson MB, Nelzen O, Risberg B, Sivertsson R. A colour Doppler ultrasound study of venous reflux in patients with chronic leg ulcers, *Eur J Vasc Endovasc Surg.* 2001. *21*(4): 353–360.

34. Bergan JJ, Pascarella L. Severe chronic venous insufficiency: Primary treatment with sclerofoam, *Semin Vasc Surg.* 2005. *18*(1): 4956.

35. Labropoulos N, Landon P, Jay T. The impact of duplex scanning in phlebology, *Dermatol Surg.* 2002. *28*(1): 15.

36. Depalma RG, Kowallek DL, Barcia TC, Cafferata HT. Target selection for surgical intervention in severe chronic venous insufficiency: Comparison of duplex scanning and phlebography, *J Vasc Surg.* 2000. *32*(5): 913–920.

37. Yamaki T, Sasaki K, Nozaki M. Preoperative duplex-derived parameters and angioscopic evidence of valvular incompetence associated with superficial venous insufficiency, *J Endovasc Ther.* 2002. *9*(2): 229–233.

38. Mekenas L, Bergan J. Venous reflux examination: Technique using miniaturized ultrasound scanning, *J Vasc Tech.* 2002. *2*(26): 139–146.

18.

SCLEROTHERAPY AND ULTRASOUND-GUIDED SCLEROTHERAPY

Paul K. Thibault

SCLEROTHERAPY

Varicose veins are a degenerative disease of the venous system where there is a defect in the strength of the vein wall with associated valvular dysfunction resulting in reflux (reverse) flow in affected areas of the superficial venous system of the legs. Usually reflux from the deep to superficial system through incompetent venous junctions and perforator veins is a major contributor to the superficial venous insufficiency. As venous disease is a chronic disease, treatment is usually directed at controlling the disease, rather than curing it. It is therefore important that interventional treatment not aggravate the condition in the long term.

Sclerotherapy refers to a method of treating varicose veins: a foreign substance, usually a chemical, is introduced into the lumen of a vein to cause endothelial necrosis and subsequent fibrosis of the vein. Apart from reducing the size of the vein to a small fibrous cord, effective sclerotherapy also eliminates the physiopathological reflux associated with varicose veins. As such, sclerotherapy is an alternative treatment to surgery and other physical endovenous ablation techniques such as endovenous laser ablation (EVLA) in the management of varicose veins. Sclerotherapy differs from the other ablative techniques in that it can be effective treatment for all types of pathological venous dilatations from major truncal varicose veins to the finest telangiectases.

Sclerotherapy for varicose veins associated with great saphenous vein (GSV) and small saphenous vein (SSV) incompetence has been traditionally relegated to treating residual varicose veins following surgical stripping or varicose veins associated with isolated perforator vein incompetence.[1] Apart from a relatively brief period of popularity of the Fegan method of sclerotherapy in the 1960s and early 1970s, surgical methods have generally been accepted as having a significantly better long-term recurrence rate compared to sclerotherapy. This has been thought to be due to the fact that traditional sclerotherapy was unable to control the proximal source of reflux—usually the saphenofemoral (SFJ) and saphenopopliteal (SPJ) junctions—adequately. In addition, preultrasound methods of sclerosing the GSV have been shown to be relatively ineffective. Some methods such as the Cloutier technique[2] administered a single, "blind" injection of a major sclerosing agent a few centimeters below the SFJ, repeated every 7 to 21 days until the GSV was occluded. Such methods have been openly discouraged as creditable methods of treating GSV or SSV incompetence as they were thought to have an inherently high risk of damaging the deep venous system or of inadvertent intra-arterial injection.

Duplex ultrasound has become the gold standard in the investigation of lower limb venous disease. As an independent investigation, duplex scanning has unrivaled relevance in the clinical decision-making process as well as being used in the serial assessment of disease progress and effectiveness of treatment.[3] Ultrasound guidance of sclerosant injections is a logical extension of the pretreatment evaluation and gives sclerotherapy the potential to rival other ablative methods in effectiveness in the treatment of varicose veins.

HISTORY OF ULTRASOUND-GUIDED SCLEROTHERAPY (UGS)

The method of ultrasonic guidance of injection into the superficial venous system was first published in 1989.[4] The method was initially used for treatment of incompetent saphenous axes, and in 1992 the method of injecting incompetent perforating veins associated with postsurgical recurrences was described.[5] Medium-term results of SFJ incompetence treated by UGS were reported by Kanter and Thibault in 1996.[6] In the late 1990s, several practitioners around the world began using sclerosant foam injected using ultrasound guidance, and the first medium-term results were reported by Cabrera in 2000.[7] Since that time UGS using microfoamed sclerosants (UGFS) has become the accepted method of UGS.[8]

PRETREATMENT ULTRASOUND MAPPING

Duplex venous scanning is the essential pretreatment investigation prior to either sclerotherapy or ultrasound-guided sclerotherapy of major varicose veins and truncal incompetence.[3] Through duplex scanning, patterns of venous incompetence will be found to be extremely variable and often unexpected. Duplex scanning involves B-mode imaging of the deep and superficial veins combined with directional pulsed Doppler assessment of blood flow. Color-duplex imaging superimposes blood flow information onto the B-mode ultrasound image, permitting visual assessment of blood flow while at the same time creating an anatomical map of the venous anatomy. The details of venous duplex examination have been described in a previous chapter and will not be dealt with here.

In short, duplex examination is able to provide an accurate anatomical and physiological map of superficial and deep venous incompetence and localize points of reflux from the deep to superficial venous system. With duplex examination a detailed map of reflux paths in the superficial system, from the proximal origin of the reflux (usually from the deep system), to a distal reentry point, can be created. This map will allow optimal decisions regarding sclerotherapy intervention and will ensure that all significant areas of reflux are addressed by treatment and, conversely, that all normal veins are preserved. Diameters of major veins and junctions are also recorded during the duplex examination. These measurements may influence various parameters of the treatment process including selection of sclerosing agent and form, and postsclerotherapy compression.

Following the duplex examination, the treatment process is then directed toward eliminating all the incompetent superficial pathways mapped out with duplex ultrasound and then, in the posttreatment phase, reexamining with duplex to ensure that the reflux pathways have not recanalized prior to complete fibrosis of the vein, which usually occurs between 6 to 12 months following initial treatment.

TECHNIQUES OF UGS

SCLEROSING AGENTS

Generally, only relatively strong sclerosants are used in UGS. In an international survey[9] of forty-four phlebologists who were known to use UGS extensively, 95% used sodium tetradecyl sulfate (STS; Fibrovein; STD Pharmaceuticals, Hereford, England), and 5% used 3% polidocanol (POL; Aethoxysclerol; Kreusler Pharma, Wiesbaden, Germany). A small minority of phlebologists used polyiodinated iodine as an alternative solution in particular circumstances, such

Table 18.1 APPROXIMATE EQUIVALENT CONCENTRATIONS OF STS AND POL REQUIRED FOR EFFECTIVE SCLEROSIS OF INCREASING CALIBER OF LOWER LIMB VEINS.

VEIN CALIBER (MM)	STS CONCENTRATION (%)	POL CONCENTRATION (%)
0.1–0.5	0.1	0.25
0.5–1.0	0.15	0.5
1.0–2.0	0.3	1.0
2.0–3.0	0.5	1.5
3.0–5.0	0.75	2.0
5.0–8.0	1.0–3.0	3.0–5.0

as in the presence of allergy to STS or at deep-to-superficial junctions. With sclerosant concentration, generally 3% STS was used, although some phlebologists use STS in various strengths from 0.75 to 2%.

In the above survey, 34% of phlebologists used foamed sclerosants, with STS again being the most common agent used as foam. It is likely that the ratio of phlebologists using foam sclerosants compared with solution has increased significantly since that survey, as the benefits of foam have become more widely known. The use of foam is described in more detail in another chapter.

STS and POL, in both solution and foam formulations have been shown to have similar efficacy, tolerability, and patient satisfaction.[10] There is good evidence however, that POL is a weaker detergent type of sclerosant than STS[11] and higher concentrations are necessary to produce complete vascular sclerosis for any given diameter of vein (Table 18.1). This is the most likely reason why many phlebologists prefer STS when performing UGS, as in general, larger truncal veins are being treated with this technique.[8]

PATIENT POSITIONING

For treatment of veins on the medial aspect of the leg, patients are placed in the supine position with the treated leg level and externally rotated at the hip. The knee is usually slightly flexed in order to relax all muscle groups. If small incompetent veins are being treated, the patient can be placed in the semireclining position in order to dilate the veins, thereby slightly assisting ultrasound visualization and subsequent injection. For treatment of veins on the posterior thigh or calf, the patient is positioned in the prone position with the foot supported by a pillow so that the knee is flexed slightly.[4] This positioning is important when injecting the SSV near the popliteal fossa, where the vein will be compressed if the knee is totally extended.

CLOSED NEEDLE TECHNIQUE

Materials

The needle size used can vary from 21 to 25 g. The most common size used are 25 g 1 1/2 inch (0.50 mm × 38 mm), as these are the smallest diameter needles that are readily visualized by B-mode ultrasound and are long enough to reach most superficial veins from the point of skin penetration. Usually the sclerosant is drawn up into a 2- or 3-ml luer lock syringe. When microfoam is used, the Tessari method[12] will also require the use of 5-ml luer lock syringe to draw up air or other gas to form the microfoam. The ratio of sclerosant to air may vary from 1:3 (wet foam) to 1:6 (dry foam).[13] Wet foam tends to have longer duration, but dry foam is a better displacer of blood. Individual practitioners will inevitably vary this ratio depending on their preferences, although Tessari and Cavezzi basing their opinion of physicochemical properties recommend the ratio of 1:4.[13]

Method

The closed needle technique is the most commonly used method.[9] With this technique, the needle is attached to the syringe containing the sclerosant at all times. A small proportion of phlebologists use an open needle technique (needle is removed to determine color/flow of blood). The procedure may be performed with the assistance of a vascular sonographer, or with the phlebologist performing both the ultrasound and the injections alone ("solo" technique).[9]

The initial injection is usually performed near to the proximal origin of the venous reflux.[5] A small proportion of practitioners inject more distally then manually "milk" the sclerosant proximally toward the proximal source of reflux using real-time ultrasound monitoring.[14] Either way, the final objective is to have the total segment of incompetent vein, from the proximal reflux point to the distal reentry point, uniformly filled with sclerosant foam. This can be observed with real-time B-mode ultrasound and will be accompanied by vasospasm of the treated vein.

The sonographer initially will localize the site of the vein to be injected in transverse view. The depth of the vein below the skin surface will be noted, as this will determine the angle of approach of the needle. The injection can then be performed either with the vein viewed in transverse section or in sagittal or longitudinal section. Approximately 50% of practitioners utilize the transverse approach solely, 33% the longitudinal approach solely, and the remainder use both approaches depending on various technical variables associated with each individual injection.[9] The transverse approach is favored by some, especially when performing the procedure "solo" because it appears to be technically easier to cannulate the vein with this method. It is therefore particularly useful when injecting smaller veins less than 3 mm in diameter. The advantages of the longitudinal approach

are: first, that the direction of flow of the sclerosant can be observed and, second, the linear array probes can be used to compress the segment of vein for a length of about 50 mm during the injection, thereby allowing better contact of the sclerosant with the vein wall at the injection site.

The imaging frequency of the transducer used may vary from 7.5 to 15 MHz, the lower frequencies are used for deeper-placed subcutaneous veins (>3 cm below the skin) and higher frequencies for more superficial veins. Commonly a 10-MHz transducer is used for its ability to imagine most subcutaneous veins adequately. Most transducers will have an indicator line or light-emitting diode (LED) that will indicate the alignment of the sagittal plane of the transducer. For either approach, the needle is inserted close to the transducer tip and along the sagittal plane of the transducer (Figure 18.1).[5] When the needle pierces the skin, the tip should be visualized by the ultrasound. Adequate amounts of ultrasound gel need to be applied to the skin to obtain optimum visualization.

As the needle is slowly inserted it appears as a reflective straight line angling toward the target vein. It is important to verify early in the procedure that the needle is being introduced in the correct sagittal plane of the transducer. When injecting in the transverse section of the vein, the transducer can be moved in small increments to align with the needle. When injecting in the longitudinal section of the vein, the direction of needle may need to be altered in small increments, to align with the sagittal plane of the transducer. For either method, the needle and vein should be imaged simultaneously at all times.

As the needle tip makes contact with the target vein, an indentation will be seen on the vein wall (Figure 18.2). At

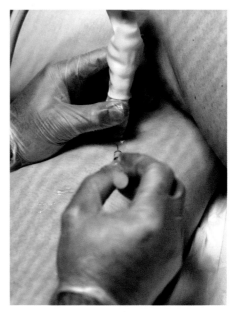

Figure 18.1   The needle is aligned directly along the longitudinal axis of the ultrasound probe prior to piercing the skin.

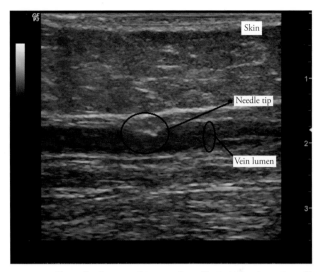

Figure 18.2   B-mode ultrasound image of needle tip indenting vein wall immediately prior to vein puncture.

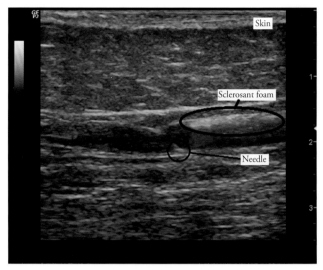

Figure 18.4   B-mode ultrasound image demonstrating initial bolus of sclerosant foam entering the vein lumen and flowing upstream initially.

this stage a little extra pressure is required to pierce the vein wall and after this occurs, the needle can be seen within the lumen (Figure 18.3) and a small amount of blood is drawn into the needle hub to confirm correct intraluminal positioning of the needle tip. A small volume (approx. 0.2 ml) of sclerosant is then injected and should be seen on the ultrasound image to be flowing into the vein (Figure 18.4). Extravasation is readily visible on the B-mode image and is manifested as a separation between the vein wall and the perivenous tissues. Should this occur, injection is stopped immediately, and the needle tip is repositioned correctly, or alternatively, the needle withdrawn and reinserted at an appropriate nearby site. When the initial small volume is seen to flow intraluminally, the remainder of the injection is then completed under continuous ultrasound imaging (Figure 18.5).

When using the longitudinal approach, during injection the direction of flow of sclerosant can be determined and with a combination probe pressure and digital pressure applied distal or proximal to the injection site, the direction of sclerosant flow can be modified to optimize the localization of the sclerosant.

The volume of sclerosant injected at any one site varies between practitioners, but usually ranges from 0.25 to 2.0 ml depending on the site and size of the vein. It is the author's preference to inject smaller quantities at multiple sites rather than larger volumes at one site, as the former technique, while equalizing the sclerosant concentration along the segment of vein,[15] minimizes the risk of overflow of sclerosant into the deep system through nearby perforating veins that can cause deep and muscular vein sclerosis and possible subsequent deep venous thrombosis (DVT).

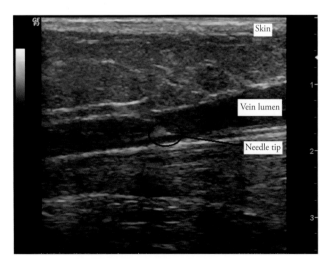

Figure 18.3   B-mode ultrasound image of needle tip clearly centered in the vein lumen. It is important to verify correct placement of the needle tip by withdrawing a small amount of blood into the hub of the needle prior to injection.

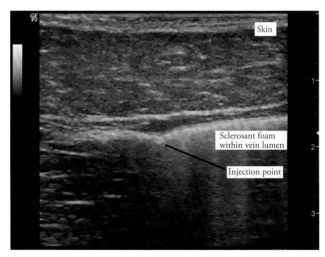

Figure 18.5   B-mode ultrasound image demonstrating uniform distribution of the sclerosant foam throughout the visualized lumen of the vein in both directions from the injection point.

When injecting the incompetent GSV or SSV, it is usual to place the first injection 5 to 10 cm distal to the incompetent SFJ or SPJ. The author uses STS 3% or POL 3% microfoam at a sclerosant:air ratio of 1:3. As the recommended maximum dose of Fibrovein is 4 ml, the maximum microfoam volume is 16 ml. If a ratio of 1:4 is used, the maximum volume becomes 20 ml. The maximum volume of POL will vary according to concentration used and patient weight (2 mg/kg/d). When using foam the author prefers to draw up 1.5 ml of foam in each syringe (so this becomes the maximum injectate volume), although many practitioners inject 2 ml at most sites.[8]

Kanter[16] compared the effect of 1 ml and 2 ml sclerosant (3% STS) injectate volumes on immediate vasospasm and later clinical outcomes after UGS. He found that 2-ml injectate volumes were less effective than 1 ml and did not reduce the number of injections given. The 2-ml injectate group received twice the volume of sclerosant and therefore some reported transient flu-like symptoms 4 to 6 hours after treatment. Hence, when injecting solution (rather than foam), it is advisable not to inject more than 1 ml at any one site. When injecting with several centimeters of visible calf perforating veins, it is advisable to inject less than 0.5 ml.[4,15]

Injections proceed distally, as previously injected segments are observed to spasm or fill with foam. Treatment end-point is when all segments of incompetent vein have undergone spasm and become incompressible to probe maneuvers. The ultrasound transducer can also be used to compress the treated vein in a rhythmical up and down motion as the vein is followed post injection to observe for uniform vasospasm. The maneuver also has the effect of uniformly distributing the sclerosant longitudinally and circumferentially along the venous endothelium, thereby accelerating the process of vasospasm.

CATHETER TECHNIQUES

Open Catheter Technique

In the early days of UGS, especially when the procedure was being developed and techniques refined, there were a number of reports of inadvertent intra-arterial injections that concerned many phlebologists.[5,17] Catheter techniques of UGS were first introduced to minimize the risk of inadvertent intra-arterial injection and the resultant extensive tissue loss that could occur. The first "open catheter" technique was described by Grondin in 1992.[18] This technique recommended a 20-gauge 44-mm cannula for cannulation of the GSV or SSV 6 to 8 cm distal to the SFJ and SPJ, which were thought to be the sites of maximum risk of inadvertent intra-arterial injection. Correct placement of the cannula could be confirmed by aspiration of nonpulsatile venous blood, ultrasound visualization of the cannula tip and finally, injection of normal saline into the vein prior to sclerosant injection. After confirmation that the cannula was correctly

inserted into the vein, the sclerosant was injected at that site as a bolus in a similar manner to that described above in the "closed" technique. The technique could be used to treat the remaining distal trunk by recannulating distal to the initial cannulation point.

Coleridge Smith[19] has described a modified version of the open cannula technique whereby he inserts multiple cannulas or 23-gauge butterfly needles into previously ultrasound-mapped varicose veins and incompetent trunks while the patient lies in the supine position. The limb being treated is then elevated to an angle of 30 degrees to empty the veins prior to injection. After the sclerosant foam is injected at each site, the progress of foam is monitored by ultrasound as described previously.

Extended Long Line Echosclerotherapy (ELLE)

The ELLE technique was first described by Parsi in 1997[20] and later by Min and Navarro.[21] This technique was developed not only to reduce the risk of intra-arterial injection, but also to improve the effectiveness of UGS especially in the treatment of larger diameter incompetent trunks by improving the delivery of the sclerosant to the venous endothelium. The method is described in detail by Parsi and Lim.[22]

Cannulation

The entry point for cannulation is selected after completion of pretreatment mapping of the superficial truncal incompetence. The ideal entry point will be at the most distal incompetent point of the axial trunk that is to be treated (GSV or SSV). For example, if the SSV is incompetent to the mid calf, the SSV would be cannulated in the mid calf; if the GSV was incompetent to the proximal calf, the GSV would be cannulated just below the knee. In the presence of significant perforator incompetence, the cannulation is done distal to the incompetent perforators. The segment of vein chosen should ideally be straight, and cannulation is easier if superficial segments of vein are chosen.

Cannulation can be performed with or without local anesthesia. If local aesthesia is used, the injection should be performed intradermally and not contain adrenaline so as to avoid causing vasoconstriction of the vein to be cannulated.

Cannula selection and penetration

The depth and lumen diameter of the selected vein is measured to assist in appropriate cannula selection. Usually 16- to 18-gauge cannulas are used with cannula lengths varying from 4 to 7 cm.

The procedure is carried out using aseptic techniques. The vein is visualized with B-mode ultrasound in the longitudinal axis, and the selected entry point is marked on the skin. A tourniquet can be applied proximal to the selected point of entry to facilitate the cannulation. Once local anesthesia is achieved, the vein is cannulated under ultrasound guidance. Successful entry of the cannula into the vein is signaled by spontaneous venous return. The tourniquet is then released and the cannula is flushed with normal saline, which is also visualized with ultrasound, ensuring correct placement. The cannula is then taped to the skin. Technically, cannulation is usually the most challenging part of this procedure.

Catheterization

The length of the selected vein is measured to assist in selection of the appropriate catheter. The selected catheter is fed through the cannula (catheter through cannula technique) and introduced into the lumen of the vein and advanced toward the junction under ultrasound guidance. Once the catheter is about 5 cm distal to the junction, the guide wire is removed. The leg is then raised to about 45 degrees to empty the vein as much as possible. It is this maneuver that is readily performed with the ELLE technique, but more difficult with the close needle technique, that theoretically will result in better contact of the sclerosant with the venous endothelium with larger truncal veins. The proximal SFJ/SPJ is then compressed (Cloutier technique)[22] and the leg is brought back to about 30 degrees while maintaining the compression on the junction. The sclerosant is then introduced as the catheter is being withdrawn. Parsi and Lim believe that a number of "pulse" injections of approximately 0.8 ml of STS 3% solution is more effective than continuous and gradual infusion of sclerosant. This is consistent with the principles of sclerosant distribution described by Guex.[15]

Special attention is given to T junctions with tributaries and perforators as the catheter is gradually withdrawn. Extra volume of sclerosant may be required at these escape points to ensure full sclerosis of these openings. Failure to sclerose the escape points may lead to partial recanalization of the vein.[6] As with the closed needle technique, the end point of the treatment include vasospasm, noncompressibility along the entire length of the treated vein, and absence of any blood flow in the vein, all confirmed with ultrasound.

There are several limitations of the ELLE technique. First, it is not useful in treating complex patterns and tortuous postsurgical recurrences. Second, it is technically difficult to treat smaller incompetent veins less than 5 mm in diameter owing to difficulty in cannulating these veins with the relatively large diameter cannula that is required for the procedure.

UGS FOR RESISTANT TELANGIECTASES AND TELANGIECTATIC MATTING

Using a high frequency ultrasound imaging transducer, Somjen et al.[23] have shown that 89% of areas of thigh telangiectases have associated incompetent reticular veins identifiable. A large proportion of these were found to be associated with deeper subcutaneous vein reflux or with perforating vein reflux. Some of the incompetent reticular veins were invisible from the surface, and these invisible reticular veins can be a cause of treatment failure when using standard techniques of sclerotherapy. Using high-frequency duplex ultrasound, Forrestal[24] has also observed incompetent reticular veins associated with resistant telangiectases and telangiectatic matting. Using ultrasound guidance, these "invisible" veins can be injected with STS 0.5–1% or POL 1%.

POSTSCLEROTHERAPY COMPRESSION TECHNIQUES

External Compression

Various forms of external compression have been recommended following sclerotherapy to varicose veins. Although Fegan[25] advised 6 weeks of continuous external compression with bandages, this is not generally required with UGS owing to the fact that the principal of the technique is that all proximal sources of reflux are controlled in the initial treatment.

The reasons for using external compression with UGS relate to increased patient comfort, reduction of symptomatic chemical phlebitis, and maintenance of optimal deep venous flow during the postinjection period. For this reason, the most commonly used compression following treatment is the application of Class II (25- to 35-mmHg) graduated compression stockings. Generally the stockings are worn during the day for 2 to 3 weeks. Some practitioners also advise their patients to wear the stockings at night for the first 3 to 4 days in order to maintain optimum deep venous flow in the early postinjection period, thereby minimizing the risk of DVT. The stocking may be removed each day for showering, without any undue adverse effects.

Internal Compression (Perivenous Compression)

This novel method has been introduced recently to improve sclerosant contact with the vein wall during the immediate postsclerotherapy period and therefore reduce the incidence of recanalization.[26] The technique was developed from the perivenous local anesthetic technique for EVLA. With this method, following each injection of the main stem (GSV or SSV) with sclerosant foam, normal saline or preferably Klein's tumescent solution[27] is injected perivenously in the compartment between the deep and superficial fascia (Figure 18.6) at 3 to 5 locations equally spaced along the axial vein in the thigh (GSV) or calf (SSV). Usually between 20 and 30 ml of tumescent solution is required, or about 5 to 10 ml at each cross-sectional segment. The injection is performed using ultrasound guidance with a cross-sectional approach using a 25g 1 1/2 inch needle. The effect is to give greater immediate compression to the vein, thereby decreasing the diameter of the already spasmed vessel by approximately another 50%, resulting in better apposition of the veins walls and more complete contact of the veins wall with the sclerosant.

The author now uses this method routinely when treating larger axial vessels (GSV and SSV) greater than 3 mm in

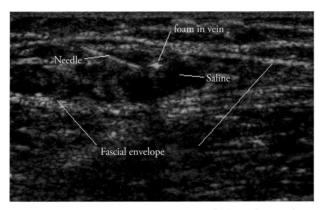

Figure 18.6 Post-UGS perivenous compression of GSV with normal saline.

diameter and early experience indicates a reduction in early recurrence and recanalization resulting in less early retreatments. In addition further benefits including reduced incidence of transient neurological episodes including migraine and chest tightness are obtained by using this method.

Many sclerotherapists now also use the tumescent compression techniques prior to injection of the sclerosant when using the cannula or catheter techniques resulting in improved sclerosis and reduced concentration and volumes of sclerosant, again resulting in reduced incidence of local adverse effects. (personal communications Parsi K, Cavezzi A).

POSTTREATMENT METHODS AND FOLLOW-UP.

Immediately after treatment, patients are advised to walk continuously for 15 to 20 minutes and are then instructed to walk for at least 45 minutes daily. This significantly improves any discomfort, which is generally minimal. Pain requiring treatment following the procedure is unusual and indicates that the patient needs to be reviewed by the phlebologist to ascertain the cause. Walking reduces superficial ambulatory pressures and ensures high flow in the deep venous system of the leg for a prolonged period at least once per day.

Patients are usually reviewed 1 to 2 weeks following treatment, at which time the venous system is reexamined with duplex ultrasound to determine (1) whether the treated veins are incompressible and have no flow and (2) the patency and flow in the deep veins.

If a treated segment of vein is found to be partially or completely patent and have persistent reflux, the segment is reinjected using ultrasound guidance. The phlebologist should be aware that lower concentrations of sclerosant may be necessary, as the vein endothelium will be partially destroyed making the vein more prone to chemical thrombophlebitis if too strong a concentration is used.

At the first post-UGS visit, once proximal closure of the treated veins has been confirmed, residual distal branch varicose veins and telangiectases may be treated with standard sclerotherapy methods. The patient is then reviewed 4–6 weeks after the initial treatment, when repeat ultrasound examination is performed and any intravascular coagula are removed through a small incision using either a 18- to 21-gauge needle or number 11 blade. Generally this procedure can be performed without any anesthesia or with local anesthetic when using the number 11 blade.

Further follow-up visits may be scheduled at 3, 6, and 12 months to ensure that there has not been recanalization of the treated vein.

ADVERSE EFFECTS OF UGS

Varcoe[9] performed a survey of forty-four experienced UGS phlebologists from seven countries and reported on their experience with adverse effects from UGS. In this survey, side effects were grouped into "minor" or "major" reactions. Minor reactions were phlebitis, pigmentation, edema, pain, minor (asymptomatic) DVT, and minor allergic reaction. Major reactions were major DVT, pulmonary embolus, and severe allergic reaction. In this survey, the incidence of major adverse effects were all less than 0.1%. Only one phlebologist reported pulmonary embolus occurring, indicating the low risk of this event. In 20 years of performing UGS, the author has not observed any pulmonary emboli following UGS and only one DVT (affecting the popliteal vein extending from a sclerosed gastrocnemius perforating vein).

Several intra-arterial injections were reported early on in the history of UGS,[4,17] and the incidence reported in the Varcoe survey was 0.01%. The risk of this event appears to be directly related to the experience and training of the phlebologist in UGS and rarely occurs in skilled hands.

The most common serious adverse effect experienced by the author has been anaphylactoid reactions to the sclerosant STS.[28] The incidence of anaphylactoid reaction in 2,686 treatment sessions was 0.15%. This reaction appears to be concentration- and volume-dependent. Interestingly, since the advent of foam this incidence has been greatly reduced. The author has not observed any anaphylactoid reactions to STS 3% foam in thc circa 2000, and Chapman-Smith[29] similarly reports zero incidence of this complication when using STS foam.

SHORT- AND LONG-TERM RESULTS

There are now are number of studies documenting the effectiveness of UGS. Most of these studies have examined the results of treating GSV incompetence, although there are several now published on SSV incompetence.

GSV INCOMPETENCE

The first reported objective ultrasound results of SFJ and GSV incompetence treated with UGS were those of Kanter and Thibault.[6] Using STS 3% solution, they reported a 76% success rate at 24 months. Cabrera et al.[7] followed-up 500 lower limbs with SFJ and GSV incompetence treated with UGS using Lauromacrogol 400 (POL) microfoam. After 3 years, 81% of treated GSVs were obliterated, and 96.5% of superficial branches disappeared. The obliteration of saphenous veins required one treatment in 86%, two in 10.5%, and three in 3.5%.

Cavezzi and Frullini[30] in a study of 106 saphenous axes or recurrent postsurgical varices achieved 95% sclerosis at 21 weeks using STS 1% or 3% sclerosant foam. There were three completely unsuccessful cases despite three treatment sessions and ten cases of early recanalization (with reflux or retrograde flow), subsequently successfully retreated with UGS.

Myers et al.[31] reported objective ultrasound results on 100 limbs (seventy-eight GSV and twenty-two SSV) after 12 months using STS or aethoxysclerol according to preference and partly determined by the diameter of the veins. All but one vein treated were less than 10 mm in diameter. UGS was successful in the first treatment in eighty-six limbs (primary success), but it was necessary to repeat treatment once in eleven and twice in three limbs to give the "secondary success." At 1 year, the cumulative primary success was 77% and the secondary success rate was 88%. During the same period, thirty-one limbs (twenty-four GSV and seven SSV) were treated surgically (primary treatment) and then with UGS for early recurrence to give a secondary success rate. In this group at 12 months cumulative primary success was 71% and the secondary success rate was 87%.

Chapman-Smith,[29] by using a regular posttreatment review with weekly ultrasound examinations initially until closure was achieved and thereafter periodical reviews and retreatment when recanalizations were detected, was able to achieve a 4% clinical recurrence at 5 years with an average of 2.53 treatments in the first year. 16.5% of patients then required an average of 2.0 treatments in the second year, and 8% of patients required average of 2.0 treatments in the third year.

Several studies have examined the effect that various clinical determinants had on UGS outcomes. Kanter[32] looked at the effects of age, gender, and vein size. He found that larger doses of STS were required to induce vasospasm in older patients, males, and those with larger veins. Regardless of gender and age, larger veins were more likely to recanalize, but were not necessarily associated with clinical recurrence. Although older patients and males tended to have larger veins, their recanalization rates were similar to younger patients and females when sufficiently higher STS doses were used to induce vasospasm. Barrett et al.[7] in a study of 115 saphenous veins treated with STS microfoam UGS confirmed a small increase in failure to close the SFJ and SPJ with increasing size of junction diameter (>10 mm), but this did not significantly alter the results with respect to clearance of visible varicosities and patient satisfaction with results.

In a separate study, Barrett et al.[33] followed 100 randomly chosen legs with varicose veins treated by UGS using STS 3% microfoam after an average of 22.5 months (range 20 to 26 months). An average number of 2.1 treatments were required to close incompetent varicose veins. Thirty-one percent of legs required a second treatment at the 3-month follow-up. Such treatments were generally for a small channel in the saphenous trunk, a small feeding vessel or perforator creating the channel, or minor residual varicosities. Success was analyzed from two perspectives: patient satisfaction and clinical and ultrasound assessment. There was an extremely high patient satisfaction, with 100% of patients stating that foam UGS had been successful in treating their varicose veins and related symptoms. Clinically, 92% had complete removal of their varicosities, with 5% developing new varicosities related generally to perforator incompetence unrelated to the treated saphenous veins. Duplex examination revealed four saphenous veins with persistent reflux.

Thibault[34] reported the 5-year recurrence rate in thirty-five limbs with GSV incompetence treated with UGS. Nine limbs (25.7%) had recurrent varicose veins clinically. Ten had persistent reflux at the SFJ, and fourteen limbs (40%) had persistent reflux at the SFJ. Comparing these results with the shorter term studies indicates that there is a slow but steady increase in cumulative recurrence with time, indicating the need for period review and retreatment when clinically indicated in this group of patients.

When comparing the results of foam UGS and solution or liquid sclerotherapy, it appears that foam is markedly superior.[35] This has been demonstrated by at least two random control trials.[36,37] For this reason, virtually all phlebologists currently use foam when treating incompetent saphenous trunks.

SSV INCOMPETENCE

Padbury and Benveniste[38] reported patient satisfaction and clinical and sonographic success in a prospective study on fifteen limbs with SSV incompetence. Primary success was achieved in all patients (SSV injected and obliterated). At 6 months, five (33%) had minor residual varices. Duplex examination at 6 months revealed one limb with a residual patent incompetent SSV. This patient had a 9-mm vein pretreatment. Patient satisfaction as gauged by the Aberdeen QoL questionnaire demonstrated an excellent response, with all patients recording a positive improvement.

PERFORATOR VEIN INCOMPETENCE

The effectiveness of UGS for incompetent perforator veins (IPVs) was reported by Thibault.[4] Thirty-six patients (thirty-eight limbs) with incompetent perforating veins were treated with UGS using STS 3% solution. The IPVs were classified according to anatomical location as thigh (n = 12), gastrocnemius (n = 13) or posterior tibial (*n* = 18). Two thigh IPVs, three posterior tibial IPVs, and one gastrocnemius IPV required repeat injection at the 6- to 8-week follow-up examination. The IPVs were then reexamined with duplex ultrasound 6 months after treatment. All (100%) the gastrocnemius IPVs remained sclerosed with no flow at 6 months, 83% of the thigh IPVs were sclerosed, and 72% of the posterior tibial IPVs remained occluded with no reflux at 6 months. The difficulty of obtaining good long-term results with posterior tibial IPVs probably relates to the high hydrostatic forces present in the distal leg.

MANAGEMENT OF POSTSURGICAL RECURRENT VARICOSE VEINS

UGS has become the preferred management of postsurgical recurrent varicose veins. There are four common sources of reflux associated with recurrence of varicose veins after surgical ligation and stripping: (1) recurrence of reflux at the SFJ or SPJ because of neovascularization or inadequate ligation; (2) incompetent thigh or calf perforating veins; (3) incompetent gastrocnemius veins; (4) persistent varicose tributaries or duplication of the GSV in the thigh, with these medial thigh veins receiving reflux from pelvic tributaries.[39] For obvious technical reasons and to avoid the risks of redo surgery (nerve and lymphatic damage) these sources of recurrent reflux are best treated with UGS.

As with primary varicose veins, there needs to be a thorough mapping of the superficial venous reflux and assessment of the deep venous system in the leg. The segments and points of reflux are then methodically treated using real-time ultrasound guidance. Standard sclerotherapy is then used to treat any residual superficial varicosities 1 to 4 weeks later.

MANAGEMENT OF VENOUS ULCERS

Foam UGS has been reported to be an effective method for accelerating healing of venous ulcers associated with superficial venous incompetence.[40] Thirteen patients with lower leg ulceration clinically suggestive of venous ulceration were confirmed to have superficial venous incompetence with or without deep venous insufficiency. The average ulcer duration was 27 months (range 3 to 96 months). The thirteen limbs were then treated with foam echosclerotherapy to all areas of superficial venous incompetence detected on duplex scanning. Nine patients had complete healing of their ulcers within 5 months of commencing treatment (Figure 18.7), two ulcers healed by 12 months, and another healed after 20 months. The remaining patient's ulceration was still improving but not fully healed at 14 months. Another case study of nine patients with 13 venous ulcers, showed rapid healing of the ulcers just 7 days after treatment.[41]

The advantage of this approach is that the underlying cause of the ulceration is being addressed, thereby reducing prolonged morbidity and cost of long-term management of

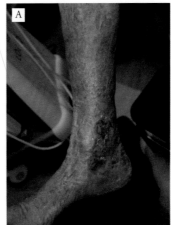
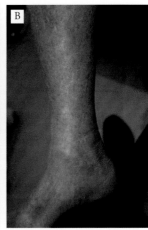

Figure 18.7. (A) Chronic venous ulcer affecting the right leg in a 90-year-old male who had had high ligation and stripping of the GSV 15 years previously. Duplex scanning revealed incompetence in the femoral, popliteal, and posterior tibial veins and associated incompetence of a medial thigh perforating vein and recurrent superficial medial thigh and calf veins. (B) Healed venous ulcer 14 weeks after two UGS treatment sessions with STS 3% sclerosant foam to the incompetent thigh perforating vein and recurrent medial thigh and calf veins. Also note the significant improvement in general skin condition following treatment.

chronic venous ulceration. UGFS is now used routinely by many phlebologists as a simple, effective means of healing venous ulcers, but randomized clinical controlled trials are needed to confirm these clinical benefits.

REFERENCES

1. Hobbs JT. Surgery and sclerotherapy in the treatment of varicose veins, *Arch Surg.* 1974. *190*: 793–796.
2. Cloutier G. Sclerose des crosses des saphenes internes et externes avec compression: Nouvelle approche, *Phlebologie.* 1976. *3*: 227–232.
3. Thibault PK. Duplex examination, *Dermatol Surg.* 1995. *21*: 77–82.
4. Knight RM, Vin F, Zygmunt JA. Ultrasonic guidance of injections into the superficial venous system. In: Davy A, Stemmer R, eds. *Phlebologie '89.* Montrouge, France: John Libbey Eurotext. 1989.
5. Thibault PK, Lewis WA. Recurrent varicose veins: Part 2: Injection of incompetent perforating veins using ultrasound guidance, *J Derm Surg Onc.* 1992. *18*: 895–900.
6. Kanter A, Thibault P. Saphenofemoral junction incompetence treated by ultrasound-guided sclerotherapy, *Dermatol Surg.* 1996. *22*: 648–652.
7. Cabrera J, Cabrera J Jr, Garcia-Olmedo MA. Treatment of varicose long saphenous veins with sclerosant in microfoam form: Long-term outcomes, *Phlebology.* 2000. *15*: 19–23.
8. Barrett JM, Allen B, Ockelford A, Goldman MP. Microfoam ultrasound-guided sclerotherapy treatment for varicose veins in a subgroup with diameters at the junction of 10mm or greater compared with a subgroup of less than 10mm, *Dermatol Surg.* 2004. *30*: 1386–1390.
9. Varcoe PF. Ultrasound guided sclerotherapy: Efficacy, adverse events, and dosing: An international survey, *ANZ J Phleb.* 2003. *7*: 17–24.
10. Rao J, Wildemore JK, Goldman MP. Double-blind prospective comparative trial between foamed and liquid POL and sodium tetradecyl sulphate in the treatment of varicose and telangiectatic leg veins, *Dermatol Surg.* 2005. *31*: 631–635.

11. Goldman MP, Kaplan RP, Oki LN. Sclerosing agents in the treatment of telangiectasia: Comparison of the clinical and histologic effects of intravascular polidocanol, sodium tetradecyl sulphate, and hypertonic saline in the dorsal rabbit ear vein model, *Arch Dermatol.* 1987. *123*: 1196–1201.

12. Tessari L, Cavezzi A, Frullini A. Preliminary experience with a new sclerosing foam in the treatment of varicose veins, *Dermatol Surg.* 2001. *27*: 58–60.

13. Cavezzi A, Tessari L. Foam sclerotherapy techniques: Different gases and methods of preparation, catheter versus direct injection, *Phlebology.* 2009. *24*: 247–251.

14. Myers KA, Jolley D, Clough A, Kirwan J. Outcome of ultrasound-guided sclerotherapy for varicose veins: Medium-term results assessed by ultrasound surveillance, *Eur J Vasc Endovasc Surg.* 2007. *33*: 116–121.

15. Guex J-J. Indications for the sclerosing agent polidocanol, *J Derm Surg Onc.* 1993. *19*: 959–961.

16. Kanter A. Clinical determinants of ultrasound-guided sclerotherapy: Part II: In search of the ideal injectate volume, *Dermatol Surg.* 1998. *24*: 136–140.

17. Biegeleisen K, Neilson RD, O'Shaughnessy A. Inadvertent intra-arterial injection complicating ordinary and ultrasound-guided sclerotherapy, *J Derm Surg Onc.* 1993. *19*: 953–958.

18. Grondin L, Soriano J. Duplex-echosclerotherapy, in the quest for the safe technique. In: Raymond-Martimbeau P, Prescott R, Zummo M, eds. *Phlebologie '92.* Paris: John Libbey Eurotext. 1992. 828–833.

19. Coleridge Smith P. Chronic venous disease treated by ultrasound guided foam sclerotherapy, *Eur J Vasc Endovasc Surg.* 2006. *32*: 577–583.

20. Parsi K. Extended long line echosclerotherapy, *Sclerotherapy of Australia Newsbulletin.* 1997. *1*: 10–12.

21. Min RJ, Navarro L. Transcatheter duplex ultrasound-guided sclerotherapy for treatment of greater saphenous vein reflux: Preliminary report, *Dermatol Surg.* 2000. *26*: 410–414.

22. Parsi K, Lim AC. Extended long line echosclerotherapy, *ANZ J Phleb.* 2000. *4*: 6–10.

23. Somjen GM, Ziegenbein R, Johnston AH, Royle JP. Anatomical examination of leg telangiectases with duplex scanning, *J Dermatol Surg.* 1993. *19*: 940–945.

24. Forrestal MD. Evaluation and treatment of venulectatic and telangiectatic varicosities of the lower extremities with duplex ultrasound (DUS)-guided injection sclerotherapy, *Dermatol Surg.* 1997. *24*: 996–997.

25. Fegan WG. Continuous compression technique of injecting varicose veins, *Lancet.* 1963. *2*: 109–112.

26. Thibault P. Internal compression (peri-venous compression) following ultrasound guided sclerotherapy to the great and small saphenous veins, *ANZ J Phlebol.* 2005. *9*: 29.

27. Venkataram J. Tumescent liposuction: A review, *J Cutan Aesthet Surg.* 2008. *1*(2): 49–57.

28. Thibault PK. Sclerotherapy of varicose veins and telangiectasias: A 2-year experience with sodium tetradecyl sulphate, *ANZ J Phleb.* 1999. *3*: 25–30.

29. Chapman-Smith P, Browne A. Prospective five-year study of ultrasound-guided foam sclerotherapy in the treatment of great saphenous vein reflux, *Phlebology.* 2009. *24*: 183–188.

30. Cavezzi A, Frullini A. The role of sclerosing foam in ultrasound guided sclerotherapy of the saphenous veins and of recurrent varicose veins: Our personal experience, *ANZ J Phleb.* 1999. *3*: 49–50.

31. Myers KA, Wood SR, Lee V. Early results for objective follow-up by duplex ultrasound scanning after echosclerotherapy or surgery for varicose veins, *ANZ J Phleb.* 2000. *4*: 71–74.

32. Kanter A. Clinical determinants of ultrasound-guided sclerotherapy outcome: Part 1: The effects of age, gender, and vein size, *Dermatol Surg.* 1998. *24*: 131–135.

33. Barrett JM, Allen B, Ockleford A, Goldman MP. Micofoam ultrasound-guided sclerotherapy of varicose veins in 100 legs, *Dermatol Surg.* 2004. *30*: 6–12.

34. Thibault PK. "5 year" follow-up of greater saphenous vein incompetence treated by ultrasound guided sclerotherapy, *ANZ J Phleb.* 2003. *7*: 5–8.

35. Hamel-Desnos C, Allaert F-A. Liquid versus foam sclerotherapy, *Phlebology.* 2009. *24*: 240–246.

36. Ouvry P, Allaert F-A, Desnos P, Hamel-Desnos C. Efficacy of polidocanol foam versus liquid in sclerotherapy of the great saphenous vein: A multicentre randomised controlled trial with a two-year follow-up, *Eur J Vasc Endovasc Surg.* 2008. *36*: 366–370.

37. Rabe E, Otto J, Schliephake D, Pannier F. Efficacy and safety of great saphenous vein sclerotherapy using standardised polidocanol foam (ESAF): A randomised controlled multicentre clinical trial, *Eur J Vasc Endovasc Surg.* 2008. *35*: 238–245.

38. Padbury A, Benveniste GL. Foam echosclerotherapy of the small saphenous vein, *ANZ J Phleb.* 2004. *8*: 5–8.

39. Thibault PK, Lewis WA. Recurrent varicose veins: Part 1: Evaluation utilizing duplex venous imaging, *J Derm Surg Onc.* 1992. *18*: 618–624.

40. Thibault S. Active treatment of venous ulceration with foam echosclerotherapy, *ANZ J Phleb.* 2004. *8*: 26.

41. Hertzman PA, Owens R. Rapid healing of chronic venous ulcers following ultrasound-guided foam sclerotherapy, *Phlebology.* 2007. *22*: 34–39.

19.

SCLEROFOAM FOR TREATMENT OF VARICOSE VEINS

Jean-Jérôme Guex

HISTORY AND BACKGROUND

Sclerofoam is not a new idea. Many authors presented their own recipes, and sometimes results, decades ago.[1] However, sclerofoam became more popular after Cabrera (in Spain) and Monfreux (in France) presented their results in the late 1990s.[2,3] After a period of reluctant observation, many surgeons previously unaccustomed to foam sclerotherapy began to express unexpected interest because it "worked amazingly well."

At that time, "evidence-based medicine" had expanded its influence over the world, and had even penetrated phlebology. The time had come for a true evaluation. The problem was the usual one in trying to apply the rules of evidence-based medicine: sclerofoam worked so well that nobody wanted to waste time to demonstrate what was obvious.

Another obstacle to testing foam sclerotherapy was the demonstration of efficacy presented by endovenous abla-tion, the VNUS Closure procedure, and endovenous laser treatment (EVLT). The subsequent combination of meth-ods frustrated any attempt to test each new technique. Despite this problem, thanks to several authors we now have evidence on which to base our medicine. A little more "medicine-based evidence" is still necessary.[4]

With all the new techniques, the problem has been that during the last 10 years treatments have evolved faster than the varicose veins of patients. The time-tested and multiply requested long-term evaluations were not feasible in the short period of time after introduction of each new tech-nique. It became obvious that new ideas sprouted before outcomes of the previous ones were harvested. The current situation is favourable to endovenous thermal ablation if a durable suppression of saphenous reflux is desired and the price not taken into account, favourable to US guided foam ablation if the cost is an important issue, knowing that the initial comfort of foam, radial tip laser, and Radio frequency is much better than that of surgery, and that at 5 years global patient's satisfaction is similar in all groups.[5]

WHAT IS SCLEROFOAM?

PREPARATION

All details of all the techniques are extensively and suffi-ciently described in the literature.[1] So we will focus on the most commonly used and well-described methods.

Sclerofoam is obtained by mixing a liquid with a gas. For sclerotherapy, detergent sclerosing agents such as polidocanol (POL) and sodium tetradecyl sulfate (STD or STS) are the most logical ingredients. The usual gas is air, although many others have been tried or are being used. Foam is obtained after repeated alternate passages from one syringe to another through a connector that may have a reduced diameter to decrease the size of each foam bubble. This has even been automated in order to standardize foam (Turbofoam, I2M, Caen, France). Foam will vary according to the nature of the sclerosing agent, POL or STS, in its initial concentration; according to the nature of the gas; and according to the ratio (volume of liquid:volume of gas) of the mixture. This and the preparation mode can modify the size of bubbles, their range of diameters, the "wetness" of the foam, and its overall stabil-ity. These characteristics probably change the power and effi-cacy, but there are so many variables that this is unclear so far.

Compared to liquid sclerosing injections, foam has sev-eral advantages: a smaller quantity of sclerosing agent to inject, no dilution with blood, and an even and homoge-neous effect along the injected vein, provided the diameter remains reasonable (see Figure 19.1).[6–8]

Another advantage of foam is its ultrasound echo-genicity. Liquid/air interfaces act as reflectors, and foam appears as an excellent contrast medium, even when only a few bubbles are present. At that stage it has the appear-ance of a cloud. Denser foam is completely opaque to ultra-sound and is completely white, with an underlying acoustic shadow. This characteristic is helpful in following foam when injected from a remote injection point.

Except in small veins, liquid sclerosants are diluted by blood and their efficacy is correct only near the injection

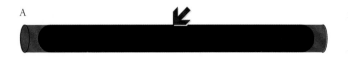

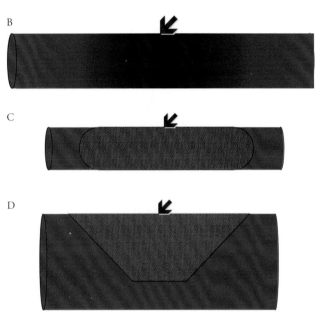

Figure 19.1   (A) In small veins (<3 mm), liquid sclerosants do not mix and replace blood. (B) In medium-sized (diameter of 4 to 12 mm) varicose veins, liquids dilute with blood, efficacy is satisfactory only near the injection site. (C) Injection of foam fills up the vein so that its efficacy is homogeneous. (D) In large veins, foam floats so its action is limited to the superficial wall, thus the importance of obtaining venous spasm.

site, where the concentration is powerful enough to initiate a sclerosing reaction. The main advantage of foam is that it does not mix with blood. It displaces blood and replaces it in the vein lumen. The concentration of active sclerosing agent along the wall is then perfectly homogeneous and even. This ensures an excellent result except when the vein is too large and, due to its low density, foam floats in contact with only the more superficial wall. Obtaining a reduction of venous diameter by any means, especially by venous spasm, is therefore of utmost importance.[8]

As derived from Tessari's method,[9] the most common method of making foam uses two 5-ml luer lock siliconized syringes. One syringe contains 1 ml of sclerosing agent at the desired concentration, the other 4 ml of (sterile, filtered) room air. Syringes are connected either by a three-way stopcock or a female/female luer lock two-way connector. Then foam is obtained by cavitation by an average of twenty back-and-forth passages from one syringe to the other. Stability of this kind of foam is correct for 1 to 2 minutes, no more.

A type of commercial foam was still undergoing clinical trials at the time of preparation of this chapter, Varisolve, based on Cabrera's initial microfoam but transformed to allow a canister-contained mixture to produce ready-made foam. This system is designed to provide standardized POL

foam that is FDA approved. Although practical interest in this foam is intense because of its proposed sanction, this is tempered by its cost. Its superiority to homemade foam remains to be demonstrated.

INJECTION

Two groups of different methods are used to inject sclerofoam. Authors usually favor one but use several, if not all, in various situations. Sclerofoam is primarily used for large veins, thus it is usually injected with duplex guidance and duplex control of efficacy.

One main difference is in the method of venous access, which can be either an open-vein access (butterfly needle, microcatheter, long catheter) or a direct puncture of the vein with the needle mounted on the syringe. Open vein access provides optimal safety since it uses devices designed for safe and durable venous infusion and allows easy continuous control of blood reflux and adequate positioning of the needle (see Box 19.1).

Open-vein access allows injection of any volume and repeat injections with additional syringes if necessary. It is important to emphasize the fact that open-vein access allows preparation of the foam at the last minute, and rapid injection of fresh foam. Short catheters and butterfly needles have almost the same utility.

Long catheters are still uncommon but may open a new perspective. The tip can be placed at any level, for example the (SFJ) junction. After positioning, the leg can be elevated and an Esmarch bandage applied. This empties the vein and then the foam is injected while pulling back the catheter. This technique, in principle, is comparable to endovenous ablation, but is much less expensive. Preliminary results are encouraging, but the technique is more complicated than open-vein access. Its advantages remain to be demonstrated.

Closed vein access is probably the most common technique, it consists in puncturing and injecting the vein with the needle mounted on the syringe. Appropriate placement of the tip of the needle is checked by gentle aspiration end observation of blood reflux into the syringe. This method requires training and skill, especially when the US probe is held by the other hand of the physician, which is our technique of choice.

VARICOSE PATTERNS WHEN CONSIDERING A SCLEROSING FOAM TREATMENT

Sclerofoam allows filling of quite a long segment of vein from a remote puncture site. Therefore, duplex scan evaluation of varicose patterns must take into account preferential channels and not just the raw mapping of eye-visible and echo-visible veins. For instance, the association of incompetent varicose medial leg and thigh tributaries joining an incompetent saphenous vein at mid thigh should be emphasized in

Box 19.1

STEP-BY-STEP ULTRASOUND-GUIDED SCLEROFOAM INJECTION WITH OPEN VENOUS ACCESS

This assumes that a preliminary duplex assessment and mapping of all veins of the lower extremities has already been carried out and that results have been carefully reviewed.

- Prepare all necessary materials on a tray:
  - 25- gauge 3/4-inch butterfly needle (for veins no deeper than 1 cm) or needle with connector, or 2.5 or 5 mL Syringe and 0.7 mm diameter needle
  - two 5-ml luer lock needles, one containing 1 ml sclerosing solution, the other 4 ml of sterile air, attached by a three-way stopcock or two-way connector
  - Adhesive tape, elasto-adhesive tape, cotton balls, medical compression stockings
  - Sterile US gel, sterile probe cover

- Map the area to treat with duplex (10-MHz probe necessary), mark possible points of injection possible points of injection

- Prepare skin

- Place needle into varicose vein under US guidance with bevel turned down

- Verify the 'flashback' or appearance of blood in the hub; secure to the skin with adhesive tape

- Prepare sclerofoam by twenty alternate passages from one syringe to the other

- Attach syringe to connector

- Place probe over needle, check position

- Inject first bubbles; check on duplex that bubbles are inside the vein or use the syringe/needle puncture:
  - Prepare foam and adapt the selected needle to the syringe
  - Place US probe longitudinally avec the vein
  - Puncture the skin and push the needle into the vein, remaining in the plane of US
  - Check the position of the tip into the vein lument, aspirate to check blood is reflux into the syringe, inject a few bubbles in order to verify needle position

- Inject sclerofoam, control filling of varicose network with duplex; if necessary massage with probe or hand to fill the desired venous network

- Check appearance of venous spasm

- Remove needle, apply cotton ball and adhesive tape

- Place foam pad (option), elasto-adhesive tape, and finally grade 2 medical stockings

- Take some time while the patient is still on the table to explain that walking is recommended, that stockings must be kept on for 24 hours, and then for 2 weeks daytime only

- Make appointment for next session (duplex evaluation and other injection if necessary).

the scan report. This is one of the best primary indications for foam sclerotherapy. This pattern requires proper assessment of diameters of both the tributary varicosity and the saphenous trunk. Many physicians consider that sclerosing the tributary is the primary aim of their injections. Others adhere to old surgical dogma that the refluxing saphenous vein must be obliterated (first or at the same time).

Current respect for the dogma of systematic elimination of reflux at the saphenofemoral junction may disappear after several years of use of endovenous ablation that preserves the junction. The next, possibly successful, heresy could be to reject saphenous trunk treatment entirely in some cases.[10]

ADVANTAGES OF SCLEROFOAM

Comparison with Other Sclerosants and with Other Methods (Surgical, Endovenous Ablation)

Choosing Sclerofoam treatment for large veins is an option. But it implies certain prerequisites and corollaries such as:

- Expertise of the treating physician

- A clear understanding and agreement between patient and physician on a treatment program requiring several sessions, additional, repeat injections, and control scans; and

- Important benefits such as ambulatory procedures without even local anesthesia but with optimal cosmetic results and cost-effectiveness.

Even today, short- and mid-term results[5,11-14] of foam sclerotherapy are not inferior to surgery or endovenous ablation. But long-term results are still under evaluation. Since repeat injections are simple and inexpensive and cause no disability, evaluation of outcomes of sclerofoam treatment should not require the same end points as surgery.[15]

Sclerofoam sclerotherapy has progressed thanks to a better understanding of pathophysiology of varicose disease, made possible by duplex ultrasound experience. For a long time, some 100 years, junctional reflux was considered as the main, if not the only, problem. All treatments up to 1990 were devoted to its eradication. More recent conceptions, however, take into account the role of the varicose reservoir. This is a necessary drainage for incompetent trunks. It allows demonstration of actual reflux. The varicose reservoir addresses different perforating veins differently. Often these are not only nonpathogenic but also necessary to drain varicose clusters (reentry perforators). This understanding of the reservoir function of refluxing varicosities is also applicable to surgical approaches. A common observation is that treating large refluxing tributaries and varicose clusters can reduce or totally suppress truncal reflux. How to decide in which cases such an approach is optimal is still undecided.

HOW MUCH TO INJECT?

The main advantage of sclerofoam is that it fills up the varicose vein without being diluted with blood. It is important to adjust the injected volume to the length and diameter of the vein. This can be estimated by a simple calculation using the formula of the cylinder:

$$V = \pi \cdot (D/2)^2 \cdot L \ (V = \text{Volume}, D = \text{Diameter}, L = \text{Length}).$$

Several results are presented in Table 19.1.

Nevertheless, it must be remembered that venous spasm will occur after injection and that massage or alternate compression and release are thought to increase spasm. The actual volume necessary for an appropriate result is probably less than that listed in the table. Duplex control of the distribution of the foam is essential and allows adapting the volume to specific conditions. From this point of view, open-vein access makes the procedure easier as it allows waiting and seeing and reinjecting if necessary.

We have recommended limiting the volume of sclerofoam as in Table 19.2. This is also recommended by the European consensus.[16]

Table 19.1 THEORETICAL VOLUME IN CM³ OF A VENOUS SEGMENT CALCULATED FROM THE FORMULA OF THE CYLINDER

VEIN DIAMETER (CM)	VEIN LENGTH (CM)							
	5	7	10	15	20	25	30	35
1.00	3.93	5.50	7.85	11.78	15.71	19.63	23.56	27.49
0.90	3.18	4.45	6.36	9.54	12.72	15.90	19.09	22.27
0.80	2.51	3.52	5.03	7.54	10.05	12.57	15.08	17.59
0.70	1.92	2.69	3.85	5.77	7.70	9.62	11.55	13.47
0.60	1.41	1.98	2.83	4.24	5.65	7.07	8.48	9.90
0.50	0.98	1.37	1.96	2.95	3.93	4.91	5.89	6.87
0.40	0.63	0.88	1.26	1.88	2.51	3.14	3.77	4.40
0.30	0.35	0.49	0.71	1.06	1.41	1.77	2.12	2.47
0.20	0.16	0.22	0.31	0.47	0.63	0.79	0.94	1.10

(From Reference 5)

SIDE EFFECTS OF SCLEROFOAM

Sclerofoam sclerotherapy shares most of its (rare) side effects with usual sclerotherapy, but some complications are more specific. Visual disturbances are frequently quoted as one of the main inconveniences of foam, but there is evidence[17] that they are related more to big bubbles than to microbubbles. When visual troubles were observed with liquid, it was mainly associated with the use of the air block technique. After sessions using only sclerofoam, we observed less than 0.25 visual adverse effects per 100 sessions.

Foam is an excellent contrast medium for ultrasound. Therefore duplex-guided sclerotherapy with foam dramatically improves the safety of sclerotherapy injections with regard to intra-arterial or extravenous injections. We observed no case of necrosis in the French registry,[17] and the number of such accidents reported by French Malpractice Insurance Company has decreased to zero these last two years.

Venous thrombosis is a complication that has been considered as one of the main drawbacks of sclerotherapy. In fact, deep venous thrombosis (DVT) has been observed in very few cases: one DVT in more than 6,000 sessions.[17] Other thrombotic complications also have been observed in other venous compartments: extension to perforating veins (two cases) and to muscular veins (three cases). Appropriate

Table 19.2 CONCENTRATIONS AND VOLUMES FOR POL FOAM

VEIN	FIRST SESSION (%)	SECOND SESSION (%)	VOLUME (CC)
Thigh GSV	2	3	Up to 8
GSV main tributary	1	1	Up to 4
SSV	2	3	Up to 4
Perforators	1	2	Up to 2
Nonsaphenous site	1	2	2 per

treatment by compression and low molecular weight heparin or nonsteroidal anti-inflammatory medications has always been successful. No pulmonary emboli have been observed in this series of over 6,000 cases. Thrombophilia is suspected in these cases but is not the only etiologic factor.

Another side effect that must be emphasized is the increased sclerosing power and the possible excessive inflammatory or phlebitic reaction produced by the foam. More than a complication, this is a manifestation of efficacy of the technique; it indicates that some serious knowledge and practice are prerequisites to its use!

After injection, some hardening of the tissues and tenderness commonly is observed, even with appropriate compression. The content of the vein is variable and unclear, sometimes made of pure blood elements, sometimes containing fibroblasts. Frequently, around the 6th week, the vein fills again with blood; this might be related to destruction of the most central layers of the venous wall and bleeding of the vasa vasorum. This inconvenience is easily cured by small thrombectomies carried out with a large needle or trocar.

The potential risk of allergy has always been mentioned in papers devoted to sclerotherapy. However, we did not observe a single case in the French registry. It makes sense to consider that foaming does not increase the risk. However, several (probably less than five) cases of lethal anaphylaxis have been reported with liquid sclerosants, and such an event must be explained to patients when obtaining consent.

The question raised by detection of bubbles in the left heart circulation is still unanswered, but several factors seem clear: passage through a patent foramen ovale is possible in certain patients. No clinical detection is possible, no pretreatment detection is required. In the case of isolated bubbles—meaning there is no cluster of microbubbles, because in the injected area they are made only of gas—the interface with blood does not carry a significant number of sclerosing agent molecules, because they have been diluted. The question of possible pulmonary sclerosis induced by bubbles is still theoretical and has not been observed clinically.

Most recent hypothesis as described by Gillet[18] and Frullini[19] consider the responsibility of endothelin. Finally, no case of sclerofoam injection followed by durable severe neurological event has been reported so far.

SCLEROFOAM IN PARTICULAR SITUATIONS

SCLEROFOAM WITH AND WITHOUT ULTRASOUND GUIDANCE

Obviously, very superficial veins do not need ultrasound guidance for access, and foam can be injected after puncture and simple observation of blood reflux. Furthermore, very superficial veins are seen only with specific high-frequency probes that are not always available. In any case, controlling the passage of the foam into upper, bigger, and deeper veins is always useful. It is also necessary to remember that in veins smaller than 3 mm, foam has no advantage over liquid. Appropriate preliminary venous mapping is required in all cases of varicose vein treatment; post treatment, ultrasound assessment of results after several days or weeks is also common practice for most phlebologists.

TRUNCAL VARICOSITIES

Truncal varicosities must be assessed carefully by duplex for their whole length. This is true especially for the great saphenous vein (GSV), because valvular incompetence is not necessarily total, and very often the terminal or preterminal valves are competent. In this situation, this part of the vein will not need to be treated. It is also necessary to remember that the saphenous trunks are always intrafascial. The frequent confusion between a varicose medial superficial tributary and the GSV trunk is responsible for some inappropriate management of varicose vein patients. What must be done and what is appropriate is different in a saphenous trunk, with its thick venous wall and distensibility limited by its intrafascial position, and in a tributary even of large diameter, with its thin venous wall, remodeling, sensitivity to sclerosing agent, and slow blood flow.

The approach to complete GSV incompetence, including the saphenofemoral junction, can be accomplished by direct puncture in the upper third of the thigh and injection of a limited amount of concentrated sclerofoam with a trend toward reduction of concentration and an increase in volume and successive injection of the distal trunk. Nobody advocates injection at the junction level anymore. Our preference is for a more distal approach, between upper and lower thirds of thigh, and US control of appropriate filling of the trunk up to the junction. Alternate compression with the probe may help to an even distribution of foam and to obtain a spasm of the vein. This approach ensures safety and comfort for patient and physician. Difference of efficacy between the two methods is unknown so far.

Due to the depth of saphenous trunks and their relative autocompression by saphenous fascia, thrombectomy after foam sclerotherapy is usually not necessary.

TRIBUTARIES

Sclerofoam power allows treatment of a vein with a mild concentration of sclerosant, which ensures a homogeneous and even reaction. Tributaries are usually more superficial than trunks, and their access is easy with butterfly needles (see Figure 19.2). If carefully used, with a lower concentration, sclerofoam decreases the incidence of matting and residual pigmentation. As explained earlier, thrombectomies may be necessary at 4 to 7 weeks.

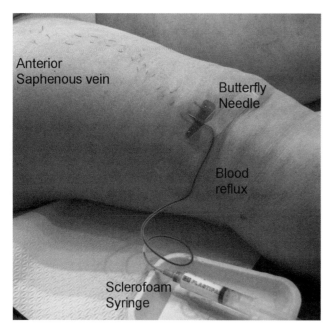

Figure 19.2 This photograph shows the butterfly needle taped in place, the foam in the syringe ready for injection, and the target vein marked for reference purposes.

Labels on figure: Anterior Saphenous vein; Butterfly Needle; Blood reflux; Sclerofoam Syringe

PERFORATORS

Perforating veins again raise a common problem: Must we get rid of all visible or identified dilated veins? Specifically, is duplex observation of reflux in a perforating vein sufficient to decide that this vein must be treated (sclerosed, ablated, and ligated)? This is not certain,[20,21] and in many cases, perforating veins act as drainage of varicose clusters (reentries), and their size decreases significantly after appropriate treatment of the varicose network situated proximally. This is especially true for the paratibial and posterior tibial perforators (lower third medial lower leg), and much less likely for perforating veins of the femoral canal (medial thigh). More precise assessment criteria are needed in order to limit treatment to what is necessary, but a first approach is to begin the treatment with the upper network (probable source of reflux) and to finish with lower elements including perforators (possible reentries).

If sclerofoam treatment of perforating veins is carried out as in other veins, special attention must be paid to avoid progression of foam into the deep network. For this reason, duplex control of foam distribution is essential. Injection directly in the perforator is dangerous due to the presence a satellite artery, whos inadvertent injection would cause a large skin necrosis. Injection of the extrafascial varices close to emergence of the perforator is recommended.

CHRONIC VENOUS INSUFFICIENCY

In case of chronic venous insufficiency, sclerofoam has demonstrated excellent results,[22] and provides dramatic improvement in skin changes. A periulcerous injection of sclerofoam appears to be a booster to wound healing.

RECURRENCES

REVAS (REcurrent Varices After Surgery) have been the subject of an international consensus conference.[23] At the time of the conference, classical sclerotherapy with liquid was presented as the method of choice for management of such cases. However, the use of foam is even more efficient and more practical.

At the saphenofemoral junction, two mechanisms have been identified: neovascularization, where small veins appear in hard scar tissue and the lymph nodes, and a persistent saphenous stump, corresponding to an inappropriate ligation and division. In the first case, direct injection with duplex guidance is possible but requires skill. A remote injection with open-vein access allows extensive filling of the recurrent network. In the second situation the objective is close to a primary treatment. Sclerofoam is the treatment of choice. Recurrent varices have unusually thin walls and are prone to easy sclerosing. There is no need for strong concentrations; 1% or less POL is usually enough.

RETICULAR AND SPIDER VEINS

Since most visual complications are observed after use of Sclerofoam and since superiority of Sclerofoam is counterbalanced by an increase of matting and pigmentation related to an increased sclerosing power, we reserve the use of Sclerofoam for telangiectasias and reticular veins to rare, individual cases.

UPPER BODY

Varicose veins of upper limbs including fingers are rare; we have treated some with sclerofoam and observed good results, and it seems unlikely that any large study will be available on this matter. Regarding sclerotherapy of hand veins in elderly patients, we do not recommend any such suppression. Ambulatory phlebectomy has been proposed, and this kind of treatment of "normal" veins is likely to be questioned if a venous access is later necessary for other medical reasons (blood tests, chemotherapy, and emergency IV injections).

Facial veins are small, foam is not needed, and liquid sclerosants are usually efficient. We have observed several good results in sclerotherapy of telangiectasias associated to venous malformations of the face.

CONTRAINDICATIONS TO SCLEROFOAM

As indicated earlier, Sclerofoam is responsible for very few side effects. However, it should be avoided in patients with severe thrombophilias, and carried out with prophylaxis in less severe thrombophilias. There is a prospective study currently in progress in France on this very matter.

Known allergy to POL or STS will not allow the use of the specific agent, but there is no crossed allergy between these agents.

Disulfiram (DCI) is a principal contraindication, but the total amount of alcohol in POL foam is so low that an effect is unlikely.

Tamoxifen (DCI) has demonstrated a potential to induce superficial venous thrombosis during sclerotherapy; therefore, injections must be postponed to the end of chemotherapy.

There is usually no emergency in treating varicose veins, so a sclerofoam treatment during pregnancy is usually not necessary. Nothing is known about effects of sclerosing molecules on embryos; the principle of precaution should be applied.

PREREQUISITES FOR CARRYING OUT FOAM SCLEROTHERAPY

Physician

- Good understanding and knowledge of venous disorders
- Good practice of duplex on veins
- Previous experience of liquid sclerotherapy
- Skill with syringes and needles
- Time devoted to training for duplex-guided injection on phantoms or beef liver
- Availability for repeat injections

Patient

- Patience
- Understanding of procedures and postprocedure care

CONCLUSIONS

Even if the physician is open to all available techniques, his personal preferences influence his management of varicose disease even before the assessment of varicose patterns. Satisfaction of the patients' main concern should be his goal, and sclerofoam will appear most of the time as the most "patient-friendly" method. In any case, carrying out such a treatment requires skill and preliminary learning and training.

Progress in sclerofoam technique is likely to revolutionize the management of varicose disease. We have always advocated an à la carte treatment of varicose veins, and it is now obvious that what we did surgically several years ago can be done with sclerofoam injections. Active, simple, inexpensive, and safe, ultrasound-guided sclerotherapy with foam is the future of varicose treatments.

REFERENCES

1. Wollmann JC. The history of sclerosing foams, *Dermatol Surg.* 2004. *30*: 694–703.
2. Cabrera J, Cabrera Garcia Olmedo JR. Nuevo método de esclerosis en las varices tronculares, *Patol Vasc.* 1995. *4*: 55–73.
3. Monfreux A. Traitement sclérosant des troncs saphéniens et leurs collatérales de gros calibre par la méthode MUS, *Phlebologie.* 1997. *50*: 351–353.
4. Knottnerus A, Dinant GJ. Medicine based evidence, a prerequisite for evidence based medicine, *Br Med J.* 1997. *315*: 1109–1110.
5. Rasmussen LH, Lawaetz M, Bjoern L, Vennits B, Blemings A, Eklof B. Randomized clinical trial comparing endovenous laser ablation, radiofrequency ablation, foam sclerotherapy and surgical stripping for great saphenous varicose veins. *Br J Surg.* 2011. *98*(8):1079–1087.
6. Guex J-J. Foam sclerotherapy: An overview of use for primary venous insufficiency, *Semin Vasc Surg.* 2005. *18*: 25–29.
7. Guex J-J. Indications for the sclerosing agent Polidocanol®, *J Derm Surg Onc.* 1993. *19*: 959–961.
8. Goldman MP, Bergan JJ, Guex JJ. *Sclerotherapy, treatment of varicose and telangiectatic leg veins,* 4e. New York; Elsevier. In press.
9. Tessari L. Nouvelle technique d'obtention de la scléromousse, *Phlebology.* 2000. *53*: 129.
10. Pittaluga P, Rea B, Barbe R. Méthode ASVAL (ablation sélective des varices sous anesthésie locale): Principes et résultats intermédiaires, *Phlebologie.* 2005 *58*: 175–181.
11. Barrett JM, Allen B, Ockelford A, Goldman MP. Microfoam ultrasound guided sclerotherapy treatment for varicose veins in a subgroup with diameters at the junction of 10 mm or greater compared with a subgroup of less than 10 mm, *Dermatol Surg.* 2004. *30*: 1386–1390.
12. Yamaki T, Nozaki M, Iwasaka S. Comparative study of duplex guided foam sclerotherapy and duplex guided liquid sclerotherapy for the treatment of superficial venous insufficiency, *Dermatol Surg.* 2004. *30*: 718–722.
13. Hamel-Desnos C, Desnos P, Wollmann JC, Ouvry P, Mako S, Allaert FA. Evaluation of the efficacy of polidocanol in the form of foam compared with liquid form in sclerotherapy of the great saphenous vein: Initial results, *Dermatol Surg.* 2003. *29*: 1170–1175; discussion 1175.
14. Barrett JM, Allen B, Ockelford A, Goldman MP. Microfoam ultrasound guided sclerotherapy of varicose veins in 100 legs, *Dermatol Surg.* 2004. *30*: 6–12.
15. Guex J-J, Isaacs MN. Comparison of surgery and ultrasound guided sclerotherapy for treatment of saphenous varicose veins: Must the criteria for assessment be the same?, *Int Angiol.* 2000. *19*(4): 299–302.
16. Rabe E, Breu F, Cavezzi A, et al.; for the Guideline Group. European guidelines for sclerotherapy in chronic venous disorders. *Phlebology.* 2013.
17. Guex J-J, Allaert FA, Gillet JL, Chleir F. Immediate and midterm complications of sclerotherapy report of a prospective multi-center registry of 12,173 sclerotherapy sessions, *J Dermatol Surg.* 2005. *31*: 123–128.
18. Gillet JL. Neurological complications of foam sclerotherapy: fears and reality. *Phlebology.* 2011. *26*(7): 277–279.
19. Frullini A, Barsotti MC, Santoni T, Duranti E, Burchielli S, Di Stefano R. Significant endothelin release in patients treated with foam sclerotherapy. *Dermatol Surg.* 2012. *38*(5): 741–747.
20. Guex J-J. Ultrasound guided sclerotherapy for perforating veins, *Hawaii Med J.* 2000. *59*(6): 261.
21. Danielsson G, Eklof B, Kistner RL. What is the role of incompetent perforator veins in chronic venous insufficiency?, *J Phleb.* 2001. *1*: 67–71.
22. Bergan JJ, Pascarella L. Severe CVI: Primary treatment with sclerofoam, *Semin Vasc Surg.* 2005. *18*: 49–56.
23. Perrin MR, Guex JJ, Ruckley CV, et al. Recurrent varices after surgery (REVAS), a consensus document, *Cardiovasc Surg.* 2000. *8*: 233–245.

20.

SCLEROSANTS IN MICROFOAM

A NEW APPROACH IN ANGIOLOGY

Juan Cabrera, Maria V. Rubia, and Juan Cabrera Jr.

INTRODUCTION

The onset of reflux and the subsequent development of varicose veins requires a connection between the triad made up of the origin of reflux, the transmission route, and the end vessel. These three elements are present in all patients with varicose veins. The origin of reflux can be identified with hand-held Doppler device or duplex ultrasound. Then it can be eliminated. It is the least important, because the absence of functioning valves in any site is of little importance if the blood cannot move in a retrograde direction. Transmission routes are anatomically highly variable but are readily identified using physical and color duplex ultrasound examinations. Their stable elimination can be confirmed by follow-up visits.

The key to therapeutic success in treating venous insufficiency lies in the complete, rigorous, and confirmed elimination of all varicose veins of leg, ankle, and foot. If this objective is not achieved, recurrence is possible. Both, endoluminal and surgical procedures, when used alone, face difficulties in completely eliminating all varicose veins in a limb. Even when these approaches are combined it is not uncommon that a few incompetent veins persist even though they are poorly developed at the time of treatment. These missed veins may lead to recurrence of varicose veins.

Sclerotherapy, a classic therapy of recognized potential[1] but limited effectiveness has entered a new era.[2,3] The drastic limitations imposed by its use in liquid form, subject to progressive dilution and inactivation in the blood and very difficult to control when within a vessel, have been overcome.

Since 1993, our experience and that of others has demonstrated the effectiveness of duplex ultrasound-guided microfoam sclerotherapy. This has been successfully used not only in patients with varicose leg veins, traditionally indicated for surgery,[4–6] but also in venous malformations that resist surgical treatment[7] and in leg ulcers caused by venous hypertension,[8,9] thus extending the limits of sclerotherapy and raising expectations for this approach. As Bergan[10] said, "foam sclerotherapy reaches its highest pinnacle of success in treating venous leg ulcers." The old concept of foam sclerotherapy has been brought back to life.

The simplistic analogy between foam and microfoam, the great ease with which foam can be produced, and the absence of available pharmaceutical grade microfoam has led to a multiplicity of efforts to use foam for sclerotherapeutic purposes. There have been numerous reports of results obtained with heterogeneous types of foam produced by various but similar homemade methods,[11–15] using a variety of application techniques. However, major differences in the physics and intravascular dynamics of foams and microfoam, especially the specific pharmaceutical grade microfoam currently in US Phase III clinical trial, suggest that a cautious view should be taken toward the use of foam. The publication of several cases of ischemic stroke after the administration of homemade foams has raised concerns about the safety of their use without following strict precautions.[16–20] At the very least, the recommendations of the Tegernsee consensus[21] should be followed on the injectable volume of homemade foams.

The drawbacks of foams include the composition of the gas mixture used, commonly atmospheric air (with a high content of low soluble Nitrogen) or even less soluble gases,[22] their high degree of coalescence and their variability in internal cohesion, and the variability in the dose of liquid sclerosant that a given volume of foam contains as well as the diameter of the bubble.[23] Microfoam has overcome these shortcomings. Nevertheless, optimization of the application technique and the development of increasingly effective safety measures remain an ongoing challenge.

MECHANISM OF ACTION

Micronization of the bubbles creates an optimal structure to endow the liquid sclerosant with the largest possible surface area and to facilitate its contact with the endothelium. The active surface area of the liquid sclerosant increases exponentially with a reduction in the diameter of the bubbles. When these sclerosant vectors possess the appropriate internal cohesion, they can physically displace the blood contained in the vessel. In this way, the liquid can be homogeneously distributed at a known concentration on an extensive endothelial surface. The ideal foam should have a specific diameter of the bubbles, gas composition, gas-liquid ratio, and internal bubble cohesion. The correct combination of these factors together with the proper application technique are all key parameters for the safety and efficacy of the procedure. Our proprietary microfoam successfully incorporates these basic elements and has, in combination with our application technique, yielded previously unmatched therapeutic outcomes with a high degree of safety.

Although some of these diverse types of foams, when compared with liquids, can be more effective in eliminating varicose veins, they may not be safer. Homemade foams may not fulfill pharmaceutical grade standards because of the gases used, the variable dose of liquid sclerosant in a given volume of foam and their even more variable physical characteristics, including those that are manufactured with a mixture of CO_2O_2. They represent a stopgap measure before the arrival of a registered and standardized product.

SAPHENOUS VEIN TREATMENT

The first step in our procedure for treating the great saphenous vein (GSV), consists in the injection of 1% polidocanol microfoam using a 20-gauge short catheter (51-mm length) placed in the vein at mid/lower third of the thigh in distal direction. With the leg raised, we inject the volume required to totally fill the GSV in the thigh (filling volume). When the microfoam is seen to arrive at the saphenofemoral junction, the injection is stopped. Approximately 10 to 20 cc are injected, depending on the dimensions of the vein (πr^2). The microfoam must remain confined to the vein to avoid filling the superficial tributaries at this high concentration, thereby preventing overdose of superficial veins and an undesirable inflammatory reaction.

We then aspirate with a syringe to see the color of the intraluminal content, repeating the injection of an appropriate volume of microfoam (renewal volume) one or two times, if necessary, until a white aspirate is obtained, indicating that the segment contains only microfoam. The renewal volume is considerably smaller than the filling volume because the vein segment already contains microfoam, and only 2 to 3 cc are needed to effectively renew the content. Excess microfoam drains into the femoral vein but is practically inactive, since it is at the proximal end of the "pneumatic piston" that displaced the blood in the vein at the first injection and has undergone major dilution and inactivation.

INTRAVASCULAR LIMITATIONS OF CIRCUMFERENTIAL COMPRESSION

Based on our observations, using color duplex ultrasound, compression stockings of 35 mmHg have no noticeable effect on the morphology or function of large varicose veins. Even when rolls of gauze or other nonelastic cylinders are placed on the varicose vein and strongly compressed by a bandage of little elasticity (Peha-Haft; Hartmann), no reduction in the diameter of trunk varicose veins is produced when the patient is in a standing position. Thus, the joint application of these compressive measures (i.e., stocking + bandage + nonelastic cylinders) does not occlude the lumen of the vessel. Since the vein preserves its dimensions, there is nothing to prevent the formation of a thrombus. For that reason, we use the proximal sclerosis approach. The involution of tributaries after the proximal occlusion (see above) is very important because it prevents the formation of a big thrombus and its undesirable side effects (Figure 20.1).

FOLLOW-UP CARE

When the patient, still wearing the compression stocking, returns to the clinic 10 to 15 days after the treatment, we verify the occlusion of the treated proximal segment and check the involution of varicose veins tributary to this segment (see Figures 20.2 and 20.3). During this second

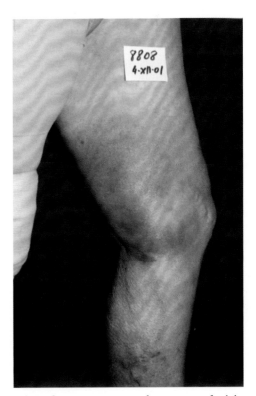

Figure 20.1 Skin inflammatory reaction after injection of polidocanol microfoam in a GSV.

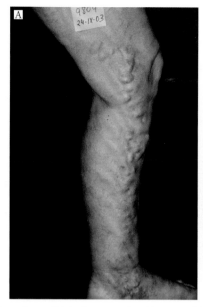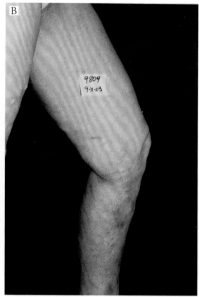

Figure 20.2A and 20.2B   Involution of superficial tributary varicosities around 15 days after closure of only the proximal segment.

treatment session, we adjust the concentration of sclerosant to the location and reduced size of these veins. The appropriate concentrations of polidocanol are between 0.18 and 0.37%, injected with a 25-gauge butterfly needle; this small diameter limits the flow of microfoam and is adjusted to the size of the injected vessels. At this point, the diminished size of the veins (by involution) allows a larger area to be treated with the same volume of microfoam. Treatment of small skin veins (thread veins) requires the use of a special approach, using fine needles (30 gauge) and lower polidocanol concentrations (0.18%). The lesser foaming capacity at these low concentrations and the high mechanical stress suffered by large bubbles when they pass through these fine needles can cause disruption of the bubbles when homemade foam is used, with most returning to their original components of gas and liquid. This is a very common cause

of complications of the foam treatment of small veins and is caused by the use of atmospheric nitrogen, with its very low solubility in blood. Micronization of the bubbles is especially necessary for treating such small vessels, whose therapy represents the bulk of the practice of many professionals.

TREATMENT EVOLUTION— PROXIMAL SCLEROSIS

After the reflex vasospasm, (see Figure 20.4) and when the patient leaves the clinic, the blood returns to fill the vessel and forms a thrombus whose size depends on the dimensions of the treated vein. Subfascial localization distant from the skin favors a recovery with moderate or few inflammatory symptoms. In other words, proximity of dilated superficial varicose veins to the skin can produce undesirable clinical symptoms and increases the risk of pigmentation. Voluminous superficial varicose veins must be treated with lower microfoam concentration and only after the size has reduced sufficiently after the proximal segment closure. The aim of this "proximal sclerosis" is not only a more stable closure of the saphenofemoral junction or of the proximal source of reflux but rather the involution of distal varicose veins. In our view, until there is a resolution of the limitations of circumferential compression, this is the most appropriate approach. In subsequent sessions, we verify by ultrasound that the treated proximal segment is occluded and the diameter of the tributary superficial veins, distal from the closed vein, has decreased significantly.

The stable occlusion of the saphenofemoral junction was a prime objective during the early years of microfoam sclerotherapy. To mimic surgical ligation and resection of the saphenofemoral junction, we aimed to close the

Figure 20.3A and 20.3B   Involution of superficial tributary varicosities 13 days after closure of only the proximal segment.

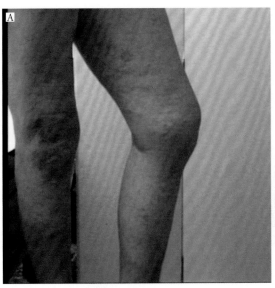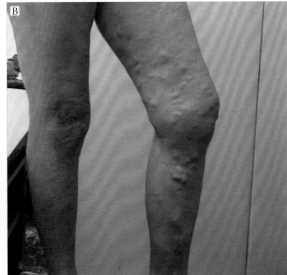

Figure 20.4A and 20.4 B   Contact of the sclerosant with the endothelium induces a severe vasospasm, a good and immediate marker of the effectiveness of the injection.

junction at the common femoral vein, monitoring its progression toward fibrosis and resorption. Nowadays, we pay little attention to the junction, which remains patent, with no reflux and excellent long-term outcomes. This is similar to the reported experience with the Venefit procedure and endovenous laser treatment (EVLT).

SAFETY MEASURES IN MICROFOAM SCLEROTHERAPY

THE CLOSED-DOOR MANEUVER

The most feared complications of sclerotherapy are intra-arterial injection and deep venous thrombosis (DVT; Table 20.1). The use of color duplex ultrasonography helps to avoid intra-arterial injection, and injection of the GSV at the thigh rules out a possible injection of the femoral artery. At other locations, the use of ultrasound-guided injection and the excellent reports warning about this issue have reduced the incidence of this complication, although the clinician must always be alert to this danger. Routine is a poor companion in sclerotherapy.

In the sclerotherapy of varicose trunk veins, DVT usually is produced by a coagulation disorder in the patient or by an error in the administration technique (see Figure 20.5). The most frequent site for this complication is in leg muscle veins. However, in our experience of treating over 10,000 GSV with microfoam sclerotherapy, we have observed no occlusion of the common femoral vein. Its high flow dilutes the sclerosant and reduces the consequences of technical failures (see Figure 20.6), such as injection of high concentrations or excessive volumes of microfoam for the size of the vessel treated. Nevertheless, in the beginning when our technique was not yet fully developed, we performed

Table 20.1 **SAFETY MEASURES**

Acknowledge limitations of perimetral compression
Previous proximal sclerosis
Limb elevation
Low polidocanol concentration: GSV: 0.7–1% Involutionated tributaries: 0.27–0.37%
Precise filling volume
Nitrogen free gases
Closed-door maneuver
Local compression (leg ulcers)

slow injections, letting the microfoam pass through the GSV without taking advantage of the mechanical action of the pneumatic piston. At that time, we observed several thromboses in the common femoral caused by bubbles that floated on the blood when the patient was in the supine position. These passed to the femoral vein in "Indian file" still loaded with sclerosant, contacting its upper endothelial wall. The limited extent of this thrombosis and its subocclusive nature ensured its rapid lysis in the very few patients with this complication. The potentially most controversial points in sclerotherapy of the saphenous reflux are perforating veins with direct connection to the deep venous system (DVS): femoral, popliteal, and medial gastrocnemius veins (see Figure. 20.7). These very common sites of reinjection carry a high risk of extending the thrombosis of the varicose vein to a more or less extensive segment of the gastrocnemius vein, which might result in further extension of the thrombus into the popliteal and superficial femoral veins.

We take two preventive measures to avoid DVT. The first one is a dual measure: a reduction in the sclerosant

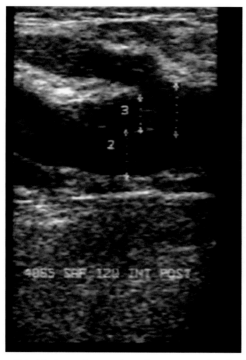

Figure 20.5　Postablation saphenous thrombus extension (PASTE) of common femoral vein with spontaneous thrombolysis. Only two cases in our experience.

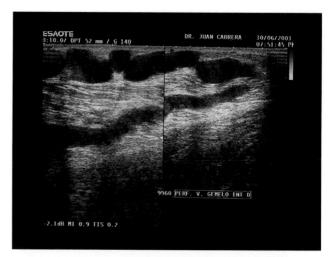

Figure 20.7　This kind of connection (perforating vein) between superficial and muscular veins increases the risk of DVT. Nothing prevents the injected sclerosant from exerting its action a little beyond the desired segment.

concentration and a strict limitation of the injected volume to the capacity of the vein to be treated (see Figure 20.8). Injections that exceed this volume and concentrations greater than 0.37% are errors of technique. The second measure is to close the gastrocnemius vein during and after the injection by taking advantage of the muscle function. We first confirm by ultrasound that muscle veins are completely closed when the patient is standing and that they remain so while the muscle contraction caused by this position persists, with complete closure of the lumen. In supine position, active dorsal flexion of the foot produces a similar result. If the patient tires, muscle vein occlusion can be achieved by passive flexion, using the hand of the clinician or assistant to exert dorsal pressure on the foot (see Figure 20.9). Active, voluntary contraction of the muscles is more effective, although many patients do not have this ability and must learn it. We routinely use active dorsal flexion during the injection of varicose leg veins, checking its effectiveness on ultrasound. If it is not effective, another variation of these maneuvers can be used (see Figure 20.10).

We also use these novel and personal "closed-door" maneuvers during the sclerosis of low perforating veins as a complementary measure to the pressure exerted on the perforating vein with fingers or ultrasound probe. We must be 100% sure that the sclerosant does not reach the DVS in an uncontrolled manner. This combination of safety measures that we have gradually developed and now applied in our daily practice has led to a dramatic reduction in complications. In our long experience, we have had only 22 cases of DVT of leg muscle veins among more than 10,000 patients.

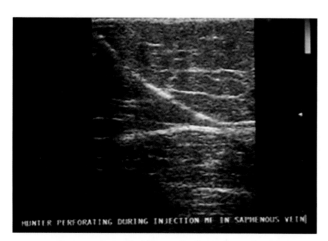

Figure 20.6　Passage of microbubbles to the femoral vein during injection of saphenous vein. This situation requires careful duplex ultrasound monitoring and clearance of the foam particles by foot flexion and extension.

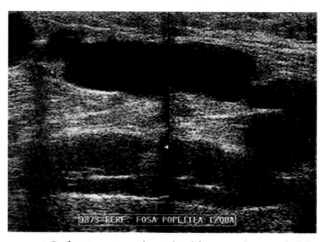

Figure 20.8　Perforating veins to the popliteal fossa must be treated while there is compression at the connection point to minimize the volume of foam drained into the deep venous system.

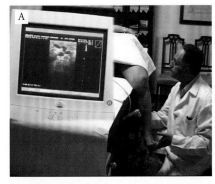 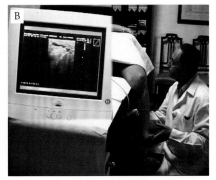

Figure 20.9A and 20.9B   Color duplex ultrasonography is used to confirm that active dorsal flexion of the foot closes the intramuscular venous segment.

In 10 of these patients, a coagulation disorder was the cause. After the introduction of these safety measures we have not observed a single DVT of muscular veins.

GAS MIXTURE AND BUBBLE SIZE

Gas solubility and bubble size are key safety elements of foams. Eckmann[24] in an "in vivo" model studied the differences in intravascular dynamics between homemade foams and Varisolve (the patented microfoam). The author demonstrated that microbubbles do not halt the arteriolar bed flow while bigger size bubbles produce its complete occlusion.

Even though foam sclerotherapy of varicose veins has become a widespread procedure, concerns were raised when ischemic stroke symptoms were reported after the use of foam sclerotherapy. The risk for cerebral gas embolism is particularly increased in patient with cardiac right-to-left shunt. At the request of the FDA a phase II clinical trial was conducted in patients with foramen ovale treated with the reformulated Varisolve with very low nitrogen level, demonstrating that this product does not produce any injury to the brain, retina, or heart[25] as demonstrated by magnetic resonance imaging with perfusion-weighted images, visual testing, and marker of myocardial ischemia.

Homemade foams are currently manufactured with the double syringe technique and a CO_2O_2 gas mixture (Table 20.2). However, these foams still contain trace amounts of nitrogen, high enough to produce symptomatic gas embolisms. In addition, they lack the key physical characteristics that define a good foam.

OTHER SAFETY MEASURES: LEG ELEVATION, ELASTIC LIGATURE, PRECISE FILLING VOLUME

Blood is the main adversary of effective contact between a known concentration of sclerosant and the endothelium of large varicose veins. The blood volume can be markedly reduced by elevating the leg, thereby decreasing the pressure and facilitating displacement of the blood by the microfoam, allowing homogeneous contact of the microfoam with the entire endothelial surface. However, leg elevation does not halt the proximal flow, and dilution of the sclerosant persists. Proximal flow can be stopped by placing an elastic ligature over the internal condyle. This ligature also avoids passage of the microfoam to varicose leg branches, which are treated at a later session with microfoam at an appropriate concentration. After the procedure, a 23-mmHg compression stocking is placed, and the patient remains resting for 10 to 15 minutes.

During the resting period, most injected bubbles drain into the general circulation, some of them are still activated bubbles. These are eventually deactivated by fixation of the

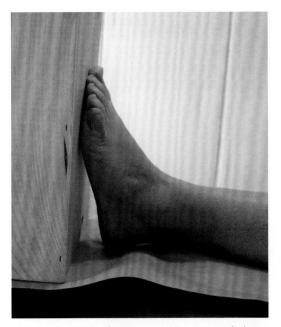

Figure 20.10   Another way to close gastrocnemius veins with the patient in the supine position is to support the ball of the foot on a flat surface while raising the heel. This maneuver is equivalent to the active contraction of the muscles while standing.

Table 20.2 **SOLUBILITY COEFFICIENTS**

Oxygen	1
CO_2	23.75
Nitrogen	0.5
Helium	0.35

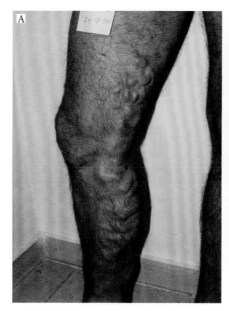
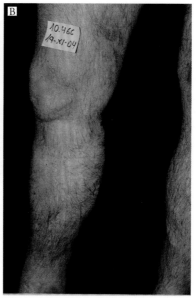

Figure 20.11A and 20.11B   Extremely voluminous and tortuous varicose veins before and after treatment (7 months).

sclerosant molecules onto the lipid rich membranes of red blood cells and venous endothelium. At the same time, the highly soluble gas is dissolved in the blood, a process that is completed in the lung thanks to its enormous vascular surface area of around 150 m². With foam, it is more critical than with microfoam to accurately determine the length of segment to be treated in order to deliver a volume that precisely matches the volume to be filled. It is not enough to let the foam float on the blood; a specific segment must be filled completely. As mentioned earlier, we test the filling of a vein segment with microfoam by reaspiration with the syringe, using the simple method described and reinjecting microfoam if necessary. This assessment of intraluminal content by aspiration cannot be used in the treatment of incompetent

leg perforating veins when the needle is close to the perforating vein, because the aspirated blood derives from the nearby DVS, and its filling should not be forced. This situation is resolved by precisely matching the volume of injected microfoam to the capacity of the vein to be treated.

In comparison to microfoam, for homemade foams the maximum volume recommended to inject is relatively small. For this reason, treatment of an extensive venous area must be performed in more sessions.

The effective safety measures that we have introduced make microfoam sclerotherapy the therapeutic procedure of choice when the anatomical and functional removal of large and complex pathological varicose veins is indicated (see Figures 20.11 and 20.12).

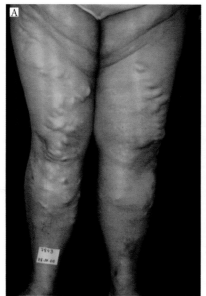
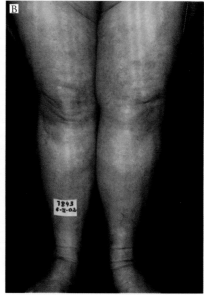

Figure 20.12   Voluminous and complex varicose veins before and after treatment.

LONG-TERM EVOLUTION — STABILITY OF OUTCOMES

The Achilles' heel of surgery is the high recurrence rate of varicose veins[26,27] together with its aggressive nature and its incomplete outcomes. In addition, varicose veins often reappear in legs that were treated only a few months earlier, even when all varicose veins were apparently successfully removed. These recurrences seem to be caused by the development of varicose veins that were not visible at the time of treatment but were nevertheless part of the varicose heritage of the patient. These incompetent veins take the place of those that were removed, maintaining hemodynamic continuity to the end vessels in leg muscles and ensuring their progression.

Besides sclerotherapy with microfoam, we know of no therapeutic procedure that can remove all types of varicose veins, in any localization and no matter their size. However, the disappearance of all varicose veins from a given area does not mean that total success has been achieved. Final victory can be claimed only when we can be reasonably sure that we have also eliminated all veins that may constitute a source of recurrence. To this end, an exhaustive color duplex ultrasound study is made at subsequent treatment sessions (at 3 to 5 months) and we treat all varicose veins revealed in the leg. Newly formed varicose veins are also identified and treated during follow-up sessions at 6, 9, and 12 months. This active follow-up approach achieves the progressive, systematic, and complete removal of varicose veins that could produce a recurrence and whose suppression is the key to long-term stability of outcomes (Table 20.3). These goals cannot be attained by surgery or endoluminal techniques when used alone. Varicose disease is considered an essentially progressive condition. Nevertheless, application of the correct treatment can markedly reduce the recurrence rate.

Our final goal is to make our outcomes stable in the long-term. Our current objectives include to improve the technique, accelerate the treatment, and make it more comfortable for the patient. The type of compression applied is of critical importance for comfort. Since we have observed no benefits from the application of a strong compression, we use stockings that exert moderate compression. The availability of a micronized, homogeneous, and reproducible foam of pharmaceutical grade is crucial, because it will allow the development of a standardized treatment protocol, facilitating the comparison of outcomes obtained by different groups (Table 20.4).

Table 20.3 **TREATMENT STRATEGY**

1° Elimination of existing varicose veins
2° Elimination of varicose heritage
3° 1-year active follow-up guarantee stable outcomes

Table 20.4 **FUTURE PERSPECTIVES**

Pharmaceutical grade microfoam
Standardized technique

OTHER INDICATIONS OF MICROFOAM

As mentioned before microfoam has been used with excellent results in patients with varicose leg ulcers and venous malformations (VM). Our results show that ultrasound-guided microfoam sclerotherapy is highly effective in achieving stable healing of venous ulcers, even in old patients. In addition, we have obtained very good results in patients with low-flow VM. In patients with medium- to small-sized VM we were able to completely eliminate the lesion. In those that presented large VM we achieved a significant clinical improvement and reduction in the size of the malformation. We have never had major complications in this group of patients.

Although we have limited experience in ultrasound-guided microfoam sclerotherapy of varicoceles, we obtained very good results and a significant improvement in sperm quality. The therapeutic approach consists in the injection of 1% polidocanol microfoam with a 21-gauge needle in the internal spermatic vein at the inguinal canal. The insertion of the needle and the administration of the microfoam takes place while the patient performs a Valsalva maneuver, allowing the microfoam to progress distally from and proximally to the point of injection, thus preventing the thrombophlebitis of the pampiniform plexus. In the follow-up session we confirm the occlusion of the varicocele by physical examination and color duplex ultrasound.

The efficacy of sclerotherapy with microfoam is now beyond doubt. It achieves the elimination of all varicose veins in all patients, with no limitations on the size, location, or morphology of the vessels treated by this method.

REFERENCES

1. Mollard JM. Chronic venous insufficiency: Prevention and drugless therapy, *Presse Med*. 1994. *23*(5): 251–258. Review.
2. Hsu TS, Weiss RA. Foam sclerotherapy: A new era, *Arch Dermatol*. 2003. *139*: 1494–1496.
3. Cabrera J, Cabrera J Jr. Nuevo método de esclerosis en las varices tronculares, *Patol Vasc*. 1995. *4*: 55–73.
4. Cabrera Garrido J. Élargissement des limites de la sclérothérapie: Nouveaux produits sclérosants, *Phlebologie*. 1997. *50*: 181–188.
5. Cabrera Garrido J. Los esclerosantes en microespuma contra la patología venosa, *Noticias Med*. 1997. *3*(653): 12–16.
6. Cabrera J, Cabrera J Jr, Garcia-Olmedo A. Treatment of varicose long saphenous veins with sclerosant in microfoam form: Long-term outcomes, *Phlebology*. 2000. *15*: 19–23.
7. Cabrera J, Cabrera J Jr, García-Olmedo A, Redondo P. Treatment of venous malformations with sclerosant in microfoam form, *Arch Dermatol*. 2003. *39*: 1409–1416.

8. Cabrera J, Redondo P, Becerra A, et al. Ultrasound-guided injection of polidocanol microfoam in the management of venous leg ulcers, *Arch. Dermatol.* 2004. *140*: 667–673.

9. Bergan JJ, Pascarella L. Severe chronic venous insufficiency: Primary treatment with sclerofoam, *Semin Vasc Surg.* 2005. *18*: 49–56.

10. Cheng VL, Shortell CK, Bergan JJ. Foam treatment of venous leg ulcers: A continuing experience. In: Bergan JJ, Shortell CK, eds. *Venous Ulcers.* Burlington, MA: Elsevier Academic Press. 2007. 215–226.

11. Monfreaux A. Traitement sclerosant des troncs sapheniens et leurs collaterales de gros calibre par la methode MUS, *Phlebologie.* 1997. *50*(3): 351.

12. Henriet JP. Three years' experience with polidocanol foam in treatment of reticular veins and varicosities, *Phlebologie.* 1999. *52*: 277.

13. Benigni JP, Sadoun S, Thirion V, et al. Telangiectasies et varices reticulaires traitement par la mousse d'Aetoxisclerol a 0.25%: Presentation d'une etude pilote, *Phlebologie.* 1999. *52*: 283–290.

14. Tessari L, Cavezzi A, Frullini A. Preliminary experience with a new sclerosing foam in the treatment of varicose veins, *Dermatol Surg.* 2001. *27*: 58–60.

15. Wollmann JC. The history of sclerosing foams, *Dermatol Surg.* 2004. *30*: 694–703.

16. Ceulen RP, Sommer A, Vernooy K. Microembolism during foam sclerotherapy of varicose veins, *N Engl J Med.* 2008. *358*(14): 1525–1526.

17. Kas A, Begue M, Nifle C, et al. Cerebellar infarction after sclerotherapy for leg varicosities, *Presse Med.* 2000. *29*(35): 1935.

18. Forlee MV, Grouden M, Moore DJ, Shanik G. Stroke after varicose vein foam injection sclerotherapy, *J Vasc Surg.* 2006. *43*(1): 162–164.

19. Bush, RG, Derrick M, Manjoney D. Major neurological events following foam sclerotherapy, *Phlebology.* 2008. *23*: 189–192.

20. Kritzinger P. Complications of foam sclerotherapy: Three case presentations, *Canad Soc Phlebology Annual Meeting.* Montreal, 2004.

21. Breu FX, Guggenbichler S. European consensus meeting on foam sclerotherapy, April, 4–6, 2003, Tegernsee, Germany, *Dermatol Surg.* 2004. *30*: 709–717.

22. García Mingo J. Foam medical system, a new technique to treat Varicose veins with foam. In: *Foam sclerotherapy state of the art.* Paris: Editions Phlebologiques Francaises. 2002. 45–50.

23. Cabrera J Jr, Garcia-Olmedo MA, Dominguez JM, Mirasol JA. Microfoam a novel pharmaceutical dosage form for sclerosants. In: *Foam sclerotherapy state of the art.* Paris: Editions Phlebologiques Francaises. 2002. 17–20.

24. Eckmann DM, Kobayashi S, Li M. Microvascular embolization following polidocanol microfoam sclerosant administration, *Dermatol Surg.* 2005. *31*(6): 636–643.

25. Regan JD, Gibson KD, Ferris B, et al. Safety of proprietary sclerosant microfoam for saphenous incompetence in patients with R-to-L shunt: Interim report, *J Vasc Interv Radiol.* 2008. *19*(Suppl): S35–S35.

26. Fischer R, Linde N, Duff C, Jeanneret C, Chandler JG, Seeber P. Late recurrent sapheno-femoral junction reflux after ligation and stripping of the greater saphenous vein, *J Vasc Surg.* 2001. *34*: 236–240.

27. Stonebridge PA, Chalmers N, Beggs I. Recurrent varicose veins: A varicographic analysis leading to a new practical classification, *Br J Surg.* 1995. *82*: 60.

21.

ULTRASOUND-GUIDED CATHETER AND FOAM THERAPY FOR VENOUS INSUFFICIENCY

Nisha Bunke-Paquette, Nicole Loerzel, and John J. Bergan

INTRODUCTION

Duplex ultrasonography is a critical tool for the phlebologist in the evaluation and treatment of venous disorders. In the initial investigation of primary and recurrent varicose veins, duplex scanning provides direct imaging, localization, and extent of venous reflux with a high sensitivity (95%) and specificity (100%).[1] Precise determination of hemodynamic patterns of insufficient veins and anatomical vein mapping help guide therapeutic options.[2-5] Ultrasound guidance and monitoring is crucial to the safety and efficacy of endovenous procedures including thermal ablation, mechanochemical ablation and chemical ablation techniques. Endovenous thermal therapies for insufficient veins include radiofrequency ablation (RFA) or endovenous laser therapy (EVLT). Ultrasonography is used to gain vein access, introduction of the wire, sheath, catheter, tumescent application, and in the immediate post-treatment evaluation for efficacy and complications such as deep venous thrombosis (DVT).[6] Mechanochemical ablation involves the use of a non-thermal, catheter-based sclerosant delivery system. A Clarivein catheter (ClariVein®, Madison, CT, USA) is introduced into the targeted vein under ultrasound guidance. The catheter's rotating wire (mechanical component) produces endothelial abrasion that is coupled with simultaneous injection of a sclerosant (chemical component). Since the heating element is absent, tumescent anesthesia is not required. Endovenous chemical ablation (ECA), also known as foam sclerotherapy or ultrasound guided foam sclerotherapy (UGFS) uses a foamed sclerosant to induce endothelial damage and sclerosis. As the name suggests, UGFS requires the use of ultrasound guidance for targeted sclerofoam treatment of incompetent veins.[7] Ultrasonography is an essential component of all endovenous treatment modalities, as well as for the pre- and post-treatment evaluation. This chapter describes the role of ultrasound imaging in the endovenous ablation procedures- techniques and procedural details are discussed elsewhere in this text.

VENOUS REFLUX EXAMINATION AND VENOUS MAPPING CONSIDERATIONS

In the pre-treatment assessment of varicose veins, a detailed duplex ultrasound study of the normal and pathologic venous anatomy (reflux) is essential. A clear graphic notation (mapping) of significant vein diameters, anomalous anatomy, superficial venous aneurysms, perforating veins, presence and extent of reflux should always be recorded during the examination (see Figure 21.1).[8,9]

The ultrasound examination is conducted with the patient standing.[10] This position has been found to dilate leg veins maximally and challenges vein valves. Sensitivity and specificity in detecting reflux are increased in examinations performed with the patient standing rather than when the patient is supine.[10,11]

The veins are scanned by moving the probe vertically up and down along their course. Duplicated segments, sites of tributary confluence, and large perforating veins and their deep venous connections are identified. Their location measured in centimeters from the floor provides a therapeutic guide. Measurements from the medial malleolus are not as precise. Transverse and longitudinal scans combined with continuous scanning are performed in order to provide a clear mapping of the venous system. Patency usually is assessed by compression of the vein with the transducer.[11] Reflux is detected by flow augmentation maneuvers such as distal compression and release of the thigh and calf or the Valsalva maneuver for only the SFJ.[11] Automated rapid inflation/deflation cuffs are cumbersome but may be used for this purpose and offer the advantage of a standardized stimulus.[12-14] Reflux greater than 500 ms is considered pathologic.[10,15]

The diameter of the SFJ and femoral vein are recorded for use in judgment for radiofrequency ablation (RFA) and endovenous laser treatments (EVLT).[16-18] Important information also is offered by the diameters of the GSV at mid

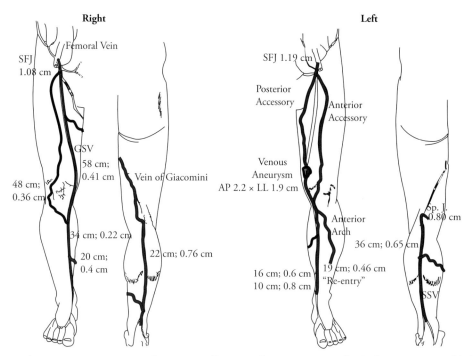

Figure 21.1   The schematic drawing represents patterns of venous insufficiency and vein mapping results. Refluxing veins are added in heavy black lines selected vein diameters should be included. Location of PVs and aneurysms can be added and distance from the floor indicated.

thigh and distal thigh. The supragenicular, infragenicular, or immediate subgenicular great saphenous vein (GSV) is often the access point for its laser or radiofrequency ablation.[18,19] Therefore the depth of the GSV, segments with tortuosity, thrombosis and anatomic variations in these regions are additional data to be recorded.

Accessory veins by definition run parallel to the GSV in the thigh (see Figure 21.1).[20] Therefore, it is imperative to map their course accurately and to note their eventual communication with GSV (see Figure 21.1). They are easily confused with the GSV, especially during continuous longitudinal scanning, when the saphenous vein appears to leave the saphenous compartment.[20] Since accessory saphenous veins can also be treated with endovenous thermal techniques, if reflux is present, their course, distance from the skin, and length of segment should be documented. The GSV is then scanned in the leg and the thigh, and tributaries to the GSV should be noted (see Figure 21.1).

The diameters of the popliteal vein and the small saphenous vein (SSV) are recorded, as well as diameters of the SSV along its course in the leg. Intersaphenous veins should also be identified, and the variability in SSV termination carefully recorded, especially if it communicates with a gastrocnemius vein. Ultrasound data regarding an incompetent SSV, such as points of termination, perforating vein connections, diameter, and proximity to nerves will help guide thereapeutic options. In transverse section, the sural nerve can be identified within the saphenous compartment. It lies in close proximity to the SSV in the distal third of the limb. Consequently, thermal ablation procedures should be used with caution on the distal leg to minimize the risk of nerve damage.[21]

The venous reflux examination also includes the mapping of exit and reentry perforating veins (PV).[22] PV reflux is detected as outward flow duration greater than 350 ms on the release phase of flow augmentation maneuver (distal compression has higher sensitivity in detecting PV reflux).[23] PVs should be accurately identified in their different locations in the leg. Their position should be measured as distance (cm) from the floor in the extended limb.[20,24]

The minimum requirements for the pre-treatment duplex ultrasound assessment are described in a Consensus Document released by the Union Internationale de Phlebologie (UIP), and are summarized in Table 21.1.[25]

ULTRASOUND MONITORING DURING EVLT AND RFA OF THE GSV AND SSV

Thermal coagulation is caused by the application of electromagnetic energy to the endothelial surface of targeted veins.[19,26,27] It has been suggested that the coagulation process in laser treatment is related to the intravascular vaporization of blood (steam) with intimal denudation and collagen fiber contraction. Vein wall thickening and rapid reorganization of the vessel to form a fibrotic cord follow.[26,27] Occlusion usually is visualized within 10 to 20 s of the laser or radiofrequency energy application.[27] These techniques have been proven to be safe and effective.[28]

Table 21.1 PREOPERATIVE DUPLEX IMAGING

1. Deep veins: assessment for patency and reflux
   - common femoral vein (CFV)
   - popliteal vein
2. Junctions: assessment for reflux (terminal valve/pre-terminal valve)
   - saphenofemoral junction (SFJ)
   - saphenopopliteal junction (SPJ)
3. Main trunks: diameter measurement and assessment of reflux (in the saphenous compartment):
   - great saphenous vein (GSV)
   - anterior accessory saphenous vein (AASV)
   - posterior accessory saphenous vein (PASV)
   - small saphenous vein (SSV)
   - thigh extension of SSV/Giacomini vein
4. Tributaries: if incompetent
5. Non-saphenous veins: if incompetent
6. Perforating veins: diameter measurement and assessment of reflux

Adapted from Reference 25.

Percutaneous introduction of the laser or radiofrequency catheter has made formerly extremely invasive therapy (SFJ ligation and GSV stripping) more acceptable to the patient in terms of posttreatment pain, number of cutaneous incisions, and postprocedural disability.[17,18]

Before the procedure, it is always recommended to rescan the patient for better identification of the venous segment to cannulate. This included imaging of the target vein for access, the saphenofemoral junction, perforators, tributaries, diameter and treatment length. In this preparatory phase some anatomic landmarks have to be clearly recognizable:

1. Femoral vein
2. SFJ
3. Saphenous compartment
4. GSV
5. Small saphenous junctional anatomy

Introduction of the introducer sheath is performed percutaneously using the Seldinger technique. The supragenicular saphenous vein is usually the access point of choice. A guidewire is readily visible on ultrasound (see Figure 21.2).[19] The intraluminal position of the sheath is ascertained by aspiration of nonpulsatile venous blood. The sheathed laser fiber or a ClosureFast catheter is advanced to a point just distal to the entrance of the epigastric vein.[19] Position of the laser fiber is confirmed by direct visualization of the red aiming beam and that of the ClosureFast catheter by ultrasound (see Figures 21.3 and 21.4).[18]

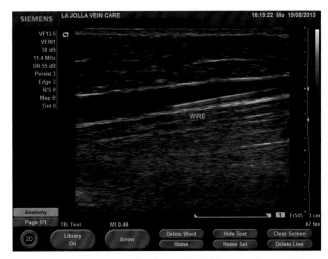

Figure 21.2 The GSV is cannulated using the Seldinger technique. This image demonstrates the introduction of a guidewire in longitudinal view, which is echogenic and can be easily visualized.

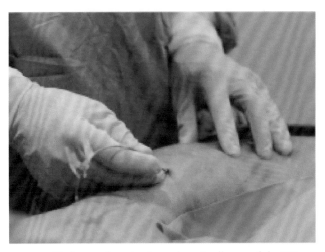

Figure 21.3 The laser catheter is advanced proximally toward the SFJ. Position of the laser fiber is confirmed by direct visualization of the red aiming beam through the skin. (Adapted from Navarro L, Min RJ, Boné C. Endovenous laser: A new minimally invasive method of treatment for varicose veins: Preliminary observations using an 810 nm diode laser, *Dermatol Surg.* 2001. *27*(2): 117).

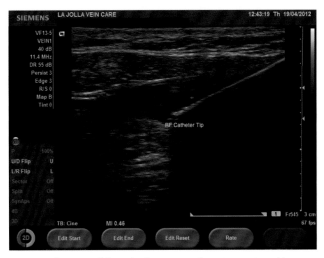

Figure 21.4 Position of the radiofrequency catheter is monitored by ultrasound visualization.

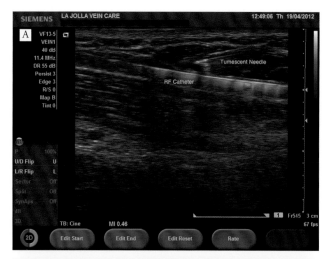

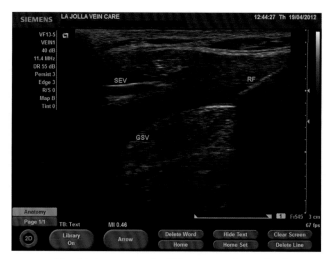

Figure 21.6 The ablation starts at the SFJ and proceeds in a distal direction. It is recommended to recheck the catheter position at the SFJ prior to the application of the energy.

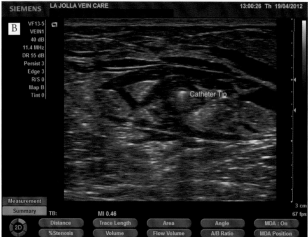

Figure 21.5 (A) Administration of the tumescent anesthesia into the saphenous compartment is monitored by ultrasound. Both the needle and catheter are visualized in longitudinal view to ensure proper placement of the solution. (B) In transverse view, tumescent infiltration within the saphenous compartment is confirmed. The administration of tumescent solution around the catheter gives an 'onion skin' appearance.

The catheter or sheath appear as a hyperechoic line in the GSV lumen.[16,17] Its placement should be 1 cm distal to the epigastric vein.[18]

Administration of the tumescent anesthesia into the saphenous compartment is monitored by ultrasound.[19] The vein is seen as "floating" in an echogenic sea of the anesthetic solution (see Figure 21.5). It is always wise to recheck the catheter position at SFJ prior to tumescent application at the tip, which may distort the image and the subsequent application of the energy (see Figure 21.6).[27] Also, forceful tumescent infiltration can advance the catheter forward.

The ablation starts at the SFJ and proceeds in a distal direction.[18] Successful obliteration is confirmed by contraction of the saphenous vein to a residual diameter of <2 mm.[18] Patency of the common femoral artery and vein are confirmed by ultrasound (see Figure 21.7). Immediately following treatment, a compressible CFV must be documented. A thrombus may be seen as a hyperechogenic core in the vessel.[16,17]

Early post treatment duplex surveillance is mandatory to evaluate for the presence or absence of DVT and efficacy of treatment. The presence of a protruding thrombus from the GSV into the CFV is termed, Post Ablation Superficial Thrombus Extension (PASTE) and can occur as a consequence of EVLT or RFA of the GSV (see Figure 21.8).[16,29] It is visualized within 3–7 days at ultrasound follow-up. Its course is typically benign.[29] Evidence of a noncompressible GSV with thickened walls and absence of flow on color ultrasound analysis are signs of successful obliteration (see Figure 21.9).[10]

MECHANOCHEMICAL ABLATION

Early results of mechanochemical ablation of the GSV and SSV are promising.[30–32] The ClariVein catheter utilizes a combination of mechanical agitation of the vessel endothelia by a rotating catheter tip and delivery of a sclerosant drug.[33] As in the thermal ablation techniques, ultrasound guidance is used for percutaneous access of a sheath, followed by a Clarivein catheter. The wire is extruded and the distal tip of the wire is positioned 2cm from the saphenofemoral junction under ultrasound guidance. Catheter wire rotation is then activated for 2-3 seconds at approximately 3500rpm. This action induces vasospasm. Since vasospasm occurs and there is no risk of thermal damage to surrounding structures, mechanochemical ablation does not require tumescent anesthesia. During rotation of the wire, a liquid sclerosant is infused simultaneously with catheter pullback. Immediately following the procedure, ultrasound is used to confirm GSV occlusion and patency of the common femoral vein using ultrasound. The same post-treatment protocol for ultrasound surveillance should be followed as for thermal endovenous procedures.

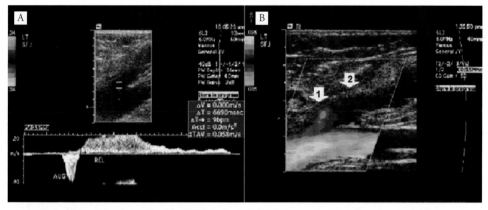

Figure 21.7   Duplex examinations (longitudinal views) of the GSV at the SFJ. (A) Pretreatment scan demonstrated an incompetent SFJ after augmentation. (B) Intraoperative color duplex interrogation showed successful occlusion of the GSV with a patent, 3-mm proximal stump (arrow 1) and absence of flow within the treated segment (arrow 2). (Adapted from Reference 16).

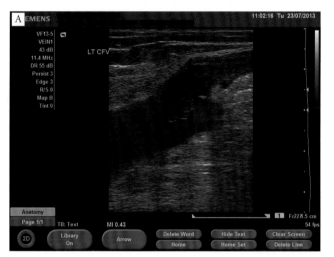
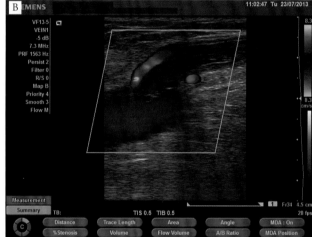

FIGURE 21.8   Early PASTE not well visualized by B-mode imaging (A) but an intraluminal filling defect is apparent (B).

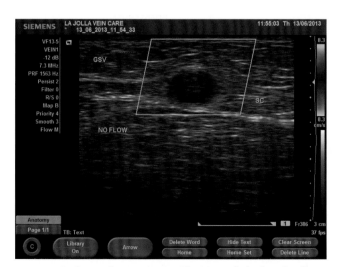

Figure 21.9   Evidence of a noncompressible GSV with thickened walls and absence of flow on color ultrasound analysis are signs of successful obliteration. SC: Saphenous compartment.

ULTRASOUND MONITORING DURING SCLEROFOAM ABLATION OF VARICOSE VEINS

Advent of foam sclerotherapy has added a new tool for the treatment of CVI. Sclerosant agents provoke endothelial damage by several mechanisms.[34] They change either the surface tension of the plasma membrane (detergents) or the intravascular pH and osmolarity. The final result is a chemical fibrosis of the treated vessel.[34]

Sclerosing foams are mixtures of gas with a liquid solution with surfactant properties. In 1993, Cabrera proposed the use of sclerosing foam, made of sodium tetradecyl sulfate or polidocanol in the treatment of varicose veins.[35] One of the intrinsic limits of liquid sclerosants in the treatment of varicose veins is dilution by the bloodstream with reduction of their efficacy.[36] Also, they are rapidly cleared by the moving bloodstream. Sclerosing foams do not mix with blood and instead remain in the vessel, continuing to strip the endothelium.[36] This persistence of the agent in the vessel causes an increased contact time with the intimal surface. Foam preparation is remarkably simple.[36] The Tessari three-way stopcock method is the most commonly used.[36,37]

As in electromagnetic ablation, the treatment starts with clear ultrasound mapping. Varicose veins can be accessed by the placement of 25-gauge butterfly needle, or the GSV or the SSV can be directly cannulated with an angiocath, an echogenic Cook needle, or a 25-gauge butterfly.[36,38,39]

Most descriptions of the technique explain direct ultrasound-guided access to the saphenous vein.[36,40] In contrast, we achieve a satisfactory and rapid obliteration of the GSV and SSV by cannulating a peripheral varicosity.[39,41] Although the saphenous vein cannot be cannulated with a catheter by way of a varicosity because of its angle of connection, there is no such obstacle to the flow of foam.

Foam functions as an efficient ultrasound contrast medium because of its air content. Its injection can be easily monitored. Its ultrasound appearance is that of a solid hyperechogenic core with an acoustic shadow projected in the tissue below (see Figure 21.10A).

Foam is introduced into a varix or the saphenous vein with the patient supine. The leg should be elevated to a 45 degree angle to exsanguinate the vein, decrease the diameter of the vein, which also reduces the amount of sclerosant needed (see Figure 21.10B).[41] Vasoconstriction and vasospasm can be induced by intermittent compression of the vein by the ultrasound transducer and by elevating the limb. Foam will be seen by ultrasound to flow distally in the elevated limb. It flows selectively through incompetent valves and is effectively blocked by competent valves. These maneuvers have the effect of prolonging the action of the foamed sclerosant on the intima, improving the efficacy of the entire treatment.

Ultrasound monitoring during foam sclerotherapy treatment increases safety as it guides treatment of targeted veins, monitors deep system involvement and helps to determine the appropriate volume of sclerofoam to be injected.[7] Ultrasound monitoring of sclerofoam can reduce the risk of reaching the deep system from the SFJ, SPJ or via perforating veins. Foam is followed as it is guided to targeted vessels while the femoral, popliteal, and deep veins of the leg are scanned throughout the entire procedure. Travel via perforating veins should be avoided. Foam particles are washed out of deep veins such as the gastrocnemius or tibial veins by flexion-extension maneuvers of the foot. Quick movements of dorsiflexion of the foot completely clear the deep veins. Despite much worry about the problem, major thrombotic events in the femoral and popliteal veins rarely have been described with use of sclerofoam. In a study of over 1,200 sclerotherapy sessions, over half of which involved foam, only a single femoral vein thrombus was encountered.[42]

Other large studies have confirmed the safety and efficacy of foam sclerotherapy.[43] Thromboses of the gastrocnemius, tibial, and peroneal veins have been reported

only occasionally.[39,44] Intra-arterial injections are uncommon because of monitoring the foam treatment of severe CVI.[39,44] Ultrasound scanning has confirmed the presence of a tangled network of varicose veins of small caliber, reticular varices, and incompetent perforating veins under lipodermatosclerotic plaques and under venous ulcers (see Figure 21.11).[39] Ultrasound monitoring is used to confirm the fact that these vessels are filled with foam during the therapeutic maneuvers. Ultrasound guidance is also used in treatment of incompetent perforating veins by direct cannulation and controlled injection of the sclerosing foam under direct visual control.[36] More often superficial peripheral veins can be directly injected with obliteration of the inciting perforator and the network of the incompetent veins.

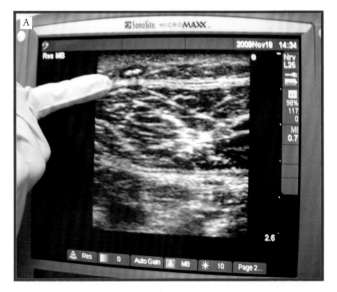

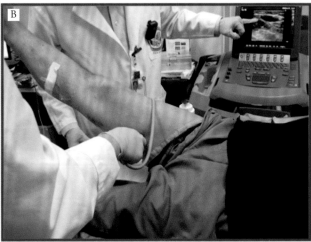

Figure 21.10   (A) Foam functions as an efficient ultrasound contrast medium because of its air content. Its injection can be easily monitored. Its ultrasound appearance is that of a solid hyperechogenic core with an acoustic shadow projected on the tissue below.

(B) Leg elevation to 45 degrees during injection of sclerofoam will help exsanguinate the vein, decrease the vein diameter which ultimately reduces the amount of sclerosant needed.

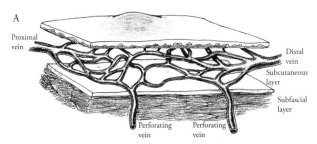

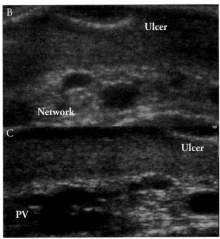

Figure 21.11   (A) There is a tangled network of varicose veins of small caliber, reticular varices, and incompetent perforating veins under lipodermatosclerotic plaques and under venous ulcers. (B) Ultrasound confirms the network of incompetent vessels beneath the wound bed. (C) Ultrasound can demonstrate the presence of IPVs relative to the wound bed. These incompetent veins are the targets for successful foam sclerotherapy.

DISCUSSION

Compression therapy and surgery have been the cornerstone of CVI treatment for years and they are still useful. New minimally invasive techniques such as radiofrequency ablation of saphenous veins, EVLT, and GSV and SSV ablation with sclerofoam of superficial varicose veins have been demonstrated to be safe, effective, and more acceptable to the patient.[18] The contribution of ultrasound in general and duplex technology in particular has given reliability to the diagnosis of CVI and has enhanced the development of these minimally invasive therapies. Intraprocedural and postprocedural duplex ultrasound monitoring offers the best control of the entire procedure with early prevention of complications (thrombosis of deep veins) and eventual minimization of failure.

CONCLUSION

Duplex ultrasound is essential in every phase of the CVI patient care. Experience, critical thinking, uniform testing, and insight in the pathology are necessary to achieve satisfactory results.

REFERENCES

1. Depalma RG, Kowallek DL, Barcia TC, Cafferata HT. Target selection for surgical intervention in severe chronic venous insufficiency: Comparison of duplex scanning and phlebography, *J Vasc Surg.* 2000. *32*(5): 913–920.
2. Labropoulos N, Touloupakis E, Giannoukas AD, Leon M, Katsamouris A, Nicolaides AN. Recurrent varicose veins: Investigation of the pattern and extent of reflux with color flow duplex scanning, *Surgery.* 1996. *119*(4):406–409.
3. Wong JK, Duncan JL, Nichols DM. Whole-leg duplex mapping for varicose veins: observations on patterns of reflux in recurrent and primary legs, with clinical correlation, *Eur J Vasc Endovasc Surg.* 2003. 25(3):267–275.
4. Coleridge-Smith P, Labropoulos N, Partsch H, Myers K, Nicolaides A, Cavezzi A. Duplex ultrasound investigation of the veins in chronic venous disease of the lower limbs—UIP consensus document. Part I. Basic principles, *Eur J Vasc Endovasc Surg.* 2006. 31(1):83–92.
5. Cavezzi A, Labropoulos N, Partsch H, Ricci S, Caggiati A, Myers K, Nicolaides A, Smith PC. Duplex ultrasound investigation of the veins in chronic venous disease of the lower limbs—UIP consensus document. Part II. Anatomy, *Eur J Vasc Endovasc Surg.* 2006. *31*(3):288–299. Epub 2005 Oct 14.
6. Labropoulos N, Abai B. Reflux testing and imaging for endovenous ablation. *Perspect Vasc Surg Endovasc Ther.* 2007. 19(1):67–70.
7. Breu FX, Guggenbichler S, Wollmann JC; Second European Consensus Meeting on Foam Sclerotherapy. Duplex ultrasound and efficacy criteria in foam sclerotherapy from the 2nd European Consensus Meeting on Foam Sclerotherapy 2006, Tegernsee, Germany, *Vasa.* 2008. *37*(1):90–95.
8. Ballard J, Bergan J, Delange M. Venous imaging for reflux using duplex ultrasonography. In: Aburahma AF, Bergan JJ (eds). *Noninvasive vascular diagnosis,* 1e. 2000. London: Springer-Verlag. Chapter 24, pp. 339–334.
9. Mekenas L, Bergan J. Venous reflux examination: Technique using miniaturized ultrasound scanning, *J Vasc Tech.* 2002. 2(26): 139–146.
10. Labropoulos N, Tiongson J, Pryor L, Tassiopoulos AK, Kang SS, Ashraf Mansour M. Definition of venous reflux in lower extremity veins, *J Vasc Surg.* 2003. 38(4): 793–798.
11. Lynch TG, Dalsing MC, Ouriel K, Ricotta JJ, Wakefield TW. Developments in diagnosis and classification of venous disorders: Noninvasive diagnosis, *Cardiovasc Surg.* 1999. *7*(2): 160–178.
12. Masuda EM, Kistner RL, Eklof B. Prospective study of duplex scanning for venous reflux: Comparison of Valsalva and pneumatic cuff techniques in the reverse Trendelenburg and standing positions, *J Vasc Surg.* 1994. *20*(5): 711–720.
13. Markel A, Meissner MH, Manzo RA, Bergelin RO, Strandness DE Jr. A comparison of the cuff deflation method with Valsalva's maneuver and limb compression in detecting venous valvular reflux, *Arch Surg.* 1994. *129*(7): 701–705.
14. Delis KT, Slimani G, Hafez HM, Nicolaides AN. Enhancing venous outflow in the lower limb with intermittent pneumatic compression: A comparative haemodynamic analysis on the effect of foot vs. calf vs. foot and calf compression, *Eur J Vasc Endovasc Surg.* 2000. *19*(3): 250–260.
15. Vasdekis SN, Clarke GH, Nicolaides AN. Quantification of venous reflux by means of duplex scanning, *J Vasc Surg.* 1989. *10*(6): 670–677.
16. Pichot O, Sessa C, Chandler JG, Nuta M, Perrin M. Role of duplex imaging in endovenous obliteration for primary venous insufficiency, *J Endovasc Ther.* 2000. *7*(6): 451–459.
17. Min RJ, Khilnani N, Zimmet SE. Endovenous laser treatment of saphenous vein reflux: Long-term results, *J Vasc Interv Radiol.* 2003. *14*(8): 991–996.
18. Sadick NS. Advances in the treatment of varicose veins: Ambulatory phlebectomy, foam sclerotherapy, endovascular laser, and radiofrequency closure, *Dermatol Clin.* 2005. 23(3): 443–455, vi.
19. Puggioni A, Kalra M, Carmo M, Mozes G, Gloviczki P. Endovenous laser therapy and radiofrequency ablation of the great saphenous

vein: Analysis of early efficacy and complications, *J Vasc Surg*. 2005. *42*(3): 488–493.

20. Caggiati A, Bergan JJ, Gloviczki P, Jantet G, Wendell-Smith CP, Partsch H. Nomenclature of the veins of the lower limbs: An international interdisciplinary consensus statement, *J Vasc Surg*. 2002. *36*(2): 416–422.

21. Ricci S, Moro L, Antonelli Incalzi R. Ultrasound imaging of the sural nerve: ultrasound anatomy and rationale for investigation. Eur *J Vasc Endovasc Surg*. 2010 May;39(5):636-41.

22. Delis KT, Husmann M, Kalodiki E, Wolfe JH, Nicolaides AN. In situ hemodynamics of perforating veins in chronic venous insufficiency, *J Vasc Surg*. 2001. *33*(4): 773–782.

23. Labropoulos N, Leon LR Jr. Duplex evaluation of venous insufficiency, *Semin Vac Surg*. 2005. *18*(1):5–9.

24. Caggiati A, Bergan JJ, Gloviczki P, Eklof B, Allegra C, Partsch H. Nomenclature of the veins of the lower limb: Extensions, refinements, and clinical application, *J Vasc Surg*. 2005. *41*(4): 719–724.

25. De Maeseneer M, Pichot O, Cavezzi A, Earnshaw J, van Rij A, Lurie F, Smith PC; Union Internationale de Phlebologie. Duplex ultrasound investigation of the veins of the lower limbs after treatment for varicose veins—UIP consensus document. *Eur J Vasc Endovasc Surg*. 2011. *42*(1):89–102.

26. Weiss RA. Comparison of endovenous radiofrequency versus 810 nm diode laser occlusion of large veins in an animal model, *Dermatol Surg*. 2002. *28*(1): 56–61.

27. Weiss RA, Weiss MA. Controlled radiofrequency endovenous occlusion using a unique radiofrequency catheter under duplex guidance to eliminate saphenous varicose vein reflux: A 2-year follow-up, *Dermatol Surg*. 2002. *28*(1): 38–42.

28. Morrison N. Saphenous ablation: What are the choices, laser or RF energy, *Semin Vasc Surg*. 2005. *18*(1): 15–18.

29. Wright D, Morrison N, Recek C, Passariello F. Post ablation superficial thrombus extension (PASTE) into the common femoral vein as a consequence of endovenous ablation of the great saphenous vein. Acta Phlebologica 2010;11:59–64.

30. Elias S, Raines JK. Mechanochemical tumescentless endovenous ablation: Final results of the initial clinical trial. Phlebology. 2012. *27*(2):67–72.

31. Boersma D, van Eekeren RR, Werson DA, van der Waal RI, Reijnen MM, de Vries JP. Mechanochemical endovenous ablation of small

32. van Eekeren RR, Boersma D, Konijn V, de Vries JP, Reijnen MM. Postoperative pain and early quality of life after radiofrequency ablation and mechanochemical endovenous ablation of incompetent great saphenous veins. *J Vasc Surg*. 2013. *57*(2):445–450.

33. Mueller RL, Raines JK. ClariVein mechanochemical ablation: background and procedural details. *Vasc Endovascular Surg*. 2013. *47*(3): 195–206.

34. Goldman M. Sclerotherapy: Treatment of varicose and telangiectatic leg veins. In: *Mechanisms of action of sclerotherapy*, 2e. 1995. St. Louis, MO: Mosby. pp. 244–279.

35. Cabrera J. Dr J. Cabrera is the creator of the patented polidocanol microfoam, *Dermatol Surg*. 2004. *30*(12 Pt 2): 1605; author reply 1606.

36. Coleridge Smith P. Saphenous ablation: Sclerosant or sclerofoam? *Semin Vasc Surg*. 2005. *18*(1): 19–24.

37. Tessari L, Cavezzi A, Frullini A. Preliminary experience with a new sclerosing foam in the treatment of varicose veins, *Dermatol Surg*. 2001. *27*(1): 58–60.

38. Cabrera J, Redondo P, Becerra A, et al. Ultrasound-guided injection of polidocanol microfoam in the management of venous leg ulcers, *Arch Dermatol*. 2004. *140*(6): 667–673.

39. Bergan JJ, Pascarella L. Severe chronic venous insufficiency: Primary treatment with sclerofoam, *Semin Vasc Surg*. 2005. *18*(1): 49–56.

40. Guex JJ. Foam sclerotherapy: An overview of use for primary venous insufficiency, *Semin Vasc Surg*. 2005. *18*(1): 25–29.

41. Bunke N, Brown K, Bergan J. Foam sclerotherapy: techniques and uses. *Perspect Vasc Surg Endovasc Ther*. 2009 *21*(2): 91–93.

42. Guex JJ, Allaert FA, Gillet JL, Chleir F. Immediate and midterm complications of sclerotherapy: Report of a prospective multicenter registry of 12,173 sclerotherapy sessions, *Dermatol Surg*. 2005. *31*(2): 123–128; discussion 128.

43. Jia X, Mowatt G, Burr JM, Cassar K, Cook J, Fraser C. Systematic review of foam sclerotherapy for varicose veins, *Br J Surg*. 2007. *94*(8):925–936.

44. Bergan JJ, Weiss RA, Goldman MP. Extensive tissue necrosis following high-concentration sclerotherapy for varicose veins, *Dermatol Surg*. 2000. *26*(6): 535–541; discussion 541–542.

22.

PRINCIPLES OF TREATMENT OF VARICOSE VEINS

Steven E. Zimmet

Treatment for venous disease has undergone rapid innovation. Despite these advances varicose vein treatment is not curative. Superficial venous insufficiency is a chronic disorder that should be viewed more as a medical than a surgical condition.[1] Nonetheless, it appears that outcomes can be optimized when certain principles of treatment are followed. This chapter discusses the development of the principles that are generally accepted today.

A history and physical and a duplex ultrasound examination are prerequisites for adequate treatment of varicose veins. Treatment of varicose veins, except when addressed by conservative or pharmacologic measures, should eliminate sources of venous hypertension. These can be gravitational, as with axial vein reflux, or hydrodynamic, due to increased compartmental pressure during muscular contraction.[2] Therefore, rational treatment depends on the delineation of sources of reflux between the deep and superficial system along with the extent of truncal and tributary incompetence. An individualized treatment plan is developed based on the findings of the evaluation and on the goals of the patient. Treatment goals may include cosmetic improvement, relief of venous-related symptoms, management of venous-related sequelae (such as edema, dermatitis, lipodermatosclerosis, ulceration, thrombophlebitis, and external bleeding), prevention of complications, and control of the disease process.

Saphenous vein reflux is the underlying primary abnormality in the majority of cases of superficial venous insufficiency. Thus, approaches to dealing with saphenofemoral junction and saphenous truncal incompetence have dominated the thinking of phlebologists. Trendelenburg described saphenofemoral junction ligation alone, without stripping of the incompetent saphenous vein, in the 1890s. The advantages of this technique over ligation and stripping are still extolled.[3] Advocates of this approach have pointed out that it preserves the saphenous trunk for possible future use as a bypass graft[4] and avoids the risk of saphenous nerve injury.[5] High ligation alone is also less invasive, quicker and simpler to perform, and associated with an easier recovery compared to vein stripping. Unfortunately, the shortcomings

of ligation alone outweigh its advantages. While it is true that such treatment routinely "spares" the saphenous trunk,[6] the use of a diseased saphenous vein as a conduit has been associated with an increased risk of graft failure.[7] Most importantly there is no longer any question that high ligation alone is coupled with persistent reflux in the saphenous trunk.[8,9] Bergan concluded in 1991 that "duplex scanning confirms the fact that high ligation alone allows persistence of distal reflux after surgical intervention."[10] It is not surprising that varicose recurrence is significantly reduced[9,11,12] and the reoperation rate is 60 to 70% less if the saphenous vein is stripped versus ligation alone.[13,14] Regarding the clinical bottom line, more patients were completely satisfied (65% versus 37%) and were recurrence-free (65% versus 17%) when the great saphenous vein (GSV) had been stripped compared with saphenofemoral ligation alone (P < 0.05 and P < 0.001 respectively).[15] The authors concluded that the addition of GSV stripping to saphenofemoral ligation and multiple avulsions results in a better overall outcome. While recurrence or residual communication with the junction in the groin was found in 80% of patients after ligation alone, 34% of limbs also had mid thigh perforator incompetence via the unstripped GSV.[16] As Neglen concluded, stripping of the GSV of the thigh is essential to minimizing recurrence due to redevelopment of incompetent communication with the saphenofemoral confluence and due to thigh perforator incompetence.[17] With the use of endovenous techniques available today, some recommend treating the entire incompetent saphenous segment rather than arbitrarily treating to the knee.[18]

At the other end of the spectrum, stripping of the entire saphenous from ankle to groin, along with stab avulsion of varices, has been practiced. This was advocated because it was assumed that reflux extended to the ankle in most patients. However, in a duplex study on over 500 legs the most common pattern was saphenous reflux from the groin to the knee (43.4%), with reflux reaching the ankle in only 1%.[19] The authors concluded that clinically diagnosed GSV reflux in the lower leg usually represented tributary varices, which joined the saphenous vein proximally. These findings, along with the high incidence of saphenous neuralgia from groin to ankle stripping, explain recommendations for "short" stripping of the GSV from groin to just below the knee. Note that such stripping would avoid the risk of saphenous nerve injury yet would disconnect mid thigh perforators, which as noted above are a common cause of recurrence when ligation alone is employed.

It is important to note that recurrence is common even after ligation and stripping of the saphenous. Inadequate surgery of the saphenofemoral junction has been claimed to be an important factor contributing to recurrence.[20] While progression of disease is another mechanism that explains some cases of recurrence, neovascularization around the junction has been established to be an important cause of recurrence after venous surgery.[12,14,21-23] Early reports suggest that endovenous ablation techniques are associated with a very low incidence of neovascularization. It may be that by avoiding groin dissection and by preserving venous drainage in normal junctional tributaries the development of neovascularization is largely avoided.[24,25]

In addition to junctional incompetence, another source of deep to superficial incompetence is via perforating veins. Ablation of the GSV doesn't address lower leg perforator incompetence directly, as most of these perforators don't drain into the GSV itself. Nonetheless, patients with superficial and perforator vein incompetence and with a normal deep venous system experienced significant improvement in air plethysmograph (APG)–measured hemodynamic parameters and clinical symptom score after superficial ablative surgery alone.[26] The authors suggested that treatment of perforator veins can be reserved for patients with persistent incompetent perforator vessels, abnormal hemodynamic parameters, or continued symptoms after superficial ablative surgery. Another study corroborated these results, but found that saphenous surgery alone failed to correct perforator reflux when there was coexistent deep venous reflux or if superficial reflux persisted postoperatively.[27]

It should be noted that a few centers advocate newer conservative surgical approaches that spare the saphenous vein. External valvuloplasty aims to restore proximal valvular competence of the GSV.[28,29] The aim of conservative hemodynamic treatment of incompetent varicose veins in ambulatory patients ("Cure Conservatrice et Hemodynamique de Insufficience Veneuse en Ambulatoire," CHIVA) is to treat varicose veins by creating a draining saphenous system by eliminating reflux points.[30] Selective ablation of the varicose veins under local anesthesia (ASVAL), based on a concept that varicose veins evolve in an ascending fashion, seeks to preserve or restore saphenous function by ablation of varices.[31] These are emerging techniques that are practiced by a few groups. Their reproducibility and long-term success remain a question.

Appropriate treatment of varicose veins begins with an accurate assessment of the underlying venous pathology and identification of sources of venous hypertension. The aims of treatment include elimination of the incompetent

connections between the deep and superficial systems as well as the obliteration of pathways of venous incompetence and incompetent varicose veins. It is clear that recurrence is reduced if the incompetent segment of the saphenous trunk is ablated. Duplex ultrasound examination reveals that the GSV is often competent and of much smaller diameter below a site of saphenous-varicose tributary connection, usually located in the thigh or proximal lower leg. Ablation of the entire GSV, from groin to ankle, is almost never required. It appears that avoiding groin dissection and preserving normal junctional drainage may prevent the development of neovascularization, an important cause of recurrence following ligation and stripping. Thus endovenous treatments, including endovenous laser, radiofrequency ablation and foam sclerotherapy, may yield the benefits of ablation of the incompetent saphenous trunk while minimizing recurrence due to neovascularization. Causes of recurrence following these endovenous treatments appear to be due primarily to failure to fully ablate incompetent saphenous veins (failure or recanalization) or due to progression of disease.

REFERENCES

1. Guex JJ, Isaacs, MN. Comparison of surgery and ultrasound guided sclerotherapy for treatment of saphenous varicose veins: Must the criteria for assessment be the same?, *Int Angiol.* 2000. *19*(4): 299–302.
2. Bergan JJ. Ambulatory surgery of varicose veins. In: Goldman MP, Bergan JJ, eds. *Ambulatory treatment of venous disease.* St. Louis, MO: Mosby. 149–154.
3. Cheatle T. The long saphenous vein: To strip or not to strip?, *Semin Vasc Surg.* 2005. *18*(1): 10–14.
4. Large J. Surgical treatment of saphenous varices, with preservation of the main great saphenous trunk, *J Vasc Surg.* 1985. *2*(6): 886–891.
5. Holme JB, Holme K, Sorensen LS. The anatomic relationship between the long saphenous vein and the saphenous nerve: Relevance for radical varicose vein surgery, *Acta Chir Scand.* 1988. *154*(11–12): 631–633.
6. Rutherford RB, Sawyer JD, Jones DN. The fate of residual saphenous vein after partial removal or ligation, *J Vasc Surg.* 1990. *12*(4): 422–426.
7. Panetta TF, Marin ML, Veith FJ, et al. Unsuspected preexisting saphenous vein disease: An unrecognized cause of vein bypass failure, *J Vasc Surg.* 1992. *15*(1): 102–110.
8. McMullin GM, Coleridge-Smith PD, Scurr JH. Objective assessment of ligation without stripping the long saphenous vein, *Br J Surg.* 1991. *78*: 1139–1142.
9. Sarin S, Scurr JH, Coleridge Smith PD. Assessment of stripping the long saphenous vein in the treatment of primary varicose veins, *Br J Surg.* 1992. *79*: 889–893.
10. Bergan JJ. Surgical procedures for varicose veins. In: Bergan JJ, Yao JST, eds. *Venous disorders.* Philadelphia: WB Saunders. 1991. 201–216.
11. Munn SR, Morton JB, Macbeth WA, McLeish AR. To strip or not to strip the long saphenous vein? A varicose vein trial, *Br J Surg.* 1981. *68*: 426–481.
12. Jones L, Braithwaite BD, Selwyn D, Cooke S, Earnshaw JJ. Neovascularisation is the principal cause of varicose vein recurrence: Results of a randomised trial of stripping the long saphenous vein, *Eur J Vasc Endovasc Surg.* 1996. *12*(4): 442–425.

13. Dwerryhouse S, Davies B, Harradine K, Earnshaw JJ. Stripping the long saphenous vein reduces the rate of reoperation for recurrent varicose veins: Five-year results of a randomized trial, *J Vasc Surg.* 1999. *29*(4): 589–592.

14. Winterborn RJ, Foy C, Earnshaw JJ. Causes of varicose vein recurrence: Late results of a randomized controlled trial of stripping the long saphenous vein, *J Vasc Surg.* 2004. *40*(4): 634–639.

15. Sarin S, Scurr JH, Coleridge Smith PD. Stripping of the long saphenous vein in the treatment of primary varicose veins, *Br J Surg.* 1994. *81*(10): 1455–1458.

16. Corbett CR, Runcie JJ, Lea TM, Jamieson CW. Reasons to strip the long saphenous vein, *Phlebologie.* 1988. *41*: 766–769.

17. Neglen P. Treatment of varicosities of saphenous origin: Comparison of ligation, selective excision, and sclerotherapy. In: Bergan JJ, Goldman MP, eds. *Varicose veins and telangiectasias: Diagnosis and treatment.* St. Louis, MO: Quality Medical. 1993. 148–165.

18. Min R, Khilnani N. Varicose veins. In: Kandarpa K, ed. *Peripheral vascular interventions.* Philadelphia: Lippincott Williams & Wilkins. 2008. 417–425.

19. Mendoza E. To the topographic anatomy of the vena saphena magna: A duplex sonographische study regarding by surgery relevant aspects, *Phlebologie.* 2001. *30*: 140–144.

20. Darke SG. Recurrent varicose veins. In: Goldman MP, Bergan JJ, eds. *Ambulatory treatment of venous disease.* St. Louis, MO: Mosby. 1996. 163–169.

21. Kostas T, Ioannou CV, Touloupakis E, et al. Recurrent varicose veins after surgery: A new appraisal of a common and complex problem in vascular surgery, *Eur J Vasc Endovasc Surg.* 2004. *27*(3): 275–282.

22. van Rij AM, Jones GT, Hill GB, Jiang P. Neovascularization and recurrent varicose veins: More histologic and ultrasound evidence, *J Vasc Surg.* 2004. *40*(2): 296–302.

23. Nyamekye I, Shephard NA, Davies B, Heather BP, Earnshaw JJ. Clinicopathological evidence that neovascularization is a cause of recurrent varicose veins, *Eur J Vasc Endovasc Surg.* 1998. *15*: 412–415.

24. Min RJ, Khilnani N, Zimmet SE. Endovenous laser treatment of saphenous vein reflux: Long-term results, *J Vasc Interv Radiol.* 2003. *14*(8): 991–996.

25. Bergan JJ, Rattner Z. Endovenous therapy: 2005, *Acta Chir Bel.* 2005. *105*(1): 12–15.

26. Mendes RR, Marston WA, Farber MA, Keagy BA. Treatment of superficial and perforator venous incompetence without deep venous insufficiency: Is routine perforator ligation necessary?, *J Vasc Surg.* 2004. *38*(5): 891–895.

27. Stuart WP, Adam DJ, Allan PL, Ruckley CV, Bradbury AW. Saphenous surgery does not correct perforator incompetence in the presence of deep venous reflux, *J Vasc Surg.* 1998. *28*(5): 834–838.

28. Lane RJ, Graiche JA, Coroneos JC, Cuzzilla ML. Long-term comparison of external valvular stenting and stripping of varicose veins, *ANZ J Surg.* 2003. *73*(8): 605–609.

29. Kim IH, Joh JH, Kim DI. Venous hemodynamic changes in the surgical treatment of primary varicose vein of the lower limbs, *Yonsei Med J.* 2004. *45*(4): 577–583.

30. Carandina S, Mari C, De Palma M, et al. Varicose vein stripping vs haemodynamic correction (Chiva): A long term randomized trial, *Eur J Vasc Endovasc Surg.* 2008. *35*: 230–237.

31. Pittaluga P, Chastane S, Rea B, Barbe R. Classification of saphenous refluxes: Implications for treatment, *Phlebology.* 2008. *23*(1): 2–9.

23.

INVERSION STRIPPING OF THE SAPHENOUS VEIN

John J. Bergan

One of the cornerstones of surgery for varicose veins is removal of the great saphenous vein (GSV) from the circulation. This can be done using minimally invasive techniques described elsewhere in this volume, but specific indications for performing saphenous surgery remain. These are largely institutional and geographic but they justify the following exposition.

Indications for intervention in primary venous insufficiency are listed in Table 23.1. Often, the appearance of telangiectatic blemishes or protuberant varicosities stimulates consultation. Ultimately, this may be the only indication for intervention.[1]

Characteristic symptoms include aching, pain, easy leg fatigue, and leg heaviness, all relieved by leg elevation,[2] and worsened on the first day of a menstrual period. Other indications for intervention for venous varicosities include superficial thrombophlebitis in varicose clusters, external bleeding from high-pressure venous blebs, or advanced changes of chronic venous insufficiency such as severe ankle hyperpigmentation, subcutaneous lipodermatosclerosis, atrophie blanche, or frank ulceration. Symptoms are frequent throughout the CEAP (clinical, etiological, anatomic, pathophysiologic) classes 1 through 6. Clinical disability scores parallel the clinical classification.[3]

Objectives of treatment should be ablation of the hydrostatic forces of axial reflux and removal of the effects of hydrodynamic forces of perforator vein reflux. The latter can be accomplished by removal of the saphenous vein in the thigh and the varicose veins without specific perforating vein interruption. In France, the two most performed procedures in the early 2000s were, respectively, high ligation + saphenous trunk stripping + tributary stab avulsion (71.9%) and high ligation + saphenous trunk stripping (17.3%). Isolated phlebectomy was done in 5.6%, high ligation + tributary stab avulsion + saphenous trunk preservation 2.8%, isolated high ligation 2.2%.[4]

Ligation of the saphenous vein at the saphenofemoral junction has been practiced widely in the belief that this would control gravitational reflux while preserving the vein for subsequent arterial bypass.[5] It is true that the saphenous vein is largely preserved after proximal ligation. Unfortunately, reflux continues and hydrodynamic forces are not controlled. Less reflux persists when the long saphenous vein has been stripped.[6] There is a better functional outcome after stripping and fewer junctional recurrences.[7] Randomized trials show efficacy of stripping compared to simple proximal ligation.[8–11]

Earlier comparisons of saphenous ligation versus stripping were flawed by today's standards. Subjective evaluation was the only means of measuring outcome for a time.[12] Duplex scanning came into use, verifying that stripping was superior to proximal ligation; this fact was supported by photoplethysmography (PPG).[13] Despite those facts, it was acknowledged that the period of disability after stripping was greater than that after simple ligation.[14] In attempts to decrease disability and improve efficacy, high tie was added to saphenous vein sclerotherapy, but foot volumetry showed that radical surgery, including stripping, produced superior results.[15]

Ultimately, attention became focused on saphenous nerve injury associated with ankle-to-groin stripping.[16,17] It was concluded that nerve injury was reduced by groin-to-ankle stripping (see Figure 23.1).[18,19] Preservation of calf veins by stripping to the knee was shown to reduce nerve injury and did not adversely affect early venous hemodynamic improvement.[20] This fact is contraintuitive, and the subject deserves further study.[21]

Table 23.1 **VARICOSE VEINS: INDICATIONS FOR INTERVENTION**

General appearance
Aching pain
Leg heaviness
Easy leg fatigue
Superficial thrombophlebitis
External bleeding
Ankle hyperpigmentation[1]
Lipodermatosclerosis
Atrophie blanche
Venous ulcer

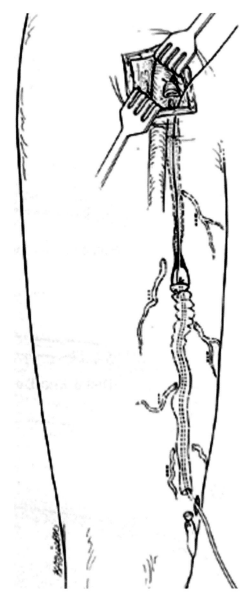

Recurrent varicose veins after surgery are acknowledged to be a major problem for patients and society.[24] Traditionally, it was thought that the most common reason for varicose recurrence was failure to perform an adequate saphenofemoral junction dissection (see Figure 23.2), or to correctly identify the saphenous vein for removal.[25] Duplex scans have clarified this situation and, instead of technical error, some investigators are convinced that new vessel growth contributes to recurrent varicose veins.[26] In particular, incomplete superficial surgery, at the saphenofemoral and saphenopopliteal junctions, is a less frequent cause of recurrent disease, and neovascular reconnection and persistent abnormal venous function are the major contributors to disease recurrence.[27]

PREOPERATIVE PREPARATION

Over the years, much space has been given to clinical examination of the patient with varicose veins. Many clinical tests have been described. Most carry the names of now-dead surgeons who were interested in venous pathophysiology. This august history notwithstanding, the Trendelenburg test, the Schwartz test, the Perthes test, and the Mahorner and

Figure 23.1   In an early attempt to improve the results of varicose vein surgery, saphenous stripping, the obturator was drawn from above downward and then retrieved through the groin incision. Postoperative appearance was improved but disability from pain, ecchymosis, and hematoma continued.

Attempts to reduce nerve injury and simultaneously clean up varicose vein surgery led to use of the hemostatic tourniquet. In a study with level 1 evidence, it was shown that use of a hemostatic cuff tourniquet during varicose vein surgery reduces perioperative blood loss, operative time, and postoperative bruising without any obvious drawbacks.[22] Villavicencio summarized this advance, saying, "This technique represents a welcome alternative to the bloody, tedious, and time-consuming traditional varicose vein surgery of the past. Complex venous surgery for extensive varicose veins of the extremities can be safely and expeditiously performed under controlled ischemia. It should be the technique of choice."[23]

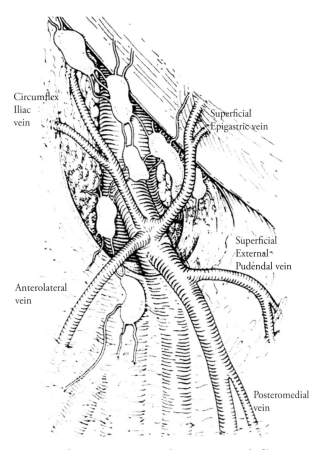

Circumflex
Iliac
vein

Superficial
Epigastric vein

Superficial
External
Pudendal vein

Anterolateral
vein

Posteromedial
vein

Figure 23.2   In the past, a proper groin dissection consisted of laying out each of the named saphenofemoral junction tributaries and dissecting them back beyond their primary tributaries. Now, this is acknowledged by most to be the strongest stimulus to neovascularization.

Ochsner modifications of the Trendelenburg test essentially are useless in preoperative evaluation of patients today.[28]

The clinical evaluation can be improved by using hand-held Doppler devices. However, preoperative evaluation is best performed by means of duplex scanning and a focused physical examination. Our protocol for duplex mapping of incompetent superficial veins has been published.[29] Although many cite cost considerations as a reason for omitting duplex evaluation, we believe that duplex scanning for venous insufficiency is in fact both simple and cost-effective. Duplex mapping defines individual patient anatomy with considerable precision and provides valuable information that supplements the physician's clinical impression.

Three principal goals must be kept in mind in planning treatment of varicose veins: (1) the varicosities must be permanently removed and the underlying cause of venous hypertension treated; (2) the repair must be done in as cosmetic a fashion as possible; (3) complications must be minimized.

Current practice of treating the source of venous hypertension, the saphenous vein alone either by endovenous laser treatment (EVLT) or VNUS technology, is inadequate. The patient's complaint, the varicose veins, must be addressed. This is as important as the physician's knowledge that the sources of venous hypertension must be addressed.

To speak of permanent removal of varicosities implies that all potential causes of recurrence have been considered and that surgery has been planned so as to address them. There are four principal causes of recurrence of varicose veins, of which three can be dealt with at the time of the primary operation.

One cause of recurrent varicosities is failure to perform the primary operation in a correct fashion. Common errors include missing a duplicated saphenous vein and mistaking an anterolateral or accessory saphenous vein for the greater saphenous vein. Such errors can be eliminated by careful and thorough groin dissection. Accordingly, failure to do a proper groin dissection has long been held to be a second principal cause of recurrent varicose veins. It is now known, however, that such dissection causes neovascularization in the groin, leading to recurrence of varicose veins.[30] A third cause of recurrent varicosities is failure to remove the GSV from the circulation. As mentioned earlier, a reason often cited for this failure is the desire to preserve the saphenous vein for subsequent use as an arterial bypass. It is clear, however, that the preserved saphenous vein continues to reflux and continues to elongate and dilate its tributaries. This produces more and larger varicosities. A fourth cause of recurrent varicosities is persistence of venous hypertension through nonsaphenous sources—chiefly, perforating veins with incompetent valves. Muscular contraction generates enormous pressures that are directed against valves in perforating veins. Venous hypertension induces a leukocyte endothelial reaction, which, in turn, incites an inflammatory response that ultimately destroys the venous valves

and weakens the venous wall.[31] The perforating veins most commonly associated with recurrent varicosities are the mid thigh perforating vein, the distal thigh perforating vein, the proximal anteromedial calf perforating vein, and the lateral thigh perforating vein, which connects the profunda femoris vein to surface varicosities.

Finally, there is a fifth cause of recurrent varicosities, which is out of control of the operating surgeon—namely, the genetic tendency to form varicosities through development of localized or generalized vein wall weakness, localized blowouts of venous walls, or stretched, elongated, and floppy venous valves.[32]

SAPHENOUS SURGERY

For varicose vein surgery to be successful, two tasks must be accomplished. The first is ablation of reflux from the deep to the superficial veins, including the saphenofemoral junction, the saphenopopliteal junction, and mid thigh varices from the Hunterian perforating vein. Accomplishment of this task is guided by the careful preoperative duplex mapping of major superficial venous reflux.

The second task is removal or destruction of all varicosities present at the time of the surgical intervention. Accomplishment of this task is guided by meticulous marking of all varicose vein clusters.

A number of options are available for surgical treatment of varicose veins. Regardless of the specific approach taken, the general technical objectives are the same: (1) ablation of the hydrostatic forces of axial saphenous vein reflux (see Figure 23.3) and (2) removal of the hydrodynamic forces of perforator vein outflow.

Ankle-to-groin stripping of the saphenous vein has been a dominant treatment of varicose veins since the early twentieth century.[33-35] One argument against routine stripping

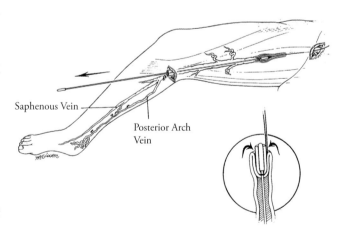

Figure 23.3   Inversion stripping of the saphenous vein was an important step forward in minimizing soft tissue trauma while accomplishing the principal objective of ablating hydrostatic venous hypertension by removing saphenous reflux. Tearing of the vein during its removal flawed its performance.

of the leg (i.e., ankle-to-knee) portion of the saphenous vein is the risk of concomitant saphenous nerve injury.[19] Another argument is that whereas the objective of saphenous vein removal is detachment of perforating veins emanating from the saphenous vein, which are seen in the thigh, the perforating veins in the leg are actually part of the posterior arch vein system rather than the saphenous vein system. This latter argument notwithstanding, preoperative ultrasonography frequently shows that the leg portion of the saphenous vein is in fact directly connected to perforating veins. Therefore, removal of the saphenous vein from ankle to knee should be a consideration in every surgical case.

OPERATIVE TECHNIQUE

The surgical approach taken must be individually tailored to each patient and each limb. Groin-to-knee stripping of the saphenous vein should be considered in every patient requiring surgical intervention.[36] In nearly all patients, this measure is supplemented by removal of the varicose vein clusters via stab avulsion or some form of sclerotherapy.

Preoperative marking, if correctly performed, will have documented the extent of varicose vein clusters and identified the clinical points where control of varices is required. Incisions can then be planned. As a rule, incisions in the groin and at the ankle should be transverse and should be placed within skin lines. In the groin, an oblique variation of the transverse incision may be appropriate. This incision should be placed high enough to permit identification of the saphenofemoral junction.

Generally, throughout the leg and the thigh, the best cosmetic results are obtained with vertical incisions. Transverse incisions are used only in the region of the knee, and oblique incisions are appropriate over the patella when the incisions are placed in skin lines.

A major cause of discomfort and occasional permanent skin pigmentation is subcutaneous extravasation of blood during and after saphenous vein stripping. Such extravasation can be minimized by applying a hemostatic tourniquet after Esmarch exsanguination of the limb. The pressure in the hemostatic tourniquet should be between 250 and 300 mm Hg, and the tourniquet should not be in place for longer than 1 hour. If a tourniquet is not used, the entire operation on one limb can be performed with the limb elevated 30 degrees so that the major varicose clusters are higher than the heart. In addition, hemostatic packing can be placed into the saphenous vein tunnel.

The practice of identifying and carefully dividing each of the tributaries to the saphenofemoral junction has been dominant since the mid-twentieth century. The rationale for this practice has been that it would be inadvisable to leave behind a network of interanastomosing inguinal tributaries. Accordingly, special efforts have been made to draw each of the saphenous tributaries into the groin incision so that

when they are placed on traction, their primary and even secondary tributaries can be controlled. The importance of these efforts has been underscored by descriptions of residual inguinal networks as an important cause of varicose vein recurrence.[37] Currently, however, this central practice of varicose vein surgery is under challenge, on the grounds that groin dissection can lead to neovascularization and hence to recurrence of varicosities (see Chapter 25).

Preoperative duplex studies have already demonstrated incompetent valves in the saphenous system, and a disposable plastic stripper can be introduced from above downward; alternatively, a metal stripper can be employed.[38] Both of these devices can be used to strip the saphenous vein from groin to knee via the inversion technique. This approach should reduce soft tissue trauma in the thigh.[39]

In the groin, the stripper is inserted proximally into the upper end of the divided internal saphenous vein and passed down the main channel through incompetent valves until it can be felt lying distally approximately 1 cm medial to the medial border of the tibia at a point approximately 4 to 6 cm distal to the level of the tibial tubercle. The saphenous vein is anatomically constant in this location, just as it is in the groin and ankle. If the saphenous vein is removed from the groin to this level, both the mid thigh perforating vein, which usually enters the saphenous vein, and the most distal incompetent perforating veins, which are in the distal third of the thigh, will be treated. A small incision is made over the palpable distal end of the stripper. The saphenous vein will subsequently be divided through this incision, and the stripper and the inverted vein will be delivered through it. In exposing the saphenous vein at knee level, the superficial fascia must be incised so as to enter the saphenous compartment. If the stripper passes unimpeded to the ankle, it can be exposed there with an exceedingly small skin incision placed in a carefully chosen skin line. Passage of the stripper from above downward to the ankle serves to confirm the absence of functioning valves, and stripping of the vein from above downward is unlikely to cause nerve damage. At the ankle, the vein should be carefully and cleanly dissected to free it from surrounding nerve fibers. If this is not done, saphenous nerve injury will result, and the patient will experience numbness of the foot below the ankle.

Stripping of the saphenous vein has been shown to produce profound distal venous hypertension. This occurs in virtually every operation, even when the limb is elevated. Therefore, after the stripper is placed, one should consider performing the stab avulsion portion of the procedure before the actual stripping maneuver.

Incisions to remove varicose clusters vary according to the size of the vein, the thickness of the vein wall, and the degree to which the vein is adhering to the perivenous tissues. In general, vertical incisions 1 to 3 mm in length are appropriate, except in areas where skin lines are obviously horizontal. Successive incisions are spaced as widely as possible. Varicosities are exteriorized by means of hooks or forceps. Particularly useful for this purpose are the specially designed vein hooks known by the names Varady dissector, Mueller hook, and Oesch hook.[40] These devices efficiently detach perforating veins from their tributary varicose clusters. Dissection of each perforating vein at the fascial level is not required, and in fact may be cosmetically undesirable. There is no need to ligate or clip the ends of each vein: the combination of leg elevation, trauma-induced venospasm, and direct pressure typically ensures adequate hemostasis. Once exteriorized, the varicosity is divided and avulsed for as long a length as possible. After avulsion, skin edges are approximated with tape or with a single absorbable monofilament suture.

Phlebectomy techniques for varicose clusters have been markedly refined by experienced workers in Europe.[41]

Once the stab avulsion portion of the procedure is complete, the previously placed stripper is pulled distally to remove the saphenous vein. Although plastic disposable vein strippers and their metallic equivalents were designed to be used with various sized olives to remove the saphenous vein, in fact, a more efficient technique is simply to tie the vein to the stripper below its tip so that the vessel can then be inverted into itself and removed distally.

To decrease oozing into the tract created by stripping, a 5-cm roller gauze soaked in a 1% lidocaine-epinephrine solution is attached to the stripper by using the ligature fastening the saphenous vein to the device (see Figure 23.4). Thus, inversion stripping is accompanied by hemostatic packing. The hemostatic pack, which lies within the saphenous vein, can be pulled into the tract with minimum tissue trauma; when it is not inverted into the vein itself, it can act as an obturator to facilitate removal of the saphenous vein without tearing. As the vein is removed by inversion, the gauze is left in place for hemostasis while the remainder of the surgical procedure is being completed.

Surgical removal of the saphenous vein on an outpatient basis still requires two incisions, one in the groin and the other near the knee. Postoperative compression bandaging is standard, and most patients experience little downtime. Some, however, do experience hematomas, pain, and extensive bruising. Varicosities recur in 15 to 30% of patients treated.[42]

EPILOGUE

Study of surgical saphenous stripping has shown that when undesirable outcomes occur, they become evident quite early. As noted earlier, it has long been accepted practice to dissect tributary vessels at the saphenofemoral junction very carefully, taking each of the vessels back beyond the primary and even the secondary tributaries if possible. In practice, however, such dissection appears to cause neovascularization in the groin. Duplex ultrasound surveillance supports this finding. It has now been amply confirmed that neovascularization causes recurrent varicose veins (see Chapter 25). Clearly, this is a significant disadvantage of standard surgical treatment of varicosities and the alternative techniques of EVLT and RFA should be considered in every case.

REFERENCES

1. Bergan JJ. Surgical management of primary and recurrent varicose veins. In: Gloviczki P, Yao JST, eds. *Handbook of venous disorders.* London: Chapman & Hall. 1996. 394–415.
2. Weiss RA, Feied CF, Weiss MA, eds. *Vein diagnosis and treatment: A comprehensive approach.* New York: McGraw-Hill. 2001.
3. Saarinen J, Heikkinen M, Suominen V, et al. Clinical disability scores and reflux in complicated and uncomplicated primary varicose veins. *Phlebology.* 2003. *18*: 73–77.
4. Perrin M, Guidicelli H, Rastel D. Surgical techniques used for the treatment of varicose veins: Survey of practice in France, *J Mal Vasc.* 2003. *28*: 277–286.
5. McMullin GM, Coleridge Smith PD, Scurr JH. Objective assessment of high ligation without stripping the long saphenous vein, *Br J Surg.* 1991. *78*: 1139–1142.
6. Butler CM, Scurr JH, Coleridge Smith PD. Prospective randomized trial comparing conventional (Babcock) stripping with inverting stripping of the long saphenous vein, *Phlebology.* 2002. *17*: 59–63.
7. Sarin S, Scurr JH, Coleridge Smith PD. Assessment of stripping the long saphenous vein in the treatment of primary varicose veins, *Br J Surg.* 1992. *79*: 889–893.
8. Dwerryhouse S, Davies B, Harradine K, Earnshaw JJ. Stripping the long saphenous vein reduces the rate of reoperation for recurrent varicose veins: Five-year results of a randomized trial, *J Vasc Surg.* 1999. *29*: 589–592.
9. Jones L, Braithwaite BD, Selwyn D, Cooke S, Earnshaw JJ. Neovascularisation is the principal cause of varicose vein recurrence: Results of a randomised trial of stripping the long saphenous vein, *Eur J Vasc Endovasc Surg.* 1996. *12*: 442–445.
10. Winterborn RJ, Foy C, Earnshaw JJ. Causes of varicose vein recurrence: Late results of a randomized controlled trial of stripping the long saphenous vein, *J Vasc Surg.* 2004. *40*: 634–639.
11. Woodyer AB, Reddy PJ, Dormandy JA. Should we strip the long saphenous vein? *Phlebology.* 1986. *1*: 221–224.
12. Rutgers PH, Kitslaar PJ. Randomized trial of stripping versus high ligation combined with sclerotherapy in the treatment of the incompetent greater saphenous vein, *Am J Surg.* 1994. *168*(4): 311–315.

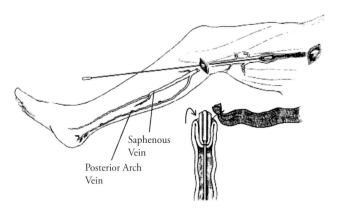

Figure 23.4   Adding a hemostatic pack to inversion stripping corrected the principal flaw in inversion stripping, the tearing of the saphenous vein. The pack acted as an obturator, which ensured total vein removal. In most instances, the pack entered the vein as it was being removed, thus minimizing the soft tissue trauma.

Saphenous Vein

Posterior Arch Vein

13. Sarin S, Scurr JH, Coleridge Smith PD. Stripping of the long saphenous vein in the treatment of primary varicose veins, *Br J Surg*. 1994. *81*: 1455–1458.

14. Jakobsen BH. The value of different forms of treatment for varicose veins, *Br J Surg*. 1979. *66*: 182–184.

15. Neglen P, Einarsson E, Eklof B. The functional long-term value of different types of treatment for saphenous vein incompetence, *J Cardiovasc Surg*. 1993. *34*: 295–301.

16. Munn SR, Morton JB, MacBeth WAAG, McLeish AR. To strip or not to strip the long saphenous vein? A varicose veins trial, *Br J Surg*. 1981. *68*: 426–428.

17. Negus D. Should incompetent saphenous veins be stripped right down to the ankle?, *Phlebologie*. 1987. *40*: 753–757.

18. Holme JB, Skajaa K, Holme K. Incidence of lesions of the saphenous nerve after partial or complete stripping of the long saphenous vein, *Acta Chir Scand*. 1990. *156*: 145–148.

19. Wellwood JM, Cox SJ, Martin A, Cockett FB, Browse NL. Sensory changes following stripping of the long saphenous vein, *J Cardiovasc Surg*. 1975. *16*: 123–124.

20. Miyazaki K, Nishibe T, Kudo F, et al. Hemodynamic changes in stripping operation or saphenofemoral ligation of the greater saphenous vein for primary varicose veins, *Ann Vasc Surg*. 2004. *18*(4): 465–469.

21. Sam RC, Silverman SH, Bradbury AW. Nerve injuries and varicose vein surgery, *Eur J Vasc Endovasc Surg*. 2004. *27*: 113–120. Review.

22. Sykes TC, Brookes P, Hickey NC. A prospective randomised trial of tourniquet in varicose vein surgery, *Ann R Coll Surg Engl*. 2000. *82*(4): 280–282.

23. Villavicencio JL, Gillespie DL, Kreishman P. Controlled ischemia for complex venous surgery: The technique of choice, *J Vasc Surg*. 2002. *36*: 881–888. *J Vasc Surg*. 2001. *34*(5): 947–951.

24. Stucker M, Netz K, Breuckmann F, Altmeyer P, Mumme A. Histomorphologic classification of recurrent saphenofemoral reflux, *J Vasc Surg*. 2004. *39*: 816–821; Discussion 822.

25. Greaney MG, Makin GS. Operation for recurrent saphenofemoral incompetence using a medial approach to the saphenofemoral junction, *Br J Surg*. 1985. *72*: 910–911.

26 Glass GM. Neovascularization in recurrence of the varicose great saphenous vein following transection, *Phlebology*. 1987. *2*: 81–91.

27. van Rij AM, Jiang P, Solomon C, Christie RA, Hill GB. Recurrence after varicose vein surgery: A prospective long-term clinical study with duplex ultrasound scanning and air plethysmography, *Eur J Vasc Endovasc Surg*. 1998. *15*: 412–415.

28. Ballard JL, Bergan JJ, DeLange M. Venous imaging for reflux using duplex ultrasonography. In: AbuRahma AF, Bergan JJ, eds. *Noninvasive vascular diagnosis*. London: SpringerVerlag. 2000. 329.

29. Mekenas LV, Bergan JD. Venous reflux examination: Technique using miniaturized ultrasound scanning, *J Vasc Technol*. 2002. *26*: 139.

30. Fischer R, Linde N, Duff C, et al. Late recurrent saphenofemoral junction reflux after ligation and stripping of the greater saphenous vein, *J Vasc Surg*. 2001. *34*: 236.

31. Ono T, Bergan JJ, Schmid-Schönbein GW, et al. Monocyte infiltration into venous valves, *J Vasc Surg*. 1998. *27*: 158.

32. Thulesius O, Ugaily-Thulesius L, Gjores JE, et al. The varicose saphenous vein, functional and ultrastructural studies, with special reference to smooth muscle, *Phlebology*. 3: 89.

33. Mayo CH. Treatment of varicose veins, *Surg Gynecol Obstet*. 1906. 2: 385.

34. Babcock WW. A new operation for extirpation of varicose veins, *NY Med J*. 1907. *86*: 1553.

35. Keller WL. A new method for extirpating the internal saphenous and similar veins in varicose conditions: A preliminary report, *NY Med J*. 1905. *82*: 385.

36. Goren G, Yellin AE. Primary varicose veins: Topographic and hemodynamic correlations, *J Cardiovasc Surg*. 1990. *31*: 672.

37. Stonebridge PA, Chalmers N, Beggs I, et al. Recurrent varicose veins: A varicographic analysis leading to a new practical classification, *Br J Surg*. 1995. *82*: 60.

38. Goren G, Yellin AE. Invaginated axial saphenectomy by a semirigid stripper: Perforate-invaginate stripping, *J Vasc Surg*. 1994. *20*: 970.

39. Bergan JJ. Saphenous vein stripping by inversion: Current technique, *Surg Rounds*. 2000. 118.

40. Bergan JJ. Varicose veins: Hooks, clamps, and suction: Application of new techniques to enhance varicose vein surgery, *Semin Vasc Surg*. 2002. *15*: 21.

41. Ricci S, Georgiev M, Goldman MP. *Ambulatory phlebectomy: A practical guide for treating varicose veins*, 2e. St Louis, MO: Mosby. 2005.

42. Darke SG. The morphology of recurrent varicose veins, *Eur J Vasc Surg*. 1992. *6*: 512.

24.

NEOVASCULARIZATION

AN ADVERSE RESPONSE TO PROPER GROIN DISSECTION

Marianne De Maeseneer

At the beginning of the twenty-first century surgical treatment of varicose veins continues to be marred by the development of recurrent varicosities. This has always been a very disappointing phenomenon for patients and surgeons alike. Most commonly recurrent reflux develops in the area of the saphenofemoral junction (SFJ), connecting with recurrent varicose veins from the thigh downward to the entire leg (Figure 24.1).[1] Even in clinical centers with a special focus on minimizing recurrence surgeons do not seem to be able to avoid such disfiguring and often disabling recurrent varicose veins.

Some causes of recurrence are obvious: insufficient understanding of venous anatomy and hemodynamics, inadequate preoperative assessment, and incorrect or insufficient surgery. However recurrence at the SFJ cannot always be explained by technical inadequacy of the original surgical intervention. Its development has also been attributed to *neovascularization* in the granulation tissue around the ligated stump.[2] Neovascularization is defined as new blood vessel formation (=angiogenesis) occurring in abnormal tissue or in an abnormal position. In some instances the growth of new blood vessels from the surrounding tissue may be induced by diffusible chemical factors (angiogenic factors). In the particular context of varicose recurrence after great saphenous vein (GSV) surgery, the term "neovascularization" describes a phenomenon of formation of new venous channels between the saphenous stump on the common femoral vein (CFV) and the residual GSV or its tributaries (Figure 24.2). Neovascularization is a distinctly uncommon finding when the true SFJ has not been divided. However, when the SFJ has been ligated properly, it is actually a marker of an anatomically correct operation, as well as the best explanation for SFJ reconnections after such an operation.

Many surgeons only start to recognize the phenomenon after having to treat patients with recurrent varicose veins some years after a previous varicose vein operation "correctly" performed by themselves. The observations with duplex ultrasound scanning at the level of the SFJ then frequently show neovascularization. Despite the fact that this frustrating phenomenon is frequently encountered, its nature and pathophysiology (hence its prevention) is poorly understood and is the subject of ongoing research.

I. A HISTORICAL PERSPECTIVE

Surgical ligation of the GSV above or below the knee has been practiced for many centuries, starting with Paulus of Aegina in AD 660. However it was not until the nineteenth century that the effect of ligation on the vein itself and on the venous hemodynamic situation became better understood.

In 1861 Langenbeck[3] described in detail what exactly happened with a vein after surgical ligation. He noticed that a vein had a very important regeneration capacity and that a new vein channel could be formed after ligation or extirpation of a piece of vein:

In one case of very large varix of the great saphena in a young man I had extirpated the enlarged vein in the length of three inches and ligated the upper and lower ends. One year later I found, in the region of the scar tissue of the extirpation, a new vein channel of the thickness of the quill of a crow's feather, which again joined the both ends of the fully functioning saphena.

Looking at his detailed description now, one and a half century later, this could be considered as the first real description of formation of new veins after ligation (which could possibly lead to recurrence of varicose veins later on).

Throughout the nineteenth century, surgical treatment of varicosity of the GSV was limited to simple ligation and transection at a site in the thigh where there were relatively few tributaries. Therefore it was obvious that, if recurrence occurred, the cause was situated at the site of ligation in the thigh. In the beginning of the twentieth century Homans[4]

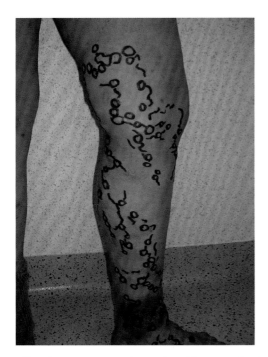

Figure 24.1   Prominent recurrent varicose veins with venous ulcer in a 32-year-old man who underwent comprehensive SFJ ligation and stripping of the GSV above the knee 8 years earlier.

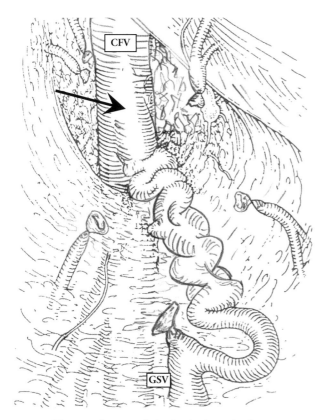

Figure 24.2   Diagram of neovascularization in the groin after correct previous ligation of the great saphenous vein (GSV) and all tributaries at the SFJ, without stripping the GSV. A new vein (arrow) is bulging at the anteromedial side of the CFV and continues downward as a very tortuous vein, connecting again with the retained GSV trunk. If the above-knee GSV has been stripped, it may connect with any other superficial vein.

introduced SFJ ligation in the groin. He advocated ligation of all tributaries to the terminal portion of the saphenous vein to prevent restoration of venous continuity through a collateral network in the groin. From that time, the theory of recurrence through preexisting collateral veins gained ascendancy over the earlier theory of recurrence through growth of new vessels. Inadequate operation by the previous surgeon was then claimed to be the main cause of recurrence. Only a minority believed that recurrence could also occur after accurately performed SFJ ligation through formation of new vessels. In explaining the genesis of this phenomenon, Sheppard[5] hypothesized that, "under the influence of the high femoral pressure, the capillaries and venules in the granulation tissue [of the newly forming scar] developed into dilated tortuous channels."

During the period 1950–1980 Glass[6,7] led surgeons to focus again on recurrence of varicose veins after surgery through "regrowth of veins." He published his clinical and experimental work concerning this problem, in 1987 mentioning the term "neovascularization" for the first time.[6] He also reported on the gross anatomy and histology at the level of the SFJ during reexploration of the groin.[7] In the majority of limbs a newly formed vessel or complex of vessels was found in connection with the former saphenous stump proximally and with varicose veins on the thigh distally. Macroscopic examination revealed several lumens in an irregular mass of vein tissue and cords or bands traversing the lumen, which suggested that the vessels were newly formed and not preexisting. Large lymph nodes were often in close proximity to them. The histology confirmed the macroscopic findings: an irregular vessel wall with a varying thickness at different points of the circumference, often with several lumens. Also typical was the presence of many small vessels close to the newly formed vessel and in neighboring lymph nodes. These studies suggested that neovascularization had played an important role in recurrent saphenofemoral incompetence after a correctly performed SFJ ligation.

II. NEOVASCULARIZATION: TODAY'S EVIDENCE

A. SONOGRAPHIC EVIDENCE

Duplex scanning can provide the necessary anatomical and functional information about the nature of recurrence and has become the investigation of choice in patients with recurrent varicose veins. Jones et al.[8] found that neovascularization at the SFJ was the commonest cause of recurrence in 113 legs 2 years after stripping of the GSV. Typical serpentine tributaries arising from the ligated SFJ were detected in 52% of limbs. Another duplex-based prospective study revealed some degree of neovascularization in 14% of 177 limbs already at one year after flush SFJ or saphenopopliteal junction (SPJ) ligation.[9] The clinical

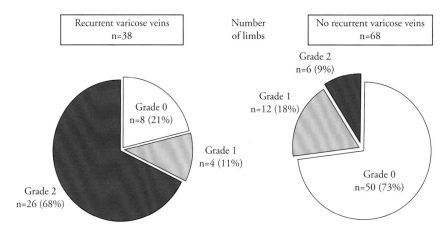

Figure 24.3   Proportional incidence of different degrees of neovascularization according to duplex ultrasound scanning of the groin at long-term follow-up in limbs with and without recurrent varicose veins. Grade 0: no neovascularization; Grade 1: tiny new vein < 4 mm; Grade 2: tortuous new connecting vein with a diameter ≥ 4 mm and with pathological reflux.

relevance of finding neovascularization on postoperative duplex ultrasound was examined in a long-term follow-up study at the same institution almost 5 years (56 months) after the varicose vein operations.[10] In 68% of limbs with clinically obvious recurrent varicose veins, neovascularization (with new veins greater than 4 mm in diameter, pathological reflux, and connected to recurrent varicose veins) was present at the site of the saphenous ligation on duplex examination, whereas in limbs without recurrent varicose veins this degree of neovascularization was only seen in 9% of cases (Figure 24.3).

B. HISTOPATHOLOGICAL EVIDENCE

Nyamekye et al.[11] provided further evidence that neovascularization was one of the causes of recurrence. Histological examination of the venous tissue blocks, excised during groin reexplorations, showed neovascularization in twenty-seven of twenty-eight blocks, characterized by vein tortuosity, small size, and mural asymmetry (Figure 24.4),

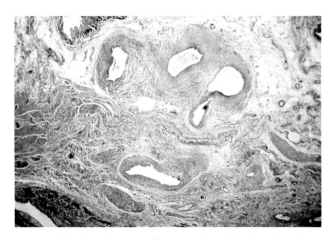

Figure 24.4   Histological section of an excised tissue block in the groin showing tortuous newly formed veins within the scar tissue (Masson's trichrome stain, original magnification 40×).

as well as lack of intramural nerves on immunohistologically S100-stained sections. The authors drew the attention to the fact that a negative demonstration of a focal structure, such as a mural nerve seen on S100-stained sections, is never entirely convincing and that a more useful tool for the diagnosis of neovascularization was not yet available. In spite of this warning, the findings of his study were cited in many instances as the final histological description of neovascularization.

The causality of recurrence was further investigated by van Rij et al.[12] by correlating findings from duplex ultrasound scans before reoperation with histological findings in specimens taken from the groin at operation and resin casts made from some of the excised tissue blocks (Figure 24.5). Neovascular channels of variable size, number, and tortuosity accounted for the ultrasound appearances in the vast majority of examined specimens. These new vessels connected to the CFV at the site of the previous SFJ. At histological examination such neovascular channels were lined by a simple squamous endothelium overlying a medial layer consisting of two to five layers of vascular smooth muscle. They lacked elastic fibers and had no distinct intimal medial boundary and no distinct adventitia. In both studies[11,12] the definition of neovascular vessels was mainly based on negative criteria: no intramural nerves, no three-layered wall structure, and lack of lumen regularity. Stücker et al.[13] added a positive criterion that scar tissue must always surround a newly formed vein (Figure 24.4).

III. RESEARCH ON THE PATHOPHYSIOLOGY OF SAPHENOFEMORAL RECURRENCE AND THE ROLE OF NEOVASCULARIZATION

The ultimate answer to the question: "is neovascularization at the ligated SFJ really important?" still has to be given. As animals do not suffer from varicose veins an animal

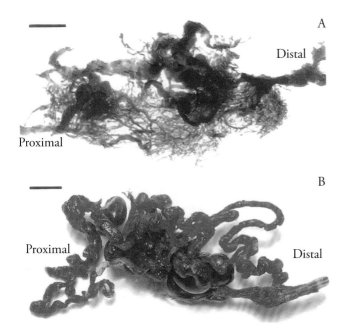

Figure 24.5   Vascular casts of recurrent refluxing SFJ specimens, showing the connecting network of vessels. In both specimens there are abundant tortuous vessels. Casts injected from the SFJ show resin present in the connecting network of vessels. Notice the variation in size of the abundant tortuous vessels in both specimens. (A) Though several channels are larger, there are more than 100 channels running in a similar proximal distal direction. (B) Three large-diameter channels dominate the cast; however, there are also small channels present in continuity. Note the injecting cannula (distal). Scale bars: A, 5 mm; B, 10 mm.

Reprinted from AM van Rij, GT Jones, GB Hill, P Jiang. Neovascularization and recurrent varicose veins: More histologic and ultrasound evidence. *J Vasc Surg* 2004. 40: 296–302, with permission from The Society for Vascular Surgery.

experiment is hardly possible to prove the existence of neovascularization. Therefore it can only be proved in an indirect way. Observations made in patients prospectively studied after varicose vein operations with duplex scan are very useful. Moreover in patients operated on because of recurrent varicose veins preoperative duplex findings can be compared with visual inspection at the previous ligation site during reexploration and histological examination of the excised tissue blocks from the scar tissue in the groin. Although findings from such studies may be suggestive for neovascularization, none of them is conclusive. This means that further observational studies will not definitely answer this question.

More fundamental research should focus on the potential pathophysiological mechanisms that could explain how new veins can develop after correct SFJ ligation: angiogenic stimulation in the free endothelium of the ligated stump,[14] transnodal lymphovenous connection,[15] dilation of small adventitial vessels in the vasa vasorum of the femoral vein, or disturbed venous drainage of the ligated tributaries of the SFJ. All of these occur on a background of the normal wound-healing process, in which angiogenesis is an important component, potentially giving rise to a more generalized, field-related neovascularization in the groin.

A. ANGIOGENIC STIMULATION IN THE FREE ENDOTHELIUM OF THE SAPHENOUS STUMP

After surgical ligation and transection of the GSV, angiogenic stimulation in the free endothelium of the ligated stump has been claimed to be one of the most important triggers for the onset of the neovascularization process. Such stump-related neovascularization might originate from hypoxia-induced activation of endothelial cells distal to the stump ligature, which could be mediated by growth factors.[14] Another cause of stump-related neovascularization could be inflammation related to ligature, particularly those of absorbable material, or to the results of dissection in the immediate area.

B. TRANSNODAL LYMPHOVENOUS CONNECTION

Lemasle et al.[15] have focused on the important role of the lymph nodes in the neighborhood of the ligated saphenous stump. Their hypothesis is that neovascularization is essentially the development of preexisting venous vessels in the inguinal lymph nodes. This physiological venous network is normally thin and competent. Due to the action of angiogenic factors it could become larger and incompetent. This could correspond with the tiny refluxing veins passing through the surrounding lymph nodes, often seen at postoperative duplex examination of the groin. In exceptional cases such lymph node vein networks can also be seen without any previous operation. Further study of the lymph nodes by means of high-definition ultrasound before and after surgery at the SFJ may help to clarify the role of lymph nodes and lymphovenous connections. In previous studies histological examination mainly focused on excised tissue blocks from the scar tissue in the groin at reoperation.[7,11–13] To improve our understanding of the histological alterations in recurrent varicosis, it might be interesting to investigate primary and recurrent varicose veins, normal vessels of the saphenofemoral area, lymph nodes, and lymph vessels of this area and compare these findings with those at other localizations.

C. DILATION OF SMALL ADVENTITIAL VESSELS IN THE VASA VASORUM

Theoretically, dilation of small adventitial vessels in the vasa vasorum of the femoral vein could be responsible for new connections between the deep and superficial venous system. It is known that the very tiny veins of the vein wall are draining their blood directly into the lumen of the vein. Venous endoscopy of the femoral vein, done to assess valve function, has occasionally shown extremely small medial or lateral orifices near the entrance of the GSV. These have been thought to be the openings of tiny tributaries that are too small to show on phlebography or duplex sonography. The observers, for this reason, cannot be certain that these are not just vasa vasorum serving the vein wall and having no external connections, but they have postulated that these tiny orifices might enlarge, to become conduits of blood refluxing to the superficial veins.

D. DISTURBED VENOUS DRAINAGE OF LIGATED TRIBUTARIES

Disturbed venous drainage of the ligated tributaries of the SFJ has also been cited as a potential pathophysiological mechanism to explain recurrence in the groin. Chandler et al.[16] have suggested that neovascularization might be driven not only by angiogenic stimuli inherent to the wound-healing process but also by localized venous hypertension, or "frustrated venous drainage" secondary to ligation of tributaries. This tributary ligation might interfere with normal venous drainage of the superficial tissues of the lower abdomen and pudendum. The presence of neovascular cross-groin collaterals (small veins passing from the anterior abdominal wall, across the groin, toward the thigh) in some cases at postoperative duplex examination or reoperation could be an illustration of this hypothesis. Moreover, the idea that localized venous hypertension might be a trigger for neovascularization is supported by the findings after endovenous treatment techniques, consisting in ablation of the saphenous vein by radiofrequency or laser energy without a groin incision. These procedures were not associated with neovascularization in the groin according to duplex scan follow-up.[17] Comparable findings were reported in a retrospective study by Pittaluga et al. 2 years after limited surgery in the groin in addition to stripping of the refluxing trunks.[18] Ligation of the GSV at a distance from the SFJ, preserving the proximal (non-refluxing) tributaries of the GSV resulted in a very low rate of neovascularization (only 1.8 %), far lower than after classic SFJ ligation. Opposite to the situation of "frustrated venous drainage" following ligation of tributaries in the groin, leaving open these tributaries could reduce the stimulus to neovascularization as the normal venous drainage of the lower abdominal and pudendal tissues is preserved. Further prospective studies will be needed to elucidate this pathophysiological issue.

E. MORE TRIGGERS INVOLVED IN DEVELOPMENT OF EARLY AND LATE RECURRENCE

Probably neovascularization at the SFJ as such is not the unique cause for the development of recurrent varicose veins after SFJ ligation surgery. Something has to happen in the periphery as well, where a refluxing vein will try to make a "joint venture" with the neovascular veins at the SFJ and vice versa, by sending out some—not yet clearly understood—chemotactic signs, which will finally result in reconnection between peripheral veins and neovascular veins. Therefore recurrence can appear *early* after the operation (sometimes already within the 1st year) if residual varicose veins or a refluxing GSV or anterior accessory saphenous trunk have been left in place: reconnection between these pathologic veins and neovascular veins could be quite evident in such situation. Recurrence developing *late* (several years) after the operation is more often primarily due to progression of the varicose disease. Neovascularization at the previous SFJ site can play a secondary role in these cases. After a few years new varicose veins develop little by little and these can connect with neovascular veins in the groin, which in the long term can become larger and refluxing. This leads to the typical clinical picture of thigh or whole-leg varicose vein recurrence several years after GSV surgery (Figure 24.1).

F. CONSTITUTIONAL RISK FACTORS

In addition to all the abovementioned pathophysiological mechanisms, constitutional risk factors, which could potentially enhance the tendency to recurrence, should also be further examined. The importance of risk factors such as female gender, left-sided disease, associated deep vein incompetence, severe chronic venous disease (C4–C6 of the CEAP classification), obesity, and subsequent pregnancies after surgery, which have all been claimed to promote recurrence, should be prospectively studied.

IV. EFFORTS TO MITIGATE NEOVASCULARIZATION-RELATED RECURRENT REFLUX

A. BARRIER TECHNIQUES TO CONTAIN NEOVASCULARIZATION

Containment involves constructing an anatomical barrier or inserting a prosthetic barrier between the ligated SFJ stump and the surrounding superficial veins in the groin. Various barrier techniques have been studied in primary as well as in recurrent varicose veins, with different rates of success. In primary GSV surgery, closing the opening in the cribriform fascia suppressed postoperative neovascularization at the SFJ after 1 year.[19] In repeat surgery at the SFJ, implantation of a patch at the level of the religated saphenous stump significantly improved the clinical and duplex scan results, after a follow-up period of 5 years.[20] In a recently published well-conducted randomized controlled trial van Rij et al. demonstrated that use of a polytetrafluoroethylene (PTFE) patch is an effective mechanical suppressant of neovascularization at the SFJ and can safely be used as a strategy to improve long-term outcome of varicose vein surgery.[21]

B. AVOIDING ENDOTHELIAL EXPOSURE AT THE GSV STUMP

Isolating the stump endothelium from the wound milieu, by oversewing the "mouth" of the ligated SFJ with a running polypropylene suture, or destroying the stump endothelium with chemical or heat cauterization have been described, all without conclusive results. A more radical approach, consisting in complete resection of the GSV stump and inversion suturing of the common femoral vein venotomy, instead of flush ligation at the level of the SFJ, did not appear to decrease neovascularization and related thigh varicose vein recurrence 2 years after GSV stripping.[22]

C. ABANDONING SFJ LIGATION

Finally, what about comprehensive *SFJ ligation*, previously considered the "sacred cow"? Although we have been taught for many decades that an accurate groin dissection with detachment of all tributaries is the ideal method to prevent recurrence from the groin, in fact, the reverse could be true. It has to be acknowledged that the importance of ligating all tributaries of the GSV in the groin is assumed rather than proved. Chandler et al.[16] attempted to define the role of extended SFJ ligation in one of the first studies on endovenous radiofrequency ablation. They compared the results of endovenous ablation with or without SFJ ligation and found no difference between the treatment options. It is now widely accepted that endovenous ablation can be safely performed without SFJ ligation with good long-term results and without inducing neovascularization at the SFJ. The same seemed to be true with an alternative surgical technique consisting of more distal ligation of the GSV with preservation of the proximal tributaries at the SFJ.[18] Therefore the old axiom that SFJ ligation with ligation of all tributaries is an essential component of the treatment of GSV insufficiency should definitely be questioned.

D. ENDOVENOUS TREATMENT METHODS

As mentioned previously, endovenous treatment does not seem to be associated with neovascularization in the groin and has now become the method of choice for treatment of primary varicose veins in many centers around the world. The results of GSV radiofrequency ablation after up to 5 years are promising, and duplex ultrasound findings confirm the absence of neovascular veins in the groin.[17,23] Endovenous laser treatment is a comparable technique developed to treat saphenous vein incompetence with very satisfying long-term results.[24] Ultrasound-guided foam sclerotherapy was introduced as a third alternative treatment method. The increased efficacy of foam, in comparison with classic sclerotherapy with liquid sclerosants, enabled treatment of varicose veins with larger diameter as well as

main superficial trunks. Encouraging results have also been obtained in patients with recurrent varicose veins.

E. IMPORTANCE OF FOLLOW-UP AFTER TREATMENT

Whatever technique has been used, serial duplex examinations remain the cornerstone of follow-up.[25] Early evaluation, 1 to 2 months after the procedure, is useful for initial quality control of the intervention. Further evaluations (at 1, 3, and 5 years) may help to understand and define the process and causes of recurrence. It has been shown that color duplex scan of the SFJ 1 year after GSV surgery has a high sensitivity and specificity. It accurately predicts which patients are more likely to have a good outcome 5 years after surgery.[26]

CONCLUSION

After proper groin dissection, neovascularization is both a marker of thoroughly performed SFJ tributary ligation and a pathway for superficial to deep reconnections. It is remarkably focused on the site of the former SFJ and it appears to arise because of stimuli that are related to healing of the surgical wound as well as to the continued (or renewed) presence of diseased superficial veins. It can be suppressed by barrier techniques but not completely eliminated. In the long term, progression of the varicose disease plays a major role in recurrence, and neovascularization takes only a secondary role. When new varicose veins develop in the thigh, they may connect with neovascular veins in the groin, and reflux from the SFJ may become obvious again.

Duplex scanning has rationalized the management of lower extremity venous disease. Thorough preoperative assessment with duplex ultrasound now leads to a well-established surgical or endovenous approach, guided by the venous anatomy of each individual patient. Duplex scanning also offers a unique opportunity to compare the posttreatment events of these two approaches with early and serial posttreatment scanning.[25] In this process, the physician will have an opportunity to assess his or her own technique and to uncover variables that might be associated with relative stability or progression to clinically relevant reconnections and new varicosities. The ultimate truth will come from knowledge of cell signaling and other molecular events that would require repeated tissue sampling, timed in accord with the evolving duplex anatomy.

ACKNOWLEDGMENTS

Section I is reprinted in part from De Maeseneer MGR. The role of postoperative neovascularisation in recurrence of varicose veins: from historical background to today's evidence, *Acta Chir Belg.* 2004. *104*: 283–289, with permission from The Royal Belgian Society of Surgeons.

Section III is reprinted in part from Fischer R, Chandler JG, De Maeseneer MG, et al. The unresolved problem of recurrent saphenofemoral reflux, *J Am Coll Surg.* 2002. *195*: 80–94, with permission from The American College of Surgeons.

REFERENCES

1. Fischer R, Chandler JG, De Maeseneer MG, et al. The unresolved problem of recurrent saphenofemoral reflux, *J Am Coll Surg.* 2002. *195*: 80–94.

2. De Maeseneer MGR. The role of postoperative neovascularisation in recurrence of varicose veins: From historical background to today's evidence, *Acta Chir Bel.* 2004. *104*: 283–289.

3. von Langenbeck B. Beitrage zur chirurgischen Pathologie der Venen, *Arch Klin Chir.* 1861. *1*: 47.

4. Homans J. The operative treatment of varicose veins and ulcers, based upon a classification of these lesions, *Surg Gynecol Obstet.* 1916. *22*: 143–158.

5. Sheppard M. A procedure for the prevention of recurrent saphenofemoral incompetence, *ANZ J Surg.* 1978. *48*: 322–326.

6. Glass GM. Neovascularization in recurrence of the varicose great saphenous vein following transection, *Phlebology.* 1987. *2*: 81–91.

7. Glass GM. Neovascularization in recurrence of varices of the great saphenous vein in the groin: Surgical anatomy and morphology, *Vasc Surg.* 1989. *23*: 435–442.

8. Jones L, Braithwaite BD, Selwyn D, Cooke S, Earnshaw JJ. Neovascularisation is the principal cause of varicose vein recurrence: Results of a randomised trial of stripping the long saphenous vein, *Eur J Vasc Endovasc Surg.* 1996. *12*: 442–445.

9. De Maeseneer MG, Ongena KP, Van den Brande F, Van Schil PE, De Hert SG, Eyskens EJ. Duplex ultrasound assessment of neovascularization after sapheno-femoral or sapheno-popliteal junction ligation, *Phlebology.* 1997. *12*: 64–68.

10. De Maeseneer MG, Tielliu IF, Van Schil PE, De Hert SG, Eyskens EJ. Clinical relevance of neovascularisation on duplex ultrasound in the long term follow up after varicose vein operation, *Phlebology.* 1999. *14*: 118–122.

11. Nyamekye I, Shephard NA, Davies B, Heather BP, Earnshaw JJ. Clinicopathological evidence that neovascularisation is a cause of recurrent varicose veins, *Eur J Vasc Endovasc Surg.* 1998. *15*: 412–415.

12. van Rij AM, Jones GT, Hill GB, Jiang P. Neovascularization and recurrent varicose veins: More histologic and ultrasound evidence, *J Vasc Surg.* 2004. *40*: 296–302.

13. Stücker M, Netz K, Breuckmann F, Altmeyer P, Mumme A. Histomorphologic classification of recurrent saphenofemoral reflux, *J Vasc Surg.* 2004. *39*: 816–821.

14. Hollingsworth SJ, Powell GL, Barker SGE, Cooper DG. Primary varicose veins: Altered transcription of VGFE and its receptors (KDR, flt-1, soluble flt-1) with sapheno-femoral junction incompetence, *Eur J Vasc Endovasc Surg.* 2004. *27*: 259–268.

15. Lemasle P, Lefebvre-Vilardebo M, Uhl JF, Vin F, Baud J. Postoperative recurrence of varices: What if inguinal neovascularisation was nothing more than the development of a pre-existing network?, *Phlebologie.* 2009. *62*: 42–48.

16. Chandler JG, Pichot O, Sessa C, Schuller-Petrovic S, Osse FJ, Bergan JJ. Defining the role of extended saphenofemoral junction ligation: A prospective comparative study, *J Vasc Surg.* 2000. *32*: 941–953.

17. Pichot O, Kabnick LS, Creton D, Merchant RF, Schuller-Petrovic S, Chandler JG. Duplex ultrasound findings two years after great saphenous vein radiofrequency endovenous obliteration, *J Vasc Surg.* 2004. *39*: 189–195.

18. Pittaluga P, Chastanet S, Guex JJ. Great saphenous vein stripping with preservation of sapheno-femoral confluence: Hemodynamic and clinical results, *J Vasc Surg.* 2008. *47*: 1300–1305.

19. De Maeseneer MG, Philipsen TE, Vandenbroeck CP, et al. Closure of the cribriform fascia: An efficient anatomical barrier against postoperative neovascularisation at the saphenofemoral junction? A prospective study, *Eur J Vasc Endovasc Surg.* 2007. *34*: 361–366.

20. De Maeseneer MG, Vandenbroeck CP, Van Schil PE. Silicone patch saphenoplasty to prevent repeat recurrence after surgery to treat saphenofemoral incompetence: Long-term follow-up study, *J Vasc Surg.* 2004. *40*: 98–105.

21. van Rij AM, Jones GT, Hill BG, et al. Mechanical inhibition of angiogenesis at the saphenofemoral junction in the surgical treatment of varicose veins, *Circulation.* 2008. *118*: 66–74.

22. Heim D, Negri M, Schlegel U, De Maeseneer M. Resecting the great saphenous stump with endothelial inversion decreases neither neovascularisation nor thigh varicosity recurrence, *J Vasc Surg.* 2008. *47*: 1028–1032.

23. Merchant RF, Pichot O, Closure Study Group. Long-term outcomes of endovenous radiofrequency obliteration of saphenous reflux as a treatment for superficial venous insufficiency, *J Vasc Surg.* 2005. *42*: 502–509.

24. Ravi R, Traylor EA, Diethrich EB. Endovenous thermal ablation of superficial venous insufficiency of the lower extremity: Single center experience with 3000 limbs treated in a 7-year period, *J Endovasc Ther.* 2009. *16*: 500–505.

25. De Maeseneer M, Pichot O, Cavezzi A, et al. Duplex ultrasound investigation of the veins of the lower limbs after treatment for varicose veins: UIP consensus document, *Eur J Vasc Endovasc Surg.* 2011. *42*: 89–102.

26. De Maeseneer MG, Vandenbroeck CP, Hendriks JM, Lauwers PR, Van Schil PE. Accuracy of duplex evaluation one year after varicose vein surgery to predict recurrence at the sapheno-femoral junction after five years, *Eur J Vasc Endovasc Surg.* 2005. *29*: 308–312.

25.

THE CHANGING IMPORTANCE OF THE SAPHENOUS VEIN

TREATING VERSUS NONTREATMENT

Paul Pittaluga, S. Chastanet, and T. Locret

INTRODUCTION

The saphenous vein (SV) has been the main target for the treatment of varices for decades. Indeed, the traditional physiopathological concept of varicose disease relies on the descending theory of evolution of the superficial venous insufficiency (SVI) that describes a development starting from junctions between the deep venous system and saphenous axes, with the reflux spreading progressively along the SV to reach the collateral veins on which the varices develop. Thus, for numerous decades, the so-called radical therapeutic principle of varicose disease has the goal of eliminating saphenous axis reflux with surgical treatment combining crossectomy with stripping (CS). The new thermal or chemical endovenous treatment techniques are based on the same physiopathological principle and have the same goal of eliminating SV reflux.

However, the analysis of the long-term results of traditional surgery, the absence of crossectomy when carrying out endovenous treatments, the recent etiopathogenic studies of SVI, and the clinical studies on the extension of the superficial venous reflux led to new physiopathological concepts of SVI that question traditional therapeutic designs focused on the treatment of the SV and the relevance of the treatment of the SV itself.

CRITICAL ANALYSIS

TRADITIONAL CONCEPT OF SVI AND THERAPEUTIC DESIGNS

Described for the first time in 1890, the concept of SVI is based on the existence of points of reflux from the deep venous network toward the superficial venous network, the principal vector of this reflux being the SV starting from the saphenofemoral junction (SFJ) according to the retrograde extension theory of the reflux.[1,2]

The saphenous reflux would progress by retrograde valvular decompensation from the ostial valve (OV) to the malleolar region, furthered by orthostatism. This venous hyperpressure progressing from the deep venous system toward the superficial system causes a dilation of the collaterals of the refluxing SV, and in some cases the appearance of skin damages of chronic venous disease.

This concept justifies the traditional surgical treatment by CS described at the start of the twentieth century.[3,4] The goal of the surgical treatment is rigorous elimination of all the reflux points, from the SFJ and all its afferents to the refluxing perforating veins (PV), by going through the resection of the SV, of course. This surgical treatment remained the gold standard for the choice of "radical" therapy of the SVI up to our time.

LONG-TERM RESULTS OF THE TRADITIONAL TREATMENT BY CS

As one of the main goals of the treatment of the SVI is to remove the varices, the presence of varices is an objective component for evaluation of the efficacy of this treatment. According to the authors, studies of results of more than 5 years report an extremely variable level of clinical varicose recurrence (6 to 93%), and of the time, the technique of the procedure, the length of follow-up, and the method of control (Table 25.1).

Analysis of the literature regarding the principal factors for recurrence shows an evolution: the oldest studies mention surgical defects, anatomical error, and tactical error,[5-8] while gradually junctional neovascularization appears as a new nosologic entity[9-12] to become the most frequent factor

Table 25.1 FREQUENCY OF RECURRENCE AFTER TRADITIONAL CROSSECTOMY AND STRIPPING OF THE SAPHENOUS VEIN

AUTHOR [REFERENCE NUMBER]	YEAR OF PUBLICATION	N	FOLLOW-UP	FREQUENCY OF RECURRENCE	MEAN OF ASSESSMENT
Fischer R [9]	2001	125	34 y	48% 60%	Clinical Ultrasound Duplex-scan
Van Rij AM [10]	2003	137	5 y	47.1% 93% 66%	Clinical Ultrasound Duplex-scan Air plethysmograph
Kostas T [11]	2004	113	5 y	25%	Clinical
Winterborn RJ [12]	2004	133	11 y	62%	Clinical

for recurrence in publications in the early 2000s.[13–15] This evolution could be attributed to the specialization in surgical training, with the enlarged practice of crossectomy, perfectly codified for vascular surgeons. Thus, the number of residual junctions has decreased, being accompanied by an increase in the frequency of inguinal neovascularization as the principal source of postsurgical recurrence.

However, in spite of a standardization of the surgical procedure, the frequency of postsurgical recurrences has not decreased, only its assumed origin has changed. Moreover, the proportion of surgical procedures carried out on recurring varices still represents approximately 20% of the volume of venous surgery in the literature with the pass of time,[16–19] even in the early 2000s, with the initial stripping including an enlarged crossectomy.

CONSERVATION OF THE SFJ AFTER ENDOVENOUS TREATMENT OR MINIMALLY INVASIVE SURGERY

The physical principle of the endovenous techniques is the delivery of endovenous thermal energy, the purpose of which is to occlude the SV, ideally leading to the elimination of the treated venous axis by resorption, thus realizing a real "ablation."[20–21]

So, in principle, the procedure is similar to that of surgical ablation by stripping, with the common purpose of eliminating the refluxing saphenous axis, based on the same 100-year-old descending theory of evolution of the SVI. Moreover, the first protocols of endovenous treatments often combined crossectomy to treat the source of the reflux.

However, the search for less invasiveness, which was the main motivation of the endovenous principle, led to avoiding the inguinal incision in order to attempt an "endovenous crossectomy," in particular with radiofrequency (RF) treatment.[21] The existence of a thromboembolic complication related to the risk of heating the femoral vein has encouraged the practitioners of endovenous techniques not to treat the subostial portion of the SFJ. Most authors agreed

that it was acceptable to preserve a stump of approximately 2 cm upstream of the OV.[22–24]

The study of the evolution of the untreated SFJ shows that it is the site of an anterograde flux from the collaterals toward the deep vein in 88 to 95.7% with a follow-up varying from 1 to 5 years.[25–30]

Thus, an effective occlusion of the SV endovenously leads to the disappearance of the junction reflux in the great majority of cases (Table 25.2).

The results obtained after RF or endovenous laser (EVL) treatment have led some authors to propose a mini-invasive surgical approach on the same principle, stripping without crossectomy (SWC), which associates the achievement of surgical stripping by invagination under tumescent local anesthesia, associated with the conservation of the SFJ by ligature of the great saphenous vein (GSV) at 2 cm from its ostium. At minimum, the results of the SWC confirm those of the RF or the EVL with abolition of the reflux of the SFJ in more than 98% of the cases after stripping of the GSV at 2 years[31] and even at 5 years.[32]

VARICOSE RECURRENCE AFTER THERMAL ENDOVENOUS TREATMENT

The series after endovenous treatment unreliably report the frequency of clinical varicose recurrence, in particular after EVL treatment where this data is often not mentioned, the principal result criterion being the closure of the SV.

On the other hand, the frequency of recurrences according to the PREVAIT definition (presence of clinical varices on a lower limb [LL] that has already been treated, whatever the mean of treatment)[33] is reported in the series with treatment by RF, with figures that vary between 22 and 30% at 3 and 5 years, while the persistence of saphenous reflux varies between 12 and 15% for these same series,[27,28,30] meaning that the majority of clinical recurrences appear while the GSV is occluded and while it no longer presents reflux.

We had reported the same observation in a surgical series in which out of 203 LL operated on for poststripping

Table 25.2 ABSENCE OF REFLUX OF THE SFJ AFTER SAPHENOUS ABLATION BY RF OR EVL TREATMENT OR BY SWC

AUTHOR [REFERENCE NUMBER]	YEAR OF PUBLICATION	N	FOLLOW-UP	TECHNIQUE	ABSENCE REFLUX JSF
Pichot [26]	2004	104	2 y	RF	95.2%
Merchant [27]	2005	406	5 y	RF	83.8%
Nicolini [28]	2005	68	3 y	RF	88%
Min RJ [25]	2003	121	2 y	EVL	93.4%
Proebstle T [29]	2006	188	1 y	EVL	95.7%
Casoni [32]	2008	62	5 y	SWC	98.4%
Pittaluga [31]	2008	195	2 y	SWC	98.2%

(From Reference 32)

recurrence, the source of reflux was a neojunction in less than 40% of the cases, while the great majority of clinical recurrences were independent of the saphenous axis that had been stripped.[34]

REVERSIBILITY OF THE REFLUX OF THE GSV AFTER PHLEBECTOMIES

Some authors have reported that simple phlebectomies could modify the hemodynamics and the diameter of the saphenous vein.[35–41] We reported our experiment with this approach through the ASVAL method (ambulatory selective varices ablation under local anesthesia) with short-term abolition of the saphenous reflux in 70% of the cases,[42] a result that remains stable with a frequency of freedom from varicose recurrence of 91.5% and 88.5% at 3 and 4 years respectively,[43,44] equivalent to or less than the frequency of freedom for recurrence after surgical[45,46] or endovenous ablation treatment of the GSV with the same follow-up.[27,28,30]

ETIOLOGY AND PATHOGENY OF ESSENTIAL VARICES

The descending theory relies on an insufficiency of the terminal valves of the SV or valves of femoral perforating veins as the origin of the insufficiency of the SV upstream of its secondary dilation.[2,47]

This theory has been predominant for a long time, but it is currently questioned by partisans of the "parietal hypothesis" with well-supported arguments. Indeed, numerous publications bring to fore the importance of parietal modifications in the etiology of the varices:

- Functional studies: presence of venous dilations under continent valves[48,49]

- Morphological studies: decrease in the elastin/collagen ratio[50,51] or increase in the connective tissue in the media[52]

- Biochemical studies: decrease in proteolytic activity, parietal hypoxia[53,54]

Thus, Labropopulos et al. confirm that "the parietal venous modifications may appear in any venous segment, whatever its localization and quality of its valves."[55]

TYPOLOGY AND EXTENSION OF THE SUPERFICIAL VENOUS REFLUX

Faced with reflux of the SV, it has been established that the ostial valve was often continent. The frequency of an isolated subostial or truncular reflux is estimated to be around 50% in the literature.[56,57] The incontinence of the ostial valve is thus not necessary for the development of distal SVI. Moreover, it is thought that the SVI is associated with a deep venous reflux in only 2 to 10% of cases.[57,58]

More and more publications mention a progression of the superficial venous reflux from the suprafascial veins.[55,56,58,59] Some authors also confirm that these observations contradict the assumption that the reflux is developed from the saphenous junction retrogradely.[60–62]

In a retrospective study based on 2,275 echo-Doppler mappings, we had noted that there was a positive correlation between the patient's age, the clinical stage of the SVI, and the extent of the superficial venous reflux, and these observations speak in favor of an anterograde or multifocal development of the superficial venous insufficiency, probably from the suprafascial venous network[63] (Figure 25.1).

In 2010, Labropoulos et al. provided additional evidence that the frequency of varicosities is lower in the saphenous trunk than in the tributaries or accessory veins. They also established a correlation between the CEAP classification and the extent of the reflux and the saphenous trunk diameter.[64]

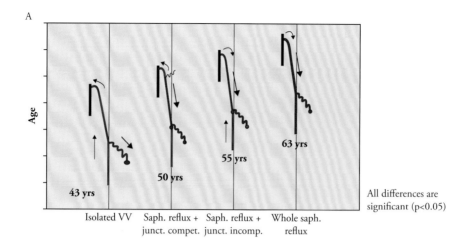

A

All differences are significant (p<0.05)

Isolated VV — Saph. reflux + junct. compet. — Saph. reflux + junct. incomp. — Whole saph. reflux

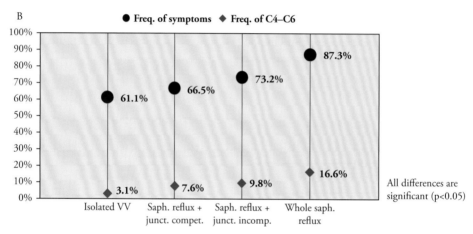

B

● Freq. of symptoms ◆ Freq. of C4–C6

All differences are significant (p<0.05)

Isolated VV — Saph. reflux + junct. compet. — Saph. reflux + junct. incomp. — Whole saph. reflux

Figure 25.1   Correlation of the venous reflux progression with age (A) and signs and symptoms (B) according to a retrospective study on 2,275 echo-Doppler mappings (From Reference 63).

QUESTIONS ABOUT THE IMPORTANCE OF THE SV

The analysis of the above studies raises several questions:

- Why does the frequency of varicose recurrences remain as high in spite of carrying out a "radical" treatment with CS of the GSV that has been perfectly codified for several decades?

- How does one explain the abolition of the reflux of the SFJ in spite of the absence of crossectomy after removal of the GSV by RF or EVL treatment or by SWC?

- How can truncular reflux of the GSV be abolished after simple phlebectomies?

- Why did more than half of the clinical recurrences observed in the medium term after treatment with RF appear while the GSV was occluded and no longer presented reflux?

- What is the physiopathological incidence in studies on the etiopathogeny of the essential varices that favor a parietal, not valvular, hypothesis of the origin of the disease?

- How does one interpret the clinical observations that report the frequent existence of a suprafascial SVI in the absence of reflux of the GSV?

QUESTIONING THE DESCENDING THEORY AND THE TREATMENT OF THE SV

It is not possible to answer these questions without questioning in depth the principle of the descending theory starting from junctions and saphenous axes. Indeed, the traditional descending theory does not enable any of the previous questions to be answered.

ON THE FREQUENCY OF RECURRENCES AFTER CS

The initial notion of a surgical defect (absence of resection of the SFJ) as the predominant explanation for the recurrence of the retrograde pathway occurring after CS, has regressed because of the extensive practice of crossectomy. The concept of inguinal neovascularization has become the predominant explanation of recurrence after CS. This neovascularization may be considered as a healing of the crossectomy zone, and some authors question its role as a recurrence factor,[65] particularly as Perrin et al.[66] report that there is only a single "source" of reflux during a poststripping recurrence in less than 10% of cases. The ablation of the saphenous axis to treat the origin of the SVI, in keeping with the descending theory, thus has very serious limits.

ON THE REVERSIBILITY OF A REFLUX OF THE SFJ AFTER RF OR EVL TREATMENT OR SWC

The absence of treatment of an SFJ that presents an ostial reflux should logically lead to the persistence of the junction reflux or at the very least to its reappearance in the medium or long term in the logic of the descending theory. However, the studies of the results of RF treatment at 5 years show that the absence of reflux at the level of the untreated SFJ is maintained when the GSV is occluded.[27,30] The results reported after SWC are similar, with an absence of reflux at the level of the SFJ in 98.2% at 2 years[31,32] and 98.4% at 5 years. Thus, the treatment of ostial reflux, a key component of the descending theory for which the irreducible corollary is the enlarged crossectomy, is solidly brought back into question.

ON THE ABOLITION OF A REFLUX OF THE GSV AFTER PHLEBECTOMIES

And yet, the descending theory of evolution following successive valvular lesions cannot explain this observed phenomenon, because a single functional valvular incompetence can explain a reversibility of the reflux.[39-44]

ON THE PROBLEM OF CLINICAL VARICOSE RECURRENCES AFTER ENDOVENOUS TREATMENT

If the endovenous techniques have shown their effectiveness for obliteration of the GSV and the elimination of the reflux of the SFJ, that has not resolved the frequency of clinical varicose recurrences that remain at about 30% at 5 years,[27,30] close to the figures obtained after CS.[45,46] Therefore, the elimination of the saphenous reflux endovenously or by stripping, even if it is a complete success, does not enable varicose recurrence to be avoided.

ON THE PROGRESSIVE ABANDONMENT OF THE VALVULAR HYPOTHESIS TO THE BENEFIT OF THE PARIETAL HYPOTHESIS

The descending theory is based on an insufficiency of the terminal valves of the SV or valves of the femoral perforating veins as being at the origin of the insufficiency of the SV by retrograde pathway. This theory is currently questioned by numerous studies[48-54] that show the existence of parietal modifications prior to valvular lesions. The parietal

hypothesis seriously contradicts the descending theory based on the successive rupture of the junctional or saphenous valves leading to "the flooding" of suprafascial collaterals.

ON THE EXISTENCE OF PRIMITIVE VARICES IN THE ABSENCE OF REFLUX OF THE SFJ, EVEN OF THE GSV

A certain number of clinical studies show that in the presence of varices not only is the SFJ competent in more than 50% of cases[56,57] but what is more, there is frequently a partially or totally competent SV.[58,59,63] Moreover, the studies that are involved with progression of reflux certainly recognize the involvement of the SV in the development of the SVI but without assigning any responsibility to the SV for it.[58-64]

NEW HEMODYNAMIC CONCEPT CALLING INTO QUESTION THE IMPORTANCE OF THE SV

This in-depth questioning of the descending theory leads to a very different hypothesis: that of ascending theory of evolution of the SVI from the suprafascial venous network, ascendingly or multifocally toward the SV. The extension of the SVI on the superficial venous network is done centripetally: the evolution begins on the suprafascial tributaries at the bottom, where the hydrostatic pressure is higher, causing the dilatation of the vein wall. This evolution initially remains within the suprafascial plane, creating a dilated and refluxing venous network and progressing following the decreasing hydrostatic pressure gradient. In addition, this refluxing network, when becomes sufficiently important, creates a "varicose reservoir" (VR) with a filling effect in the intrafascial saphenous axis, causing functional incompetence of the saphenous valves, then a dilatation of the SV, evolving anterogradely up to the SFJ also following the decreasing hydrostatic pressure gradient.[61,62]

The concept of the ascending theory makes it possible to outline answers to the questions mentioned previously:

ON THE FREQUENCY OF RECURRENCES AFTER CS

Treatment as specific as CS cannot eradicate varicose recurrence, which would be more or less irreducible because of the natural evolution of the disease starting from the collateral veins themselves.

ON THE REVERSIBILITY OF A REFLUX OF THE SFJ AFTER RF OR EVL TREATMENT OR BY SWC

Since reflux of the SFJ is a consequence of the reflux upstream, it can be understood that abolition of the reflux of the GSV by RF or EVL treatment or by SWC could restore an antero-grade flow with it by virtue of the anastomosis of the collaterals of the SFJ that have an anterograde flow. The enlarged crossectomy, removing an important physiological drainage pathway of the inguinal region could even be deleterious, as the very low rate of neovascularization appears to demonstrate after preservation of the SFJ (0 to 1.7%)[26–28, 31] in contrast to the surgical series with crossectomy (20 to 52%).[46,65]

ON THE ABOLITION OF A REFLUX OF THE GSV AFTER PHLEBECTOMIES

According to the ascending theory, the ablation of the VR may lead to abolition of the saphenous reflux with the elimination of the filling effect and the disappearance of the functional incompetence of the saphenous valves.[39–44] Furthermore, Lurie suggested the possibility of functional insufficiency of the saphenous valves in the absence of any anatomical lesions. The closing of the valves would be caused by the existing pressure in the valvular sinus, which pressure would increase in direct proportion to the velocity of the anterograde flow. If this velocity fails to reach a critical value that allows pressure to reach a level sufficient to close the valve, the valve will not close.[67] This is why a reflux may be present that passes through healthy valves when a patient is in the decubitus position, because the velocity of the anterograde flow is slight. Because ablation of the VR makes it possible to improve the saphenous hemodynamics, it may also make it possible to eliminate a functional valvular insufficiency by increasing the anterograde velocity.

ON THE PROBLEM OF CLINICAL VARICOSE RECURRENCES AFTER ENDOVENOUS TREATMENT

In spite of the abolition of the reflux of the GSV, the natural evolution of the SVI is not affected in the medium or long term, and the varices appear again more or less obviously

according to a personal evolution factor. Thus, the endovenous treatments or the mini-invasive surgery can decrease the aggressiveness of the initial treatment compared with the CS, but its prognosis would not be changed in the medium or long term, with an irreducible rate of clinical recurrences (Table 25.3).

ON THE PROGRESSIVE ABANDONMENT OF THE VALVULAR HYPOTHESIS TO THE BENEFIT OF THE PARIETAL HYPOTHESIS

The parietal etiopathogenic hypothesis of the origin of the SVI gets its clinical illustration with the development of the disease starting from suprafascial veins, the wall of which is most fragile, causing an initial extension within this suprafascial network.

ON THE EXISTENCE OF PRIMITIVE VARICES IN THE ABSENCE OF REFLUX OF THE SFJ, EVEN THE GSV

The GSV is the superficial vein, the wall of which is thickest and most muscular, protected moreover by the doubling of the subcutaneous fascia in which it flows.[63,64] Thus, it could logically be the last to be decompensated, which makes it possible to explain the presence of a suprafascial SVI with an absent or partial reflux in the GSV.

PERSPECTIVES

NEW THERAPIES

The ascending theory validates the new therapeutic approaches:

• The RF or EVL treatment with conservation of the SFJ, which is no longer considered to be the origin of the

Table 25.3 **FREQUENCY OF VARICES RECURRENCES (PREVAIT [REFERENCE 34])** AFTER CS, ENDOVENOUS ABLATION BY RF, SWC, AND ASVAL

AUTHOR [REFERENCE NUMBER]	YEAR OF PUBLICATION	FOLLOW-UP	TECHNIQUE	REVAS
Van Rij AM [10]	2003	5 y	CS	47.1%
Kostas T [11]	2004	5 y	CS	25%
Merchant [27]	2005	5 y	RF	27.4%
Nicolini [28]	2005	3 y	RF	22.8%
Pittaluga [31]	2003	2 y	SWC	6.7%
Casoni [32]	2008	5 y	SWC	11.1%
Pittaluga [43]	2006	4 y	ASVAL	11.5%
(From Reference 32)				

SVI, and which even becomes a useful functional entity for venous drainage of the inguinal region.

- Foam echosclerotherapy, which makes it possible to have great flexibility in treatment adaptation according to the evolutive stage of the patient since it will be capable of treating the GSV but also the VR.

- Mini-invasive surgery, whether it is ablative (SWC) for the same reasons as RF or EVL treatment, or conservative (ASVAL) since it limits the treatment to the VR, starting point of the SVI according to the ascending theory.

NEW STRATEGIES FOR TREATMENT

However, apart from the ASVAL, all the new SVI treatments up to now, whether they are surgical, thermal, or chemical, have the goal of obliterating the refluxing SV, which is the principal, and sometimes only, criterion for evaluation of the result of these techniques in the literature.

The traditional descending theory bases its entire therapeutic position on the presence of a saphenous reflux with its elimination as a goal, without real analysis of the subtleties of this reflux (reflux of the junction, extent of the reflux, hemodynamic profile) or analysis of the relationship of this reflux to the patient's complaint. Thus, the result is assessed on the quality of the elimination of the saphenous reflux. It is paradoxical to observe that one could consider that treatment by stripping, RF, or EVL is a success because the saphenous reflux no longer exists, while varices or symptoms are present.

If we accept the ascending theory as an explanation of the SVI in the majority of cases, the treatment of the SV can no longer be considered to be the goal with priority or even the only goal of the therapy. It is the treatment of the VR that becomes the treatment goal with priority.[43,68]

In addition, the ascending theory leads to the question of treatment of varices preserving the SV in earlier stages, especially for young patients, which might avoid or slow down the progression to the higher stages of disease, toward skin damage.[64] Obviously the answer to this question requires longitudinal cohort studies.

Much work remains to be done, because if the VR is an essential component for the treatment and prognosis of the SVI, it is indispensable to integrate it as an assessment criterion in all studies of treatment of the SVI. However, there are no reliable means currently for assessing the VR.

CONCLUSION

The traditional descending physiopathological description can no longer be considered to be the only explanation of the SVI. More and more it appears that the evolution of the SVI develops from the distal network ascendingly or multifocally toward the saphenous axes. Thus, the systematic treatments of ablation of the saphenous vein or crossectomy are widely questioned. Treatment should be focused on the VR and personalized according to the hemodynamic and clinical checkup, but also according to the wish of the patient. The scientific studies necessary to validate the different therapeutic choices are indispensible with a long-term follow-up.

REFERENCES

1. Trendelenburg F. Ueber die Unterbindung der Vena Saphena magna bei Unterschenkel Varicen, *Beitr Klin Chir.* 1890–1891. *7*: 195–210.
2. Ludbrook J, Beale G. Femoral venous valves in relation to varicose veins, *Lancet.* 1962. *1*: 79–81.
3. Mayo CH. Treatment of varicose vein, *Surg Gyn Obst Br J Surg.* 1906. *2*: 385–388.
4. Babcock WW. A new operation for the extirpation of varicose veins of the leg, *New York Med J.* 1907. *86*: 153–156.
5. Rivlin S. The surgical cure of primary varicose veins, *Br J Surg.* 1975. *62*: 913–917.
6. Royle JP. Recurrent varicose vein, *World J Surg.* 1986. *10*(6): 944–953.
7. Couffinhal C. Récidive de varices après chirurgie: Définition, epidémiologie, physiopathologie: Traitement chirurgical des récidives post-opératoire de varices. In Kieffer E, Bahnini A, eds. *Chirurgie des veines des membres inférieurs.* Paris: AERCV. 1990. 227–238.
8. Negus D. Recurrent varicose veins: A national problem, *Br J Surg.* 1993. *80*: 823–824.
9. Fischer R, Linde N, Duff C, Jeanneret C, Chandler JG, Seeber P. Late recurrent saphenofemoral junction reflux after ligation and stripping of the greater saphenous vein, *J Vasc Surg.* 2001. *34*: 236–240.
10. van Rij AM, Jiang P, Solomon C, Christie RA, Hill GB. Recurrence after varicose vein surgery: A prospective long-term clinical study with duplex ultrasound scanning and air plethysmography, *J Vasc Surg.* 2003. *38*: 935–943.
11. Kostas T, Ioannou CV, Touloupakis E, et al. Recurrent varicose veins after surgery: A new appraisal of a common and complex problem in vascular surgery, *Eur J Vasc Endovasc Surg.* 2004. *2*: 275–282.
12. Winterborn RJ, Foy C, Earnshaw JJ. Causes of varicose vein recurrence: Late results of a randomized controlled trial of stripping the long saphenous vein, *J Vasc Surg.* 2004. *40*: 634–639.
13. van Rij AM, Jones GT, Hill GB, Jiang P. Neovascularization and recurrent varicose veins: More histologic and ultrasound evidence, *J Vasc Surg.* 2004. *40*: 296–302.
14. De Maeseneer MG. The role of postoperative neovascularisation in recurrence of varicose veins: From historical background to today's evidence, *Acta Chir Bel.* 2004. *104*: 283–289. Review.
15. De Maeseneer MG, Vandenbroeck CP, Van Schil PE. Silicone patch saphenoplasty to prevent repeat recurrence after surgery to treat recurrent saphenofemoral incompetence: Long-term follow-up study, *J Vasc Surg.* 2004. *40*: 98–105.
16. Puppinck P, Chevalier J, Espagne P, Habi K, Akkari J. Traitement chirurgical des récidives post-opératoire de varices. In: Kieffer E, Bahnini A, eds. *Chirurgie des veines des membres inférieurs.* Paris: AERCV. 1990. 239–254.
17. Bradbury AW, Stonebridge PA, Ruckley CV, Beggs I. Recurrent varicose veins: Correlation between pre-operative clinical and hand-held Doppler ultrasonic examination and anatomical findings at surgery, *Br J Surg.* 1993. *80*: 849–851.
18. Darke SG. The morphology of recurrent varicose veins, *Eur J Vasc Surg.* 1992. *6*: 512–517.
19. Fischer R, Chandler JG, Stenger D, Puhan MA, De Maeseneer MG, Schimmelpfennig L. Patient characteristics and physician-determined

variables affecting saphenofemoral reflux recurrence after ligation and stripping of the great saphenous vein, *J Vasc Surg.* 2006. *43*: 81–87.

20. Navarro L, Min RJ, Bone C. Endovenous laser: A new minimally invasive method of treatment for varicose veins: Preliminary observations using an 810 nm diode laser, *Dermatol Surg.* 2001. *27*(2): 117–122.

21. Chandler JG, Pichot O, Sessa C, Schuller-Petrovic S, Kabnick LS, Bergan JJ. Treatment of primary insufficiency by endovenous saphenous vein obliteration, *Vasc Surg.* 2000. *38*: 201–214.

22. Manfrini S, Gasbarro V, Danielsson G, et al. Endovenous management of saphenous vein reflux: Endovenous Reflux Management Study Group, *J Vasc Surg.* 2000. *32*: 330–342.

23. Min RJ, Zimmet SE, Isaacs MN, Forrestal MD. Endovenous laser treatment of the incompetent greater saphenous vein, *J Vasc Interv Radiol.* 2001. *12*: 1167–1171.

24. Guex JJ, Min RJ, Pittaluga P. Traitement de l'insuffisance veineuse de la grande saphène par laser endoveineux: Technique et indication, *Phlebologie.* 2002. *55*: 239–243.

25. Min RJ, Khilnani N, Zimmet SE. Endovenous laser treatment of saphenous vein reflux: Long-term results. *J Vasc Interv Radiol.* 2003. *14*: 991–996.

26. Pichot O, Kabnick LS, Creton D, Merchant RF, Schuller-Petroviae S, Chandler JG. Duplex ultrasound scan findings two years after great saphenous vein radiofrequency endovenous obliteration, *J Vasc Surg.* 2004. *39*: 189–195.

27. Merchant RF, Pichot O. Long-term outcomes of endovenous radio-frequency obliteration of saphenous reflux as a treatment for superficial venous insufficiency, *J Vasc Surg.* 2005. *42*: 502–509.

28. Nicolini P, Closure® Group. Treatment of primary varicose veins by endovenous obliteration with the VNUS Closure® system: Results of a prospective multicentre study, *Eur J Vasc Endovasc Surg.* 2005. *29*: 433–439.

29. Proebstle TM, Moehler T, Herdemann S. Reduced recanalization rates of the great saphenous vein after endovenous laser treatment with increased energy dosing: Definition of a threshold for the endovenous fluence equivalent, *J Vasc Surg.* 2006. *44*: 834–839.

30. Creton D et le Groupe Closure®. Oblitération tronculaire saphène par le procédé radiofréquence Closure®: Résultats à 5 ans de l'étude prospective multicentrique, *Phlebologie.* 2006. *59*: 67–72.

31. Pittaluga P, Chastanet S, Guex JJ. Great saphenous vein stripping with preservation of the sapheno-femoral confluence: Hemodynamic and clinical results, *J Vasc Surg.* 2008. *47*: 1300–1305.

32. Casoni P. *Is crossectomy still the first obligatory step in varicose vein surgery? Five year follow up in 124 legs without inguinal dissection: Randomized study.* 22th Annual meeting of the American College of Phlebology, Marco Island, FL, November 8, 2008.

33. Eklöf B, Perrin M, Delis K, Rutherford RB, VEIN-TERM Transatlantic Interdisciplinary. Updated terminology of chronic venous disorders: The VEIN-TERM Transatlantic Interdisciplinary consensus document, *J Vasc Surg.* 2009. *48*: 498–501.

34. Pittaluga P. Chirurgie des récidives variqueuses: Les mauvais résultats, *Phlebologie* 2004. *1*. 47–53.

35. Muller R. Traitement des varices par phlébectomie ambulatoire, *Phlebologie.* 1966. *19*: 277–279.

36. Ricci S, Georgiev M, Goldman MP. Phlebectomy: Vein avulsion. In Ricci S, Georgiev M, Goldman MP, eds. *Ambulatory phlebectomy*, 2e. Boca Raton, FL: Taylor and Francis. 2005. 121–133.

37. Large J. Surgical treatment of saphenous varices, with preservation of the main great saphenous trunk, *J Vasc Surg.* 1985. *2*: 886–891.

38. de Ross KP, Nieman FH, Neumann HA. Ambulatory phlebectomy versus compression sclerotherapy: Results of a randomized controlled trial, *Dermatol Surg.* 2003. *29*: 221–226.

39. Vidal-Michel JP, Bourrel Y, Emsallem J, Bonerandi JJ. Respect chirurgical des crosses saphènes internes modérement incontinentes par "effet siphon" chez les patients variqueux, *Phlebologie.* 1993. *1*: 143–147.

40. Creton D. Diameter reduction of the proximal long saphenous vein after ablation of a distal incompetent tributary, *Dermatol Surg.* 1999. *25*: 394–397.

41. Zamboni P, Cisno C, Marchetti F, Quaglio D, Mazza P, Liboni A. Reflux elimination without any ablation or disconnection of the saphenous vein: A haemodynamic model for venous surgery, *Eur J Vasc Endovasc Surg.* 2001. *21*: 361–369.

42. Pittaluga P, Rea B, Barbe R. Méthode ASVAL (ablation sélective des varices sous anesthésie locale): Principes et résultats préliminaires, *Phlebologie.* 2005. *2*: 175–181.

43. Pittaluga P, Chastanet S. Saphenous vein preservation: Is it the new gold standard? In: Becquemin JP, Alimi YS, eds. *Updates and controversies in vascular surgery.* Turin, Italy: Minerva Medica. 2007. 392–399.

44. Pittaluga P, Chastanet S, Réa B, Barbe R. Midterm results of the surgical treatment of varices by phlebectomy with conservation of a refluxing saphenous vein, *J Vasc Surg.* 2009. *50*: 107–118.

45. Rutgers PH, Kitslaar PJ. Randomized trial of stripping versus high ligation combined with sclerotherapy in the treatment of the incompetent greater saphenous vein, *Am J Surg.* 1994. *168*: 311–315.

46. Jones L, Braithwaite BD, Selwyn D, Cooke S, Earnshaw JJ. Neovascularisation is the principal cause of varicose vein recurrence: Result of a randomised trial of stripping the long saphenous vein, *Eur J Vasc Endovasc Surg.* 1996. *12*: 442–445.

47. Moore HD. Deep venous valves in the aetiology of varicose veins, *Lancet.* 1951. *2*: 7–10.

48. Psaila JV, Melhuish J. Viscoelastic properties and collagen content of the long saphenous vein in normal and varicose veins, *Br J Surg.* 1989. *76*: 37–40.

49. Clarke H, Smith SR, Vasdekis SN, Hobbs JT, Nicolaides AN. Role of venous elasticity in the development of varicose veins, *Br J Surg.* 1989. *76*: 577–580.

50. Jurukova Z, Milenkov C. Ultrastructural evidence for collagen degradation in the walls of varicose veins, *Exp Mol Pathol.* 1982. *37*: 37–47.

51. Rose SS, Ahmed A. Some thoughts on the aetiology of varicose veins, *J Cardiovasc Surg.* 1986. *27*: 534–543.

52. Porto LC, da Silveira PR, de Carvalho JJ, Panico MD. Connective tissue accumulation in the muscle layer in normal and varicose saphenous veins, *Angiology.* 1995. *46*: 243–249.

53. Gandhi RH, Irizarry E, Nackman GB, Halpern VJ, Mulcare RJ, Tilson MD. Analysis of the connective tissue matrix and proteolytic activity of primary varicose veins, *J Vasc Surg.* 1993. *18*: 814–820.

54. Lengyel I, Acsády G. Histomorphological and pathobiochemical changes of varicose veins: A possible explanation of the development of varicosis, *Acta Morphol Hung.* 1990. *38*: 259–267.

55. Labropoulos N, Giannoukas AD, Delis K, et al. Where does venous reflux start?, *J Vasc Surg.* 1997. *26*: 736–742.

56. Abu-Own A, Scurr JH, Coleridge Smith PD. Saphenous vein reflux without incompetence at the saphenofemoral junction, *Br J Surg.* 1994. *81*: 1452–1454.

57. Labropoulos N, Leon M, Nicolaides AN, Giannoukas AD, Volteas N, Chan P. Superficial venous insufficiency: Correlation of anatomic extent of reflux with clinical symptoms and signs, *J Vasc Surg.* 1994. *20*: 953–958.

58. Myers KA, Ziegenbein RW, Zeng GH, Matthews PG. Duplex ultrasonography scanning for chronic venous disease: Patterns of venous reflux, *J Vasc Surg.* 1995. *21*: 605–612.

59. Engelhorn CA, Engelhorn AL, Cassou MF, Salles-Cunha SX. Patterns of saphenous reflux in women with primary varicose veins, *J Vasc Surg.* 2005. *41*: 645–651.

60. Labropoulos N, Leon L, Kwon S, et al. Study of the venous reflux progression, *J Vasc Surg.* 2005. *41*: 291–295.

61. Hebrant J, Colignon A. *La varicose: Nouvelle hypothèse étiologique, nouvelle approche thérapeutique* [Varices: New etiological hypothesis, new therapeutic approach]. Open communications session, Société Française de Phlébologie, Paris, December 10, 2005.

62. Bernardini E, De Rango P, Piccioli R, et al. Development of primary superficial venous insufficiency: the ascending theory. Observational and hemodynamic data from a 9-year experience. *Ann Vasc Surg.* 2010. *24*: 709–720.

63. Pittaluga P, Chastanet S. Classification of saphenous refluxes: Implications for treatment, *Phlebology.* 2008. *23*: 2–9.

64. Labropoulos N, Kokkosis A, Spentzouris G, Gasparis A, Tassiopoulos A. The distribution and significance of varicosities in the saphenous trunks, *J Vasc Surg.* 2010. *51*: 96–103.

65. Egan B, Donnelly M, Bresnihan M, Tierney S, Feeley MJ. Neovascularization: An "innocent bystander" in recurrent varicose veins, *Vasc Surg.* 2006. *44*: 1279–1284.

66. Perrin MR, Labropoulos N, Leon LR Jr. Presentation of the patient with recurrent varices after surgery (REVAS), *J Vasc Surg.* 2006. *43*: 327–334.

67. Lurie F. *New investigations for venous valve insufficiency: Perspective for early detection.* 9th Annual Meeting of the European Venous Forum, Barcelona, Spain, June 26, 2008.

68. Pittaluga P, Chastanet S. The lesser importance of the saphenous vein in therapy of varicose veins. In: Bergan JJ, ed. *Foam sclerotherapy.* London: Royal Society of Medicine Press. 2008. 163–176.

26.

PRINCIPLES OF AMBULATORY PHLEBECTOMY

Jose I. Almeida and Jeffrey K. Raines

Ambulatory phlebectomy (AP) is a surgical procedure designed to allow outpatient removal of bulging varicose veins. This treatment originally was described and performed by Aulus Cornelius Celsus (56 BC–AD 30) in ancient Rome.[1] However, the art of AP was revived, redefined, and practiced by the sagacious Swiss dermatologist Robert Muller in 1956. Prior to Muller's reintroduction of AP, veins were removed with relatively large incisions and ligation of venous ends. Muller developed the stab avulsion method that is now in widespread use. Characteristics of Muller's AP technique are absence of venous ligatures, exclusive use of local infiltration anesthesia, immediate ambulation after surgery, 2-mm incisions, absence of skin sutures, and a postoperative compression bandage kept in place for 2 days, then replaced with daytime compression stockings for 3 weeks.

It is of interest that after its introduction, the medical-scientific community exhibited minimal interest in Muller's AP procedure. Muller published his first manuscript on AP in 1966;[2] however, AP did not gain popularity in the United States until the American surgeon Gabriel Goren published his findings in 1991.[3] In contemporary vein centers, AP is a common office-based procedure performed with local anesthesia. Unless the patient's history suggests other comorbidities, hematologic or other laboratory investigations are not generally required.

INDICATIONS

AP is indicated for the removal of varicose venous tributaries, when visible and palpable on the surface of the skin. AP is simple to perform, is well tolerated, and can be used in conjunction with other treatment modalities. The most important concept for the practitioner treating varicose veins to understand is that simple vein removal, without proper diagnostic evaluation, will not yield good results. It is critical to recognize that bulging veins usually are associated with an underlying source of venous hypertension, and treatment of the source is as important as the vein removal

itself. Prior to performing AP the treating physician must perform a thorough evaluation with duplex ultrasound imaging to identify the source of venous hypertension and its most proximal point of reflux. To prevent recurrence, the refluxing source in continuity with the varicose veins should be eliminated prior to undergoing AP.

The most common source of ambulatory venous hypertension is an incompetent superficial system, usually the great saphenous vein (GSV). An incompetent GSV, in continuity with a bulging venous tributary, commonly is encountered in patients presenting with venous disease. However, venous hypertension also may originate from deep veins, perforating veins, or any combination of superficial, perforating, and deep systems. If a source of ambulatory venous hypertension is identified during the preoperative studies, it should be treated either prior to or at the same time as AP. There are many techniques available to treat axial or perforator vein incompetence that are beyond the scope of this essay. Briefly, superficial axial vein reflux may be corrected by surgical, thermal, or chemical means.

PREOPERATIVE MAPPING

Mapping is done prior to commencing AP and is a critical step in the procedure. It must be comprehensive. The key to success is accurate marking of the surface bulges with an indelible marker in the standing position (see Figure 26.1). Marking is performed in the standing position because hydrostatic pressure is no longer active when the patient is supine. Stated differently, bulging veins disappear when patients lie flat because the local venous pressure decreases to near 0 mmHg. We prefer mapping these veins using visual inspection and palpation; other investigators prefer transillumination mapping.[4] Precise mapping provides a blueprint for the operator to locate veins with ease, careless mapping provides a poor blueprint and results in suboptimal surgical results. Patients should avoid placing moisturizing lotions on their legs the morning before surgery as this promotes

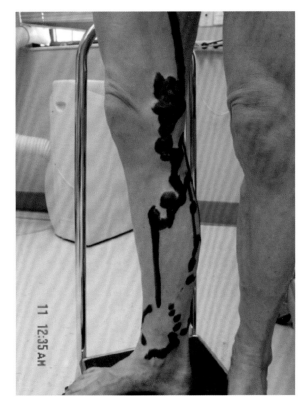

Figure 26.1 Mapping.

smudging during the preoperative surgical scrubbing process, thereby undermining the quality of the blueprint.

ANESTHESIA

Tumescent anesthesia provides a safe, easy to administer, and comfortable anesthetic technique for use with ambulatory phlebectomy. The technique of tumescent anesthesia involves infiltration of the subcutaneous compartment with relatively large volumes of a dilute mixture of a buffered local anesthetic solution. Preparation of the tumescent solution is easily accomplished. Our preparation requires a 50-cc vial of 1% lidocaine with added 1:100,000 mg of epinephrine mixed with 500 cc of Ringer's lactate. This gives a 0.1% preparation of lidocaine with epinephrine, which is delivered with a 30-cc syringe and 20-gauge needle subdermally, under pressure, until the characteristic *peau d'orange* effect is seen on the skin.

This form of anesthesia requires no specialized training or expensive equipment and offers several intraoperative as well as postoperative advantages not found in traditional local anesthesia. Not only is excellent anesthesia provided to relatively large areas of the leg, but the tumescent fluid hydrodissects the subcutaneous fat. It enters perivenous tissues under pressure, thus facilitating vein extraction. This has led to use of this technique not only in AP, but also in surgical stripping[5] and thermal ablation of the GSV.

Originally developed by Klein[6] in 1987 for use in liposuction, the technique of tumescent anesthesia for use in ambulatory phlebectomy was introduced by Cohn[7] in 1995. Surprisingly, as the concentration of lidocaine was lowered during the developmental stages of the technique, it was observed that the anesthetic effect was augmented until a threshold 0.04% was reached. Klein has shown through clinical studies involving assays of lidocaine in peripheral blood, that doses well above the manufacturer's recommendation are safe. The widely held dogma that lidocaine administration should be limited to 7 mg/kg was based on extrapolated data from procainamide levels. This dogma was rigidly adhered to from 1948 because of recommendations from the manufacturer. It is now known through Klein's work that a dose of 35 mg/kg of dilute lidocaine solution is well tolerated.[8] Further documentation and years of safe use have made it the standard for anesthesia in liposuction surgery. However, the authors have found that exceeding 7 mg/kg is rarely necessary to complete a unilateral lower extremity endovenous thermal ablation with concomitant AP.

Infiltrating solutions should contain epinephrine in appropriate concentrations to reduce the incidence of hematoma and induce a more gradual absorption of lidocaine into the bloodstream. When general anesthesia is used for this surgery (i.e., dry technique), there is no infiltration of local anesthetic or vasoconstrictor agents. This results in blood loss and significant pain. Other advantages of tumescent anesthesia include the ability to anesthetize large areas of the body without toxicity, positive effect on intravascular fluid status, avoidance of general anesthesia, less pain, and shorter postoperative recovery time.[8]

Infections are rare after liposuction and AP with tumescent anesthesia, and usually are confined to an incision site.[9] Infections have not been seen in our practice since we began office-based AP surgery with tumescent anesthesia. The reason for the low rate of infection is not clear, although there are reports of lidocaine concentration-dependent bacteriostatic and bactericidal activity. Pathogens commonly found on the skin may be sensitive to this activity.[10]

SURGICAL TECHNIQUE

INCISIONS

Access to varicose veins is accomplished with a sharp instrument using small stab incisions (see Figure 26.2). Incisions of 1–3 mm in length are usually sufficient to extirpate even the largest veins. The methods and required tools are simple and basic. The most popular instruments for creating incisions are number 11 scalpel blades, 18-gauge needles, and 15-degree ophthalmologic Beaver blades. Incision length should correspond to vein size, but is rarely larger than 3 mm. Small varicose veins are extracted through an

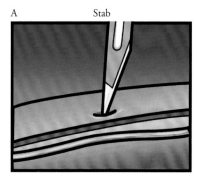

A   Stab

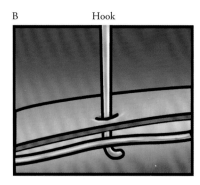

B   Hook

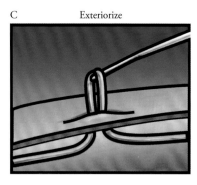

C   Exteriorize

Figure 26.2   Stab incisions.

Hooking the target vein through the small incision is the next step (see Figure 26.2). There are many instruments available on the market to accomplish this goal, ranging from inexpensive to very expensive. Most operators use hooks to elevate the vein from the wound whereas others reach into the wound and grasp the vein with fine hemostats. The most popular hooks are medical grade with the developer's name used for identification (i.e., Muller, Oesch, Tretbar, Ramelet, Verady, and Dortu-Mortimbeau). However, we prefer hooks manufactured for crocheting; they are readily available, come in a variety of sizes, and are suitable for autoclave sterilization between uses.

Using a hook of choice, the vein is exteriorized from the wound (see Figure 26.2). Hooks need not be introduced into the wound deeper than 2–3 mm and should be inserted gently and deliberately to avoid unnecessary trauma to the wound margins. Gentle probing and "searching" for the target vein with the hook are routinely necessary and should be done with great care. Once a segment of vein is exteriorized from the wound it is extracted. The vein is grasped with fine hemostatic clamps, and using gentle traction in a circular motion the vein is teased out of the wound. Dissection of the vein from its perivenous investments greatly facilitates its extraction. Perivenous tissue issuing from the wound is excised at the skin level. This tissue should never be forcefully pulled out of the wound. Care should be taken during extraction not to enlarge the wound, especially in the elderly.

When traction is applied to the vein, the skin adjacent to the wound will momentarily depress downward. Attention to this detail gives the operator an idea of where to place the next incision. The depression represents the point at which the vein will avulse. The next incision is made near the area of depressed skin and the process is repeated sequentially until all the venous bulges have been addressed. Although all bulges should be marked during the mapping procedure, not all the marks need to be incised if the operator takes care in identifying the skin depressions described earlier. In some cases, segments as large as 12 inches may be removed from a single site (see Figure 26.3). Segmental extraction of very small portions of varicose veins can make the operation quite tedious; in some cases this cannot be avoided.

If vein exteriorization proves difficult, it is better to make larger incisions rather than traumatize the wound's edges since this may cause visible scars. In order to reduce the number of incisions, the incisions are made one at a time. If avulsion proves difficult and the vein breaks, it is more convenient to make more incisions than to increase effort and in return lose time.[11] One should also keep in mind that the skin in elderly patients is thin and easily damaged if not handled properly. This is especially true in the ankle, foot, and popliteal areas.[12]

18-gauge needle puncture, and larger veins are removed through 2-mm incisions made with a number 11 scalpel blade. The incisions are oriented vertically on most areas of the lower extremity. Horizontal incisions are preferred around the knees and ankles.

Widening of incisions with a hemostat should be avoided because this results in an increased potential for unsightly scars and/or wound infections. If wound margins are traumatized this may lead to increased pigmentation in the postoperative scar. There have been anecdotal reports of "tattooing" the skin when the incision is placed through the indelible ink mark made during the preoperative mapping process. This has not been the experience of the authors.

Reimbursement for AP has been established with Current Procedural Terminology (CPT) codes. Insurance carriers base the remuneration for services on the number of stab incisions; therefore, it is important to count the total number of incisions made during each case and document this information in the clinical record.

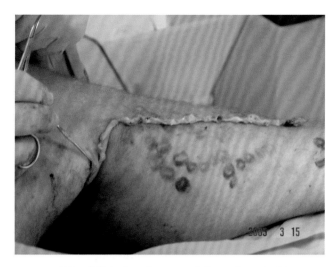

Figure 26.3   Vein of Michaelangelo extracted via one 2-mm incision.

Several areas of the lower extremity are more challenging when attempting to hook a vein. Areas of previous surgery and the anterior aspect of the knee have thick skin and fibrous underlying tissue, which can make the hooking process difficult. There is a paucity of subcutaneous fat in the pretibial areas and dorsum of the foot that can also prove challenging. With experience one learns to distinguish between the vein wall, which is elastic, and the connective perivenous tissue, which is not. Ultrasound-guided vein hooking is useful for deeper or more difficult veins. AP is not the best technique for removal of the GSV or SSV; we prefer endovenous thermal ablation for these veins.

Avulsion of venous segments treated by AP is not associated with significant bleeding when tumescent anesthesia is used. Hemostasis is achieved with gentle pressure over the incision site. The epinephrine in the anesthetic solution enhances the hemostasis process. When extracting larger veins with the stab-avulsion technique, significant force may be required and some minor bleeding may be encountered. Using digital pressure over the wound with a gloved finger generally controls bleeding. Placing the patient in the Trendelenburg position may also augment hemostasis.

Varicose veins are sometimes outflow tracts for perforating veins; therefore, avulsion of varicose veins can disconnect underlying perforators. A perforator may be recognized by its perpendicular course and by the fact that the patient reports discomfort or pain upon traction of the perforator. The perforator is pulled until it yields, and then avulsed. Bleeding is controlled with digital compression. However, in areas difficult to compress (i.e., thigh) or when perforators are very large, ligation is preferred.[11]

INCISION CLOSURE

The wounds may be left open, or closed with simple sutures or adhesive tape. Whether to close or not close wounds is a matter of judgment. Most operators leave the wounds open

and allow spontaneous healing. This technique results in little or no scarring and also has the advantage of allowing drainage of blood and anesthetic fluid into the overlying compressive dressing. A single suture to close wounds near the foot and ankle may be required because of the elevated venous pressure in the upright position in these locations. Frequent postprocedural ambulation will aid in decreasing ambulatory venous pressure in these dependent locations. Adhesive tapes are associated with a high incidence of skin blistering; therefore, these must be used with caution.

COMPRESSION BANDAGE

Careful application of the postoperative dressing cannot be overstated. Careless dressing placement can lead to hematomas, blisters, nerve injury, ischemia, and bleeding. The limb is wrapped circumferentially from foot to groin with a compression dressing and removed after 48 hours. The dressing should be applied with graduated pressure; the amount of pressure should decrease as one proceeds from foot to groin. During placement of the compressive bandage, it is important to pad the lateral fibular head to avoid pressure-induced injury to the deep and superficial peroneal nerves, which can lead to footdrop. Patients are encouraged to ambulate immediately after the procedure to minimize thromboembolic complications.

Application of a compressive dressing in obese patients is especially critical because the dressing has a tendency to unravel. There is a tendency to apply this dressing tightly, but this can lead to undue pressure, blistering, and/or skin necrosis.

POSTPROCEDURE ISSUES

The patients ambulate from the office with a three-layer compression bandage after 10 minutes of postoperative observation. Very little postoperative discomfort is the norm, and is usually easily managed with nonsteroidal antiinflammatory agents. When the bandage is removed in the office on postoperative day 2, some minor leakage of blood and tumescent anesthesia may be seen in cases where the wounds are left open. These areas are covered with small bandages until dry. We perform a duplex ultrasound at the postoperative visit to exclude the presence of deep vein thrombosis.

Some ecchymosis is to be expected, rarely resulting in permanent discoloration of the skin. Indurated areas are commonly seen and usually decompress without incident over a period of weeks. Firm subcutaneous inflammatory nodules can form directly under the incision, and these, too, are self-limiting. We give the patient 3 days of postoperative antibiotic prophylactic therapy. After the compression bandage is removed on postoperative day 2, we have the patients wear graduated compression stockings (20–30 mmHg) for 2 weeks during the daytime.

COMPLICATIONS

Complications from AP in experienced hands are rare and, when they do occur, are minor.[12] The Miami Vein Center to date has performed more than 1,500 AP procedures in the office environment. Complications have been limited to hyperpigmentation, telangiectatic matting, seroma, transient paresthesia, superficial phlebitis, blistering, and "missed veins" requiring repeat treatment. Each of these complications occurred in less than 0.5% of cases.

A multicenter study performed in France evaluated 36,000 phlebectomies. The most frequently encountered complications were telangiectasias (1.5%), blister formation (1%), phlebitis (0.05%), hyperpigmentation (0.03%), postoperative bleeding (0.03%), temporary nerve damage (0.05%), and permanent nerve damage (0.02%).[13]

STAGING OF SURGERY

Prior to the advent of endovenous ablation, high ligation and stripping of the GSV usually relegated venous surgery to the operating room. However, with the development of minimally invasive, catheter-based interventions, venous surgery is a simple office procedure.

Complete surgical removal of varicose veins may be achieved in a single session or in separate sessions. Endovenous ablation and AP are suitable for the office, and in the author's practice, routinely are performed together. The advantage of this combination technique is that patients can expect all varicose veins to disappear after a 1-hour procedure.

We feel that in order to become a complete vein surgeon, the individual must become facile with all of the available tools. The operator should enter the procedure room with a complete plan of action. The duplex ultrasound device must be an extension of the surgeon's eyes. Duplex ultrasound is essential for managing the patient preoperatively, intraoperatively, and postoperatively. Combining endovenous thermal ablation, AP, and sclerotherapy techniques with accurate imaging will allow the development of a complete treatment algorithm.

We do not look at AP as a solitary procedure, but as part of the armada in the treatment of venous disease. We usually perform endovenous thermal ablation of the saphenous trunk at the same setting as AP because bulging varicose veins are usually in continuity with a refluxing axial vein such as the GSV. Sclerotherapy is also often used simultaneously with AP when the refluxing axial vein is tortuous. This is often the case when the anterior accessory saphenous vein is incompetent or when we treat recurrent varicose veins after previous high ligation and stripping. We try to keep the sites of AP remote from the sites of sclerotherapy for fear of extravasation of sclerosant from fractured vein ends into the subcutaneous tissues. All procedures are guided with duplex ultrasound to get a "roadmap underneath the skin."

Varicosities in continuity with a refluxing truncal vein (e.g., the GSV), and not in continuity with any perforating veins, will diminish in size after endovenous ablation. Therefore, some patients will not require further treatment. However, in review of our last 1,000 cases of endovenous thermal ablation of the saphenous vein, AP was performed concomitantly in 86% of cases.

Some operators delay AP until 4 weeks following endovenous ablation. The argument for this strategy is to allow the bed of varicosities distal to a refluxing axial vein to shrink in size and number. Then, fewer incisions will be required for vein removal at the time of AP.

If the patient returns in the postoperative period and points out veins that were missed during AP, a redo procedure generally is not required. Sclerotherapy, with or without ultrasound guidance, can be performed 4 to 6 weeks postoperatively to remove any missed veins. As a general rule, we prefer not to combine AP with ultrasound-guided sclerotherapy of varicose veins, unless the sites are distant from one another. As stated earlier, leakage of sclerosant from fractured vein ends is undesirable. If redo phlebectomy is required, we allow 3 months to elapse; this allows the inflammatory response to improve at the original AP sites.

AVOIDING NONTARGET TISSUES

If the treating physician heeds several important suggestions, complications will rarely be encountered. The venous surgeon must have a thorough command of neurovascular anatomy to avoid injury to nontarget tissues such as arteries and nerves. Knowledge of the course of the common femoral artery, superficial femoral artery, popliteal artery, and anterior and posterior tibial arteries will keep the surgeon from injuring these structures while probing to exteriorize a varicose vein. It would be very difficult, although not impossible, to injure the profunda femoris or peroneal arteries during AP. As stated earlier, the hook rarely needs to plunge deeper than 3 mm to contact the target vein.

The saphenous and sural nerves are particularly prone to injury below the knee because of their proximity to the GSV and small saphenous vein (SSV). If the saphenous or sural nerves are displaced by the hook, the patient usually will complain of shooting pain into the foot. This is a sign for the surgeon to gently release the structure and replace it *in situ*. The femoral, obturator, sciatic, tibial, and peroneal (common, deep, and superficial) nerves are deep and generally not disturbed in the hands of a competent surgeon. However, when placing the postoperative compression bandage, the deep peroneal nerve can be injured if the lateral fibular head is not properly padded. Occasionally, hair-sized sensory cutaneous nerves are encountered and inadvertently extracted during the course of AP. They are recognized as small threads and the patient will feel acute sharp pain. The pain usually dissipates after 2 to 5 minutes without treatment. If this occurs in the ankle and foot area, chances are that the patient will develop postoperative paresthesias or areas of dysesthesia that in most cases will be temporary.[14]

TREATMENT OF VARICOSE VEINS FROM NONSAPHENOUS ORIGINS

Bulging varicose veins on the surface of the skin can originate from different sources. Identification of these sources is important because this influences the treatment plan. Varicosities on the medial aspect of the thigh and calf are usually the result of GSV incompetence. In order to minimize the chance for recurrence, the GSV must be eliminated from the circulation. This concept has been substantiated in several prospective randomized clinical trials involving patients who were treated with or without saphenectomy by conventional vein stripping.[15–18] The recurrence rates for limbs without saphenectomy were much higher than those with saphenectomy. Of course, now thermal ablation techniques with either radiofrequency or laser have proven to be the method of choice for eliminating the GSV from the circulation.[19,20]

Varicosities on the anterior thigh usually result from anterior accessory saphenous vein (AASV) incompetence. These veins usually course over the knee and into the lower leg. SSV reflux produces varicosities on the posterior calf. When also present on the posterior thigh, the surgeon must consider a cranial extension of the SSV, which can be identified with duplex ultrasound imaging. Cranial extensions may enter the GSV (Giacomini vein) or enter the femoral vein directly.

In cases where no "feeding source" is found, phlebectomy of the varicosities may be all that is required. Labropoulos[21] has shown that varicose veins may result from a primary vein wall defect and that reflux may be confined to superficial tributaries throughout the lower limb. Without great and small saphenous trunk incompetence, perforator and deep-vein incompetence, or proximal obstruction, his data suggest that reflux can develop in any vein without an apparent feeding source. This is often the case when bulging reticular veins are seen along the course of the lateral leg. This lateral subdermic complex and its vein of Albanese are often dilated and bulging in elderly patients. The underlying source of venous hypertension is usually perigeniculate perforating veins, not easily identifiable with duplex imaging. AP using an 18-gauge needle stab incision and a small crochet hook for exteriorization of the vein is an excellent procedure for this clinical problem. Perforating veins of the thigh or calf also may become incompetent and be sources of ambulatory venous hypertension. These can be treated by

a variety of techniques including ligation, subfascial endoscopic perforator surgery (SEPS), and ultrasound-guided sclerotherapy (UGS).

AP VERSUS POWERED PHLEBECTOMY

In a published prospective comparative randomized trial comparing AP with the new technique of transillumination-powered phlebectomy (TriVex), there was no difference in operating time. Although an incision ratio of 7:1 favored TriVex, there was no perceived cosmetic benefit among the patient groups. There was a higher number of recurrences in the TriVex group (21.2%; 7 of 33) compared with the AP group (6.2%; 2 of 32) at 52 weeks postoperatively. Assessment of pain scores showed no difference between groups.[22] These findings have been supported by other investigators.[23–27]

It is important to point out that all Trivex procedures were performed in the hospital under general anesthesia, and the cost of disposable equipment used for the TriVex procedure was $314 per patient. Because the trend for venous surgery is office-based, with local anesthesia, TriVex will likely fall into disfavor in the future if modifications for office use are ignored.

AP VERSUS COMPRESSION SCLEROTHERAPY

The combination of compression therapy with intravenous injection of a sclerosing agent for the treatment of varicose veins was introduced in 1953.[28] Early studies indicated compression sclerotherapy (Sclero) would be an efficient addition to varicose vein surgery practiced at that time Although ambulatory phlebectomy was "invented" around the same period,[2] this technique required considerable time to become well established worldwide. There is one randomized controlled trial on recurrence rates and other complications after Sclero and AP. A total of ninety-eight operations were randomized to either AP (n = 49) or Sclero (n = 49) in a total of eighty-two lateral accessory varicose veins (LAVs). In this study, polidocanol was used in a 3% solution (Aethoxysclerol; Kreussler & Co., Wiesbaden, Germany), which is equivalent to 1.5% sodium tetradecyl sulfate. One year after Sclero, twelve LAVs had recurred (25%), and only one postphlebectomy LAV (2.1%). After 2 years, the difference in recurrence was even larger because another six recurrences developed, making a total of eighteen recurrences in the Sclero group (37.5%) and only one recurrence in the AP group (2.1%). The authors of the study concluded that AP is the treatment of choice for LAV.[29]

AP FOR OTHER AREAS
OF THE BODY

FOOT

In recent years there have been several publications on the use of AP for the treatment of varicose veins of the foot and ankle region.[30–32] There are patients who present with serious phlebologic complaints of varicosities of the foot and ankle region that can be alleviated through simple treatment. The venous anatomy of the foot with many parallel veins is complicated; however, safe treatment is possible.

The skin of the foot is thin and fibrotic. Further, there is minimal subcutaneous fat, less protection against trauma of the skin, and important underlying tissues such as tendons, tendon sheaths, and joints. There are more small nerve branches that can be damaged by the hook. As in the popliteal space, there is greater risk of injuring an artery. Moreover, it is possible to grasp and avulse a tendon.

EYELID

Many ophthalmic plastic surgeons and dermatologic surgeons experienced in sclerotherapy avoid the use of this agent near the eye or use it in substantially lower concentrations and volumes. This is due to fear that the solution may travel to unintended areas of venous circulation such as the central retinal vein, choroidal vortex veins, or even the cavernous sinus via valveless anastomoses.[33] Blindness has been reported following STS injection into a venous malformation partially located in the orbit.[34]

Ambulatory phlebectomy of the periocular vein avoids the concerns regarding thrombotic phenomena within ocular, orbital, or cerebral veins possibly associated with periocular vein sclerotherapy. Weiss[35] reported excellent results for ten patients who underwent removal of periocular reticular blue veins by AP. A single puncture with an 18-gauge needle sufficed in most cases. It is important to attempt to remove the entire segment, as partial resection may lead to recurrence. The use of postoperative compression for 10 minutes reduces the incidence of bruising. The puncture sites typically disappear quickly without leaving scars.

HANDS

In general, inquiries about hand vein treatment come from elderly women who find them unsightly. Often, they have had prior facelift surgery and worry that their hands need rejuvenation to complement the face. Our initial consultation stresses the importance of hand veins for reasons of intravenous access, furthermore, removal of these veins may require central venous access should the patient be hospitalized in the future. If attempts to dissuade the patient fail, we recommend AP as the procedure of choice for hand vein removal. It is performed identical to leg vein treatment, and closely resembles treating the dorsum of foot because of the thin skin overlying the area. Results have been excellent.

OFFICE-BASED AP WITH
TUMESCENT ANESTHESIA

Although there are reports of death and serious complications with tumescent anesthesia, these have largely been found in the plastic surgery literature.[36] Complications are described when tumescent anesthesia is used in conjunction with intravenous sedation, and/or general anesthesia.[37] Coldiron et al. recently studied State of Florida data over a 4-year period to help clarify actual adverse events occurring in the office setting. There were seventy-seven events reported to the Florida Agency for Health Care Administration (ACHA) from March 1, 2000, to March 1, 2004. Liposuction performed under general anesthesia was the most frequent procedure reported. Five reported deaths and fourteen transfer incidents occurred as a complication of liposuction (with or without another associated procedure) under general anesthesia or deep sedation. According to the Florida data, there were no problems associated with liposuction using dilute or tumescent anesthesia.[38] Similarly, a malpractice claims study by Coleman and colleagues study supported the safety of office-based liposuction performed by dermatologists using tumescent anesthesia for small-volume fat removal.[39] In addition, Housman and colleagues surveyed 261 dermatologic surgeons performing a total of 66,570 liposuction procedures and found a low rate of serious adverse events (0.68 per 1000) and no reports of associated deaths.[40] All three studies support the safety of tumescent liposuction performed by dermatologists in an office setting.

Because the tumescent anesthetic technique for venous procedures has been adopted from the liposuction community, we feel these data are relevant to subcutaneous venous surgery using dilute tumescent anesthesia. There have been no adverse events reported to the Florida ACHA as a result of varicose vein surgery using tumescent anesthesia.

Advantages of office-based surgery are ease of scheduling for doctor and patient, less paperwork (unnecessary duplication of information and record keeping), no waiting for other surgeons to finish their operations, elimination of travel time, and cost containment for the health care system. Furthermore, a staff that performs the same procedures daily is more streamlined and safe.

CONCLUSION

Ambulatory phlebectomy is elegant by its mere simplicity. It is effective and safe with acceptable cosmetic results (see Figure 26.4). AP is a perfect complement to endovenous thermal ablation of the saphenous veins. With this combination, patients can expect all varicose veins to vanish

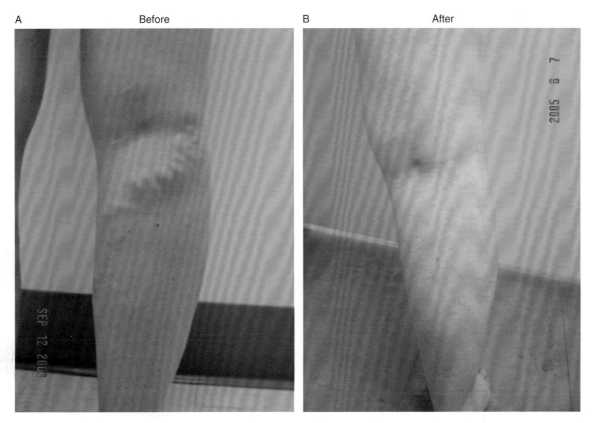

A   Before   B   After

Figure 26.4   Before and after photos.

following a 1-hour procedure that employed only local anesthesia, in the comfort of a physician's office.

REFERENCES

1. Celsus AC. *Medicinae libri octo, patavii: Typis seminarii apud joannem manfre, liber septimus.* 1749. 473–474.
2. Muller R. Traitement des varices par la phlebectomie ambulatoire, *Phlebologie.* 1966. *19*: 277–279.
3. Goren G, Yellin AE. Surgery for varicose veins: The ambulatory stab avulsion phlebectomy, *Am J Surg.* 1991. *162*: 166–174.
4. Weiss RA, Goldman MP. Transillumination mapping prior to ambulatory phlebectomy, *Dermatol Surg.* 1998. *24*: 447–450.
5. Proebstle TM, Paepcke U, Weisel G, Gass S, Weber L. High ligation and stripping of the long saphenous vein using the tumescent technique for local anaesthesia, *Dermatol Surg.* 1998. *24*: 149–153.
6. Klein JA. The tumescent technique for liposuction surgery, *Am J Cosmet Surg.* 1987. *4*: 263–267.
7. Cohn MS, Seiger E, Goldman S. Ambulatory phlebectomy using the tumescent technique for local anaesthesia, *Dermatol Surg.* 1995. *21*: 315–318.
8. Klein JA. Tumescent technique for local anaesthesia improves safety in large-volume liposuction, *Plast Reconstr Surg.* 1993. *92* 1085–1098.
9. Keel D, Goldman MP. Tumescent anaesthesia in ambulatory phlebectomy: Addition of epinephrine, *Dermatol Surg.* 1999. *25*: 371–372.
10. Schmid RM, Rosenkranz HS. Antimicrobial activity of local anaesthetics: Lidocaine and procaine, *J Infect Dis.* 1970. *121*: 597.
11. Ricci S. Ambulatory phlebectomy: Principles and evolution of the method, *Dermatol Surg.* 1998. *24*: 459–464.
12. Olivencia JA. Complications of ambulatory phlebectomy: Review of 1,000 consecutive cases, *Dermatol Surg.* 1997. *23*: 51–54.
13. Gauthier Y. Incidents and complications. In: Dortu J, Raymond-Martimbeau P, eds. *Ambulatory Phlebectomy/Phlebectomie Ambulatoire.* Houston: PRM Editions. 1993. 109–112.
14. Ramelet AA. Complications of ambulatory phlebectomy, *Dermatol Surg.* 1997. *23*: 947–954.
15. Jones L, Braithwaite BD, Selwyn D, Cooke S, Earnshaw JJ. Neovascularisation is the principal cause of varicose vein recurrence: Results of a randomized trial of stripping the long saphenous vein, *Eur J Vasc Endovasc Surg.* 1996. *12*(4): 442–445.
16. Winterborn RJ, Foy C, Earnshaw JJ. Causes of varicose vein recurrence: Late results of a randomized controlled trial of stripping the long saphenous vein, *J Vasc Surg.* 2004. *40*(4): 634–639.
17. Dwerryhouse S, Davies B, Harradine K, Earnshaw JJ. Stripping the long saphenous vein reduces the rate of reoperation for recurrent varicose veins: Five-year results of a randomized trial, *J Vasc Surg.* 1999. *29*(4): 589–592.
18. Sarin S, Scurr JH, Coleridge Smith PD. Stripping of the long saphenous vein in the treatment of primary varicose veins, *Br J Surg.* 1994. *81*(10): 1455–1458.
19. Min RJ, Khilnani N, Zimmet SE. Endovenous laser treatment of saphenous vein reflux: Long-term results, *J Vasc Interv Radiol.* 2003. *14*(8): 991–996.
20. Merchant RF, Pichot O, Myers KA. Four-year follow-up on endovascular radiofrequency obliteration of great saphenous reflux, *Dermatol Surg.* 2005. *31*(2): 129–134.
21. Labropoulos N, Kang SS, Mansour MA, Giannoukas AD, Buckman J, Baker WH. Primary superficial vein reflux with competent saphenous trunk, *Eur J Vasc Endovasc Surg.* 1999. *18*(3): 201–206.
22. Aremu MA, Mahendran B, Butcher W, et al. Prospective randomized controlled trial: Conventional versus powered phlebectomy, *J Vasc Surg.* 2004. *39*(1): 88–94.
23. Spitz GA, Braxton JM, Bergan JJ. Outpatient varicose vein surgery with transilluminated powered phlebectomy, *Vasc Surg* 2000. *34*: 547–555.

24. Arumugasamy M, McGreal G, O'Connor A, Kelly C, Bouchier-Hayes D, Leahy A. The technique of transilluminated powered phlebectomy: A novel minimally invasive system for varicose vein surgery, *Eur J Vasc Endovasc Surg*. 2002. *23*: 180–182.

25. Scavée V, Theys S, Schoevaerdts JC. Transilluminated powered miniphlebectomy: Early clinical experience, *Acta Chir Belg*. 2001. *101*: 247–249.

26. Cheshire N, Elias SM, Keagy B, et al. Powered phlebectomy (TriVex) in treatment of varicose veins, *Ann Vasc Surg*. 2002. *16*: 488–494.

27. Scavée V, Lesceu O, Theys S, Jamart J, Louagie Y, Schoevaerdts JC. Hook phlebectomy versus transilluminated powered phlebectomy for varicose vein surgery: Early results, *Eur J Vasc Endovasc Surg*. 2003. *25*: 473–475.

28. Fegan WG. Continuous compression technique for injecting varicose veins, *Lancet* 1963. *20*(2): 109–109.

29. De Roos KP, Nieman FH, Neumann HA. Ambulatory phlebectomy versus compression sclerotherapy: Results of a randomized controlled trial, *Dermatol Surg*. 2003. *29*(3): 221–226.

30. Olivencia JA. Ambulatory phlebectomy of the foot: Review of 75 patients, *Dermatol Surg*. 1997. *23*: 279–280.

31. Muller R. Traitement des varices du pied par la phlebectomie ambulatoire, *Phlebologie*. 1990. *43*: 317–318.

32. Constancias-Dortu I. Indications therapeutiques de la phlebectomie ambulatoire, *Phlebologie*. 1987. *40*: 853–858.

33. Fante RG, Goldman MP. Removal of periocular veins by sclerotherapy, *Ophthalmology*. 2001. *108*: 433–434.

34. Siniluoto TM, Svendsen PA, Wikholm GM, Fogdestam I, Edstrom S. Percutaneous sclerotherapy of venous malformations of the head and neck using sodium tetradecyl sulphate (sotradecol), *Scand J Plast Reconstr Surg Hand Surg*. 1997. *31*: 145–150.

35. Weiss RA, Ramelet AA. Removal of blue periocular lower eyelid veins by ambulatory phlebectomy, *Dermatol Surg*. 2002. *28*(1): 43–45.

36. Rao RB, Ely SF, Hoffman RS. Deaths related to liposuction, *N Engl J Med*. 1999. *340*: 1471–1475.

37. Hanke CW, Bernstein G, Bullock S. Safety of tumescent liposuction in 15,336 patients, *Dermatol Surg*. 1995. *21*: 459–462.

38. Coldiron B, Fisher AH, Adelman E, et al. Adverse event reporting: Lessons learned from 4 years of Florida office data, *Dermatol Surg*. 2005. *31*(9): 1079–1093.

39. Coleman W, Hanke C, Lillis P, et al. Does the location of the surgery or the specialty of the physician affect malpractice claims in liposuction?, *Dermatol Surg*. 1999. *25*: 343–347.

40. Housman TS, Lawrence N, Mellen BG, et al. The safety of liposuction: Results of a national survey, *Dermatol Surg*. 2002. *28*: 971–978.

27.

TRANSILLUMINATED POWERED PHLEBECTOMY

Nick Morrison

Transilluminated powered phlebectomy (TIPP) is also known by the trade name TriVex. TIPP is a mechanical method used to remove tributary varicose veins that would normally be excised with the traditional techniques of stab avulsion and hook phlebectomy. The indications for TIPP are the same as for traditional phlebectomy. The TriVex system consists of a transilluminator/irrigator (Figure 27.1) and a powered resector (Figure 27.2).

The operation is generally performed under general, spinal, or laryngeal mask airway anesthesia.[1] Reports on the use of local tumescent anesthesia have also appeared.[2]

The transilluminator/irrigator is placed subcutaneously to provide visualization of the varicose veins and instillation of the tumescent fluid (Figure 27.3). The varicosities are removed using the powered resector with its rotating blade on suction mode (Figure 27.4). Later modifications of the technique including the use of larger blades and slower speeds seemed to cause less tissue trauma.[3]

Complications include hematoma, subcutaneous scarring, bruising, and hyperpigmentation among the most notable. Both over-resecting and shearing through tissue cause subcutaneous scarring and bruising.

The reported advantages of the TIPP technique compared to traditional open surgery are shorter procedure time, decreased number of incisions, similar patient satisfaction, and similar complication rates, when compared with traditional methods.[4-6] Cheshire et al reported the average phlebectomy time as 14 minutes and the median number of incisions as three.[7] Improved results with experience was expected and was reported by a number of investigators.[4,5,8] And in a Swedish report, Akesson described satisfactory results in eighteen of twenty-one patients undergoing TIPP.[9] Proponents acknowledge that the learning curve leads from poorer early cosmetic results to improved results with experience.[10]

However, some more recent reports have questioned the reported advantages of TIPP compared to

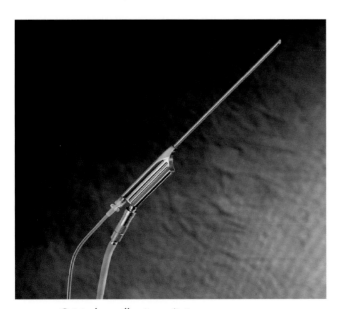

Figure 27.1   Original transilluminator/irrigator.

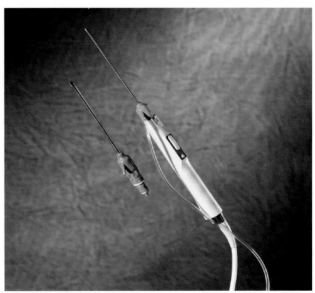

Figure 27.2   Original powered resector.

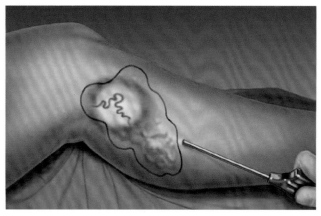

Figure 27.3 Instillation of tumescent fluid.

microphlebectomy. Scavee noted that "no trial has proven any significant advantage of TIPP technique when compared with conventional surgery, except for the number of surgical incisions, although TIPP procedure seems to be shorter than conventional surgery, particularly for the extensive or recurrent varicose veins."[11] And Luebke and Brunwall reported a "significant statistical advantage of TIPP technique over the conventional treatment, only for number of incisions, mean cosmetic score and duration of the procedure. However the TIPP technique seemed to be faster only for extensive varicose veins. There was, however, a significantly reduced incidence of calf hematoma after hook phlebectomy compared to TIPP, and TIPP procedure was associated with a worse mean pain score."[12]

In a randomized clinical trial comparing traditional microphlebectomy with TIPP, Chetter et al reported that while TIPP had the advantage of fewer surgical incisions, it was associated with more extensive bruising, prolonged pain, and reduced early postoperative quality of life than microphlebectomy.[13]

And in a letter to the editor regarding Akesson's report, Stefano Ricci pointed out that TIPP was complicated, expensive to deliver, dangerous because of excessive

tissue removal, and "cosmetically insufficient" since 15% of patients (3/21) had "remaining problems," a figure much higher than with microphlebectomy.[14]

For many reasons, enthusiasm for TIPP has waned.

CONCLUSIONS

Endovenous thermal ablation and TIPP are generally safe. Technical challenges, intraoperative and postoperative adverse events, and sequelae are infrequent and generally are seen less frequently with endovenous thermal ablation than with more traditional surgical procedures.

Differences in methods of follow-up examination, and in definitions of successful ablation, may help explain differences in results between published reports and those seen in the provider's own clinical setting. Only long-term follow-up will show where these minimally invasive methods belong in the therapeutic armamentarium of the treatment of chronic venous insufficiency of the lower extremity. While some surgeons have expressed the view that none of these techniques has yet been shown to improve on conventional surgery in the long term, the patient's perception has uniformly been that minimal invasion is better.

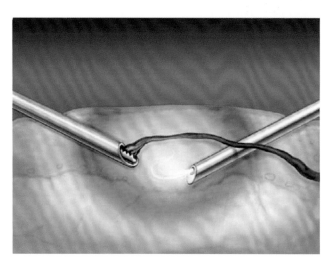

Figure 27.4 Resection of varicosities.

REFERENCES

1. Spitz GA, Braxton JM, Bergan JJ. Outpatient varicose vein surgery with transilluminated powered phlebectomy, *Vasc Endovascular Surg.* 2000. *34*: 547–555.
2. de Zeeuw R, Wittens C, Loots M, Neumann M. Transilluminated powered phlebectomy accomplished by local tumescent anaesthesia in the treatment of tributary varicose veins: Preliminary clinical results, *Phlebology.* 2007. *22*(2): 90–94.
3. Elias SM, Frasier KL. Minimally invasive vein surgery: Its role in the treatment of venous stasis ulceration, *Am J Surg.* 2004. *188*(1A Suppl): 26–30.
4. Ray-Chaudhuri SB, Huq Z, Souter RG, McWhinnie D. A randomized controlled trial comparing transilluminated powered phlebectomy with hook avulsions: An adjunct to day surgery?, *J One Day Surg.* 2003. *13*(2): 24–27.

5. Aremu M, Mahendran B, Butcher W, et al. Prospective randomized controlled trial: Conventional versus powered phlebectomy, *J Vasc Surg.* 2004. *39*(1): 88–94.

6. Scavee V, Lesceu O, Theys S, Jamart J, Louagie Y, Schoevaerdts JC. Hook phlebectomy versus transilluminated powered phlebectomy for varicose vein surgery: Early results, *European J Vasc Endovascular Surg.* 2003. *25*(5): 473–475.

7. Cheshire N, Elias SM, Keagy B, et al. Powered phlebectomy (TriVexTM) in treatment of varicose veins, *Ann Vasc Surg.* 2002. *16*(4): 488–494.

8. Franz RW, Knapp ED. Transilluminated powered phlebectomy surgery for varicose veins: A review of 339 consecutive patients, *Ann Vasc Surg.* 2009. *23*(3): 303–309.

9. Akesson H. Transilluminated powered phlebectomy: A clinical report, *Phlebology.* 2008. *23*: 295–298.

10. Elias SM, Frasier KL. Minimally invasive vein surgery, *Mt Sinai J Med.* 2004. *71*(1): 42–46. Review.

11. Scavee V. Transilluminated powered phlebectomy: Not enough advantages? Review of the literature, *Eur J Vasc Endovasc Surg.* 2006. *31*(3): 316–319.

12. Luebke T, Brunkwall J. Meta-analysis of transilluminated powered phlebectomy for superficial varicosities, *J Cardiovasc Surg (Torino).* 2008. *49*(6): 757–764.

13. Chetter IC, Mylankal KJ, Hughes H, Fitridge R. Randomized clinical trial comparing multiple stab incision phlebectomy and transilluminated powered phlebectomy for varicose veins, *Br J Surg.* 2006. *93*(2):169–174.

14. Ricci S. Letter regarding article titled "Transilluminated powered phlebectomy: a clinical report," *Phlebology.* 2009. *24*: 189.

28.

LASER AND RADIOFREQUENCY ABLATION

Nick Morrison

TREATMENT OBJECTIVES

Superficial venous disorders are nonlethal disease processes, treatment of which is held to a higher standard with respect to the risk of complications than in the treatment of a life-threatening disease. The objective of treatment will be the ablation of venous incompetence, whatever its source—axial, tributary, or perforator vein reflux. Achieving this objective will nearly always involve a combination of approaches to the different sources of reflux, such as ablation of the great, small, and/or major tributary veins, removal of other incompetent tributaries from the venous circulation, and interruption/correction of reflux in perforator veins. Therapeutic intervention should promote improved venous function using the most cosmetically appropriate methods available, while being mindful of the need to minimize the risk of complications.

SUPERFICIAL VENOUS ABLATION

The indications and contraindications for endovenous ablation procedures are essentially the same for any superficial venous ablative procedure. Indications should include: symptoms and physical signs of venous insufficiency; duplex scan showing a patent proximal vein with reflux greater than 0.5 s; patent deep venous system; vein conducive to instrumentation; and a fully mobile patient. Contraindications may include patients with arteriovenous malformations, restricted ambulation, and deep venous obstruction. A duplex scan of the entire deep and superficial system, performed by a qualified sonographer, is mandatory prior to any intervention. Specific indications/contraindications will be amplified in relation to specific techniques.

ENDOVENOUS THERMAL ABLATION

INTRODUCTION

Since 2000, endovenous thermal ablation has been reported to be a safe and effective method of removing the great saphenous vein (GSV) from the venous circulation, with faster recovery and better cosmetic results than either the traditional or perforate invagination (PIN) stripping procedures.[1-10] The ClosureFAST radiofrequency (RF) system (Covidien, Mansfield, Massachusetts) results in segmental destruction of the vein wall by means of conductive heating. Another RF system is available in Europe (Olympus Celon RFITT Olympus Medical Systems, Hamburg, Germany), but clinical data regarding this device in English literature are scarce. Various laser generators produce wavelengths of 808 to 1500 nm to induce vein wall destruction with conduction and/or convective heating.

Extensive international experience with endovenous thermal ablation has resulted in widespread adoption by phlebologists, particularly in the United States. As a result of this experience successful ablation of additional veins such as the small saphenous vein (SSV), major tributaries such as the anterior or posterior accessory saphenous vein (AASV, PASV), and perforator veins have been reported.[11-19] As with a stripping procedure, it is important to treat the incompetent distal saphenous vein, tributaries, and *persistently* incompetent perforator veins in order to eliminate all major sources of venous insufficiency.[20]

OUTCOME LITERATURE

Prospective randomized studies directly comparing RF ablation with stripping, reported by Lurie,[21,22] Stotter,[23] and Rautio et al.[1] demonstrated successful ablation, with patient-reported outcomes of less painful recovery and faster return to work with RF than with stripping. Five-year data published in 2005 from the VNUS registry suggest that the Closure procedure is effective in occluding target veins and abolishing reflux.[11] In this report, vein occlusion was documented by duplex ultrasound in 87.1% of legs at 1 year; 88.2% at 2 years, 83.5% at 3 years, 84.9% at 4 years, and 87.2% at 5 years. A major deficiency of this report is lack of life-table analysis, as the statistical analysis effectively ignores all patients lost to follow-up, thus skewing success rates. Although early reports are encouraging for the newer generation RF system, it must be noted that few peer-reviewed publications have thus far examined the success and complications.[24]

Similar rates of successful ablation are found in the laser thermal ablation literature, mostly single-center series reports, from the early reports of Min[5] and Proebstle[25] showing 93% and 100% success respectively, to the well-documented series of Myers[6,9] reporting 76% primary success at 4 years by life-table analysis, and 97% secondary success when ultrasound-guided foam sclerotherapy is used in those patients with recurrent vein patency.

TECHNICAL EQUIPMENT

RF GENERATOR

The RF ClosureFAST system destroys the vein wall with segmental conductive heating resulting in fibrotic occlusion of the target vein. The heat generated has shown tissue penetration of 1.5 mm, and in the absence of dilute local anesthetic surrounding the vein, heating of surrounding tissues can occur also by means of conduction. The addition of the local anesthetic mitigates damage to the surrounding tissue by conducted heat.[26]

LASER GENERATOR

The first laser generators introduced were in the range of 800- to 1,000-nm wavelengths. More recently somewhat higher wavelengths from 1,300 nm to 1,500 nm have been used. There remains some controversy regarding the mechanism of vein wall destruction, that is, whether it occurs by direct contact or indirectly via steam bubbles.[25,27,28] It is theorized that the higher wavelength lasers result in less postoperative bruising and discomfort for patients because the primary chromophore for the lower wavelength lasers is the hemoglobin in intravascular blood, while for the higher wavelength lasers it is water contained in the vein wall. Consequently the higher wavelength lasers may produce fewer vein wall perforations because less energy is necessary to target the vein wall; this may lead to a more comfortable recovery period than with the lower wavelength lasers.[29] But

most phlebologists can agree that all commonly used laser generators are highly effective.

RF CATHETER

Early in the RF experience, treatment of veins larger than 12 mm in diameter was not recommended. However, experience has demonstrated that given adequate ultrasound-guided deposition of dilute local anesthetic completely surrounding the target vein, successful treatment of veins much larger than 12 mm is quite feasible.[30] The 7Fr ClosureFAST catheters (Figure 28.1) for treatment of truncal veins, and the ClosureRFS for perforator veins, both have a central lumen allowing for infusion of fluid (often heparinized saline) or a guide wire to assist advancement of the catheter to the uppermost limit of the intended treatment.

LASER FIBERS

Fiber size is generally 200 to 600 μm, with a bare-tipped fiber most commonly used. Other radial-emitting fibers,[31] tulip-shaped catheters[8,10] and jacketed fibers have been developed to avoid direct vein wall contact and to promote a uniform delivery of laser energy, and therefore presumably reduce the incidence of vein wall perforations during thermal ablation.

CONTRAINDICATIONS

Absolute exclusion criteria include arteriovenous malformations, restricted ambulation, and deep venous obstruction. Relative exclusion criteria might also include: vein tortuosity; veins less than 2 mm or greater than 25 mm; partial obstruction of the proximal vein; and known thrombophilia.

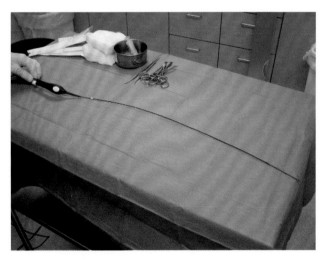

Figure 28.1 ClosureFAST catheter.

PROCEDURE

Many practitioners have preferred to perform these procedures in the hospital surgical or radiological suites, frequently under general or regional anesthesia or using conscious sedation. More recently, in the U.S. a variety of factors have combined to encourage displacement of the endovenous ablation procedure out of the hospital and into the office setting under local anesthesia. Furthermore, while the thermal ablation procedure is often performed on veins other than the GSV, the technical details remain quite similar for other veins and for laser ablation.

After obtaining informed consent, patients may be given oral or intravenous sedation prior to the procedure. Antibiotic and/or anticoagulation prophylaxis is not generally used in the U.S., unless specific indications for them are present. The patient is placed on an adjustable operating table (with Trendelenberg capability), and the course of the target vein is mapped. The insertion site is chosen to maximize treatment length and to assure facile access. Placing the patient in a semi-erect position will help dilate the vein and enhance successful cannulation.

The distal portions of the great and/or small saphenous vein may be treated with endovenous thermal ablation if the practitioner is highly skilled in the delivery of ultrasound-guided local anesthetic and the patient is aware of the potentially increased risk of paresthesia from damage to the saphenous or sural nerve, which is in close proximity to these veins distally. Thermal ablation of the most proximal portion of the SSV nearest the saphenopopliteal junction (SPJ) should be avoided to reduce the risk of common peroneal or posterior tibial nerve damage, with the disastrous result of foot drop.

Access to the vein may be achieved using an ultrasound-guided, percutaneously placed needle, or via microincision and hooking of the vein for direct venapuncture. If the percutaneous method is used, Nitropaste may be helpful at the proposed insertion site prior to the sterile surgical prep to improve access by dilating the vein and preventing venospasm. It is sometimes appropriate to choose a primary access site and a more proximal, larger diameter, secondary (backup) access site in case access at the primary site is unsuccessful. Perivenous or intramural hematoma from unsuccessful attempts at cannulation may render that portion of the vein technically inaccessible, leading to the need for a secondary site. As the practitioner's ultrasound-guided technical skills improve, even veins as small as 2 mm in diameter or less, or more than 25 mm in diameter, can be successfully cannulated and treated.

The first attempt at cannulation of the vein is the most likely to be successful, so the insertion site should be carefully chosen to make access as ergonomically advantageous as possible. Just below the knee, the GSV is relatively anterior, and with the patient's operative leg externally rotated, this site becomes more advantageous than in the distal or mid thigh. And even though the saphenous nerve is closer to the vein in this area, the catheter/fiber sheath will prevent treatment of this portion of vein, and thus reduce the risk of nerve damage. The insertion site for the SSV is usually at the junction of the middle and distal third of the calf.

Following removal of the Nitropaste, the leg is cleansed with an antiseptic. The operative area is isolated with sterile drapes. After infiltration of local anesthetic at the insertion site, an introducer needle is inserted into the vein under ultrasound guidance; or a small incision is made and the vein is withdrawn through the skin incision with a phlebectomy hook. After advancement of a guide wire into the vein, a sheath is advanced into the vein. If desired, the tip of the sheath can be positioned near the deep venous junction, just below the entrance of the superficial epigastric vein into the GSV, or to the point at which the SSV angulates to join the popliteal vein; position of the sheath is confirmed by ultrasound. Alternatively, a shorter sheath may be used and the bare catheter/fiber advanced to the area of the deep venous junction. Occasionally, passage of the catheter/fiber may be impeded by vein tortuosity. Usually straightening of the leg or manipulation of the catheter/fiber by external compression will allow advancement. If these maneuvers are unsuccessful, a guide wire threaded through the RF catheter and beyond the point of difficulty, with subsequent advancement of the catheter over the guide wire will allow appropriate positioning of the tip of the catheter. Segmental stenosis from previous sclerotherapy will sometimes also impede advancement of the catheter/fiber. In this case, or if the vein is so tortuous as to not allow passage of the catheter, a second cannulation, with another insertion kit, will allow treatment of first the proximal and then the distal segments of the vein.

Using ultrasound guidance, high-volume dilute anesthetic solution is then injected into the saphenous compartment (Figure 28.2) from the insertion site to below the deep venous junction. The patient is sometimes placed in

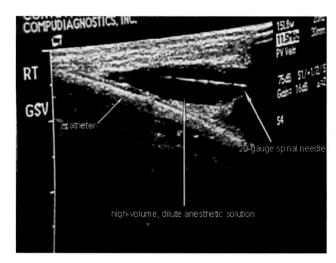

Figure 28.2   GSV, with catheter inside, compressed by local anesthetic solution.

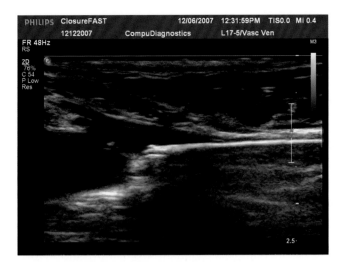

Figure 28.3   RF catheter in GSV with tip just inferior to entrance of the superficial epigastric vein and SFJ.

a moderate Trendelenberg position to enhance a bloodless vein, and the final position of the tip of the catheter/fiber is confirmed by ultrasound (Figures 28.3 and 28.4), below the entrance of the superficial epigastric vein in the GSV (or alternatively, 2 cm below the saphenofemoral junction [SFJ]), and 2 to 3cm below the SPJ. The anesthetic solution is finally injected into the tissue surrounding the proximal 3 to 4 cm of the vein. Alternatively, one may use regional (femoral nerve block) or general anesthesia, but both are far less commonly used in the United States than internationally. The advantages of tumescent anesthesia are the patient's ability to ambulate immediately after the procedure (possibly reducing the risk of venous stasis and consequent deep vein thrombosis), and the protection of the delicate tissues surrounding the treated vein (possible reducing the incidence of postoperative paresthesia or neuropraxia). The maximum volume of local anesthetic is not accurately known, but with the use of 0.1% xylocaine with epinephrine

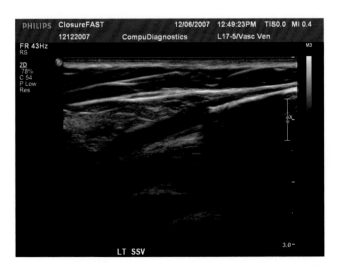

Figure 28.4   RF catheter tip within small saphenous vein (SSV) where SSV angulates to join popliteal vein at the SPJ, 2 to 3 cm from the SPJ.

solution, it is thought that a dose less than 45 mg/kg lidocaine (less than 3,100 mL in a 70 kg patient) is safe.[32]

The withdrawal of the ClosureFAST RF catheter is in 6.5-cm segments after a 7-cm section has been treated, while with the Olympus system, the rate is reportedly 1 cm/s. Withdrawal rate of laser fibers depends on the equipment and the energy delivered, but will range from 1 to 4 mm/s. Laser energy delivery is usually reported as linear endovenous energy density (LEED) in joules per centimeter (J/cm) and ranges from 50 to 150 J/cm. In general, the higher the energy delivered, not only the higher the occlusion rate but also the higher the complication rate, while the converse also appears to be true.

On conclusion of the procedure, patients may then be placed in compression therapy, for example, short-stretch bandages or graduated compression hose (thigh-high or panty—patient's preference); some use eccentric compression with firm pads. Although level-1 evidence is lacking, most phlebologists maintain compression for at least several days, if not longer, to enhance patient comfort and reduce ecchymosis and the risk of superficial thrombophlebitis. Adjunctive SFJ ligation is thought to be not only unnecessary but also meddlesome and it increases the risk of recurrence through neovascularization.

FOLLOW-UP

Because of the possibility of incomplete ablation or recurrent patency of the treated vein, and the need for adjunctive treatment of the distal saphenous veins, the refluxing tributaries or *persistently* incompetent large perforator veins, color-flow Doppler ultrasound, interviews, and physical examinations at appropriate intervals are needed to assure a successful outcome. At a minimum, patients should be examined at 1 week, 6 months, and 1 year following thermal ablation of the target vein. More frequent follow-up visits will often reveal the need for adjunctive treatment earlier in the postoperative course, and result in more complete treatment of the venous insufficiency with better and sustained resolution of the patient's symptom complex. It is not appropriate to merely ablate the proximal portion of an incompetent vein and expect resolution of every patient's symptoms and varicosities. Unless one is committed to a program of meticulous follow-up and adjunctive treatment, the practitioner and the patient will be left with unsatisfactory results.

COMPLICATIONS

Authors from the American Venous Forum and the Society for Interventional Radiology have proposed guidelines for reporting of results and complications following endovenous ablation techniques by which it is hoped some standardization of outcome reporting will result.[33]

Complications may be divided into intraoperative and postoperative adverse events. Intraoperative adverse events can be technical challenges and adverse patient events (Table 28.1). The technical challenges one may encounter are: difficult access (venospasm, access location); and problems threading the catheter/fiber (vein tortuosity, aneurysmal segments), or sclerosis from previous sclerotherapy. Adverse patient events that can occur are: dysrrhythmia or vagal reaction (often because of anxiety); saphenous nerve pain, or transient heat (inadequate anesthetic infiltration).

Postoperative adverse events (or expected sequelae) include bruising, paresthesia, infection, intramural hematoma, skin burn, superficial thrombophlebitis, lymphedema, and deep vein thrombosis (Table 28.2). Bruising is nearly always minimal, and of less than 2 weeks' duration. Unlike following groin-to-ankle stripping, paresthesia following endovenous ablation is usually mild, short-lived, and limited to the distal thigh. It is seen in 2 to 23% of patients,[2,22,24,34] and its rate of occurrence appears to be inversely related to the experience of the practitioner with ultrasound-guided techniques. Infection and skin burns are rare, occurring in less than 0.1% of patients. These are avoided with good sterile technique and accurately placed and adequate ultrasound-guided anesthetic volume to protect the structures in close proximity to the vein, and to separate the skin from the underlying vein. Superficial thrombophlebitis is seen in less than 5% of cases,[11,24,35] and responds to the usual clinical measures of anti-inflammatory medication, compression, and ambulation. Lymphedema has not been reported, but we have seen it in our own center, and is believed to be most commonly caused from unrecognized impaired lymphatic drainage usually present prior to any procedures. Treatment of this complication (or more likely sequela) will include therapeutic lymphatic massage, compression with multilayered low-stretch bandages, compression hose, and exercise.

Deep vein thrombosis is the most significant complication, and is generally reported to occur in less than 1% of the patients (depending on the duplex scanning interval and the quality of the examination).[2,24] Most reported cases are calf vein thrombosis, and if stability is demonstrated by serial duplex examinations, these are of limited clinical significance.

Table 28.1 INTRAOPERATIVE ADVERSE EVENTS

TECHNICAL CHALLENGES	ADVERSE PATIENT EVENTS
Difficult access	Painful insertion
Dysrrhythmia	
Trouble threading introducer wire/ catheter	Vagal reaction
Treatment interruption (with ClosurePLUS)	Transient heat
Unable to reinsert catheter	Saphenous nerve pain
GSV tortuosity	
Aneurysmal segments	

Table 28.2 POSTOPERATIVE ADVERSE EVENTS

(or expected sequelae)
Bruising
Paresthesia
Skin burn
Superficial thrombophlebitis
Lymphedema
Deep vein thrombosis
Infection

Therapy is usually as an outpatient, with compression, ambulation, and anti-inflammatory medication. Several reports of SFJ or SPJ thrombus extensions have been published.[14,19,35] These appear to be of an entirely different character than those seen in association of spontaneous superficial thrombophlebitis of the GSV or SSV. Clinically relevant sequelae of these types of thromboses are rare, and if demonstrated to be resolving by serial duplex examination, can be treated expectantly. More extensive proximal thromboses do occur, however, and should be aggressively searched for and treated,[36] including with percutaneous pharmacomechanical treatment if prudent.

One complication, of interest because of its relative absence, is neovascularization. Neovascularization is commonly seen following the traditional surgical high ligation procedure, wherein all tributaries of the great saphenous vein are carefully dissected and divided.[37] It is thought to be secondary to "frustrated" venous drainage from the abdominal wall and perineum. The ultrasound picture of neovascularization, seen as grape-like clusters of veins in the groin, is quite characteristic (Figure 28.5). Whether this is actually the development of new veins, or simply enlargement of previously existing veins, the result is recurrent reflux in veins of the thigh and lower leg. The endovenous ablation procedure

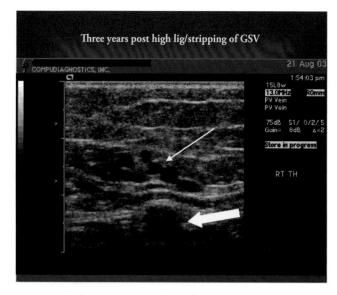

Figure 28.5   Block arrow: common femoral vein; Line arrow: neovascularization.

deliberately avoids a groin incision and leaves the superficial epigastric vein intact, which, it is believed, has resulted in fewer reports of neovascularization at the 5-year interval.[11]

DISCUSSION

Considerable confusion in the literature exists regarding the definition of successful treatment, the means used to detect treatment failures, and the reporting of results. Agreement on the very definition of success has not yet been achieved, being variably reported as: sonographic absence of the target vein;[30] no flow in treated segment;[38] absence of visible reflux;[38] segmental patency of no more than 5 cm without reflux;[39] and resolution of symptoms.[2] Extensive advancements in the technology of ultrasound since the early 2000s have allowed far more critical evaluation of clinical results than was possible in the past. As a result of these advancements, it is now possible to more readily identify incompletely ablated veins. Recurrent patency can occur anywhere in the thermally ablated portion of the vein, either along its length or segmentally. Segmental recurrent patency is usually seen at the site of an incompetent perforator or a refluxing tributary. And because there are likely to be closed segments above and/or below the patent segment, distal compression of the closed portion of the vein to identify reflux is futile. Likewise, using Valsalva's maneuver to identify proximal patency is unreliable and lacks reproducibility. The use of more sensitive duplex ultrasound equipment and critical ultrasound examination of treated veins brings into question earlier reports in which success is defined as "absence of visible reflux" or "resolution of symptoms." Indeed, many patients will experience temporary resolution of symptoms following an incomplete ablation procedure, only to have those symptoms recur when reflux becomes clinically significant.

Identification of recurrent patency, incomplete ablation, or treatment failures is ultimately dependent on the sensitivity of the ultrasound equipment used for postoperative examination, the expertise of the sonographer, and the vigor with which the examination is conducted. In a study of ultrasound equipment from our center reported at the Union Internationale De Phlebologie (UIP) meeting in 2003, five different ultrasound machines commonly used in vascular laboratories were evaluated. Six patients with moderate reflux were examined by the same registered vascular technologist, using all five machines. The sensitivity of each machine was found to be: 100% (for the control machine); and 85%, 77%, 69%, and 62% for the other four machines (Figure 28.6). In other words, reflux was *not* identified in 15%, 23%, 31%, and 38% of the veins known to have reflux. Since identification of flow is directly related to the sensitivity of the duplex machine, it is reasonable to assume that following patients for postoperative results will be greatly influenced by the equipment used for the examinations. Further, the expertise and independence of the sonographer, the extent of their superficial venous experience, and the

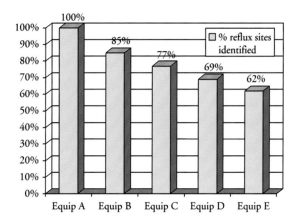

Figure 28.6 Comparison of sensitivity of duplex equipment.

care with which the examination is conducted are all factors of paramount importance in critical reporting of results.

No consensus has been established on such critical reporting issues as: duration of follow-up and duplex-scanning intervals; quality and sensitivity of duplex equipment used for follow-up examination of a treated vein; and training and experience of the duplex operator.

Thorough Duplex examination for successful ablation of a vein should include gray scale, compression, and color flow Doppler. Patients often have ultrasound-guided foam sclerotherapy for distal segments of the treated vein, refluxing tributaries of the treated vein, and incompetent perforators. Such foam sclerotherapy has had an unexpected effect on critical analysis of successful ablation. The ablated vein that remains sonographically identifiable long after it should have disappeared, but that by all of the duplex ultrasound criteria noted above is completely occluded, is commonly found to have foam within the vein following injection of a tributary, perforator, or distal segment. This further calls into question even the most critical examination techniques. Whether these minimally patent segments will become clinically significant is unknown at this time. But certainly patients who complain of localized pain in the area of a previously ablated vein deserve very careful examination to identify an incompletely ablated segment.

Adjunctive treatment in order to remove all sources of insufficiency from the venous circulation is thought by most to be mandatory. Adjunctive treatment may include such things as: endovenous ablation (thermal or chemical) of the incompetent accessory saphenous or major saphenous tributaries, and/or *persistently* incompetent perforators; ambulatory (micro)phlebectomy; and visual sclerotherapy. These techniques will help to achieve the greatest resolution of the patient's varicosities and symptoms.

It has been reported that most incompletely ablated veins will be seen in the first few months following treatment, since failure rates do not steadily increase over time.[11] However, we have identified patients more than 6 years following apparently successful ablation with recurrent symptoms and partially patent segments. Thus, it is necessary to perform thorough follow-up of these patients for 1 year, and then either yearly or certainly with recurrent symptoms.

The total cost of performing the procedure in-office in the United States under local anesthesia, exclusive of the provider's time, is generally between US$400 and $1100, depending on the equipment used.

REFERENCES

1. Rautio T, Ohinmaa A, Perala J, et al. Endovenous obliteration versus conventional stripping operation in the treatment of primary varicose veins: A randomized controlled trial with comparison of the costs, *J Vasc Surg.* 2002. *35*: 958–965.
2. Rautio T, Perala J, Wiik H, Juvonen T, Haukupuro K. Endovenous obliteration with radiofrequency resistive heating for greater saphenous vein insufficiency: A feasibility study, *J Vasc Interv Radiol.* 2002. *13*: 569–575.
3. Almeida JI, Raines JK. Radiofrequency ablation and laser ablation in the treatment of varicose veins, *Ann Vasc Surg.* 2006. *20*: 547–552.
4. Desmyttere J, Grard C, Wassmer B, Mordon S. Endovenous 980-nm laser treatment of saphenous veins in a series of 500 patients, *J Vasc Surg.* 2007. *46*: 1242–1247.
5. Min RJ, Khilnani NM, Zimmett SE. Endovenous laser treatment of saphenous vein reflux: Long-term results, *J Vasc Interv Rafiol.* 2003. *14*: 991–996.
6. Myers K, Fris R, Jolley D. Treatment of varicose veins by endovenous laser therapy: Assessment of results by ultrasound surveillance, *Med J Austral.* 2006. *185*: 199–202.
7. Rasmussen LH, Bjoern L, Lawaetz M, et al. Randomized trial comparing endovenous laser ablation of the great saphenous vein with high ligation and stripping in patients with varicose veins: Short term results, *J Vasc Surg.* 2007. *46*: 308–315.
8. Vuylsteke M, Van den Bussche D, Audenaert EA, Lissens P. Endovenous laser obliteration for the treatment of primary varicose veins, *Phlebology.* 2006. *21*(2): 80–87.
9. Myers K, Jolly D. Outcome of endovenous laser therapy for saphenous reflux and varicose veins: Medium-term results assessed by ultrasound surveillance, *Eur J Vasc Endovasc Surg.* 2009. *37*(2): 239–245.
10. Vuylsteke M, Van Dorpe J, Roelens J, De Bo T, Mordon S, Fourneau I. Intraluminal fibre-tip centring can improve endovenous laser ablation: A histological study, *Eur J Vasc Endovasc Surg.* 2010. *40*(1):110–116.
11. Merchant RF, Pichot O. Long-term outcomes of endovenous radiofrequency obliteration of saphenous reflux as a treatment for superficial venous insufficiency, *J Vasc Surg.* 2005. *42*: 502–509.
12. Elias S, Peden E. Ultrasound-guided percutaneous ablation for the treatment of perforating vein incompetence, *Vascular.* 2007. *15*(5): 281–289.
13. Gibson KD, Ferris BL, Polissar N, Neradilek B, Pepper D. Endovenous laser treatment of the short saphenous vein: Efficacy and complications, *J Vasc Surg.* 2007. *45*(4): 795–801; discussion 801–803.
14. Hingorani AP, Ascher E, Marks N, et al. Predictive factors following radio-frequency stylet ablation of incompetent perforating veins, *J Vasc Surg.* 2009. *50*: 844–848.
15. Theivacumar NS, Beale RJ, Mavor AI, Gough MJ. Initial experience in endovenous laser ablation (EVLA) of varicose veins due to small saphenous vein reflux, *Eur J Vasc Endovasc Surg.* 2007. *33*(5): 614–618.
16. Timperman PE, Sichlau M, Ryu RK. Greater energy delivery improves treatment success of endovenous laser treatment of incompetent saphenous veins, *J Vasc Interv Radiol.* 2004. *10*: 1061–1063.
17. Timperman PE. Prospective evaluation of higher energy great saphenous vein endovenous laser treatment, *J Vasc Interv Radiol.* 2005. *16*: 791–794.
18. Timperman PE. Endovenous laser treatment of incompetent below-knee great saphenous vein, *J Vasc Interv Radiol.* 2007. *18*: 1495–1499.
19. Hingorani A, Ascher E, Markevich N, et al. Deep venous thrombosis after radiofrequency ablation of greater saphenous vein: A word of caution, *J Vasc Surg.* 2004. *40*: 500–504.
20. Weiss RA, Feied CF, Weiss MA. *Vein diagnosis and treatment.* New York: McGraw-Hill Medical. 2001. 211–221.
21. Lurie F, Creton D, Eklof B, et al. Prospective randomised study of endovenous radiofrequency obliteration (closure) versus ligation and vein stripping (EVOLVeS): Two-year follow-up, *Eur J Vasc Endovasc Surg.* 2005. *29*: 67–73.
22. Lurie F, Creton D, Eklof B, et al. Prospective randomised study of endovenous radiofrequency obliteration (closure) versus ligation and stripping in a select patient population (EVOLVeS study), *J Vasc Surg.* 2003. *38*: 207–214.
23. Stotter L, Schaaf I, Bockelbrink A. Comparative outcomes of radiofrequency endoluminal ablation, invagination stripping, and cryostripping in the treatment of great saphenous vein insufficiency, *Phlebology.* 2006. *21*(2): 60–64.
24. Proebstle T, Vago B, Alm J, Gockeritz O, Lebard C, Pichot O. Treatment of the incompetent great saphenous vein by endovenous radiofrequency powered segmental thermal ablation: First clinical experience, *J Vasc Surg.* 2008. *47*(1): 151–156.
25. Proebstle TM, Lehr HA, Kargl A, et al. Endovenous treatment of the greater saphenous vein with a 940-nm diode laser: Thrombotic occlusion after endoluminal thermal damage by laser-generated steam bubbles, *J Vasc Surg.* 2002. *35*(4): 729–736.
26. Lumdsen A, Peden E. Clinical use of the new VNUS ClosureFAST radiofrequency catheter, *Endovasc Today.* 2007. (Suppl): 7–10.
27. Fan CM, Rox-Anderson R. Endovenous laser ablation: Mechanism of action, *Phlebology.* 2008. *23*(5): 206–213.
28. Bush RG. Regarding endovenous treatment of the greater saphenous vein with a 940-nm diode laser: Thrombolytic occlusion, *J Vasc Surg.* 2003. *36*: 242.
29. Goldman M, Mauricio M, Rao J. Intravascular 1320-nm laser closure of the great saphenous vein: A 6- to 12-month follow-up study, *Dermatol Surg.* 2004. *30*: 1380–1385.
30. Merchant R, Pichot O, Myers KA. Four years follow-up on endovascular radiofrequency obliteration of saphenous reflux, *Dermatol Surg.* 2005. *31*: 129–134.
31. Schwarz T, von Hodenberg E, Furtwangler C, Rastan A, Zeller T, Neumann FJ. Endovenous laser ablation of varicose veins with the 1470-nm diode laser, *J Vasc Surg.* 2010. *51*(6): 1474–1478.
32. Klein J. Maximum safe lidocaine dosage for tumescent anesthesia without liposuction is 45mg/kg: Abstract of presentation, 16th World Congress of Union Internationale de Phlebologie, Monaco, September, 2009.
33. Kundu S, Lurie F, Millward SF, et al. Recommended reporting standards for endovenous ablation for the treatment of venous insufficiency: Joint statement of the American Venous Forum and the Society of Interventional Radiology, *J Vasc Surg.* 2007. *46*: 582–589.
34. Weiss R, Weiss M. Controlled radiofrequency endovenous occlusion using a unique radiofrequency catheter under duplex guidance to eliminate saphenous varicose vein reflux: A 2-year follow-up, *Dermatol Surg.* 2002. *28*: 38–42.
35. Puggioni A, Kalra M, Carmo M, Mozes G, Gloviczki P. Endovenous laser therapy and radiofrequency ablation of the great saphenous vein: Analysis of early efficacy and complications, *J Vasc Surg.* 2005. *42*: 488–493.
36. Mozes G, Kalra M, Carmo M, Swenson L, Gloviczki P. Extension of saphenous thrombus into the femoral vein: A potential complication of new endovenous ablation techniques, *J Vasc Surg.* 2005. *41*: 130–135.
37. Perrin M. Endovenous therapy for varicose veins of the lower extremities (in French). *Ann Chir.* 2004. *129*: 248–257.
38. Pichot O, Kabnick LS, Creton D, Merchant RF, Schuller-Petrovic, Chandler JG. Duplex ultrasound scan findings two years after great saphenous vein radiofrequency endovenous obliteration, *J Vasc Surg.* 2004. *39*(1): 189–195.
39. Pichot O, Sessa C, Chandler JG, Nuta M, Perrin M. Role of duplex imaging in endovenous obliteration for primary venous insufficiency, *J Endovasc Ther.* 2000. *7*: 451–459.

29.

TREATMENT OF SMALL SAPHENOUS VEIN REFLUX

Kenneth Myers, Amy Clough, Stefania Roberts, and Damien Jolley

Venous anatomy in relation to small saphenous reflux is far more complicated than that relative to great saphenous reflux. The pathophysiology of small saphenous disease is poorly understood. There is no consensus as how to best treat small saphenous reflux, largely because of the lack of objective information regarding outcome. The few reports available show poor results after traditional surgery, so that there is a swing to endovenous treatment. Discussion will be largely based on findings from duplex ultrasound scanning.

EMBRYOLOGY

In the embryo, there are three venous plexuses of the lower limb: the axial, preaxial, and postaxial plexuses.[1,2] The three plexuses meet at the popliteal vein. The future small saphenous vein (SSV) and thigh extension (TE) derive from the postaxial venous plexus that accompanies the postaxial nerve (posterior femoral cutaneous nerve). What is now termed the vein of Giacomini is an anastomosis between the pre- and postaxial plexuses. Variations in the popliteal fossa presumably reflect whether or not the postaxial plexus maintains a connection with the popliteal vein.

ANATOMY

SSV

The SSV is always present and frequently continues as the TE. It is duplicated in less than 5% of limbs. There is a variable connection, if any, between the SSV and deep veins, and variable terminations of the TE. These patterns were well described by Giacomini in 1873[3,4] and have now been clearly defined by ultrasound.[5-9] Current terminology is described in a consensus document.[10]

The SSV originates from the lateral marginal vein of the foot and courses proximally on the posterior aspect of the calf, usually in the midline between the bellies of the gastrocnemius muscle. It turns deep to join the popliteal or femoral vein at the saphenopopliteal junction (SPJ) in approximately 75% of limbs but continues on as the TE without an SPJ in the remainder (SEE Figure 29.1). The SSV joins gastrocnemius veins rather than the popliteal vein in up to one-third of limbs, usually at or near the SPJ.[10] It is distinguished from tributaries on ultrasound by the observation that it lies in a fascial compartment from above the ankle, just as for the great saphenous vein (GSV).[10]

SPJ

The SPJ is the proximal end of the SSV above the preterminal valve otherwise referred to as the small saphenous arch. The SPJ is rudimentary or absent in approximately 25% of limbs (see Figure 29.1). When present, it usually lies within 4 cm above the knee crease. However, in approximately 25%

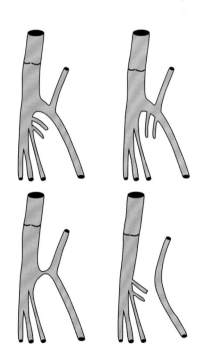

Figure 29.1 Presence or absence of an SPJ and variations in the destination of gastrocnemius veins.

of limbs it is above this level and then joins the proximal popliteal or femoral vein.[10] A low termination in the upper calf joining the gastrocnemius veins or GSV occurs in about 1%.[8,11] Ultrasound shows that the junction is at the posterior aspect of the popliteal vein in just 15%, and it joins on the medial or lateral side in approximately 85% and even anteriorly in 1% of limbs.[11]

TE AND VEIN OF GIACOMINI

The TE is present in approximately 70% of limbs and is frequently as large as the SSV. The TE passes upward in a groove between the semitendinosis and biceps femoris muscles in a fascial compartment just as for the SSV and GSV.[4,10] It usually extends to the middle or upper thigh and terminates in almost equal proportions into deep or superficial veins.[8] Giacomini clearly showed that what is now termed the TE may terminate in veins in the buttocks, posterior thigh perforators, or superficial tributaries (see Figure 29.2).[3,4] A communication of the TE with the posterior circumflex thigh vein to connect to the GSV is now termed the vein of Giacomini.[10] The terminal TE pierces the deep fascia if it passes to deep veins but passes superficial to the membranous fascia if it forms the vein of Giacomini.[10] Valves may be oriented in the TE to allow normal flow either cephalad or caudal[3] so that pathological "reflux" is defined as bidirectional flow.

GASTROCNEMIUS VEINS

Gastrocnemius veins drain from the medial and lateral gastrocnemius muscles, and the medial are larger than the lateral gastrocnemius veins. They have a variable pattern.[12]

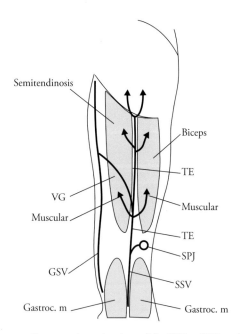

Figure 29.2 Course and terminations of the SSV and TE at the back of knee and thigh. (VG—vein of Giacomini).

Multiple veins draining from each muscle venous plexus most frequently join to form a pair of veins, which then become a single main trunk before joining the deep veins. The main trunk varies from 0.5 to 5.5 cm in length and usually has at least one valve. Drainage is to the popliteal vein in over 85% of limbs and to crural veins in the remainder. The main gastrocnemius veins can enter the popliteal vein separate to the SSV or with a conjoint junction.

ACCOMPANYING NERVES AND ARTERIES

Ricci and colleagues have studied the anatomy of the sural nerve by ultrasound.[13] It lies close to the SSV in the distal third of leg with a highly variable and more distant relationship in the proximal calf. It usually lies lateral to the SSV within the fascial space. The sural nerve does not share a common association of the perivenous and perineural fasciae as frequently occurs with the GSV and saphenous nerve.[14] The sural nerve has two accompanying arteries. Both the sural nerve and its arteries lying in close proximity to the SSV can be damaged by any form of intervention.[15–17]

The posterior tibial nerve lies lateral to the SSV in two-thirds and medial in one-third of legs, and the peroneal nerve almost always lies medially.[18,19] The posterior tibial nerve lies close to the SSV near the SPJ and often twines around the vein. These major nerves are prone to trauma during surgery to ligate the vein at the SPJ.

PATHOLOGY

The larger proportion of limbs with varicose disease have superficial reflux with or without deep reflux, with deep reflux alone uncommon (see Table 29.1).

REFLUX IN THE SSV TERRITORY

Approximately one-third of all limbs with saphenous disease have reflux in the SSV.[9] The prevalence of SSV reflux increases with greater clinical severity of disease

Table 29.1 **AN ULTRASOUND STUDY OF PROPORTIONS OF LIMBS WITH REFLUX IN THE SUPERFICIAL AND DEEP VEINS IN RELATION TO THE CLINICAL SEVERITY OF VENOUS DISEASE**

VENOUS REFLUX	C2–3 NUMBER	%	C4–6 NUMBER	%	TOTAL NUMBER	%
Superficial alone	1,626	89%	65	42%	1,691	85%
Superficial and deep	172	9%	73	47%	245	12%
Deep alone	29	2%	16	11%	45	3%
Total	1,827		154		1,981	
(Myers and colleagues—unpublished data)						

SUPERFICIAL REFLUX	C2–3 NUMBER	%	C4–6 NUMBER	%	TOTAL NUMBER	%
GSV alone	1,255	70%	65	47%	1,320	68%
SSV alone	242	13%	31	23%	273	14%
GSV & SSV	301	17%	42	30%	343	18%
Total	1,798		138		1,936	

(Myers and colleagues—unpublished data)

Table 29.4 AN ULTRASOUND STUDY OF THE
FREQUENCY OF ASSOCIATION BETWEEN REFLUX IN
THE TE OR VEIN OF GIACOMINI AND REFLUX IN THE
GSV OR SSV

SAPHENOUS REFLUX	NUMBER	NUMBER WITH TE REFLUX	% WITH TE REFLUX
GSV alone	922	6	1%
SSV alone	138	23	17%
GSV & SSV	166	47	28%
Total	1,226	76	6%

(From Reference 2)

(see Table 29.2). The SPJ is competent in approximately one-third of limbs with SSV reflux with other incompetent connections to the SSV from popliteal perforators, pelvic veins, GSV, or thigh veins (see Table 29.3). Cavezzi and colleagues found with ultrasound that most limbs show reflux after release of calf compression but that a few show flow through the SPJ during calf compression, particularly where the destination for flow is into the TE.[5]

SSV reflux is a significant risk factor for recurrence of venous ulceration.[7] Ulcers associated with GSV reflux may be on any aspect of the leg, but ulceration over the lateral aspect of the ankle usually is associated with SSV reflux, often without associated pigmentation or eczema.[20]

BIDIRECTIONAL FLOW IN THE TE AND VEIN OF GIACOMINI

This is far more likely to occur in association with SSV than GSV reflux (see Table 29.4).[4] Saphenopopliteal incompetence can result in distal to proximal flow from the SSV to GSV or thigh tributaries. Saphenofemoral or pelvic vein incompetence can result in proximal to distal flow to the SSV through the vein of Giacomini and TE (see Figure 29.3 and Table 29.5).

REFLUX IN THE GASTROCNEMIUS VEINS

Reflux in gastrocnemius veins is reasonably common. It may be symptomatic, causing aching from calf congestion, frequently without evidence of superficial varicose veins.

MECHANISMS FOR DISEASE

It is now widely accepted that saphenous reflux is not initiated by retrograde pressures and that there is an antegrade progression of disease from tributaries into the saphenous veins with secondary incompetence at the saphenous junctions.[21] However, most of this evidence comes from studies of GSV disease.

If ultrasound is used to demonstrate SSV reflux then it is also found that there are one or more intact valves in deep veins above the SPJ or at the junction itself in most limbs. Calf compression or cuff inflation during scanning causes approximately 20 to 30 ml of blood to reflux from deep veins to the SSV if the SPJ is incompetent. This equates to the volume in a 5 to 10 cm length of deep vein above and below the junction, approximately the distance expected between competent valves. There is no large central pool of blood for reflux into the SSV in most patients.

The pathophysiology of blood accumulating in the SSV and its tributaries is undoubtedly more complex than reflux alone. It is probable that an ultrasound examination bears little relation to everyday hemodynamics during standing and walking, which are poorly understood. There is probably a complex interaction of antegrade and retrograde flow through the SSV and deep veins, and flow in either direction through some calf perforators in the presence of disease.

Accordingly, it is naive to anticipate that simple interruption at the junction would restore normal venous function. This suggests that destruction of the entire diseased segment of SSV and TE is required for best results from treatment. This is not common surgical practice.

Table 29.3 AN ULTRASOUND STUDY OF THE
SOURCES AND DESTINATIONS OF REFLUX INTO
THE SSV TERRITORY

DISTAL DESTINATION	PROXIMAL CONNECTIONS				
	SSV ONLY	SSV & VG	VG ONLY	SSV TRIBUTARIES	TOTAL PROXIMAL CONNECTIONS
SPJ only	169	11	5	1	186 (56%)
SPJ & VG	10	–	–	–	10 (3%)
VG only	54	–	–	1	55 (17%)
GSV tributaries	55	–	–	2	57 (17%)
Perforators	11	–	–	–	11 (3%)
Unknown	15	–	–	–	15 (4%)
Total distal destinations	314 (94%)	11 (4%)	5 (1%)	4 (1%)	

(From Reference 3)

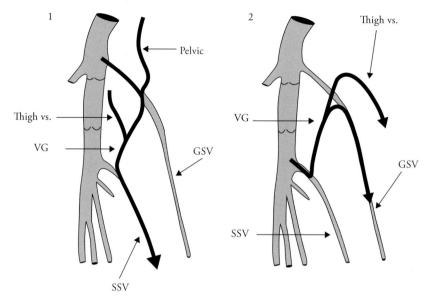

Figure 29.3 Reflux through the vein of Giacomini from the GSV territory to the SSV (1) and from the SSV to the GSV territory (2).

DIAGNOSIS

CLINICAL

Inspection, palpation, and the percussion test may reveal a dilated SSV or tributaries behind the knee in the SSV territory, but provide no information regarding the SPJ. Tourniquet tests are of little value for reflux into the SSV if there are competent valves in deep veins above the SPJ preventing deep reflux, as is usually the case. Even if there is full-length deep reflux, it is difficult to be sure that a tourniquet selectively occludes superficial veins and not deep veins. Interpreting results in patients with combined GSV and SSV reflux is almost impossible.

CONTINUOUS-WAVE (CW) DOPPLER

The handheld CW Doppler probe is considered by many to be a convenient way to record popliteal vein or SSV reflux,

Table 29.5 **AN ULTRASOUND STUDY OF THE SOURCES AND DESTINATIONS FOR REFLUX THROUGH THE TE OR VEIN OF GIACOMINI FROM PROXIMAL SOURCES TO THE SSV OR FROM THE DISTAL SSV TO PROXIMAL DESTINATIONS**

SOURCE OF REFLUX	DESTINATION OF REFLUX	NUMBER WITH TE REFLUX	% WITH TE REFLUX
GSV	SSV	15	20%
Thigh veins	SSV	18	24%
Pelvic veins	SSV	20	26%
Total distal reflux			70%
SSV	GSV	18	24%
SSV	Thigh veins	5	6%
Total proximal reflux			30%

(From Reference 2)

but it will provide false-positive results that could lead to unnecessary popliteal fossa exploration in at least 10% of patients.[22] CW Doppler cannot define variations in anatomy and in particular the information required regarding the SPJ. CW Doppler is widely used to exclude SSV reflux because it has a low false-negative rate, but this seems pointless if the policy is to perform routine duplex ultrasound scanning.

DUPLEX ULTRASOUND SCANNING

Anatomy needs to be defined before treating SSV reflux. However, results are reliable only if performed by specialist vascular sonographers or sonologists. Principles relating to preoperative ultrasound evaluation have been described in a consensus document.[23] Many surgeons now routinely request a duplex ultrasound scan prior to treatment for varicose veins.[24] A survey from the Vascular Surgical Society of Great Britain and Ireland found that 90% of surgeons obtained duplex scans in all patients with suspected SSV reflux.[25] In addition, approximately 60% routinely obtained a further scan to mark the SPJ and SSV immediately before surgery. A British report found that the preoperative scan did not improve outcome after SSV surgery, but the recurrence rate was high with or without preoperative scanning.[26]

Our technique is to examine with the patient standing or tilted on a table with the knee slightly flexed and weight taken on the opposite side. We prefer to test for reflux with manual calf compression and release.

The routine scan for the SSV territory in our practice is to examine for:

- Incompetence at the SPJ and reflux in the SSV;

- Reflux in the popliteal vein proximal and distal to the SPJ;

- Reflux in gastrocnemius veins; and

- Alternative connections including the TE or vein of Giacomini, popliteal fossa perforators, intersaphenous veins, or pelvic veins traced to the buttocks or perineum.

  If there is reflux then we note:

- Diameters at the SPJ and along the SSV and TE;

- The level of the SPJ in relation to the skin crease on the posterior aspect of the knee;

- The position of the SSV in relation to the midline axis in the popliteal fossa—midline, lateral, or medial;

- A common insertion of SSV and gastrocnemius veins into the popliteal vein;

- Alternative destinations for reflux including the TE or vein of Giacomini, or tributaries; and

- Venography and varicography

A minority of surgeons use this technique prior to or at the start of the operation, to confirm the presence of SSV reflux and to define the anatomy.

TREATMENT FOR SSV REFLUX

Reflux in the SSV or TE can be treated by surgery, ultrasound-guided sclerotherapy (UGS), endovenous laser ablation (EVLA), or endovenous mechanical ablation (ClariVein). We have found no reference to specific treatment of SSV reflux by radiofrequency closure.

Surgery appears to be the most frequently recommended treatment for SSV reflux in most countries,[24] but many phlebologists now prefer endovenous techniques. Repeat surgery for recurrent SSV reflux to remove the saphenous stump or other connections is technically demanding and prone to complications from damage to the popliteal vein or adjacent nerves, and it is our practice to always recommend endovenous treatment for recurrence.

It is not known whether perforators with valvular incompetence are an avenue for outward flow into superficial varicose veins or whether perforators act as safety valves for blood to escape from diseased superficial veins to be removed through normal functioning deep veins. Accordingly, there is debate as to whether or not they should be interrupted during treatment.

Gastrocnemius vein reflux can be treated by flush ligation at the junction with the popliteal vein or excision of the terminal SSV if the gastrocnemius veins drain to the SSV. However, recurrence after ligation is common because of failure to ligate all connections or revascularization.[27] Recently, treatment by EVLA has been described.[28]

SURGERY

Surgery is usually directed toward dividing the SPJ, presupposing that reflux through the junction causes varicose veins in the SSV territory. Ultrasound is required prior to surgery, for if an operation is to be performed to ligate the SSV flush with the popliteal vein then it is necessary to know that the junction is present as well as its exact location and any other variations in anatomy.

TECHNIQUE

A survey of members of the Vascular Surgical Society of Great Britain and Ireland found that most surgeons performed flush ligation and that few extensively exposed the popliteal vein unless surgery was for recurrent SSV reflux.[25] There was a degree of caution about the extent of surgery, for only 15% routinely stripped the SSV and approximately one-quarter simply ligated the vein, while over one-half avulsed or excised as much as possible within the operation field. Practice patterns in other countries do not appear to have been documented.

The operation usually is performed under general anesthesia, although spinal anesthesia or popliteal nerve and posterior nerve of thigh blocks can be used. Most surgeons operate with the patient prone, which requires intubation for general anesthesia. A transverse popliteal fossa incision is favored by most, although an incision for a high SPJ can be disfiguring.

Each surgeon has a favored technique:

- **Flush ligation and division** require precise identification of the point where the SSV joins the deep vein. It is important not to leave a stump, particularly if it includes a tributary.

- **Excision of the terminal SSV** within the operation field is preferred by many to eliminate tributaries near the junction that could contribute to recurrence. Care must be taken to identify and ligate the gastrocnemius veins if they join the SSV.

- **Retrograde stripping** to mid calf or further, now favoring invagination stripping. There is no evidence as to whether stripping reduces recurrence rates or increases risk of sural nerve damage, or whether invagination reduces the incidence of nerve injury.

- **Antegrade stripping** from the ankle. The presence of the stripper in the SSV at the junction makes it easier to identify the veins. Care must be taken to avoid damage to the sural nerve during the distal dissection.

OUTCOME

The small number of prospective studies published that used ultrasound for surveillance after SSV surgery show disturbingly high recurrence rates. Van Rij and colleagues reported that recurrence rates at 3 weeks and 3 years were 23% and 52% respectively compared to 1% and 25% respectively after GSV surgery.[29] Smith and colleagues studied thirty-seven limbs treated by SSV ligation with excision within the popliteal fossa and showed that the recurrence rate at 12 months was 38% (due to inadequate surgery in 27% and neovascularization in 11%).[26] Another British report found an "ideal" outcome in only 39% of 67 limbs at 6 weeks, with persistent SSV reflux from tributaries in 20% and an intact patent SPJ in 36%.[30] A Dutch study found that only five of thirty-two limbs treated by SSV ligation were completely controlled at 3 months, with persisting reflux into adjacent tributaries in fourteen and a patent junction in thirteen limbs.[31] There is a need for larger prospective objective studies using ultrasound surveillance for outcome after ligation alone or ligation and stripping.

Sites for recurrence after SSV surgery have been defined by retrospective ultrasound studies. Tong and Royle showed an intact SSV to be the most common finding, with varices from the popliteal vein to residual SSV in the remainder.[32]

COMPLICATIONS

The risk of deep vein thrombosis after SSV surgery has not been defined. Many surgeons use deep vein thrombosis prophylaxis selectively prior to varicose vein surgery, but few use it routinely. Nerve injury after venous surgery is the most common reason for medicolegal claims in vascular surgical practice.[33] A survey from the Vascular Surgical Society of Great Britain and Ireland found that nerve injury is perceived to be more likely after SSV surgery since two-thirds of surgeons were more likely to warn of this complication for SSV surgery compared to GSV surgery.[25] However, the incidence of sural or popliteal nerve injuries after SSV surgery has not been determined and may be low.[34] Damage to the sural nerve during SSV surgery probably results from straying away from the vein during dissection.

ULTRASOUND-GUIDED SCLEROTHERAPY (UGS)

TECHNIQUE

Techniques are described in Chapter 18, and our technique has been presented in detail elsewhere.[35] This chapter will summarize particular features relating to SSV reflux in our practice. UGS has been used by our group to treat 264 SSV systems in 207 patients. We favor aethoxysklerol or sodium tetradecyl sulfate in varying concentrations. The sclerosant may be used as liquid or as foam, and foam may be made with air or a CO_2/O_2 mixture. Injection is made as far distal

in the vein as possible, controlling communications to deep veins at the SPJ or through large perforators with a finger or the ultrasound probe.

POSTOPERATIVE MANAGEMENT AND SURVEILLANCE

All limbs are bandaged or compressed with class II stockings continuously for 24 hours and then compressed with stockings during the day for 1 to 2 weeks. However, a recent study showed no difference in outcome according to whether or not compression stockings were worn.[36] Patients are reviewed with ultrasound at 3 to 7 days to confirm occlusion of the treated veins and to exclude deep vein thrombosis. They are then followed by ultrasound surveillance at 6 weeks, semiannually for 2 years, then annually.

STATISTICAL METHODS

We used Kaplan-Meier methods to generate survival curves for time to failure (primary or secondary). Univariable and multivariable survival hazard ratios and their confidence intervals were computed using Cox regression methods, with veins clustered within patient to account for within-patient similarities. We classed each continuous predictor variable into two groups using its median value. These were: age (55 yrs), diameter (4 mm), concentration of sclerosant (1.5%), foam volume (5 ml). We used Stata Release 11 for all computations and statistical graphs.[37]

OUTCOME

In our series, the primary success rate at 4 years after UGS for SSV reflux determined by ultrasound surveillance using Kaplan-Meier analysis was 46%, with a secondary success rate of 62% with repeat UGS as required for clinical recurrence (see Figure 29.4). Patients should be told that

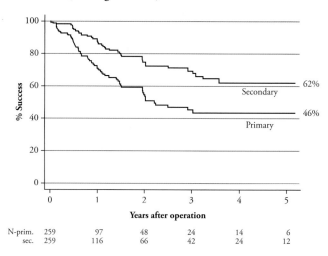

Figure 29.4   Kaplan-Meier analysis of primary and secondary success rates from ultrasound surveillance for UGS for SSV reflux.

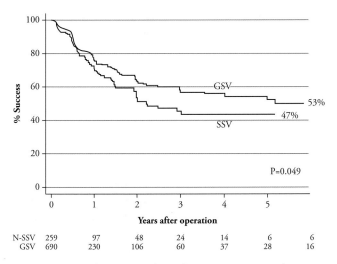

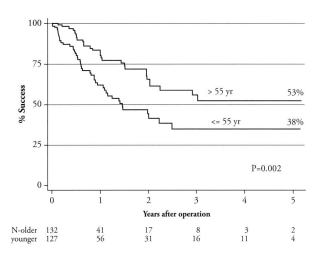

Figure 29.5   Kaplan-Meier analysis of primary success rates from ultrasound surveillance for UGS for GSV and SSV reflux.

Figure 29.6   Kaplan-Meier analysis of primary success rates from ultrasound surveillance for UGS for SSV reflux according to the patients' ages.

future repeat treatment by UGS may be required. These results were significantly worse than for patients treated for GSV reflux (see Figure 29.5); the reason is not apparent. Multivariate Cox regression analysis showed significantly worse results for patients younger than 55 years and veins greater than 4 mm diameter but no worse according to other patient or vein characteristics or technique (See Table 29.6 and Figures 29.6 and 29.7). A large, multicenter European study has shown a relatively small incidence of complications including migraine, visual disturbance, chest pressure, and thromboembolic events.[38] The few reported transient strokes appear to have all followed treatment of the GSV.

In our practice, concern regarding long-term results for surgery has made UGS the preferred treatment for older

patients with small-diameter refluxing SSVs or their tributaries, while EVLA or ClariVein are preferred for younger patients with larger diameter veins.

EVLA

Techniques are described in Chapter 28 and our technique has been presented in detail elsewhere.[39] This section will summarize particular features relating to SSV reflux in our practice. EVLA has been used by our group for 164 limbs of 146 patients with SSV reflux using 810-nm and 1500-nm systems. The procedure is performed with perivenous tumescent anesthesia injected into the saphenous compartment along the vein. Perivenous fluid injection provides a

Table 29.6 **MULTIVARIATE ANALYSIS OF COVARIATES THAT MIGHT AFFECT OUTCOME AFTER UGS FOR SSV REFLUX.**

VARIABLE	HAZARD RATIO	STANDARD ERROR	P	95% CIS	
Sex	0.83	0.28	0.589	0.43	1.61
Side	0.90	0.20	0.649	0.59	1.39
CEAP	1.58	0.63	0.254	0.72	3.45
Primary/ Recurrent	0.71	0.35	0.490	0.27	1.88
Foam/Liquid	2.02	1.20	0.234	0.63	6.45
Sclerosant	0.92	0.45	0.872	0.36	2.39
Concentration	0.73	0.28	0.414	0.35	1.55
Volume	1.38	0.38	0.241	0.80	2.38
Age	0.44	0.12	0.004	0.25	0.76
Diameter vein	1.95	0.50	0.009	1.18	3.21

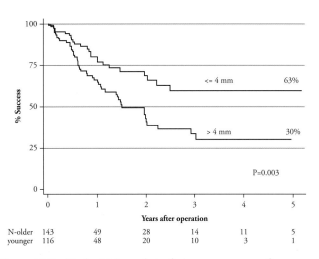

Figure 29.7   Kaplan-Meier analysis of primary success rates from ultrasound surveillance for UGS for SSV reflux according to the vein diameters.

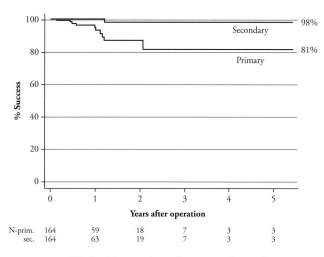

N-prim. 164   59   18   7   3   3
  sec.   164   63   19   7   3   3

Figure 29.8   Kaplan-Meier analysis of primary and secondary success rates from ultrasound surveillance for EVLA for SSV reflux.

heat sink and compresses the vein onto the probe as well as producing anesthesia. Residual tributaries are treated by UGS but can be well treated by ambulatory phlebectomy. Postoperative management and surveillance are identical to that after UGS.

OUTCOME

The cumulative primary success rate at 3 years from serial ultrasound studies using Kaplan-Meier analysis was 81%, and the secondary success rate with UGS for recurrences was 98% (see Figure 29.8). Multivariate analysis showed no significant effects from patient or vein characteristics, or from technique. The only complications encountered were permanent partial sural nerve palsy in one limb and asymptomatic minor extension of a tongue of thrombus into the popliteal vein in another. Arteriovenous fistula has been reported as a rare complication.[15,16] Others have found excellent patient satisfaction and return to work at a mean 4 days after EVLA for the SSV.[40] These results persuade us to favor EVLA for SSV reflux where the vein has been shown to be straight and of diameter greater than an arbitrary 4 to 5 mm.

CONCLUSIONS

The hemodynamics of SSV reflux are poorly understood. The concept of a "source" of reflux from a deep venous pool does not seem to be valid at this stage. The variable anatomy and reflux patterns are probably responsible for the wide variation in treatment techniques and poor results from surgery. Better techniques need to be defined to improve surgical outcome if it is to remain the preferred technique for treatment. Otherwise, new endovenous techniques will replace surgery as experience grows.

REFERENCES

1. Uhl J-F, Gillot C. Embryology and three-dimensional anatomy of the superficial venous system of the lower limbs, *Phlebology*. 2007. *22*: 194–206.
2. Barberini F, Cavallini A, Caggiati A. The thigh extension of the small saphenous vein: A hypothesis about its significance, based on morphological, embryological, and anatomo-comparative reports, *Ital J Anat Embryol*. 2006. *111*: 187–198.
3. Georgiev M, Myers KA, Belcaro G. Giacomini's observations on the superficial veins of the abdominal limb and principally the external saphenous, *Int Angiol*. 2001. *20*: 225–233.
4. Georgiev M, Myers KA, Belcaro G. The thigh extension of the lesser saphenous vein: From Giacomini's observations to ultrasound scan imaging, *J Vasc Surg*. 2003. *37*: 558–563.
5. Cavezzi A, Tarabini C, Collura M, Sigismondi G, Barboni MG, Carigi V. Hemodynamique de la jonction sapheno-poplitee: Evaluation par echo-doppler couleur, *Phlebologie*. 2002. *55*: 309–316.
6. Caggiati A. Fascial relationships of the short saphenous vein, *J Vasc Surg*. 2001. *34*: 241–246.
7. Myers KA, Wood SR, Lee V, Koh P. Variations of connections to the saphenous systems in limbs with primary varicose veins: A study of 1481 limbs by duplex ultrasound scanning, *J Phlebology*. 2002. *2*: 11–17.
8. Delis KT, Knaggs AL, Khodabakhsh P. Prevalence, anatomic patterns, valvular competence, and clinical significance of the Giacomini vein, *J Vasc Surg*. 2004. *40*: 1174–1183.
9. Lin JC, Iafrati MD, O'Donnell TF Jr, Estes JM, Mackey WC. Correlation of duplex ultrasound scanning-derived valve closure time and clinical classification in patients with small saphenous vein reflux: Is lesser saphenous vein truly lesser?, *J Vasc Surg*. 2004. *39*: 1053–1058.
10. Cavezzi A, Labropoulos N, Partsch H, et al. Duplex ultrasound investigation of the veins in chronic venous disease of the lower limbs: UIP consensus document: Part II: Anatomy, *Eur J Vasc Endovasc Surg*. 2006. *31*: 288–299.
11. Lemasle P, Lefebvre-Vilardebo M, Tamisier D, Baud JM, Cornu-Thenard A. Confrontation echo-chirurgicale de la terminaison de la saphene externe dans le cadre de la chirurgie d'exerese: Resultats preliminaires, *Phlebologie*. 1995. *47*: 321–327.
12. Aragãoa JA, Reisa FP, Pittab GBB, Miranda F, Poli de Figueiredob LF. Anatomical study of the gastrocnemius venous network and proposal for a classification of the veins, *Eur J Vasc Endovasc Surg*. 2006. *31*: 439–442.
13. Ricci S, Moro L, Antonelli Incalzi R. Ultrasound imaging of the sural nerve: Ultrasound anatomy and rationale for investigation, *Eur J Vasc Endovasc Surg*. 2010. *39*(5): 636–641.
14. Murakami G, Negishi N, Tanaka K, Hoshi H, Sezai Y. Anatomical relationship between saphenous vein and cutaneous nerves, *Okajimas Folia Anat Jpn*. 1994. *71*: 21–33.
15. Timperman PE. Arteriovenous fistula after endovenous laser treatment of the short saphenous vein, *J Vasc Interv Radiol*. 2004. *15*: 625–627.
16. Theivacumar NS, Gough MJ. Arterio-venous fistula following endovenous laser ablation for varicose veins, *Eur J Vasc Endovasc Surg*. 2009. *38*(2): 234–236.
17. Theivacumar NS, Beale RJ, Mavor AI, Gough MJ. Initial experience in endovenous laser ablation (EVLA) of varicose veins due to small saphenous vein reflux, *Eur J Vasc Endovasc Surg*. 2007. *33*: 614–618.
18. Schweighofer G, Mühlberger D, Brenner E. Back to the basics: The anatomy of the small saphenous vein: Part 1: Fascial and neural relations, saphenofemoral junction, and valves, *J Vasc Surg*. 2010. *51*(4):982–989.
19. Tuveri M, Borsezio V, Argiolas R, Medas F, Tuveri A. Ultrasonographic venous anatomy at the popliteal fossa in relation to tibial nerve course in normal and varicose limbs, *Chir Ital*. 2009. *61*: 171–177.

20. Bass A, Chayen D, Weinmann EE, Ziss M. Lateral venous ulcer and short saphenous vein insufficiency, *J Vasc Surg.* 1997. *25*: 654–657.

21. Caggiati A, Rosi C, Heyn R, Franceschini M, Acconcia MC. Age-related variations of varicose veins anatomy, *J Vasc Surg.* 2006. *44*: 1291–1295.

22. Darke SG, Vetrivel S, Foy DM, Smith S, Baker S. A comparison of duplex scanning and continuous wave Doppler in the assessment of primary and uncomplicated varicose veins, *Eur J Vasc Endovasc Surg.* 1997. *14*: 457–461.

23. Coleridge-Smith P, Labropoulos N, Partsch H, Myers K, Nicolaides A, Cavezzi A. Duplex ultrasound investigation of the veins in chronic venous disease of the lower limbs: UIP consensus document: Part I: Basic principles, *Eur J Vasc Endovasc Surg.* 2006. *31*: 83–92.

24. Lees TA, Beard JD, Ridler BM, Szymanska T. A survey of the current management of varicose veins by members of the Vascular Surgical Society, *Ann R Coll Surg Engl.* 1999. *81*: 407–417.

25. Winterborn RJ, Campbell WB, Heather BP, Earnshaw JJ. The management of short saphenous varicose veins: A survey of the members of the vascular surgical society of Great Britain and Ireland, *Eur J Vasc Endovasc Surg.* 2004. *28*: 400–403.

26. Smith JJ, Brown L, Greenhalgh RM, Davies AH. Randomised trial of pre-operative colour duplex marking in primary varicose vein surgery: Outcome is not improved, *Eur J Vasc Endovasc Surg.* 2002. *23*: 336–343.

27. Juhan C, Barthelemy P, Alimi Y, Di Mauro P. Recurrence following surgery of the gastrocnemius veins, *J Mal Vasc.* 1997. *22*: 326–329.

28. Chapman-Smith P. Endovenous laser treatment (EVLA) of gastrocnemius vein reflux with 1320nm: 2 case reports, *Int Angiol.* 2009. *28*(Suppl 1): 130.

29. van Rij AM, Jiang P, Solomon C, Christie RA, Hill GB. Recurrence after varicose vein surgery: A prospective long-term clinical study with duplex ultrasound scanning and air plethysmography, *J Vasc Surg.* 2003. *38*: 935–943.

30. Rashid HI, Ajeel A, Tyrell MR. Persistent popliteal fossa reflux after saphenopopliteal disconnection, *Br J Surg.* 2002. *89*: 748–751.

31. Spronk S, Boelhouwer RU, Veen HF, den Hoed PT. Subfascial ligation of the incompetent short saphenous vein: Technical success measured by duplex sonography, *J Vasc Nurs.* 2003. *21*: 92–95.

32. Tong Y, Royle J. Recurrent varicose veins after short saphenous vein surgery: A duplex ultrasound study, *Cardiovasc Surg.* 1996. *4*: 364–367.

33. Campbell WB, France F, Goodwin HM. Research and audit committee of the vascular surgical society of Great Britain and Ireland: Medico-legal claims in vascular surgery, *Ann R Coll Surg Engl.* 2002. *84*: 181–184.

34. Sam RC, Silverman SH, Bradbury AW. Nerve injuries and varicose vein surgery, *Eur J Vasc Endovasc Surg.* 2004. *27*: 113–120.

35. Myers KA, Jolley D, Clough A, Kirwan J. Outcome of ultrasound-guided sclerotherapy for varicose veins: Medium-term results assessed by ultrasound surveillance, *Eur J Vasc Endovasc Surg.* 2007. *33*: 116–121.

36. Hamel-Desnos CM, Guias BJ, Desnos PR, Mesgard A. Foam sclerotherapy of the saphenous veins: Randomised controlled trial with or without compression, *Eur J Vasc Endovasc Surg.* 2010. *39*(4):500–507.

37. StataCorp. *Stata: Release 11: Statistical software.* College Station, TX: StataCorp LP. 2009.

38. Gillet JL, Guedes JM, Guex JJ, et al. Side-effects and complications of foam sclerotherapy of the great and small saphenous veins: A controlled multicentre prospective study including 1,025 patients, *Phlebology.* 2009. *24*: 131–138.

39. Myers KA, Jolley D. Outcome of endovenous laser therapy for saphenous reflux and varicose veins: Medium-term results assessed by ultrasound surveillance, *Eur J Vasc Endovasc Surg.* 2009. *37*: 239–245.

40. Trip-Hoving M, Verheul JC, van Sterkenburg SM, de Vries WR, Reijnen MM. Endovenous laser therapy of the small saphenous vein: Patient satisfaction and short-term results, *Photomed Laser Surg.* 2009. *27*: 655–658.

30.

CLASSIFICATION AND TREATMENT OF RECURRENT VARICOSE VEINS

Michel Perrin

INTRODUCTION

Recurrent varices after operative treatment are a common, complex, and costly problem both for the patients and for the physicians who treat venous diseases. To deal with this problem, in Paris in 1998 an international consensus meeting was held, which proposed guidelines for the definition and description of REcurrent Varices After Surgery (REVAS).[1] In this article ninety-four references were listed.[1] Since 1998, more than 100 new articles in English and French have been published on the topic.[2–113]

Nowadays classical surgery is no longer the most frequent operative procedure used for treating varicose vein. On the one hand chemical and thermal ablation and on the other mini-invasive surgery including CHIVA (French acronym for ambulatory conservative hemodynamic management of varicose veins)[15] and ASVAL (French acronym for tributary varices phlebectomy under local anesthesia)[86] are currently taking over high ligation plus stripping.

DEFINITIONS

The term "operative treatment" encompasses open surgery with and without conservation of the saphenous trunk as well as all kinds of endovenous procedures including thermal and chemical ablation.

The following definitions were published in 2009 in the VEIN-TERM transatlantic interdisciplinary consensus document.[114]

Recurrent varices: Reappearance of varicose veins in an area previously treated successfully

Residual varices: Varicose veins remaining after treatment

PREVAIT: **PRE**sence of **V**arices (residual or recurrent) **A**fter operat**I**ve **T**reatment

The concept of PREVAIT was developed for two reasons: First, it is frequently difficult to classify correctly the results of initial procedures done by others and consequently to differentiate recurrent varices from residual varices. Second, REVAS, the previous concept, was limited to patients previously treated by surgery, nowadays all kinds of operative treatment should be assessed by the same protocol.

EPIDEMIOLOGY AND SOCIOECONOMIC CONSEQUENCES

PREVALENCE AND INCIDENCE OF PREVAIT

The most documented outcomes are provided by classical surgery, but most studies are retrospective. In a 34-year follow-up[41] varicose veins were present in 77% of the lower limbs examined and were mostly symptomatic. Fifty-eight percent were painful, 83% had a tired feeling, and 93% showed a reappearance of edema.

Two prospective studies concerning classical surgery are available with a follow-up of 5 years.[63,107] In both, the patients had preoperative duplex scanning (DS) and were treated by high ligation, saphenous trunk stripping, and stab avulsion.

In the Kostas et al. series, 28 patients out 100 had PREVAIT. True recurrent varices were present in eight limbs (8/28, 29%), primarily caused by neovascularization; new varicose veins as a consequence of disease progression were seen in seven limbs (7/28, 25%), residual veins were found in three limbs (3/28, 11%) mainly due to tactical errors (e.g. failure to strip the great saphenous vein), and complex patterns were identified in ten limbs (10/28, 36%).[63]

In the Van Rij et al. series 127 limbs (CEAP class C_2–C_6) were evaluated postoperatively by clinical exam, DS and air plethysmography (APG). Clinical varices recurrence was progressive from 3 months onward (13.7%) to 5 years (51.7%). Corresponding to clinical changes, there was a progressive deterioration in venous function measured by APG and recurrence of reflux evaluated by DS.[107]

These studies showed that recurrence of varicose veins after surgery in high-skilled centers is common. However, the clinical condition of most affected limbs remains improved. Progression of the disease and neovascularization are responsible for more than half of the recurrences. Rigorous evaluation of patients and assiduous surgical technique might reduce recurrence resulting from technical and tactical failures.

A prospective study concerning recurrence after radiofrequency procedure (ClosurePlus) has been reported. At 5-year PREVAIT is estimated at 27.4%.[73] There is presently no long-term data on ClosureFast.

After endovenous laser (EVL) treatment the longest follow-up has been reported by the Italian group.[2] They claim a PREVAIT rate of 6% at 36 months.

Hamel-Desnos et al.[52] reported a 36% and 37% recanalization rate at 2-year follow-up with 3% and 1% ultrasound-guided foam sclerotherapy (USGFS) one injection with respectively 1% and 3% polidocanol foam.

SOCIOECONOMIC CONSEQUENCES

There are no available published socioeconomic data on PREVAIT. When redo surgery is performed, its cost is higher than first-time surgery because of the number of peri- and postoperative complications. In one observational study 40% of patients had complications.[54]

MECHANISMS AND PHYSIOPATHOLOGY

Several possible mechanisms have been implicated in recurrence of varices. These have been classified into four groups: tactical errors, technical errors, neovascularization, and progression of the disease.

TACTICAL ERRORS

Nonidentified refluxive connections between the deep and superficial system, that is, saphenofemoral junction (SFJ), saphenopopliteal junction (SPJ), and perforators that have not been initially treated.

Identified or nonidentified superficial incompetent veins that have not been treated.

TECHNICAL ERRORS

Identified refluxive connections between the deep and superficial system, that is, SFJ, SFP, and perforators were scheduled to be treated, but surgery was incorrectly performed, and the reflux persists.

Identified superficial incompetent veins were scheduled to be treated, but surgery was incorrectly or incompletely performed.

It must be kept in mind that both tactical or/and technical errors do not always lead to REVAS.

NEOVASCULARIZATION

PREVAIT after surgery or endovenous obliteration cannot always be attributed to tactical errors or technical inadequacy. Many clinical and instrumental studies have indicated that postoperative neovascularization may frequently occur (Figure 30.1). Tiny new venous vessels developing in the granulation tissue mainly around the SFJ and/or/ the SPJ may enlarge and connect deep to superficial veins, causing clinically obvious recurrence after a few years. Neovascularization is more frequent after open surgery.

Because in several endovenous obliteration DS studies postoperative neovascularization is infrequent or absent, it has been suggested that the absence of high ligation can explain this phenomenon insofar as neoangiogenesis is a normal process in tissue healing. Furthermore, the persistence of draining tributaries in the saphenous stump may play a role.

But in one study neovascularization was identified at 1-week follow-up by DS both after RF and endovenous laser (EVL) respectively in 2.2% and 7.1% of cases.[66]

PROGRESSION OF THE DISEASE

Varicosity is a progressive disorder, and new territories are affected by the evolution of the disease.

PATHOLOGY

Two studies investigating the cause of the most frequent recurrence, that at the SFJ, and taking account of the pathology have been reported. Their conclusions are contradictory. In a German study, the most frequent pattern identified (68%) was a persistent stump related to a possible nonflush high ligation, but surprisingly a valve was identified in only eighteen out of sixty-three cases with a single channel.[99] Conversely, van Rij et al. found multiple vessels in 94% at the stump site at the SFJ and concluded that neovascularization was the most frequent cause of recurrence.[108] This conclusion was in accordance with their previous clinical study.[107] Geier et al. emphasized that the only tool valid for the identification of neovascularization remains the histologic and immunohistochemical work-up of the resected vein.[45] But, this work-up is rarely performed. Consequently, the real cause of recurrence remains debatable in many studies.

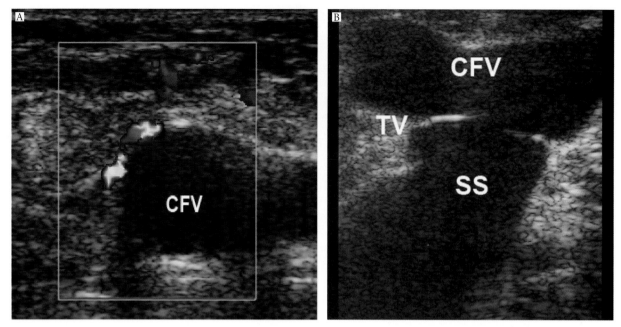

Figure 30.1   Neovascularization identified by color duplex ultrasound. (A) The saphenofemoral junction after flush ligation of the SFJ. CFV, common femoral vein. (B) At initial surgery the incompetent termination of the small saphenous vein had been tied flush to the popliteal vein (PV). Neovascularization has developed, and very small veins connect the remaining varicose network to the popliteal vein at the site of the previous SPJ and are identified by duplex scanning after the compression-decompression maneuver.

CLASSIFICATION

Many classifications other than REVAS have been developed concerning recurrences,[115,116] but they have not been widely used. At the consensus meeting held in 1998 we decided to use both the previously reported CEAP classification and a specific REVAS classification.[1] This new classification was intended to serve everyday clinical practice as well as research studies into epidemiology, clinical status, and treatment of recurrent varicose veins. A survey was undertaken in order to test its intraobserver and interobserver reproducibility.[84] The conclusion of this study was that intraobserver reproducibility is quite satisfactory, and making slight changes in the answers to one question, might increase interobserver reproducibility. However, the fact that interobserver reproducibility was less than intraobserver reproducibility reflects conditions of real life, and especially interobserver differences. Such interobserver differences may arise from interobserver technical differences, but this finding emphasizes the need for validating a duplex scanning protocol and a standardizing duplex scan reports (see below, "Investigations")

The REVAS classification (Table 30.1) includes six items: *T* is for *topographic* sites of REVAS; *S* for *sources* of reflux; *R* for degree of *reflux*; *N* for *nature* of sources (*Nss* for same site of previous surgery, and *Nds* for different sites); *P* for contribution from a *persistent* incompetent saphenous trunk; and *F* for possible contributory *factors* (*Fg* for general and *Fs* for specific factors).

This classification has been used only for REVAS, but it might be used for any kind of recurrence after operative treatment in combination with the CEAP classification. Nevertheless it looks that a new classification—PREVAIT classification—not yet drawn up might be a better tool.

DIAGNOSIS

MODES OF PRESENTATION

Patients who have previous nonconservative treatment may consult their physicians for various reasons: *unsightly recurrent varicose veins* or related emotional problems that are especially common in female patients, *discomfort* (in other words venous-related symptoms), *appearance* of cutaneous or subcutaneous changes, *concerns* about the health risk related to their veins, or *limitation* of activity. Also PREVAIT may be found at routine follow-up.

MEDICAL HISTORY

Family and Personal History

Family history of varicose veins and personal history including pregnancies, hormone therapy, superficial thrombophlebitis, deep vein thrombosis, and so forth, should be recorded.

Previous Treatment

The date of previous treatment(s) for varicose veins must be reported, as well as the age of the patient at the time of operative treatment, occurrence of new pregnancies after initial

REVAS Classification sheet

Date of examination ☐☐ ☐☐ ☐☐☐☐
                    Day Month Year

Patient Rename:
First name or given name ☐☐☐☐☐☐☐☐☐☐☐☐☐☐
Last name or family name ☐☐☐☐☐☐☐☐☐☐☐☐☐☐

✓ Topographical sites of REVAS
Since more than one territory may be involved, several boxes may be ticked

Groin   ☐ 1
Thigh   ☐ 2
Popliteal fossa   ☐ 3
Lower leg including ankle and foot   ☐ 4
Other   ☐ 5

✓ Source(s) of recurrence
Since more than one Source may be involved, several boxes may be ticked

No source of reflux   ☐ 0
For petvic or abdominal   ☐ 1
Saphenofemoral junction   ☐ 2
Thigh perforator(s)   ☐ 3
Saphenopopliteal junction   ☐ 4
Popliteal perforator   ☐ 5
Gastrocnemius vein(s)   ☐ 6
Lower leg perforator(s)   ☐ 7

✓ Reflux
Only one box can be ticked

PROBABLE   Clinical significance **R+**   ☐ 1
UNLIKE   Clinical significance **R−**   ☐ 2
UNCERTAIN Clinical significance **R?**   ☐ 3

✓ Nature of sources
Only one box can be ticked

N classifies the source as to whether or not it is the site of previous surgery and describes the cause of recurrence.

● N Ss is for same site   ☐
Only one box can be ticked

Technical failures   ☐ 1
Tactical failures   ☐ 2
Neovascularization   ☐ 3
Uncertain   ☐ 4
Mixed   ☐ 5

● N Ds is for different (new) site   ☐
Only one box can be ticked

Persistent   ☐ 1
(Known to have been present at the time of previous surgery)

New   ☐ 2
(Known to have been absent at the time of previous surgery)

Uncertain/not known   ☐ 3
(insufficient information at the time of previous surgery)

✓ Contribution from persistent incompetent saphenous trunks
Since more than one territory may be involved several boxes may be ticked

AK great saphenous (above knee)   ☐ 1
BK great saphenous (below knee)   ☐ 2
SSV short saphenous   ☐ 3
0 neither/other   ☐ 4
Comment:_____
_____
_____
_____
_____

✓ Possible contributory factors
Several boxes may be ticked

General factors
Family history   ☐ 1
Obesity   ☐ 2
Pregnancy*   ☐ 3
Oral contraceptive   ☐ 4
Lifestyle factors**   ☐ 5
* Pregnancy since the intial operation
**Prolonged standing, lack of exercise, chair siting

Specific factors
Several boxes may be ticked

Primary deep vein reflux   ☐ 1
Post-thrombotic syndrome   ☐ 2
Iliac vein compression   ☐ 3
Angiodysplasia   ☐ 4
Lymphatic insufficiency   ☐ 5
Caly pump dysfunction   ☐ 6

Table 30.1   The REVAS classification includes six items as demonstrated on this intake sheet.

treatment, and the name of therapist and the place of the operation in order to retrieve the operative record; postoperative complications; and date of the onset of PREVAIT and reappearance of symptoms. Other treatment received after initial operative treatment, such as veinoactive drugs, use of compression stockings, and leg elevation must also be documented.

PHYSICAL EXAMINATION

Presence and intensity of the various vein-related symptoms have to be noted: pain, throbbing, heaviness, itching, feeling of swelling, night cramps, heat or burning sensations or restless legs.

Some data are available on patients presenting PREVAIT, including severity of leg symptoms and clinical disability scores.[65,81,83,97] In an international REVAS survey, there was a statistical difference in terms of the presence or absence of symptoms between CEAP class C_2 and C_3–C_6 ($P = 0.0001$).[81] Conversely in a Finnish series, there was no difference between the C_2–C_3 group and the C_4–C_6 group except itching ($P < 0.001$).[97]

Inspection and palpation allow the C of the CEAP (clinical, etiological, anatomic, pathophysiologic) classification to be completed, but other signs such as corona phlebectatica should also be identified, and edema should be quantified. The presence of scars on the lower limb must be noted, especially at the groin or popliteal fossa. Neurological abnormalities and particularly numbness must be documented. Efficiency of the calf pump has to be assessed and particularly degree of ankle motion. Arterial pulses should be checked and ankle brachial index calculated. A general examination including abdominal palpation should be performed, and possible obesity can be identified by body mass index calculation.

INVESTIGATION

Many investigations have been used in the past to assess REVAS. At the moment there is a large consensus for recommending DS in all cases of PREVAIT. This investigation provides anatomical and hemodynamic data including

- The topographical sites of recurrence that can be mapped,

- The possible sources of reflux from the deep venous system to the superficial (Figures 30.2 and 30.3),

- The intensity or degree of reflux, and

- The nature of sources keeping in mind that causes have to be classified differently if recurrence occurs in a site previously treated or not.

In addition, DS gives information on perforator and deep venous systems.

One problem remains: a standardized DS investigation protocol was not universally used by the different investigators. But recently a consensus document has been published on postoperative DS that provides a precise investigation methodology as well as a better and more precise description of the anatomical and hemodynamic anomalies

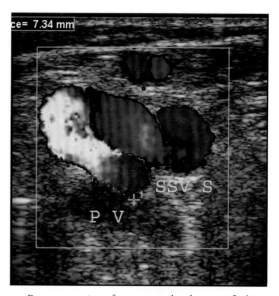

Figure 30.3   Recurrent varices after surgery related to a nonflush resection of the SPJ. The postoperative duplex scanning identified reflux in the SSV stump, which feeds the varicose network after the compression-decompression maneuver. SSV S, short saphenous vein stump; PV, popliteal vein.

according to the operative treatment modalities, surgery or endovenous treatment.[117]

In few select cases ascending venography in three-dimensional imaging may give complementary valuable information. PREVAIT related to refluxive pelvic varices is better investigated by selective descending phlebography (Figure 30.4). Other investigations such as air plethysmography and ambulatory pressure measurement may be useful for research studies but not for daily practice.

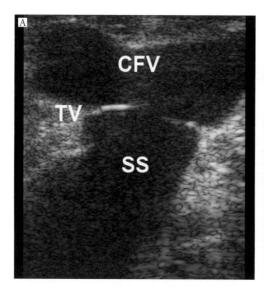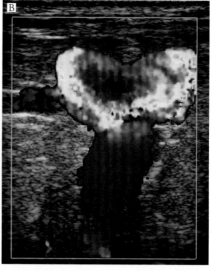

Figure 30.2   Recurrent varices after surgery related to a nonflush resection of the saphenofemoral junction in a patient with an incompetent terminal valve. (A) B-mode ultrasound. The terminal valve is identified at the saphenofemoral junction. (B) Same patient; color duplex ultrasound. Massive reflux induced by a Valsalva maneuver. CFV, common femoral vein; TV, terminal valve; SS, saphenous stump.

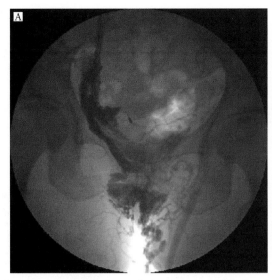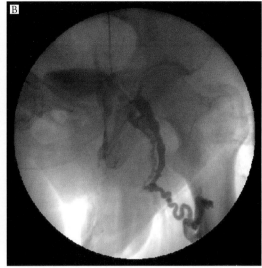

Figure 30.4   Selective pelvic venography at Valsalva maneuver. (A) Reflux through the internal pudendal vein feeding contralateral GSV. (B) Reflux through the obturator vein feeding nonsaphenous vein network.   (Courtesy Drs. Monedero and Zubicoa)

QUALITY-OF-LIFE QUESTIONNAIRES

To determine whether PREVAIT affect patients quality of life, the health-related quality-of-life score of patients can been used in different ways for clinical studies. Beresford[9] compared patients presenting recurrence after conventional surgery versus patients with untreated varicose veins. No survey has compared operated patients with or without PREVAIT after endovenous ablation.

TREATMENT

METHODS

Compression

Compression in varicose veins is frequently recommended and improves both symptoms and signs, but it does not cure the disease.

Drugs

In varicose veins phleboactive drugs are prescribed mainly to improve edema and symptoms. The most commonly used are flavonoids, but others exist.

Operative Procedures

Operative procedures share the same goals: (1) to supress reflux from deep to superficial systems when present, (2) to supress varices, and (3) in some specific cases to suppress deep vein abnormality to prevent new recurrences.

The final goals are multiple: decrease the ambulatory venous pressure, prevent worsening of chronic venous disorders, avoid further recurrences and of course improve patients' in terms of cosmetic appearance, symptoms and signs.

Ultrasound-Guided Sclerotherapy

Sclerotherapy has been used for a very long time for treating REVAS, but ultrasound-guided sclerotherapy (USGS) has improved the efficacy. Different protocols have been used, but no comparative study with other operative treatment is available. Recently polidocanol foam has entered the ring, but currently no consensus exists on the techniques, doses, concentrations, or sclerosing agents for PREVAIT.

Nevertheless one of the main advantages of sclerotherapy with or without foam is that the process is cheap, simple, less invasive, and repeatable. USGFS can both obliterate the refluxive varices and suppress most of the leak points between deep and superficial venous system including pelvic, SFJ or SPJ, and perforator reflux as well as varices not connected to the deep venous system

Open Surgery

Procedures can be classified into three groups according to their objective, and should be used in combination.

GROUP 1: TECHNIQUES THAT AIM TO ELIMINATE REFLUX FROM DEEP TO SUPERFICIAL SYSTEMS   At the SFJ or SPJ, if the site has previously been operated and depending on the extent of postoperative fibrosis, redo surgery may be difficult. It is recommended that the deep vein be approached first in order to avoid dissection of scar tissues, lymphatic nodes, and cavernoma. The last does not need to be ablated. Flush ligation of the stump is then performed and can be completed by patch interposition at the SFJ for avoiding new recurrence.[24,25] Complications following re-exploration of the groin are common.[54] No data are available concerning redo surgery at the SPJ.

The second procedure of this group is perforator ligation. When severe cutaneous and subcutaneous changes are present, subfascial endoscopic perforator surgery (SEPS) is the favored technique.

GROUP 2: PROCEDURES TO SUPRESS THE REFLUX-ING VARICES   According to the location and type of varicose veins, various techniques can be used. Stab avulsion and phlebectomy are the most used techniques. Stripping is sometimes used for treating the residual saphenous trunk.

GROUP 3: PROCEDURES TO SUPPRESS DEEP VEIN REFLUX   Valvuloplasty and valve transfer are used to suppress deep vein reflux, as several studies have demonstrated that primary deep axial reflux is frequently associated with REVAS.[118,119] Primary obstruction represented by iliac vein compression is also probably guilty in PREVAIT, but no data are available on this possible cause.

Embolization and Coils of the Pelvic and Gonadic Veins

In patients whose varices are fed by pelvic or gonadic reflux this procedure is less invasive than direct ligation.

RESULTS

Compression and Drugs

We have no specific data on the efficacy of compression treatment and drugs in PREVAIT patients.

Chemical Ablation

The value of REVAS treatment by USGFS has been assessed in several studies. The Birmingham study has the longest follow-up and is fully documented in terms of ultrasound investigation.[21]

There is no data concerning USGFS in treatment of PREVAIT after thermal or chemical ablation, but it seems reasonable to state that results should be as good as after surgery.

Surgery

Surprisingly very few data are available on the results provided by redo surgery in patients investigated preoperatively with DS.

We reported a series of 145 limbs with a 5- to 6-year follow-up.[120] All had major reflux from the deep system at the SFJ or SPJ feeding recurrent varices that were treated by surgery. Postoperative sclerotherapy was performed in all patients during the first 2 years. An external audit revealed a global objective improvement of 85%, but there was better improvement of signs and symptoms than cosmetic appearance.

The results of two studies using an interposition patch for treating recurrence at the SFJ have been published. Creton,[17] using this procedure without resection of the groin cavernoma but with combined resection of varices (saphenous trunks and/or tributaries) had only 4.2% recurrences at the SFJ at 4.9 years mean follow-up (range 3 to 7 years) in 119 extremities. Nevertheless, 22.6% of patients had diffuse varices, with a new site of incompetence between the deep and superficial systems.

De Maeseneer[24,25] has compared the results at 5 years of two nonrandomized groups with and without patch, respectively group 1 and 2 in a prospective study. All patients had recurrent SFJ incompetence. At 5-year follow-up, recurrent thigh varicosities were observed in 58% of group 2 versus 26% of group 1.

Thermal Ablation

Only one series reported a randomized control trial in patients with recurrent varices initially treated by isolated SFJ ligation and presenting a persistent reflux at the SFJ and in the patent GSV trunk.[56] Radiofrequency caused less pain and bruising and was performed more quickly than traditional open surgery.

Pelvic and Gonadal Vein Embolization

At 6-month follow-up, 90% of 215 patients treated by embolization of gonadal and pelvic veins were significantly improved in both signs and symptoms, but relief of pelvic pain or lower limb symptoms or signs were not evaluated separately (Figure 30.5).[69]

INDICATIONS

Indications for treating patients with recurrent varices.
    Patients can be roughly divided into two groups:

1. Patients complaining of symptoms or aesthetic concerns, or presenting with signs of chronic venous disease (C_2–C_6). In all cases these patients need to be investigated by DS.

2. Subjects attending a routine follow-up. The decision whether to undertake DS or not depends on the presenting complaint and physical findings. In practice, DS is almost always done.

ASYMPTOMATIC

When hemodynamic or anatomic abnormalities are found in *asymptomatic* patients without severe signs who are not concerned by their minor varices as cosmetic problems the decision to treat depends of the severity of the noninvasive findings. In all cases follow-up is required, because abnormal DS findings precede symptoms and signs.

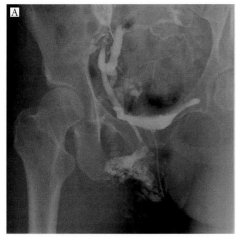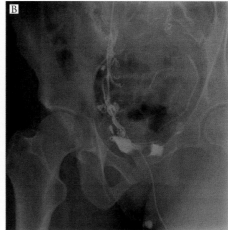

Figure 30.5   Venography using brachial access and internal iliac vein tributary vein catheterization. (A) Reflux filling both pelvic varices and lower-limb varicose veins is identified after injection into internal pudendal vein and Valsalva maneuver. (B) Same patient after embolization. No more reflux into internal vein and no lower limb varices. (Courtesy Drs. Monedero and Zubicoa)

SYMPTOMATIC

In *symptomatic* patients presenting with recurrent varices and hemodynamic anomalies, operative treatment must be considered.

Although there is no randomized controlled trial comparing redo surgery to chemical ablation, there is a consensus for treating recurrences with USGFS as first-line treatment[21,60,84] for reasons discussed above. In very few cases when duplex scanning reveals an intact and large incompetent saphenous stump at the SFJ or SPJ with a massive reflux filling the varicose network, redo surgery at the junction should be considered in combination with USGFS.

In patients with severe disease $(C_{4b}-C_6)$ with PREVAIT and primary deep vein axial reflux, USGFS and valvuloplasty in association must be considered in active patients reluctant to wear lifelong compression or with recurrent ulcer.

GUIDELINES FOR PROSPECTIVE STUDIES

In order to know the prevalence and annual incidence of PREVAIT after nonconservative treatment we need prospective studies well documented in detail from the outset of surgical treatment as in the series by Kostas et al. and van Rij et al.[63,107] These studies may give information on:

–   The value of routine postoperative scanning in the early detection of persisting reflux;

–   The relationship between hemodynamics and clinical recurrence; and

–   The possible role of compression therapy or/and complementary postoperative sclerotherapy in preventing recurrence.

Table 30.2 THE VENOUS CLINICAL SEVERITY SCORE

CHARACTERISTIC	ABSENT = 0	MILD = 1	MODERATE = 2	SEVERE = 3
Pain	None	Occasional/nonanalgesia restricting	With moderate activity/analgesia use	Daily pain, limitations to activities or regular analgesia
Varicose Veins > 4 mm	None	Few	Multiple GSV	Extensive GSV and SSV
Venous Edema	None	Evening/Ankle	Afternoon/Above knee	Morning/ requiring elevation
Skin Pigmentation	None	Limited/Brown	Diffuse lower 1/3/ purple	Wide/purple
Inflammation	None	Mild cellulitis in marginal area	Moderate involving most of gaiter area	Severe cellulitis or significant eczema
Induration	None	Focal <5 cm	Medial or lateral less than lower 1/3	1/3 of leg or more
Number of active ulcers	None	1	2	3
Active ulcer duration	<3 months	>3 months	<12 months	> 12 months
Active ulcer diameter	None	<2 cm	2-6 cm	>6 cm
Compression	None or noncompliant	Intermittent use	Compression stockings worn most days	Compression stockings worn daily

These studies may use both the updated CEAP and REVAS classification or better a PREVAIT classification to be established a specific quality of life questionnaire and venous clinical severity score (Table 30.2).[121]

CONCLUSION

PREVAIT is a frequent condition frustrating both patients and physicians that has been poorly evaluated. In order to build a scientifically convincing evidence base and to achieve a greater degree of comparability between studies, an international consensus on conformity is required.

REFERENCES

1. Perrin M, Guex JJ, Ruckley CV, et al. Recurrent varices after surgery (REVAS), a consensus document, *Cardiovasc Surg*. 2000. *8*: 233–245.
2. Agus B, Mancini S, Magi G. The first 1000 cases of Italian Endovenous-Laser Working Group (IEWG): Rational, and long terms outcomes for the 1999–2003 period, *Int Angiology*. 2006. *25*: 209–215.
3. Ali SM, Callam MJ. Results and significance of colour duplex assessment on the deep venous system in recurrent Varicose veins, *Eur J Vasc Endovasc Surg*. 2007. *34*: 97–101.
4. Allaf N, Welch M. Recurrent varicose veins: Inadequate surgery remains a problem, *Phlebology*. 2005. *20*: 138–140.
5. Allegra C, Antignani PL, Carlizza A. Recurrent varicose veins following surgical treatment: Our experience with five years follow-up, *Eur J Vasc Endovasc Surg*. 2007. *33*: 751–756.
6. Belcaro G, Nicolaides AN, Cesarone NM, et al. Flush ligation of the sapheno-femoral junction vs simple distal ligation: A randomised, 10-year, follow-up: The safe study, *Angeiologie*. 2002. *54*: 19–23.
7. Belcaro G, Cesarone NM, Di Renzo A, et al. Foam sclerotherapy, surgery, sclerotherapy, and combined treatment for varicose veins: A 10-year, prospective, randomised, controlled trial (VEDICO trial), *Angiology*. 2003. *54*: 307–315.
8. Bhatti TS, Whitman B, Harradine K, Cooke SG, Heather BP, Earnshaw JJ. Causes of re-recurrence after polytetrafluoroethylene patch saphenoplasty for recurrent varicose veins, *Br J Surg*. 2000. *87*: 1356–1360.
9. Beresford T, Smith JJ, Brown L, Greenhalgh RM, Davies AH. A comparison of health-related quality of life of patients with primary and recurrent varicose veins, *Phlebology*. 2003. *18*: 35–37.
10. Blomgren L, Johansson G, Dahlberg-Akerman A, et al. Recurrent varicose veins: Incidence, risk factors, and groin anatomy, *Eur J Vasc Endovasc Surg*. 2004. *27*: 269–274.
11. Blomgren L, Johansson G, Dahlberg-Akerman A, Thermaenius P, Bergqvist D. Changes in superficial and perforating vein reflux after varicose vein surgery, *J Vasc Surg*. 2005. *42*: 315–320.
12. Bountourouglou DG, Azzam M, Pathmarajh M, Young P, Geroulakos G. Ultrasound guided foam sclerotherapy combined with sapheno-femoral ligation compared to surgical treatment of varicose veins: Early results of a randomised controlled trial, *Eur J Vasc Endovasc Surg*. 2006. *31*: 93–100.
13. Bridget M, Donnelly M, Tierney S. Recurrent varicose veins after surgery, *Bri J Surg*. 2006. *38*: 49.
14. Campanello M, Hammarsten J, Forsberg C, Bernland P, Henrikson O, Jensen J. Standard stripping versus long saphenous vein saving surgery for primary varicose veins: A prospective, randomized study with the patients as their own controls, *Phlebology*. 1996. *11*: 45–49.
15. Carandina S, Mari C, De Palma M, et al. Stripping vs haemodynamic correction (CHIVA): A long term randomised trial, *Eur. J Vasc Endovasc Surg*. 2008. *35*: 230–237.

16. Creton D. Surgery of great saphenous vein recurrences: The presence of diffuse varicose veins without a draining residual saphenous trunk is a factor of poor prognosis for long-term results, *JP* 2002. *2*: 83–89.
17. Creton D. Surgery for recurrent saphenofemoral incompetence using expanded polytetrafluoroethylene patch interposition in front of the femoral vein: Long-term outcome in 119 extremities, *Phlebology*. 2002. *16*: 93–97.
18. Creton D. 125 réinterventions pour récidives variqueuses poplitées après exérèse de la petite saphène. Hypothèses anatomiques et physiologiques du mécanisme de la récidive, *JMV*. 1999. *24*: 30–36.
19. Creton D, Uhl JF. La sclérothérapie à la mousse dans la chirurgie des varices: Résultats précoces: 130 cas, *Phlebologie*. 2005. *58*: 343–348.
20. Creton D. A nondraining saphenous system is a factor of poor prognosis for long-term results in surgery of great saphenous vein recurrences, *Dermatol Surg*. 2004. *30*(5): 744–749.
21. Darvall KAL, Batev GR, Adam DJ, Silverman SH, Bradbury AW. Duplex ultrasound outcomes following ultrasound-guided foam sclerotherapy of symptomatic recurrent great saphenous varicose veins, *Eur J Vasc Endovasc Surg*. 2011. *42*: 107–114.
22. De Maeseneer MG. The role of postoperative neovascularisation in recurrence of varicose veins: From historical background to today's evidence, *Acta Chir Bel*. 2004. *104*: 281–287.
23. De Maeseneer MG, Tielliu IF, Van Schil PE, De Hert SG, Eyskens EJ. Clinical relevance of neovascularization on duplex ultrasound in long term follow up after varicose vein operation, *Phlebology*. 1999. *14*: 118–122.
24. De Maeseneer MG, Giuliani DR, Van Schil PE, De Hert SG. Can interposition of a silicone implant after sapheno-femoral ligation prevent recurrent varicose veins, *Eur J Vasc Endovasc Surg*. 2002. *24*: 445–449.
25. De Maeseneer MG, Vandenbroeck CP, Van Schil PE. Silicone patch saphenoplasty to prevent repeat recurrence after surgery to treat recurrent saphenofemoral incompetence: Long-term follow-up study, *J Vasc Surg*. 2004. *40*: 98–105.
26. De Maeseneer MG. *Recurrent varicose veins after surgery*. Thesis, University of Antwerp. 2005.
27. De Maeseneer MG, Vandenbroeck CP, Hendriks JM, Lauwers PR, Van Schil PE. Accuracy of duplex evaluation one year after varicose vein surgery to predict recurrence at the sapheno-femoral junction after five years, *Eur J Vasc Endovasc Surg*. 2005. *29*: 308–312.
28. De Maeseneer MG, Ongena KP, Van den Brande F, Van Schil PE, De Hert SG, Eyskens EJ. Duplex ultrasound assessment of neovascularisation after saphenofemoral or sapheno-popliteal junction ligation, *Phlebology*. 1997. *12*: 64–68.
29. De Maeseneer MG, Philipsen TE, Vandenbroeck CP, et al. Closure of the cribriform fascia: An efficient anatomical barrier against postoperative neovascularisation at the saphenofemoral junction? (A prospective study), *Eur J Vasc Endovasc Surg*. 2007. *34*: 361–366.
30. Dwerryhouse S, Davies B, Harradine K, Earnshaw JJ. Stripping the long saphenous vein reduces the rate of reoperation for recurrent varicose veins, *J Vasc Surg*. 1999. *29*: 589–592.
31. Edwards AG, Donaldson D, Bennets C, Mitchell DC. The outcome of recurrent varicose veins surgery: The patient's perspective, *Phlebology*. 2005. *20*: 57–59.
32. Egan G, Donnelly M, Bresnilhan M, Tierney S, Feeley M. Neovascularization: An innocent bystander in recurrent varicose veins, *J Vasc Surg*. 2006. *44*: 1279–1284.
33. Einarsson E, Eklöf B, Neglén P. Sclerotherapy or surgery as treatment for varicose veins: A prospective randomized study, *Phlebology*. 1993. *8*: 22–26.
34. El Wajew Y, Giannoukas CJ, Juvarna SK, Chan P. Saphenofemoral venous channels associated with recurrent varicose veins are not neovascular, *Eur J Vasc Endovasc Surg*. 2004. *28*: 590–594.
35. Englund R. Duplex scanning for recurrent varicose veins, *ANZ J Surg*. 1996. *66*(9): 618–620.
36. Farrah J, Shami SK. Patterns of incompetence in patients with recurrent varicose veins: A duplex ultrasound study, *Phlebology*. 2001. *16*: 34–37.
37. Fassiadis N, Kianifard B, Holdstock JM, Hiteley MS. A novel approach to the treatment of recurrent varicose veins, *Int Angiol*. 2002. *21*(3): 275–276.

38. Ferrara F, Bernbach HR. La sclérothérapie des varices récidivées, *Phlebologie*. 2005. *58*: 147–150.

39. Fischer R, Chandler JG, De Maeseneer MG, et al. The unresolved problem of recurrent saphenofemoral reflux, *J Am Coll Surg*. 2002. *195*: 80–94.

40. Fischer R, Linde N, Duff C, Jeanneret C, Chandler JG, Seeber P. Late recurrent saphenofemoral junction reflux after ligation and stripping of the greater saphenous vein, *J Vasc Surg*. 2001. *34*: 236–240.

41. Fischer R, Linde N, Duff C. Cure and reappearance of symptoms of varicose veins after stripping operation: A 34 year follow-up, *J Phlebology*. 2001. *1*: 49–60.

42. Fischer R, Chandler JG, Stenger D, Puhan MA, De Maeseneer MG, Schimmelpfennig L. Patients characteristics and physician-determined variables affecting saphenofemoral reflux recurrence after ligation and stripping of the great saphenous vein, *J Vasc Surg*. 2006. *43*: 81–87.

43. Frings N, Nelle A, Tran P, Fischer R, Krug W. Reduction of neoreflux after correctly performed ligation of the saphenofemoral junction: A randomized trial, *Eur J Vasc Endovasc Surg*. 2004. *28*: 246–252.

44. Geir B, Stücker M, Hummel T, et al. Residual stumps associated with inguinal varicose vein recurrence: A multicenter study, *Eur J Vasc Endovasc Surg*. 2008. *36*: 207–210.

45. Geier B, Olbrich S, Barbera L, Stücker M, Mumme A. Validity of the macroscopic identification of neovascularization at the saphenofemoral junction by the operating surgeon, *J Vasc Surg*. 2005. *41*: 64–68.

46. Geier B, Mumme A, Hummel H, Marpe B, Stücker M, Asciutto G. Validity of duplex-ultrasound in identifying the cause of groin recurrence after, *J Vasc Surg*. 2009. *49*: 968–972.

47. Gibbs PJ, Foy DM, Darke SG. Reoperation for recurrent saphenofemoral incompetence: A prospective randomised trial using a reflected flap of pectineus fascia, *Eur J Vasc Endovasc Surg*. 1999. *18*: 494–498.

48. Gillet JL, Perrin M. Exploration echo-Doppler des récidives variqueuses post-chirurgicales, *Angeiologie*. 2004. *56*: 26–31.

49. Gillet JL. Traitement des récidives chirurgicales de la jonction saphèno-fémorale et saphéno-poplitée par echo-sclérose, *Phlebologie*. 2003. *56*: 241–245.

50. Glass GM. Prevention of saphenofemoral and sapheno popliteal recurrence of varicose veins by forming a partition to contain neovascularisation, *Phlebology*. 1998. *18*: 494–498.

51. Haas E, Burkhardt T, Maile N. Recurrence rate by neovascularisation following a modification of long saphenous vein operation in the groin: A prospective randomized duplex-ultrasound controlled study, *Phlebologie*. 2005. *34*: 101–104.

52. Hamel-Desnos C, Ouvry P, Benigni JP, et al. Comparison of 1% and 3% polidocanol foam in ultrasound guided sclerotherapy of the great saphenous vein: A randomized, double-blind trial with 2-year-follow-up: The 3/1 study, *Eur J Vasc Endovasc Surg*. 2007. *34*: 723–729.

53. Hartman K, Klode J, Pfister R, et al. Recurrent varicose veins: Sonography-based re-examination of 210 patients 14 years after ligation and saphenous stripping, *VASA*. 2006. *35*: 21–26.

54. Hayden A, Holdsworth J. Complications following re-exploration of the groin for recurrent varicose veins, *Ann R Coll Surg Engl*. 2001. *83*: 272–273.

55. Heim M, Negri M, Schlegel U, De Maeseneer M. Resecting the great saphenous stump with endothelial inversion decreases neither neovascularization nor thigh varicosity recurrence, *J Vasc Surg*. 2008. *47*: 1028–1032.

56. Hinchliffe RJ, Uhbi J, Beech A, Ellison J, Braithwaite BD. A prospective randomised controlled trial of VNUS Closure versus surgery for the treatment of recurrent long saphenous varicose veins, *Eur J Vasc Endovasc Surg*. 2006. *31*: 212–218.

57. Jones L, Braithwaite BD, Selwyn D, Cooke S, Earnshaw JJ. Neovascularisation is the principal cause of varicose vein recurrence: Results of a randomised trial of stripping the long saphenous vein, *Eur J Vasc Endovasc Surg*. 1996. *12*: 442–445.

58. Jiang P, van Rij AM, Christie R, et al. Recurrent varicose veins: Patterns of reflux and clinical severity, *Cardiovasc Surg*. 1999. *7*: 322–329.

59. Kakkos SK, Bountouroglou DG, Azzam M, Kalodiki E, Daskapoulos M, Geroulakos G. Effectiveness and safety of ultrasound-guided foam sclerotherapy for recurrent varicose veins: Immediate results, *J Endovasc Ther*. 2006. *13*: 357–364.

60. Kambal A, De'ath AD, Albon H, Watson A, Shandall A, Greenstein D. Endovenous laser ablation for persistent and recurrent venous ulcers after varicose vein surgery, *Phlebology*. 2008. *23*: 193–195.

61. Khaire HS, Crowson MC, Parnell A. Colour flow duplex in the assessment of recurrent varicose veins, *Ann R Coll Surg Engl*. 1996. *78*: 139–141.

62. Kianifard B, Holdstock JM, Whiteley MS. Radiofrequency ablation (VNUS closure) does not cause neo-vascularisation at the groin at one year: Results of a case controlled study, *Surgeon*. 2006. *4*: 71–74.

63. Kostas T, Loannou CV, Toulouopakis E, et al. Recurrent varicose veins after surgery: A new appraisal of a common and complex problem in vascular surgery, *Eur J Vasc Endovasc Surg*. 2004. *27*: 275–282.

64. Kostas T, Loannou C, Veligrantakis M, Pagonidis C, Katsamouris A. The appropriate length of great saphenous vein stripping should be based on the extent of reflux and not on the intent to avoid saphenous nerve injury, *J Vasc Surg*. 2007. *46*: 1234–1241.

65. Kotoed SC, Qvamme GM, Schroeder TV, Jakobsen BH. Causes of need for reoperation following surgery for varicose veins in Denmark, *Ugeskr Laeger*. 1999. *8*: 779–783.

66. Labropoulos N, Touloupakis E, Giannoukas AD, Leon M, Katsamouris A, Nicolaides AN. Recurrent varicose veins: Investigation of the pattern and extent of reflux with color flow duplex scanning, *Surgery*. 1996. *119*: 406–409.

67. Labropoulos N, Bhatti A, Leon L, Borge M, Rodriguez H, Kalman P. Neovascularization after great saphenous ablation, *Eur J Vasc Endovasc Surg*. 2006. *31*: 219–222.

68. Lane RJ, Cuzilla ML, Coroneos JC, Phillips MN, Platt JT. Recurrence rates following external valvular stenting of the saphenofemoral junction: A contralateral stripping of the great saphenous vein, *Eur J Vasc Endovasc Surg*. 2007. *34*: 595–603.

69. Leal Monedero J, Zubicoa Ezpeleta S, Castro Castro J, Calderón Ortiz M, Sellers Fernández G. Embolization treatment of recurrent varices of pelvic origin, *Phlebology*. 2006. *21*: 3–11.

70. Lemasle PH, Lefebvre-Villardebo M, Uhl JF, Vin F, Baud JM. Récidive variqueuse post-opératoire: Et si la neovascularisation inguinale n'était que le développement d'un réseau pré-existant, *Phlebologie*. 2009. *62*: 42–48.

71. Lurie F, Creton D, Eklof B, et al. Prospective randomized study of endovenous radiofrequency obliteration (Closure) versus ligation and vein stripping (EVOLVeS): Two-year follow-up, *Eur J Vasc Endovasc Surg*. 2005. *29*: 67–73.

72. McDonagh B, Sorenson S, Gray C, et al. Clinical spectrum of recurrent postoperative varicose veins and efficacy of sclerotherapy management using the compass technique, *Phlebology*. 2003. *18*: 173–185.

73. Merchant RF, Pichot O. Longterm outcomes of endovenous radiofrequency obliteration of saphenous reflux as a treatment for superficial venous insufficiency, *J Vasc Surg*. 2005. *42*: 502–509.

74. Mikati A. Indications et resultants de la ligature coelioscopique des veines perforantes incontinentes dans les récidives variqueuses compliquées, *Phlebologie*. 2010. *63*: 59–67.

75. Mouton WG, Bergner M, Zehnder T, von Wattenwyl R, Naef M, Wagner HE. Recurrence after surgery for varices in the groin is not dependent on body mass index, *Swiss Med Wkly*. 2008. *138*(11–12): 186–188.

76. O'Hare JL, Parkin D, Vandenbroeck CP, Earnshaw JJ. Mid term results of ultrasound guided foam sclerotherapy for complicated and uncomplicated varicose veins, *Eur J Vasc Endovasc Surg*. 2008. *36*: 109–113.

77. Pavei P, Vecchiato M, Spreafico G, et al. Natural history of recurrent varices undergoing reintervention: A retrospective study, *Dermatol Surg*. 2008. *34*: 1676–1682.

78. Perala J, Rautio T, Biancari F, et al. Radiofrequency endovenous obliteration versus stripping of the long saphenous vein in the management of primary varicose veins: 3-year outcome of a randomized study, *Ann Vasc Surg*. 2005. *19*: 1–4.

79. Perrin M. Recurrent varicose veins after surgery, *Phlebolymphology*. *31*: 14–20.

80. Perrin M. Recurrent varices after surgery, *Hawaii Med J.* 2000. *59*: 214–216.

81. Perrin M, Labropoulos N, Leon LR. Presentation of the patient with recurrent varices after surgery (REVAS), *J Vasc Surg.* 2006. *43*: 27–34.

82. Perrin M, Gillet J-M. Management of recurrent varices at the popliteal fossa after surgical treatment, *Phlebology.* 2008. *23*: 64–68.

83. Perrin M. Le profil du patient REVAS: Résultats d'une enquête internationale, *Angeiologie.* 2006. *58*: 44–45. In French.

84. Perrin M, Allaert FA. Intra-and inter-observer reproducibility of the recurrent varicose veins after surgery (REVAS) classification, *Eur J Vasc Endovasc Surg.* 2006. *32*: 326–333.

85. Perrin M, Gillet JL. Récidive de varices à l'aine et à la fosse poplitée après traitement chirurgical, *J Mal Vasc.* 2006. *31*: 236–246.

86. Pittaluga P, Chastanet S, Rea B, Barbe R. Midterm results of the surgical treatment of varices by phlebectomy with conservation of a refluxing saphenous vein, *J Vasc Surg.* 2009. *50*: 107–118.

87. Pittaluga P, Chastanet S, Locret T, Rousset O. Retrospective evaluation of the need of a redo surgery at the groin for the surgical treatment of varicose vein, *J Vasc Surg.* 2010. *51*: 1442–1450.

88. Pourhassan S, Zarras K, Mackrodt HG, Stock W. Recurrent varicose veins: Surgical procedure-results, *Zentralbl Chir.* 2001. *126*(7): 522–525.

89. Rashid HI, Ajeel A, Tyrrell MR. Persistent popliteal fossa reflux following saphenopopliteal disconnection, *Br J Surg.* 2002. *89*: 748–751.

90. Reich-Schupke S, Mumme A, Altmeyer P, Stuecker M. Decorin expression with stump recurrence and neovascularization after varicose vein surgery: A pilot study, *Dermatol Surg.* 2011. *37*: 480–485.

91. Rassmussen LH, Bjoern L, Lawaetz M, Blemings A, Lawaetz B, Eklof B. Randomized trial comparing endovenous laser ablation of the great saphenous vein with ligation and stripping in patients with varicose veins: Short-term results, *J Vasc Surg.* 2007. *46*: 308–315.

92. Rasmussen LA, Lawaetz M, Bjoern L, Vennits B, Blemings A, Eklof B. Randomized clinical trial comparing endovenous laser ablation, radiofrequency ablation, foam sclerotherapy, and surgical stripping for great saphenous varicose veins, *Br J Surg.* 2011. *98*: 1079–1087.

93. Rewerk S, Noppeney T, Winkler M, Willeke F, Duczek C, Meyer AJ. Pathogenese der Primär- und Rezidiv-varikosis an der Magna-Krosse (Die Rolle von VEGF und VEGF-Rezeptor), *Phlebologie.* 2007. *36*: 137–142.

94. Roka F, Binder M, Bohler-Sommeregger K. Mid-term recurrence rate of incompetent perforating veins after combined superficial vein surgery and subfascial endoscopic perforating vein surgery, *J Vasc Sur.* 2006. *44*(2): 359–363.

95. Rutgers PH, Kitslaar PJEHM. Randomized trial of stripping versus high ligation combined with sclerotherapy in the treatment of the incompetent greater saphenous vein, *Am J Surg.* 1994. *168*: 311–315.

96. Rutherford EE, Kanifard B, Cook SJ, et al. Incompetent perforating veins are associated with recurrent varicose veins, *Eur J Vasc Endovasc Surg.* 2001. *21*: 458–460.

97. Saarinen J, Suominen V, Heikinen M, et al. The profile of leg symptoms, clinical disability, and reflux in legs with previously operated varices, *Scand J Surg.* 2005. *94*: 51–55.

98. Stonebridge P, Chalmers N, Beggs I. Recurrent varicose veins: A varicographic analysis leading to a new practical classification, *Br J Surg.* 1995. *82*: 60–62.

99. Stücker M, Netz K, Breuckmann F, Altmeyer P, Mumme A. Histomorphologic classification of recurrent saphenofemoral reflux, *J Vasc Surg.* 2004. *39*: 816–822.

100. Theivacumar NS, Dellagrammaticas D, Darwood RJ, Mavor AID, Gough MJ. Fate of the great saphenous vein following endovenous laser ablation: Does re-canalisation mean recurrence, *Eur J Vasc Endovasc Surg.* 2008. *36*: 211–215.

101. Theivacumar NS, Gough MJ. Endovenous laser ablation (EVLA) to treat recurrent varicose veins, *Eur J Vasc Endovasc Surg.* 2011. *41*: 691–696.

102. Tsang FJ, Davis M, Davies AH. Incomplete saphenopopliteal ligation after short saphenous vein surgery: A summation analysis, *Phlebology.* 2005. *20*: 106–109.

103. Turton EPL, Scott DJA, Richards SP, et al. Duplex derived evidence of reflux after varicose vein surgery: Neo reflux or neovascularisation, *Eur J Vasc Endovasc Surg.* 1999. *17*: 230–233.

104. van Groenendael L, van der Vliet A, Flinkenflögel L, Roovers EA, van Sterkenburg SMM, Reijnen MMPJ. Treatment of recurrent varicose veins of the great saphenous vein by conventional surgery and endovenous laser, *J Vasc Surg.* 2009. *50*: 1106–1113.

105. van Neer PAFA, Kessels AGH, de Haan MW, et al. Residual varicose veins below the knee are not related to incompetent perforating veins, *J Vasc Surg.* 2006. *44*: 1051–1054.

106. van Neer P, de Haan MW, de Veraart JCJM, Neuman AM. Recurrent varicose veins below the knee after varicose vein surgery, *Phlebologie.* 2007. *36*: 132–136.

107. van Rij AM, Jiang P, Solomon C, Christie RA, Hill GB. Recurrence after varicose vein surgery: A prospective long-term clinical study with duplex ultrasound scanning and air plethysmography, *J Vasc Surg.* 2003. *38*: 935–943.

108. van Rij AM, Jones GT, Hill GB, Jiang P. Neovascularization and recurrent varicose veins: More histologic and ultrasound evidence, *J Vasc Surg.* 2004. *40*: 296–302.

109. Vin F, Chleir F. Aspect échographique des récidives variqueuses postopératoires du territoire de la veine petite saphène, *Ann Chir.* 2001. *126*: 320–324.

110. Winterborn RJ, Foy C, Earnshaw JJ. Causes of varicose vein recurrence: Late results of a randomized controlled trial of stripping the long saphenous vein, *J Vasc Surg.* 2004. *40*: 634–639.

111. Winterborn RJ, Earnshaw JJ. Randomized trial pf PTFE patch for recurrent great Saphenous varicose veins, *Eur J Vasc Endovasc Surg.* 2007. *34*: 367–373.

112. Wong JKF, Duncan JL, Nichols DM. Whole-leg duplex mapping for varicose veins: Observation on patterns of reflux in recurrent and primary legs, with clinical correlation, *Eur J Vasc Endovasc Surg.* 2003. *25*: 267–275.

113. Wright D, Rose KG, Young E, McCollum CN. Recurrence following varicose vein surgery, *Phlebology.* 2002. *16*: 101–105.

114. Eklof B, Perrin M, Delis KT, Rutherford RB, Gloviczki P. Updated terminology of chronic venous disorders: The VEIN-TERM transatlantic interdisciplinary consensus document, *J Vasc Surg.* 2009. *49*: 498–501.

115. Browse NL, Burnand KG, Irvine AT, Wilson NM. *Disease of the veins*, 2e. London: Arnold. 1999. 191–248.

116. Stonebridge PA, Chalmers N, Beggs I, et al. Recurrent varicose veins: A varicographic analysis leading to a new practical classification, *Br J Surg.* 1999. *82*: 60–62.

117. De Maeseneer M, Pichot O, Cavezzi A, et al. Duplex ultrasound investigation of the veins of the lower limbs after treatment for varicose veins: UIP Consensus Document, *Eur J Vasc Endovasc Surg.* 2011. *42*: 89–102.

118. Almgren B, Eriksson I. Primary deep vein incompetence in limbs with varicose veins, *Acta Chir Scand.* 1989. *155*: 445–460.

119. Guarnera G, Furgiuele S, Di Paola FM, Camilli S. Recurrent varicose veins and primary deep venous insufficiency: Relationship and therapeutic implications, *Phlebology.* 1995. *10*: 98–10.

120. Perrin M, Gobin JP, Grossetete C, Henri F, Lepretre M. Valeur de l'association chirurgie itérative-sclérothérapie après échec du traitement chirurgical des varices, *J Mal Vasc.* 1993. *18*: 314–319. In French.

121. Vasquez MA, Rabe E, McLafferty RB, et al. Revision of the venous clinical severity score: Venous outcomes consensus statement: Special communication of the American Venous Forum Ad Hoc Outcomes Working Group, *J Vasc Surg.* 2010. *52*: 1387–1396.

122. Darke SG, Baker SJA. Ultrasound-guided foam sclerotherapy for the treatment of varicose veins, *Br J Surg.* 2006. *93*: 969–974.

123. Coleridge Smith P. Chronic venous disease treated by ultrasound guided foam sclerotherapy, *Eur J Vasc Endovasc Surg.* 2006. *32*: 577–583.

124. Bergan JJ, Le Cheng V. Treatment of recurrent varicose veins by sclerosant foam. In: Bergan JJ, Le Cheng V, eds. *Foam Sclerotherapy.* London: Royal Society of Medicine Press. 2008. 193–198.

31.

USE OF SYSTEM-SPECIFIC QUESTIONNAIRES

A. C. Shepherd, Meryl Davis, and Alun H. Davies

The introduction of minimally invasive, endovenous therapies has revolutionized the treatment of varicose veins over the last decade. In the United Kingdom between 2008 and 2009, approximately 37,000 procedures were performed, of which approximately 18,000 (49%) were combined procedures, 2,000 (5%) were open procedures, 7,000 (19%) were endovenous ablation procedures, and 6,000 (16%) were injection sclerotherapy; the remainder were unspecified.[1] Data from questionnaire surveys and venous registries[2] support a movement away from traditional inpatient surgery toward minimally invasive outpatient treatments, a trend that appears set to continue.[3-6] The Edinburgh vein study described the incidence of varicose veins as 40% in men and 32% in women with the incidence increasing with age.[7] Although the number of varicose vein procedures performed has declined in recent years,[1,8] the morbidity attributable to venous disease and its complications is considerable and estimated at £600 million to the National Health Service (NHS) per annum. Despite good evidence that the treatment of varicose veins is both beneficial in terms of quality-of-life improvements that are cost effective,[9-11] recent introduction of rationing the treatment of varicose veins in a number of health care trusts has led many to question the assessment of outcomes following treatment, in order to ensure that resources are allocated efficiently.

QUALITY OF LIFE

Health is defined by the World Health Organization as "a state of complete physical, mental and social well being and not merely the absence of disease"; and measuring health and improving quality of life is of major importance throughout all branches of medicine. In 1997 Beattie et al.[12] suggested that the ideal quality-of-life measure should be:

- Equally applicable to any disease process or outcome,
- Equally applicable across all levels of illness and degrees of invalidity, and

- Of proven validity, with a high level of convergence within patient groups, when applied across geographic, linguistic, and cultural boundaries.

Currently there is no quality-of-life tool that is sufficiently sensitive to detect clinically significant changes and fulfill all of the above criteria; and a number of different generic health care questionnaires have been developed. In recent years the most popular tools for the measurement of venous disease have included the Nottingham Health Profile (NHP), the EuroQol (EQ-5D), and the short form 36 (SF36). The EQ-5D and SF36 are also validated in other major languages and are widely accepted internationally. Although applicable across a spectrum of disorders to allow a comparison of health-related quality of life across populations of patients with different diseases, these generic tools are frequently insufficiently sensitive to detect clinically significant changes in specific disease processes over time. For this reason, disease-specific quality-of-life tools have been designed, in order to be sensitive to these key dimensions in quality of life that are affected by the disease. In 2007 the American Venous Forum (AVF) published a consensus of recommended reporting standards specific to endovenous ablation of varicose veins, which supported the use of a combination of disease-specific and generic quality-of-life questionnaires.[13]

MEASUREMENT OF OUTCOMES

In developing an outcome measure, the concepts of validity, reliability, and responsiveness are vital.

Validity is the extent to which a questionnaire measures what is intended. This is frequently evaluated by comparing a new measure with an established one (criterion validity). In the absence of a gold standard, a construct's validity can be measured; this allows comparison of a new tool with objective or clinical findings.

Table 31.1 THE VENOUS CLINICAL SEVERITY SCORE

CHARACTERISTIC	ABSENT = 0	MILD = 1	MODERATE = 2	SEVERE = 3
Pain	None	Occasional/nonanalgesia restricting	With moderate activity/analgesia use	Daily pain, limitations to activities or regular analgesia
Varicose Veins > 4 mm	None	Few	Multiple GSV	Extensive GSV and SSV
Venous Edema	None	Evening/Ankle	Afternoon/Above knee	Morning/requiring elevation
Skin Pigmentation	None	Limited/Brown	Diffuse lower 1/3/purple	Wide/purple
Inflammation	None	Mild cellulitis in marginal area	Moderate involving most of gaiter area	Severe cellulitis or significant eczema
Induration	None	Focal <5cm	Medial or lateral less than lower 1/3	1/3 of leg or more
Number of active ulcers	None	1	2	3
Active ulcer duration	<3 months	>3 months	<12 months	> 12 months
Active ulcer diameter	None	<2 cm	2–6 cm	>6 cm
Compression	None or noncompliant	Intermittent use	Compression stockings worn most days	Compression stockings worn daily

Reliability is the degree to which measurements on the same individual are similar under different conditions. Test-retest comparisons are the most appropriate method for assessing reliability if the instrument is intended as an evaluative tool. Reliability can also be assessed using internal consistency; this checks the extent to which similar questions give consistent replies.

Responsiveness considers whether the tool is sensitive to assess measurable change. If meaningful comparisons are to be made then a standardized measure of responsiveness is required. The standardized response mean represents the mean change in score over two points in time divided by the standard deviation of the score differences and allows such a comparison.[14]

SYSTEM-SPECIFIC TOOLS

CLINICAL SCORING SYSTEMS

Consistent and accurate diagnosis and classification of clinical signs and symptoms are required before posttreatment responses can be analyzed. The CEAP (for clinical, etiological, anatomical, pathophysiological) classification, originally developed in 1994, was included in the international recommendations for the reporting standards in venous disease published in 1995.[15] It was further modified in 2004[16] and is available in several major languages and has now been adopted worldwide by the vascular community. The CEAP classification is purely descriptive and is not a quantifiable scoring system, nor is it sensitive to changes following intervention, and for this reason the Venous Clinical Severity Score (VCSS), Venous Segmental Disease Score (VSDS), and Venous Disability Score (VDS) were designed, based on the CEAP classification.[17] The VCSS is a simple clinical

scoring system is based around ten clinical domains with a potential maximum score of 30 (see Table 31.1). It has been used in the assessment of treatment outcomes and in clinical trials.[18,19] It is currently under revision, in order to modify the language with the aim of further evaluating the criteria in certain categories to make it more easily applicable to patients without affecting the sensitivity, and therefore making it an easier tool for clinicians to use as part of their routine practice as well as in clinical reserach.[20] The VSDS assesses the anatomical and pathophysiological components of the CEAP. The scores are allocated based on reflux or obstruction observed in eleven venous segments on venous imaging—usually color duplex. The VDS is a score ranging from 0 to 3 based on the degree of impairment to daily activities and reliance on compression. At present the VSDS and VDS are infrequently used in clinical practice and clinical trials.

In order to fully evaluate and compare different treatments or results from different publications, there is the need for standardization of the severity of venous disease, both from a clinical and function perspective.

Currently there are several system- or disease-specific instruments for measuring health-related quality of life in patients with varicose veins or chronic venous disease of the lower limb.

SYSTEM-SPECIFIC QUESTIONNAIRES

ABERDEEN VARICOSE VEIN QUESTIONNAIRE (AVVQ)

The Aberdeen Varicose Vein Questionnaire was originally designed by Garratt et al. as a postal questionnaire.[21] It consists of thirteen questions relating to varicose veins including observable signs, symptoms experienced, the use of compression hosiery, the effect of varicose veins on daily activities, and concerns regarding cosmesis, scores range from 0 (no disease) to 100 (severe disease). The original paper surveyed 373 patients with varicose veins selected from a hospital and general practice setting. A comparison was made with 900 members of the general population, selected randomly from the electoral register in Aberdeen, who were sent a similar questionnaire without the condition-specific tool. A high correlation with the SF36 generic health profile confirmed the validity of the questionnaire and illustrated that the perceived health of patients with varicose veins was significantly lower than that of the general population.[21] In 1999 the AVVQ was shown to be responsive to changes following surgery in a cohort of 137 consecutive patients with primary varicose veins.[22] Based on data collected from the AVVQ, SF36, and twenty-five questions that focused on symptoms and concerns, it was concluded that the AVVQ was a valid measure of quality of life for patients pre- and postsurgery. It also confirmed that patients had a significant improvement in quality of life following surgery. Since its introduction, the AVVQ has become a well-established and valid tool for measuring quality of life and has been used in numerous clinical trials and cohort studies to assess improvements following surgery and endovenous thermal ablation procedures in patients with varicose veins.[18,23-26] At present it is validated in English only.

CHRONIC VENOUS INSUFFICIENCY QUESTIONNAIRE (CIVIQ)

The original version of the CIVIQ was developed from a cross-sectional observational study in over 2,000 patients, of whom over 50% had a diagnosis of venous insufficiency based on clinical signs and reported symptoms. The CIVIQ2 was devised following a second analysis using a questionnaire of 20 equally weighted questions on the 1,001 patients with venous disease based on 4 criteria including physical, psychological, and social concerns as well as pain. The CIVIQ2 questionnaire has been shown to be appropriate, specific, and reliable for the assessment of chronic lower limb venous insufficiency.[27] And since its original publication in 1996 it has been shown to be reliable and responsive in the assessment of patients with chronic venous insufficiency, following venous outflow stenting in a study to 870 patients[28] and has also been successfully used to evaluate improvement following endovenous thermal ablation procedures for varicose veins in a number of clinical trials.[29,30] In recent years its use has becoming increasingly popular.

THE CHARING CROSS VENOUS ULCERATION QUESTIONNAIRE (CXVUQ)

The CXVUQ was designed to assess quality of life specifically in patients with venous leg ulceration. An ulcer-specific

questionnaire was designed with questions relating to physical discomfort, the effects on daily activities and social activities, emotional consequences, and perspectives regarding dressings and mobility. It was validated with the SF36 in a group of ninety-eight patients,[31] it has found to be reliable and responsive to treatment in this patient group, however is not designed for use in patients without venous ulceration.

VENOUS INSUFFICIENCY EPIDEMIOLOGY AND ECONOMIC STUDY (VEINS)

The Veins Questionnaire was developed over 10 years from an international prospective cohort study of 5,688 outpatients with chronic venous disease, that evaluated epidemiological factors and outcomes. The questionnaire consists of two separate categories: The VEINES quality-of-life questionnaire (VEINES QoL) consists of twenty-five items relating to the impact of chronic venous disease on quality of life. The VEINES symptom questionnaire (VEINS-SYM) consists of ten questions evaluating symptoms. Together they form a questionnaire of thirty-five different items with two summary scores. It was originally validated in English, French, French Canadian, and Italian and has been shown to be acceptable, reliable, valid, and responsive in patients with deep venous thrombosis.[32] It has also been shown to correlate with the SF36 and the CEAP[33] classification as further evidence of its validity, and in a study of 1,313 patients the VEINES QoL was found to be more sensitive to quality-of-life changes associated with varicose veins in combination with venous disorders than the SF36.[34] It was also suggested that in patients with varicose veins alone, cosmetic concerns and quality of life/relief of symptoms should be considered separately. In addition to the assessment of deep venous thrombosis the VEINES questionnaire has been used to evaluate a wide spectrum of venous disorders from telangiectasia, to varicose veins, edema and skin changes, and leg ulceration in patients from the original VEINES study population and responsiveness in an additional 1516 patients following treatment, where treatment outcomes were correlated with quality of life.[35]

SPECIFIC QUALITY OF LIFE AND OUTCOME RESPONSE-VENOUS (SQOR-V)

The SQOR-V questionnaire was developed by a French-American collaboration and published in 2007.[36] The aim was to develop a patient-reported outcome measure that would fully evaluate symptoms, impairment to activities, cosmetic concerns, and the psychological impact of the disease including concerns regarding risk to health. The authors proposed that existing disease-specific tools were insufficiently sensitive to fully evaluate venous symptoms experienced by patients with supposedly mild disease of clinical CEAP class C0–C3, and designed the questionnaire in order to evaluate this particular group of patients. Forty-six questions were carefully composed to evaluate symptoms, with a rating scale of 1 to 5 instead of yes/no answers in order to improve accuracy and sensitivity. Questions are divided into 5 domains, each with a possible total score of 20, giving a possible range of scores from 20 (no disease) to 100 (severe disease). It was originally developed in English and then translated into French, in which it was initially validated, along with the SF12 and a Center for Epidemiologic Studies-Depression scale (CES-D) in a group of 202 patients. It has been shown to have internal consistency, reducibility, structural validity, convergent validity, and clinical validity[36] and has now been validated in several other languages including English and Spanish. To date there have been few published studies of the SQOR-V, however early data collected in an English-speaking population suggest that it is responsive to change following endovenous thermal ablation treatments in patients of C2–C4 disease, and correlates with the AVVQ and VCSS scores.[37] Larger studies are awaited to support it's widespread use and superior sensitivity in this target patient group.

DIFFICULTIES WITH DISEASE-SPECIFIC QUALITY OF LIFE

Because the symptoms of venous insufficiency are notoriously difficult to determine and assess,[38,39] finding a single outcome measure that has sufficient scope to encompass the wide spectrum of symptoms experienced at the extremes of venous disease while remaining sensitive enough to evaluate improvements following intervention in those with milder disease is challenging, and at present no single solution exists. At present the majority of published clinical studies rely on a number of different disease-specific, generic, and clinical-outcome measures, making comparison among different techniques and patient groups difficult. In recent years there has been a move away from the use of surrogate outcome measures of anatomical and hemodynamic function to evaluate treatments and toward functional and in particular disease-specific, quality-of-life outcomes, which are though to be more truly representative of the patients' experience. The routine use of patient-reported outcome measures has several drawbacks, including being time-consuming and open to bias from patients and physicians, however they are likely to gain increasing popularity in the future. Already in 2009 Patient Reported Outcome Measures (PROMs) for hip and knee replacements and in hernia and varicose vein surgery have been introduced in many NHS trusts in the UK. Patients are requested to complete a preoperative disease specific and generic quality-of-life questionnaire. For varicose veins this is based on the EQ-5D and the AVVQ and they are then sent a postal questionnaire at 3 months

following their intervention. The data is collected centrally and will be used in the clinical evaluation and assessment of the performance of treatment centers and research into the clinical and cost-effectiveness of treatments.[40]

CONCLUSION

The AVVQ was one of the first disease-specific tools designed for the evaluation of varicose veins and remains the most popular to date, however, a number of newer questionnaires are gaining in popularity. At present there is no single tool that can be used in isolation, and consideration should be given to the population under investigation. With the introduction of rationing for venous interventions, accurate and appropriate measurement of outcomes to support the cost-effectiveness of treatments are of paramount importance. The cost-effectiveness of treatments is calculated in quality-adjusted life years (QALYs), a measure of disease burden and at present is calculated based on generic quality of life tools. In the future the assessment of the disease burden attributable to chronic venous disease is likely to become increasingly important in order to justify the allocation of resources, and therefore the need arises for the development of a disease specific tool in order to assess disease burden.

REFERENCES

1. http://www.hscic.gov.uk/hes. Main Procedures and Interventions. 2008–2009.
2. Database updates from the International Venous Registry (IVR). March 2009; In press.
3. Edwards AG, Baynham S, Lees T, Mitchell DC. Management of varicose veins: A survey of current practice by members of the Vascular Society of Great Britain and Ireland, Ann R Coll Surg Engl. 2009. 91(1): 77–80.
4. Lindsey B, Campbell WB. Rationing of the treatment of varicose veins and the use of new treatment methods: A survey of practice in the United Kingdom, Eur J Vasc Endovasc Surg. 2006. 32(4): 472.
5. Shepherd AC, Gohel MS, Lim CS, Hamish M, Davies AH. Endovenous ablation for varicose veins: Overtaking or overrated?, Phlebology. 2010. 25: 38–43.
6. Winterborn RJ, Corbett CR. Treatment of varicose veins: The present and the future: A questionnaire survey, Ann R Coll Surg Engl. 2008. 90(7): 561–564.
7. Evans CJ, Allan PL, Lee AJ, Bradbury AW, Ruckley CV, Fowkes FG. Prevalence of venous reflux in the general population on duplex scanning: The Edinburgh vein study, J Vasc Surg. 1998. 28(5): 767–776.
8. Lim CS, Gohel MS, Shepherd AC, Davies AH. Secondary care treatment of patients with varicose veins in National Health Service England: At least how it appeared on a National Health Service website, Phlebology. 2010. 25(4): 184–189.
9. Michaels JA, Campbell WB, Brazier JE, et al. Randomised clinical trial, observational study, and assessment of cost-effectiveness of the treatment of varicose veins (REACTIV trial), Health Technol Assess. 2006. 10(13): 1–196, iii–iv.
10. Gohel MS, Barwell JR, Earnshaw JJ, et al. Randomized clinical trial of compression plus surgery versus compression alone in chronic venous ulceration (ESCHAR study): Haemodynamic and anatomical changes, Br J Surg. 2005. 92(3): 291–297.

11. Ratcliffe J, Brazier JE, Campbell WB, Palfreyman S, MacIntyre JB, Michaels JA. Cost-effectiveness analysis of surgery versus conservative treatment for uncomplicated varicose veins in a randomized clinical trial, *Br J Surg*. 2006. *93*(2): 182–186.

12. Beattie DK, Golledge J, Greenhalgh RM, Davies AH. Quality of life assessment in vascular disease: Towards a consensus, *Eur J Vasc Endovasc Surg*. 1997. *13*(1): 9–13.

13. Kundu S, Lurie F, Millward SF, et al. Recommended reporting standards for endovenous ablation for the treatment of venous insufficiency: Joint statement of the American Venous Forum and the Society of Interventional Radiology, *J Vasc Surg*. 2007. *46*(3): 582–589.

14. Katz JN, Larson MG, Phillips CB, Fossel AH, Liang MH. Comparative measurement sensitivity of short and longer health status instruments, *Med Care*. 1992. *30*(10): 917–925.

15. Porter JM, Moneta GL. Reporting standards in venous disease: An update: International Consensus Committee on Chronic Venous Disease, *J Vasc Surg*. 1995. *21*(4): 635–645.

16. Eklof B, Rutherford RB, Bergan JJ, et al. Revision of the CEAP classification for chronic venous disorders: Consensus statement, *J Vasc Surg*. 2004. *40*(6): 1248–1252.

17. Rutherford RB, Padberg FT Jr., Comerota AJ, Kistner RL, Meissner MH, Moneta GL. Venous severity scoring: An adjunct to venous outcome assessment, *J Vasc Surg*. 2000. *31*(6): 1307–1312.

18. Darwood RJ, Theivacumar N, Dellagrammaticas D, Mavor AI, Gough MJ. Randomized clinical trial comparing endovenous laser ablation with surgery for the treatment of primary great saphenous varicose veins, *Br J Surg*. 2008. *95*(3): 294–301.

19. Vasquez MA, Wang J, Mahathanaruk M, Buczkowski G, Sprehe E, Dosluoglu HH. The utility of the Venous Clinical Severity Score in 682 limbs treated by radiofrequency saphenous vein ablation, *J Vasc Surg*. 2007. *45*(5): 1008–1014; discussion 1015.

20. Vasquez MA, Munschauer CE. Venous Clinical Severity Score and quality-of-life assessment tools: Application to vein practice, *Phlebology*. 2008. *23*(6): 259–275.

21. Garratt AM, Macdonald LM, Ruta DA, Russell IT, Buckingham JK, Krukowski ZH. Towards measurement of outcome for patients with varicose veins, *Qual Health Care*. 1993. *2*(1): 5–10.

22. Smith JJ, Garratt AM, Guest M, Greenhalgh RM, Davies AH. Evaluating and improving health-related quality of life in patients with varicose veins, *J Vasc Surg*. 1999. *30*(4): 710–719.

23. Mekako AI, Hatfield J, Bryce J, Lee D, McCollum PT, Chetter I. A nonrandomised controlled trial of endovenous laser therapy and surgery in the treatment of varicose veins, *Ann Vasc Surg*. 2006. *20*(4): 451–457.

24. MacKenzie RK, Paisley A, Allan PL, Lee AJ, Ruckley CV, Bradbury AW. The effect of long saphenous vein stripping on quality of life, *J Vasc Surg*. 2002. *35*(6): 1197–1203.

25. Rasmussen LH, Bjoern L, Lawaetz M, Blemings A, Lawaetz B, Eklof B. Randomized trial comparing endovenous laser ablation of the great saphenous vein with high ligation and stripping in patients with varicose veins: Short-term results, *J Vasc Surg*. 2007. *46*(2): 308–315.

26. Rautio T, Ohinmaa A, Perala J, et al. Endovenous obliteration versus conventional stripping operation in the treatment of primary varicose veins: A randomized controlled trial with comparison of the costs, *J Vasc Surg*. 2002. *35*(5): 958–965.

27. Launois R, Reboul-Marty J, Henry B. Construction and validation of a quality of life questionnaire in chronic lower limb venous insufficiency (CIVIQ), *Qual Life Res*. 1996. *5*(6): 539–554.

28. Neglen P, Hollis KC, Olivier J, Raju S. Stenting of the venous outflow in chronic venous disease: Long-term stent-related outcome, clinical, and hemodynamic result, *J Vasc Surg*. 2007. *46*(5): 979–990.

29. Almeida JI, Kaufman J, Gockeritz O, et al. Radiofrequency endovenous ClosureFAST versus laser ablation for the treatment of great saphenous reflux: A multicenter, single-blinded, randomized study (RECOVERY study), *J Vasc Interv Radiol*. 2009. *20*(6): 752–759.

30. Lurie F, Creton D, Eklof B, et al. Prospective randomized study of endovenous radiofrequency obliteration (closure procedure) versus ligation and stripping in a selected patient population (EVOLVeS Study), *J Vasc Surg*. 2003. *38*(2): 207–214.

31. Smith JJ, Guest MG, Greenhalgh RM, Davies AH. Measuring the quality of life in patients with venous ulcers, *J Vasc Surg*. 2000. *31*(4): 642–649.

32. Kahn SR, Lamping DL, Ducruet T, et al. VEINES-QOL/Sym questionnaire was a reliable and valid disease-specific quality of life measure for deep venous thrombosis, *J Clin Epidemiol*. 2006. *59*(10): 1049–1056.

33. Kahn SR, M'Lan CE, Lamping DL, Kurz X, Berard A, Abenhaim LA. Relationship between clinical classification of chronic venous disease and patient-reported quality of life: Results from an international cohort study, *J Vasc Surg*. 2004. *39*(4): 823–828.

34. Kurz X, Lamping DL, Kahn SR, et al. Do varicose veins affect quality of life? Results of an international population-based study, *J Vasc Surg*. 2001. *34*(4): 641–648.

35. Lamping DL, Schroter S, Kurz X, Kahn SR, Abenhaim L. Evaluation of outcomes in chronic venous disorders of the leg: Development of a scientifically rigorous, patient-reported measure of symptoms and quality of life, *J Vasc Surg*. 2003. *37*(2): 410–419.

36. Guex JJ, Zimmet SE, Boussetta S, Nguyen C, Taieb C. Construction and validation of a patient-reported outcome dedicated to chronic venous disorders: SQOR-V (specific quality of life and outcome response: venous), *J Mal Vasc*. 2007. *32*(3): 135–147.

37. Shepherd AC, Gohel MS, Lim CS, Hamish M, Davies AH. The use of disease-specific quality-of-life tools in patients with varicose veins: Abstract published from American College of Phlebology 22nd Annual Congress, Marco Island, FL, November 6–9, 2008. *Phlebology*. 2009. *24*: 89.

38. Bradbury A, Evans C, Allan P, Lee A, Ruckley CV, Fowkes FG. What are the symptoms of varicose veins? Edinburgh vein study cross sectional population survey, *Br Med J*. 1999. *318*(7180): 353–356.

39. Campbell WB, Decaluwe H, Boecxstaens V, et al. The symptoms of varicose veins: Difficult to determine and difficult to study, *Eur J Vasc Endovasc Surg*. 2007. *34*(6): 741–744.

40. http://www.hscic.gov.uk/proms. Patient Reported Outcome Measures (PROMs). 2009.

32.

PELVIC CONGESTION SYNDROME

DIAGNOSIS AND TREATMENT

Graeme D. Richardson

INTRODUCTION

Pelvic congestion syndrome (PCS) is still treated with skepticism by the medical community, and in most instances is called "the female varicocoele."

PCS is a distinct clinical entity in relatively young multiparous women characterized by chronic pelvic pain in the setting of pelvic venous varicosities. The syndrome, first described as a vascular condition by Taylor in 1949[1] was more recently shown by Hobbs[2] to be the result of venous engorgement of the pelvis due to gross dilatation and incompetence of one or both of the ovarian veins. In a series of fifty symptomatic patients with either pelvic or vulval varicose veins assessed by our ultrasound techniques in Wagga Wagga, the cause was found to be ovarian vein reflux in 71% of cases, more often the left than the right (24:9). These cases could well be described as the female varicocoele. Saphenofemoral tributaries were the only cause of vulval varicose veins in approximately 10% of cases, and the remainder were assumed to be caused by internal iliac reflux alone. The latter probably accounts for at least 10% of the cases of PCS. In addition, it seems likely that segmental pelvic vein reflux accounts for a further 10% of cases. Many patients with recurrent leg varicose veins are found to have a significant component of their problem from the pelvis. Seeking symptoms of PCS, a history of vulval varicose veins of pregnancy, and looking for a contribution from the pelvis in all patients presenting with leg varicosities will result in a greater awareness of a common yet poorly understood clinical problem.

ETIOLOGY

Although rarely seen in nulliparous teenagers and young women, when one may assume the cause is identical to male varicocoele, this condition largely follows pregnancy. Vulval varicose veins are said to occur in 2 to 7% of pregnancies.[3,4] These become larger in subsequent pregnancies, although they often disappear in the postpartum period. Usually after three pregnancies some varicose veins remain in the vulva, upper medial thigh, perianal, or gluteal regions. Probably the majority of cases are related to massive enlargement of the ovarian veins draining the pregnant uterus, perhaps associated with internal iliac vein compression. Perhaps after pregnancy some ovarian veins do not return to normal size, and the limited one or two valves at the upper end of the ovarian veins may become incompetent. Maybe segmental reflux occurs in tributaries of the internal iliac veins such as the uterine veins, and the round ligament veins, and can be responsible for persisting pelvic varicosities, even though we are unable to demonstrate ovarian vein or main trunk internal iliac vein reflux. We have often demonstrated this segmental reflux in our pelvic ultrasound assessment.

Compression syndromes are a further cause of left ovarian vein reflux, particularly superior mesenteric artery compression of the left renal vein and retro aortic left renal vein with compression. Compression of the left common iliac vein by the right common iliac artery can produce internal iliac reflux.

While hormonal and psychiatric factors have at times been implicated in the symptomatology, exacerbation of symptoms with menstruation, sexual activity, and ovulation suggests increased arterial flow to the pelvis at these times results in pooling of venous blood in the pelvic varicosities. This results in pressure in the pelvis alone, or if there are pelvic escape veins some or all of the pressure is transmitted to the vulva, buttock, or leg varicosities.

If large pelvic veins persist in the broad ligament, typical pelvic symptoms occur. Associated with these varicosities there may be pelvic escape through either the internal iliac tributaries, namely obturator or internal pudendal, or the round ligament into the vulva and upper medial thigh (Figure 32.1A), or posteriorly into the buttock and posterior thigh, sometimes including varices of the vein of the sciatic nerve, producing sciatica. These veins usually feed into either the long or short saphenous system, and if these are not treated at the time of treatment of long or

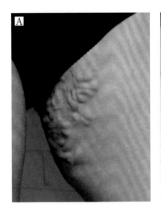
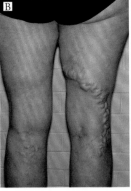

Figure 32.1 (**A**) Residual vulval varices. (**B**) Vulval to posterior thigh to lateral calf varices.

short saphenous varicose veins, then they cause recurrent varicose veins. A typical pattern is posterior vulval veins coursing posteriorly into the short saphenous via the vein of Giacomini (Figure 32.1B).

DIAGNOSIS

Clinical suspicion of PCS relies on typical symptoms, namely pelvic heaviness or deep pelvic pain, which is present before the period, on Day 1 and sometimes Day 2 of menstruation, midcycle, and post coitus. The latter is particularly noticeable on standing up immediately after having had morning intercourse. This aching may persist for several hours through the day. The pelvic heaviness is particularly severe after long periods of standing. Many patients complain of dyspareunia and many are aware of vulval and leg varicosities that are worse at the time of their pelvic symptoms. Commonly there are bladder symptoms related to perivesical varicosities causing frequency or a difficulty in starting the flow of urine. Many patients have symptoms of irritable bowel syndrome.

The diagnosis of PCS is often delayed until investigations looking for endometriosis, inflammatory bowel disease, urinary tract disease, or pelvic inflammatory disease have proved negative. It is common for patients to have suffered marital stress and dissatisfaction with their treating doctor's lack of interest in their condition.

INVESTIGATIONS

All patients with symptoms consistent with PCS are carefully examined to exclude other causes of pelvic pathology, and then undergo standard pelvic ultrasound and duplex ultrasound assessment of the pelvic, ovarian, and when appropriate, groin and lower limb veins. Earlier reports have advocated venography to demonstrate pelvic varices, either by use of vulval varicography,[5] transuterine venography,[6,7] periosseous[8] venography, or selective ovarian venography.[9,10] These techniques are invasive and may, in some cases,

invalidate assessment for reflux. For example, if a catheter is selectively placed adjacent to or inside the orifice of the right or left ovarian vein, it may pass the only valve present, and injection will then demonstrate "reflux." Varicography can demonstrate the anatomy of vulval and buttock varices and the relevant pelvic escape veins, but not the physiology of reflux (Figure 32.2).More recently, magnetic resonance imaging (MRI) and multislice computed tomography (CT) have been used to detect pelvic varices[11] in the assessment of chronic pelvic pain. Dynamic MRI techniques are currently being developed in Madrid (personal communication) that can show ovarian vein reflux but will need to be compared with ultrasound techniques for cost and reliability.

ULTRASOUND ASSESSMENT

PCS is confirmed on transvaginal ultrasound by finding excessive pelvic varicose veins in the broad ligament, which we would grade as mild (<5 mm), moderate (5–7 mm), or marked (8–10 mm), depending on the diameter, and whether these pelvic varicosities are found to distend when the patient is tilted head up by 60 degrees on a motorized ultrasound examination table. Our ultrasound assessment begins with the patient presenting after 6 hours of fasting and with a full bladder. Fasting reduces gut motility, and the full bladder enables standard gynecological pelvic ultrasound. A full bladder however compresses pelvic varicosities, which may be visible by transabdominal ultrasound after voiding. Transvaginal ultrasound then follows, and having confirmed PCS, we examine the ovarian veins and the internal iliac veins, including anterior and posterior divisions. The round ligament veins and saphenofemoral tributaries are also assessed.

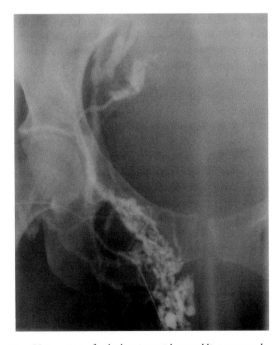

Figure 32.2 Varicogram of vulval varices with round ligament and obturator pelvic escape veins.

In Wagga Wagga, windows were developed to assess ovarian vein incompetence using transabdominal duplex ultrasound and color flow Doppler (3.5 or 5 MHz transducer).[12] We demonstrated the ability to locate ovarian veins and assess reflux in 93% of cases,[13] which compares well with the 92% visualization shown by Lechter[14] using venography. The left ovarian vein is found by first locating the left renal vein as it passes under the superior mesenteric artery. The ultrasound window is through the left lobe of the liver and the pancreas. The ovarian vein is located by following the left renal vein laterally and rotating the transducer through 90 degrees (Figure 32.3A). A retroaortic left renal vein, duplicated renal vein, or large ureteric veins are noted if present. It is important not to confuse accessory renal veins or the inferior mesenteric vein for the ovarian vein. The right ovarian vein is found using a window through the liver or gallbladder, by following the inferior vena cava upward to where the right ovarian vein enters it anterolaterally at a very acute angle. Sampling by color and wave form is taken about 2 cm below the termination of the ovarian veins (Figure 32.3B). The criterion for incompetence in the ovarian vein is reversed flow when lying down, sitting, or standing without augmentation. Treatment either by surgery, or more recently endovascular methods, is based on the ultrasound findings.

LAPAROSCOPY

Laparoscopy is sometimes required to exclude other possible causes for pelvic pain, such as endometriosis or pelvic inflammatory disease in patients who have pelvic varices on ultrasound assessment. We do this with the patient's gynecologist. Laparoscopy involves using an extra left iliac fossa port to retract the sigmoid colon. The patient, who initially is head down for gynecological laparoscopy, is then tilted head up, and the ovarian and broad ligament veins are seen to distend rapidly if reflux is present.

VENOGRAPHY

Many centers rely on clinical findings, then proceed to selective venography for confirmation, and then to endovascular treatment. Ultrasound confirmation of excessive pelvic varicose veins by transvaginal ultrasound, even if ultrasound assessment for ovarian vein reflux is not possible, should prevent unnecessary invasive venography, and assist in provision of informed consent, should a patient be referred to an interventional radiologist for venography with a view to coils with or without sclerotherapy. Left renal venography is followed by selective ovarian venography (Figures 32.4 and 32.5). If indicated by ultrasound findings, we may do selective iliac venograms.

TREATMENT

Various methods have been used to treat the symptoms of pelvic congestion, including psychotherapy, ovarian suppression,[15] intravenous dihydroergotamine,[16] and bilateral oophorectomy with hysterectomy.[17] Ovarian vein ligation has been performed to eliminate reflux since 1985, as either a bilateral procedure (Lechter,[14] Hobbs[2]), or unilateral based on ultrasound assessment (Richardson 1989). The long-term results of such treatment have been poorly investigated. It is important that any assessment of treatment of venous conditions have at least a 5-year follow-up. In recent years, however, endovascular ablative techniques have been popularized and similarly must be adequately assessed.

As many of these patients have associated leg varicosities, a treatment plan is required. The pelvic veins are only treated if there are pelvic symptoms, or if they significantly contribute to the leg varicosities. In these cases the pelvic veins are treated initially, and the response of symptoms is determined over a period of 2 to 3 months before treating the vulval or leg varicosities. In a few instances, the veins can reduce in size such that sclerotherapy of the residual

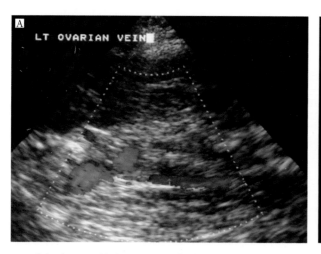 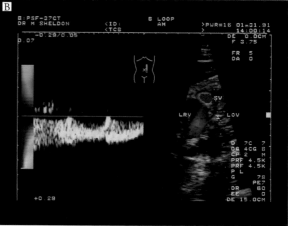

Figure 32.3 (A) Ultrasound left ovarian vein (red) and left renal vein (blue). (B) Ultrasound left ovarian vein and left renal vein with waveform showing reflux.

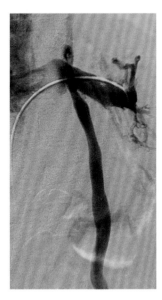

Figure 32.4 Left renal venogram with reflux into a large left ovarian vein. Note the narrow upper end, which helps prevent embolization of coils.

vulval or leg veins might be appropriate, rather than surgical treatment.

Ovarian Vein Incompetence

As most cases involve treatment of the left ovarian vein, the choice of treatment is between surgery and endovascular ablation techniques. Laparoscopic treatment has been investigated, and although it is possible to clip the upper end of the ovarian veins, it is currently not possible to remove a segment, nor would it be easy to deal with nearby tributaries.

Surgery

Ovarian vein ligation has been performed on 120 patients since 1989 by the author. It involves a "sympathectomy"

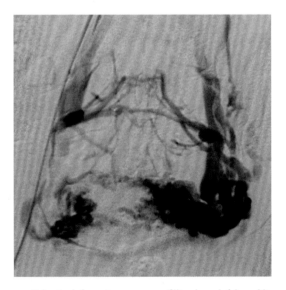

Figure 32.5 Selective left ovarian venogram filling large left broad ligament varices, with crossover to the right broad ligament, and drainage via the right ovarian vein and both iliac veins, also showing presacral veins.

incision with a muscle-splitting extraperitoneal approach to the ureter and the adjacent ovarian vein, which is ligated carefully using nonabsorbable material at the level of the pelvic brim. The ligature is then used for traction to enable further multiple ligations upward to finish at approximately 2 cm from the left renal vein. A narrow Dever retractor is useful to expose this uppermost portion. There is significant risk of major hemorrhage if the ovarian vein is not handled gently. This surgery requires approximately 2 days' hospitalization and 2 weeks' discomfort, which for a mother of young children is a considerable inconvenience compared with outpatient endovascular treatment. When choosing the most appropriate method of ovarian vein ablation, we accept that surgical ligation is complete, and provided all tributaries have been ligated, should produce long-term ablation of the ovarian vein. It can be performed by any general surgeon and requires no special equipment. It does however produce a scar and discomfort. I should reiterate that I would only ligate an ovarian vein that was shown to reflux on ultrasound assessment. Other surgeons have routinely ligated both ovarian veins.[14,2] It would seem unwise to ligate a draining vein that did not reflux. Some surgeons have advocated an even more extensive dissection to include the ovarian pedicle.[18] There is no evidence to suggest a more limited operation such as the Wagga Wagga technique has inferior results.

SURGICAL RESULTS

Long-term results in a series of seventy-two patients treated until June 1995 in Wagga Wagga certainly encourage one to treat patients based on the ultrasound findings of ovarian vein reflux.[19] These patients were sent questionnaires and were assessed independently by a surgical registrar for their quantitative response of symptoms to surgical treatment using visual analogue scales.[20] Sixty-seven of the seventy-two patients responded with a mean follow-up of thirty-three months (range 4 to 71) with a mean age of thirty-five years and mean pregnancies of 3.1. Pelvic heaviness was found to improve significantly (>50%) in 70% of patients, and in 56% of patients this was almost complete. Thirteen percent reported little or no improvement, and when these were subsequently investigated, including further ultrasound and venography, no ovarian reflux could be found, and in all cases alternative diagnoses such as irritable bowel syndrome were present. Dyspareunia was present preoperatively in 82% of cases, and 84% of these improved; 50% of these patients reported complete recovery.

Postintercourse pelvic aching was present in 75% of patients and improved in 70% of cases, with 64% having complete recovery. Bladder symptoms of frequency and obstruction improved in 45% of patients, and some of the 20% of patients who preoperatively were aware of bowel spasm improved. Two patients had normal pregnancies subsequent to ovarian vein ligation with no development of vulval veins in the pregnancy and no recurrence of symptoms.

Ovarian Endovascular Ablation

There have been several reports of single or a few case reports of successful treatment by ovarian vein embolization.[21–24] Thus far, there has been no standardization of the techniques used by several centers, but in all instances coils of various diameters and lengths have been used. In some centers sclerotherapy has been used, but in the Dutch[23] experience, sclerotherapy was contraindicated because of a perceived risk of entering the portal system. A team in Vancouver, which has a very large experience of treatment of male varicocoele using similar techniques, has utilized a combination of coils and glue (personal communication).

Since January 1999 we have been using endovascular techniques. We prefer to use an inguinal approach, and when cannulation of the ovarian vein is difficult, would use a guiding catheter and still use the groin, rather than a jugular or brachial approach. Our technique uses stainless steel coils with attached synthetic fibers (Cook), choosing a diameter to oversize by 2 to 3 mm the ovarian vein diameter. In addition, sclerosant has been used with 2 ml of 3% aethoxysklerol diluted with about 1 to 2 ml of contrast so that the spread of sclerosant can be clearly seen on the screen to avoid spillover into the left renal vein. Air is added and the syringe shaken to produce coarse bubbles. Our hope is that the sclerosant will help obliterate pelvic and broad ligament varices. By causing spasm we may help prevent migration of the coils. In no instances have we seen any contrast pass beyond the ovarian vein or broad ligament veins. While preparing the sclerosant as a foam would seem desirable, the contrast is further diluted and less visible than with coarse bubbles, and we are less sure of its spread. In an attempt to reduce the cost to the patient, we have tried to use the minimum number of coils to achieve the following principles. The first coil is deployed at the level of the pelvic brim just above where it crosses the ureter. Depending on the anatomy of the ovarian vein, we aim to place a coil across junctions or selectively coil major tributaries. We try to have good cross-section coverage of the vein by varying the deployment, and we aim to have the highest point above all incompetent tributaries, and within 2 to 3 cm of the left renal vein. Usually two long (20-cm) coils suffice, with occasional shorter coils in tributaries or at the upper end of the vein. We are aiming for the highest and longest possible ablation.

Our approach has been via the right femoral vein and having confirmed ovarian vein reflux by a selective left renal venogram, a guide wire is passed down the ovarian vein to the pelvis, and a catheter advanced to the level of the pelvic brim. Approximately one-third of the 2 ml of sclerosant is injected slowly, with the patient holding her breath with Valsalva as long as possible. In male varicocoele patients, this is combined with compression at the level of the external ring to avoid the sclerosant passing into the scrotum.

There are risks to endovascular techniques including embolization, migration and perforation of coils, irritation of nerves such as the genitofemoral, and the possibility of later recanalization. There have been reports of recanalization resulting in recurrent symptoms requiring later surgical treatment.

Internal Iliac Veins

Where patients are shown to have significant internal iliac vein reflux as a cause for the pelvic congestion syndrome, surgical treatment to ligate the main branch or selectively the anterior division has been performed on a few patients in our series and by others.[18] There are risks to the surrounding structures, such as ureteric and iliac vessels. There are also significant risks to endovascular treatment of the internal iliac system, being a very large vein at its junction with the external iliac vein. The shape of the vein encourages embolization. In one case, we have deployed a coil into the anterior division together with sclerotherapy. When the patient has ovarian and internal iliac vein reflux on ultrasound assessment, we have only treated the ovarian vein. Thus far we have not needed to treat the internal iliac vein because of a disappointing result.

Vulval Varicosities

Having treated the ovarian vein, these improve and can be treated by avulsion techniques by minor surgery, or at the time of dealing with the long or short saphenous varicosities. Large round ligament veins can be ligated as they emerge from the external inguinal ring. Sclerotherapy of residual minor vulval varicosities is possible, and the author has on many occasions used 2% aethoxysklerol. To apply adequate compression after the sclerotherapy I use cotton balls covered by tape and the patient wears a firm support, such as bicycle pants, in an attempt to provide as much compression as practical. Side effects from the sclerotherapy have been surprisingly few.

Ureteric Vein Reflux

Inevitably unusual cases will appear associated with venous anomalies. We have treated several cases with large refluxing ureteric veins that are tortuous and feed into the ovarian vein usually in the lower third of the abdomen. They are often difficult to cannulate for coil treatment. Sometimes the ovarian vein joins a lower renal vein branch, or a large lumbar vein rather than the renal vein, and sometimes the ovarian or the renal vein is duplicated. In all cases coming to endovascular treatment we have to be prepared for such anomalies and devise the best treatment strategy.

Other Causes of Pelvic Congestion

Some patients present with congestion symptoms or minor vulval varices, yet we are unable to demonstrate ovarian or internal iliac incompetence. As with most venous disease, there is variability related to long periods of standing and the menstrual cycle. Repeat ultrasound studies show this, and we try to perform studies when symptoms are maximal. There remain patients in whom there clearly are significant pelvic varices but no source of reflux. Some of these are due to venous obstruction associated with collateral venous pathways. We have observed patients with both fixed and intermittent reflux of internal iliac veins associated with common iliac vein obstruction. In some cases this is postural, when recumbent there is reversed flow, and is associated with 1- to 2-mm anteroposterior (AP) diameter where the right common iliac artery crosses the left common iliac vein. Perhaps some of these patients would benefit from a venous stent. A retroaortic left renal vein has frequently been associated with PCS and rarely left renal vein obstruction following surgical ligation. I avoid ablation of the ovarian vein in these patients with collateral drainage of the kidney.

Segmental Pelvic Vein Reflux

There remains a group of patients where we cannot demonstrate a definite cause. It appears quite feasible that some very large pelvic veins in pregnancy don't shrink and thus produce segmental reflux in uterine and broad ligament veins. These patients and others whose symptoms fail to resolve after ovarian or iliac vein ablation, are best treated by hysterectomy.

COMPARISON OF RESULTS OF COIL AND SURGICAL TREATMENT OF OVARIAN REFLUX

Patients treated by surgery from 1989 until 1998, and endovascular treatment from 1999 until June 2002 were studied using a questionnaire with visual analogue scales. Statistical analysis of pelvic heaviness and overall satisfaction showed no difference between endovascular and surgical treatment.[25] Both treatments resulted in statistically significant improvement after treatment. A decision to treat in both groups was based on clinical findings and ultrasound assessment, and there was no statistical difference in the presenting features of patients in either the surgical or the endovascular series.

Patients undergoing coil treatment were also subjected to follow-up ultrasound studies at 6 weeks and 6 months as well as abdominal radiographs. There was no evidence of coil migration in thirty-four patients. Early ultrasounds showed two clots in broad ligament veins, no significant

reduction in diameter at 6 to 10 weeks, but some evidence of reduction by 6 months.

Long-term results of endovascular treatment have not yet been reported. Recanalization remains possible but should be amenable to further endovascular treatment. While the great majority of patients tolerate coil treatment with little discomfort, with anxious patients it is more difficult to cannulate the femoral vein, and spasm of the ovarian vein could lead to perforation. Patients have far less loin discomfort than after surgery, but it seems excessive exercise should be restricted. A few patients have severe pain, and this could be due to thrombosis of the ovarian vein or perforation.

Patient satisfaction justifies ablation of an ovarian vein shown by ultrasound to reflux.

Provided endovascular ovarian vein ablation can be delivered safely and at reasonable cost, then there are definite advantages over surgical treatment. Complications can occur from either method. The incidence of long-term recanalization is unknown.

There is no evidence that endovascular treatment produces better results than surgery. Provided patients are prepared to accept the scar, pain, hospitalization, and other potential complications of an operation, at this point one cannot say surgical treatment has been superseded.

REFERENCES

1. Taylor HC, Wright H. Vascular congestion and hyperaemia, *Am J Obst Gynecol.* 1949. *57*: 211–230.
2. Hobbs JT. The pelvic congestion syndrome, *Br J Hosp Med.* 1990. *43*: 200–206.
3. Dodd H, Wright AP. Vulval varicose veins in pregnancy, *Br Med J.* 1959. *1*: 831–832.
4. Dixon JA, Mitchell WA. Venographic and surgical observations in vulvar varicose veins, *J Surg Gynaecol Obstet.* 1970. *131*: 458–464.
5. Craig O, Hobbs JT. Vulval phlebography in the pelvic congestion syndrome, *Clin Radiol.* 1974. *24*: 517–525.
6. Heiner G, Siegel T. Zur Frage des Iokalen Kontrast Mittel Schadigung bei der Uterus Phlebography, *Z Cl Gynak.* 1925. *87*: 829.
7. Chidakel N, Ediundh KO. Transuterine phlebography with particular reference to pelvic varicosities, *Acta Radiol.* 1968. *7*: 1–12.
8. Lea Thomas M, Hobbs JT. Vulval phlebography in the pelvic congestion syndrome, *Clin Radiol.* 1974. *25*: 517.
9. Ahlberg NE, Bartley O, Chidakel N. Retrograde contrast filling of the left gonadal vein, *Acta Radiol.* 1965. *3*: 385.
10. Chidakel N. Female pelvic veins demonstrated by selective renal phlebography with particular reference to pelvic varicosities, *Acta Radiol.* 1968. *7*: 193–209.
11. Gupta A, McCarthy S. Pelvic varices as a cause of pelvic pain: MRI appearance, *Magn Reson Imaging.* 1994. *12*(4): 679–681.
12. Richardson GD, Beckwith TC, Sheldon M. Ultrasound windows to abdominal and pelvic veins, *Phlebology.* 1991. *6*: 111–125.
13. Richardson GD, Beckwith TC, Sheldon M. Ultrasound assessment in the treatment of pelvic varicose veins. Presented at the American Venous Forum, Fort Lauderdale, FL, 1991.
14. Lechter A. Pelvic varices: Treatment, *J Cardiovasc Surg.* 1985. *26*: 111.
15. Farquhar CM, Rogers V, Franks S, Pearce S, Wadsworth J, Beard RW. A randomized controlled trial of medroxyprogesterone acetate and

pschycotherapy for the treatment of pelvic congestion, *Br J Obstet Gynaecol.* 1989. *96:* 1153–1162.

16. Reginald PW, Beard RW, Kooner JS, et al. Intravenous dihydroergotamine to relieve pelvic congestion with pain in young women, *Lancet.* 1987. *330*(8555): 351–353.

17. Beard RW, Kennedy RG, Gangar KE, et al. Bilateral oophorectomy and hysterectomy in the treatment of intractable pelvic pain associated with pelvic congestion, *Br J Obstet Gynaecol.* 1991. *98:* 988–992.

18. Gomez ER, Villavicencio JL, Conaway CW, et al. The management of pelvic varices by combined retroperitoneal ligation and sclerotherapy (Abstract). European American Venous Symposium, Washington, DC, 1987.

19. Richardson GD, Beckwith TC, Mykytowycz M, Lennox AF. Pelvic congestion syndrome: Diagnosis and treatment, *ANZ J Phlebol.* 1999. *3*(2): 51–56.

20. Scott J, Huskisson EC. Graphic representation of pain, *Pain.* 1976. *2:* 175–184.

21. Edwards RD, Robertson IR, McLean AB, Hemingway AP. Case report: Pelvic pain syndrome: Successful treatment of a case by ovarian vein embolization, *Clin Radiol.* 1993. *47:* 429–431.

22. Sichlau MJ, Yao JST, Vagelzang RL. Transcatheter embolotherapy for the treatment of pelvic congestion syndrome, *Obstet Gynecol.* 1994. *83:* 892–896.

23. Boomsma J, Potocky V, Kievit C, Vertrulsdonek J, Gooskens V, Weemhof R. Phlebography and embolization in women with pelvic vein insufficiency, *MedicaMundi.* 1998. *42*(2): 22–29.

24. Cordts P, Eclavea A, Buckley P, DeMaioribus C, Cockerill M, Yeager T. Pelvic congestion syndrome: Early clinical results after transcatheter ovarian vein embolisation, *Vasc Surg.* 1998. *5:* 862–868.

25. Richardson GD, Driver B. Ovarian vein ablation: Coils or surgery?, *Phlebology.* 2005. *21*(1): 16–23.

PART III

VENOUS THROMBOEMBOLISM

33.

THE EPIDEMIOLOGY OF VENOUS THROMBOEMBOLISM IN THE COMMUNITY

IMPLICATIONS FOR PREVENTION AND MANAGEMENT

John A. Heit

INTRODUCTION

The epidemiology of venous thromboembolism (VTE) in the community has important implications for prevention and management. This chapter describes the incidence, survival, recurrence, complications, and risk factors for deep vein thrombosis of the leg, pelvis, or arm, and its complication, pulmonary embolism. The epidemiology of thrombosis affecting other venous circulations (e.g., cerebral sinus, mesenteric, renal, hepatic, portal) is beyond the scope of this review. Since population-based studies of venous thromboembolism epidemiology are most generalizable to the reader's individual patients, this chapter focuses on data provided from studies that included the complete spectrum of the disease from well-described populations.

THE INCIDENCE OF DEEP VEIN THROMBOSIS AND PULMONARY EMBOLISM

The average annual incidence rates of venous thromboembolism among white Americans during the 25-year period 1966 to 1990 (age- and sex-adjusted to the 1980 US white population), was 117 per 100,000 person-years.[1] The venous thromboembolism incidence over the 7-year period 1991 to 1997 (117.7 per 100,000; similarly adjusted, but to the 2000 US white population), had not changed significantly compared with the 10-year period 1981 to 1990 (116.7 per 100,000; see Figure 33.1). Based on the 1991–1997 rates, 249,000 incident venous thromboembolism cases occur annually among US whites. The incidence appears to be similar or higher among African Americans and lower among Asian Americans and Native Americans.[2–6] Assuming that the 1991 to 1997 age- and sex-specific venous thromboembolism incidence among blacks (black or African American alone) is comparable to whites, and adjusting for the different age and sex distribution of black Americans, the overall age- and sex-adjusted venous thromboembolism incidence was 77.6 per 100,000. Based on this incidence, 27,000

incident venous thromboembolism cases occur annually among US blacks, for a total of over 275,000 new venous thromboembolism cases per year in the United States.

Venous thromboembolism is predominantly a disease of older age.[1,7,8] In the absence of a central venous catheter[9] or thrombophilia,[10] venous thromboembolism is rare prior to late adolescence.[1,11] The age- and sex-adjusted venous thromboembolism incidence rate for persons age 15 years or older is 149 per 100,000.[1] Incidence rates increase exponentially with age for both men and women and for both deep vein thrombosis and pulmonary embolism (see Figures 33.2 and 33.3).[1,8] The overall age-adjusted incidence rate is higher for men (130 per 100,000) than women (110 per 100,000; male:female sex ratio is 1.2:1).[1] Incidence rates are somewhat higher in women during the childbearing years, whereas incidence rates after age 45 years are generally higher in men. Pulmonary embolism accounts for an increasing proportion of venous thromboembolism with increasing age for both genders.[1]

SURVIVAL AFTER DEEP VEIN THROMBOSIS AND PULMONARY EMBOLISM

Survival after venous thromboembolism is worse than expected, and survival after pulmonary embolism is much worse than after deep vein thrombosis alone (see Table 33.1).[12–14] The risk of early death among patients with symptomatic pulmonary embolism is 18-fold higher compared with patients with deep vein thrombosis alone.[12] Pulmonary embolism is an independent predictor of reduced survival for up to 3 months. For almost one-quarter of pulmonary embolism patients, the initial clinical presentation is sudden death. Independent predictors of reduced early survival after venous thromboembolism include increasing age, male gender, lower body mass index, confinement to a hospital or nursing home at venous thromboembolism onset, congestive heart failure, chronic lung disease, serious neurological disease, and

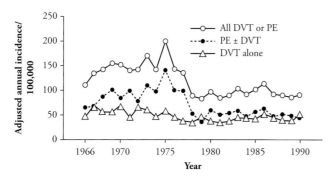

Figure 33.1 Age- and sex-adjusted annual incidence of all venous thromboembolism, deep vein thrombosis (DVT) alone, and pulmonary embolism with or without deep vein thrombosis (PE ± DVT). (From Reference 1)

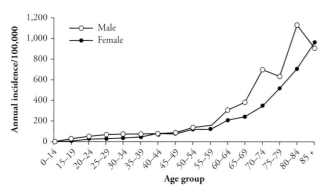

Figure 33.2 Annual incidence of venous thromboembolism by age and gender. (From Reference 1)

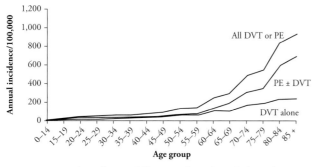

Figure 33.3 Annual incidence of all venous thromboembolism, deep vein thrombosis (DVT) alone, and pulmonary embolism with or without deep vein thrombosis (PE ± DVT) by age. (From Reference 1)

active malignancy.[8,12,13] Additional clinical predictors of poor early survival after pulmonary embolism include syncope and arterial hypotension.[15] Evidence of right heart failure based on clinical examination, plasma markers (e.g., cardiac troponin T, brain natriuretic peptide),[16,17] or echocardiography[13] predicts poor survival among normotensive pulmonary embolism patients. Pulmonary embolism patients with these characteristics should receive aggressive anticoagulation therapy, and possibly thrombolytic therapy in selected cases.[18,19]

Table 33.1 SURVIVAL (%) AFTER DEEP VEIN THROMBOSIS VERSUS PULMONARY EMBOLISM

TIME	DEEP VEIN THROMBOSIS ALONE	PULMONARY EMBOLISM
0 days	97.0	76.5
7 days	96.2	71.1
14 days	95.7	68.7
30 days	94.5	66.8
90 days	91.9	62.8
1 year	85.4	57.4
2 years	81.4	53.6
5 years	72.6	47.4
8 years	65.2	41.5

(From Reference 12)

VENOUS THROMBOEMBOLISM RECURRENCE

Venous thromboembolism recurs frequently; about 30% of patients develop recurrence within the next 10 years (see Table 33.2, Figure 33.4).[20] The hazard of recurrence varies with the time since the incident event and is highest within the first 6 to 12 months. However, even at 10 years the hazard of recurrent venous thromboembolism never falls to zero. Although active therapeutic anticoagulation is effective in preventing recurrence,[21–23] the duration of anticoagulation does not affect the risk of recurrence once primary therapy for the incident event is stopped.[24–26] These data suggest that for a subset of patients, venous thromboembolism is a chronic disease with episodic recurrence; indefinite secondary prophylaxis may be warranted for this patient subset.[21–23,26,27] Independent predictors of recurrence include male gender,[20,28,29] increasing patient age and body mass index, neurological disease with extremity paresis, and active malignancy (see Table 33.3).[8,20,30–33] Additional predictors include "idiopathic" venous thromboembolism,[22,24,33] a lupus anticoagulant or antiphospholipid antibody,[22,34] antithrombin, protein C or protein

Table 33.2 CUMULATIVE INCIDENCE AND HAZARD OF VENOUS THROMBOEMBOLISM RECURRENCE

	VENOUS THROMBOEMBOLISM RECURRENCE	
TIME TO RECURRENCE	CUMULATIVE RECURRENCE %	HAZARD OF RECURRENCE PER 1,000 PERSON-DAYS (±SD)
0 days	0.0	0
7 days	1.6	170 (30)
30 days	5.2	130 (20)
90 days	8.3	30 (5)
180 days	10.1	20 (4)
1 year	12.9	20 (2)
2 years	16.6	10 (1)
5 years	22.8	6 (1)
10 years	30.4	5 (1)

(From Reference 20)

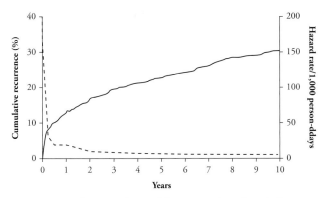

Figure 33.4   Cumulative incidence of first venous thromboembolism recurrence (—), and the hazard of first recurrence per 1000 person-days (- - -).   (From Reference 20)

S deficiency,[35] and possibly persistent residual deep vein thrombosis.[36] Prolonged secondary prophylaxis with anticoagulation therapy should be considered for patients with these characteristics. Although the incident event type (deep vein thrombosis alone vs. pulmonary embolism) is not a predictor of recurrence, patients with recurrence are significantly more likely to recur with the same event type as the incident event type.[37,38] Because the 7-day case fatality rate is significantly higher for recurrent pulmonary embolism (34%) compared to recurrent deep vein thrombosis alone (4%),[38] prolonged anticoagulation should be considered for incident pulmonary embolism, especially for patients with chronically reduced cardiopulmonary functional reserve.

COMPLICATIONS OF VENOUS THROMBOEMBOLISM

The major complications of venous thromboembolism are venous stasis syndrome (e.g., postthrombotic syndrome, including dependent leg swelling and pain, stasis pigmentation and dermatitis, and dermatoliposclerosis) and venous ulcer, and chronic thromboembolic pulmonary hypertension. The overall incidence of venous stasis syndrome and venous ulcer is 76.1 and 18.0 per 100,000 person-years,

Table 33.3 **INDEPENDENT PREDICTORS OF VENOUS THROMBOEMBOLISM RECURRENCE**

CHARACTERISTIC	HAZARD RATIO	95% CI
Age*	1.17	1.11, 1.24
Body Mass Index†	1.24	1.04, 1.47,
Neurologic Disease with Extremity Paresis	1.87	1.28, 2.73
Active Malignancy		
Malignancy with Chemotherapy	4.24	2.58, 6.95
Malignancy without Chemotherapy	2.21	1.60, 3.06

*per decade increase in age.
†per 10 kg/m² increase in body mass index.
(From Reference 20)

respectively.[39] Venous thromboembolism patients have a 17-fold increased risk of venous stasis syndrome.[39] The 20-year cumulative incidence of venous stasis syndrome after venous thromboembolism and after proximal deep vein thrombosis are about 25% and 40%, respectively.[32,40] Risk factors for venous stasis syndrome include the venous thromboembolism event type (deep vein thrombosis, with or without pulmonary embolism) and deep vein thrombosis location (proximal deep vein thrombosis). The 20-year cumulative incidence of venous ulcer is 3.7%.[40] The risk for venous ulcer is increased 30% per decade of age at the incident venous thromboembolism.[40] Venous thromboembolism accounts for about 12% of all venous stasis syndrome occurring in the community.[39]

The incidence of chronic thromboembolic pulmonary hypertension over the 21-year period 1976 to 1996 was 6.5 per million person-years.[41] Over this same time period, the incidence of acute pulmonary embolism was 485.6 per million person-years. Thus, the vast majority of acute pulmonary emboli do not progress to chronic thromboembolic pulmonary hypertension. Applying these incidence rates to the 2000 US white population, approximately 1,367 new chronic thromboembolic pulmonary hypertension cases occur in the United States annually.

RISK FACTORS FOR VENOUS THROMBOEMBOLISM

In order to improve survival, avoid recurrence, prevent complications, and reduce health care costs, the occurrence of venous thromboembolism must be reduced. To accomplish this, persons at risk for venous thromboembolism first must be identified. Independent risk factors for venous thromboembolism include patient age, surgery, trauma, hospital or nursing home confinement, active malignant neoplasm with or without concurrent chemotherapy, central vein catheterization or transvenous pacemaker, prior superficial vein thrombosis, varicose veins among the young, and neurological disease with extremity paresis; patients with chronic liver disease have a reduced risk (see Table 33.4).[42,43] The incidence of venous thromboembolism increases significantly with age for both idiopathic and secondary venous thromboembolism, suggesting that the risk associated with advancing age may be attributable to the biology of aging rather than simply an increased exposure to venous thromboembolism risk factors with advancing age.[44] Compared to residents in the community, hospitalized residents have over a 150-fold increased incidence of acute venous thromboembolism.[45] Hospitalization and nursing home residents together account for almost 60% of incident venous thromboembolism events occurring in the community.[46] Thus, hospital confinement provides an important opportunity to significantly reduce venous thromboembolism incidence. Of note, hospitalization for medical illness and

Table 33.4 INDEPENDENT RISK FACTORS FOR DEEP VEIN THROMBOSIS OR PULMONARY EMBOLISM

BASELINE CHARACTERISTIC	ODDS RATIO	95% CI
Institutionalization with or without recent surgery		
Institutionalization without recent surgery	7.98	4.49, 14.18
Institutionalization with recent surgery	21.72	9.44, 49.93
Trauma	12.69	4.06, 39.66
No malignancy	1.0	
Malignancy without chemotherapy	4.05	1.93, 8.52
Malignancy with chemotherapy	6.53	2.11, 20.23
Prior central venous catheter or transvenous pacemaker	5.55	1.57, 19.58
Prior superficial vein thrombosis	4.32	1.76, 10.61
Neurologic disease with extremity paresis	3.04	1.25, 7.38
Serious liver disease	0.10	0.01, 0.71

(From Reference 42)

hospitalization for surgery account for almost equal proportions of venous thromboembolism (22% and 24%, respectively), emphasizing the need to provide prophylaxis to both of these risk groups. Nursing home residents independently account for over one-tenth of all venous thromboembolism disease in the community.[46]

The risk among surgery patients can be further stratified based on patient age, type of surgery, and the presence of active cancer.[47,48] The risk of postoperative venous thromboembolism increases with advancing patient age,[49] especially for surgery patients that are 65 years of age or older.[48] High-risk surgical procedures include neurosurgery; major orthopedic surgery of the leg; thoracic, abdominal, or pelvic surgery for malignancy; renal transplantation; and cardiovascular surgery.[48] Obesity[49-51] and poor American Society of Anesthesiology physical status[51] are risk factors for venous thromboembolism after total hip arthroplasty. Other independent risk factors for venous thromboembolism after major surgery (after controlling for active cancer) include intensive care unit (ICU) length of stay greater than 6 days, immobility, and infection.[49] The risk from surgery may be less with neuraxial (spinal or epidural) anesthesia compared to general anesthesia.[52] Risk factors for venous thromboembolism among patients hospitalized for acute medical illness may include active cancer and prior venous thromboembolism.[53] After controlling for active cancer, additional independent risk factors include increasing patient age and body mass index, prior superficial vein thrombosis, chronic renal disease, neurological disease with extremity paresis, fracture and immobility,[54] and possibly infection.[53]

Active cancer accounts for almost 20% of incident venous thromboembolism events occurring in the community.[46] The risk appears to be higher for patients with pancreatic cancer, lymphoma, malignant brain tumors, cancer of the liver, leukemia, and colorectal and other digestive cancers.[55,56] Cancer patients receiving immunosuppressive or cytotoxic chemotherapy are at even higher risk for venous thromboembolism,[42] including therapy with L-asparaginase, thalidomide, or tamoxifen.

A central venous catheter or transvenous pacemaker now accounts for 9% of incident venous thromboembolism occurring in the community.[46] Prior superficial vein thrombosis is an independent risk factor for subsequent deep vein thrombosis or pulmonary embolism remote from the episode of superficial thrombophlebitis.[42] The risk of deep vein thrombosis imparted by varicose veins is uncertain and appears to vary by patient age.[42] Long-haul (>6 h) air travel is associated with a slightly increased risk for venous thromboembolism that is preventable with elastic stockings.[57] Coenzyme A reductase inhibitor (statin) therapy may provide a 20 to 50% risk reduction for venous thromboembolism.[58] However, the risk associated with atherosclerosis, or other risk factors for atherosclerosis, remains uncertain.[59-61] Body mass index, current or past tobacco smoking, chronic obstructive pulmonary disease, and renal failure are not independent risk factors for venous thromboembolism after controlling for other risk factors (e.g., surgery, hospitalization, trauma).[42] The risk associated with congestive heart failure, independent of hospitalization, is low.[42,43] Among women, additional risk factors for venous thromboembolism include oral contraceptive use and hormone therapy[62] and therapy with the selective estrogen receptor modulator, raloxifene, and pregnancy and the postpartum period.[43,63] Compared to nonpregnant women of childbearing age, the venous thromboembolism risk among pregnant women is increased over four-fold.[64] The annual venous thromboembolism incidence is five-fold higher among postpartum compared to pregnant women (511.2 versus 95.8 per 100,000), and the incidence of deep venous thrombosis is three-fold higher than pulmonary embolism (151.8 versus 47.9 per 100,000). Pulmonary embolism is relatively uncommon during pregnancy compared to postpartum (10.6 versus 159.7 per 100,000).

Other conditions associated with venous thromboembolism include heparin-induced thrombocytopenia, myeloproliferative disorders (especially polycythemia rubra vera and primary thrombocythemia), intravascular coagulation and fibrinolysis/disseminated intravascular coagulation (ICF/DIC), nephrotic syndrome, paroxysmal nocturnal hemoglobinuria, thromboangiitis obliterans (Buerger's disease), thrombotic thrombocytopenic purpura, Bechet's syndrome, systemic lupus erythematosus, inflammatory bowel disease, Wegener's granulomatosis, homocystinuria, and possibly hyperhomocysteinemia.[65,66]

THE GENETIC EPIDEMIOLOGY OF VENOUS THROMBOEMBOLISM

Recent family-based studies indicate that venous thromboembolism is highly heritable and follows a complex mode of inheritance involving environmental interaction.[67-69] Inherited reductions in plasma natural anticoagulants (e.g., antithrombin, protein C, or protein S) have long been recognized as uncommon but potent risk factors for venous thromboembolism.[70,71] More recent discoveries of impaired downregulation of the procoagulant system (e.g., activated protein C resistance, Factor V Leiden),[72-74] increased plasma concentrations of procoagulant factors (e.g., factors I [fibrinogen], II [prothrombin], VIII, IX, and XI),[75-79] increased basal procoagulant activity,[80-82] impaired fibrinolysis,[83] and altered innate immunity[84] have added new paradigms to the list of inherited or acquired disorders predisposing to thrombosis (thrombophilia). These plasma hemostasis-related factors or markers of coagulation activation both correlate with increased thrombotic risk and are highly heritable.[85-89] Inherited thrombophilias interact with such clinical risk factors (e.g., environmental risk factors) as oral contraceptives,[90] pregnancy,[91] hormone therapy,[92] and surgery[93] to increase the risk of incident venous thromboembolism. Similarly, genetic interaction increases the risk of incident[94] and recurrent venous thromboembolism.[95-99] These findings support the hypothesis that an acquired or familial thrombophilia may predict the subset of exposed persons who actually develop symptomatic venous thromboembolism. Although the clinical utility of diagnostic testing for an inherited or acquired thrombophilia remains controversial, such studies hold the potential for further identifying individual patients at high and low risk for incident and recurrent venous thromboembolism, targeting prophylaxis to those who would benefit most, and, ultimately, reducing the occurrence of venous thromboembolism.

REFERENCES

1. Silverstein MD, Heit JA, Mohr DN, Petterson TM, O'Fallon WM, Melton LJ III. Trends in the incidence of deep vein thrombosis and pulmonary embolism: A 25-year population-based study, *Arch Intern Med*. 1998. *158*: 585–593.

2. White RH, Zhou H, Romano PS. Incidence of idiopathic deep venous thrombosis and secondary thromboembolism among ethnic groups in California, *Ann Intern Med*. 1998. *128*: 737–740.

3. Klatsky AL, Armstrong MA, Poggi J. Risk of pulmonary embolism and/or deep venous thrombosis in Asian-Americans, *Am J Card*. 2000. *85*(11): 1334–1337.

4. Stein PD, Kayali F, Olson RE, Milford CE. Pulmonary thromboembolism in Asians/Pacific Islanders in the United States, *Am J Med*. 2004. *116*: 435–442.

5. Hooper WC, Holman RC, Heit JA, Cobb N. Venous thromboembolism hospitalizations among American Indians and Alaska Natives, *Thromb Res*. 2002. *108*(5–6): 273–278.

6. Stein PD, Kayali F, Olson RE, Milford CE. Pulmonary thromboembolism in American Indians and Alaskan Natives, *Arch Intern Med*. 2004. *164*: 1804–1806.

7. Stein PD, Hull RD, Kayali F, Ghali WA, Alshab AK, Olson RE. Venous thromboembolism according to age: Impact of an aging population, *Arch Intern Med*. 2004. *164*: 2260–2265.

8. Cushman M, Tsai AW, White RH, et al. Deep vein thrombosis and pulmonary embolism in two cohorts: The Longitudinal Investigation of Thromboembolism Etiology, *Am J Med*. 2004. *117*: 19–25.

9. Massicote MP, Dix D, Monagle P, Adams M, Andrew M. Central venous catheter related thrombosis in children: Analysis of the Canadian Registry of Venous Thromboembolic Complications, *J Pediatr*. 1998. *133*: 770–776.

10. Tormene D, Simioni P, Prandoni P, et al. The incidence of venous thromboembolism in thrombophilic children: A prospective cohort study, *Blood*. 2002. *100*(7): 2403–2405.

11. van Ommen CH, Heijboer H, Büller HR, Hirasing RA, Heijmans HSA, Peters M. Venous thromboembolism in childhood: A prospective two-year registry in The Netherlands, *J Pediatr*. 2001. *139*: 676–681.

12. Heit JA, Silverstein MD, Mohr DN, Petterson TM, O'Fallon WM, Melton LJ III. Predictors of survival after deep vein thrombosis and pulmonary embolism: A population-based cohort study, *Arch Intern Med*. 1999. *159*: 445–453.

13. Goldhaber SZ, Visani L, De Rosa M. Acute pulmonary embolism: Clinical outcomes in the International Cooperative Pulmonary Embolism Registry (ICOPER), *Lancet*. 1999. *353*: 1386–1389.

14. Janata K, Holzer M, Domanovits H, et al. Mortality of patients with pulmonary embolism, *Wiener Klinische Wochenschrift*. 2002. *114*(17–18): 766–772.

15. Konstantinides S, Geibel A, Olschewski M, et al. Association between thrombolytic treatment and the prognosis of hemodynamically stable patients with major pulmonary embolism: Results of a multicenter registry, *Circulation*. 1997. *96*: 882–888.

16. Pruszczyk P, Bochowicz A, Torbicki A, et al. Cardiac troponin T monitoring identifies high-risk group of normotensive patients with acute pulmonary embolism, *Chest*. 2003. *123*: 1947–1952.

17. Kucher N, Printzen G, Doernhoefer T, Windecker S, Meier B, Hess OM. Low pro-brain natriuretic peptide levels predict benign clinical outcome in acute pulmonary embolism, *Circulation*. 2003. *107*(12): 1576–1578.

18. Wan S, Quinlan DJ, Agnelli G, Eikelboom JS. Thrombolysis compared with heparin for the initial treatment of pulmonary embolism: A meta-analysis of the randomized controlled trials, *Circulation*. 2004. *110*: 755–759.

19. Konstantinides S, Geibel A, Heusel G, Heinrich F, Kasper W. Heparin plus alteplase compared with heparin alone in patients with submassive pulmonary embolism, *N Engl J Med*. 2002. *347*: 1143–1150.

20. Heit JA, Mohr DN, Silverstein MD, Petterson TM, O'Fallon WM, Melton LJ III. Predictors of recurrence after deep vein thrombosis and pulmonary embolism: A population-based cohort study, *Arch Intern Med*. 2000. *160*: 761–768.

21. Schulman S, Granqvist S, Holmstrom M, et al. The duration of oral anticoagulant therapy after a second episode of venous thromboembolism, *N Engl J Med*. 1997. *336*: 393–398.

22. Kearon C, Gent M, Hirsh J, et al. A comparison of three months of anticoagulation with extended anticoagulation for a first episode of idiopathic venous thromboembolism, *N Engl J Med*. 1999. *340*(12): 901–907.

23. Agnelli G, Prandoni P, Becattini C, et al. Extended oral anticoagulant therapy after a first episode of pulmonary embolism, *Ann Intern Med*. 2003. *139*: 19–25.

24. Agnelli G, Prandoni P, Santamaria MG, et al. Three months versus one year of oral anticoagulant therapy for idiopathic deep venous thrombosis, *N Engl J Med*. 2001. *345*: 165–169.

25. Pinede L, Ninet J, Duhaut P, et al. Comparison of 3 and 6 months of oral anticoagulant therapy after a first episode of proximal deep vein thrombosis or pulmonary embolism and comparison of 6 and 12 weeks of therapy after isolated calf deep vein thrombosis, *Circulation*. 2001. *103*: 2453–2460.

26. van Dongen CJJ, Vink R, Hutten BA, Büller HR, Prins MH. The incidence of recurrent venous thromboembolism after treatment with vitamin K antagonists in relation to time since first event: A meta-analysis, *Arch Intern Med*. 2003. *163*: 1285–1293.

27. Kyrle PA, Eichinger S. The risk of recurrent venous thromboembolism: The Austrian Study on Recurrent Venous Thromboembolism, *Wiener Klinische Wochenschrift*. 2003. *115*(13–14): 471–474.

28. Kyrle PA, Minar E, Bialonczyk C, Hirschl M, Weltermann A, Eichinger S. The risk of recurrent venous thromboembolism in men and women, *N Engl J Med*. 2004. *350*: 2558–2563.

29. Baglin T, Luddington R, Brown K, Baglin C. High risk of recurrent venous thromboembolism in men, *J Thromb Haemost*. 2004. *2*: 2152–2155.

30. Hansson PO, Sörbo J, Eriksson H. Recurrent venous thromboembolism after deep vein thrombosis, *Arch Intern Med*. 2000. *160*: 769–774.

31. Prandoni P, Lensing AW, Piccioli A, et al. Recurrent venous thromboembolism and bleeding complications during anticoagulant treatment in patients with cancer and venous thrombosis, *Blood*. 2002. *100*: 3484–3488.

32. Prandoni P, Lensing AW, Cogo A, et al. The long-term clinical course of acute deep venous thrombosis, *Ann Intern Med*. 1996. *125*(1): 1–7.

33. Baglin T, Luddington R, Brown K, Baglin C. Incidence of recurrent venous thromboembolism in relation to clinical and thrombophilic risk factors: Prospective cohort study, *Lancet*. 2003. *362*(9383): 523–526.

34. Schulman S, Svenungsson E, Granqvist S, Duration of Anticoagulation Study Group. Anticardiolipin antibodies predict early recurrence of thromboembolism and death among patients with venous thromboembolism following anticoagulant therapy, *Am J Med*. 1998. *104*: 332–338.

35. van den Belt AGM, Sanson BJ, Simioni P, et al. Recurrence of venous thromboembolism in patients with familial thrombophilia, *Arch Inter Med*. 1997. *157*: 227–232.

36. Prandoni P, Lensing AW, Prins MH, et al. Residual venous thrombosis as a predictive factor of recurrent venous thromboembolism, *Ann Intern Med*. 2002. *137*(12): 955–960.

37. Murin S, Romano PS, White RH. Comparison of outcomes after hospitalization for deep venous thrombosis or pulmonary embolism, *Thromb Haemost*. 2002. *88*: 407–414.

38. Heit JA, Farmer SA, Petterson TM, Ballman KV, Melton LJ III. Venous thromboembolism event type (PE ± DVT vs. DVT alone) predicts recurrence type and survival, *Blood*. 2002. *100*(11): 149a (Abstract 560).

39. Heit JA, Rooke TW, Silverstein MD, et al. Trends in the incidence of venous stasis syndrome and venous ulcer: A 25-year population-based study, *J Vasc Surg*. 2001. *33*: 1022–1027.

40. Mohr DN, Silverstein MD, Heit JA, Petterson TM, O'Fallon WM, Melton LJ III. The venous stasis syndrome after deep venous thrombosis or pulmonary embolism: A population-based study, *Mayo Clin Proc*. 2000. *75*: 1249–1256.

41. Dunn WF, Heit JA, Farmer SA, Petterson TM, Ballman KV. *The incidence of chronic thromboembolic pulmonary hypertension (CTEPH): A 21-year population-based study (Abstract P2927).* European Respiratory Society 13th Annual Congress, Vienna, Austria, September 27–October 1, 2003.

42. Heit JA, Silverstein MD, Mohr DN, Petterson TM, O'Fallon WM, Melton LJ III. Risk factors for deep vein thrombosis and pulmonary embolism: A population-based case-control study, *Arch Intern Med*. 2000. *160*: 809–815.

43. Samama MM. An epidemiologic study of risk factors for deep vein thrombosis in medical outpatients, *Arch Intern Med*. 2000. *160*: 3415–3420.

44. Kobbervig CE, Heit JA, Petterson TM, Bailey KR, Melton LJ III. The effect of patient age on the incidence of idiopathic vs. secondary venous thromboembolism: A population-based cohort study (abstract 3516), *Blood*. 2004. *104*(11): 957a.

45. Heit JA, Melton LJI, Lohse CM, et al. Incidence of venous thromboembolism in hospitalized patients versus community residents, *Mayo Clin Proc*. 2001. *76*: 1102–1110.

46. Heit JA, O'Fallon WM, Petterson TM, et al. Relative impact of risk factors for deep vein thrombosis and pulmonary embolism: A population-based study, *Arch Intern Med*. 2002. *162*: 1245–1248.

47. Geerts WH, Pineo GF, Heit JA, et al. Prevention of venous thromboembolism: The seventh ACCP conference on antithrombotic and thrombolytic therapy, *Chest*. 2004. *126*: 338S–400S.

48 White RH, Zhou H, Romano PS. Incidence of symptomatic venous thromboembolism after different elective or urgent surgical procedures, *Thromb Haemost*. 2003. *90*: 446–455.

49. Heit JA, Petterson TM, Bailey KR, Melton LJ III. Risk factors for venous thromboembolism among patients hospitalized for major surgery: A population-based case-control study, *J Thromb Haemost*. 2005. 3(Suppl 1).

50. White RH, Gettner S, Newman JM, Romano PS. Predictors of rehospitalization for symptomatic venous thromboembolism after total hip arthroplasty, *N Engl J Med*. 2000. *343*: 1758–1764.

51. Mantilla CB, Horlocker TT, Schroeder DR, Berry DJ, Brown DL. Risk factors for clinically relevant pulmonary embolism and deep venous thrombosis in patients undergoing primary hip or knee arthroplasty, *Anesthesiology*. 2003. *99*(3): 552–560.

52. Sharrock NE, Haas SB, Hargett MJ, Urguhart B, Insall JN, Scuderi G. Effects of epidural anesthesia on the incidence of deep vein thrombosis after total knee replacement, *J Bone Joint Surg*. 1991. *73A*: 502–506.

53. Alikhan R, Cohen AT, Combe S, et al. Risk factors for venous thromboembolism in hospitalized patients with acute medical illness, *Arch Intern Med*. 2004. *164*: 963–968.

54. Heit JA, Petterson TM, Bailey KR, Melton LJ III. Risk factors for venous thromboembolism among patients hospitalized for acute medical illness: A population-based case-control study, *J Thromb Haemost*. 2005. *3*(8): 1611.

55. Heit JA, Petterson TM, Bailey KR, Melton LJ III. The influence of tumor site on venous thromboembolism risk among cancer patients: A population-based study (abstract 2596), *Blood*. 2004. *104*(11): 711a.

56. Levitan N, Dowlati A, Remick SC, et al. Rates of initial and recurrent thromboembolic disease among patients with malignancy versus those without malignancy, *Medicine*. 1999. *78*: 285–291.

57. Dalen J. Economy class syndrome: Too much flying or too much sitting? *Arch Intern Med*. 2003. *163*: 2674.

58. Ray JG, Mamdani M, Tsuyuki RT, Anderson DA, Yeo EL, Laupacis A. Use of statins and the subsequent development of deep vein thrombosis, *Arch Intern Med*. 2001. *161*: 1405–1410.

59. Prandoni P, Bilora F, Marchiori A, et al. An association between atherosclerosis and venous thrombosis, *N Engl J Med*. 2003. *348*(15): 1435–1441.

60. Tsai AW, Cushman M, Rosamond WD, Heckbert SR, Polak JF, Folsom AR. Cardiovascular risk factors and venous thromboembolism incidence, *Arch Intern Med*. 2002. *162*: 1182–1189.

61. Petterson TM, Agmon Y, Meissner I, Khandheria BK, Heit JA. Atherosclerosis as a risk factor for venous thromboembolism: A population-based cohort study (abstract 2584), *Blood*. 2004. *104*(11): 708a.

62. Gomes MPV, Deitcher SR. Risk of venous thromboembolic disease associated with hormonal contraceptives and hormone replacement therapy, *Arch Intern Med*. 2004. *164*: 1965–1976.

63. Rosendaal FR. Risk factors for venous thrombotic disease, *Thromb Haemost*. 1999. *82*: 610–619.

64. Heit JA, Kobbervig CE, James AH, Petterson TM, Bailey KR, Melton LJ III. Trends in the incidence of deep vein thrombosis and pulmonary embolism during pregnancy or postpartum: A 30-year population-based study, *Ann Intern Med*. 2005. *143*: 697–706.

65. Key NS, McGlennen RC. Hyperhomocyst(e)inemia and thrombophilia, *Arch Path Lab Med*. 2002. *126*: 1367–1375.

66. Tsai AW, Cushman M, Tsai MH, et al. Serum homocysteine, thermolabile variant of methylene tetrahydrofolate reductase (MTHFR), and venous thromboembolism: Longitudinal Investigation of Thromboembolism Etiology (LITE), *Am J Hematol*. 2003. *72*: 192–200.

67. Souto J, Almasy L, Borrell M, et al. Genetic susceptibility to thrombosis and its relationship to physiological risk factors: The GAIT

study: Genetic analysis of idiopathic thrombophilia, *Am J Hum Genet*. 2000. *67*(6): 1452–1459.

68. Larsen TB, Sorensen HT, Skytthe A, Johnsen SP, Vaupel JW, Christensen K. Major genetic susceptibility for venous thromboembolism in men: A study of Danish twins, *Epidemiology*. 2003. *14*(3): 328–332.

69. Heit JA, Phelps MA, Ward SA, Slusser J, Petterson TM, de Andrade M. Familial segregation of venous thromboembolism, *J Thromb Haemost*. 2004. *2*: 731–736.

70. Sanson BJ, Simioni P, Tormene D, et al. The incidence of venous thromboembolism in asymptomatic carriers of a deficiency of antithrombin, protein C, or protein S: A prospective cohort study, *Blood*. 1999. *94*(11): 3702–3706.

71. Folsom AR, Aleksic N, Wang N, Cushman M, Wu KK, White RH. Protein C, antithrombin, and venous thromboembolism incidence: A prospective population-based study, *Arterioscler Thromb Vasc Biol*. 2002. *22*: 1018–1022.

72. Folsom AR, Cushman M, Tsai MY, et al. A prospective study of venous thromboembolism in relation to factor V Leiden and related factors, *Blood*. 2002. *88*: 2720–2725.

73. Juul K, TybjærgHansen A, Schnohr P, Nordestgaard BG. Factor V Leiden and the risk for venous thromboembolism in the adult Danish population, *Ann Intern Med*. 2004. *140*: 330–337.

74. Heit JA, Sobell JL, Li H, Sommer SS. The incidence of venous thromboembolism in Factor Leiden carriers: A population-based cohort study, *J Thromb Haemost*. 2005. *3*(2): 305–311.

75. van Hylckama Vlieg A, Rosendaal FR. High levels of fibrinogen are associated with the risk of deep venous thrombosis mainly in the elderly, *J Thromb Haemost*. 2003. *1*(12): 2677–2678.

76. Folsom AR, Cushman M, Tsai MY, Heckbert SR, Aleksic N. Prospective study of the G20210A polymorphism in the prothrombin gene, plasma prothrombin concentration, and incidence of venous thromboembolism, *Am J Hematol*. 2002. *71*: 285–290.

77. Koster T, Blann AD, Briët E, Vandenbroucke JP, Rosendaal FR. Role of clotting factor VIII in effect of von Willebrand factor on occurrence of deep-vein thrombosis, *Lancet*. 1995. *345*: 152–155.

78. van Hylckama Vlieg A, van der Linden IK, Bertina RM, Rosendaal FR. High levels of factor IX increase the risk of venous thrombosis, *Blood*. 2000. *95*: 3678–3682.

79. Meijers JCM, Tekelenburg WLH, Bouma BN, Bertina RM, Rosendaal FR. High levels of coagulation factor XI as a risk factor for venous thrombosis, *N Engl J Med*. 2000. *342*: 696–701.

80. Tripodi A, Chantarangkul V, Martinelli I, Bucciarelli P, Mannucci PM. A shortened activated partial thromboplastin time is associated with the risk of venous thromboembolism, *Blood*. 2004. *104*: 3631–3634.

81. Folsom AR, Cushman M, Heckbert SR, Rosamond WD, Aleksic N. Prospective study of fibrinolytic markers and venous thromboembolism, *J Clin Epidemiol*. 2003. *56*: 598–603.

82. Cushman M, Folsom AR, Wang L, et al. Fibrin fragment D-dimer and the risk of future venous thrombosis, *Blood*. 2003. *101*: 1243–1248.

83. Lisman T, de Groot PG, Meijers JCM, Rosendaal FR. Reduced plasma fibrinolytic potential is a risk factor for venous thrombosis, *Blood*. 2005. *105*: 1102–1105.

84. Reitsma PH, Rosendaal FR. Activation of innate immunity in patients with venous thrombosis: The Leiden Thrombophilia Study, *J Thromb Haemost*. 2004. *2*: 619–622.

85. Souto J, Almasy L, Borrell M, et al. Genetic determinants of hemostasis phenotypes in Spanish families, *Circulation*. 2000. *101*(13): 1546–1551.

86. de Lange M, Snieder H, Ariëns RA, Spector TD, Grant PJ. The genetics of haemostasis: A twin study, *Lancet*. 2001. *357*(9250): 101–105.

87. Ariëns R, de Lange M, Snieder H, Boothby M, Spector T, Grant P. Activation markers of coagulation and fibrinolysis in twins: Heritability of the prethrombotic state, *Lancet*. 2002. *359*: 667–671.

88. Vossen CY, Hasstedt SJ, Rosendaal FR, et al. Heritability of plasma concentrations of clotting factors and measures of a prethrombotic state in a protein C-deficient family, *J Thromb Haemost*. 2004. *2*: 242–247.

89. Morange PE, Tregouet DA, Frere C, et al. Biological and genetic factors influencing plasma factor VIII levels in a healthy family population: Results from the Stanislas cohort, *Brit J Haematol*. 2004. *128*: 91–99.

90. van Hylckama Vlieg A, Rosendaal FR. Interaction between oral contraceptive use and coagulation factor levels in deep venous thrombosis, *J Thromb Haemost*. 2003. *1*: 2186–2190.

91. Martinelli I, De Stefano V, Taioli E, Paciaroni K, Rossi E, Mannucci PM. Inherited thrombophilia and first venous thromboembolism during pregnancy and puerperium, *Thromb Haemost*. 2002. *87*(5): 791–795.

92. Cushman M, Kuller LH, Prentice R, et al. Estrogen plus progestin and risk of venous thrombosis, *JAMA*. 2004. *292*: 1573–1580.

93. Lindahl TL, Lundahl TH, Nilsson L, Anderson CA. APC-resistance is a risk factor for postoperative thromboembolism in elective replacement of the hip or knee: A prospective study, *Thromb Haemost*. 1999. *81*: 18–21.

94. Libourel EJ, Bank I, Meinardi JR, et al. Cosegregation of thrombophilic disorders in factor V Leiden carriers: The contributions of factor VIII, factor XI, thrombin activatable fibrinolysis inhibitor and lipoprotein(a) to the absolute risk of venous thromboembolism, *Haematologica*. 2002. *87*: 1068–1073.

95. Lindmarker P, Schulman S, Sten-Linder M, Wiman B, Egberg N, Johnsson H. The risk of recurrent venous thromboembolism in carriers and non-carriers of the G1691A allele in the coagulation factor V gene and the G20210a allele in the prothrombin gene, *Thromb Haemost*. 1999. *81*(5): 684–689.

96. Meinardi JR, Middeldorp S, de Kam PJ, et al. The incidence of recurrent venous thromboembolism in carriers of factor V Leiden is related to concomitant thrombophilic disorders, *Brit J Haematol*. 2002. *116*: 625–631.

97. Kyrle PA, Minar E, Hirschl M, et al. High plasma levels of factor VIII and the risk of recurrent venous thromboembolism, *N Engl J Med*. 2000. *343*: 457–462.

98. Weltermann A, Eichinger S, Bialonczyk C, et al. The risk of recurrent venous thromboembolism among patients with high factor IX levels, *J Thromb Haemost*. 2003. *1*(1): 28–32.

99. Eichinger S, Minar E, Bialonczyk C, et al. D-dimer levels and risk of recurrent venous thromboembolism, *JAMA*. 2003. *290*(8): 1071–1074.

34.

FUNDAMENTAL MECHANISMS IN VENOUS THROMBOSIS

Jose A. Diaz, Daniel D. Myers Jr., and Thomas W. Wakefield

INTRODUCTION

Venous thromboembolism (VTE) comprises deep vein thrombosis (DVT) and pulmonary embolism (PE). VTE occurs worldwide, in all age groups and socioeconomic populations in North America and Western Europe.[1,2] In a recent study by Heit et al., the estimated total annual number of VTE events in the United States exceeded 900,000.[3] Symptomatic VTE accounted for two-thirds of the cases reported. Interestingly, no changes in the incidence of VTE were noted during this 25-year cohort study.[3] Thus, VTE and its sequelae remain an important health care problem that demands coordination between the efforts of clinicians, surgeons, and investigators. In this setting, venous thrombosis research plays a pivotal role in the process of elucidating the intrinsic mechanisms involved in thrombogenesis and thrombus resolution. Only by understanding VTE pathophysiology will we be able to identify potential therapeutic targets to aid the patient population affected by VTE. In this chapter, the authors will summarize the mechanisms involved in VTE as well as potential therapeutic targets.

PATHOPHYSIOLOGY

ENDOTHELIUM

The endothelium forms the inner cell lining of all blood vessels in the body and is a spatially distributed organ. In an average individual, the endothelium weighs approximately 1 kg and covers a total surface area of 4,000 to 7,000 square meters.[4] The endothelium has been described as a primary determinant of pathophysiology or as a target for collateral damage in most, if not all, disease processes.[1,4] Endothelial cells (ECs) play a critical role in the balance between procoagulant and anticoagulant mechanisms in healthy individuals. The ECs' anticoagulant properties involve supporting local fibrinolysis, in which coagulation (platelet activation and adhesion) and inflammation (leukocyte activation) remain suppressed.[5] In contrast, a procoagulant effect is observed during states of EC activation and disturbance, either physical (vascular trauma) or functional (sepsis; Figure 34.1).[5]

It is widely known that, under normal conditions, cellular blood components interact with the vessel wall promoting vascular repair. Activated or dysfunctional ECs trigger a mechanism of rapid deposition of platelets, erythrocytes, leukocytes, and insoluble fibrin, which establishes a mechanical barrier to blood flow, termed thrombosis.[4]

INFLAMMATION AND THROMBOGENESIS

Arterial thrombosis requires EC disruption with collagen exposure, as it occurs in atherosclerotic plaque rupture.[6] On the contrary, in venous thrombosis the ECs are "intact" (at least at the initiation of the thrombus formation), and no collagen exposition is needed in order to generate thrombi.[6] ECs play a pivotal role in venous thrombosis. Thus, during a normal EC response to a stimulus, the balance between anticoagulant and procoagulant mechanism is altered toward the ECs procoagulant activity.[1,7,8] Inflammation and vein thrombosis were linked in a publication by Stewart, Ritchie, and Lynch in 1974 demonstrating leukocyte migration into the vein wall with an intact layer of ECs.[9] Since then, several studies demonstrated the interaction between inflammation and thrombosis.[5,10–13] The question of what alters the EC toward a procoagulant effect is fundamental to understanding the pathophysiology of VTE. Inflammatory cytokines such as tumor necrosis factor alpha (TNF-α), interleukin 1 (IL-1). and interleukin 6 (IL-6), induce EC activation and contribute to venous thrombosis[8,14] (Figure 34.2). Once ECs are activated, cell interaction between ECs, leukocytes, monocytes, and platelets occurs.[5,6,10,15]

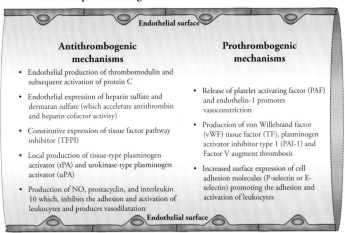

Anti- and pro-thrombogenic mechanisms of endothelial surface

Endothelial surface

Antithrombogenic mechanisms

- Endothelial production of thrombomodulin and subsequent activation of protein C

- Endothelial expression of heparin sulfate and dermatan sulfate (which accelerate antithrombin and heparin cofactor activity)

- Constitutive expression of tissue factor pathway inhibitor (TFPI)

- Local production of tissue-type plasminogen activator (tPA) and urokinase-type plasminogen activator (uPA)

- Production of NO, prostacyclin, and interleukin 10 which, inhibits the adhesion and activation of leukocytes and produces vasodilatation

Prothrombogenic mechanisms

- Release of platelet activating factor (PAF) and endothelin-1 promotes vasoconstriction

- Production of von Willebrand factor (vWF) tissue factor (TF), plasminogen activator inhibitor type 1 (PAI-1) and Factor V augment thrombosis

- Increased surface expression of cell adhesion molecules (P-selectin or E-selectin) promoting the adhesion and activation of leukocytes

Endothelial surface

Figure 34.1   Anti- and prothrombogenic mechanisms of the endothelial surface. One of the main functions of the ECs is to maintain the balance between the procoagulant and anticoagulant mechanisms in healthy individuals. The anticoagulant properties of the ECs involve supporting local fibrinolysis, suppressing coagulation and inflammation. The procoagulant effect of the ECs is observed during states of EC activation and/or disturbance.

P-Selectin, P-Selectin Receptor, Leukocytes, and Platelets in Vein Thrombosis

Selectins are cell adhesion molecules that have critical roles in inflammation and thrombogenesis[5,10,16] (Figure 34.3). P-selectin is involved in leukocyte rolling and adhesion, an early inflammatory mechanism that facilitates leukocyte transmigration.[9,16] Animal studies that utilized rat and mouse thrombosis models have demonstrated the upregulation of P-selectin in the vein wall at 6 hours after thrombus induction.[16] Thus, it has been shown that P-selectin is a common molecule that links inflammation and thrombosis in vivo. The P-selectin receptor, P-selectin glycoprotein ligand 1 (PSGL-1), is a glycoprotein expressed on the surface of leukocytes and platelets that plays a critical role in the recruitment of leukocytes and platelets into inflamed tissue. The interaction of PSGL-1 with P-selectin (the EC P-selectin:PSGL-1-leukocyte complex and the EC P-selectin:PSGL-1-platelet complex) promotes rolling and adhesion of leukocytes and platelets respectively, which ultimately results in increased vein wall cell infiltration[17,18] (Figure 34.3).

It is widely known that the initiation of inflammation and/or the thrombosis processes occurs, chronologically, almost immediately after EC activation. This could be possible only if the ECs have stored P-selectin that could be released upon stimulation, as secretory cells do.[15] Weibel-Palade bodies (WPBs) are the EC-specific storage organelles for regulated secretion of von Willebrand factor (vWF) and P-selectin on their cell surface membrane.[15,19–21] Wagner et al. demonstrated that the increase in the number

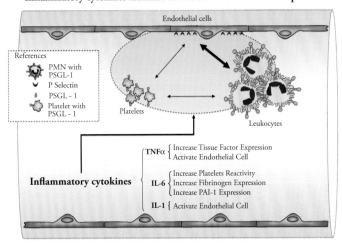

Inflammatory cytokines facilitate initiation of vein thrombosis process

Endothelial cells

References
- PMN with PSGL-1
- P Selectin
- PSGL - 1
- Platelet with PSGL - 1

Platelets

Leukocytes

Inflammatory cytokines

TNFα { Increase Tissue Factor Expression / Activate Endothelial Cell

IL-6 { Increase Platelets Reactivity / Increase Fibrinogen Expression / Increase PAI-1 Expression

IL-1 { Activate Endothelial Cell

Figure 34.2   Inflammatory cytokines such us tumor necrosis factor alpha (TNF-α)and interleukins 1 and 6 (IL-1 and IL-6), induce EC activation and contribute to venous thrombosis. Once ECs are activated, cell interaction between ECs, leukocytes, and platelets occurs.

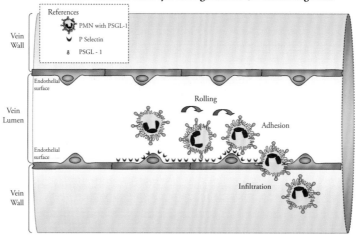

P-selectin facilitates leukocyte rolling, adhesion, and transmigration

Figure 34.3   P-selectin is involved in leukocyte rolling and adhesion, an early inflammatory mechanism that facilitates leukocyte transmigration. The interaction of P-selectin glycoprotein Ligand 1 with P-selectin on ECs and leukocytes promotes rolling and adhesion of leukocytes and platelets, which ultimately results in increased vein wall cell infiltration.

of P-selectin molecules present on the EC surface is due to its release from the WPB.[15,21] Thus, the exocytosis of WPBs initiates a rapid translocation of P-selectin to the EC surface, resulting in the EC's adhesiveness for leukocytes and platelets (Figure 34.4).

The role of platelets in arterial thrombosis is well known, but how platelets participate in venous thrombosis remains unclear. Platelets are anucleate circulating blood particles derived from bone marrow megakaryocytes, initially called plates.[2] Osler, Hayam, and Bizzonero initially described them as small particles in the blood until the Wright blood staining method clearly identified the platelets.[2] The

megakaryocytes extend their cytoplasm into the bone marrow sinusoid and release a small portion of cytoplasm containing alpha granules and dense granules surrounded by a bilipid membrane into the blood circulation.

Under physiological conditions, circulating platelets are resting or nonactivated and express PSGL-1.[15,22] The platelet's PSGL-1 allows an EC-platelet interaction.[15,17] Once activated, platelets excrete the contents of the granules, which increases their adhesiveness and ultimately potentiates platelet aggregation.[22] Particularly, alpha granules contain P-selectin, and its expression on platelet surface favors leukocyte-platelet crosstalk as a direct consequence

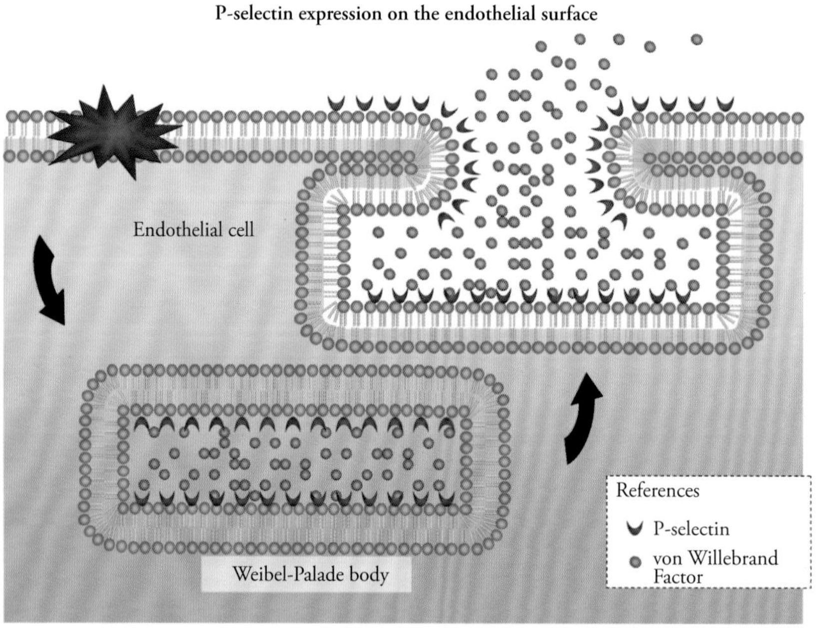

P-selectin expression on the endothelial surface

Figure 34.4   Weibel-Palade bodies are the endothelial-specific storage organelle for regulated secretion of von Willebrand factor and P-selectin onto its membrane. Thus the exocytosis of WPBs initiates a rapid translocation of P-selectin to the endothelial surface, resulting in augmented endothelial adhesiveness for leukocytes and platelets.

of platelet activation.[15,17] In addition, it has been shown that platelets release a greater amount of P-selectin than ECs.[15] Thus, once platelets are attached to the vein wall, the concentration of P-selectin available increases dramatically, improving the leukocyte recruitment efficiency of the vein wall.[15] It was elegantly demonstrated by Frenette et al. in a mouse model that platelets roll on the vein wall, as leukocytes do, when EC activation occurs.[17]

Microparticles

Circulating cell-derived microparticles (MPs) contribute to coagulation and amplification of thrombosis. They are present in the blood of healthy individuals and increase under certain circumstances including DVT.[2,23] MPs are defined as small vesicles (less than 1 micrometer) consisting of a plasma membrane surrounding a small amount of cytoplasm that contains cell-specific surface molecules.[24,25] In thrombogenesis, MPs are associated with ECs, leukocytes, and platelets, carrying membrane proteins that characterize their cell of origin.[2,24,26] ECs, leukocytes, and platelets have a very well structured plasma membrane characterized by a controlled transverse lipid distribution termed "rafts."[27] The activation of these cells promotes a general membrane content redistribution, during which rafts concentrate in areas of the cell that will ultimately produce MPs (Figure 34.5).[27] Therefore, the MP membrane is rich in lipid rafts.[27] Also, lipid raft–derived MPs concentrate tissue factor (TF).[27] The fusion of MPs with activated platelets promotes thrombus formation in a TF-dependent manner. In addition to TF, the expression

of prothrombinase activity on the membrane and PSGL-1 are involved in the procoagulant activity of MPs.[5,28]

During inflammation, the activation of ECs upregulates the expression of P-selectin on their surface, leading to the formation of the EC P-selectin: PSGL-1-leukocyte complexes. These complexes stimulate the production of MPs from leukocytes, particularly monocytes, along with platelets and ECs. In addition, the accumulation of leukocyte markers expressed on the surface of MPs in the growing thrombus is mediated by the P-selectin:PSGL-1 complex.[5] The MP concentration increases dramatically at the area of vein wall injury and inflammation.[10] MPs also possess a phosphatidylserine-rich anionic surface capable of assembling complexes of the coagulation cascade. Another molecule expressed on the MPs' membrane surfaces is PSGL-1, which then can bind to upregulated P-selectin on platelet surfaces in the thrombus. There is even evidence that the macrophage-1 antigen (Mac-1) on leukocyte-derived MPs can allow interactions between MPs and inactivated platelets using "glycoprotein I b (platelet) alpha polypeptide" (GP1bα), resulting in further platelet activation with P-selectin upregulation.[29,30] All of these events, which are occurring in the area of thrombus formation, lead to thrombus amplification. The increase of circulating MPs with the onset of inflammation adds to the proposed mechanisms linking vein wall inflammation and thrombogenesis.

Platelet-Activating Factor (PAF) and Endothelin-1(ET-1) Play a Role in Inflammation

PAF, also known as PAF-acether or AGEPC (acetyl-glyceryl-ether-phosphorylcholine), is produce by EC, macrophages, mast cells, and leukocytes.[31] One of the central functions of PAF during inflammation is to activate the leukocytes adhered to the vessel wall via the adhesion molecules expressed by ECs.[31,32] ET-1 is a 21-amino-acid peptide produced in a variety of tissues including endothelial and smooth muscle cells.[33] ET-1 receptors include ET_A and ET_B.[33,34] Specific locations have also been proposed for ET-1 receptors: vein EC (ET_{B1}) and vein vascular smooth muscle cell (ET_{B1}).[33] When ET-1 binds to its receptors (which are Gq-proteins) on the vascular smooth muscle, this induces an increase of inositol 1,4,5 phosphate levels, leading to calcium release and subsequent muscle contraction.[33] Particularly, it has been shown that endothelial dysfunction and inflammation contribute to overproduction of ET-1 in humans.[35] In addition, ET_A is expressed in inflammatory cells.[35] Future directions include elucidating the role of PAF and ET-1 in venous thrombosis.

Molecules That Participate as Inhibitors of Coagulation: Natural Anticoagulants

Circulating inhibitory molecules regulating the process of thrombogenesis include: antithrombin III (ATIII),

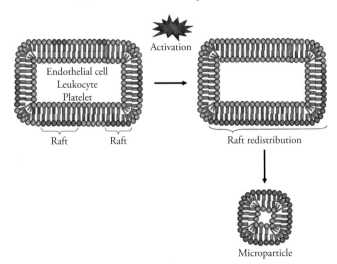

Rafts re-distribution and microparticle formation

Activation

Endothelial cell
Leukocyte
Platelet

Raft   Raft

Raft redistribution

Microparticle

Figure 34.5 ECs, leukocytes, and platelets have a very well structured plasma membrane characterized by rafts. Rafts are a particular membrane structure with a controlled transverse protein-lipid distribution. The activation of these cells promotes a general membrane raft redistribution that concentrates in areas of the cell that will ultimately produce MPs. Therefore, the MP membrane is rich in lipid rafts.

protein C, protein S, and tissue factor pathway inhibitor (TFPI). Antithrombin III, a plasma glycoprotein synthesized in the liver, is a serine protease inhibitor (SERPIN) structurally related to other plasma protease inhibitors such as alpha 1-antichymotrypsin, alpha 2-antiplasmin, and heparin cofactor II.[2] Antithrombin III acts as a pseudosubstrate for the inhibition of intrinsic pathway (Factors IIa [thrombin], IXa, Xa, XIa, XIIa) and extrinsic pathway (Factor VII), kallikrein, and plasmin.[2] Other targets of antithrombin III include trypsin and the C1s subunit, which are involved in the classical complement pathway.[36] The plasma half-life of antithrombin III is 60 to 70 hours, while the thrombin:antithrombin (TAT) complex is cleared by the liver and its inhibitory activity is increased by heparin.[1,36]

Protein C, a vitamin K–dependent plasma glycoprotein, is synthesized as a single chain and cleaved prior to secretion by the liver.[37] Plasma protein C consists of a two-chain molecule, light and heavy chain. Its plasma half-life is 6 to 7 hours.[2] Once protein C binds to its receptor, EC protein C receptor, it is activated by the thrombin:thrombomodulin complex on the EC surface, resulting in activated protein C (APC).[2,38] In the presence of calcium and protein S, APC inactivates Factor Va and Factor VIIIa of the "protein C anticoagulant pathway"[2] (Figure 34.6).

Protein S, a vitamin K–dependent plasma glycoprotein, is synthesized by the liver, the endothelial, cells and the megakaryocytes.[39] Protein S is a cofactor of APC in the protein C anticoagulant pathway.[38] In addition, protein S exhibits APC-independent anticoagulant activity by binding to Factors Va, VIIIa, and Xa.[1] In serum, protein S is found in two forms: free (active) and bound (inactive) protein. Almost 70% of protein S circulates bound to a complement protein (C4b-binding protein).[2] The remaining protein S circulates as "free protein S," which has a half-life of 96 hours, and acts as a cofactor for protein C.[1]

TFPI is a single chain plasma polypeptide that inhibits Factor Xa and TF:Factor VIIa complex catalytic activity.[40,41] Plasma contains a minor fraction of TFPI, 20 to 30 % of intravascular distribution, which is largely bound to lipoproteins.[2,40] The major proportion of TFPI (60 to 70%) is normally bound to the vascular endothelium.[40] This pool of TFPI is released into the blood flow after an injection of heparin.[1,40,41]

Finally, prostacyclin and nitric oxide (NO) are secreted by ECs.[42] These compounds synergistically contribute to vessel homeostasis by reducing the tone and growth of vascular smooth muscle cells, platelet aggregation, and leukocyte adhesion to endothelium, and thus decreasing the vessel's susceptibility to form thrombus.[2,42] Interestingly, Osanai et al. demonstrated that vessel homeostasis might be maintained through an increase in prostacyclin production in vascular ECs when nitric oxide (NO) synthesis is impaired.[43] The endothelial NO synthase (eNOS) function has been widely studied in arterial ECs, but there is also evidence suggesting that decreased NO production may play a role in the development of venous disease.[44–46]

PLASMINOGEN ACTIVATORS AND THROMBOLYSIS

Venous thrombosis is a dynamic process, with thrombus formation (thrombogenesis) and dissolution (thrombolysis) occurring almost simultaneously under normal conditions in a healthy individual.[1] Thrombolysis depends on multiple physiological processes, including fibrinolysis.[47] In response to thrombus formation, natural anticoagulants such as protein C and protein S are activated.[37,39] Similarly, circulating plasminogen is activated to plasmin, which is the main fibrinolytic enzyme.[5,47] The substrates of plasmin substrates include fibrin, fibrinogen, other coagulation

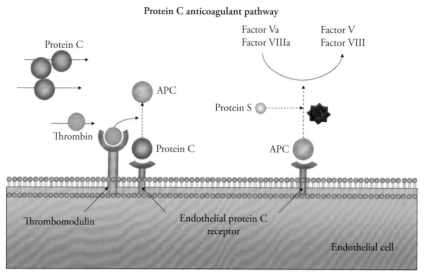

Protein C anticoagulant pathway

Figure 34.6   Protein C anticoagulant pathway. Once protein C binds to its receptor, endothelial protein C receptor, it is cleaved by the thrombin:thrombomodulin complex on the endothelial surface, resulting in activated protein C (APC). In the presence of calcium and protein S, APC inactivates Factor Va and Factor VIIIa.

factors, procollagenases, and latent transforming growth factor beta (TGFβ).[47] In addition, plasmin interferes with vWF-mediated platelet adhesion by proteolysis of GpIb.[48]

Plasminogen activators are serine proteases that activate plasminogen by the proteolytic cleavage of a single arginine-valine peptide bond.[47] Plasminogen activator inhibitor-type 1 (PAI-1) is the primary inhibitor of the plasminogen activators, both tissue type plasminogen activator (t-PA) and urokinase type plasminogen activator (u-PA), and hence of fibrinolysis.[5,47,49] The primary function of PAI-1 is to inhibit plasminogen activators from converting plasminogen to plasmin, which is responsible for initiating fibrinolysis.[2] PAI-1 is produced by the EC but is also secreted in an active form by the liver and adipose tissue.[47,50] Increased PAI-1 levels are found in various disease states such as cancer, obesity, and metabolic syndrome.[51] Thus, it has been suggested that the increased occurrence of thrombosis in patients with these conditions could be associated with elevated PAI-1 levels.[51] PAI-1 elevation appears to synergize with Factor V Leiden genetic abnormalities.[5] Elevated PAI-1 may suppress fibrinolysis and increase thrombosis, hence increasing the clinical manifestations of VTE, although studies on the role of elevated levels of PAI-1 in venous thrombosis have been contradictory.[52] Particularly, it has been published that increased serum levels of PAI-1 and impaired fibrinolysis is associated with hyperlipidemia in humans.[53] This relationship suggests that hyperlipidemic patients have an increased risk to develop cardiovascular diseases, including VTE related to impaired fibrinolysis.[53]

Polymorphism in the PAI-1 gene has been suggested to be associated with an increased risk of VTE.[54,55] Human studies have evaluated the role of genetic polymorphisms, particularly the 4G/5G insertion/deletion in the promoter region, which affects transcription rates. The highest levels of PAI-1 have been noted in those individuals carrying the 4G/4G polymorphism.[55] Akar et al. reported an increased odds ratio of 5.5× for DVT with the 4G allele. This increase was even greater when the 4G allele coexisted with Factor-V-Leiden.[55] Another study, by Zoller et al., showed an 8.14× increased risk of PAI-1 elevation in individuals carrying the 4G allele in combination with other thrombophilic markers, while PE was increased in 4G/4G patients with protein S deficiency (odds ratio 4.5×).[54]

Fibrin degradation products (FDPs) result from the action of plasmin on deposited fibrin. FDPs include the fragment E and fragment D, which, during physiological thrombolysis, are released as a covalently linked dimer, the D-dimer.[5] Clinically, the level of circulating D-dimers is used as a surrogate marker for the diagnosis of ongoing DVT and/or PE.[56] In addition, the presence of elevated D-dimer levels after successful treatment of DVT has a high positive predictive value for recurrent VTE.[5] D-dimer levels may also aid in the diagnosis of disseminated intravascular coagulation.

THROMBUS RESOLUTION AND VEIN WALL REMODELING

DVT resolution is a fibrotic process that mimics wound healing. This process involves profibrotic growth factors, collagen deposition, and matrix metalloproteinase (MMP) expression and activation.[57] The kinetics of leukocytes in the vein wall follows the same pattern as that observed in thrombi.[57] Thus, immediately after thrombus formation, an early influx of polymorphonuclear (PMN) cells is followed by a migration of monocytes.[5] Leukocyte migration, first from the blood into the vein wall and then from the vein wall into the thrombus, follow a specific sequence of events leading to thrombus resolution.[5] The first cell type that migrates as described above is the PMN leukocyte.[5,8-10] PMNs are essential for early thrombus resolution as they promote both fibrinolysis and collagenolysis.[5] In support of this concept, a study using a rat model of stasis DVT showed that neutropenia increased both thrombi size, at 2 and 7 d, and intrathrombus collagen deposition. It also significantly lowered intrathrombus levels of both uPA and MMP-9.[58]

Chronologically, the second cell type observed in the thrombus is the monocyte.[59] Monocytes are important cells in the chronic stages of thrombus resolution.[59] Monocyte influx into the thrombus is detected at day 8, after thrombus generation, which correlates with elevated levels of monocyte chemotactic protein-1 (MCP-1), a CC chemokine that promotes monocyte chemotaxis and activation.[5] MCP-1 has been associated with DVT resolution.[5] In a study using a mouse model of stasis thrombosis, chronic stages of thrombus resolution were tested using target deleted CC receptor-2 (CCR-2 KO) mice.[60] In this study, late impairment of thrombus resolution appeared to be mediated via impaired MMP-2 and MMP-9 activity.[5,60]

Thrombus resolution involves a number of proinflammatory factors that are released into the local environment. These factors include IL-1β and TNFα.[5,8,14] It has been suggested that these mediators are released by leukocytes and smooth muscle cells found within the resolving thrombus, although the specific mechanisms involved in this process have yet to be elucidated. Henke et al. observed that elastinolysis occurs early in a mouse model of stasis-induced DVT.[60] In this model, the evaluation of elastinolysis was determined by tensiometry and was associated with an increase in vein wall stiffness. Elastinolysis persisted for 14 d, together with elevated MMP-2 and MMP-9 activity.[60] In the same model, vein wall collagenolysis was observed within the first 7 d, representing an acute response to injury.[60]

The elevation of profibrotic mediators, including TGFβ, IL-13, and MCP-1, have been associated with early biomechanical injury during DVT.[61] These mediators are present in the vein wall, and thrombus and may drive the fibrotic response.[61] Exogenous MCP-1 may accelerate DVT resolution as it also promotes organ fibrosis in vivo.[61] TGFβ is also present in the thrombus and is activated during thrombolysis.[61] This factor appears to be critical in the mechanisms promoting vein wall fibrosis. In mice, late fibrosis has been associated with a significant increase in vein wall collagen after stasis thrombogenesis.[57] Increased gene expression and activity of collagen types I and III, MMP-2, and MMP-9 has also been observed.[10,57] Thus, vein wall injury is associated with active matrix remodeling that seems to promote net fibrosis.[57]

Myers et al. demonstrated that inhibition of the inflammatory response can decrease vein wall fibrosis.[16] These data add to the evidence of the close interaction between inflammation and fibrosis.[16] In another study using an inferior vena cava stenosis model in rats, animals were treated with either low molecular weight heparin or an oral P-selectin inhibitor starting 2 d after thrombus initiation.[18] In this study, the P-selectin inhibitor significantly decreased vein wall injury (independent of thrombus size), which was assessed by vein wall tensiometry (stiffness), intimal thickness score, IL-13 levels, MCP-1 levels, and platelet-derived growth factor-β levels.[18]

In summary, venous thrombosis is a complex and dynamic process that involves at least two phases: thrombus formation and thrombus resolution.

Thrombus formation: Inflammation appears to be closely involved in thrombus formation. ECs, platelets, and leukocytes (PMNs and monocytes) are the main circulatory elements involved in venous thrombosis. Inflammatory cytokines orchestrate this early phase. Thus, preventive or prophylaxis therapeutic approaches should be directed to these potential targets.

Thrombus resolution: Vein wall remodeling is a complex process that varies as the thrombus ages. Profibrotic mediators play an important role in this phase, leading to fibrosis. The severity of this fibrosis will determine the outcome after an episode of DVT (i.e., postthrombotic syndrome or thrombus recanalization with or without valve insufficiency). Novel therapeutic approaches aimed to alleviate postthrombotic cell wall damage and focused on the sequence of events occurring during thrombus aging are warranted.

REFERENCES

1. Kitchens CS, Alving BM, Kessler CM. *Consultative hemostasis and thrombosis.* Philadelphia: W.B. Saunders. 2002.
2. Heith JA. Thrombophilia: Clinical and laboratory assessment and management. In: Kitchens CS, Alving BM, Kessler CM, eds. *Consultative hemostasis and thrombosis*, 2e. Philadelphia: W.B. Saunders. 2002. 213–244.
3. Silverstein MD, Heit JA, Mohr DN, Petterson TM, O'Fallon WM, Melton LJ 3rd. Trends in the incidence of deep vein thrombosis and pulmonary embolism: A 25-year population-based study, *Arch Intern Med.* 1998. *158*(6): 585–593.
4. Aird WC. Endothelium. In: Kitchens CS, Alving BM, Kessler CM, eds. *Consultative hemostasis and thrombosis*, 2e. Philadelphia: W.B. Saunders. 2002. 35–42.
5. Wakefield TW, Myers DD, Henke PK. Mechanisms of venous thrombosis and resolution, *Arterioscler Thromb Vasc Biol.* 2008. *28*(3): 387–391.
6. Mackman N, Tilley RE, Key NS. Role of the extrinsic pathway of blood coagulation in hemostasis and thrombosis, *Arterioscler Thromb Vasc Biol.* 2007. *27*(8): 1687–1693.
7. Gamble JR, Harlan JM, Klebanoff SJ, Vadas MA. Stimulation of the adherence of neutrophils to umbilical vein endothelium by human recombinant tumor necrosis factor, *Proc Natl Acad Sci U S A.* 1985. *82*(24): 8667–8671.
8. Schleimer RP, Rutledge BK. Cultured human vascular endothelial cells acquire adhesiveness for neutrophils after stimulation with interleukin 1, endotoxin, and tumor-promoting phorbol diesters, *J Immunol.* 1986. *136*(2): 649–654.
9. Stewart GJ, Ritchie WG, Lynch PR. Venous endothelial damage produced by massive sticking and emigration of leukocytes, *Am J Pathol.* 1974. *74*(3): 507–532.
10. Myers DD, Wakefield TW. Inflammation-dependent thrombosis, *Front Biosci.* 2005. *10*: 2750–2757.
11. Collins T, et al. Transcriptional regulation of endothelial cell adhesion molecules: NF-kappa B and cytokine-inducible enhancers, *FASEB J.* 1995. *9*(10): 899–909.
12. Chen W, et al. Anti-inflammatory effect of docosahexaenoic acid on cytokine-induced adhesion molecule expression in human retinal vascular endothelial cells, *Invest Ophthalmol Vis Sci.* 2005. *46*(11): 4342–4347.
13. Murase T, et al. Gallates inhibit cytokine-induced nuclear translocation of NF-kappaB and expression of leukocyte adhesion molecules in vascular endothelial cells, *Arterioscler Thromb Vasc Biol.* 1999. *19*(6): 1412–1420.
14. Kasthuri RS, Key NS. Disseminated intravascular coagulation and other microangiopathies. In: Key N, Makris M, O'Shaughnessy D, Lillicrap, D, eds. *Practical hemostasis and thrombosis*, 2e. Chapel Hill, NC: Wiley-Blackwell. 2009. 123–134.
15. Wagner DD and Frenette PS, The vessel wall and its interactions, *Blood.* 2008. *111*(11): 5271–5281.
16. Myers D Jr., et al. Selectins influence thrombosis in a mouse model of experimental deep venous thrombosis, *J Surg Res.* 2002. *108*(2): 212–221.
17. Frenette PS, et al. Platelets roll on stimulated endothelium in vivo: an interaction mediated by endothelial P-selectin, *Proc Natl Acad Sci U S A.* 1995. *92*(16): 7450–7454.
18. Myers DD Jr., et al. Treatment with an oral small molecule inhibitor of P selectin (PSI-697) decreases vein wall injury in a rat stenosis model of venous thrombosis, *J Vasc Surg.* 2006. *44*(3): 625–632.
19. McEver RP, et al. GMP-140, a platelet alpha-granule membrane protein, is also synthesized by vascular endothelial cells and is localized in Weibel-Palade bodies, *J Clin Invest.* 1989. *84*(1): 92–99.
20. Wagner DD, Olmsted JB, Marder VJ. Immunolocalization of von Willebrand protein in Weibel-Palade bodies of human endothelial cells, *J Cell Biol.* 1982. *95*(1): 355–360.
21. Bonfanti R, et al. PADGEM (GMP140) is a component of Weibel-Palade bodies of human endothelial cells, *Blood.* 1989. *73*(5): 1109–1112.
22. Jung SM, Moroi M. Platelet collagen receptors. In: Kenzo T, Davie EW, Ikeda Y, et al., eds. *Recent advances in thrombosis and hemostasis 2008.* Tokyo: Springer. 2008. 231–242.
23. Enjeti AK, Lincz LF, Seldon M. Microparticles in health and disease, *Semin Thromb Hemost.* 2008. *34*(7): 683–691.
24. Blann A, Shantsila E, Shantsila A. Microparticles and arterial disease. *Semin Thromb Hemost.* 2009. *35*(5): 488–496.
25. Ahn ER, et al. Differences of soluble CD40L in sera and plasma: implications on CD40L assay as a marker of thrombotic risk, *Thromb Res.* 2004. *114*(2): 143–148.
26. Nomura S, Ozaki Y, Ikeda Y. Function and role of microparticles in various clinical settings, *Thromb Res.* 2008. *123*(1): 8–23.
27. Del Conde I, et al. Tissue-factor-bearing microvesicles arise from lipid rafts and fuse with activated platelets to initiate coagulation, *Blood.* 2005. *106*(5): 1604–1611.
28. Satta N, et al. Monocyte vesiculation is a possible mechanism for dissemination of membrane-associated procoagulant activities

and adhesion molecules after stimulation by lipopolysaccharide, *J Immunol*. 1994. *153*(7): 3245–3255.

29. Pluskota E, et al. Expression, activation, and function of integrin alphaMbeta2 (Mac-1) on neutrophil-derived microparticles, *Blood*. 2008. *112*(6): 2327–2335.

30. Andrews RK, Berndt MC. Microparticles facilitate neutrophil/platelet crosstalk, *Blood*. 2008. *112*(6): 2174–2175.

31. Tjoelker LW, Stafforini DM. Platelet-activating factor acetylhydrolases in health and disease, *Biochim Biophys Acta*. 2000. *1488*(1–2): 102–123.

32. Zimmerman GA, et al. Juxtacrine intercellular signaling: another way to do it, *Am J Respir Cell Mol Biol*. 1993. *9*(6): 573–577.

33. Watts SW. Endothelin Receptors: what's new and what do we need to know?, *Am J Physiol Regul Integr Comp Physiol*. 2010. *298*(2):R254–260.

34. Ram CV. Possible therapeutic role of endothelin antagonists in cardiovascular disease, *Am J Ther*. 2003. *10*(6): 396–400.

35. Mencarelli M, et al. Endothelin receptor A expression in human inflammatory cells, *Regul Pept*. 2009. *158*(1–3): 1–5.

36. Perry DJ. Antithrombin and its inherited deficiencies, *Blood Rev*. 1994. *8*(1): 37–55.

37. Kottke-Marchant K, Comp P. Laboratory issues in diagnosing abnormalities of protein C, thrombomodulin, and endothelial cell protein C receptor, *Arch Pathol Lab Med*. 2002. *126*(11): 1337–1348.

38. Fukudome K. Structure and function of the endothelial cell protein C receptor. In: Kenzo T, Davie EW, Ikeda Y, et al., eds. *Recent advances in thrombosis and hemostasis 2008*. Tokyo: Springer. 2008. 211–217.

39. Goodwin AJ, et al. A review of the technical, diagnostic, and epidemiologic considerations for protein S assays, *Arch Pathol Lab Med*. 2002. *126*(11): 1349–1366.

40. Broze GJ Jr. Tissue factor pathway inhibitor, *Thromb Haemost*. 1995. *74*(1): 90–93.

41. Sandset PM. Tissue factor pathway inhibitor (TFPI)—an update, *Haemostasis*. 1996. *26* Suppl 4: 154–165.

42. Sessa WC. eNOS at a glance, *J Cell Sci*. 2004. *117*(Pt 12): 2427–2429.

43. Osanai T, et al. Cross talk between prostacyclin and nitric oxide under shear in smooth muscle cell: role in monocyte adhesion, *Am J Physiol Heart Circ Physiol*. 2001. *281*(1): H177–H182.

44. Higman DJ, et al. Smoking impairs the activity of endothelial nitric oxide synthase in saphenous vein, *Arterioscler Thromb Vasc Biol*. 1996. *16*(4): 546–552.

45. Higman DJ, Greenhalgh RM, Powell JT. Smoking impairs endothelium-dependent relaxation of saphenous vein, *Br J Surg*. 1993. *80*(10): 1242–1245.

46. Broeders MA, et al. Endogenous nitric oxide protects against thromboembolism in venules but not in arterioles, *Arterioscler Thromb Vasc Biol*. 1998. *18*(1): 139–145.

47. Kojima S. Regulation of cellular uPA activity and its implication in pathogenesis of diseases. In: Kenzo T, Davie EW, Ikeda Y, et al., eds. *Recent advances in thrombosis and hemostasis 2008*. Tokyo: Springer. 2008. 301–313.

48. Adelman B, et al. Plasmin effect on platelet glycoprotein Ib-von Willebrand factor interactions, *Blood*. 1985. *65*(1): 32–40.

49. Rijken DC, Lijnen HR. New insights into the molecular mechanisms of the fibrinolytic system, *J Thromb Haemost*. 2009. *7*(1): 4–13.

50. Binder BR, et al. Plasminogen activator inhibitor 1: physiological and pathophysiological roles, *News Physiol Sci*. 2002. *17*: 56–61.

51. Alessi MC, Juhan-Vague I. PAI-1 and the metabolic syndrome: links, causes, and consequences, *Arterioscler Thromb Vasc Biol*. 2006. *26*(10): 2200–2207.

52. Crowther MA, et al. Fibrinolytic variables in patients with recurrent venous thrombosis: a prospective cohort study, *Thromb Haemost*. 2001. *85*(3): 390–394.

53. Puccetti L, et al. Dyslipidemias and fibrinolysis, *Ital Heart J*. 2002. *3*(10): 579–586.

54. Zoller B, Garcia de Frutos P, Dahlback B. A common 4G allele in the promoter of the plasminogen activator inhibitor-1 (PAI-1) gene as a risk factor for pulmonary embolism and arterial thrombosis in hereditary protein S deficiency, *Thromb Haemost*. 1998. *79*(4): 802–807.

55. Akar N, et al. Effect of plasminogen activator inhibitor-1 4G/5G polymorphism in Turkish deep vein thrombotic patients with and without FV1691 G-A, *Thromb Res*. 2000. *97*(4): 227–230.

56. Nordenholz KE, Mitchell AM, Kline JA, Direct comparison of the diagnostic accuracy of fifty protein biological markers of pulmonary embolism for use in the emergency department, *Acad Emerg Med*. 2008. *15*(9): 795–799.

57. Deatrick KB, et al. Vein wall remodeling after deep vein thrombosis involves matrix metalloproteinases and late fibrosis in a mouse model, *J Vasc Surg*. 2005. *42*(1): 140–148.

58. Varma MR, et al. Deep vein thrombosis resolution is not accelerated with increased neovascularization, *J Vasc Surg*. 2004. *40*(3): 536–542.

59. Shantsila E, Lip GY. The role of monocytes in thrombotic disorders. Insights from tissue factor, monocyte-platelet aggregates and novel mechanisms, *Thromb Haemost*. 2009. *102*(5): 916–924.

60. Henke PK, et al. Targeted deletion of CCR2 impairs deep vein thrombosis resolution in a mouse model, *J Immunol*. 2006. *177*(5): 3388–3397.

61. Thanaporn P, et al. P-selectin inhibition decreases post-thrombotic vein wall fibrosis in a rat model, *Surgery*. 2003. *134*(2): 365–371.

35.

CONGENITAL AND ACQUIRED HYPERCOAGULABLE SYNDROMES

Jocelyn A. Segall and Timothy K. Liem

INTRODUCTION

A fine balance exists between anticoagulant, procoagulant, and fibrinolytic factors. Intravascular thrombosis represents a shift in this balance, and may occur as the result of many factors in conjunction with a congenital or acquired abnormality in coagulation. An understanding of the differing hypercoagulable syndromes is important to appreciate the complexity of hemostasis and the factors that may offset normal clotting and anticoagulant mechanisms (see Figure 35.1). In addition, methods of prophylaxis and treatment of venous thromboembolism (VTE) are increasingly being stratified based, in part, on the presence or absence of a thrombophilic state. The presence of a hypercoagulable state does not imply that the patient will have thrombosis of a vessel. It does suggest that the individual is at a higher risk for thrombosis especially when the other factors of Virchow's triad (endothelial injury and stasis) are involved.[1]

CONGENITAL VERSUS ACQUIRED HYPERCOAGULABLE STATES

Some congenital hypercoagulable states place the individual at higher risk for thrombosis than others. Most genetic abnormalities in existence have clinically imperceptible consequences.[2,3] Additionally, some individuals have multiple genetic abnormalities, increasing their risk of thrombosis.[4] The common congenital hypercoagulable disorders are listed in Table 35.1.

Many causes exist for acquired hypercoagulable states, and some congenital hypercoagulable states may exist as acquired states as well. For instance, protein C and protein S deficiencies may occur secondary to decreased protein production from liver failure, sepsis, and/or malnutrition and increased protein loss secondary to nephrotic syndrome and inflammatory states.[5] In addition, hyperhomocysteinemia may occur because of enzymatic defects or because of

deficiencies in Vitamins B_6 and B_{12} and folate. The acquired hypercoagulable disorders are listed in Table 35.2.

THE CONGENITAL HYPERCOAGULABLE DISORDERS

ANTITHROMBIN DEFICIENCY

Antithrombin is a serine protease inhibitor of thrombin and also inhibits factors IXa, Xa, XIa, and XIIa. Thrombin is irreversibly bound by antithrombin and prevents thrombin's action on fibrinogen, on factors V, VIII, and XIII, and on platelets.[6] This anticoagulant is synthesized in the liver and endothelial cells, and has a half-life of 2.8 days.[7] Antithrombin deficiency has a prevalence of 1:5,000 with more than 100 genetic mutations and an autosomal dominant inheritance pattern.[8] Homozygotes typically die in utero, whereas heterozygotes typically have an antithrombin level that is 40 to 70% of normal.

Antithrombin deficiency is associated with lower extremity venous thrombosis as well as mesenteric venous thrombosis, and there are two clinical types. Individuals with Type I deficiency have a reduced number and function of antithrombin, and individuals with Type II have normal production but a reduction in function. Additionally, the heparin-binding site of the antithrombin may be mutated.[9] The risk of thrombosis increases as the functional antithrombin activity decreases to less than 80% of normal levels. The highest risk for thrombosis occurs when the activity is less than 60% of normal.[1]

The most common presentation in those with antithrombin deficiency is deep venous thrombosis (DVT) with or without pulmonary embolism.[10] The frequency of thromboembolism is unusual before the late teenage years and plateaus around the age of 40.[11] Thromboembolism may occur spontaneously but is often precipitated by other factors such as pregnancy, oral contraceptive use, estrogen replacement, trauma, surgery, or infection.[12]

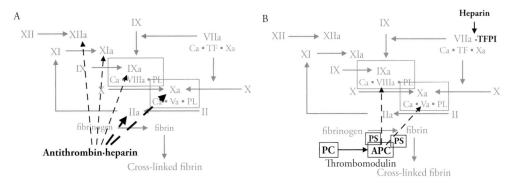

Figure 35.1   The coagulation cascade (light gray) and the sites of action for the natural anticoagulants (black). PC = protein C, APC = activated protein C. Protein S (PS) is a cofactor for the inhibition of factors V and VIII. TFPI (tissue factor pathway inhibitor) levels increase severalfold in response to heparin. TFPI binds to factor VIIa, inhibiting the conversion of factor X to Xa, and factor IX to IXa.

Table 35.1 **THE MOST COMMON CONGENITAL HYPERCOAGULABLE DISORDERS**

CONGENITAL HYPERCOAGULABLE DISORDERS
Antithrombin Deficiency
Protein C Deficiency
Protein S Deficiency
Factor V Leiden
Prothrombin G20210A Polymorphism
Hyperhomocysteinemia
Dysfibrinogenemia and Abnormal Fibrinogens

Table 35.2 **ACQUIRED HYPERCOAGULABLE DISORDERS**

ACQUIRED HYPERCOAGULABLE DISORDERS	
Heparin-Induced Thrombocytopenia/ Heparin-Induced Thrombocytopenia and Thrombosis Syndrome	Hyperfibrinogenemia Nephrotic Syndrome Renal Failure
Lupus Anticoagulant/Antiphospholipid Antibody Syndrome	Vasculitis Malignancy
Smoking	Thrombocythemia
Warfarin	Homocysteinemia
Pregnancy	Sepsis
Oral Contraceptive Pills/Hormone Replacement Therapy	Obesity Immobility
Mechanical Injury/Trauma/Surgery	
Diabetes Mellitus	
Hyperlipidemia	
Polycythemia vera	

Antithrombin deficiency should be suspected in a patient with spontaneous thrombosis, in a patient who cannot be anticoagulated adequately on heparin or in a patient who develops thrombosis while on heparin. To detect this deficiency, antithrombin levels should be measured when the patient has not been exposed to heparin.[13,14]

PROTEIN C AND PROTEIN S DEFICIENCY

Protein C is a vitamin K–dependent anticoagulant protein that, once activated by thrombin, will inactivate factors Va and VIIIa, thereby inhibiting the generation of thrombin.[4] Additionally, activated Protein C (APC) stimulates the release of tissue-type plasminogen activator (t-PA). It is produced in the liver and is the dominant endogenous anticoagulant with an 8-h half-life. Protein C deficiency has a prevalence of 1 in 200–300 with more than 150 mutations and an autosomal dominant inheritance.[4,7] Similar to antithrombin deficiency, protein C deficiency has two types: Type I is associated with decreased production and function and Type II is associated with a low functional level.[8] Type I deficiency predominates.

Protein S is also a vitamin K–dependent anticoagulant protein that is a cofactor to APC. The actions of protein S are regulated by complement C4b binding protein and only the free form of protein S serves as an APC cofactor.[15] Additionally, protein S appears to have independent anticoagulant function by directly inhibiting procoagulant enzyme complexes.[7,16] The prevalence of protein S deficiency is about 1:500 with an autosomal dominant inheritance. Three types of protein S deficiencies exist: Type I is associated with low levels of free and total protein S antigen and decreased APC activity; Type II has normal levels of protein S antigen but low levels of APC cofactor activity; and Type III has normal to low levels of total protein S, low free protein S, and an increased proportion of protein S bound to complement C4b.[8] In addition, many patients with protein S deficiency also have resistance to APC, which may be the reason for the thrombosis.[1]

Clinically, protein C and protein S deficiencies are essentially identical. With homozygous protein C and protein S deficiencies, infants typically will succumb to purpura fulminans, a state of unrestricted clotting and fibrinolysis. In heterozygotes, venous thromboses may occur at an early age especially in the lower extremity.[17] Thrombosis may also occur in mesenteric, renal, and cerebral veins. Protein C and protein S deficiencies usually become clinically evident when the levels of these proteins are less than 50% of normal.

Plasma protein C and S concentrations may be obtained to diagnose deficiencies of these proteins. Antigen and activity levels of protein C are measured, whereas for protein S, only antigen levels are measured. These measurements should be made prior to starting anticoagulation therapy with either heparin or warfarin.[8,13,18]

FACTOR V LEIDEN MUTATION AND APC RESISTANCE

Factor V is a glycoprotein synthesized in the liver. With Factor V Leiden, a point mutation occurs when arginine is substituted by glutamine at position 506. This point mutation causes the activated Factor V to be resistant to inactivation by APC, thus causing a procoagulant state. The mutation appears almost exclusively in the Caucasian population, and inheritance is autosomal dominant. The relative risk of a thromboembolic event in a heterozygous carrier is increased five- to seven-fold over the general population and increased up to eighty-fold in a homozygous carrier.[4] The risk of thrombosis also increases with combined genetic defects and/or additional acquired risk factors and will exceed the sum of the separate risks.[15]

Clinically, patients may present with DVT in the lower extremities, or less commonly in the portal vein, cerebral vein, or superficial venous system. Laboratory testing for the diagnosis of APC resistance and Factor V Leiden may be performed using functional clotting-based assays or by genetic testing. Factor V Leiden is the most common cause for APC resistance. Other less common causes include Factor V Cambridge, HR2 haplotype, Factor V Hong Kong, and Factor V Liverpool. The functional clotting-based assays include a modified activated partial thromboplastin time (aPTT) test, which dilutes the patient's plasma in Factor V–deficient plasma or incorporates dilute Russell's viper venom in the assay. The presence of APC resistance is then determined by measuring the aPTT in the presence and absence of APC. This modified test may be used in the presence of heparin, warfarin, and lupus anticoagulant. The genetic test relies on DNA amplification using PCR and is the most reliable test.[18]

PROTHROMBIN G20210 POLYMORPHISM

Prothrombin (Factor II) is a zymogen synthesized in the liver and dependent on vitamin K. When prothrombin is activated, it forms thrombin (Factor IIa). A single mutation where adenine is substituted for guanine occurs at the 20210 position. The mechanism for increased thrombotic risk is not well understood, but individuals with this genetic variant have supranormal levels of prothrombin. The mutation is inherited as an autosomal dominant trait and is associated with both arterial and venous thrombosis. Like Factor V Leiden, this mutation occurs almost exclusively in the Caucasian population. Individuals with the prothrombin gene variant are typically heterozygous.[7] Heterozygosity

confers a two-fold increase in the risk of thrombosis, and homozygosity confers approximately a ten-fold increase in the risk of thrombosis.[13]

Clinically, patients may present with DVT of the lower extremity, cerebral venous thrombosis, and arterial thrombosis. The risk of thrombosis increases in the presence of other genetic coagulation defects and with acquired risk factors.[1,7] Detection of the prothrombin G20210 polymorphism is by genetic analysis alone, as no correlation exists between functional prothrombin levels and those individuals with the genetic mutation.[13]

HYPERHOMOCYSTEINEMIA

Homocysteine is an amino acid formed during the metabolism of methionine and may be elevated secondary to inherited defects in two enzymes that are part of the conversion of homocysteine to cysteine. The two enzymes involved are N^5,N^{10}–methylene tetrahydrofolate reductase (MTHFR) or cystathionine beta-synthase. Hyperhomocysteinemia has been shown to increase the risk of atherosclerosis, atherothrombosis, and venous thrombosis.

Elevated plasma homocysteine levels cause various dysfunctions of endothelial cells leading to a prothrombotic state. With the oxidation of homocysteine, superoxide radicals are formed, which cause endothelial damage, smooth muscle proliferation, and activation of platelets and leukocytes. Additionally, hyperhomocysteinemia augments factor V and VII activity and decreases the activation of protein C, indirectly stimulates platelet aggregation, decreases the production of endothelium-derived nitric oxide, and interferes with the binding of t-PA.[1,19]

In patients with unexplained VTE, homocysteine levels should be measured. Levels may be measured by obtaining a fasting plasma homocysteine or after giving a standardized methionine-loading test. In patients who have been given the loading dose of methionine, hyperhomocysteinemia is present if the level of homocysteine is two standard deviations above the mean.

In patients with hyperhomocysteinemia, folate, B_6, and/or B_{12} can be given with normalization of homocysteine levels after several weeks of therapy. Whether this treatment has any affect on the prothombotic effects of hyperhomocysteinemia remains to be proven.[19]

ACQUIRED HYPERCOAGULABLE DISORDERS

There exist far more known causes of acquired hypercoagulable disorders than inherited disorders. Additionally, several of the congenital hypercoagulable states may be seen as acquired states attributable to a change in the production or consumption of various factors. Many of the common causes of acquired hypercoagulable disorders will be discussed.

HEPARIN-INDUCED THROMBOCYTOPENIA (HIT) AND HEPARIN-INDUCED THROMBOCYTOPENIA AND THROMBOSIS SYNDROME (HITTS)

Approximately 2 to 3% of patients who undergo heparin therapy will develop HIT or HITTS. Patients with HIT will have thrombocytopenia (characterized by a platelet count less than 100,000/mm³ or a decrease in the baseline count by more than 30%), will be resistant to anticoagulation with heparin, and may develop arterial or venous thromboses.

Two types of HIT exist. The first type is not associated with an immune mediated response and typically is seen in the first few days after initiation of heparin therapy. Typically, platelet levels do not fall below 100,000/mm³. Type II is immune-mediated with patients producing immunoglobulin G (IgG) antibodies against complexes of heparin and platelet factor 4. Antibody formation usually occurs between the 5th and 10th day after the first heparin exposure. The formation of these immune complexes creates a hypercoagulable state by activating platelets and the endothelium.[8,20]

Antibodies may develop against any form of heparin, and the formation of antibodies is independent of the age or sex of the patient, the route of administration of heparin, or the amount of heparin administered. Clinically, a patient will have a declining platelet count, may have an increasing resistance to anticoagulation therapy with heparin, and may develop a new thrombosis. Laboratory testing may be performed, which includes testing for antibodies to heparin.[1] Functional assays to detect platelet aggregation or activation in the presence of heparin-associated antibodies are well established. Enzyme-linked immunosorbent assays (ELISA) are readily available, but there is up to 40% discordance in the results of these antigenic assays, when compared with the functional platelet aggregation tests. The ELISA may detect IgM and IgA varieties, whereas platelet aggregation assays detect only the IgG antibodies.

The treatment of HIT includes the prompt discontinuation of heparin or low molecular weight heparin, and the administration of alternative anticoagulants, such as recombinant hirudin or argatroban (both direct thrombin inhibitors). Danaparoid (a low molecular weight heparinoid), has been used in the past as an alternative anticoagulant in patients with HIT. However, danaparoid production was discontinued in 2002 because of a shortage in the drug substance. Fondaparinux (a pentasaccharide that inactivates factor Xa via an antithrombin-dependent mechanism) has had recent success as another alternative anticoagulant. As with hirudin and argatroban, there are no reliable agents that can reverse the anticoagulant effect of fondaparinux. Hirudin and fondaparinux are metabolized primarily via renal excretion, whereas argatroban is metabolized primarily by the liver.

Patients with heparin-induced thrombocytopenia are at high risk for the development of subsequent thromboses, and the discontinuation of heparin alone is usually not sufficient. Warfarin may be used for prolonged anticoagulation in patients with acute thromboses, but its initiation should be delayed until the platelet count has substantially recovered. In addition, warfarin therapy should overlap with the administration of a direct thrombin inhibitor until the platelet count normalizes.

LUPUS ANTICOAGULANT/ ANTIPHOSPHOLIPID ANTIBODY SYNDROME

The term "antiphospholipid syndrome" was developed to describe the clinical manifestations of a hypercoagulable state associated with antiphospholipid antibodies. The most commonly identified antiphospholipid antibodies are lupus anticoagulant, anticardiolipin antibody, and anti-β_2-glycoprotein I antibodies.[21]

This syndrome is divided into primary and secondary syndromes. The primary syndrome occurs in patients without associated autoimmune disorders, and the secondary syndrome occurs in patients with systemic lupus erythematosus (SLE) and/or other autoimmune disorders. The procoagulant effects of the antiphospholipid antibodies leading to thrombosis include inhibition of the APC pathway, inhibition of antithrombin activity, inhibition of anticoagulant activity of β_2-glycoprotein I, inhibition of fibrinolysis, potentiation of platelet activation, and enhanced platelet activation, among others.[8,21]

Antiphospholipid antibodies are found in 1 to 5% of the population, and their prevalence increases with age. Among patients with SLE, the prevalence of antiphospholipid antibodies is much higher, with 12 to 30% having anticardiolipin antibodies and 15 to 34% having lupus anticoagulant antibodies. In patients with SLE and an antiphospholipid antibody, 50 to 70% may develop the antiphospholipid syndrome.[1] In order for the diagnosis of antiphospholipid syndrome to be made, the patient must meet the criteria of the international consensus statement. A definitive diagnosis may be made if the patient has at least one of the clinical criteria and one of the laboratory criteria. The consensus statement is defined in Table 35.3.[22]

Clinically, the most common manifestation of the antiphospholipid syndrome is DVT of the legs. Arterial thrombosis also may be seen but less often than venous thrombosis. Laboratory tests to detect the antiphospholipid antibodies include the aPTT test, performed with and without exogenous normal plasma to detect the presence of an inhibitor. Other tests include the kaolin clotting time, and dilute Russell's viper venom time (dRVVT). ELISA tests are performed to detect anticardiolipin antibodies and anti-β_2-glycoprotein I antibodies.[21]

Table 35.3 CRITERIA FOR THE CLASSIFICATION OF THE ANTIPHOSPHOLIPID SYNDROME

INTERNATIONAL CONSENSUS STATEMENT ON PRELIMINARY CRITERIA FOR THE CLASSIFICATION OF THE ANTIPHOSPHO-LIPID SYNDROME
Clinical Criteria:
Vascular thrombosis: 1 or more clinical episodes of arterial, venous, or small vessel thrombosis, occurring within any tissue or organ.
Complications of Pregnancy:
1 or more unexplained deaths of morphologically normal fetuses at or after the 10th week of gestation; or
1 or more premature births of morphologically normal neonates at or before the 34th week of gestation; or
3 or more unexplained consecutive spontaneous abortions before the 10th week of gestation.
Laboratory Criteria:
Anticardiolipin antibodies
Anticardiolipin IgG or IgM antibodies present at moderate or high levels in the blood on 2 or more occasions at least 6 weeks apart.
Lupus anticoagulant antibodies
Lupus anticoagulant antibodies detected in the blood on 2 or more occasions at least 6 weeks apart.

(From Reference 22)

Aspirin and hydroxychloroquine have been used in subsets of patients with the antiphospholipid syndrome for prophylaxis against thrombotic events. The treatment of established VTE in these patients consists of acute heparinization and longer-term (possibly lifelong) vitamin K antagonists. The optimal intensity of warfarin anticoagulation (international normalized ratio [INR] 2.0–2.9 versus 3.0–3.9) has not been determined.[21]

WARFARIN-INDUCED SKIN NECROSIS

This disorder is the most severe nonhemorrhagic complication of oral anticoagulation. Although rare, it seems to show a predilection for perimenopausal obese women who are being anticoagulated. Venules and capillaries within the subcutaneous fat and overlying skin thrombose, leading to necrosis. This typically is seen in the subcutaneous fat of the breasts, thighs, buttocks, and legs. Clinically, the patient may initially have paresthesias, which are then followed by painful, erythematous lesions. When hemorrhagic bullae are present, this is indicative of full thickness skin necrosis.

The pathogenesis for this process is the depletion of protein C prior to the other vitamin K–dependent coagulation factors. As the half-life of protein C is only 8 h, its rapid depletion causes a transient hypercoagulable state until the rest of the vitamin K–dependent factors also are reduced to levels that produce anticoagulation.

The primary treatment is prevention with heparin or low molecular weight heparin anticoagulation for the first 48 to 72 h of anticoagulation with warfarin. If skin necrosis develops, warfarin needs to be discontinued, and anticoagulation may continue with heparin or a direct thrombin inhibitor.[8]

SURGERY/TRAUMA

The risk of thrombosis is dependent on the type of surgery and the presence of additional risk factors. This risk may persist for up to several months after surgery. Patients who are at particularly high risk include those who undergo hip fracture surgery, hip or knee arthroplasty, neurosurgical procedures, and patients with major trauma. Injury to tissues and vessels during the procedure may enhance thrombogenesis.[8,23] Operative dissection, thermal injuries, and soft tissue trauma activate the coagulation cascade by inducing tissue factor release, thereby increasing the thrombogenic risk.

With a major traumatic injury, risk for venous thrombosis is highest in patients with spinal injuries, pelvic fractures, and lower extremity fractures. The risk of thrombosis also increases with greater injury severity. In part, this may be due to the accompanying systemic inflammatory response (another prothrombotic state, covered later).

PREGNANCY

During pregnancy, there is an associated hypercoagulable state due to the increase in factors I, VII, VIII, IX, X, XI, and XII. Additionally, platelet counts increase and concentrations of protein S and antithrombin decrease. The fibrinolytic system also may be inhibited secondary to the increased production of plasminogen-activated inhibitors 1 and 2 by the placenta. Compounding this risk is the degree of stasis that occurs as a result of compression of the lower extremity veins by the gravid uterus. In the postpartum period, the risk for thrombosis is up to five times greater than during pregnancy. Approximately 2 months after delivery, the coagulation and fibrinolytic systems will return to normal.[1]

The risk of thrombosis is increased further in pregnant women who have a genetic risk for thrombosis. Depending on the inherited thrombophilia, a woman with a thrombophilia who becomes pregnant may have a risk of venous thrombosis up to eight times higher than those without a thrombophilia.[4] In addition, women with a genetic risk for thrombosis are also at an increased risk for fetal loss and preeclampsia. Many women with a history of thrombophilia or thromboembolism are treated with heparin, low molecular weight heparin, and/or aspirin while pregnant.[24]

ORAL CONTRACEPTIVE-RELATED THROMBOSIS

Oral contraceptives are among the drugs most frequently used by women. The use of oral contraceptives initially was associated with a three-fold increased risk of venous thrombosis. With the decrease in the amount of estrogen placed in the pill, a subsequent decrease in the incidence of venous thrombosis was seen. With lower levels of estrogen, the risk of thrombosis is 1.5 to 2 times that over control patients.

Additionally, newer oral contraceptives using newer progesterones have shown an increased risk of thromboembolism.[25]

The risk for venous thrombosis is highest during the 1st year of use of the oral contraceptive, and the risk is not cumulative with prolonged use. Once the pill is discontinued, the risk returns to baseline for that patient.[25,26]

Oral contraceptives influence the plasma levels of nearly every protein involved in coagulation. Factors VII, VIII, IX, X, and XI increase, and the natural anticoagulants antithrombin and protein S decrease. However, oral contraceptive administration is associated with elevated protein C, α_1-antitrypsin, and fibrinolytic proteins, producing an antithrombotic effect. Additionally, the pill has been associated with an acquired APC resistance occurring within 3 days of initiation of the pill and reversing with discontinuation. This resistance has been shown to have a more pronounced increase in those women using third-generation oral contraceptives. The combination of APC resistance, increased prothrombin levels, and decreased protein S levels produces a net prothrombotic affect and confers the prothrombotic risk of oral contraceptives.[27,28]

In women with inherited thrombophilias who also take oral contraceptives, the risk for thrombosis increases thirty- to fifty-fold. For example, women who take oral contraceptives and are heterozygous for the Factor V Leiden mutation have been shown to have an increased risk of venous thrombosis by a factor of approximately thirty-five. This increased relative risk for venous thrombosis is in the same order of magnitude as patients who are homozygous for the Factor V Leiden mutation (almost fifty-fold increased risk). The women who have other inherited thrombophilias also appear to have a remarkably increased risk.[4,25]

HORMONE REPLACEMENT THERAPY–RELATED THROMBOSIS

Historically, hormone replacement therapy (HRT) has been used to reduce the progression of osteoporosis, relieve the symptoms of menopause, and reduce the cardiovascular risk profile. Several studies including the Heart Estrogen/Progestin Replacement Study (HERS) and the Women's Health Initiative (WHI) have shown an increased risk of VTE with the use of HRT. A two- to four-fold increased risk, compared with nonusers, has been shown.[26,29]

Similar to oral contraceptives, the risk of VTE is highest during the first year of HRT. Once HRT is discontinued, the risk of thrombosis returns to baseline. Additionally, increasing age has been associated with an increased risk of venous thrombosis. Several studies also have shown an increased risk in patients using HRT who had lower extremity fractures, recent surgery, previous VTE, cancer, and obesity.[29] Also similar to oral contraceptive pills, patients on HRT with thrombophilias have a significantly increased risk of VTE.[4] The coagulation factor changes that occur as a result of hormone replacement therapy are similar to those changes that occur with oral contraceptive pills, but to a lesser degree.

SYSTEMIC INFLAMMATORY RESPONSE (SIR) AND SEPSIS

With the SIR, cytokines and other inflammatory mediators are released causing a prothrombotic state. Specifically, tumor necrosis factor α (TNFα) and interleukin-1α (IL-1α) are increased. These factors activate the coagulation cascade, cause an increase in tissue factor expression, and decrease levels of protein C and protein S. Fibrinogen synthesis also will increase as part of the inflammatory response. Additionally, the inflammatory response is enhanced by thrombin, which augments leukocyte adhesion and activates platelets. Platelet activation in turn, further promotes tissue factor expression and increases cytokine release. All these factors contribute to the hypercoagulable state seen with SIRs and sepsis and predispose the patient to thrombosis.[30]

MALIGNANCY

VTE is a common complication of cancer. In 10% of patients who present with an idiopathic VTE, malignancy will be discovered. The majority of thrombotic episodes occur spontaneously, although patients with cancer often have other concurrent risk factors (inherited thrombophilias, immobilization, major surgical procedures, chemotherapy, and central venous catheters) that place them at high risk for VTE.

Tissue factor and cancer procoagulant are produced by tumor cells. The cancer procoagulant directly activates factor X independently of factor VII. Additionally, tumor cells produce proteins that may regulate the fibrinolytic system. These proteins impair fibrinolytic activity, leading to a prothrombotic state.[31] Tumor cells also produce various cytokines and affect the coagulation cascade and induce a thrombogenic state in a similar manner as SIRS. TNF-α and IL-1β are released by cancer cells and induce tissue factor expression and downregulate thrombomodulin. Furthermore, tumor cells activate other cytokines and several different types of leukocytes, which also increase tissue factor expression and activate platelets. The interaction of all these processes lead to a prothrombotic condition.[31]

TESTING FOR INHERITED THROMBOPHILIC CONDITIONS

We perform testing for inherited thrombophilic conditions in the following clinical circumstances: idiopathic DVT, recurrent DVT, DVT with young age at onset, and venous thromboses in unusual locations (mesenteric or portal venous thrombosis, cerebral vein thrombosis). Many hospitals provide testing with a "hypercoagulable panel." However, the clinician should ascertain that the following tests are performed: antithrombin activity, protein C activity, protein S activity, testing for either APC resistance or Factor V Leiden, prothrombin gene mutation, homocysteine levels, anticardiolipin antibody and lupus anticoagulant testing, and factor VIII activity. Antithrombin, protein C, and protein S levels may be depressed by the presence of acute thrombosis. Protein C and S may be similarly affected by warfarin administration. Therefore, an abnormal test result drawn during these time periods does not necessarily signify the presence of an inherited thrombophilic condition. Repeat testing is required.

OTHER ACQUIRED HYPERCOAGULABLE CONDITIONS AND TREATMENT STRATIFICATION

Patients are predisposed to thrombosis via many other clinical conditions. These conditions may affect the coagulation cascade, the fibrinolytic system, and/or platelet function, thereby increasing the risk of thrombosis. With two or more conditions that predispose to thrombosis, the patient is at a higher risk for suffering a thrombosis.

The objectives for treating acute VTE include the prevention of death from pulmonary embolism, reduction of lower extremity symptoms, prevention of the postphlebitic syndrome, and prevention of recurrent VTE. By limiting the propagation of thrombus, anticoagulation potentially has a role in achieving all of these objectives. Initial anticoagulation with unfractionated heparin or low molecular weight heparin, followed by 6 weeks to 6 months of oral vitamin K antagonists has been the mainstay of therapy. More recently, the American College of Chest Physicians Consensus Statement has stratified the type and duration of anticoagulation, based in part on the whether the patient has a concurrent thrombophilic condition (see Table 35.4).[32] In general, the overall trend is to extend the duration of anticoagulation, especially in patients with recurrent DVT, antiphospholipid syndrome, and patients with multiple thrombophilic conditions. In patients with malignancy and VTE, the recommended duration of low molecular weight heparin therapy has been extended to 3 to 6 months, followed by long-term vitamin K antagonists.

CONCLUSION

A clear understanding of the various conditions and situations in which a patient may have a hypercoagulable state is important for the ability to manage and appropriately treat patients in whom the risk of thrombosis exists. Once that risk is recognized, appropriate observation, prophylaxis, and treatment may ensue. It must be recognized that the number of acquired disease processes that predispose patients to thrombosis far outweighs the number of patients with congenital thrombophilias. Although a large portion

Table 35.4 AMERICAN COLLEGE OF CHEST PHYSICIANS RECOMMENDATIONS FOR DURATION OF ANTICOAGULATION FOR VENOUS THROMBOEMBOLISM[32]

CLINICAL SUBGROUP	TREATMENT DURATION
First episode DVT/transient risk	UH/LMWH followed by 3 mos VKA
First episode DVT/concurrent cancer	3–6 mos LMWH
Indefinite anticoagulation until cancer resolves	
First episode idiopathic DVT	UH/LMWH followed by 6–12 mos VKA (suggest indefinite)
First episode DVT/ thrombophilia antithrombin deficiency protein C and S deficiency factor V leiden prothrombin 20210 homocysteinemia factor VIII elevation (>90th %)	UH or LMWH followed by 6–12 mos VKA (suggest indefinite if idiopathic)
First episode DVT/ thrombophilia Antiphospholipid antibodies 2 or more thrombophilias	UH or LMWH followed by 12 mos VKA (suggest indefinite)
Recurrent DVT	UH or LMWH followed by indefinite VKA

UH = unfractionated heparin, LMWH = low-molecular-weight heparin, VKA = vitamin K antagonist.

of the population may have a thrombosis, few thromboses are caused by an inherited thrombophilia alone.

REFERENCES

1. Silver D, Vouyouka A. The caput medusae of hypercoagulability, *J Vasc Surg*. 2000. *31*: 396–495.
2. Franco RF, Reitsma PH. Genetic risk factors of venous thrombosis, *Hum Genet*. 2001. *109*: 369.
3. Rosendaal FR. Venous thrombosis: A multicausal disease, *Lancet*. 1993. *353*: 1167.
4. Seligsohn U, Lubetsky A. Genetic susceptibility to venous thrombosis, *N Engl J Med*. 2001. *344*: 1222–1231.
5. Henke PK, Schmaier A, Wakefield TW. Vascular thrombosis due to hypercoagulable states, *Rutherford Vascular Surgery*. 2005. 568–578.
6. Whiteman T, Hassouna HI. Hypercoagulable states, *Hematol Oncol Clin North Am*. 2000. *14*(2): 355–377.
7. Bick RL. Prothrombin G20210A mutation, antithrombin, heparin cofactor II, protein C, and protein S defects, *Hematol Oncol Clin N Am*. 2003. *17*: 9–36.
8. Johnson CM, Mureebe L, Silver D. Hypercoagulable states: A review, *Vasc Endovasc Surg*. 2005. *39*: 123–133.
9. Rosenberg RD, Aird WC. Vascular-bed-specific hemostasis and hypercoagulable states, *N Engl J Med*. 1999. *340*: 1555–1564.
10. Bick RL. Clinical relevance of antithrombin III, *Semin Thromb Hemost*. 1982. *8*: 276.
11. Thaler E, Lechner K. Antithrombin III deficiency and thromboembolism *Clin Haematol*. 1981. *10*: 369–390.
12. Candrina R, Goppini A. Antithrombin III Deficiency, *Blood Rev*. 1988. *2*: 239–250.

13. Mannucci PM. Laboratory detection of inherited thrombophilia: A historical perspective, *Semin Thromb Hemost.* 2005. *31*: 5–10.
14. De Moerloose P, Bounameaux HR, Mannucci PM. Screening tests for thrombophilic patients: Which tests, for which patient, by whom, when and why?, *Semin Thromb Hemost.* 1998. *24*: 321–327.
15. Nicolaes GAF, Dahlback B. Activated protein C resistance (FVLeiden) and thrombosis: Factor V mutations causing hypercoagulable states, *Hematol Oncol Clin N Am.* 2003. *17*: 37–61.
16. Koppelman SJ, Hackeng TM, Sixma JJ, et al. Inhibition of the intrinsic factor X activating complex by protein S: Evidence for specific binding of protein S to factor VIII, *Blood.* 1995. *86*: 1062–1071.
17. Allaart CF, Poort SR, Rosendaal FR, et al. Increased risk of venous thrombosis in carriers of hereditary protein C deficiency defect, *Lancet* 1993. *341*: 134–138.
18. Hertzberg MS. Genetic testing for thrombophilia mutations, *Semin Thromb Hemost.* 2005. *31*: 33–38.
19. Coppola A, Davi G, De Stefano V, et al. Homocysteine, coagulation, platelet function, and thrombosis, *Semin Thromb Hemost.* 2000. *26*: 243–254.
20. Warkentin TE, Kelton JG. Temporal aspects of heparin-induced thrombocytopenia, *N Engl J Med.* 2001. *344*: 1286–1292.
21. Levine JS, Branch DW, Ruach J. The antiphospholipid syndrome, *N Engl J Med.* 2002. *346*: 752–763.
22. Wilson WA, Ghavari AE, Koike T, et al. International consensus statement on preliminary classification criteria for de finite antiphospholipid syndrome: Report of an international workshop, *Arthritis Rheum.* 1999. *42*: 1309–1311.
23. Kyrle PA, Eichinger S. Deep vein thrombosis, *Lancet.* 2005. *365*: 1163–1174.
24. Pabinger I, Vormittag R. Thrombophilia and pregnancy outcomes, *J Thromb Haemo.* 2005. *3*: 1603–1610.
25. Bloemenkamp KWM. Epidemiology of oral contraceptive related thrombosis, *Thromb Res.* 2005. *115*(Suppl 1): 1–6.
26. Rosendaal FR, Van Hylckama Vlieg A, Tanis BC, et al. Estrogens, progestogens, and thrombosis, *J Thromb Haemo.* 2003. *1*: 1371–1380.
27. Rosing J. Mechanisms of OC related thrombosis, *Thromb Res.* 2005. *115*(Suppl 1): 81–83.
28. Vandenbroucke JP, Rosing J, Bloemenkamp KWM, et al. Oral contraceptives and the risk of venous thrombosis, *N Engl J Med.* 2001. *344*: 1527–1535.
29. Walker ID. Hormone replacement therapy and venous thromboembolism, *Thromb Res.* 2005. *115*(Suppl 1): 88–92.
30. Esmon CT. Inflammation and thrombosis, *J Thromb Haemo.* 2003. *1*: 1343–1348.
31. Prandoni P, Falanga A, Piccioli A. Cancer and venous thromboembolism, *Lancet.* 2005. *6*: 401–410.
32. Buller HR, Agnelli G, Hull RD, et al. Antithrombotic therapy for venous thromboembolic disease: The seventh ACCP conference on antithrombotic and thrombolytic therapy, *Chest.* 2004. *126*: 401S–428S.

36

NEW WAYS TO PREVENT VENOUS THROMBOEMBOLISM

INHIBITION OF FACTOR XA AND THROMBIN

David Bergqvist

In prevention of postoperative venous thromboembolism one of the low molecular weight heparins has been dominating the market since the early 1990s. There is, however, room for improvement, especially in patients undergoing high-risk surgery such as major orthopedic surgery and surgery for abdominal/pelvic malignancies. For the clinician, and for the patient, new methods should be either more effective or safer than low molecular weight heparins and be more cost-effective or easier to administer (i.e., be available for oral administration). The latter is especially true as long-term prophylaxis will undoubtedly increase in volume.

The various low molecular weight heparins have a rather complex mechanism of action, inhibiting activated factor X to a higher degree than inhibiting thrombin. This has been considered necessary for the good prophylactic effect.

In search of new agents overcoming some of the drawbacks with heparins, there have been two important developments within the field of antithrombotic substances. One development was to use the heterogeneous heparin molecule as a basis, and, working with the relation between structure and function, Lindahl et al. in Uppsala, Sweden,[1,2] defined the specific antithrombin-binding pentasaccharide sequence. The research group of Choay in Paris was able to synthesize this pentasaccharide as fondaparinux—a selective Xa inhibitor.[3,4] The other development was to synthesize small direct thrombin inhibitors, knowing the pivotal role thrombin plays within the hemostatic system and knowing that the thrombin inhibitor hirudin (originally from the saliva of medicinal leeches) had a good thromboprophylactic effect.[5] Many attempts have been made to synthesize such small selective thrombin inhibitors and the first with clinical documentation was ximelagatran/melagatran.[6–8] However, this substance was withdrawn shortly after approval because of liver toxicity.[9]

These two new ways of preventing venous thromboembolism with molecules that are more selective and structurally more homogeneous have been investigated in large clinical trial programs and both have got an approval in major orthopedic surgery.

When evaluating new thromboprophylactic substances and principles in the clinical setting, there should ideally be a three-step research program:

1. Studies on mechanism of action, pharmacokinetics, and pharmacodynamics.
2. Proof of principle with phlebographic evaluation of the antithrombotic effect in high risk
   a. major orthopedic surgery
   b. major abdominal/pelvic surgery (especially cancer)
3. Proof of clinical importance in
   a. large studies with a simple protocol on clinical venous thromboembolism
   b. meta-analyses.

Regarding step 2, although elective hip surgery is a well-established clinical model, it is important also to evaluate other high-risk surgical procedures. This is to make conclusions and clinical use more generalizable. From a practical point of view it is not ideal to have different prophylactic programs for various surgical procedures in a hospital or a surgical department. Prophylaxis must be simple to obtain widespread and well-accepted use. The manufacturers of the substances discussed in this chapter have first focused on and obtained approval for major orthopedic surgery.

FONDAPARINUX

Fondaparinux is a synthetic analogue of the natural pentasaccharide sequence of the heparin molecule, which mediates its interaction with antithrombin.[4] The molecular weight is 1,728 D, with a very high batch-to-batch consistency. The reversible binding, to a specific site on antithrombin, results in a 300-fold increase in the rate of factor Xa inhibition by antithrombin. After subcutaneous administration with a 100% bioavailability, the peak plasma level is obtained in about 2 h with an elimination half-life of about 17–21 h, longer in elderly, which allows once-daily administration.[9,10] The elimination is mainly unchanged through the renal route. The drug is therefore contraindicated in patients with renal failure, defined by a creatinine clearance of less than 30 ml/min. If used there is a potential for bleeding complications. A peak steady state plasma level is reached after 3–4 d (dose 2.5 mg daily). There is no specific antidote to fondaparinux, but in case of emergency recombinant factor VIIa may be used.[11] This could be the case in accidental overdosing with clinical hemorrhage.

A large phase III clinical program was performed to evaluate the effect of fondaparinux in major orthopedic surgery of the lower limbs. The studies conducted used various acronyms: EPHESUS (European Pentasaccharide Hip Elective SUrgery Study with 2,309 patients[12]), PENTATHLON (PENTAsaccharide in Total Hip Replacement Surgery with 2,275 patients[13]), PENTAMAKS (PENTAsaccharide in MAjor Knee Surgery with 1,049 patients[14]) and PENTHIFRA (PENTasaccharide in HIp FRActure surgery with 1,711 patients[15]). The studies were consistently performed using 2.5 mg fondaparinux daily starting postoperatively. The comparator was enoxaparin: in EPHESUS and PENTHIFRA with 40 mg once daily with preoperative start as used in Europe and in PENTATHLON and PENTAMAKS with 30 mg twice daily with postoperative start as used in North America. Phlebography was used for end-point assessment and the studies were evaluated in a meta-analysis.[16] The primary efficacy outcome is summarized in Table 36.1, the common odds reduction being 55% in favor of fondaparinux (p < 0.001). The incidence of symptomatic venous thromboembolism was low without difference between the groups (0.6% in the fondaparinux group and 0.4% in the enoxaparin group; p = 0.25). Fatal pulmonary embolism was diagnosed in two and three patients respectively. The beneficial effect of fondaparinux was consistent regarding sex, age, body mass index, type of anesthesia, use of cement for fixation of prosthesis, and duration of the surgical procedure.

There were 2.7% adjudicated major bleedings in the fondaparinux group versus 1.7 in the enoxaparin group (p = 0.008). This difference was mainly due to a difference in bleeding index, whereas fatal bleedings, bleedings in critical organs, and bleeding leading to reoperation did not differ. There was a significant relation between the incidence of major bleeding and the timing of the first injection of fondaparinux (between 3 and 9 h postoperatively, p = 0.008), whereas the thromboprophylactic effect was not influenced by timing (p = 0.67). Thrombocytopenia was not reported (there is no binding to platelet factor 4).[17] In the PENTHIFRA Plus study[18] the effect of prolonged prophylaxis with fondaparinux was evaluated in patients undergoing hip fracture surgery. All 656 patients received fondaparinux for 6 to 8 d, whereafter they were randomized to placebo or fondaparinux for another 19 to 23 d. Venous thromboembolism (bilateral phlebography or symptomatic venous thromboembolism) differed significantly, being 35% in the placebo group and 1.4% in the fondaparinux group, a

Table 36.1 FREQUENCY OF VENOUS THROMBOEMBOLISM UP TO DAY 11 (PERCENT WITHIN BRACKETS).

	FONDAPARINUX (N = 2,682)	ENOXAPARIN (N = 2,703)
Venous thromboembolism	182 (6.8)	371 (13.7)
Any DVT	174 (6.5)	363 (13.5)
Any proximal DVT	35 (1.3)	81 (2.9)

(From Reference 17)

reduction that is highly remarkable. The effect was also significant when symptomatic venous thromboembolism was used as end point (2.7% vs. 0.3%; p = 0.02).

In a multicenter, double-blind study (PEGASUS trial) on 2,048 patients undergoing high-risk abdominal surgery, fondaparinux was noninferior to dalteparin.[17] In the subgroup operated on for cancer the difference was significant in favor of fondaparinux (Table 36.2).

In another trial in elective abdominal surgery (APOLLO study) fondaparinux combined with intermittent pneumatic compression was significantly more effective than intermittent compression alone. The frequency of venous thromboembolism was reduced from 5.3 to 1.7% (p < 0.004).[19] Major bleeds occurred in 0.2% and 1.6% respectively (p = 0.006); none of them fatal or in a critical organ.

Fondaparinux is safe, the main concern being bleeding, which in some studies have been significantly higher than with the comparator. One important finding in a post hoc analysis of the orthopedic trials was the significantly increased frequency of major bleeding when the first fondaparinux injection was given within 6 h after wound closure instead of more than 6 h after (3.2% vs. 2.1 %; p = 0.045).[16] In case of serious bleeding complications recombinant factor VIIa may be used to reverse the anticoagulant effect, also adding tranexamic acid.[11,20]

Thrombocytopenia is seen at a similar frequency as following low molecular weight heparins, and there are no reports of heparin-induced thrombocytopenia (HIT). There does not seem to be an increase in liver enzymes.

RIVAROXABAN

Rivaroxaban is an oral direct factor Xa inhibitor with a molecular mass of 436 D. The bioavailability exceeds 80%.

Table 36.2 FONDAPARINUX IN HIGH-RISK ABDOMINAL SURGERY (PEGASUS). VENOGRAPHIC DVT.

	FONDAPARINUX	DALTEPARIN
Primary efficacy analyses	47/1,027 (4.6%)	62/1,021 (6.1%)
Patients with cancer	37/696 (4.7%)	55/712 (7.7%)

(From Reference 20)

The half-life is 7–11 h, and it is to about 65% excreted via the kidneys.

Three phase II trials[21-23] and four phase III clinical trials (The RECORD program)[24-27] have evaluated its efficacy and safety in orthopedic surgery. As comparator enoxaparin has been used. The two phase II trials were designed to allow pooling of the results, which showed that rivaroxaban in a total daily dose of 5–20 mg had the most favorable balance between effect and safety.[28]

In RECORD 1 rivaroxaban was shown superior to enoxaparin in reducing the primary end point of any DVT, nonfatal pulmonary embolism, or death (1.1% vs. 3.7 % respectively; p < 0.001), but not in symptomatic venous thromboembolism (0.3% vs. 0.5%). In RECORD 2 both total and symptomatic venous thromboembolism were significantly lower in the patients treated with rivaroxaban (2.0% vs. 9.3% and 0.2% vs. 1.2% respectively, p = 0.004), but the study did not compare similar prophylactic routines, rivaroxaban given for 35 d versus enoxaparin for 12 d. In the RECORD 3 and 4 rivaroxaban was superior to enoxaparin. The incidence of major and clinically significant nonmajor hemorrhage was increased across the rivaroxaban treatment groups, although not statistically significant. The RECORD trials with 12,500 patients demonstrated a more than 50% reduction compared with enoxaparin in the composite primary efficacy end point (symptomatic venous thromboembolism and death). Bleeding did not differ from that in the enoxaparin groups.

APIXABAN

Apixaban is a reversible direct oral factor Xa inhibitor. It has a bioavailability of 51–85% and reaches a Tmax after 3 h. The half life is 9–14 h, 25% being excreted by the kidneys and 65% via feces.

In the ADVANCE program apixaban was tested against enoxaparin in major orthopedic surgery with altogether around 11,600 patients. The apixaban dose is 2.5 mg twice daily. ADVANCE 1 and 2 used elective knee arthroplasty as the study population.[29-30]

In the American way of dosing enoxaparin (30 mg × 2) apixaban was noninferior, but when the European administration was used (40 mg × 1) apixaban was significantly better than enoxaparin. In both studies prophylaxis was given for 10–14 d. In ADCANCE 3[31] extended prophylaxis was studied in patients undergoing total hip replacement, 40 mg, and again apixaban was superior (1.4% vs. 2.9%). In all three studies apixaban prophylaxis started 12–24 h post surgery. In ADVANCE 1, major bleeding was significantly lower in the apixaban group.

The ADVANCE 2 and 3 studies have been pooled in an analysis, apixaban being more effective than enoxaparin 40 mg once daily.[32] Bleeding did not differ.

In the ADOPT study[33] the patient group consisted of medically ill patients (congestive heart failure, acute respiratory failure, infection, acute rheumatic disorder, or inflammatory bowel disease) with additional risk factors: age greater than or equal to 75 years, previous venous thromboembolism, cancer, body mass index greater than or equal to 30, estrogen therapy, or chronic heart or respiratory failure. Of 4,495 available patients 2.7% of apixaban patients and 3.1% of enoxaparin patients reached the primary composite efficacy outcome (30-d death related to venous thromboembolism, pulmonary embolism, symptomatic DVT, or proximal DVT detected with bilateral ultrasonography). Major bleeding was significantly more common in the apixaban patients (0.5% vs. 0.2%).

DABIGATRAN

Dabigatran etixilate is the oral prodrug form of the active direct factor IIa (thrombin) inhibitor dabigatran. Absorption and conversion are rapid. It is a small (molecular mass 472 D) synthetic molecule, the oral bioavailability being around 6.5%. The half-life in patients is 14–17 h, 85% being excreted via the kidneys.[34]

Data from two phase II[35,36] and three phase III clinical trials, RE-NOVATE, RE-MODEL, and RE-MOBILIZE[37-39] have been published. They deal with efficacy and safety in major orthopedic surgery. The RE-NOVATE and RE-MODEL studies compared two dabigatran dose regimens (150 mg and 220 mg once daily starting with half the dose 1–4 h postoperatively) with the European regimen of enoxaparin (40 mg × 1) in patients operated on with total hip or total knee replacement. In both trials dabigatran was as effective and safe as enoxaparin. In the RE-MOBILIZE trial in total knee replacement dabigatran in the same doses was less effective than the American regimen of enoxaparin (30 mg × 2), but safety was similar. The three phase III trials have been meta-analyzed with the total of 8,210 patients.[40] No significant differences were seen between dabigatran 220 mg once daily and enoxaparin in any of the end points regarding thrombosis prevention and safety.

LIMITATIONS OF NEW ANTICOAGULANTS

There are no available antidotes to dabigatran, rivaroxaban, or apixaban. This is a concern in patients who may require urgent reversal of the effect for emergency surgical procedures, in the case of trauma or a hemostatic emergency such as cerebral bleeding or overdosage.

There is still very limited experience in patients with decreased renal function as well as in pregnancy.

With the liver toxicity of ximelagatran such an effect has been a concern with the new oral substances, but so far there is no indication that this may be a problem.

CONCLUDING REMARKS

Today, there are synthetic substances inhibiting very well defined steps or specific factors in the hemostatic system, showing a clear effect in prevention of postoperative venous thromboembolism in major orthopedic surgery. Apart from being of practical importance, the principal mechanisms of action are of great theoretical interest. The target for optimal clotting factor inhibition is still a matter for discussion.

The substances have been extensively evaluated in clinical studies of high quality with large sample sizes. The effect is at least as effective as or more effective than today's dominating prophylactic method (low molecular weight heparin). Data are largely lacking on prophylaxis in nonorthopedic surgery, but the few results there are seem promising.

Another direct oral factor Xa inhibitor—apixaban[41]—has also recently been evaluated in a large phase III program (ADVANCE), the effect being promising at least comparable to enoxaparin, which has led to approval as prophylaxis in major orthopedic surgery in several countries.

One important issue in studies on new anticoagulants in surgical prophylaxis is the definition of bleeding and the impact that has on major bleeding outcome.[42,43] None of the new oral substances have any specific antidote. Another concern with the oral substances is the question of compliance outside a strict trial situation. This is important to evaluate as an oral substance would be of value in situations where extended out-of-hospital prophylaxis is indicated.[44]

The new anticoagulants are indeed promising, but it is important to study other risk groups than orthopedic surgery and to follow the effect in routine clinical care outside strict clinical trial situations. Heparins and low molecular weight heparins also have nonanticoagulant effects, which are used therapeutically, and whether the new substances can totally replace heparins needs to be shown.[45]

REFERENCES

1. Lindahl U, Backstrom G, Hook M, Thunberg L, Fransson LA, Linker A. Structure of the antithrombin-binding site in heparin, *Proc Natl Acad Sci USA.* 1979. *76*(7): 3198–3202.
2. Lindahl U, Bäckström G, Thunberg L, Leider I. Evidence from a 3-0-suphated D-glucosamine residence in the antithrombin binding sequence of heparin, *Proc Natl Acad Sci USA.* 1980. *77*: 6651–6655.
3. Choay J, Petitou M, Lormeau J, Sinay P, Casa B, Gatti G. Structure-activity relationship in heparin: A synthetic pentasaccharide with high affinity for antithrombin III and eliciting high antifactor Xa activity, *Biochem Bioph Res Co.* 1983. *116*: 492–499.
4. Petitou M, Lormeau JC, Choay J. Chemical synthesis of glycosaminoglycans: New approaches to antithrombotic drugs, *Nature.* 1991. *350*(Suppl 6319): 30–33.
5. Eriksson BI, Wille-Jorgensen P, Kalebo P, et al. A comparison of recombinant hirudin with a low-molecular-weight heparin to prevent thromboembolic complications after total hip replacement, *N Engl J Med.* 1997. *337*(19): 1329–1335.
6. Gustafsson D, Elg M. The pharmacodynamics and pharmacokinetics of the oral direct thrombin inhibitor ximelagatran and its active metabolite melagatran: A mini-review, *Thromb Res.* 2003. *109*(Suppl 1): S9–S15.
7. Crowther MA, Weitz JI. Ximelagatran: The first oral direct thrombin inhibitor, *Expert Opin Investig Drugs.* 2004. *13*(4): 403–413.
8. Eriksson BI, Dahl OE. Prevention of venous thromboembolism following orthopaedic surgery: Clinical potential of direct thrombin inhibitors, *Drugs.* 2004. *64*(6): 577–595.
9. Bauer KA, Hawkins DW, Peters PC, et al. Fondaparinux, a synthetic pentasaccharide: The first in a new class of antithrombotic agents: The selective factor Xa inhibitors, *Cardiovasc Drug Rev.* 2002. *20*(1): 37–52.
10. Boneu B, Necciari J, Cariou R, et al. Pharmacokinetics and tolerance of the natural pentasaccharide (SR90107/Org31540) with high affinity to antithrombin III in man, *Thromb Haemost.* 1995. *74*(6): 1468–1473.
11. Bijsterveld NR, Moons AH, Boekholdt SM, et al. Ability of recombinant factor VIIa to reverse the anticoagulant effect of the pentasaccharide fondaparinux in healthy volunteers, *Circulation.* 2002. *106*(20): 2550–2554.
12. Lassen MR, Bauer KA, Eriksson BI, Turpie AG. Postoperative fondaparinux versus preoperative enoxaparin for prevention of venous thromboembolism in elective hip-replacement surgery: A randomised double-blind comparison, *Lancet.* 2002. *359*(9319): 1715–1720.
13. Turpie AG, Bauer KA, Eriksson BI, Lassen MR. Postoperative fondaparinux versus postoperative enoxaparin for prevention of venous thromboembolism after elective hip-replacement surgery: A randomised double-blind trial, *Lancet.* 2002. *359*(9319): 1721–1726.
14. Bauer KA, Eriksson BI, Lassen MR, Turpie AG. Fondaparinux compared with enoxaparin for the prevention of venous thromboembolism after elective major knee surgery, *N Engl J Med.* 2001. *345*(18): 1305–1310.
15. Eriksson BI, Bauer KA, Lassen MR, Turpie AG. Fondaparinux compared with enoxaparin for the prevention of venous thromboembolism after hip-fracture surgery, *N Engl J Med.* 2001. *345*(18): 1298–1304.
16. Turpie AG, Eriksson BI, Lassen MR, Bauer KA. A meta-analysis of fondaparinux versus enoxaparin in the prevention of venous thromboembolism after major orthopaedic surgery, *J South Orthop Assoc.* 2002. *11*(4): 182–188.
17. Agnelli G, Bergqvist D, Cohen A, Gallus A, Gent M. PEGASUS investigations: Postoperative fondaparinux versus preoperative dalteparin for prevention of venous thromboembolism in hip-risk abdominal surgery: A randomized double-blind trial, *Br J Surg.* 2005. *92*: 1212–1220.
18. Eriksson BI, Lassen MR. Duration of prophylaxis against venous thromboembolism with fondaparinux after hip fracture surgery: A multicenter, randomized, placebo-controlled, double-blind study, *Arch Intern Med.* 2003. *163*(11): 1337–1342.
19. Turpie AG, Bauer KA, Caprini JA, Comp PC, Gent M, Muntz JE. Fondaparinux combined with intermittent pneumatic compression vs. intermittent pneumatic compression alone for prevention of venous thromboembolism after abdominal surgery: A randomized, double-blind comparison, *J Thromb Haemost.* 2007. *5*(9): 1854–1861.
20. Huvers F, Slappendel R, Benraad B, van Hellemondt G, van Kraaij M. Treatment of postoperative bleeding after fondaparinux with rFVIIa and tranexamic acid, *Neth J Med.* 2005. *63*(5): 184–186.
21. Turpie AG, Fisher WD, Bauer KA, et al. BAY 59-7939: An oral, direct factor Xa inhibitor for the prevention of venous thromboembolism in patients after total knee replacement: A phase II dose-ranging study, *J Thromb Haemost.* 2005. *3*(11): 2479–2486.
22. Eriksson BI, Borris LC, Dahl OE, et al. A once-daily, oral, direct Factor Xa inhibitor, rivaroxaban (BAY 59-7939), for thromboprophylaxis after total hip replacement, *Circulation.* 2006. *114*(22): 2374–2381.
23. Eriksson BI, Borris L, Dahl OE, et al. Oral, direct Factor Xa inhibition with BAY 59-7939 for the prevention of venous thromboembolism after total hip replacement, *J Thromb Haemost.* 2006. *4*(1): 121–128.

24. Eriksson BI, Borris LC, Friedman RJ, et al. Rivaroxaban versus enoxaparin for thromboprophylaxis after hip arthroplasty, *N Engl J Med.* 2008. *358*(26): 2765–2775.

25. Kakkar AK, Brenner B, Dahl OE, et al. Extended duration rivaroxaban versus short-term enoxaparin for the prevention of venous thromboembolism after total hip arthroplasty: A double-blind, randomised controlled trial, *Lancet.* 2008. *372*(9632): 31–39.

26. Lassen MR, Ageno W, Borris LC, et al. Rivaroxaban versus enoxaparin for thromboprophylaxis after total knee arthroplasty, *N Engl J Med.* 2008. *358*(26): 2776–2786.

27. Turpie AG, Lassen MR, Davidson BL, et al. Rivaroxaban versus enoxaparin for thromboprophylaxis after total knee arthroplasty (RECORD4): A randomised trial, *Lancet.* 2009. *373*(9676): 1673–1680.

28. Fisher WD, Eriksson BI, Bauer KA, et al. Rivaroxaban for thromboprophylaxis after orthopaedic surgery: Pooled analysis of two studies, *Thromb Haemost.* 2007. *97*(6): 931–937.

29. Lassen MR, Raskob GE, Gallus A, Pineo G, Chen D, Portman RJ. Apixaban or enoxaparin for thromboprophylaxis after knee replacement, *N Engl J Med.* 2009. *361*(6): 594–604.

30. Lassen MR, Raskob GE, Gallus A, Pineo G, Chen D, Hornick P. Apixaban versus enoxaparin for thromboprophylaxis after knee replacement (ADVANCE-2): A randomised double-blind trial, *Lancet.* 2010. *375*(9717): 807–815.

31. Lassen MR, Gallus A, Raskob GE, Pineo G, Chen D, Ramirez LM. Apixaban versus enoxaparin for thromboprophylaxis after hip replacement, *N Engl J Med.* 2010. *363*(26): 2487–2498.

32. Raskob GE, Gallus AS, Pineo GF, et al. Apixaban versus enoxaparin for thromboprophylaxis after hip or knee replacement: Pooled analysis of major venous thromboembolism and bleeding in 8464 patients from the ADVANCE-2 and ADVANCE-3 trials, *J Bone Joint Surg Br.* 2012. *94*(2): 257–264.

33. Goldhaber SZ, Leizorovicz A, Kakkar AK, et al. Apixaban versus enoxaparin for thromboprophylaxis in medically ill patients, *N Engl J Med.* 2011. *365*(23): 2167–2177.

34. Stangier J, Stahle H, Rathgen K, Fuhr R. Pharmacokinetics and pharmacodynamics of the direct oral thrombin inhibitor dabigatran in healthy elderly subjects, *Clin Pharmacokinet.* 2008 *47*(1): 47–59.

35. Eriksson BI, Dahl OE, Ahnfelt L, et al. Dose escalating safety study of a new oral direct thrombin inhibitor, dabigatran etexilate, in patients undergoing total hip replacement: BISTRO I, *J Thromb Haemost.* 2004. *2*(9): 1573–1580.

36. Eriksson BI, Dahl OE, Buller HR, et al. A new oral direct thrombin inhibitor, dabigatran etexilate, compared with enoxaparin for prevention of thromboembolic events following total hip or knee replacement: The BISTRO II randomized trial, *J Thromb Haemost.* 2005. *3*(1): 103–111.

37. Eriksson BI, Dahl OE, Rosencher N, et al. Dabigatran etexilate versus enoxaparin for prevention of venous thromboembolism after total hip replacement: A randomised, double-blind, non-inferiority trial, *Lancet.* 2007. *370*(9591): 949–956.

38. Eriksson BI, Dahl OE, Rosencher N, et al. Oral dabigatran etexilate vs. subcutaneous enoxaparin for the prevention of venous thromboembolism after total knee replacement: The RE-MODEL randomized trial, *J Thromb Haemost.* 2007. *5*(11): 2178–2185.

39. Ginsberg JS, Davidson BL, Comp PC, et al. Oral thrombin inhibitor dabigatran etexilate vs North American enoxaparin regimen for prevention of venous thromboembolism after knee arthroplasty surgery, *J Arthroplasty.* 2009. *24*(1): 1–9.

40. Wolowacz SE, Roskell NS, Plumb JM, Caprini JA, Eriksson BI. Efficacy and safety of dabigatran etexilate for the prevention of venous thromboembolism following total hip or knee arthroplasty: A meta-analysis, *Thromb Haemost.* 2009. *101*(1): 77–85.

41. Raghavan N, Frost CE, Yu Z, et al. Apixaban metabolism and pharmacokinetics after oral administration to humans, *Drug Metab Dispos.* 2009. *37*(1): 74–81.

42. Hull R, Yusen RD, Bergqvist D. Assessing the safety profiles of new anticoagulants for major orthopedic surgery thromboprophylaxis, *Clin Appl Thrombos Hemostas.* 2009. *15*(4): 377–388.

43. Bergqvist D. Bleeding profiles of anticoagulants, including the novel oral direct thrombin inhibitor ximelagatran: Definitions, incidence, and management. *Eur J Haematol.* 2004. *73*(4): 227–242.

44. Bergqvist D, Agnelli G, Cohen AT, et al. Duration of prophylaxis against venous thromboembolism with enoxaparin after surgery for cancer, *N Engl J Med.* 2002. *346*(13): 975–980.

45. Lever R, Page CP. Novel drug development opportunities for heparin, *Nat Rev Drug Discov.* 2002. *1*(2): 140–148.

37.

DIAGNOSIS OF DEEP VENOUS THROMBOSIS

David A. Frankel and Warner P. Bundens

BACKGROUND

Patients with one or more of Virchow's triad of stasis, hyper-coagulability, or vein wall abnormalities are susceptible to thrombosis.[1] Lower limb deep venous thrombosis (DVT) is a common and potentially serious problem. Over five million occur in the United States annually, and approximately 10% become pulmonary emboli.[2,3] Ninety percent of pulmonary emboli originate from lower limb DVTs.[4,5] Furthermore, DVT can also result in permanent venous obstruction, that is, chronic DVT, and/or damage to venous valves leading to postphlebitic chronic venous insufficiency. Timely and accurate diagnosis can aid significantly in the reduction of morbidity and mortality.

The clinical presentation of DVT can range from silent, with no symptoms or physical findings, to phlegmasia cerula dolens and venous gangrene. However, the sensitivity and specificity of symptoms and physical findings such as pain, tenderness, swelling, redness, or a positive Homan's sign range from 30 to 80%. The clinical diagnosis of DVT is not reliable with an overall accuracy of only approximately 50%.[6-10] Thus, when DVT is suspected or it is part of a differential diagnosis, an accurate and objective test that can rule in or rule out DVT is indicated.

Though this chapter is devoted to the diagnosis of thrombosis in the deep leg veins, one should keep DVT in mind when seeing a patient with superficial thrombophlebitis. The clinical diagnosis of thrombophlebitis of a superficial vein is accurate. One should be aware, however, that multiple studies have shown that approximately 20% of patients will also have an occult DVT.[11-16] The extent of thrombus in superficial veins usually extends further than is evident clinically, and in up to one-third of cases the thrombus will eventually extend into the deep system via the saphenofemoral junction or communicating veins.[17-19]

The traditional "gold standard" of objective testing is ascending contrast phlebography. Compared with autopsy findings it has a 97% sensitivity and 95% specificity.[20] The test, however, is costly, invasive, uncomfortable, and associated with definite risks. One of the "particularly unwelcome"

complications is a 2 to 3% risk of the contrast agents actually causing DVT.[9] For decades, trends have been toward less invasive and in the case of ultrasonography, less expensive methods of studying patients suspected of having DVT. For years, radioactive fibrinogen scanning and impedance plethysmography were widely used but were supplanted by duplex ultrasonography as scanners became widely available and multiple studies showed acceptable accuracy. Currently, duplex ultrasonography is still the most commonly used method of testing for lower limb DVT, though other methodologies are being increasingly used in selected settings.

DUPLEX ULTRASONOGRAPHY

The combination of B-mode imaging and the pulse Doppler into one instrument, the Duplex, was originally done as an aid to arterial diagnosis. It soon became evident that it could also be used for venous investigations of both obstruction and reflux. Since 1990s the hardware technology has improved the quality of the B-mode imaging dramatically. Color-coded flow displays as well as "power Doppler" are now available in most instruments. These two modes are often helpful for locating veins and outlining intraluminal defects.

The possible duplex findings with a lower limb DVT are listed in Table 37.1. Virtually all vascular labs use the first criteria, the inability to collapse a vein with probe pressure (Figures 37.1 and 37.2), as the primary diagnostic method. Some use only this finding.[21] Meta-analysis has shown this sign to be 95% sensitive and 98% specific for proximal leg DVTs. When all the criteria of Table 37.1 are used the sensitivity is 98% and specificity 94%.[22]

Although the accuracy of this noninvasive, readily available, and relatively low cost test is impressive, one should realize most data reflect findings in patients with femoral and/or popliteal vein disease. The majority of patients with symptomatic DVTs have thrombus in these veins.[23,24] In some cases the thrombus may also involve the iliac or calf veins. Duplex examination may not detect

Table 37.1 DUPLEX FINDINGS OF LOWER-LIMB DVT

MODE	FINDING	IMPLICATION
B-Mode Image	Unable to coapt vein walls with probe pressure	Intraluminal thrombus
	Visible thrombus	Thrombus, possibly old
	Vein enlarged	Acute thrombus
Pulse Doppler	No spontaneous flow	Occlusive thrombus
	No augmentation of flow with distal limb compression	Obstruction distal to probe
	No flow variation with respiration	Obstruction proximal to probe
Color Flow or Power Doppler	Intraluminal defect	Nonocclusive thrombus
Combined	Increased flow velocity and size of surrounding veins	Being used as collaterals

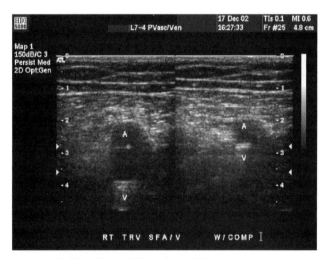

Figure 37.1 Duplex of normal femoral vein. Vein can be completely collapsed with probe pressure.

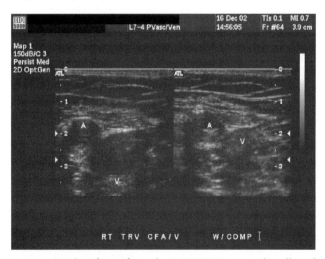

Figure 37.2 Duplex of acute femoral vein DVT. Vein cannot be collapsed with probe pressure. Also note, vein is enlarged, thrombus is echolucent and is partially compressible, which are signs of acute thrombus.

the full extent of thrombosis in these instances, but at least the diagnosis of DVT will be made and, presumably, appropriate treatment given. One must realize, however, that isolated calf vein DVT are common and isolated iliac thrombi do occur. Duplex is not as accurate in these instances. In a study of postoperative orthopedic patients, 24% of the symptomatic and 88% of the asymptomatic patients had isolated calf thrombi. In the symptomatic group, duplex imaging was 85% sensitive and 86% specific, but in the asymptomatic group sensitivity was 16% and specificity 99%.[25]

Isolated iliac vein thrombosis is often reported as being rare. However, most series from which data comes do not include patients who are at increased risk for this problem (i.e., those who are pregnant or have pelvic conditions such as tumors, trauma, or recent surgery). The true incidence of isolated pelvic vein thrombosis is unknown but probably higher than previous estimates. Most vascular labs do not routinely scan iliac veins as part of a lower extremity DVT study. Those that do find the study unsatisfactory because of excessive bowel gas in 20% of patients.[26] The primary sign used in the leg, the ability to coapt vein walls with probe pressure, is usually not possible. Many labs use indirect signs such as lack of flow variation with respiration in the proximal femoral ("common femoral") vein, or a 50% increase in proximal femoral vein diameter with the Valsalva maneuver. The accuracy of these methods varies greatly in the literature.[27–30] Magnetic resonance venography is a more reliable diagnostic modality in these patients.

In addition to the ability to diagnose the presence of a deep vein thrombosis, duplex ultrasonography usually provides information as whether the thrombus is acute or chronic. Criteria are listed in Table 37.2. The finding of a partially compressible thrombus is the most common reliable sign of an acute DVT, as "free floating" thrombi (i.e., thrombi that appear to be moving within the vein lumen) are only occasionally seen. Many clinicians use the criteria

Table 37.2 DUPLEX CRITERIA FOR DIFFERENTIATING ACUTE VERSUS CHRONIC THROMBUS.

CHARACTERISTIC	ACUTE		CHRONIC	
Degree of Occlusion	Total	++	Partial	++
Free Floating	Free	++++	Stationary	+
Clot Compressibility	Soft	++++	Firm	+
Surface Character	Smooth	++	Irregular	++
Echogenicity	Faint or None	++	Bright	++
Homogeneity	Homogen.	++	Heterogen.	++
Collaterals	Absent	+	Present	++
Recanalization	Absent	+	Present	++++

++++ = Diagnostic +++ = Good ++ = Fair + = Poor
Modified from Karkow, Ruoff, Cranley, B-Mode Imaging. In: Kempczinski RF, Yao JS, eds. *Practical noninvasive vascular diagnosis*. Chicago: Year Book Medical Publishers. 1982.

of the degree of echogenicity of a thrombus to determine age. While the echogenicity of thrombus does increase with time, it is also dependent on the duplex settings and is only a fair indication of age.[31-34]

Determination of the thrombus age is particularly important when a clinician is faced with the presentation of a patient with a past history of DVT who presents with the complaint of new or increasing leg pain and/or swelling with no past studies available for comparison. Because 10 to 20% of acute DVTs may become chronic, determining whether the patient has a new thrombus, or new thrombus in addition to chronic thrombus or some other cause of the leg symptoms such as chronic venous insufficiency can be challenging. When thrombus is found, application of the Table 37.2 age criteria are reliable, but one should realize there may be both acute and chronic thrombi in conjunction (i.e., "new on old"). In these cases one should look for partially compressible thrombus (i.e., acute, at either the proximal or distal ends of the old DVT).

Duplex examination can also be used to help determine the cause of leg pain and/or swelling when a DVT is not found. Intramuscular hematomas sometimes with associated muscle tears, ruptured and unruptured Baker's cysts, and venous reflux disease are common causes of symptoms that may mimic DVT and can often be identified by duplex ultrasonography if one keeps them in mind.

D-DIMER

Eighty to 90% of all duplex exams ordered are negative for DVT.[35-37] It would therefore be clinically sensible and cost-effective to adopt the use of a blood test to rule in or rule out DVT and negate the need for more complicated and expensive testing. Over the last decade, the ability to detect circulating D-dimer using monoclonal antibody tests, and red cell and latex agglutination has received considerable attention as a diagnostic adjunct in the detection of DVT. D-dimers are degradation products that result from the action of plasmin on cross-linked fibrin specifically in the final step of thrombus generation. Thus the presence of D-dimer is an indication of the initiation of blood clotting. Other conditions that can cause an elevated D-dimer include infection, inflammation, cancer, vasculitis, pregnancy, trauma, hemorrhage, and postsurgical states.

Several laboratory methods are currently available for D-dimer testing (Table 37.3). Though the enzyme-linked immunosorbent assay (ELISA) is the most sensitive, it is also the most expensive and time consuming. The red blood cell and latex agglutination tests are less expensive and much quicker, taking minutes as opposed to hours, and are thus more attractive as clinical tools for management of patients with suspected DVT. As can be seen from the table, however, the low specificity makes a positive test virtually useless for ruling in DVT.

Table 37.3 SENSITIVITY AND SPECIFICITY OF DIFFERENT D-DIMER TESTS.

METHOD	SENSITIVITY (%)	SPECIFICITY (%)
ELISA	96	39
Red Blood Cell Agglutination	88	64
Latex Agglutination	87	60

Figures represent averages from the literature.[35-38] The results include subjects with both possible pulmonary embolism and/or DVT.

A negative test, however, may be a useful aid in ruling out DVT. Numerous studies have reported sensitivities of D-dimer but there are limitations to drawing conclusions from these. Different methodologies were used, heterogeneous populations were tested, and many studies combined patients with pulmonary emboli and/or DVT. Other studies have shown varying sensitivity in relation to the timing of testing and to the location and or extent of DVT.[38-41] Overall, D-dimer on its own has not proven to be an effective test to make the diagnosis of DVT.

In 1999, the American Thoracic Society recommended duplex ultrasonography or impedence plethysmography for all patients with suspected DVT,[42] and in many institutions, this is current practice. Recent evidence points out that the use of a D-dimer blood test and a pretest probability score can safely exclude DVT and obviate the need for further diagnostic testing in a large proportion of cases.[43,44] The 2006 Institute for Clinical Systems Improvement (ICSI) reviewed the most recent literature and put forth an algorithm for the diagnosis of DVT. They first recommend determining the clinical pretest probability of DVT using the Wells score (Table 37.4)[45] and then using either form

Table 37.4 WELLS SCORE. A MODEL FOR THE PREDICTION OF THE CLINICAL PRETEST PROBABILITY OF DVT.

SCORE

1 Active cancer (treatment ongoing or within previous 6 months or palliative)
1 Paralysis, paresis, or recent plaster immobilization of lower extremity
1 Recently bedridden for more than three days or major surgery within four weeks
1 Localized tenderness along the distribution of the deep venous system
1 Entire leg swollen
1 Calf swollen by more than 3 cm when compared with asymptomatic leg (measured 10 cm below tibial tuberosity)
1 Pitting edema (greater in the symptomatic leg)
1 Collateral superficial veins (nonvaricose)
-2 Alternative diagnosis as likely or greater than that of DVT
If both legs are symptomatic, score the more severe side.
High risk = scored 3 or more
Moderate risk = 1 or 2
Low risk = 0 or less

(From Reference 45)

(agglutination or ELISA) of D-dimer test to determine which patients need to proceed to duplex ultrasonography. All patients with either a moderate or high Wells score should undergo duplex ultrasonography.[46] The presence of a DVT, however, cannot be excluded by a negative duplex in these higher risk patients and a D-dimer test is helpful. A negative D-dimer makes DVT very unlikely, whereas a positive D-dimer then warrants repeat ultrasonography within 1 week or sooner if symptoms progress.

Conversely, all patients with a low pretest probability undergo D-dimer measurement. Those with a positive D-dimer are recommended to undergo duplex ultrasonography. Those with a low pretest probability and a negative D-dimer do not require any further diagnostic testing. This algorithm is most effective in the outpatient setting, as many inpatient conditions will cause D-dimer elevation.

Newer pretest probability scoring algorithms have been described, including the modified Wells score and the Hamilton score,[47] which stratify patients into only two groups based on the likelihood of having DVT. Unfortunately, a standardized algorithm using a single pretest probability scoring system and a single D-dimer assay has not been developed. The trend, however, is toward the use of a pretest probability score in combination with a D-dimer assay to safely rule out DVT and avoid a large number of unnecessary and costly diagnostic examinations.

MAGNETIC RESONANCE VENOGRAPHY

The quality of magnetic resonance venography (MRV) has steadily improved since its introduction in the early 1990s. It is now a powerful technology that is often used as a "problem solver." Various techniques are used, including spin echo and gradient-recalled echo. Intravenous gadolinium can be used to enhance images and can aid in determination of the age of the thrombus. Absence of imaging of a vein or an intraluminal filling defect indicate the presence of DVT. Examiners must be cognizant, however, of known flow artifacts that can be mistaken for thrombus. Images can be viewed in axial, coronal, or sagittal planes, and postprocessing techniques are available that can be used to produce 3D images with removal of background structures for improved ease of viewing.

MRV has been shown to highly accurate. Sensitivities of 97% and specificities of 100% have been demonstrated along with excellent interobserver variability for iliac, femoral, and below knee DVT.[48,49] Several authors now consider MRV to be the study of choice for pelvic vein DVT. Compared with conventional contrast venography it is not only noninvasive and avoids the use of ionizing radiation, but it also has demonstrated better ability to show the proximal extent of femoral and iliac vein thrombi. An added advantage is that it may show underlying pathology that contributed to the formation of the DVT such as pelvic masses or left iliac vein compression by the right common iliac artery.[50]

The limitations of MRV include expense and lack of portability and, in some cases, availability. Also, some patients with implanted metal devices, claustrophobia, and inability to remain still are not suitable for this exam. Gadolinium must be used with caution in patients with renal impairment due to the risk of nephrogenic systemic fibrosis.[51]

COMPUTERIZED TOMOGRAPHIC VENOGRAPHY

Computerized tomographic venography has many of the same advantages as MRV when compared with duplex sonography. It does, however, involve the use of ionizing radiation and intravenous iodinated contrast agents for imaging peripheral veins. In imaging peripheral and pelvic veins, the accurate timing of image acquisition in relation to contrast injection is often difficult, and multiple runs may be necessary to acquire all of the desired veins. In larger veins one can also be faced with the inflow of noncontrast blood from a branch vein into a vein with blood containing contrast, which creates a "wash in" artifact that can be mistaken for thrombus. For these reasons MRV is usually considered a more appropriate modality when duplex testing is felt to be inadequate. However, some do employ a technique known as combined computerized tomographic venography and pulmonary arteriography (CCTVPA). Computerized tomographic pulmonary arteriography (CTPA) has become the test of choice in many centers for suspected pulmonary emboli. Katz et al. reported that by waiting for 3 to 3.5 min after the injection of contrast that is used for CTPA, one can then scan the veins from the diaphragm to the calves. The scanning can be a survey with cuts taken every 4 cm or a continual helical imaging. The latter though involves considerably more radiation to the subject.[52] Thus, with this technique, one study can not only answer the question of whether or not there is a pulmonary embolus and its extent but also often find the source of the embolus and the amount of residual thrombus in the veins. 97% sensitivity and 100% specificity has been reported for CCTVPA in comparison with ultrasonography, and a large study has shown that in patients with lower limb DVT 23% extended into the iliac veins or the inferior vena cava.[53]

SUMMARY

It is well documented that the clinical diagnosis of lower limb DVT is unreliable. Fortunately, there are a number of methodologies available that can objectively rule in or rule out the presence of DVT with accuracies very close to the "gold standard" of conventional contrast phlebography.

They are also less invasive, safer, and usually less costly. Duplex utrasonography, with its high accuracy and absent risk, remains the most common diagnositic modality, however, the use of a pretest probability score along with D-dimer measurement can safely obviate the need for this study in low-risk patients. This new algorithm for diagnosis is slowly being adopted in practice. This chapter has presented a brief overview of the currently available technologies and diagnostic strategies, which continue to evolve and improve.

REFERENCES

1. Virchow R. Die Cellularpathologic. In: *Ihrer Begrundung auf Physiologische und Pathologische Gewebelehere*. Berlin: Hirschewald. 1858.
2. Moser K. Pulmonary embolism. In: Murray J, Nadel J, eds. *Respiratory medicine*, 2e. Philadelphia: WB Saunders. 1994. 653.
3. Anderson FA Jr, Wheeler HB, Goldberg RJ, et al. A population-based perspective of the hospital incidence and case-fatality rates of deep vein thrombosis and pulmonary embolism, *Arch Intern Med*. 1991. *151*: 933–938.
4. Matzdorff A, Green D. Deep vein thrombosis and pulmonary embolism: Prevention, diagnosis, and treatment, *Geriatrics*. 1992. *47*: 48–63.
5. Sperry K, Key C, Anderson R. Toward a population-based assessment of death due to pulmonary embolism in New Mexico, *Hum Pathol*. 1990. *21*: 159–165.
6. Diamond P, Macciocchi S. Predictive power of clinical symptoms in patients with presumptive deep venous thrombosis, *AM J Phys Med Rehabil*. 1997. *76*: 49–51.
7. Kahn S. The clinical diagnosis of deep venous thrombosis: Integrating incidence, risk factors, and symptoms and signs, *Arch Intern Med*. 1998. *158*: 2315–2323.
8. Robinson K, Anderson D, Gross M. Accuracy of screening compression ultrasonography and clinical examination for the diagnosis of deep vein thrombosis after total hip or knee arthroplasty, *Can J Surg*. 1998. *41*: 368–373.
9. Weinmann E, Salzman E. Deep-vein thrombosis, *New Engl J Med*. 1994. *331*: 1630–1641.
10. Oudega R, Moons K, Hoes A, Arno W. Limited value of patient history and physical examination in diagnosing deep vein thrombosis in primary care, *Fam Pract*. 2005. *22*: 86–91.
11. Jorgensen J, Hanel K, Morgan A, Hunt J. The incidence of deep venous thrombosis in patients with superficial thrombophlebitis of the lower limbs, *J Vasc Surg*. 1993. *18*: 70–73.
12. Prountjos P, Bastounis E, Hadjinikolaou L, Felekuras E, Bala P. Superficial venous thrombosis of the lower extremities co-existing with deep venous thrombosis, *Int Angiol*. 1991. *10*: 63–65.
13. Lutter K, Kerr T, Roedersheimer L, Lohr J, Sampson M, Cranley J. Superficial thrombophlebitis diagnosed by duplex scanning, *Surgery*. 1991. *110*: 42–46.
14. Skillman J, Kent K, Porter D, Kim D. Simultaneous occurrence of superficial and deep thrombophlebitis in the lower extremity, *J Vasc Surg*. 1990. *11*: 818–824.
15. Bergqvist D, Jaroszewski H. Deep vein thrombosis in patients with superficial thrombophlebitis of the leg, *Brit Med J*. 1986. *292*: 658–659.
16. Guex J. Thrombotic complications of varicose veins: A literature review of the role of superficial venous thrombosis, *Dermatol Surg*. 1996. *22*: 378–382.
17. Markovic M, Lotina S, Davidovic L, et al. Acute superficial thrombophlebitis: Modern diagnosis and therapy, *Srp Arh Celok Lek*. 1997. *125*: 261–266.
18. Salzman E. Venous thrombosis made easy, *New Engl J Med*. 1986. *314*: 847–848.
19. Mattos M, Londrey G, Leutz D, et al. Color-flow duplex scanning for the surveillance and diagnosis of acute deep venous thrombosis, *J Vasc Surg*. 1992. *15*: 366–376.
20. Lund F, Diener L, Ericsson J. Postmortem intraosseous phlebography as an aid in studies of venous thromboembolism, *Angiology*. 1969. *20*: 155.
21. Lensing A, Preandoni P, Brandjes D, et al. Detection of deep-vein thrombosis by real-time B-mode ultrasonography, *N Engl J Med*. 1989. *320*: 342–345.
22. Wheeler H, Anderson F. Use of noninvasive tests as the basis for treatment of deep vein thrombosis. In: Bernstein EF, ed. *Vascular diagnosis*, 4e. St Louis: Mosby. 1993. 867.
23. Markel A, Manzo R, Bergelin R, Strandness D. Acute deep vein thrombosis: Diagnosis, localization, and risk factors, *J Vasc Med Biol*. 1991. *3*: 432–439.
24. Markel A, Manzo R, Bergelin R, Strandness D. Pattern and distribution of thrombi in acute venous thrombosis, *Arch Surg*. 1992. *127*: 305–309.
25. Sumner D, Mattos M. Diagnosis of deep vein thrombosis with real-time color and duplex scanning. In: Bernstein EF, ed. *Vascular diagnosis*, 4e. St Louis: Mosby. 1993. 794–795.
26. Messina L, Sarpa M, Smith M, Greenfield L. Clinical significance of routine imaging of iliac and calf veins by color flow duplex scanning in patients suspected of having lower extremity deep venous thrombosis, *Surgery*. 1993. *114*: 921–927.
27. Polak J, O'Leary D. Deep venous thrombosis in pregnancy: Noninvasive diagnosis, *Radiology*. 1988. *166*: 377–379.
28. Effeney D, Friedman M, Gooding G. Iliofemoral venous thrombosis: Real-time ultrasound diagnosis, normal criteria, and clinical application, *Radiology*. 1984. *150*: 787–792.
29. Duddy M, McHugo J. Duplex ultrasound of the common femoral vein in pregnancy and puerperium, *Brit J Radiol*. 1991. *64*: 785–791.
30. Bach A, Hann L. When the common femoral vein is revealed as flattened on spectral Doppler sonography: Is it a reliable sign for the diagnosis of proximal venous obstruction, *Am J Roentgenol*. 1997. *168*: 733–736.
31. Wright D, Shepard A, McPharlin M, Ernst B. Pitfalls in lower extremity venous duplex scanning, *J Vasc Surg*. 1990. *11*: 675–679.
32. Van Gemmeren D, Fobbe F, Ruhnke-Trautmann M, et al. Diagnostik tiefer Beinvenenthrombosen mit der farbcodierten Duplexsonographie und sonographische Altersbestimmung der Thrombose, *Arch Kardiol*. 1991. *80*: 523–528.
33. Salles-Cuna S, Fowlkes J, Wakefield T. B-mode quantification of deep vein thrombi, *J Vasc Tech*. 1994. *18*: 207–209.
34. Fowlkes J, Streiter R, Downing L, et al. Ultrasound echogenicity in experimental venous thrombosis, *Ultrasound in Med Biol*. 1998. *24*: 1175–1182.
35. Lensing AW, Prandoni P, Prins MH, Büller HR. Deep-vein thrombosis, *Lancet*. 1999. *353*: 479–485.
36. Ten Cate-Hoek AJ, Prins MH. Management studies using a combination of D-dimer test result and clinical probability to rule out venous thromboembolism: A systematic review, *J Thromb Haemost*. 2005. *3*: 2465–2470.
37. Wells PS, Owen C, Doucette S, Fergusson D, Tran H. Does this patient have deep vein thrombosis?, *JAMA*. 2006. *295*: 199–207.
38. Turkstra F, van Beek E, Buller H. Observer and biological variation of a rapid whole blood D-dimer test, *Thromb Haemost*. 1998. *79*: 91–93.
39. Bounameaux H, Cirafici P, de Moerloose P, et al. Measurement of D-dimer in plasma as diagnostic aid in suspected pulmonary embolism, *Lancet*. 1991. *337*: 196–200.
40. Quinn D, Fogel R, Smoth C, et al. D-dimers in the diagnosis of pulmonary embolism, *Am J Respir Crit Care*. 1999. *159*: 1445–1449.
41. Chapman C, Akhtar N, Campbell S, et al. The use of D-dimer assay by enzyme imunnoassay and latex agglutination techniques in the diagnosis of deep vein thrombosis, *Clin Lab Haematol*. 1990. *12*: 37–42.

42. Tapson V, Carroll B, Davidson B, et al. ATS guidelines: Diagnostic approach to acute venous thromboembolism, *Am J Respir Crit Care Med.* 1999. *160*: 1043–1066.

43. Yamaki T, Nozaki M, Sakurai H, Takeuchi M, Soejima K, Kono T. Prospective evaluation of a screening protocol to exclude deep vein thrombosis on the basis of a combination of quantitative D-dimer testing and pretest clinical probability score, *J Am Coll Surg.* 2005. *201*(5): 701–709.

44. Schutgens P, Ackermark FJLM, Haas HK, et al. Combination of a normal D-dimer concentration and a non-high pretest clinical probability score is a safe strategy to exclude deep venous thrombosis, *Circulation.* 2003. *107*: 593–597.

45. Wells PS, Anderson DR, Bormanis J, et al. Value of assessment of pretest probability of deep vein thrombosis in clinical management, *Lancet.* 1997. *350*: 1795–1798, 1326–1330.

46. *Health care guideline: Venous thromboembolism.* Institute for Clinical Systems Improvement. Revised February 2006. Available at www. icsi.org. Accessed on September 27, 2006.

47. Subramaniam R, Chou T, Heath R, Allen R. Importance of pretest probability score and D-dimer assay before sonography for lower limb deep venous thrombosis, *Am J Roentgenol.* 2006. *186*: 206–212.

48. Fraser D, Moody A, Morgan P, et al. Diagnosis of lower limb deep venous thrombosis: A prospective blinded study of magnetic resonance direct thrombus imaging, *Ann Intern Med.* 2002. *136*: 89–98.

49. Spritzer C, Arata M, Freed K. Isolated pelvic deep vein thrombosis: Relative frequency as detected with MR imaging, *Radiology.* 2001. *219*: 521–525.

50. Fraser D, Moody A, Martel A, Morgan P. Re-evaluation of iliac compression syndrome using magnetic resonance imaging in patients with acute deep venous thromboses, *J Vasc Surg.* 2004. *40*: 604–611.

51. Kuo P, Kanal E, Abu-Alfa A, Cowper S. Gadolinium-based MR contrast agents and nephrogenic systemic fibrosis, *Radiology.* 2007. *242*: 647–649.

52. Katz D, Hon M. Current DVT imaging, *Tech in Vasc Intervent Radiol.* 2004. *7*: 55–62.

53. Cham D, Yankelevitz D, Shaham D, et al. Distribution of suspected pulmonary embolism, *Radiology.* 2002. *225*: 384 (abstr).

38.

THROMBOTIC RISK ASSESSMENT

A HYBRID APPROACH

Joseph A. Caprini

INTRODUCTION

Venous thromboembolism (VTE) is one of the most common, yet highly preventable, causes of in-hospital death. In response to this problem, the implementation of an appropriate, targeted thromboprophylaxis strategy has been described as the most important single factor for improving patient safety.[1] Both medical and surgical patients are at risk of VTE. It has been calculated that without prophylaxis, the incidence of hospital-acquired deep venous thrombosis (DVT) is approximately 10 to 40% among medical patients and general surgery patients, and 40 to 60% following major orthopedic surgery.[2] In patients subjected to autopsy, approximately 10% of all deaths in the hospital are attributed to pulmonary embolism (PE),[3] with most patients who suffer a fatal embolus dying within the initial 30-minute period. This small window for effective treatment, combined with its frequently asymptomatic nature, explains the high fatality rate associated with this condition.[4] VTE is also responsible for a significant number of long-term health problems: Prandoni et al. have shown that 30% of patients with symptomatic DVT will suffer recurrent VTE in the 8 years following an event,[5] while almost a third of patients who suffer a DVT will go on to develop long-term venous insufficiency complications in the lower leg, also known as "postthrombotic syndrome" (PTS). This condition may result in chronic leg swelling, discomfort, dermatitis, and leg ulcers, which can reduce the patient's quality of life and have an economic impact frequently overlooked in DVT cost assessment.[6]

Clinically proven methods of prophylaxis have been shown to prevent a significant proportion of clinically significant VTE events. Yet despite the publication of regularly updated consensus guidelines,[2,7–10] VTE prophylaxis is still under- or inappropriately prescribed in a high proportion of patients, leaving them at significant risk of serious complication due to PE or DVT.[11,12]

Effective VTE risk assessment is therefore critical in targeting and optimizing prophylaxis, and for the subsequent improvement in patient outcomes. There is an urgent need for a clear, easy-to-use risk assessment model based on information in the patient's medical history and clinical examination. Although there has been, and continues to be, a great deal of clinical research into VTE, it is unlikely that there will ever be sufficient high-quality clinical evidence to guide decisions on prophylaxis in every group of patients—medical and surgical. With each patient representing a unique clinical situation with their own combination of risk factors, it can be difficult to determine the level of VTE risk, and the appropriate intensity of thromboprophylaxis. This review considers the reasons contributing to underuse of prophylaxis, and discusses a "hybrid approach" combining risk assessment scoring with the application of current treatment guidelines. The results of an audit from the author's hospital and a real-world case study are also detailed to illustrate key issues.

POOR ADHERENCE TO PROPHYLAXIS GUIDELINES

Consensus groups such as the American College of Chest Physicians (ACCP) and the THRIFT Consensus Group regularly publish guidelines on the prevention and treatment of VTE in both surgical and nonsurgical patients.[2,7–10] While the recommendations from these groups are based on clinical evidence from trials and meta-analyses that are stratified clearly according to patient risk, VTE prophylaxis is still suboptimal in many patients,[11–17] and the rates of total and proximal DVT remain high.

US surveys of prophylaxis use indicate that the percentage of surgical patients receiving prophylaxis ranges from 38 to 94% depending on the type of procedure.[11,15,18,19] One particular study documenting adherence to the 1995 ACCP guidelines in surgical patients found that 25% of patients undergoing high-risk major abdominal surgery did not receive any form of VTE prophylaxis.[11] Furthermore, in a retrospective analysis by Arnold et al. looking at cases of VTE in a US cohort of surgical and medical patients, it was found that one out of six VTE events could have been prevented if physicians had followed the ACCP guidelines.[12] Inadequate prophylaxis was most often attributable to the fact that no prophylactic measures were prescribed.

Surprisingly, a tendency has been reported for prophylaxis to be administered less frequently with increasing risk level.[20] Why this occurs is unknown, although it may reflect physician concerns that the risk of complications due to anticoagulant therapy may be greater in very high-risk patients.

SUBOPTIMAL PROPHYLAXIS IN ACTION

The extent of the prophylaxis problem was highlighted in a recent study by the author's group.[14] Carried out to test the performance of current VTE risk assessment, the primary objective was to determine the percentage of a surgical patient population falling into one of three risk categories (moderate, high, and highest risk; Table 38.1). The study also sought to identify whether patients were receiving appropriate prophylaxis based on their risk level, and to compare the degree of compliance with prophylaxis guidelines with that found and reported for the same hospital in 1991. A total of 157 patients undergoing neurosurgery, cardiovascular surgery, general surgery, gynecological surgery, or orthopedic surgery (other than arthroplasty) were included in the study. Each patient had a detailed preoperative VTE risk assessment, and the type and duration of prophylaxis prescribed to each patient was recorded and compared with their individual risk score. In-hospital outcomes for all patients were carefully monitored, and patients were followed up by telephone after a month.

The study found that 19% (30 out of 157) of patients were not prescribed any prophylactic measures despite the existence of several risk factors. This was even more surprising considering that the majority of patients were in the highest risk category, and therefore at greatest need of prophylaxis. Clinically overt VTE appeared in two out of seventy-three (2.7%) patients in the highest risk category,

both of whom had not received appropriate prophylaxis, while a total 57% of patients were shown to have received inadequate prophylaxis according to the ACCP guidelines.[2] Comparison of these results with our previous thromboprophylaxis audit performed in 1991 (Table 38.1) indicates no improvement in compliance with treatment guidelines; indeed, in the group at highest risk of VTE, only 30% of patients received appropriate prophylaxis in 2002 compared with 70% in the same category in 1991.

UNDERUSE OF PROPHYLAXIS— WHY IS THERE A PROBLEM?

MISCONCEPTION OF RISK

Although the serious implications to health are now well accepted—both in the short and long term—a large part of the problem can be attributed to the clinically silent nature of VTE. For surgical patients there is a low incidence of clinically apparent VTE in the perioperative period, thus it is rare for an individual surgeon to witness an acute PE or major DVT event in one of their patients. Studies have shown that a significant proportion of symptomatic thromboembolic complications occur after discharge from hospital,[21-23] with a survey of California orthopedic surgeons finding that 76% of VTE events were diagnosed following discharge from hospital after total hip replacement (THR), and 48% after total knee replacement (TKR).[24] The current trend toward shorter hospital stays serves to accentuate this problem, whereby the need for and benefits of thromboprophylaxis can be difficult to appreciate for a physician who rarely sees the problem. Extended prophylaxis has value in preventing not only sudden death but also all of the other complications of VTE responsible for significant morbidity and mortality.

Although the majority of trials in VTE have studied surgical patients, medical patients are also at significant risk of thrombotic disease.[2] Fewer than a third of patients who suffer a fatal PE have recently undergone surgery,[25] and as many

Table 38.1 ADHERENCE WITH ACCP CONSENSUS GUIDELINES: AN AUDIT OF HOSPITAL PRACTICE

	MODERATE RISK (2 RISK FACTORS)	HIGH RISK (3-4 RISK FACTORS)	HIGHEST RISK (5 OR MORE RISK FACTORS)
Total (2002)	9/157 (6%)	43/157 (27%)	105/157 (67%)
Prophylaxis guidelines followed	7/9 (78%)	28/43 (65%)	32/105 (30%)
Prophylaxis guidelines not followed	2/9 (22%)	15/43 (35%)	73/105 (70%)
	Low (0–1 risk factors)	Moderate (2–4 risk factors)	High risk (more than 4 risk factors)
Total (1991)	185/538 (34%)	261/538 (49%)	92/538 (17%)
Prophylaxis guidelines followed	18/185 (10%)	110/261 (42%)	70/92 (76%)
Prophylaxis guidelines not followed	167/185 (90%)	151/261 (58%)	22/92 (24%)

Modified from Reference 14 with permission from Blackwell Publishing.

as one in twenty hospitalized patients with multiple clinical conditions go on to develop PE.[26] The average overall incidence of DVT in medical patients is 10% to 20%,[2] but this rises in certain patient groups. For example, stroke is associated with a 20 to 50% risk of VTE complications without prophylaxis,[2] while VTE is thought to occur in 20 to 40% of patients with an acute myocardial infarction.[27] Cancer is also a well-known thrombotic risk factor due to the hypercoagulable state induced by the malignancy, with treatments for the disease, such as surgery and chemotherapy, serving to further compound the risk.[2,28] Despite current guidelines stating that medical patients can be at significant risk of VTE and should receive thromboprophylaxis, a survey from the International Medical Prophylaxis Registry on Venous Thromboembolism (IMPROVE) of acutely ill medical patients recently revealed that fewer than 40% of patients enrolled in the registry received prophylaxis.[13]

SAFETY CONCERNS

Another factor underlying the suboptimal use of pharmacological prophylaxis is overestimation of the bleeding risk associated with anticoagulant prophylaxis. For example, a survey of orthopedic surgeons in the United Kingdom found that almost half (48%) had discontinued the use of low molecular weight heparin (LMWH) for TKR or THR due to concern over bleeding complications.[29] However, numerous randomized, placebo-controlled, double-blind trials and further meta-analyses of prophylaxis with LMWH and unfractionated heparin (UFH) during major surgery have demonstrated that both types of heparin prophylaxis are extremely effective in preventing VTE at the expense of no increase, or a very small increase, in the rate of major bleeding.[30-35] Although LMWH and UFH are associated with an increased risk of wound hematomas,[30,33,34] major bleeding complications are extremely uncommon, and the consequences of VTE are potentially much more severe—thereby outweighing any justification for withholding heparin prophylaxis.

LMWH is at least as safe and effective as UFH.[31,34,36,37] LMWH has been associated with a lower risk of major bleeding complications; one particular study of patients undergoing abdominal surgery reported a 23% reduction in the frequency of major bleeding events in patients who received LMWH compared with UFH, although this difference was not significant. The study also observed significantly fewer severe bleeds and wound hematomas.[30] LMWH exhibits minimal binding with plasma proteins, endothelial cells, and platelet factor IV, providing a more predictable clinical response than UFH as well as reducing the likelihood of causing heparin-induced thrombocytopenia (HIT).[38,39] With an incidence of 1 to 5%, immune HIT is an uncommon but serious complication of heparin therapy, and is often cited as a reason for caution in prescribing heparin prophylaxis. Of 665 patients who received prophylaxis with

either UFH or LMWH during elective THR, 18 patients developed HIT, and the majority of these patients were in the UFH group (4.8% versus 0.6%; p < 0.001).[39]

While the benefits of LMWH thromboprophylaxis have been shown in numerous studies, suboptimal use may arise from additional safety concerns combined with a misconception of risk. Clinical issues remain unanswered and may contribute to physician hesitation to pharmacologic prophylaxis, for example, optimal dosing and the need for monitoring in patients with severe obesity or renal insufficiency.[37]

LACK OF AWARENESS OF THE PROBLEM

Physicians frequently cite informal, retrospective surveys of their own clinical service or personal experience to explain why they believe the rate of VTE is low.[40] There also appears to be poor awareness of the diverse range of clinical signs and symptoms that can be attributed to thrombosis and the fact that these relatively minor symptoms can be extremely common (Table 38.2). Many physicians fail to realize that what they are seeing may be an indicator of an otherwise silent thrombotic event requiring further investigation, which can therefore be attributed to a lack of prophylaxis.

COST OF SUBOPTIMAL PROPHYLAXIS

Pharmacological prophylaxis undoubtedly incurs a significant cost, both in terms of the drugs themselves and, with UFH and oral anticoagulants, an increase in nursing time and laboratory monitoring. However, the economic

Table 38.2 CLINICAL SIGNS, SYMPTOMS, OR EVENTS THAT MAY BE ASSOCIATED WITH VTE IN CLINICAL PRACTICE

- Leg pain
- Leg swelling
- Chest pain
- Shortness of breath
- Transient orthostatic hypotension
- Decreased level of consciousness presumed to be narcotic excess
- Fainting spell
- Hypoxia
- Follow-up of patient for readmission or death 90 d postoperatively
- Sudden death
- Death without autopsy
- Postoperative stroke due to patent foramen ovale
- Suspected myocardial infarction
- Failure to thrive, sinking spell, or "the dwindles"
- Postthrombotic syndrome during physical examination of the legs (standing) 5 years postoperatively
- Postoperative pneumonia

consequences of withholding prophylaxis are often overlooked. In addition to the short-term costs of delayed hospital discharge due to an acute VTE event or patient readmission for DVT, failure to prevent VTE increases the risk of long-term morbidity due to PTS and recurrent thrombosis. Patients with symptomatic DVT have a high risk of recurrent VTE that persists for at least 8 years, and which may increase with comorbidities such as cancer.[5] Estimates based on a recent cost-of-illness study conducted by our group suggest that in the United States, the annual per-patient cost of severe PTS is $3,816 in the first year and $1,677 thereafter, while the cost of DVT and PE complications were estimated at $3,798 and $6,604, respectively.[41] Therefore, prevention of DVT can have an enormous impact on both the patient's quality of life and the long-term cost of care.

Mechanical methods of prophylaxis provide a cheaper alternative to pharmacological methods taken on a direct cost-per-patient basis, but this must be balanced with issues of safety and efficacy. Mechanical devices, such as intermittent pneumatic compression (IPC) and graduated compression stockings (GCS), do not increase the risk of bleeding and can offer important protection in some groups of patients for whom anticoagulant therapy is contraindicated or is impractical because of their clinical status (e.g., trauma patients). One early study comparing five methods of thromboprophylaxis found that antistasis modalities performed well compared to the drug modalities (UFH, dextran, and aspirin), with the lowest incidence of DVT events reported in the IPC group.[42] A subsequent study evaluating the effectiveness of combining a pharmacologic drug with an antistasis modality reduced the incidence of DVT to just 1.5% in a group of 328 surgical patients.[43] The value of combination therapy has been further highlighted in the more recent APOLLO trial, which compared the use of IPC plus fondaparinux with IPC alone in 1,300 high-risk abdominal surgery patients in North America.[44] IPC was chosen on the basis of a survey that found approximately half of clinicians in the United States use this modality for the prevention of thrombosis in general surgery patients. IPC showed 5% incidence of DVT by venography—and is therefore itself an effective modality. A 1.7% incidence was reported for IPC plus fondaparinux. A benefit is also suggested when mechanical methods are combined with LMWH.[2] In a review of trials comparing the use of GCS alone or in combination with LMWH in high-risk surgical patients (general and orthopedic), combination therapy was found to be more effective than pharmacological methods alone.[45]

Overall, however, mechanical means of prophylaxis have been less extensively studied than pharmacological methods, and are generally considered less efficacious than anticoagulants for the prevention of DVT. While there is evidence supporting the efficacy of mechanical devices in low-risk patients,[2] they do not provide adequate prophylaxis in those at high-risk. The most recent ACCP guidelines recommend combination therapy for high-risk patients with multiple risk factors, and that, in general, mechanical prophylaxis be used primarily in patients who are at high risk of bleeding or as an adjunct to anticoagulant-based prophylaxis.[2]

THE BIGGEST PROBLEM: LACK OF CLEAR DATA?

There are established international guidelines based on level-1 evidence that estimate the incidence of VTE in various populations, and then assess in as scientific a way as possible the efficacy and safety of prophylactic methods based on sound prospective randomized trials. However, only a small subset of what is done in medicine has been tested in appropriate, well-designed studies. Appropriate trials for every clinical situation have not been, and probably never will be, carried out for every situation.

When clinical data are either lacking or insufficient to guide treatment, the physician has to use clinical reasoning to identify the approach that best fits the patient and the pathology involved. It can be frustrating to see patients not being given effective prophylaxis simply because there are "no data available." Such individuals may be at very high risk of a thrombotic event, but there is no clear treatment path because their clinical situations have yet to be subjected to randomized prospective trials. So how do we ensure such patients are treated appropriately?

MATCHING RISK WITH PROPHYLACTIC STRATEGY

Routine screening of patients for symptomatic DVT is logistically difficult, and both clinically and economically inefficient.[2] Equally, reliance on clinical surveillance to identify early symptoms or signs of DVT is inadequate to prevent clinically important VTE events: the first manifestation of VTE may be a fatal PE.

Thrombotic risk assessment allows patients to be stratified according to their overall VTE risk and thromboprophylaxis to be tailored appropriately, but it is a complex task that must take into account both *exposing* risk factors relating to the clinical situation (e.g., duration/type/site of surgery, type of anesthesia, concomitant illness, presence of infection, etc.), and *predisposing* factors unique to the individual patient (e.g., age, thrombophilic abnormalities, history/family history of DVT, etc.). Many patients have more than one VTE risk factor and are considered to be at increased risk due to their cumulative effect[46–48] (although interestingly, a recent paper from the MEDENOX study reported an insignificant relationship between the number of VTE events and the number of risk factors).[49] Risk assessment models (RAMs) have been developed with the intention of simplifying and standardizing the scoring of VTE risk, and to allow optimization of prophylactic strategies.

Unfortunately, there has been a history of poor compliance with RAMs, with a common complaint from physicians being that they are overly complicated and logistically difficult to implement in their own clinical setting. Many early VTE risk-scoring systems also relied on diagnostic information not readily available from clinical examination (e.g., laboratory values such as euglobulin lysis levels), which has led to reluctance among many doctors to implement such systems.

A simple, clinically validated, easy-to-use RAM based on factors in the patient's medical history and clinical examination is needed, and has the potential to be widely adopted. The model should be used to stratify patients according to risk and the treatment strategy applied in conjunction with academic guidelines where available, that is, the "hybrid approach" to risk assessment.

A RAM developed by our team and implemented in our hospital overcomes the complexities and practical constraints associated with previous models (Table 38.3).[50] The model includes clear lists of risk factors with a simple accompanying scoring system, which allows patients to be assigned to one of the four VTE risk categories identified in the ACCP guidelines (low, moderate, high, very high), and an appropriate prophylaxis regimen to be recommended (Table 38.4). This RAM represents a thorough history and physical relative to thrombotic risk. The following case study highlights the value of a simple RAM in determining the prophylactic action required for a patient whose risk of VTE is not easily categorized according to current guidelines.

CASE STUDY

Patient history

A 65-year-old man with a body mass index (BMI) > 30 kg/m², who received irradiation treatment for prostate cancer 5 years earlier, was found to have a 2-cm³ carcinoma of the cecum during routine colonoscopy. The patient had been suffering from inflammatory bowel disease for many years was taking a statin for elevated cholesterol levels, had mild hypertension with treatment and was on a baby aspirin daily. The patient underwent a laparoscopically assisted colon resection that lasted 2 h 30 min. The patient did well postoperatively and was discharged 6 d later. The path report confirmed the presence of an early cancer without signs of metastasis.

There are no specific data based on prospective randomized trials on VTE risk and prophylaxis in a group of individuals with this exact combination of risk factors. That is not to say there are no relevant data because it is known that age > 60 years, BMI > 30 kg/m², inflammatory bowel disease, a history of cancer, and abdominal surgery for colon cancer are all risk factors for the patient developing a VTE.[2] What form of prophylaxis should this patient receive given his risk factor profile?

TREATMENT

The patient received 5,000 U of heparin preoperatively and during the operation, the patient was protected with pneumatic compression devices and elastic stockings to reduce stasis of blood in the legs during and immediately following the procedure. In addition, a prophylactic LMWH was administered once daily for a month starting 24 h postoperatively. No complications were reported during a 90-d follow-up period.

This approach may be considered extreme, and is endorsed at the present time by only a minority of physicians in the United States and worldwide.

So what is the clinical basis of this treatment strategy?

LINKING THERAPY AND RISK

Based on clinical research to date, a patient undergoing a surgical procedure with more than five risk factors has a 40 to 80% chance of developing a VTE, and this is associated with a 0.2 to 5% rate of fatality from a PE.[2] According to the RAM shown in Table 38.3, the patient described in the case study presented with five VTE risk factors, which clearly placed him in the highest risk category (age, cancer, obesity, abdominal surgery, and IBD; Table 38.4). Based on clinical trial data, in abdominal surgery cancer patients 1 month of daily LMWH injections were done. Although there may be concerns about the expense, the risk of bleeding or other adverse events, these are small compared to the ≤5% risk of a fatal event in this patient group (five factors; see Table 38.4). Few passengers would board a plane knowing there to be up to a 5% risk of a fatal crash, which begs the question as to why an individual would choose not to use effective prophylaxis when there are no clinical data contraindicating such an approach.

Furthermore, often overlooked in this equation is the impact of postoperative thrombosis. While postoperative DVT can occur asymptomatically in the lower limbs, if part of a clot breaks off, it may embolize to the right atrium. Right-to-left shunt may then occur through a patent foramen ovale that temporarily opens due to atrial dilation in response to the thrombus. Known as a "paradoxical embolism," this allows the clot to pass into the systemic circulation, whereupon it may lodge in the brain and lead to nonhemorrhagic stroke. In such cases, not only is there a 50% chance of residual damage, including paralysis due to stroke, but 20% of patients may die (Salinger, *Disease-a-Month* Feb-Mar, 2005). Is this a risk worth taking in postoperative patients simply because they may be perceived to be at low risk? Finally, these patients will probably not be fully ambulatory while hospitalized and during the first week post discharge.

ACCUMULATING EVIDENCE YET ABSENCE OF GUIDELINES

In situations for which specific data are not available, a conservative approach should be followed, and physicians must

Table 38.3 EXAMPLE OF A PRACTICAL, EASY-TO-USE, VTE RAM

Thrombosis risk factor assessment

Patient's name: _____   Age: _____   Gender: _____   Weight: _____

Each factor represents 1 point:

- Age 41 to 60 years
- Minor surgery planned
- History of prior major surgery (<1 month)
- Varicose veins
- History of inflammatory bowel disease
- Swollen legs (current)
- Obesity (BMI > 25 kg/m2)
- Acute myocardial infarction
- Congestive heart failure (<1 month)
- Sepsis (<1 month)
- Serious lung disease including pneumonia (<1 month)
- Abnormal pulmonary function (chronic obstructive pulmonary disease)
- Medical patient currently on bed rest
- Other risk factors (specify)

Each factor represents 2 points:

- Age 60 to 74 years
- Arthroscopic surgery
- Malignancy (present or previous)
- Major surgery (>45 min)
- Laparoscopic surgery (>45 min)
- Patient confined to bed (>72 h)
- Immobilizing plaster cast (<1 month)
- Central venous access catheter

Each factor represents 3 points:

- Age > 75 years
- History of DVT/PE
- Family history of thrombosis*
- Positive Factor V Leiden
- Positive prothrombin 20210A
- Elevated serum homocysteine
- Positive lupus anticoagulant
- Elevated anticardiolipin antibodies
- Heparin-induced thrombocytopenia
- Other congenital or acquired thrombophilia

If yes, enter type: _____

*Most frequently missed risk factor

Each factor represents 5 points:

- Elective major lower extremity arthroplasty
- Hip, pelvis, or leg fracture (<1 month)
- Stroke (<1 month)
- Multiple trauma (<1 month)
- Acute spinal cord injury (paralysis; <1 month)

(continued)

Table 38.3 (CONTINUED)

For women only (each factor represents 1 point):

- Oral contraceptives or hormone-replacement therapy
- Pregnancy or postpartum (<1 month)
- History of unexplained stillborn infant, recurrent abortion (≥3), premature birth with toxemia or growth-restricted infant

TOTAL RISK FACTOR SCORE _____

Prophylaxis safety considerations: Check box if answer is "YES"

Anticoagulants: Factors associated with increased bleeding

- Is patient experiencing any active bleeding?
- Does patient have (or has patient had history of) heparin-induced thrombocytopenia?
- Is patient's platelet count < 100,000/mm^3?
- Is patient taking oral anticoagulants, platelet inhibitors (e.g.., nonsteroidal anti-inflammatory drugs, clopidogrel)
- Is patient's creatinine clearance abnormal? If yes, please indicate value

If any of the above boxes are checked, the patient may not be a candidate for anticoagulant therapy and should consider alternative prophylactic measures.

Intermittent pneumatic compression

- Does patient have severe peripheral arterial disease?
- Does patient have congestive heart failure?
- Does patient have an acute superficial/deep vein thrombosis?

If any of the above boxes are checked, the patient may not be a candidate for intermittent compression therapy and should consider alternative prophylactic measures.

use reason where level-1 evidence is lacking. For example, in terms of our exact case study patient, no clear guidelines exist to guide management. Yet looking at the literature, we see a strong case for prolonged prophylaxis. Two studies using the LMWHs dalteparin[51] and enoxaparin[52] have shown that prolonging LMWH prophylaxis for a further 3 weeks is effective in preventing DVT after major abdominal surgery in patients with cancer with no increase in bleeding complications. Meta-analysis of these two studies confirmed that prolonging LMWH for an additional 3 weeks following discharge significantly reduces the risk of late-occurring VTE by 62%.[53] An increased dose of the LMWH dalteparin from 2,500 IU to 5,000 IU once daily for 7 d significantly reduced the incidence of VTE in cancer patients, with no increase in bleeding complications, a result of particular significance given that cancer patients are at increased risk for bleeding.[54] Long-term LMWH (dalteparin 200 IU/kg for 6 months) has also been shown to be more effective than an oral anticoagulant in reducing recurrent VTE in cancer patients with no increased risk for bleeding,[55] while further studies suggest benefits of LMWH for improved cancer survival.[56,57] This improved survival is thought to be associated

Table 38.4 **PROPHYLAXIS DECISION-MAKING TOOL (BASED ON VTE RISK SCORES)**

TOTAL VTE RISK SCORE	INCIDENCE OF DVT (%)	RISK LEVEL	RECOMMENDED PROPHYLACTIC REGIMEN	RISK OF FATAL PE WITHOUT PROPHYLAXIS (%)
0–1	<10	Low	No specific measures; early ambulation	<0.01
2	10–20	Moderate	LWMH (≤3,400 U once daily) or LDUH, (5,000 U bid) or GCS* or IPC	0.1–0.4
3–4	20–40	High	LMWH (>3,400 U daily), LDUH (5,000 U tid) or oral anticoagulant alone or in combination with GCS or IPC	0.4–1.0
≥ 5	40–80	Highest	LMWH (>3,400 U daily) or LDUH (5,000 U tid) or oral anticoagulant alone or in combination with GCS or IPC	0.2–5

*Combining GCS with other prophylactic methods (LDUH, LMWH, or IPC) may give better protection.

The total risk score guides the physician to the most appropriate prophylactic treatment; risk categories correspond to the ACCP guidelines.[2]

bid, twice daily; DVT, deep venous thrombosis; GCS, graduated compression stockings; IPC, intermittent pneumatic compression; LDUH, low-dose unfractionated heparin; LMWH, low molecular weight heparin; PE, pulmonary embolism; tid, three times daily; VTE, venous thromboembolism.

(Modified with permission from Reference 2).

with the antiangiogenic properties of LMWH that inhibit tumor progression.[58]

THE IMPORTANCE OF WEIGHTING RISK FACTORS

Without accounting for all risk factors, inadequate prophylaxis may result. While the aim is to develop a practicable RAM that overcomes the hindering complexities of its predecessors, this must not be at the expense of oversimplification. For instance, in its categorization of risk groups, the current ACCP guidelines lists patients >60 years undergoing surgery as a high-risk group, with IPC as an acceptable sole means of prophylaxis.[2] Is this misleading when we note the increased incidence of VTE in cancer patients (up to 6 times higher than individuals without a malignancy[59]) and see that LMWH or UFH are presented as the mainstays of prophylaxis in this group? By assigning 6 points to such a patient (2 each for surgery, cancer, and age >60 years) as suggested in our RAM, the patient would clearly be placed in the highest risk group, underlining the importance of weighting the factors. In this case the IBD and obesity reinforce placing this patient in the highest risk group. Another key element was studied by Borow and Goldson[42] where incidence of venographic DVT was found to be related to surgery duration (20% at 1–2 h, 46.7% at 2–3 h, 62.5% at >3 h). In this same study, age was also stratified (40–60, 61–70, 61–70, >71 years), a weighting that is also employed in our RAM and further validates the weighted scoring system. The incidence of DVT in those over 71 is more than 60% compared to only 20% for ages 40–60. We are currently in the process of implementing the RAM in the electronic record and adding a reminder to encourage prophylaxis. The aim is to build on the positive results (a 41% reduced risk of VTE at 90 d) shown with the electronic alert developed by Kucher et al.[60] by combining it with a stratified approach to prophylaxis methods using weighted risk factors.

VALIDATION OF THE CAPRINI RAM

Since 2007, several important validation studies have appeared using the scoring system and correlating the score with the subsequent development of clinically evident imaging-proven VTE. In the first study Seruya[61] performed 1,156 operations over a 2-year period and applied the risk score to all of these patients. The authors identified 173 operations (15%) involving 120 patients with a risk score greater than 4. Nine patients suffered a VTE (7.5%) including one nonfatal PE. All patients received prophylaxis with either physical, pharmacologic, or combined modalities. The authors suggested that combined physical and pharmacologic prophylaxis be used in patients with a score greater than 4 along with outpatient LMWH. No clinical VTE events occurred in patients with a score of less than 4.

A major validation study reported from the University of Michigan involved 8,216 surgical patients. A retrospective score was obtained using the Caprini risk template based on electronic medical records, the pharmacy database, and hospital coding records. The score was compared to the 30-d incidence of clinically evident imaging-proven VTE events.[62]

Risk level was significantly associated with VTE (1.9; 1.3–2.6, $P < 0.01$). The bivariate probit model demonstrated significant correlation between the probability of VTE and lack of adherence to prophylaxis guidelines (0.299, $P = 0.013$). The overall incidence of acquired VTE within 30 days was 1.44%. The incidence was associated with an increase in risk level; of the patients in the highest risk level, 1.94% acquired a VTE; of the high-risk patients, 0.97%; moderate-risk patients, 0.70%; and low-risk patients, 0%. The difference between high and highest risk levels was statistically significant ($P < 0.001$).

Further score breakdown revealed that patients with a score of 5–6 had a 1.33% VTE incidence, those with a score of 7–8 had a VTE incidence of 2.58%, and this percentage rose to 6.51% in those with a score of 9 or above. Many of us feel that these data are critical because the score can be correlated with the eventual development of clinically significant VTE events.

Another recent validation study involving the Caprini score involved over 1,126 patients in the Venous Thromboembolism Prevention Study (VTEP) in five tertiary care centers involving plastic surgery patients.[63] They included 1,126 historic control patients.

The overall VTE incidence was 1.69%. Approximately 1 in 9 (11.3%) patients with Caprini score >8 had a VTE event. Patients with Caprini score >8 were significantly more likely to develop VTE when compared with patients with Caprini score of 3 to 4 (odds ratio [OR] 20.9, p_0.001), 5 to 6 (OR9.9, p_0.001), or 7 to 8 (OR4.6, p_0.015). Among patients with Caprini score 7 to 8 or Caprini score >8, VTE risk was not limited to the immediate postoperative period (postoperative days 1-14). In these high-risk patients, more than 50% of VTE events were diagnosed in the late (days 15-60) postoperative period.

The authors conclude that "The Caprini RAM effectively risk-stratifies plastic and reconstructive surgery patients for VTE risk. Among patients with Caprini score >8, 11.3% have a postoperative VTE when chemoprophylaxis is not provided. In higher risk patients, there was no evidence that VTE risk is limited to the immediate postoperative period." This allows the clinician to recommend continued prophylaxis for those with high scores. Unfortunately, the ACCP guidelines contain little data regarding out-of-hospital prophylaxis except for certain very specific orthopedic and abdominal surgery patients. The vast majority of patients seen in clinical practice have not been included in these trials so without risk scores the clinician has very little data to formulate an outpatient plan.

We are becoming aware that the vast majority of VTE events occur following hospital discharge. The GLORY orthopedic registry, according to the authors, has shown the following:

The cumulative incidence of venous thromboembolism within three months of surgery was 1.7% in the THR and 2.3% in the TKR patients. The mean times to venous thromboembolism were 21.5 days (SD 22.5) for THR, and 9.7 days (SD 14.1) for TKR. It occurred after the median time to discharge in 75% of the THR and 57% of the TKA patients who developed venous thromboembolism. Of those who received recommended forms of prophylaxis, approximately one-quarter (26% of THR and 27% of TKR patients) were not receiving it seven days after surgery, the minimum duration recommended at the time of the study. The risk of venous thromboembolism extends beyond the usual period of hospitalization, while the duration of prophylaxis is often shorter than this. According to the authors, practices should be re-assessed to ensure that patients receive appropriate durations of prophylaxis.[64]

Another large, real-world database—the RIETE registry—indicates that 77% of patients develop VTE following hospital discharge, and in 55% of these individuals the thrombotic event occurred after anticoagulant prophylaxis was stopped.[65] The million-women study also has shown the following, according to the authors:

Compared with not having surgery, women were 70 times more likely to be admitted with venous thromboembolism in the first six weeks after an inpatient operation (relative risk 69.1, 95% confidence interval 63.1 to 75.6) and 10 times more likely after a day case operation (9.6, 8.0 to 11.5). The risks were lower but still substantially increased 7–12 weeks after surgery (19.6, 16.6 to 23.1 and 5.5, 4.3 to 7.0, respectively). This pattern of risk was similar for pulmonary embolism (n=2487) and deep venous thrombosis (n=3529).[66]

As can be seen from all of these data, the ongoing use of prophylaxis is becoming increasingly important and can be guided by risk scores until further studies are done.

SUMMARY

High-quality clinical data are unlikely to be available to guide thromboprophylactic decisions in all clinical situations, particularly for medical patients, in whom VTE has been less extensively studied. Thorough and up-to-date academic guidelines are available and are the foundation for treatment regimens; however, with new trial data constantly emerging, there will always be some disparity between the guidelines and clinical practice.

Despite the availability of effective methods of prophylaxis, both surgical and nonsurgical patients continue to be placed at risk of VTE and its potentially fatal complications, such as PE or stroke, through the underuse of thromboprophylaxis. Prophylaxis is also being prescribed inappropriately, with patients at highest risk often receiving ineffective treatment due to misconceptions of VTE risk and concerns about the safety of anticoagulant therapy.

Where firm recommendations are available, the physician should treat according to the evidence, but where evidence is lacking, the physician should assess each patient based on their medical and clinical status and use a risk factor model to help stratify patients according to risk. Now that the scoring system has been validated, an additional guide to ongoing prophylaxis is available. Using this "hybrid approach," which combines clinical guidelines and intelligent clinical practice, more patients should receive appropriate prophylactic treatment tailored to their individual risk.

REFERENCES

1. Shojania KG, Duncan BW, McDonald KM, et al. Making health care safer: A critical analysis of patient safety practices [Summary], *Evid Rep Technol Assess.* 2001. *43*: i–x, 1–668.
2. Geerts WH, Pineo GF, Heit JA, et al. Prevention of venous thromboembolism: The Seventh ACCP Conference on Antithrombotic and Thrombolytic Therapy, *Chest.* 2004. *126*: 338S–400S.
3. Lindblad B, Eriksson A, Bergqvist D. Autopsy-verified pulmonary embolism in a surgical department: Analysis of the period from 1951 to 1968, *Br J Surg.* 1991. *78*: 849–852.
4. Hyers TM. Venous thromboembolism, *Am J Respir Crit Care Med.* 1999. *159*: 1–14.
5. Prandoni P, Lensing AW, Cogo A, et al. The long-term clinical course of acute deep venous thrombosis, *Ann Intern Med.* 1996. *125*: 1–7.
6. Bergqvist D, Jendteg S, Johansen L, et al. Cost of long-term complications of deep vein thrombosis of the lower extremities: An analysis of a defined patient population in Sweden, *Ann Intern Med.* 1997. *126*: 454–457.
7. Nicolaides AN, Bergqvist D, Hull RD, et al. Prevention of venous thromboembolism: International Consensus Statement (guidelines according to scientific evidence), *Int Angiol.* 1997. *16*: 3–38.
8. Nicolaides AN, Breddin HK, Fareed J, et al. Prevention of venous thromboembolism: International Consensus Statement (guidelines according to scientific evidence), *Int Angiol.* 2001. *20*(1): 1–37.
9. Thromboembolic Risk Factors (THRIFT) Consensus Group. Risk of and prophylaxis for venous thromboembolism in hospital patients, *Br Med J.* 1992. *305*: 567–574.

10. Second Thromboembolic Risk Factors (THRIFT II) Consensus Group. Risk of and prophylaxis for venous thromboembolism in hospital patients, *Phlebology.* 1998. *13*: 87–97.

11. Stratton MA, Anderson FA, Bussey HI, et al. Prevention of venous thromboembolism: Adherence to the 1995 American College of Chest Physicians consensus guidelines for surgical patients, *Arch Intern Med.* 2000. *160*: 334–340.

12. Arnold DM, Kahn SR, Shrier I. Missed opportunities for prevention of venous thromboembolism: An evaluation of the use of thromboprophylaxis guidelines, *Chest.* 2001. *120*: 1964–1971.

13. Anderson FA, Tapson VF, Decousus H, et al. IMPROVE, a multinational observational cohort study of practices in prevention of venous thromboembolism in acutely ill medical patients: A comparison with clinical study populations, *Blood.* 2003. *102*: 3l9a.

14. Caprini JA, Glase C, Martchev D, et al. Thrombosis risk factor assessment in surgical patients: Compliance with chest consensus guidelines, *J Thromb Haemost.* 2003. *1*(Suppl 1): CD125.

15. Friedman R, Gallus A, Cushner F, et al. Compliance with ACCP Guidelines for Prevention of Venous Thromboembolism: Multinational findings from the Global Orthopaedic Registry (GLORY). *Blood.* 2003. *102*: 165a.

16. Panju A, Kahn SR, Geerts W, et al. Utilization of venous thromboprophylaxis in acutely ill medical patients in Canada: Results from the Canadian Registry (CURVE), *Blood.* 2003. *102*: 498a.

17. Caprini JA, Arcelus JI. State-of-the-art venous thromboembolism prophylaxis, *Scope on Phlebology and Lymphology.* 2001. *1*: 228–240.

18. Anderson FA Jr, Audet A-M, St John R. Practices in the prevention of venous thromboembolism, *J Thromb Thrombolysis.* 1998. *5*: S7–S11.

19. Bratzler DW, Raskob GE, Murray CK, et al. Underuse of venous thromboembolism prophylaxis for general surgery patients: Physician practices in the community hospital setting, *Arch Intern Med.* 1998. *158*: 1909–1912.

20. Ahmad HA, Geissler A, MacLellan DG. Deep venous thrombosis prophylaxis: Are guidelines being followed?, *ANZ J Surg.* 2002. *72*: 331–334.

21. Huber O, Bournameaux H, Borst F, Rohner A. Postoperative pulmonary embolism after hospital discharge: An underestimated risk, *Arch Surg.* 1992. *127*: 310–313.

22. Bergqvist D. Long-term prophylaxis following orthopedic surgery, *Haemostasis.* 1993. *23*(Suppl 1): 27–31.

23. Trowbridge A, Boese CK, Woodruff B, et al. Incidence of posthospitalization proximal deep venous thrombosis after total hip arthroplasty: A pilot study, *Clin Orthop.* 1994. *299*: 203–208.

24. White RH, Romano PS, Zhou H, et al. Incidence and time course of thromboembolic outcomes following total hip or knee arthroplasty, *Arch Intern Med.* 1998. *158*: 1525–1531.

25. Lindblad B, Sternby NH, Bergqvist D. Incidence of venous thromboembolism verified by necropsy over 30 years, *Br Med J.* 1991. *302*: 709–711.

26. Baglin TP, White K, Charles A. Fatal pulmonary embolism in hospitalised medical patients, *J Clin Pathol.* 1997. *50*: 609–610.

27. Gensini GF, Prisco D, Falciani M, et al. Identification of candidates for prevention of venous thromboembolism, *Semin Thromb Hemost.* 1997. *23*: 55–67.

28. Kakkar AK, Williamson RC. Prevention of venous thromboembolism in cancer using low-molecular-weight heparins, *Haemostasis.* 1997. *27*: 32–37.

29. McNally MA, Cooke EA, Harding ML, Mollan RA. Attitudes to, and utilization of, low molecular weight heparins in joint replacement surgery, *JR Coll Surg Edinb.* 1997. *42*: 407–409.

30. Kakkar VV, Cohen AT, Edmonson RA, et al. Low molecular weight versus standard heparin for prevention of venous thromboembolism after major abdominal surgery: The Thromboprophylaxis Collaborative Group, *Lancet.* 1993. *341*: 259–265.

31. Koch A, Bouges S, Ziegler S, et al. Low molecular weight heparin and unfractionated heparin in thrombosis prophylaxis after major surgical intervention: Update of previous meta-analyses, *Br J Surg.* 1997. *84*: 750–759.

32. Clagett GP, Reisch JS. Prevention of venous thromboembolism in general surgical patients: Results of a meta-analysis, *Ann Surg.* 1988. *208*: 227–240.

33. Collins R, Scrimgeour A, Yusuf S, Peto R. Reduction in fatal pulmonary embolism and venous thrombosis by perioperative administration of subcutaneous heparin: Overview of results of randomized trials in general, orthopedic, and urologic surgery, *N Engl J Med.* 1988. *318*: 1162–1173.

34. Nurmohamed MT, Rosendaal FR, Buller HR, et al. Low molecular weight heparin versus standard heparin in general and orthopedic surgery: A meta-analysis, *Lancet.* 1992. *340*: 152–156.

35. Jorgensen LN, Wille-Jorgensen P, Hauch O. Prophylaxis of postoperative thromboembolism with low molecular weight heparins, *Br J Surg.* 1993. *80*: 689–704.

36. Mismetti P, Laporte S, Darmon JY, Buchmüller, Decousus H. Meta-analysis of low molecular weight heparin in the prevention of venous thromboembolism in general surgery, *Br J Surg.* 2001. *88*: 913–930.

37. Hirsh J, Raschke R. Heparin and low-molecular-weight heparin: The Seventh ACCP Conference on Antithrombotic and Thrombolytic Therapy, *Chest.* 2004. *126*: 188S–203S.

38. Warkentin TE, Levine MN, Hirsh J, et al. Heparin-induced thrombocytopenia in patients treated with low-molecular weight heparin or unfractionated heparin, *N Engl J Med.* 1995. *332*: 1330–1335.

39. Warkentin TE, Roberts RS, Hirsh J, Kelton JG. An improved definition of immune heparin-induced thrombocytopenia in postoperative orthopedic patients, *Arch Intern Med.* 2003. *163*: 2518–2524.

40. Geerts WH, Heit JA, Clagett GP, et al. Prevention of venous thromboembolism: The Sixth ACCP Conference on Antithrombotic and Thrombolytic Therapy. *Chest.* 2001. *119*: 132S–175S.

41. Caprini JA, Botteman MF, Stephens JM, et al. Economic burden of long-term complications of deep vein thrombosis after total hip replacement surgery in the United States, *Value Health.* 2003. *6*: 59–74.

42. Borow M, Goldson HJ. Postoperative venous thrombosis: Evaluation of five methods of treatment, *Am J Surg.* 1981. *141*(2): 245–251.

43. Borow M, Goldson HJ. Prevention of postoperative deep vein thrombosis and pulmonary emboli with combined modalities, *Am Surg.* 1983. *49*(11): 599–605.

44. Turpie AG, Bauer, Caprini J, et al. Fondaparinux with intermittent pneumatic compression (IPC) versus IPC alone in the prevention of VTE after major abdominal surgery: Results of the APOLLO Study, *J Thromb Haem.* 2005. *3*(Suppl 1): P1046.

45. Agu O, Hamilton G, Baker D. Graduated compression stockings in the prevention of venous thromboembolism, *Br J Surg.* 1999. *86*: 992–1004.

46. Wheeler HB. Diagnosis of deep vein thrombosis: Review of clinical evaluation and impedance plethysmography, *Am J Surg.* 1985. *150*: 7–13.

47. Flordal PA, Bergqvist D, Burmark US, et al. Risk factors for major thromboembolism and bleeding tendency after elective general surgery operations: The Fragmin Multicentre Study Group, *Eur J Surg.* 1996. *162*: 783–789.

48. Caprini JA, Arcelus JI, Hasty JH, et al. Clinical assessment of venous thromboembolic risk in surgical patients, *Semin Thromb Hemost.* 1991. *17*: 304–312.

49. Alikhan R, Cohen AT, Combe S, et al. Risk factors for venous thromboembolism in hospitalized patients with acute medical illness: Analysis of the MEDENOX study, *Arch Intern Med.* 2004. *164*: 963–968.

50. Caprini JA, Arcelus JI, Reyna JJ. Effective risk stratification of surgical and nonsurgical patients for venous thromboembolic disease, *Semin Hematol.* 2001. *38*(2 Suppl 5): 12–19.

51. Rasmussen MS, Jorgensen L, Wille-Jorgensen, et al. Prolonged prophylaxis with dalteparin after major abdominal surgery, *Thromb Haemost*. 2001. OC1733.

52. Bergqvist D, Agnelli G, Cohen AT, et al. Duration of prophylaxis against venous thromboembolism with enoxaparin after surgery for cancer, *N Engl J Med*. 2002. *346*: 975–980.

53. Rasmussen MS. Preventing thromboembolic complications in cancer patients after surgery: A role for prolonged thromboprophylaxis, *Cancer Treat Rev*. 2002. *28*: 141–144.

54. Bergqvist D, Burmark U, Flordal P, et al. Low molecular weight heparin started before surgery as prophylaxis against deep vein thrombosis: 2500 versus 5000 XaI units in 2070 patients, *Br J Surg*. 1995. *82*: 496–501.

55. Lee AYY, Levine MN, Blaer RI, et al. Low-molecular-weight heparin versus a coumarin for the prevention of recurrent venous thromboembolism in patients with cancer, *N Eng J Med*. 2003. *349*: 146–153.

56. von Tempelhoff G-F, Harenberg J, Niemann F, et al. Effect of low molecular weight heparin (Certoparin) versus unfractionated heparin on cancer survival following breast and pelvic cancer surgery: A prospective randomized double-blind trial, *Int J Oncol*. 2000. *16*: 815–824.

57. Lee AYY, Rickles FR, Julian JA, et al. Randomized comparison of low molecular weight heparin and coumarin derivatives on the survival of patients with cancer and venous thromboembolism, *J Clin Oncol*. 2005. *23*(10): 1–7.

58. Mousa SA, Mohamed S. Anti-angiogenic mechanisms and efficacy of the low molecular weight heparin, tinzaparin: Anti-cancer efficacy, *Oncol Rep*. 2004. *12*(4): 683–688.

59. Heit JA, Silverstein MD, Mohr DN, et al. Risk factors for deep vein thrombosis and pulmonary embolism: A population-based case-control study, *Arch Intern Med*. 2000. *160*: 809–815.

60. Kucher N, Koo S, Quiroz R, et al. Electronic alerts to prevent venous thromboembolism among hospitalized patients, *N Engl J Med*. 2005. *352*: 969–977.

61. Seruya MS, Venturi ML, Iorio ML, Davison SP. Efficacy and safety of venous thromboembolism prophylaxis in highest risk plastic surgery patients, *Plast Reconstr Surg*. 2008. *122*: 1701–1708.

62. Bahl V, Hu HM, Henke P. A validation study of a retrospective venous thromboembolism risk scoring method, *Ann Surg*. 2010. *251*: 344–350.

63. Pannucci CJ, Bailey SH, Dreszer G, et al. Validation of the Caprini Risk Assessment Model in plastic and reconstructive surgery patients, *J Am Coll Surg*. 2011. *212*: 105–112.

64. Warwick D, Friedman RJ, Agnelli G, et al. Insufficient duration of venous thromboembolism prophylaxis after total hip or knee replacement when compared with the time course of thromboembolic events: Findings from the Global Orthopaedic Registry, *J Bone Joint Surg Br*. 2007. *89*: 799–807.

65. Arcelus JI, Monreal M, Caprini JA, Guisado JG, Soto MS. Clinical presentation and time-course of postoperative venous thromboembolism: Results from the RIETE Registry, *Thromb Haemost*. 2008. *99*: 546–551.

66. Sweetland S, Green J, Liu B, Berrington de González A. Duration and magnitude of the postoperative risk of venous thromboembolism in middle aged women: Prospective cohort study, *Br Med J*. 2009. *339*: b4583. doi:10.1136/bmj.b4583.

39.

VENOUS THROMBOEMBOLISM PROPHYLAXIS IN THE GENERAL SURGICAL PATIENT

J. I. Arcelus and J. A. Caprini

INTRODUCTION

Patients undergoing major surgery are at a twenty-fold increased risk for development of venous thromboembolism (VTE), an often asymptomatic condition that encompasses both deep venous thrombosis (DVT) and pulmonary embolism (PE).[1] Kakkar and colleagues demonstrated in 1975 that the observed rate of DVT by an isotopic technique in general surgery patients who did not receive VTE prophylaxis was nearly 30%.[2] A meta-analysis of randomized trials in general, orthopedic, and urologic surgery conducted 30 years later reported similar results (27% incidence of DVT and 3.4% incidence of fatal PE).[3] Pooled data from more than fifty trials published between 1970 and 1985 showed that the overall postoperative incidence of DVT as assessed by fibrinogen uptake test (FUT), a study in which radiolabeled fibrinogen is incorporated into newly formed thrombi, and/or contrast venography ranges from 19 to 29% in untreated patients who undergo general surgery.[4] Rates of total and fatal PE were approximately 1.6% and 0.9%, respectively. The majority of patients included in this pooled analysis underwent elective gastrointestinal surgery, although some study populations also included patients who had undergone gynecologic, thoracic, urologic, or vascular surgery.

In the United States, DVT is reported to affect up to 145 individuals per 100,000 per year in the general population, and it is accompanied by PE in up to 69 individuals per 100,000.[5] Approximately 11 to 16% of all symptomatic VTE diagnosed in European or North American countries occurred in patients who underwent surgery several weeks before, and almost half of them were general surgical patients.[6] Because of the strong data demonstrating the high risk of VTE in general surgery patients, clinical studies without prophylaxis are no longer performed in this patient population and, thus, the current risk of VTE is unknown. The incidence of VTE in this patient population without prophylaxis was approximately 30% in studies done in the 1970s and 1980s.[2,3] With pharmacologic prophylaxis, the incidence ranges from 4.6 to 8%. Despite the seriousness of the condition and its high prevalence, it has been demonstrated that 25 to 62% of general surgery patients do not receive any form of prophylaxis, as opposed to standard therapy in clinical trials.[7,8] Furthermore, a recent epidemiologic study shows that only 59% of surgical patients at high risk to develop postoperative VTE received appropriate prophylaxis according to ACCP recommendations.[9] Clearly, there is a need to improve venous thrombosis prevention in general surgery patients at high thrombotic risk.

Postoperative VTE is difficult to diagnose because it is often asymptomatic or, when symptoms are present, they usually are nonspecific. Symptoms of DVT include leg pain, swelling, and heaviness. Symptoms of PE include chest pain, shortness of breath, tachypnea, transient orthostatic hypotension, fainting spell, hypoxia, and sudden death. Although many surgeons may feel that they do not often see VTE postoperatively, many most likely see these signs of VTE often, but overlook their possible connection to VTE. Actually, in 70 to 80% of patients who died from a PE confirmed by autopsy, this diagnosis was not even considered prior to a patient's death.[10,11]

The prevention of VTE is important because both symptomatic and asymptomatic VTE are associated with long-term consequences, even when the condition is diagnosed and treated. A common, serious complication associated with DVT is postthrombotic syndrome (PTS). PTS is characterized by permanent vein damage that results in chronic leg swelling that worsens during the day, which may be accompanied by the presence of varicose veins, edema, skin discoloration, and skin ulcerations. In a prospective inception cohort study of 528 patients with venography-confirmed DVT, 19% of whom were postoperative, the cumulative incidence of PTS at 2, 5, and 8 years following initial diagnosis and treatment was 24.5%, 29.6%, and 29.8%, respectively.[12] PTS also represents a significant economic impact of DVT. It has been estimated that 15 million Americans are afflicted with PTS and that 2 million work days are lost annually due to the condition. Recurrent DVT or PE is also a common clinical consequence of VTE. The cumulative incidence of recurrent VTE after 2, 5, and 8 years of follow-up in the above mentioned study by Prandoni was 17.2%, 24.3% and 29.7%, respectively. A rare but serious consequence that is associated with symptomatic and asymptomatic DVT is fatal PE. It has been estimated that less than 50% of patients are alive 1 year following an acute PE.[13] According to the results of the RIETE registry, the mortality of acute PE is around 12% in the first 3 months after diagnosis.[6] In addition, almost 4% of patients who survive an acute PE will develop chronic pulmonary hypertension.[14]

PE is also associated with embolic stroke in patients with patent foramen ovale (PFO), a condition estimated to be present in 10% to nearly 30% of the general population.[15,16] PE can lead to elevated pressures in the right side of the heart, which can lead to expansion of PFO. A clot or part of a clot can move from the right to left chamber of the heart through the expanded PFO, causing cerebral and peripheral ischemic events characteristic of paradoxical embolism (passage of a clot from a vein to an artery).[17] These serious, disabling, and sometimes fatal consequences of VTE underscore the importance of prevention in patients at risk, including patients undergoing general surgery.

Although a high incidence of VTE has been demonstrated in general surgery patients, risk for VTE varies among general surgery patients, and different methods of prophylaxis are appropriate for different levels of risk. An optimal approach to risk assessment and VTE prophylaxis should combine evidence-based and clinical practice guidelines with clinical experience where a lack of science exists. Several risk factor assessment models have been proposed to predict VTE risk preoperatively, but only one of them has been validated prospectively.[18–22]

RISK FACTORS FOR VTE

Although the risk for VTE is increased in most patients undergoing major general surgery, the relative risk for postoperative development of this complication varies among individual patients based on numerous factors, including the length of immobilization following surgery, the type of surgery performed, and the presence of comorbid conditions (Table 39.1).[1,23,24] Important patient-specific or intrinsic risk factors for VTE include age greater than 40 years, ethnicity, cancer, and body mass index (BMI) over 25. A recent retrospective study in general surgery patients found that, while a steady rise in the incidence of VTE is seen between 40 and 75 years of age, this increase does not continue above the age of 75 years.[23]

Among the extrinsic or exposing risk factors related to the hospital admission, immobilization for an extended period of time is a well-established risk factor for VTE, and early mobilization following surgery has been shown to lower the risk for postoperative VTE.[25] There is also strong evidence that the type of surgical procedure a patient undergoes is predictive of the risk for postoperative VTE. Major general surgery (usually defined as abdominal or thoracic

Table 39.1 **RISK FACTORS FOR VTE**

Patient Factors	
• Age >40 years	• Pregnancy
• Prolonged immobility	• Puerperium
• Obesity	• High-dose estrogen therapy
• History of DVT or PE	• Varicose veins
Medical/Surgical Risk Factors	
• Major surgery (especially involving the abdomen, pelvis, lower extremities)	• Acute respiratory failure
• Malignancy (especially pelvic, abdominal, metastatic)	• Congestive heart failure
• Myocardial infarction	• Inflammatory bowel disease
• Stroke	• Nephrotic syndrome
• Fractures of the pelvis, hip, or leg	• Pacemaker wires
• Polycythemia	• Paraproteinemia
• Paroxysmal nocturnal hemoglobinuria	• Behcet's disease
Hypercoagulable States	
• Lupus anticoagulant and antiphospholipid antibodies	• Disorders of plasminogen and plasminogen activation
• Homocystinemia	• HIT
• Dysfibrinogenemia	• Protein C deficiency
• Myeloproliferative disorders	• Protein S deficiency
• Antithrombin deficiency	• Hyperviscosity syndromes
• Factor V Leiden	• Prothrombin gene mutation 20210A
• Disseminated intravascular coagulation	

operations that require general anesthesia lasting >45 minutes) is associated with a high risk of VTE. Orthopedic surgery is also associated with a high risk for VTE. In a retrospective study of more than 1 million surgery patients, the incidence of symptomatic VTE was highest among patients who underwent orthopedic surgery of the hip or knee as well as those who had invasive neurosurgery involving brain incision, excision, or biopsy. Other procedures associated with a substantially increased risk for VTE included major vascular surgery, small or large bowel resection, gastric bypass, radical cystectomy, kidney transplantation, and below-the-knee amputation. A low risk of VTE was reported with radical neck dissection, inguinal hernia repair, appendectomy, laparoscopic cholecystectomy, transurethral prostatectomy, repair of a cystocoele or rectocoele, cruciate ligament repair, and thyroid or parathyroid surgery.[23]

Certain medical conditions, including congestive heart failure, chronic obstructive pulmonary disease, recent myocardial infarction, stroke, nephrotic syndrome, inflammatory bowel disorder, and systemic lupus erythematosus are known to increase the risk for VTE.[13] There is a particularly strong association between cancer and VTE.[26,27]

Cancer patients undergoing surgery have a two- to five-fold increased risk for postoperative VTE, compared with noncancer patients undergoing the same procedures.[28] In addition, among patients with DVT, those with cancer have a more than two-fold higher risk for VTE recurrence than those without cancer. In a retrospective study of 986 patients who underwent venous ultrasonography because of suspected DVT, 12% of patients with confirmed DVT were subsequently found to have cancer.[29] The likelihood for development of VTE in cancer patients is increased among those with more advanced clinical disease, and varies by tumor type. Malignancies stemming from the uterus, brain, ovary, pancreas, stomach, kidneys, and colon are among those that have been associated with the highest relative risk for VTE.[30] In a prospective multicenter registry from Italy including more than 2,300 patients undergoing surgery for cancer, PE was the main cause of postoperative death. In a multivariable analysis from this study, five independent risk factors of VTE were identified: age above 60 years, previous VTE, advanced cancer, anesthesia longer than 2 h, and bed rest longer than 3 d.[31]

Acquired or inherited thrombophilia disorders can also increase risk of VTE. A mutation in the factor V gene, known as Factor V Leiden, is the most common cause of familial thrombophilia.[32] This mutation can increase the risk of VTE fifty- to eighty-fold over that of the general population in individuals who are homozygous for the mutation and three-fold in heterozygous individuals. The second most common cause of familial thrombophilia is the prothrombin 20210A mutation. This mutation is associated with a three-fold increase in the risk for VTE. Another thrombophilia disorder is antiphospholipid antibody syndrome, including lupus anticoagulants and anticardiolipin antibodies. Thromboembolic events are reported in approximately one-third of antiphospholipid-positive patients. The risk of recurrent thrombosis in these patients ranges from 22 to 69%.[33] Other thrombophilia disorders include hyperhomocysteinemia; protein C, protein S, and antithrombin deficiencies; and elevated levels of coagulation factors, including factors II, VIII, IX, and XI. Detection of these disorders is critical for identification of a patient's true risk for VTE and should be a factor in a patient's decision regarding whether or not to undergo elective surgery.

VTE PROPHYLAXIS

Aside from early and frequent mobilization, the American College of Chest Physicians does not recommend specific measures for general surgical patients at low risk for VTE (Figures 39.1 and 39.2).[34] Pharmacologic methods such as unfractionated heparin (UFH) at doses of 5,000 U bid or low molecular weight heparin (LMWH) at doses lower than 3,400 U qd are recommended for the prevention of VTE in patients at moderate risk (risk factor score of 2).

For patients at high risk (risk factor score of 3–4), both UFH at doses of 5,000 U tid or LMWH (>3,400 U qd) in combination with intermittent pneumatic compression (IPC) boots are recommended for protection against VTE. For patients at highest risk for VTE (risk factor score ≥ 5), pharmacologic therapy using high-dose UFH or LMWH doses are always recommended in the absence of contraindications, and the adjunctive use of mechanical prophylaxis is also recommended.[34]

NONPHARMACOLOGIC INTERVENTIONS FOR THE PREVENTION OF VTE

Nonpharmacologic VTE prevention strategies are often appealing because they tend to be associated with a low risk for bleeding; however, they have not been as extensively studied as pharmacologic prophylaxis. It is recommended that early and frequent ambulation be a routine part of postoperative care in all patients unless there is an absolute contraindication.[34] Although early mobilization following surgery has been shown to significantly lower the risk for postoperative VTE, it is recommended as the sole method of prophylaxis only for low-risk patients: those under 40 years of age without any additional risk factors for VTE who are undergoing minor surgery (outpatient surgery lasting less than 45 minutes). For surgical patients at moderate risk for VTE (major surgery with two additional risk factors), mechanical methods of prophylaxis, including graduated compression stockings (GCS) and IPC, have been very safe and effective modalities and have been very well accepted in the United States, particularly in patients at high risk for bleeding complications. A recent epidemiologic study has shown that around 10% of surgical patients at high risk for VTE had contraindications for the use of anticoagulants.[9]

The results of IPC have been variable, depending on the type of surgery, patient's risk factors, and end points used to detect DVT. Overall, most studies show that IPC reduces the incidence of DVT in general surgery, urology, neurosurgery, and orthopedic surgery. The systematic review by Roderick et al.[35] identified nineteen trials assessing IPC as monotherapy in 2,255 patients undergoing different types of surgery. The results show that IPC significantly reduced the incidence of DVT from 23.4% (268/1,147) in the control group to 10.1% (112/1,108) in the IPC group, a 66% odds reduction (p < 0.0001). There was no evidence that sequential compression devices were more protective than uniform compression machines, as their odds reductions were 65% (six trials) and 66% (twelve trials), respectively.

A meta-analysis of the literature has reviewed fifteen randomized controlled trials with a total of sixteen treatment groups comparing IPC with controls in 2,270 surgical patients with objective diagnosis of DVT by imaging techniques. In comparison to no prophylaxis, IPC reduced

A1: Each Risk Factor Represents 1 Point	B: Each Risk Factor Represents 2 Points
○ Age 40-59 years	○ Age 60-74 years
○ Minor surgery planned	○ Major surgery (> 60 minutes)*
○ History of prior major surgery	○ Arthroscopic surgery (> 60 minutes)*
○ Varicose veins	○ Laparoscopic surgery (> 60 minutes)*
○ History of inflammatory bowel disease	○ Previous malignancy
○ Swollen legs (current)	○ Morbid obesity (BMI > 40)
○ Obesity (BMI > 30)	
○ Acute myocardial infarction (< 1 month)	**C: Each Risk Factor Represents 3 Points**
○ Congestive heart failure (< 1 month)	○ Age 75 years or more
○ Sepsis (< 1 month)	○ Major surgery lasting 2-3 hours*
○ Serious lung disease incl. pneumonia (< 1 month)	○ BMI > 50 (venous stasis syndrome)
○ Abnormal pulmonary function (chronic obstructive pulmonary disease)	○ History of SVT, DVT/PE
	○ Family history of DVT/PE
○ Medical patient currently at bed rest	○ Present cancer or chemotherapy
○ Leg plaster cast or brace	○ Positive Factor V Leiden
○ Central venous access	○ Positive Prothrombin 20210A
○ Blood transfusion (< 1 month)	○ Elevated serum homocysteine
○ Other risk factor/s _____	○ Positive Lupus anticoagulant
	○ Elevated anticardiolipin antibodies
	○ Heparin-induced thrombocytopenia (HIT)
	○ Other thrombophilia- Type_____

A2: For Women Only (Each Represents 1 Point)	D: Each Risk Factor Represents 5 Points
○ Oral contraceptives or hormone replacement therapy	○ Elective major lower extremity arthroplasty
○ Pregnancy or postpartum (<1 month)	○ Hip, pelvis or leg fracture (< 1 month)
○ History of unexplained stillborn infant, recurrent spontaneous abortion (≥ 3), premature birth with toxemia of pregnancy or growth restricted infant	○ Stroke (< 1 month)
	○ Multiple trauma (< 1 month)
	○ Acute spinal cord injury (paralysis) (< 1month)
	○ Major surgery lasting over 3 hours*

TOTAL RISK FACTOR SCORE:

Figure 39.1   Thrombosis risk factor assessment scoring sheet.

the risk of DVT by 60% (RR 0.40; 95% CI 0.29–0.56; p < 0.001).[36]

Although there is strong evidence supporting the use of IPC alone in moderate-risk patients, it has not been studied as thoroughly as pharmacologic agents and is only recommended as an adjunctive therapy in surgery patients at high and highest risk for VTE or when anticoagulants are contraindicated.[34]

GCS have also been shown in meta-analyses to substantially reduce the incidence of lower extremity DVT in patients who have undergone general surgery.[37] A systematic review from the Cochrane Collaboration analyzed seven randomized controlled trials in surgery patients (four general surgery, one gynecologic surgery, one neurosurgery, one orthopedic surgery). The incidence of lower-limb DVT in patients who used GCS was significantly reduced, compared with those who did not use this intervention (15% vs. 29%, $P < 0.00001$).[38] In a meta-analysis of eleven studies that investigated the prophylactic efficacy of GCS in patients who had undergone moderate-risk surgery (nine abdominal surgery, one gynecologic surgery, and one neurosurgery), elastic stockings reduced the risk for lower limb DVT by

68%.[37] The current evidence suggests that GCS is effective in moderate-risk general surgery patients, but there is little data exploring the efficacy of this intervention in high-risk general surgery patients or surgery patients with cancer.

The main limitations of GCS include the lack of international standardization of their pressure profiles and the difficulty of fitting patients with unusual leg sizes or shapes. Patient compliance may be another limiting issue, especially with thigh-length stockings, as discussed above. The most common reasons for noncompliance by patients and nurses were that stockings were not reapplied after cleaning or bathing, or were removed because patients complained from itching or heat. Compression stockings should not be used in patients with peripheral arterial disease. Therefore, lack of foot pulses or an ankle-brachial index lower than 0.8 should be considered contraindications for their use, as well as in patients with massive leg edema associated with cardiac failure. Infectious dermatitis and fragile skin secondary to diabetes are other contraindications to the use of GCS.

Clinical trials have shown that combining GCS or IPC with pharmacologic prophylaxis, such as heparin, results in better protection against VTE than either of these

VTE risk and suggested prophylaxis for surgical patients

Total Risk Factor Score	Incidence of DVT	30-day Proven DVT Incidence*	Risk Level	Prophylaxis Regimen
0-1	< 10%	0%	Low Risk	No specific measures; early ambulation
2	10-20%	0.7%	Moderate Risk	IPC, LDUH (5000U BID), or LWMH (<3400 U)
3-4	30-40%	0.97%	High Risk	IPC, LDUH (5000U TID), or LMWH (>3400U or FXa I
5 or more	40-80% 1-5% mortality	1.94%	Highest Risk	Pharmacological: LDUH, LMWH (>3400 U), Warfarin, or FXa I alone or in combination with IPC

*30-day post-discharge clinically evident imaging proven DVT
IPC - Intermittent Pneumatic Compression; LDUH - Low Dose Unfractionated Heparin LMWH - Low Molecular Weight Heparin FXa I - Factor X Inhibitor

Prophylaxis Safety Considerations: Check box if answer is 'YES'

Anticoagulants: Factor Associated with Increased Bleeding

○ Is patient experiencing any active bleeding?
○ Does patient have (or has had history of) heparin-induced thrombocytopenia?
○ Is patient's platelet count <100,000/mm3?
○ Is patient's taking oral anticoagulants, platelet inhibitors (e.g., NSAIDS, Clopidogre, Salicylates)?
○ Is patient's creatinine clearance abnormal? If yes, please indicate value _____.

If any of the above boxes are checked, then patient may not be a candidate for anticoagulant therapy and you should consider alternative prophylactic measures such as IPC or FP.

Intermittent Pneumatic Compression (IPC)

○ Does patient have severe peripheral arterial disease?
○ Does patient have congestive heart failure?
○ Does patient have an acute superficial/deep vein thrombosis?

If any of the above boxes are checked, then patient may not be a candidate for intermittent compression therapy and you should consider alternative prophylactic measures. (IVC filter?)

Figure 39.2 Categories for risk for VTE in patients undergoing general surgery and recommended prophylactic regimens.

approaches used alone.[38] The incidence of DVT was only 1.5% in a group of 328 surgical patients who received a pharmacologic and antistasis agent, compared with 26.8% in a control group who did not receive prophylaxis.[39] In a study in cardiac patients (N = 2,551) randomized to receive subcutaneous heparin alone or in combination with IPC, the incidence of PE was 62% lower (1.5% vs. 4%) in those who received combination therapy (P < 0.001).[40] Similarly, a review of the literature shows that combined modalities are more effective than single modalities in patients undergoing different types of surgery, with a mean reduction in the incidence of postoperative VTE of 69%.[41]

Further support for the benefit of combined mechanical and pharmacological prophylaxis for the prevention of VTE came from the APOLLO study. In this double-blind, placebo-controlled trial, patients undergoing major abdominal surgery (N = 1,309) received IPC with or without the Factor Xa inhibitor fondaparinux.[42] Combined IPC and fondaparinux therapy produced a significant reduction in the incidence of all VTE from 5.3% (IPC alone) to 1.7% (P = 0.004). The rates of proximal DVT were also significantly reduced in the combined therapy group from 1.7% (IPC alone) to 0.2% (P = 0.037). Patients receiving fondaparinux treatment had significantly more

major bleeding episodes than IPC alone (1.6% vs. 0.2%, P = 0.006); however, none of these was fatal or involved critical organs. In addition, a major bleeding rate of 1.6% is comparable to the major bleeding rates observed with abdominal surgery (colorectal surgery) with enoxaparin and UFH.[43] Although patients might be at a higher risk for bleeding with the addition of pharmacological anticoagulation treatments, combined therapy has been shown to be significantly more effective for the prevention of VTE following major surgery than mechanical prophylaxis alone.

Inferior vena cava (IVC) filters are not routinely used for the prevention of DVT, but rather for the prevention of PE in patients who either fail or have contraindications to other prophylactic therapies, particularly anticoagulants. Prophylactic use of IVC filters is indicated for patients with an absolute contraindication to anticoagulation, serious complication while on anticoagulation (i.e., hemorrhage, thrombocytopenia, or drug reaction), or documented failure on anticoagulation. In addition, IVC filters can be effective in patients with pelvic fractures or closed head injuries who are at high risk for thrombosis or have had a previous thrombosis.

IVC filters are generally safe, and have been shown to reduce the incidence of PE and fatal PE to 2.6–3.8% and

0.3–1.9%, respectively, in patients at risk for VTE.[44] An increase in recurrent DVT has been observed with IVC filters by Decousus and colleagues, who demonstrated a reduction in symptomatic and asymptomatic PE at 12 days from 4.8 to 1.1% in patients with proximal DVT who received filters, but at 2 years the incidence of recurrent DVT was significantly increased in these patients (20.8% vs. 11.6%, P =0.02).[45] However, 8-year follow-up on these patients was analyzed and while the significant reduction in the incidence of PE was maintained (P = 0.01), at 8 years there were no significant differences in recurrent DVT (P = 0.08), PTS, or overall mortality with and without filters. Several types of IVC filters are available, but the Greenfield filter is the only filter with good long-term follow-up.[46] Although relatively rare, other complications associated with IVC filter placement and long-term use include migration of the filter, postfilter caval thrombosis, and PTS.[47]

In summary, nonpharmacologic or mechanical prophylaxis modalities can be very effective in reducing the incidence of DVT in general surgery patients at moderate risk for VTE. However, they have not been as extensively studied as pharmacologic agents and are not recommended as the sole method of prophylaxis in patients at higher risk for VTE. However, in conjunction with pharmacologic agents, mechanical prophylaxis can be very effective in reducing the incidence of VTE in these patients. On the other hand, mechanical prophylaxis with GCS or IPC is recommended in patients at high VTE risk who cannot receive anticoagulants because of a high risk for bleeding.[34]

PHARMACOLOGIC THERAPIES FOR THE PREVENTION OF VTE

Commonly used pharmacologic therapies for prevention of VTE in patients undergoing general surgery include subcutaneous UFH and LMWH (including enoxaparin, dalteparin, fraxiparine, and tinzaparin). Low-dose subcutaneous UFH was the first pharmacologic agent to be widely investigated for prevention of VTE in patients undergoing general surgery. In the 1970s, Kakkar and colleagues demonstrated that this therapy significantly reduced the risk for both DVT and PE in this patient population. In a landmark prospective randomized study of 4,121 patients undergoing major surgery (primarily abdominal, gynecologic, or urologic surgery), UFH prophylaxis reduced the incidence of DVT from 25 to 8% (P < 0.005).[2] Patients treated with UFH also had a significantly reduced incidence of PE (P < 0.005) and death from PE (P < 0.005) compared with control patients.

A subsequent meta-analysis of forty-six trials by Collins and colleagues that included 16,000 patients who had undergone general, orthopedic, or urologic surgery confirmed Kakkar's results, with a DVT incidence of 27% without prophylaxis compared with 10.6% with UFH and

an incidence of fatal PE of 3.4% and 1.7%, respectively.[3] The incidence of DVT was 8% (95% CI, 7% to 8%) with UFH following general surgery in a recent meta-analysis of forty-seven clinical studies. It has been suggested that the administration of 5,000 U of UFH tid is more effective than 5,000 U bid, without increased bleeding, but no direct comparison studies have been conducted. In general, UFH can be given twice daily in moderate- to high-risk patients, but should be given three times daily in higher risk patients.

Although UFH is effective for prevention of DVT and PE in general surgery patients, bleeding complications associated with this therapy present a serious safety concern. Cancer patients may be at higher risk for hemorrhagic complications with UFH than noncancer patients.[48] Another limitation of UFH is its association with heparin-induced thrombocytopenia (HIT). UFH used at therapeutic doses has been associated with up to a 5% incidence of HIT, an antibody-mediated process characterized by a dramatic drop in platelets.[49] In 20% of cases, HIT develops into thrombosis. UFH can also cause osteopenia by binding to osteoblasts, which stimulates osteoclast activation and results in bone breakdown when used long-term. The short half-life of UFH (0.5–2 h) relative to other anticoagulants is another limitation of UFH because it necessitates more frequent dosing; however, the short half-life can also be an advantage in the case of bleeding complications or for the management of patients with renal failure. Another advantage of UFH is that an antidote, protamine sulfate, is available for situations where immediate reversal is required, although reversal is not without risks.

LMWHs appear to be at least as effective as UFH for the prevention of DVT in clinical trials of patients undergoing general surgery (Figure 39.3).[50] Overall, the residual incidence of VTE in abdominal surgery patients receiving LMWH ranges from about 5 to 15%, with the highest rates in patients with cancer.[51] The incidence of DVT with LMWHs following general surgery was 6% (95% CI, 6% to 7%) in a recent meta-analysis of twenty-one clinical studies. Available LMWHs appear to be similarly effective for the prevention of VTE. Both enoxaparin and dalteparin have been shown to reduce the incidence of DVT in patients undergoing general surgery to rates of approximately 6 to 8%; however, direct comparison studies have not been conducted.[52,53]

LMWHs appear to be effective in VTE prophylaxis, even in patients with cancer. The incidence of VTE in patients with cancer given enoxaparin was slightly lower than that observed in patients given UFH (14.7% vs. 18.2%) in a study of patients undergoing abdominal surgery for malignant disease (N = 1,115).[51] In addition, when patients undergoing planned curative surgery for abdominal or pelvic cancer were given LMWH for 6 to 10 d and then randomized to receive extended prophylaxis with LMWH or placebo for 21 d, the incidence of venographically demonstrated VTE at 3 months was significantly reduced (5.5% vs. 13.8%,

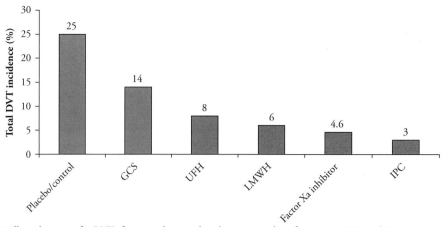

*All incidences are for DVT after general surgery based on meta-analyses from Geerts WH et al (2001) except the incidence for Factor Xa inhibitor, which includes venographically proven DVT, symptomatic DVT, and PE and is based on the results from Agnelli G et al (2005).

Figure 39.3   Incidence of VTE with currently available prophylactic therapies following general surgery.*   *All incidences are for DVT after general surgery based on meta-analyses from Reference 4 except the incidence for Factor Xa inhibitor, which includes venographically proven DVT, symptomatic DVT, and PE and is based on the results from Reference 72.

$P = 0.01$) with extended prophylaxis.[54] There was no significant increase in bleeding with extended prophylaxis. These results suggest that LMWH is at least as effective as UFH in general surgery patients with cancer and that extended prophylaxis with LMWH is safe and can significantly reduce the incidence of VTE in general surgery patients with cancer. Recent meta-analyses demonstrate that extending prophylaxis with LWMW for 28 d after abdominal cancer surgery reduces the risk of postoperative VTE by more than 50% compared to standard prophylaxis for 7–10 d.[55,56]

It has been suggested that survival may be increased in patients with cancer who receive LMWH compared with UFH, although the reason for this is not clear. In women with previously untreated breast and pelvic cancer who had undergone primary surgery, those who received LMWH (n = 160) had significantly better long-term survival at 650 d than those who received UFH (n = 164, $P = 0.0066$).[57] A significant survival benefit (12.6% vs. 27%, $P = 0.041$) was also observed with LMWH in a subset of patients with cancer who were treated for DVT with a LMWH or UFH.[58,59] In a randomized controlled study where patients with advanced cancer (N = 385) were randomized to receive a LMWH once daily for 1 year or placebo, there was no significant difference in survival at 1, 2, or 3 years; however, in a subset of patients with a better prognosis, survival was significantly ($P = 0.03$) improved at 2 and 3 years (78% vs. 55% and 60% vs. 36%, respectively).[60] These results suggest that there may be some survival benefit of LMWH in patients with cancer, particularly those at early stages of malignancy.[61]

Although there is some evidence that LMWH therapy may lead to fewer bleeding complications than observed with UFH, results from clinical studies have been inconsistent, and bleeding remains an important safety concern associated with LMWH, particularly when it is used at higher doses.[50,51,53,62–65] Advantages of LMWH over UFH

include specific binding to ATIII, better bioavailability at low doses, no monitoring required, and a longer half-life (4 h vs. 0.5–2 h), allowing for once-daily dosing in some patients. However, a long half-life can sometimes be a disadvantage in the case of bleeding complications. In addition, LMWHs are incompletely reversed by protamine sulfate.[66] Other disadvantages of LMWHs include renal excretion, precluding use in patients with renal failure, and increased cost relative to UFH. Furthermore, LMWHs also carry a risk for HIT and should not be used in patients at risk for HIT, although they appear to be associated with a lower incidence than UFH.[49]

NEWER ANTICOAGULANTS: SELECTIVE FACTOR XA INHIBITORS

Fondaparinux is a novel synthetic pentasaccharide that selectively binds to antithrombin III with selective neutralization of factor Xa.[67] It has demonstrated better efficacy than LMWH in VTE prophylaxis following total joint replacement[68–70] and hip fracture surgery[71] and has been evaluated for VTE prophylaxis in patients undergoing general surgery. In the Pentasaccharide in General Surgery Study (PEGASUS) study, the efficacy and safety of postoperative fondaparinux (2.5 mg once daily) was compared with that of the LMWH dalteparin started preoperatively in high-risk abdominal surgery patients.[72] This multicenter, randomized, double-blind study included 2,900 high-risk abdominal surgery patients, in which high risk was defined as patients older than 60 years of age or older than 40 years of age with 1 or more risk factors including cancer, obesity (BMI > 30 for men and 28.6 for women), history of VTE, heart failure (NYHA grade III or IV), chronic obstructive pulmonary disease, or inflammatory bowel disease. PEGASUS showed that the rates of VTE (venographically proven DVT, symptomatic DVT, or fatal or nonfatal PE) up to day 10 among patients treated with fondaparinux and dalteparin were 4.6% and 6.1% ($P = 0.14$), respectively, representing a 24.5% reduction in the incidence of VTE in favor of fondaparinux (Figure 39.4A). At postoperative day 32, symptomatic DVT was seen in 0.8% of patients treated with fondaparinux and 1.0% of patients who received dalteparin. The difference in the incidence of major bleeding between the two treatment groups was not significant (3.4% fondaparinux vs. 2.4% dalteparin, $P = 0.12$). These results demonstrate that fondaparinux is at least as effective as, if not more than, UFH and LMWH in preventing VTE in general surgery patients. Based on this data, fondaparinux was recently approved for VTE prevention in abdominal surgery patients undergoing general anesthesia for more than 45 minutes who are over 40 years of age and have additional risk factors. A post hoc analysis was performed to compare the effects of the two therapies in the 68% of the evaluable study population who underwent surgery for cancer. In the cancer subpopulation, fondaparinux significantly reduced the incidence of VTE compared with dalteparin from 7.7% to 4.7% ($P = 0.02$), representing a 39% reduction in the incidence of VTE (Figure 39.4B). The incidence of major bleeding was similar between groups (3.4% fondaparinux vs. 2.5% dalteparin). These preliminary findings suggest that postoperative fondaparinux is at least as effective and safe as preoperative dalteparin for the prevention of VTE after abdominal surgery, and significantly more effective than dalteparin in cancer patients undergoing the same procedures.

Another advantage of fondaparinux is that, unlike UFH and LMWH, it has not been associated with HIT. Because the fondaparinux molecule does not bind to platelet factor 4, it cannot form the complex that reacts with the platelet-activating antibody and it does not cross-react with HIT antibodies from patients with confirmed type II HIT.[73,74] Fondaparinux has also been shown to be safe for extended prophylaxis (4 weeks) although this was shown in patients who had undergone hip fracture surgery, not in general surgery patients. In addition, because fondaparinux does not interfere with thrombin binding, it has no negative effect on wound healing. Further, fondaparinux has a 17-h half-life, which allows for once-daily dosing and there is no dose alteration required in patients weighing less than 50 kg or renally impaired patients. However, no antidote is available and a long half-life can also be a disadvantage in the case of bleeding complications. Fondaparinux is renally excreted and should not be used in patients with kidney failure and should be avoided in patients undergoing neuraxial anesthesia, as there is the potential for epidural hematoma formation.

In summary, there are a variety of agents available for the prevention of VTE in patients undergoing general surgery. No one agent is optimal for all patients. Different agents should be used in patients at different levels of risk, and patient characteristics and comorbid conditions can make one agent more appropriate than another in a certain patient. The stratification of general surgery patients by risk for VTE can guide surgeons in their selection of appropriate VTE prophylaxis.

RISK STRATIFICATION

The risk for VTE ranges from low to very high in patients undergoing general surgery. Risk category placement is dependent on the presence of factors that influence the risk for VTE, including type of surgery, age, immobilization, and comorbidities. It has been demonstrated that up to 36% of general surgery patients had three or more risk factors, placing them in the high or highest risk groups.[75] These are groups in which pharmacologic VTE prophylaxis is strongly recommended. The number of factors that can influence the risk of VTE and the variety of agents available for VTE prophylaxis can make risk assessment and management difficult.

Risk stratification has been suggested as a means of determining the risk for VTE in patients undergoing surgery and for guiding the selection of appropriate prophylactic measures. Risk assessment models, like the one pictured in Figure 39.1, can be used to assign each patient a total risk factor score, which can then be used to categorize patients into one of four risk categories (low, moderate, high, and

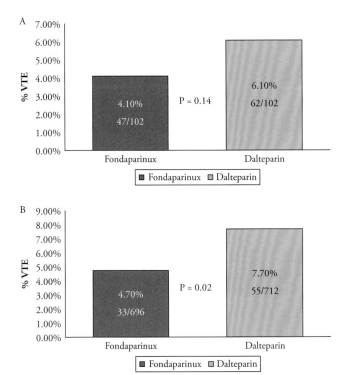

Figure 39.4 (A) VTE reduction with fondaparinux versus dalteparin in high-risk abdominal surgery patients. (B) VTE reduction with fondaparinux versus dalteparin in high-risk abdominal surgery patients with cancer.

highest).[76] An appropriate method of VTE prophylaxis can be chosen based on the patient's level of risk, taking into consideration any contraindications to prophylaxis that may be present (Figure 39.2).

This risk assessment model has recently been validated in a series of 8,216 surgical patients as part of the National Surgical Quality Improvement Program (NSQIP).[22] Patients had risk scores calculated by administrative data using the electronic medical record and these were correlated with clinically evident imaging-proven VTE events at 30 d. Statistically significant correlation of these VTE events with the risk score occurred, including identifying a low-risk group where the risk of anticoagulation is greater than the anticipated clinical incidence of VTE. In those with a very high score (>8), the 30-d proven VTE risk was 6.5%. This score enables the clinician to suggest continuing prophylaxis beyond hospital discharge for these thrombosis-prone individuals.

The incidence of VTE in patients in the low-risk category (one risk factor) is so low that prophylactic measures would most likely not further reduce the risk. Thus, no measures above early and frequent ambulation are recommended in this patient population (Figure 39.2). Elastic stockings and IPC reduce the incidence of DVT to 14% and 3% (Figure 39.3), respectively, and can be used alone in moderate-risk patients (two risk factors). Although IPC has been shown to reduce the incidence of DVT to 3% following general surgery, it has not been extensively studied in general surgery and is not recommended as the sole method of prophylaxis in patients at greater than moderate risk for VTE.

Subcutaneous UFH (5,000 U bid), LMWH (≤3,400 U qd), or fondaparinux (2.5 mg qd) can be used in patients at moderate and high risk (Figure 39.2). In patients at the highest risk for VTE (≥5 risk factors) higher doses of both subcutaneous UFH (5,000 U tid) and LMWH (>3,400 U qd) or fondaparinux (2.5 mg qd) should be used. Although fondaparinux has not been as extensively studied as UFH or LMWHs in general surgery patients, the results of the above-mentioned PEGASUS study suggest that fondaparinux is effective for VTE prophylaxis in this patient population and may be particularly effective in patients in the highest risk category. In addition, for patients at highest risk for VTE, mechanical prophylaxis combined with pharmacologic prophylaxis can be more effective than pharmacologic prophylaxis alone. The recent APOLLO trial results emphasize the value of combined prophylaxis since in that trial the incidence of venographically positive DVT was 1.7% in moderate and high-risk general surgery patients.[42]

As an alternative to a risk assessment model, it has been suggested that appropriate thromboprophylactic measures be used in all but very low risk general surgery patients. In a recent editorial comment, Goldhaber suggests using pharmacological prophylaxis for all hospitalized patients, according to easily implemented protocols. For those patients with contraindications to receive anticoagulants, mechanical methods should be used.[77]

CONCLUSIONS

Although the development of VTE is relatively common in the postoperative setting and is a common cause of sudden postoperative death, VTE prophylaxis remains underutilized. Because VTE is often asymptomatic, or when present, symptoms are nonspecific, surgeons may feel that they do not often see VTE in their practice. However, signs of VTE include leg pain, leg swelling, chest pain, shortness of breath, transient orthostatic hypotension, narcotic excess, fainting spell, hypoxia, sudden death, postoperative stroke, suspected myocardial infarction, PTS at 5 years, and postoperative pneumonia, and most surgeons would agree that many of these conditions are relatively common following surgery.

Due to the significant morbidity and mortality that is associated with VTE, the risk of VTE must be considered in all general surgery patients. In this population, nearly 40% of patients are at high or highest risk for VTE (three or more risk factors) and, therefore, require pharmacologic VTE prophylaxis. Risk stratification schemes may help to guide intensity of clot-preventing measures. Risk stratification schemes like the one in Figure 39.1 may be helpful for assessing VTE risk in general surgery patients. Together with the consideration of any contraindications or precautions, risk stratification can be used to guide surgeons in selection of the optimal prophylactic therapy for each patient.

Clinical data suggest that using nonpharmacologic measures, such as GCS and IPC, can be effective in low and moderate-risk patients and can further enhance protection against VTE in high-risk patients when used in combination with pharmacologic agents. Pharmacologic therapies, including UFH and LMWH, are recommended for use in all high-risk (three or more risk factors) general surgery patients. In addition, fondaparinux is an important treatment option for higher risk patients undergoing abdominal surgery. It has been demonstrated that extended pharmacologic prophylaxis (up to 4 weeks) can significantly reduce the incidence of VTE events compared with prophylaxis for 1 week. Based on these data, it is suggested that high-risk patients receive extended pharmacologic prophylaxis.

UFH is the least expensive pharmacologic agent and is safe for use in patients with renal failure and those undergoing neuraxial anesthesia. However, it is associated with HIT and must be given three times daily in patients at high risk for VTE. LMWH has been shown to be at least as safe and effective as UFH, is associated with a lower incidence of HIT, can be given once or twice daily, and may improve survival in patients with cancer. LMWH should be used with caution in patients with renal failure or in those undergoing neuraxial anesthesia. Prophylactic administration of a novel factor Xa inhibitor, fondaparinux, has been shown to be as safe and at least as effective as UFH and LMWH for the prevention of VTE after abdominal surgery, and significantly more effective than LMWH in cancer surgery patients. In addition, there is an apparent lack of association with HIT with fondaparinux, and it can be given once daily. Fondaparinux has a long half-life, allowing for once-daily dosing, but this can be a disadvantage in the event of bleeding complications. It cannot be used in patients with renal failure or those undergoing neuraxial anesthesia.

There is no one method of VTE prophylaxis that is optimal for every patient. The benefits and risks of each agent should be considered for each patient so that the safest, most effective therapy is initiated. As yet, little is known as to the appropriate duration of these measures; however, in selected patients at high risk for VTE, extended prophylaxis is recommended.

REFERENCES

1. Heit JA, Silverstein MD, Mohr DN, et al. The epidemiology of venous thromboembolism in the community, *Thromb Haemost.* 2001. *86*(1): 452–463.
2. Kakkar VV, Corrigan TP, Fossard DP, et al. Prevention of fatal postoperative pulmonary embolism by low doses of heparin: An international multicentre trial, *Lancet.* 1975. *2*: 45–51.
3. Collins R, Scrimgeour A, Yusuf S, et al. Reduction in fatal pulmonary embolism and venous thrombosis by perioperative administration of subcutaneous heparin: Overview of results of randomized trials in general, orthopaedic, and urologic surgery, *N Engl J Med.* 1988. *318*: 1162–1173.
4. Geerts WH, Heit JA, Clagett GP, et al. Prevention of venous thromboembolism, *Chest.* 2001. *119*: 132S–175S.
5. Silverstein MD, Heit JA, Mohr DN, et al. Trends in the incidence of deep vein thrombosis and pulmonary embolism: A 25-year population-based study, *Arch Intern Med.* 1998. *158*: 585–593.
6. Arcelus JI, Monreal M, Caprini JA, et al. Clinical presentation and time-course of postoperative venous thromboembolism: Results from the RIETE registry, *Thromb Haemost.* 2008. *99*: 546–551.
7. Bratzler DW, Raskob, GE, Murray CK, Bumpus LJ, Piatt DS. Underuse of venous thromboembolism prophylaxis for general surgery patients: Physician practices in the community hospital setting, *Arch Intern Med.* 1998. *158*: 1909–1912.
8. Stratton MA, Anderson FA, Bussey HI, et al. Prevention of venous thromboembolism: Adherence to the 1995 American College of Chest Physicians consensus guidelines for surgical patients, *Arch Intern Med.* 2000. *160*: 334–340.
9. Kakkar AK, Cohen AT, Tapson VF, et al. Venous thromboembolism risk and prophylaxis in the acute care hospital setting (ENDORSE survey): Findings in surgical patients, *Ann Surg.* 2010. *251*: 330–338.
10. Stein PD, Henry JW. Prevalence of acute pulmonary embolism among patients in a general hospital and at autopsy, *Chest.* 1995. *108*: 978–981.
11. Sandler DA, Martin JF. Autopsy proven pulmonary embolism in hospital patients: Are we detecting enough deep vein thrombosis?, *J R Soc Med.* 1989. *82*: 203–205.
12. Prandoni P, Villalta S, Bagatella P, et al. The clinical course of deep vein thrombosis: Prospective long-term follow-up of 528 patients symptomatic patients, *Haematologica.* 1997. *82*: 423–428.
13. Heit JA, Silverstein MD, Mohr DN, et al. Predictors of survival after deep vein thrombosis and pulmonary embolism: A population-based, cohort study, *Arch Intern Med.* 1999. *159*: 445–453.
14. Pengo V, Lensing AWA, Prins MH, et al. Incidence of chronic thromboembolic pulmonary hypertension after pulmonary embolism, *N Engl J Med.* 2004. *350*: 2257–2264.
15. Lechat P, Mas JL, Lascaul G, et al. Prevalence of patent foramen ovale in patients with stroke, *N Engl J Med.* 1988. *318*: 1148–1152.
16. Hagen PT, Scholz DG, Edwards WD. Incidence and size of patent foramen ovale during the first 10 decades of life: An autopsy study of 965 normal hearts, *Mayo Clin Proc.* 1984. *59*: 17–20.
17. Konstantinides S, Geibel A, Kasper W, Olschewski M, Blumel L, Just H. Patent foramen ovale is an important predictor of adverse outcome in patients with major pulmonary embolism, *Circulation.* 1998. *97*: 1946–1951.
18. Nicolaides AN, Irving D. Clinical factors and the risk of deep venous thrombosis. In: Nicolaides AN, ed. *Thromboembolism: Aetiology, advances in prevention and management.* Lancaster, UK: MTP. 1975. 193–204.
19. Clayton JK, Anderson JA, McNicol GP. Preoperative prediction of postoperative deep vein thrombosis, *Br Med J.* 1976. *2*: 910–912.
20. Crandon AJ, Peel KR, Anderson JA, Thompson V, McNicol GP. Postoperative deep vein thrombosis: Identifying high-risk patients, *Br Med J.* 1980. *281*: 343–344.
21. Cofrancesco E, Cortellaro M, Corradi A, Ravasi F, Bertocchi F. Coagulation activation markers in the prediction of venous thrombosis after elective hip surgery, *Thromb Haemost.* 1997. *77*: 267–269.
22. Bahl V, Hu H, Henke PK, Wakefield TW, Campbell DA Jr, Caprini JA. A validation study of a retrospective venous thromboembolism risk scoring method based on the Caprini Risk Assessment Model, *Ann Surg.* 2010. *251*: 344–350.
23. White RH, Zhou H, Romano PS. Incidence of symptomatic venous thromboembolism after different elective or urgent surgical procedures, *Thromb Haemost.* 2003. *90*: 446–455.
24. Heit JA, Silverstein MD, Mohr DN, et al. Risk factors for deep vein thrombosis and pulmonary embolism: A population-based case control study, *Arch Intern Med.* 2000. *160*: 809–815.
25. White RH, Gettner S, Newman JM, Trauner KB, Romano PS. Predictors of rehospitalization for symptomatic venous thromboembolism after total hip arthroplasty, *N Engl J Med.* 2000. *343*(24): 1758–1764.
26. Rickles FR, Levine MN. Epidemiology of thrombosis in cancer, *Acta Haematol.* 2001. *106*(1–2): 6–12.
27. Khorana AA, Connolly GC. Assessing risk of venous thromboembolism in the patient with cancer, *J Clin Oncol.* 2009. *27*: 4839–4847.
28. Bergqvist D. Risk of venous thromboembolism in patients undergoing cancer surgery and options for thromboprophylaxis, *J Surg Oncol.* 2007. *95*: 167–174.
29. Cornuz J, Pearson SD, Creager MA, et al. Importance of findings on the initial evaluation for cancer in patients with symptomatic idiopathic deep venous thrombosis, *Ann Intern Med.* 1996. *125*(10): 785–793.
30. Thodiyil PA, Kakkar AK. Variation in relative risk of venous thromboembolism in different cancers, *Thromb Haemost.* 2002. *87*: 1076–1077.
31. Agnelli G, Bolis G, Capussotti L, et al. A clinical outcome-based prospective study on venous thromboembolism after cancer surgery: The Aristos Project, *Ann Surg.* 2006. *243*: 89–95.
32. Dahlback B. New molecular insights into the genetics of thrombophilia: Resistance to activated protein C caused by Arg506 to Gln mutation in factor V as a pathogenic risk factor for venous thrombosis, *Thromb Haemost.* 1995. *74*: 139–148.
33. Khamashta MA, Cuadrado MJ, Mujic F, Taub NA, Hunt BJ, Hughes GR. The management of thrombosis in the antiphospholipid-antibody syndrome, *N Engl J Med.* 1995. *332*: 993–997.
34. Geerts WH, Bergqvist D, Pineo GF, et al. Prevention of venous thromboembolism: American College of Chest Physicians evidence-based clinical practice guidelines (8th edition), *Chest.* 2008. *133*: 381–453.
35. Roderick P, Ferris G, Wilson K, et al. Towards evidence-based guidelines for the prevention of venous thromboembolism: Systematic

reviews of mechanical methods, oral anticoagulation, dextran, and regional anaesthesia as thromboprophylaxis, *Health Technol Asses.* 2005. *9*(49): iii–iv, ix–x, 1–78.

36. Urbankova J, Quiroz R, Kucher N, Goldhaber SZ. Intermittent pneumatic compression and deep vein thrombosis prevention: A meta-analysis in postoperative patients, *Thromb Haemost.* 2005. *94*(6): 1181–1185.

37. Wells PS, Lensing AWA, Hirsh J. Graduated compression stockings in the prevention of postoperative venous thromboembolism, *Arch Intern Med.* 1994. *154*: 67–72.

38. Amaragiri SV, Lees TA. Elastic compression stockings for prevention of deep vein thrombosis (Cochrane Review), In: *The Cochrane Library*, Issue 2, 2004. Chichester, UK: John Wiley & Sons, Ltd.

39. Borow M, Goldson HJ. Prevention of postoperative deep venous thrombosis and pulmonary emboli with combined modalities, *Am Surg.* 1983. *49*: 599–605.

40. Ramos R, Salem BI, De Pawlikowski MP, Coordes C, Eisenberg S, Leidenfrost R. The efficacy of pneumatic compression stockings in the prevention of pulmonary after cardiac surgery, *Chest.* 1996. *109*: 82–85.

41. Kakkos SK, Caprini J, Nicolaides AN, Reddy D. Combined modalities in the prevention of venous thromboembolism: A review of literature, *Phlebology.* 2006. *21*(Suppl): 1–6.

42. Turpie AG, Bauer KA, Caprini JA, Comp PC, Gent M, Muntz JE. Fondaparinux combined with intermittent pneumatic compression vs. intermittent pneumatic compression alone for prevention of venous thromboembolism after abdominal surgery: A randomized, double-blind comparison, *J Thromb Haemost.* 2007. *5*(9): 1854–1861.

43. McLeod RS, Geerts WH, Sniderman KW, et al. Subcutaneous heparin versus low-molecular-weight heparin as thromboprophylaxis in patients undergoing colorectal surgery: results of the Canadian colorectal DVT prophylaxis trial: A randomized, double-blind trial. *Ann Surg.* 2001. *233*: 438–444.

44. Streiff MB. Vena caval filters: A comprehensive review, *Blood.* 2000. *95*(12): 3669–3677.

45. Decousus H, Leizorovicz A, Parent F, et al. A clinical trial of vena caval filters in the prevention of pulmonary embolism in patients with proximal deep-vein thrombosis: Prevention du Risque d'Embolie Pulmonaire par Interruption Cave Study Group, *N Engl J Med.* 1998. *338*: 409–415.

46. Greenfield LJ, Michna BA. Twelve-year clinical experience with the Greenfield vena caval filter, *Surgery.* 1988. *104*: 706–712.

47. Athanasoulis CA, Kaufman JA, Halpern EF, et al. Inferior vena caval filters: Review of a 26-year single-center clinical experience, *Radiology.* 2000. *216*(1): 54–66.

48. Krauth D, Holden A, Knapic N, et al. Safety and efficacy of long-term oral anticoagulation in cancer patients, *Cancer.* 1987. *59*: 983–985.

49. Warkentin TE, Levine MN, Hirsh J, et al. Heparin-induced thrombocytopenia in patients treated with low-molecular-weight heparin or unfractionated heparin, *N Engl J Med.* 1995. *332*: 1330–1335.

50. Mismetti P, Laporte S, Darmon JY, et al. Meta-analysis of low molecular weight heparin in the prevention of venous thromboembolism in general surgery, *Br J Surg.* 2001. *88*(7): 913–930.

51. ENOXACAN Study Group. Efficacy and safety of enoxaparin versus unfractionated heparin for prevention of deep vein thrombosis in elective cancer surgery: A double-blind randomized multicenter trial with venographic assessment, *Br J Surg.* 1997. *84*: 1099–1103.

52. Bergqvist D, Burmark US, Flordal PA, et al. Low molecular weight heparin started before surgery as prophylaxis against deep vein thrombosis: 2500 versus 5000 XaI units in 2070 patients, *Br J Surg.* 1995. *82*(4): 496–501.

53. Nurmohamed MT, Verhaeghe R, Haas S, et al. A comparative trial of a low molecular weight heparin (enoxaparin) versus standard heparin for the prophylaxis of postoperative deep vein thrombosis in general surgery, *Am J Surg.* 1995. *169*(6): 567–571.

54. Bergqvist D, Agnelli G, Cohen AT, et al. Duration of prophylaxis against venous thromboembolism with enoxaparin after surgery for cancer, *N Engl J Med.* 2002. *346*: 975–980.

55. Bottaro FJ, Elizondo MC, Doti C, et al. Efficacy of extended thrombo-prophylaxis in major abdominal surgery: What does the evidence show? A meta-analysis, *Thromb Haemost.* 2008. *99*(6): 1104–1111.

56. Rasmusen MS, Jorgensen LN, Wille-Jorgensen PW. Prolonged thromboprophylaxis with low molecular weight heparin for abdominal or pelvic surgery, *Cochrane Database Syst Rev.* 2009. *1*: CD004318.

57. von Tempelhoff GF, Harenberg J, Niemann F, Hommel G, Kirkpatrick CJ, Heilmann L. Effect of low molecular weight heparin (Certoparin) versus unfractionated heparin on cancer survival following breast and pelvic cancer surgery: A prospective randomized double-blind trial, *Int J Oncol.* 2000. *16*: 815–824.

58. Green D, Hull RD, Brant R, Pineo GF. Lower mortality in cancer patients treated with low-molecular-weight versus standard heparin, *Lancet.* 1992. *339*: 1476.

59. Hull RD, Raskob GE, Pineo GF, et al. Subcutaneous low-molecular-weight heparin compared with continuous intravenous heparin in the treatment of proximal-vein thrombosis, *N Engl J Med.* 1992. *326*: 975–982.

60. Kakkar AK, Levine MN, Kadziola Z, et al. Low molecular weight heparin, therapy with dalteparin, and survival in advanced cancer: The Fragmin advanced malignancy outcome study (FAMOUS), *J Clin Oncol.* 2004. *22*: 1944–1948.

61. Kuderer N, Ortel TL, Francis CW. Impact of venous thromboembolism and anticoagulation on cancer and cancer survival, *J Clin Oncol.* 2009. *27*: 4902–4911.

62. Verhaeghe R. Comparison of enoxaparin versus unfractionated heparin in general surgery: SURGEX-Study Group, *Eur J Surg.* 1994. *571*(Suppl): 35.

63. Koch A, Bouges S, Ziegler S, Dinkel H, Daures JP, Victor N. Low molecular weight heparin and unfractionated heparin in thrombosis prophylaxis after major surgical intervention: Update of previous meta-analyses, *Br J Surg.* 1997. *84*(6): 750–759.

64. Bergqvist D, Matzsch T, Burmark US, et al. Low molecular weight heparin given the evening before surgery compared with conventional low-dose heparin in prevention of thrombosis, *Br J Surg.* 1988. *75*: 888–891.

65. Bergqvist D, Burmark US, Frisell J, et al. Low molecular weight heparin once daily compared with conventional low-dose heparin twice daily: A prospective double-blind multicentre trial on prevention of postoperative thrombosis, *Br J Surg.* 1986. *73*: 204–208.

66. Sugiyama T, Itoh M, Ohtawa M, Natsuga T. Study on neutralization of low molecular weight heparin (LHG) by protamine sulfate and its neutralization characteristics, *Thromb Res.* 1992. *68*: 119–129.

67. Bauer KA. Fondaparinux sodium: A selective inhibitor of factor Xa, *Am J Health Syst Pharm.* 2001. *58*(Suppl 2): S14–S17.

68. Lassen MR, Bauer KA, Eriksson BI, Turpie AG. Postoperative fondaparinux versus preoperative enoxaparin for prevention of venous thromboembolism in elective hip-replacement surgery: A randomised double-blind comparison, *Lancet.* 2002. *359*: 1715–1720.

69. Turpie AG, Bauer KA, Eriksson BI, Lassen MR. Postoperative fondaparinux versus postoperative enoxaparin for prevention of venous thromboembolism after elective hip-replacement surgery: A randomised double-blind trial, *Lancet.* 2002. *359*: 1721–1726.

70. Bauer KA, Eriksson BI, Lassen MR, Turpie AG. Fondaparinux compared with enoxaparin for the prevention of venous thromboembolism after elective major knee surgery, *N Engl J Med.* 2001. *345*: 1305–1310.

71. Eriksson BI, Bauer KA, Lassen MR, Turpie AG. Fondaparinux compared with enoxaparin for the prevention of venous thromboembolism after hip-fracture surgery, *N Engl J Med.* 2001. *345*: 1298–1304.

72. Agnelli G, Bergqvist D, Cohen AT, Gallus AS, Gent M. Randomized clinical trial of postoperative fondaparinux versus perioperative

dalteparin for prevention of venous thromboembolism in high-risk abdominal surgery, *Br J Surg.* 2005. *92*(10): 1212–1220.

73. Amiral J. [Platelet factor 4, target of anti-heparin antibodies: application to biological diagnosis of heparin-induced thrombopenia]. *Ann Med Intern* (Paris). 1997. *148*(2): 142–149. Review. French.

74. Ahmad S, Walenga JM, Jeske WP, Cella G, Fareed J. Functional heterogeneity of antiheparin-platelet factor 4 antibodies: implications in the pathogenesis of the HIT syndrome. *Clin Appl Thromb Hemost.* 1999. 5 Suppl 1: S32–S37.

75. Anderson FA Jr, Wheeler HB, Goldberg RJ, Hosmer DW, Forcier A. The prevalence of risk factors for venous thromboembolism among hospital patients, *Arch Intern Med.* 1992. *152:* 1660–1664.

76. Caprini JA, Arcelus JI, Reyna JJ. Effective risk stratification of surgical and nonsurgical patients for venous thromboembolic disease, *Semin Hematol.* 2001. *38*(2 Suppl 5): 12–19.

77. Goldhaber SZ. Venous thromboembolism: An ounce of prevention, *Mayo Clin Proc.* 2005. *80:* 725–726.

40.

CONVENTIONAL TREATMENT OF DEEP VENOUS THROMBOSIS

Graham F. Pineo and Russell D. Hull

INTRODUCTION

Deep venous thrombosis (DVT) and/or pulmonary embolism (PE) can be considered manifestations of the same clinical entity, venous thromboembolism (VTE). There is mounting evidence that patients who present with PE have a worse prognosis than do patients who present with symptomatic DVT; recurrence is more likely to be fatal in patients who initially present with PE.[1] Patients who present with symptomatic PE have been shown to have recurrent episodes of PE rather than DVT.[2,3] Apart from these differences, the initial and long-term treatment for patients with either DVT or PE is the same with the possible exception of the use of thrombolytic therapy for patients with submassive or massive PE. Indeed, the recommendations for treatment of DVT and PE are similar in the recent chapter "Antithrombotic Therapy for Venous Thromboembolic Disease" in the ninth ACCP Conference on Anti-Thrombotic and Thrombolytic Therapy.[4]

The objectives for the treatment of patients with VTE are to prevent death from PE, to prevent recurrent VTE, and to prevent the postthrombotic syndrome.

In addition to the significant morbidity and decreased quality of life of patients[5] suffering from severe postthrombotic syndrome, particularly with venous ulcers, this syndrome is associated with very significant health care costs. The use of graduated compression stockings has been shown to significantly decrease the incidence of the postthrombotic syndrome,[6,7] but many patients still do not have these devices prescribed or do not comply with their use. In more recent years more attention has been paid to factors that predispose to the development of the postthrombotic syndrome, which still affects a significant proportion of patients who develop proximal DVT. These factors include recurrent ipsilateral proximal DVT,[8] increased thrombus burden as measured by venography or ultrasonography,[9] poor oral anticoagulant therapy during the treatment period,[10] and early ambulation.[11]

The initial anticoagulant treatment of VTE usually consists of either intravenous or subcutaneous unfractionated heparin (UFH) or low molecular weight heparin (LMWH) with long-term anticoagulation with a Vitamin K antagonist such as warfarin or acencoumarol commencing in conjunction with the heparins. This chapter will review the conventional treatment of VTE.

UNFRACTIONATED HEPARIN THERAPY

HEPARIN THERAPY

Unfractionated heparin has been used extensively to prevent and treat VTE. However, more recently LMWHs have replaced UFH for the treatment of VTE in most cases either entirely or predominantly in the out of hospital setting. However, there are patients in whom UFH by continuous infusion continues to be used primarily because the anticoagulant effect can be reversed by stopping the intravenous infusion and/or administering protamine sulfate.[12] Such patients include critically ill patients in the intensive care unit or cardiovascular unit, patients who may be candidates for interventions requiring interruption of anticoagulant therapy, for example, for surgical procedures or thrombolysis or in patients with severe renal failure.[12] In some countries, UFH is the anticoagulant of choice for patients suffering PE who are hemodynamically unstable.

The anticoagulant activity of UFH depends on a unique pentasaccharide, which binds to antithrombin III (ATIII) and potentiates the inhibition of thrombin and activated factor X (Xa) by ATIII.[12–14] About one-third of all heparin molecules contain the unique pentasaccharide sequence.[12–14] It is the pentasaccharide sequence that confers the molecular high affinity for ATIII.[12–14] In addition, heparin catalyzes the inactivation of thrombin by another plasma cofactor (cofactor II) that acts independently of ATIII.[12]

Heparin has a number of other effects.[13] These include the release of tissue factor pathway inhibitor; binding to numerous plasma and platelet proteins, endothelial cells, and leucocytes; suppression of platelet function; and an increase in vascular permeability. The anticoagulant response to a standard dose of UFH varies widely between patients. This makes it necessary to monitor the anticoagulant response of UFH, using either the activated partial thromboplastin time (APTT) or heparin levels, and to titrate the dose to the individual patient.[12]

The simultaneous use of initial UFH and LMWH has become clinical practice for all patients with VTE who are medically stable.[12] Exceptions include patients who require immediate medical or surgical intervention, such as in thrombolysis or insertion of a vena cava filter, or patients at very high risk of bleeding. Heparin is continued until the international normalized ratio (INR) has been within the therapeutic range (2 to 3) for 2 consecutive days.[12]

It has been established from experimental studies and clinical trials that the efficacy of UFH therapy depends on achieving a critical therapeutic level of UFH within the first 24 h of treatment.[15–17] Data from double blind clinical trials indicate that failure to achieve the therapeutic APTT threshold by 24 h was associated with a 23.3% subsequent recurrent VTE rate, compared with a rate of 4–6% for the patient group who were therapeutic at 24 h.[16,17] The recurrences occurred throughout the 3-month follow-up period and could not be attributed to inadequate oral anticoagulant therapy.[16] The critical therapeutic level of UFH, as measured by the APTT, is 1.5 times the mean of the control value or the upper limit of the normal APTT range.[15–17] This corresponds to a UFH blood level of 0.2 to 0.4 U/ml by the protamine sulfate titration assay, and 0.35 to 0.70 by the antifactor Xa assay. It is vital for each laboratory to establish the minimal therapeutic level of UFH, as measured by the APTT, that will provide a UFH blood level of at least 0.35 U/ml by the antifactor Xa assay for each batch of thromboplastin reagent being used, particularly if a new batch of reagent is provided by a different manufacturer.[12]

Numerous audits of UFH therapy indicate that administration of intravenous UFH is fraught with difficulty, and that the clinical practice of using an ad hoc approach to UFH dose-titration frequently results in inadequate therapy. The use of a prescriptive approach or protocol for administering intravenous UFH therapy has been evaluated in two prospective studies in patients with VTE.[18,19] Both protocols were shown to achieve therapeutic UFH levels in the vast majority of patients. Using the weight-based nomogram there were fewer episodes of recurrent VTE as compared with standard care. Continued use of the weight-based nomogram has been shown to be similarly effective.[20]

Adjusted-dose subcutaneous UFH has been used in initial treatment of VTE.[21] Four randomized clinical trials compared the efficacy of subcutaneous UFH with subcutaneous LMWH in patients with proven VTE.[22–25] Prandoni et al. confirmed the importance of achieving the therapeutic range by 24 h for UFH.[22] Nomograms have been developed for subcutaneous UFH.[26] The largest of these trials compared subcutaneous UFH dose adjusted with the use of APTT by means of a weight-adjusted algorithm with fixed dose LMWH for the initial treatment of patients with VTE, 16% of whom presented with PE.[25] Subcutaneous UFH was shown to be similar to fixed dose LMWH in terms of efficacy and safety.[25]

COMPLICATIONS OF HEPARIN THERAPY

The main adverse effects of UFH therapy include bleeding, thrombocytopenia, and osteoporosis. Patients at particular risk are those who have had recent surgery or trauma, or who have other clinical factors that predispose to bleeding on heparin, such as peptic ulcer, occult malignancy, liver disease, hemostatic defects, weight, age > 65 years, and female gender.

The management of bleeding on heparin will depend on the location and severity of bleeding, the risk of recurrent VTE, and the APTT; heparin should be discontinued temporarily or permanently. Patients with recent VTE may be candidates for insertion of an inferior vena cava filter. If urgent reversal of heparin effect is required, protamine sulfate can be administered.[12]

Heparin-induced thrombocytopenia (HIT) is a well-recognized complication of UFH therapy, usually occurring within 5 to 10 d after heparin treatment has started.[27,28] Approximately 1 to 2% of patients receiving UFH will experience a fall in platelet count to less than the normal range or a 50% fall in the platelet count within the normal range. In the majority of cases, this mild to moderate thrombocytopenia appears to be a direct effect of heparin on platelets and is of no consequence. However, approximately 0.1 to 0.2% of patients receiving UFH develop an immune thrombocytopenia mediated by immunoglobulin G (IgG) antibody directed against a complex of platelet factor 4 (PF4) and heparin.[29] In some cases neutrophil acting peptide 2 (NAP-2) and interlukin 8 (IL-8) also play a role in pathogenesis.

The incidence of HIT is lower with the use of LMWH;[29–31] however the clinical manifestations may be as severe than those seen with UFH.[31,32] Furthermore, the nadirs of the platelet count and onset and duration of thrombocytopenia have been shown to be somewhat different.[32] Recently, delayed onset of HIT has been described with the onset being as long as several weeks after the end of exposure to heparin, thus, making this syndrome sometimes more difficult to diagnose.[33] Furthermore, the incidence and severity of HIT varies among different patient populations, being more prevalent in patients having cardiac or orthopedic procedures than in medical patients.[29] The development of thrombocytopenia may be accompanied by arterial or DVT, which may lead to serious consequences such as death or limb amputation.[23,29]

When a clinical diagnosis of HIT is made, heparin in all forms must be stopped immediately.[27,34] In most centers the confirmatory laboratory test is an ELISA assay for the PF4-heparin complex, but where possible this should be confirmed with a functional assay, such as the serotonin release assay.[27,35] In those patients requiring ongoing anticoagulation, an alternative form of anticoagulation must be undertaken immediately because of the high incidence of thrombosis when heparin is stopped.[35] Some authorities recommend the use of alternative anticoagulants in all patients once a diagnosis is made. The most common alternative agents are the specific antithrombin argatroban[27,36,37] or the direct thrombin inhibitor lepirudin.[27,38,39] Both agents are given by intravenous infusion. Lepirudin is renally excreted[27,38,39] and has the disadvantage that with prolonged use antibodies develop and some of these can have serious deleterious effects, including anaphylaxis.[40–42] Argatroban is metabolized in the liver.[35,36] Both agents can be used in conjunction with vitamin K antagonists, but it should be noted that argatroban by itself increases the INR beyond that observed with warfarin alone, and this must be taken into account in controlling the vitamin K antagonist.[37] The alternative antithrombotic agents should be continued until the platelet count is at least back to 100×10^9/L and/or the INR is therapeutic for 2 consecutive days.[35] Danaparoid has been used in the past but is no longer available for many countries. The pentacharide fondaparinux has been used as an alternative antithrombotic agent in HIT patients and it has the advantage that it is given by a once daily subcutaneous injection.[43,44] Insertion of an inferior vena cava filter is seldom indicated.

Osteoporosis has been reported in patients receiving UFH in dosages of 20,000 U/day (or more) for more than 6 months.[12] Demineralization can progress to the fracture of vertebral bodies or long bones, and the defect may not be entirely reversible.[12] Laboratory and clinical studies indicate that the incidence of osteoporosis with use of long-term LMWH is low.[12]

LMWH FOR THE INITIAL TREATMENT OF VTE

Heparin currently in use clinically is polydispersed unmodified heparin, with a mean molecular weight ranging from 10 to 16 kDa. Low molecular weight derivatives of commercial heparin have been prepared that have a mean molecular weight of 4–5 kDa.[45,46]

The LMWHs commercially available are made by different processes (such as nitrous acid, alkaline, or enzymatic depolymerization) and they differ chemically and pharmacokinetically.[45,46] The clinical significance of these differences, however, is unclear, and there have been very few studies comparing different LMWHs with respect to clinical outcomes.[46] The doses of the different LMWHs have been established empirically and are not necessarily

interchangeable. Therefore, at this time, the effectiveness and safety of each of the LMWHs must be tested separately.[46]

The LMWHs differ from UFH in numerous ways. Of particular importance are the following: increased bioavailability(>90% after subcutaneous injection), prolonged half-life and predictable clearance enabling once- or twice-daily injection, and predictable antithrombotic response based on body weight permitting treatment without laboratory monitoring.[12,45,46] Other possible advantages are their ability to inactivate platelet-bound factor Xa, resistance to inhibition by PF4, and their decreased effect on platelet function and vascular permeability (possibly accounting for less hemorrhagic effects at comparable antithrombotic doses).

Subcutaneous unmonitored LMWH has been compared with continuous intravenous heparin in a number of clinical trials for the treatment of proximal venous thrombosis or PE using long-term follow-up as an outcome measure.[47–54] These studies have shown that LMWH is at least as effective and safe as unfractionated heparin in the treatment of proximal venous thrombosis. Pooling of the most methodologically sound studies indicates a significant advantage for LMWH in the reduction of major bleeding and mortality.[55] LMWH used predominantly out of hospital was as effective and safe as intravenous UFH given in hospital.[52,53,56] Economic analysis of treatment with LMWH versus intravenous heparin demonstrated that LMWH was cost-effective for treatment in hospital[57] as well as out of hospital. As these agents become more widely available for treatment, they have replaced intravenous UFH in the initial management of most patients with VTE. LMWH is now the recommended agent for initial treatment of VTE (ACCP).[4]

There has been a hope that the LMWHs will have fewer serious complications, such as bleeding,[46] heparin-induced thrombocytopenia,[12,27,58] and osteoporosis,[57] when compared with unfractionated heparin. Evidence is accumulating that these complications are indeed less serious and less frequent with the use of LMWH.

Recent reviews suggest the absolute risk for heparin-induced thrombocytopenia with LMWH was 0.2%, and with UFH the rise was 2.6%. Accordingly there is an advantage in this regard using LMWH.[58]

In obese patients the clinician should review the pharmacopeia recommendations for the particular LMWH agent being used concerning dosage guidelines.[12] For patients with significant renal impairment the clinician should review the pharmacopeia guidelines for dosage modifications for the individual LMWH agent. In patients with severe renal failure it may be preferable to use unfractionated heparin.[12]

LONG-TERM LMWH

The use of LMWH for the long-term treatment of acute VTE has been evaluated in randomized clinical trials.[59–61] Two studies[60,61] indicate that long-term treatment with subcutaneous LMWH for 3–6 months is at least as effective as, and in cancer patients more effective than, adjusted doses of oral vitamin K antagonist therapy (INR, 2.0–3.0) for preventing recurrent VTE. LMWH was also associated with less bleeding complications than vitamin K antagonists treatment, because of a reduction in minor bleeding.[61] The ACCP Consensus panel states: "For most patients with deep vein thrombosis and cancer, we suggest treatment with LMWH over vitamin-K antagonist for at least the first 3 months of long-term treatment."[4]

VITAMIN K ANTAGONIST—WARFARIN

The anticoagulant effect of warfarin is mediated by the inhibition of the vitamin K-dependent γ-carboxylation of coagulation factors II, VII, IX, and X.[62,63] This results in the synthesis of immunologically detectable but biologically inactive forms of these coagulation proteins. Warfarin also inhibits the vitamin K–dependent γ-carboxylation of proteins C and S. Protein C circulates as proenzyme that is activated on endothelial cells by the thrombin-thrombomodulin complex to form activated protein C. Activated protein C in the presence of protein S inhibits activated factor VIII and activated factor V activity.[62,63] Therefore, vitamin K antagonists such as warfarin create a biochemical paradox by producing an anticoagulant effect through the inhibition of procoagulants (factors II, VII, IX, and X) and a potentially thrombogenic effect by impairing the synthesis of naturally occurring inhibitors of coagulation (proteins C and S). Heparin and warfarin treatment should overlap by 4–5 d when warfarin treatment is initiated in patients with thrombotic disease.[63]

The anticoagulant effect of warfarin is delayed until the normal clotting factors are cleared from the circulation, and the peak effect does not occur until 36–72 hours after drug administration.[63] During the first few days of warfarin therapy the prothrombin time (PT) reflects mainly the depression of factor VII, which has a half-life of 5–7 h.[64,65] Equilibrium levels of factors II, IX, and X are not reached until about 1 week after the initiation of therapy.[65] The use of small initial daily doses (e.g., 5–10 mg) is the preferred approach for initiating warfarin treatment.[63,66,67]

The dose-response relationship to warfarin therapy varies widely between individuals and, therefore, the dose must be carefully monitored to prevent overdosing or underdosing. A number of drugs interact with warfarin.[62,63] Critical appraisal of the literature reporting such interactions indicates that the evidence substantiating many of the claims is limited.[68] Nonetheless, patients must be warned against taking any new drugs without the knowledge of their attending physician.[69]

LABORATORY MONITORING AND THERAPEUTIC RANGE

The laboratory test most commonly used to measure the effects of warfarin is the one-stage PT test. The PT is sensitive to reduced activity of factors II, VII, and X but is insensitive to reduced activity of factor IX. Confusion about the appropriate therapeutic range has occurred because the different tissue thromboplastins used for measuring the PT vary considerably in sensitivity to the vitamin K–dependent clotting factors and in response to warfarin.[70,71]

To promote standardization of the PT for monitoring oral anticoagulant therapy, the World Health Organization (WHO) developed an international reference thromboplastin from human brain tissue and recommended that the PT ratio be expressed as the *international normalized ratio* or INR.[63] The INR is the PT ratio obtained by testing a given sample using the WHO reference thromboplastin. For practical clinical purposes, the INR for a given plasma sample is equivalent to the PT ratio obtained using a standardized human brain thromboplastin known as the Manchester Comparative Reagent, which has been widely used in the UK.[63]

Warfarin is administered in an initial dose of 5 to 10 mg per day for the first 2 days. The daily dose is then adjusted according to the INR.[66,67] Heparin therapy is discontinued on the 4th or 5th day following initiation of warfarin therapy, provided the INR is prolonged into the recommended therapeutic range (INR 2 to 3).[63] Because some individuals are either fast or slow metabolizers of the drug, the selection of the correct dosage of warfarin must be individualized. Therefore, frequent INR determinations are required initially to establish therapeutic anticoagulation.

Once the anticoagulant effect and patient's warfarin dose requirements are stable, the INR should be monitored at regular intervals throughout the course of warfarin therapy for VTE. However, if there are factors that may produce an unpredictable response to warfarin (e.g., concomitant drug therapy), the INR should be monitored frequently to minimize the risk of complications due to poor anticoagulant control.[63] Several warfarin nomograms and computer software programs are now available to assist care givers in the control of warfarin therapy. Also, there is increasing interest in the use of self-testing with portable INR monitors and, in selective cases, self-management of oral anticoagulant therapy.[63]

LONG-TERM TREATMENT OF VTE USING VITAMIN K ANTAGONISTS

Patients with established venous thrombosis or PE require long-term anticoagulant therapy to prevent recurrent disease. Vitamin K-antagonist therapy is highly effective[4,63] and is preferred in most but not all patients Adjusted-dose, subcutaneous heparin or body weight adjusted LMWHs have been used for the long-term treatment of patients in whom oral anticoagulant therapy proves to be very difficult to control,[59] and LMWH is the preferred treatment in patients with DVT and cancer.[4,60,61]

The preferred intensity of the anticoagulant effect of treatment with vitamin K antagonists has been confirmed by the results of randomized trials.[63,71] The results of two recent randomized trials[72,73] indicate that although low-intensity warfarin therapy is more effective than placebo, it is less effective than standard-intensity therapy (INR 2–3), and does not reduce the incidence of bleeding complications.[72,73] Additional important evidence regarding the intensity of anticoagulant therapy with vitamin K antagonists is provided by a recent randomized trial by Crowther et al.,[74] who compared standard-intensity warfarin therapy (INR 2–3) with high-intensity warfarin therapy (INR 3.1–4.0) for the prevention of recurrent thromboembolism in patients with persistently positive antiphospholipid antibodies and a history of thromboembolism (venous or arterial). The high-intensity warfarin therapy (INR 3.1–4.0) did not provide improved antithrombotic protection. The high-intensity regimen has been previously shown to be associated with a high risk (20%) of clinically important bleeding in a series of randomized trials[74–76] in patients with DVT. The evidence outlined above provides the basis for the recommendation of an INR of 2.0–3.0 as the preferred intensity of anticoagulant treatment with vitamin K antagonists.

The safety of oral anticoagulant treatment depends heavily on the maintenance of a narrow therapeutic INR range.[63,77] The importance of maintaining careful control of oral anticoagulant therapy is evident and may be enhanced with the use of anticoagulant management clinics if oral anticoagulants are going to be used for extended periods of time.[63]

DURATION OF ANTICOAGULANT THERAPY AND RECURRENT VTE

The appropriate duration of oral anticoagulant treatment for VTE using a vitamin K antagonist has been evaluated by multiple randomized clinical trials.[4,78–84] Treatment should be continued for at least 3 months in patients with a first episode of proximal vein thrombosis or PE secondary to a transient (reversible) risk factor (grade 2C).[4] Stopping treatment at 4 to 6 weeks resulted in an increased incidence of recurrent VTE during the following 6 to 12 months (absolute risk increase 8%). In contrast, treatment for 3 to 6 months resulted in a low rate of recurrent VTE during the following 1 to 2 years (annual incidence 3%).

Patients with a first episode of idiopathic VTE should be treated for at least 3 months[4] (grade 2B), and considered for indefinite anticoagulant therapy. This decision should be individualized, taking into consideration the estimated risk of recurrent VTE, risk of bleeding, and patient compliance and preference. Indefinite therapy is recommended for patients in whom risk factors for bleeding are absent and in whom good anticoagulant control can be achieved (grade 1B).[4] If indefinite anticoagulant treatment is given, the risk-benefit of continuing such treatment should be reassessed at periodic intervals.

A variety of prothrombotic conditions or markers reportedly are associated with an increased risk of recurrent VTE. These conditions include deficiencies of the naturally occurring inhibitors of coagulation such as antithrombin, protein C, and protein S, specific gene mutations including Factor V Leiden and prothrombin 20210A, elevated levels of coagulation factor VIII, elevated levels of homocysteine, and the presence of antiphospholipid antibodies. The presence of residual DVT assessed by compression ultrasonography,[85–87] elevated levels of plasma D-dimer after discontinuation of anticoagulant treatment,[88–89] and male gender[90,91] have been associated with an increased incidence of recurrent thromboembolism. No randomized trials have been performed, a priori, in these subgroups of patients with thrombophilic conditions to evaluate the risk-benefit of different durations of anticoagulant treatment, so no definitive recommendations can be made.

For patients with a first episode of VTE and documented antiphospholipid antibodies or two or more thrombophilic conditions (e.g., combined Factor V Leiden and prothrombin 20210A gene mutations), indefinite anticoagulant treatment should be considered.[4] For patients with a first episode of VTE who have documented deficiency of antithrombin, protein C, or protein S, or the Factor V Leiden or prothrombin 20210A gene mutation, hyperhomocysteinemia, or high factor VIII levels (>90th percentile), the duration of treatment should be individualized after the patients have completed at least 3 months of anticoagulant therapy. Some of these patients also may be candidates for indefinite therapy.[4]

Oral vitamin K antagonist treatment should be given indefinitely for most patients with a second episode of unprovoked VTE[4] (grade 1B), because stopping treatment at 3 to 6 months in these patients results in a high incidence (21%) of recurrent VTE during the following 4 years. The risk of recurrent thromboembolism during 4-year follow-up was reduced by 87% (from 21% to 3%) by continuing anticoagulant treatment; this benefit is partially offset by an increase in the cumulative incidence of major bleeding (from 3% to 9%).[81]

Use of LMWH for long-term treatment of VTE has been evaluated in clinical trials.[59–61] The studies indicate that long-term treatment with subcutaneous LMWH for 3 to 6 months is at least as effective as, and in cancer patients is more effective than, an oral vitamin K antagonist adjusted to maintain the INR between 2.0 and 3.0. LMWH also was associated with less bleeding complications because of a reduction in minor bleeding. Therefore, patients with VTE and concurrent cancer should be treated with LMWH for the first 3 to 6 months of long-term treatment (grade 2B).[4,60,61] The patients then should receive anticoagulation indefinitely or until the cancer resolves. The regimens of LMW heparin that are established as effective for long-term treatment are dalteparin 200 U/kg once daily for 1 month, followed by 150 U/kg daily thereafter, or tinzaparin 175 U/kg once daily.

ADVERSE EFFECTS OF ORAL ANTICOAGULANTS

The major side effect of oral anticoagulant therapy is bleeding.[63,70,77] A number of risk factors have been identified that predispose to bleeding on oral anticoagulants.[77,92,93] The most important factor influencing bleeding risk is the intensity of the INR[70,77,92,93] Other factors include a history of bleeding, previous history of stroke or myocardial infarction, hypertension, renal failure, diabetes, and a decreased hematocrit.[92] Efforts have been made to quantify the bleeding risk according to these underlying clinical factors.[92,93] Introduction of a multicomponent intervention combining patient education and alternative approaches to the maintenance of INR resulted in a reduced frequency of major bleeding in the patients in this group.[92] Furthermore, patients in the intervention group were within the therapeutic INR a significantly greater amount of time than were patients in the standard care group. In a retrospective cohort study of patients with an INR greater than 6.0, it was shown that a prolonged delay in the return of the INR to the therapeutic range was seen in patients who had an INR over 4.0 when two doses of warfarin were withheld, patients with an extreme elevation of the INR, and older age patients, particularly those with a decompensated congestive heart failure and active cancer.[93] Numerous randomized clinical trials have demonstrated that clinically important bleeding is higher when the targeted INR increases above 4.5 or 5.[70,93,94] There is a strong negative relationship between the percentage of time that patients are within the targeted INR and both bleeding and recurrent thrombosis.

Oral anticoagulant therapy in elderly patients presents further problems.[95,96] Many of these patients require long-term anticoagulants because of their underlying clinical conditions that increase with age, while they are more likely to have underlying causes for bleeding including the development of cancer, intestinal polyps, renal failure, and stroke, and they are more prone to having frequent falls. The daily requirements for warfarin to maintain the therapeutic INR also decreases with age, presumably because of decreased clearance of the drug. Therefore, before initiating oral anticoagulant treatment in elderly patients, the risk/benefit ratio of treatment must be considered. If they are placed on oral anticoagulant therapy, careful attention to the INR is required.

Patients with cancer are more likely to bleed on oral anticoagulant treatment.[97] Compared with patients on oral anticoagulants who do not have cancer, patients with cancer have a higher incidence of both major and minor bleeding and anticoagulant withdrawal is more frequently due to bleeding. Patients with cancer have a higher thrombotic complication rate and a higher bleeding rate regardless of the INR, whereas bleeding in noncancer patients was seen only when the INR was greater than 4.5. Safer and more effective anticoagulant therapy is required for the treatment of VTE in patients with cancer.[97]

MANAGEMENT OF OVERANTICOAGULATION

The approach to the patient with an elevated INR depends on the degree of elevation of the INR and the clinical circumstances.[63,98,99] Options available to the physician include temporary discontinuation of warfarin treatment, administration of vitamin K[99,100] or administration of blood products such as fresh frozen plasma (FFP) or prothrombin concentrate[101] to replace the vitamin K–dependent clotting factors, or administration of activated Factor VII.[102] If the increase is mild and the patient is not bleeding, no specific treatment is necessary other than reduction in the warfarin dose. The INR can be expected to decrease during the next 24 h with this approach. With more marked increase of the INR in patients who are not bleeding, treatment with small doses of vitamin K, (e.g., 1 mg), given either orally or by subcutaneous injection should be considered.[98–100] With very marked increase of the INR, particularly in a patient who is either actively bleeding or at risk for bleeding, the coagulation defect should be corrected. Vitamin K can be given intravenously slowly, subcutaneously, or orally.[98–100] Where possible, the oral route is preferred. If ongoing anticoagulation with warfarin is planned, then repeated small doses of vitamin K should be given so that there is no problem with warfarin resistance.[63,98]

FFP remains the most widely used factor replacement for more urgent reversal of warfarin, but it takes time to thaw and for cross-matching if group-specific plasma is to be given.[98] Anticoagulation can be more rapidly reversed with the use of prothrombin complex concentrates given intravenously.[98,101] Recombinant activated Factor VII has been used to control life-threatening bleeding, especially where other more effective agents are not readily available.[98,102]

Coumarin-induced skin necrosis is a rare but serious complication that requires immediate cessation of oral anticoagulant therapy.[98] It usually occurs between 3 and 10 d after therapy has commenced, is commoner in women, and most often involves areas of abundant subcutaneous tissues, such as the abdomen, buttocks, thighs, and breast. The mechanism of coumarin-induced skin necrosis, which is associated with microvascular thrombosis, is uncertain but appears to be related, at least in some patients, to depression of the protein C level. Patients with congenital deficiencies of protein C may be particularly prone to the development of coumarin skin necrosis.

MANAGEMENT OF PATIENTS ON LONG-TERM ORAL ANTICOAGULANTS REQUIRING SURGICAL INTERVENTION

Physicians are commonly confronted with the problem of managing oral anticoagulants in individuals who require temporary interruption of treatment for surgery or other invasive procedures. In the absence of data from randomized clinical trials, recommendations can only be made based on cohort studies, retrospective reviews, and expert opinions.[103–105] The most common conditions requiring long-term anticoagulant therapy are atrial fibrillation, mechanical or prosthetic heart valve replacement, and VTE. For each of these conditions, the risk of arterial thromboembolism or VTE when anticoagulants have been discontinued must be weighed against the risk of bleeding if UFH or LMWH is applied before or after the surgical procedure, or if oral anticoagulant therapy is continued at the therapeutic level.[106–109] The possible choices based on the risk-benefit assessment in the individual patient include (1) discontinuing warfarin for 3–5 d before the procedure to allow the INR to return to normal and then restarting therapy shortly after surgery, (2) lowering the warfarin dose to maintain an INR in the lower or subtherapeutic range during the surgical procedure, and (3) discontinuing warfarin and treating the patient with LMWH before and after the surgical procedure, until warfarin therapy can be reinstituted.[109]

ANTICOAGULANT THERAPY DURING PREGNANCY

LMWH does not cross the placenta, and these agents have become the treatment of choice for VTE in pregnancy and LMWH is recommended over UFH for both prevention and treatment of VTE in pregnancy.[110] Data from retrospective studies and systematic reviews indicate that the risk of bleeding and recurrent thrombosis is low and the development of osteoporosis with these agents is less than is seen with UFH.[110–113] Also, the risk of HIT is lower with LMWH.[110] There is still some uncertainty whether the regimens for LMWH established as effective for initial and long-term therapy in nonpregnant patients, who do not require anticoagulant monitoring, can be generalized to pregnant patients. While some studies indicate that there are no major changes in the peak anti-Xa levels over the course of pregnancy in most patients treated with therapeutic LMWH regimens,[114] others advocate periodic measurement of factor Xa levels with dose adjustment to maintain therapeutic anti-Xa levels.[115,116] Evidence-based guidelines for antithrombotic therapy during pregnancy are available.[110]

In patients treated with adjusted-dose LMWH or UFH, therapy should be discontinued 24 h before induction of labor or cesarean section.[110] Following delivery patients with acute VTE during pregnancy should receive warfarin therapy for a minimum total duration of three months.[110]

FONDAPARINUX AND RELATED COMPOUNDS

Fondaparinux, a synthetic indirect inhibitor of factor Xa which markedly increases the activity of antithrombin, has been studied in a wide variety of patients for the prevention and treatment of VTE. Fondaparinux is rapidly absorbed following subcutaneous injection.[116] The elimination half-life is 17–21 h in healthy subjects and is prolonged in patients over the age of 75 years. About 77% of the drug is excreted unchanged in the urine, and drug levels increase with increasing renal impairment.[116] Therefore fondaparinux is contraindicated in patients with severe renal insufficiency (creatinine clearance [CrCL] < 30 ml/minute) and should be used with caution in anyone with mild-moderate renal failure. It should also be used with caution in patients weighing less than 50 Kg. and in those over age 75. Based on the results of clinical trials, fondaparinux has been approved as a substitute for UFH or LMWH for the initial treatment of VTE.[117,118] Fondaparinux has not replaced LMWH for the initial treatment of VTE in most countries mainly because of the prolonged half-life, the concern about using it in patients with renal insufficiency, and the fact that the anticoagulant effect cannot be blocked. Fondaparinux has been used off label for the treatment of HIT.[44]

NEW ORAL ANTICOAGULANTS

Recently, there has been much interest in developing new oral antithrombotic agents that may be able to replace Warfarin. The most advanced agents are specific inhibitors of activated factor X (Factor Xa) or thrombin (factor 2).[119,120] These agents have the advantage that they can be given by the oral route once or twice daily and they require no laboratory monitoring, and in most cases the same dose is taken by all patients. The agents most advanced are the Factor Xa inhibitors rivaroxaban (Xarelto, Bayer/Johnson and Johnson) and apixaban (Eliquis, BMS/Pfizer) and the thrombin inhibitor (2A inhibitor) dabigatran etexilate (Pradaxa/Pradaxa, Boehringer-Ingelheim International).

Factor Xa Inhibitors

Rivaroxaban
Rivaroxaban is a direct inhibitor of Factor Xa.[119,121] It has about 80% absorbability with peak blood levels appearing in 2–3 h. The terminal half-life is 7–11 h. About 30% of rivaroxaban is eliminated unchanged by the kidneys, one-third is metabolized by the liver via CYP3A4-dependent and CYP3A4-independent pathways and excreted in feces, and the remainder is metabolized to inactive metabolites.[121,122] Following oral dosing of rivaroxaban there is a direct relationship between pharmacodynamic effects and the degree of renal impairment.[122] Therefore, rivaroxaban should be used with caution in patients with moderate renal impairment, CrCL of 30–49 ml/min, and is contraindicated in patients with CrCL < 30 ml/min.[121] Inhibitors of CYP3A4 and P-glycoprotein can increase the drug concentration of rivaroxaban and are contraindicated. The pharmacokinetic/pharmacodynamic (PK/PD) profile of rivaroxaban is predictable and dose-dependent. There is no change in PK/PD

with age, body weight, and gender. In clinical trials there has been no evidence of liver or other toxicity and no increase in the incidence of vascular events such as myocardial infarction, stroke, or peripheral disorders.[121,122]

Rivaroxaban prolongs the APTT and PT in an unpredictable fashion, and these laboratory tests cannot be used for monitoring drug effect.[123,124] The most reliable test for detecting drug levels when required, for example, if urgent surgical intervention is required or to check for drug compliance, is a modified PT using an PT reagent that has been calibrated for rivaroxaban such as neoplastin.[124] There is no specific blocker for rivaroxaban at this time, although search for an antibody with these properties is underway.[121] Various agents like FFP or Factor VIIa do not reverse the anticoagulant effect of rivaroxaban, but at least in healthy individuals, the infusion of prothrombin complex concentrates (PCCs) can effectively correct the abnormal coagulation tests.[125,126] It has yet to be shown that PCCs are effective in stopping bleeding in human patients who are actively bleeding.

Apixaban

Apixaban is a direct inhibitor of Factor Xa with an oral availability of approximately 50% for doses up to 10 mg. Peak levels of apixaban appear in 3–4 h, about 87% of the drug is protein-bound and the terminal half-life is 8–12 h.[119,127] As with rivaroxaban, apixaban inhibits both free and clot-bound Factor Xa. Multiple routes of elimination of apixaban include renal excretion of about 27% with the rest being mainly oxidative metabolism via the hepatic/gastrointestinal route.[128,129] As with rivaroxaban, potent inhibitors of the CYP3A4 and P-glycoprotein pathways such as ketoconazole and ritonavir are contraindicated, but there are no other major drug interactions.[127,130] Apixaban dose adjustment is not required in patients with mild-moderate renal impairment, but it is contraindicated in patients with severe impairment (i.e., CrCL 15–29 ml/min).[127] No dose adjustments are required for age (>65 years) or for weight.[127] In clinical trials there has been no evidence of hepatic or other toxicities and no increase in the incidence of myocardial infarction or stroke.[127]

The most reliable laboratory test for apixaban drug effect is the modified PT using a reagent that is calibrated for apixaban as for rivaroxaban.[124,131] There is no specific inhibitor for apixaban. As with rivaroxaban, infusion of either FFP or Factor VIIa is not effective. Although PCCs have not been studied in humans it is anticipated that they should have the same benefit as with rivaroxaban.[126]

Factor 2a Inhibitor

Dabigatran etexilate is a prodrug with an oral availability of about 6.5%.[119,132] After absorption, dabigatran etexilate is rapidly converted in the liver to dabigatran. Peak blood levels are seen within 2 h, and the terminal half-life is 14–17 h. Dabigatran is eliminated primarily via the kidneys, with about 80% of the drug being excreted unchanged in the urine.[132–134] Dabigatran has predictable PK/PD profiles with no influence of weight or gender and no food interactions.[119,132–134] Dabigatran is not metabolized by the CYP3A4 pathway, but inhibitors or inducers of P-glycoprotein can affect drug levels. Drugs like amiodarone, verapamil, and clarithramycin should either not be used or used with caution. Because of the high proportion of dabigatran excreted by the kidney, the drug is contraindicated in patients with a CrCL < 30 ml/min and should be used with caution in those with CrCL of 30–49 ml/min. It is recommended that CrCL measurements be made before starting dabigatran and periodically during treatment, particularly in elderly patients with borderline renal function.[132,134–135]

Dabigatran treatment has been complicated by troublesome dyspepsia, which has led to discontinuation of therapy in some of the clinical trials with this agent as compared with warfarin.[136] Taking the drug with food has been helpful in reducing this problem. There has been the suggestion that tartaric acid contained in the capsule with the purpose of enhancing absorption by lowering the pH in the stomach may contribute to the development of dyspepsia and the higher incidence of bleeding from the upper gastrointestinal tract that has also been observed. Patients taking dabigatran have also had a higher incidence of lower gastrointestinal tract bleeding, which may be related to the high concentration of active dabigatran that is excreted in the feces.[135] A higher rate of myocardial infarction has been observed in clinical trials of dabigatran as compared with warfarin or enoxaparin treatment.[136,137] A meta-analysis of seven clinical trials involving dabigatran supported the findings of individual trials.[138] A secondary analysis of a Phase III trial with dabigatran (Re-LY) in patients with atrial fibrillation showed that patients with a history of coronary artery disease did not have a higher risk of events while on dabigatran than those patients without such a history.[139] Since the widespread use of dabigatran for the prevention of stroke in atrial fibrillation there have been reports of excessive bleeding in the medical literature as well as concern about not being able to block the anticoagulant effect of the drug in cases of trauma or patients experiencing severe bleeding. Patients who are elderly and who have borderline renal function that may deteriorate rapidly seem to be most at risk for excessive bleeding.

There is no specific blocker of the anticoagulant effect of dabigatran at this time.[132] There is promising evidence that an antibody developed against dabigatran and a hapten can rapidly and completely reverse the anticoagulant effect of dabigatran in experimental animals after intravenous infusion.[140] The administration of FFP, PCCs, and Factor VIIa[126,132] has no benefit, but a clinical trial demonstrated that hemodialysis for 2 h could decrease the dabigatran blood levels by 60%.[141] Therefore, at this time hemodialysis is the only effective treatment in patients on dabigatran who experience uncontrolled bleeding or require emergency surgery. The blood test best suited for detecting the drug effect of dabigatran is the dilute thrombin time, and this test should be available in most treatment centers.[142]

When any of these drugs must be discontinued for periprocedural reasons such as surgery or insertion of a pacemaker it is recommended that the drug should be stopped in time to allow 4–5 drug half-lives before surgery, particularly if no or minimal drug effect is required.[125] For dabigatran that would be 3 d before surgery if the CrCL is >50 ml/min and 4–5 d for a CrCL 30–49 ml/min. For rivaroxaban and apixaban, in patients with mild or moderate renal impairment (CrCL > 50 ml/min), the last dose would be 3 d before surgery.[125] In patients where mild-moderate anticoagulant effect may be acceptable the drug may be continued for an extra day before discontinuing. When the drugs are to be resumed it is recommended that they be delayed for 48 h after major surgery and 24 h after minor surgery. In all cases a determination of the risk of thrombosis must be weighed against the risk of bleeding.[125]

In patients undergoing total hip or total knee replacement surgery all of these new oral agents have been compared with enoxaparin either 40 mg once daily beginning 12 h prior to surgery, or 30 mg twice a day beginning 12–24 h postoperatively.[143–149] These procedures carry a high risk for VTE, and because of the nature of the procedure there is a significant risk of bleeding. Therefore agents that can be shown to be effective and safe in this setting show promise for the prevention and treatment of VTE in other settings. To date clinical trials in patients undergoing total hip or total knee replacement with the Factor Xa inhibitors rivaroxiban (Bayer Health Care)[143–145] and apixaban (BMS-Pfizer)[147–149] and the anti-factor 2a agent dabigatran (Boehringer-Ingelheim) have been published.[146] Rivaroxiban, apixaban, and dabigatran have been approved by a number of agencies and are used in a number of countries; rivaroxaban has been approved by the FDA for the prevention of VTE following total hip or knee replacement.

All three agents have been compared to standard vitamin K antagonist therapy for the prevention of stroke in atrial fibrillation (AF)[150–152] and for the initial and/or extended treatment of VTE.[153–156] At this time dabigatran and rivaroxaban are available for use in several countries for the prevention of stroke in AF, and apixaban is under review by the regulatory agencies. Dabigatran and rivaroxaban are under review for the treatment of DVT and PE.

In the RECOVER study, dabigatran etexilate 150 mg bid was compared with standard Warfarin therapy with an INR target of 2–3.[153] In patients presenting with VTE who had an initial course of parenteral therapy usually with LMWH for 8–11 d. Treatment continued for 6 months and there was a follow up of 30 d. Dabigatran was shown to be noninferior to standard therapy in the prevention of recurrent VTE or VTE related death, and the incidence of major bleeding was comparable. However, the incidence of combined major and nonmajor, clinically relevant bleeding was significantly less with dabigatran.[153] Two studies on the extended treatment of VTE with dabigatran showed that the results for efficacy and safety can be extrapolated to another 16 months (mean) of treatment (RE-MEDY)[154] and that dabigatran reduces the risk of recurrence by 90% compared to placebo (RE-SONATE).[155] In the latter case there was an increase in clinically relevant bleeding.

In the EINSTEIN DVT and PE studies, rivaroxaban 15 mg bid for 3 weeks followed by 20 mg/d was compared with standard warfarin therapy with an INR target of 2–3.[156,157] There was no initial use of LMWH in the rivaroxaban arm, although patients were ineligible if they had received a therapeutic dose of LMWH, fondaparinux, or UFH for more than 48 h or if they had received more than a single dose of a vitamin K antagonist before randomization. Treatment continued for 3, 6, or 12 months. In the EINSTEIN-DVT trial rivaroxaban was shown to be noninferior to warfarin in the prevention of recurrent VTE with similar bleeding rates.[156] In parallel, rivaroxaban was compared with placebo in the prevention of recurrent VTE for an additional 6–12 months in patients who had completed 6–12 months treatment of VTE.[126] Rivaroxaban significantly reduced the incidence of recurrent VTE, but there was increased (nonsignificant) major bleeding.[156]

In the EINSTEIN-PE study rivaroxaban was shown to be noninferior to warfarin in the prevention of recurrent VTE.[157] The rates of the principal safety end point of the composite of major and nonmajor, clinically relevant bleeding were similar, but the rates of major bleeding alone were significantly reduced by rivaroxaban.[157]

THROMBOLYSIS AND/OR MECHANICAL FRAGMENTATION FOR THE TREATMENT OF PROXIMAL DVT

In the past there has been a limited role for the use of systemic thrombolysis in the treatment of DVT.[98] More recently clinical trials on the use of catheter-directed thrombolysis (CDT) with or without mechanical thrombus fragmentation in patients with extensive iliofemoral venous thrombosis have been shown to improve vein patency and venous valve function in the initial and follow-up period in a number of these patients.[158–161] There is also evidence that CDT can reduce the incidence of the postthrombotic syndrome and improve quality of life in these patients.[98,161] Finally, operative thrombectomy has been shown to improve vein patency with less leg swelling and fewer venous ulcers compared with anticoagulation alone.[162] Patients who are candidates for these more invasive approaches to therapy include those with ileofemoral DVT of <14 days' duration particularly if venous gangrene is imminent, good functional status, and low risk of bleeding. In all circumstances the initial treatment is followed by long-term anticoagulant therapy.[98,162] CDT may cause less major bleeding and in particular lower incident of intercranial hemorrhage than systemic thrombolysis, but further studies are required. At this time the ACCP recommendation is for anticoagulation therapy alone over CDT, systemic thrombolysis, or venous thrombectomy.[98]

INFERIOR VENA CAVA FILTER

Insertion of a removable or permanent inferior vena cava (IVC) filter is indicated for patients with acute VTE and an absolute contraindication to anticoagulant therapy or in some patients with objectively documented recurrent VTE during adequate anticoagulant therapy.[4,163–167] Although IVC filters have not been shown to decrease mortality, they can effectively prevent important PE.[98,163,164] In follow-up studies, although there is a decreased incidence of PE, there is an increased incidence of recurrent DVT and IVC filter thrombosis in patients with indwelling IVC filters.[98,166] There is also evidence that IVC filter use may increase the incidence of the postthrombotic syndrome.[168] Long-term anticoagulant therapy should be started as soon as safely possible after placement of an IVC filter and continued for the duration of treatment as for patients without an IVC filter.[4,98]

REFERENCES

1. Douketis JD, Foster GA, Crowther MA, et al. Clinical risk factors and timing of recurrent venous thromboembolism during the initial 3 months of anticoagulant therapy, *Arch Intern Med.* 2000. *160*: 3431–3436.
2. Douketis JD, Kearon C, Bates B, Duk EK, Ginsberg JS. Risk of fatal pulmonary embolism in patients with treated venous thromboembolism, *JAMA.* 1998. *279*: 458–462.
3. Heit JA, Mohr DN, Silverstein MD, et al. Predictors of recurrence after deep vein thrombosis and pulmonary embolism: A population-based cohort study, *Arch Intern Med.* 2000. *160*: 761–768.
4. Kearon C, Akl EA, Comerota AJ, et al. Antithrombotic therapy for venous thromboembolic disease: American College of Chest Physicians Evidence-Based Clinical Practice Guidelines (9th Edition), *Chest.* 2012. *141*(2): e419S–e494S.
5. Kahn SR, M'Lan CE, Lamping DL, et al. The influence of venous thromboembolism on quality of life and severity of chronic venous disease, *J Thromb Haemost.* 2004. *2*: 2146–2151.
6. Brandjes DPM, Büller HR, Heijboer H, et al. Randomised trial of effect of compression stockings in patients with symptomatic proximal-vein thrombosis, *Lancet.* 1997. *349*: 759–762.
7. Prandoni P, Lensing AWA, Prins MH, et al. Below-knee elastic compression stockings to prevent the post-thrombotic syndrome: A randomized, controlled trial, *Ann Intern Med.* 2004. *141*: 249–256.
8. Kahn SR, Kearon C, Julian JA, et al. Predictors of the post-thrombotic syndrome during long-term treatment of proximal deep vein thrombosis, *J Thromb Haemost.* 2005. *3*: 718–723.
9. Hull RD, Marder VJ, Mah AF, et al. Quantitative assessment of thrombus burden predicts the outcome of treatment for venous thrombosis: A systematic review, *Am J Med.* 2005. *118*: 456–464.
10. Van Dongen CJJ, Prandoni P, Frulla M, et al. Relation between quality of anticoagulant treatment and the development of the postthrombotic syndrome, *J Thromb Haemost.* 2005. *3*: 939–942.
11. Partsch H, Kaulich M, Maycr W. Immediate mobilisation in acute vein thrombosis reduces post-thrombotic syndrome, *Int Angiol.* 2004. *23*: 206–212.
12. Hirsh J, Bauer KA, Donati MG, et al. Parenteral anticoagulants: American College of Chest Physicians Evidence-Based Clinical Practice Guidelines (8th Edition), *Chest.* 133(6): 141S–159S.
13. Lane DA. Heparin binding and neutralizing protein. In: Lane DA, Lindahl U, eds. *Heparin: Chemical and biological properties, clinical applications.* London: Edward Arnold. 1989. 363–391.
14. Rosenberg RD, Lam L. Correlation between structure and function of heparin, *Proc Natl Acad Sci.* 1979. *76*: 1218–1222.
15. Gallus A, Jackaman J, Tillett J, Mills W, Wycherley A. Safety and efficacy of warfarin started early after submassive venous thrombosis or pulmonary embolism, *Lancet.* 1986. *2*: 1293–1296.
16. Hull RD, Raskob GE, Rosenbloom D, et al. Heparin for 5 days as compared with 10 days in the initial treatment of proximal venous thrombosis, *N Engl J Med.* 1990. *332*: 1260–1264.
17. Hull RD, Raskob GE, Rosenbloom D, et al. Optimal therapeutic level of heparin therapy in patients with venous thrombosis, *Arch Intern Med.* 1992. *152*: 1589–1595.
18. Hull RD, Raskob GE, Brant RF, et al. The relation between the time to achieve the lower limit of the APTT therapeutic range and recurrent venous thromboembolism during heparin treatment for deep-vein thrombosis, *Arch Intern Med.* 1997. *157*: 2562–2568.
19. Raschke RA, Reilly BM, Guidry JR, et al. The weight based heparin dosing nomogram compared with a "standard care" nomogram, *Ann Intern Med.* 1993. *119*: 874–881.
20. Raschke R, Hirsh J, Guidry JR. Suboptimal monitoring and dosing of unfractionated heparin in comparative studies with low-molecular-weight heparin, *Ann Int Med.* 2003. *138*: 720–723.
21. Van Den Belt AG, Prins MG, Lensing AW, et al. Fixed dose subcutaneous low molecular weight heparins versus adjusted dose unfractionated heparin for venous thromboembolism, *Cochrane Database Syst Rev.* 2004. *4*: CD001100.
22. Prandoni IP, Carnovali M, Marchiori A, et al. Subcutaneous adjusted-dose unfractionated heparin vs fixed-dose low-molecular-weight heparin in the initial treatment of venous thromboembolism, *Arch Intern Med.* 2004. *164*(10): 1077–1083.
23. Lopaciuk S, Meissner AJ, Filipecki S, et al. Subcutaneous low molecular weight heparin versus subcutaneous UFH in the treatment of DVT: A Polish multicenter trial, *Thromb Haemost.* 1992. *68*: 14–18.
24. Belcaro G, Nicolaides AN, Cesarone MR, et al. Comparison of low-molecular-weight heparin, administered primarily at home, with UFH, administered in hospital, and subcutaneous heparin, administered at home for deep-vein thrombosis, *Angiology.* 1999. *50*: 781–787.
25. Writing Committee for the Galilei Investigators. Subcutaneous adjusted-dose UFH vs fixed-dose low-molecular-weight heparin in the initial treatment of venous thromboembolism, *Arch Intern Med.* 2004. *164*: 1077–1083.
26. Prandoni P, Bagatella P, Bernardi E, et al. Use of an algorithm for administering subcutaneous heparin in the treatment of deep vein thrombosis, *Ann Intern Med.* 1998. *129*: 299–302.
27. Warkentin TE, Greinacher A, Koster A, et al. Treatment and prevention of heparin induced thrombocytopenia: American College of chest Physicians Evidence-Based Clinical Practice Guidelines (8th Edition), *Chest.* 2008. *133*(6): 340S–380S.
28. Warkentin TE. Review: Heparin-induced thrombocytopenia: Pathogenesis and management, *Br J Haematol.* 2003. *121*: 535–555.
29. Amiral J, Peynaud-Debayle E, Wolf M, Bridey F, Vissac AM, Meyer D. Generation of antibodies to heparin-PF4 complexes without thrombocytopenia in patients treated with unfractionated or low-molecular-weight heparin, *Am J Hematol.* 1996. *52*: 90–95.
30. Ahmad S, Untch B, Haas S, et al. Differential prevalence of anti-heparin-PF4 immunoglobulin subtypes in patients treated with clivarin and heparin: Implications in the HIT pathogenesis, *Mol Cell Biochem.* 2004. *258*: 163–170.
31. Gruel Y, Pouplard C, Nguyen P, et al. Biological and clinical features of low-molecular-weight heparin-induced thrombocytopenia, *Br J Haematol.* 2003. *121*: 786–792.
32. Girolami B, Prandoni P, Stefani PM, et al. The incidence of heparin-induced thrombocytopenia in medical patients treated

with low molecular weight heparin: A prospective Cohort Study, *Blood*. 2003. *101*: 2955–2959.

33. Rice L, Attisha WK, Drexler A, Francis FL. Delayed-onset heparin-induced thrombocytopenia, *Ann Intern Med*. 2002. *136*: 210–215.

34. Wirth SM, Macaulay TE, Armitstead JA, et al. Evaluation of a clinical scoring scale to direct early appropriate therapy in heparin-induced thrombocytopenia, *J Oncol Pharm Pract*. 2009. *16*(3): 161–166.

35. Hirsh J, Heddle N, Kelton JG. Treatment of heparin-induced thrombocytopenia: A critical review, *Arch Intern Med*. 2004. *164*: 361–369.

36. Lewis BE, Wallis DE, Leya F, Hursting MJ, Kelton JG. Argatroban anticoagulation in patients with heparin-induced thrombocytopenia, *Arch Intern Med*. 2003. *163*: 1849–1856.

37. Matthai WH Jr, Hursting MJ, Lewis BE, Kelton JG. Argatroban anticoagulation in patients with a history of heparin-induced thrombocytopenia, *Thromb Research*. 2005. *116*: 121–126.

38. Greinacher A, Eichler P, Lubenow N, Kwasny H, Luz M. Heparin-induced thrombocytopenia with thromboembolic complications: Meta-analysis of two prospective trials to assess the value of parenteral treatment with lepirudin and its therapeutic aPTT range, *Blood*. 2000. *96*: 846–851.

39. Call JT, Deliargyris EN, Sane DC. Direct thrombin inhibitors in the treatment of immune-mediated heparin-induced thrombocytopenia, *Semin Thromb Hemost*. 2004. *30*: 297–304.

40. Gtrinsvhrt S, Rivhlrt P. Anaphylactic and anaphylactoid reactions associated with lepirudin in patients with heparin-induced thrombocytopenia, *Circulation*. 2003. *108*: 2062–2065.

41. Greinacher A, Lubenow N, Eichler P. Anaphylactic and anaphylactoid reactions associated with lepirudin in patients with heparin-induced thrombocytopenia, *Circulation*. 2003. *108*: 2062–2065.

42. Harenberg J, Jorg I, Fenyvesi T, Piazolo L. Treatment of patients with a history of heparin-induced thrombocytopenia and anti-lepirudin antibodies with argatroban, *J Thromb Thrombolys*. 2005. *19*: 65–69.

43. Savi P, Chong BH, Greinacher A, et al. Effect of fondaparinux on platelet activation in the presence of heparin-independent antibodies: A blinded comparative multicenter study with unfractionated heparin, *Blood*. 2005. *105*: 139–144.

44. Warkentin TE, Sheppard JI, Schulman S, et al. Fondaparinux treatment of acute heparin-induced thrombocytopenia confirmed by serotonin-release assay: A 30 month, 16-patient case series, *J Thromb Haemost*. 2011. *9*(12): 2389–2396.

45. Barrowcliffe TW, Curtis AD, Johnson EA, Thomas DP. An international standard for low molecular weight heparin, *Thromb Haemost*. 1988. *60*: 1–7.

46. Weitz JI. Low molecular weight heparins, *N Engl J Med*. 1997. *337*: 688–698.

47. Hull RD, Raskob GE Pineo GF. Subcutaneous low molecular weight heparin compared with continuous intravenous heparin in the treatment of proximal vein thrombosis, *N Engl J Med*. 1992. *326*: 975–988.

48. Lopaciuk S, Meissner AJ, Filipecki S, et al. Subcutaneous low molecular weight heparin versus subcutaneous unfractionated heparin in the treatment of deep vein thrombosis: A Polish multicentre trial, *Thromb Haemost*. 1992. *68*: 14–18.

49. Simonneau G, Charbonnier B, Decousus H, et al. Subcutaneous low molecular weight heparin compared with continuous intravenous unfractionated heparin in the treatment of proximal deep vein thrombosis, *Arch Intern Med*. 1993. *153*: 1541–1546.

50. Simonneau G, Sors H, Charbonnier B, et al. A comparison of low molecular weight heparin with unfractionated heparin for acute pulmonary embolism, *N Engl J Med*. 1997. *337*: 663–669.

51. Decousus H, Leizoravicz A, Parent F, et al. A clinical trial of vena caval filters in the prevention of pulmonary embolism in patients with proximal deep vein thrombosis, *N Engl J Med*. 1998. *338*: 409–415.

52. Levine M, Gent M, Hirsh J, et al. A comparison of low molecular weight heparin administered primarily at home with unfractionated heparin administered in the hospital for proximal deep vein thrombosis, *N Engl J Med*. 1996. *334*: 677–681.

53. Koopman MMW, Prandoni P, Piovella F, et al. Treatment of venous thrombosis with intravenous unfractionated heparin administered in the hospital as compared with subcutaneous low molecular weight heparin administered at home, *N Engl J Med*. 1996. *334*: 682–687.

54. Hull RD, Raskob GE, Brant RF, et al. Low-molecular-weight heparin versus heparin in the treatment of patients with pulmonary embolism: American-Canadian Thrombosis Study Group, *Arch Intern Med*. 2000. *160*: 229–236.

55. Gould MK, Dembitzer AD, Doyle RL, et al. Low-molecular-weight heparins compared with unfractionated heparin for treatment of acute deep venous thrombosis: A meta-analysis of randomized, controlled trials, *Ann Intern Med*. 1999. *130*: 800–809.

56. Columbus Investigators. Low-molecular-weight heparin in the treatment of patients with venous thromboembolism, *N Engl J Med*. 1997. *337*: 657–662.

57. Shaughnessy SG, Young E, Deschamps P, et al. The effects of low molecular weight and standard heparin on calcium loss from fetal rat calvaria, *Blood*. 1995. *86*: 1368–1373.

58. Martel N, Lee J, Wells PS. Risk for heparin-induced thrombocytopenia with unfractionated and low-molecular-weight heparin thromboprophylaxis: A meta-analysis, *Blood*. 2005. *106*: 270–215.

59. van der Heijden JF, Hutten BA, Büller HR, et al. Vitamin K antagonists or low-molecular-weight heparin for the long term treatment of symptomatic venous thromboembolism, *Cochrane Database Syst Rev*. 2002. *1*: CD002001.

60. Lee AY, Levine MN, Baker BI, et al. For the CLOT Investigators: Low-molecular-weight heparin versus coumarin for the prevention of recurrent venous thromboembolism in patients with cancer, *N Engl J Med*. 2003. *349*: 146–153.

61. Hull R, Pineo GF, Brant RR, et al. For the LITE Trial Investigators, Long-term low-molecular-weight heparin versus usual care in proximal-vein thrombosis patients with cancer, *Am J Med*. 2006. *119*: 1062–1072.

62. Freedman MD. Oral anticoagulants: Pharmacodynamics, clinical indication, and adverse effects, *J Clin Pharmacol*. 1992. *32*: 196–209.

63. Ansell J, Hirsh J, Hylek E, et al. Pharmacology and management of the vitamin K antagonists: *American College of Chest Physicians Evidence-Based Clinical Practice Guidelines* (8th Edition), *Chest*. 2008. *133*: 160S–198S.

64. Wessler S, Gitel SN. Warfarin: From bench to bedside, *N Engl J Med*. 1984. *311*: 645–652.

65. Zivelin A, Rao LV, Rapaport SI. Mechanism of the anticoagulant effect of warfarin as evaluated in rabbits by selective depression of individual procoagulant vitamin K-dependent clotting factors, *J Clin Invest*. 1993. *92*: 2131–2140.

66. Crowther MA, Ginsberg J, Kearon C, et al. A randomized trial comparing 5-mg and 10-mg warfarin loading doses, *Arch Intern Med*. 1999. *154*: 46–48.

67. Wells PS, Le Gal G, Tierney S, et al. Practical application of the 10mg warfarin initiation nomogram, *Blood Coagul Fibrinolysis*. 2009. *20*(6): 403–408.

68. Holbrook AM, Pereira JA, Labiris R, et al. Systematic overview of warfarin and its drug and food interactions, *Arch Intern Med*. 2005. *165*: 1095–1106.

69. Ramsay NA, Kenny MW, Davies G, Patel JP. Complimentary and alternative medicine use among patients starting warfarin, *Brit J Haemost*. 2005. *130*: 777–780.

70. Poller L, Taberner DA. Dosage and control of oral anticoagulants: An international collaborative survey, *Br J Haematol*. 1982. *51*: 479–485.

71. Hull RD, Hirsh J, Jay R, et al. Different intensities of oral anticoagulant therapy in the treatment of proximal-vein thrombosis, *N Engl J Med*. 1982. *307*: 1676–1681.

72. Ridker P, Goldhaber SZ, Danielson E, et al. Long-term low-intensity warfarin therapy with conventional-intensity warfarin therapy for the prevention of recurrent venous thromboembolism, *N Engl J Med.* 2003. *348*: 1425–1434.

73. Kearon C, Ginsberg JS, Kovacs MH, et al. Comparison of low-intensity warfarin therapy with conventional-intensity warfarin therapy with conventional-intensity warfarin therapy for long-term prevention of recurrent venous thromboembolism, *N Engl J Med.* 2003. *349*: 631–639.

74. Crowther MA, Ginsberg JS, Kovacs MH, et al. A comparison of two intensities of warfarin for the prevention of recurrent thrombosis in patients with the antiphospholipid antibody syndrome, *N Engl J Med.* 2003. *349*: 1133–1138.

75. Hull RD, Delmore TJ, Genton E, et al. Warfarin sodium versus low-dose heparin in the long-term treatment of venous thrombosis, *N Engl J Med.* 1979. *301*: 855–858.

76. Hull RD, Delmore TJ, Carter C, et al. Adjusted subcutaneous heparin versus warfarin sodium in the long-term treatment of venous thrombosis, *N Engl J Med.* 1982. *306*: 189–194.

77. O'Donnell M, Hirsh J. Establishing an optimum therapeutic range for coumarins, filling in the gaps, *Arch Intern Med.* 2004. *164*: 588–590.

78. Research Committee of the British Thoracic Society. Optimum duration of anticoagulation for deep-vein thrombosis and pulmonary embolism, *Lancet.* 1992. *340*: 873–876.

79. Schulman S, Rhedin A-S, Lindmarker P, et al. A comparison of six weeks with six months of oral anticoagulant therapy after a first episode of venous thromboembolism, *N Engl J Med.* 1995. *332*: 1661–1665.

80. Levine M, Hirsh J, Gent M, et al. Optimal duration of oral anticoagulant therapy: A randomized trial comparing four weeks with three months of warfarin in patients with proximal deep-vein thrombosis, *Thromb Haemost.* 1995. *74*: 606–611.

81. Schulman S, Granqvist S, Holmström M, et al. The duration of oral anticoagulant therapy after a second episode of venous thromboembolism, *N Engl J Med.* 1997. *336*: 393–398.

82. Kearon C, Gent M, Hirsh J, et al. A comparison of three months of anticoagulation with extended anticoagulation for a first-episode of idiopathic venous thromboembolism, *N Engl J Med.* 1999. *340*: 901–907.

83. Agnelli G, Prandoni P, Santamaria M, et al. Three months versus one year of oral anticoagulant therapy for idiopathic deep-venous thrombosis, *N Engl J Med.* 2001. *345*: 165–169.

84. Campbell IA, Bentley DP, Prescott RJ, et al. Anticoagulation for three versus six months in patients with deep vein thrombosis or pulmonary embolism, or both: Randomized trial. *Br Med J.* 2007. *334*(7595): 674.

85. Kearon C. A conceptual framework for two phases of anticoagulant treatment of venous thromboembolism, *J Thromb Haemost.* 2012. *10*: 507–511.

86. Young L, Ockelford P, Milne D, et al. Post-treatment residual thrombus increases the risk of recurrent deep vein thrombosis and mortality, *J Thromb Haemost.* 2006. *4*(9): 1919–1924.

87. Siragusa S, Malato A, Anastasio R, et al. Residual vein thrombosis to establish duration of anticoagulation after a first episode of deep vein thrombosis: The Duration of Anticoagulation based on Compression UltraSonography (DACUS) study, *Blood.* 2008. *179*(5): 417–426.

88. Palareti G, Cosmi B, Vigano D'Angelo S, et al. D-dimer testing to determine the duration of anticoagulant therapy, *N Engl J Med.* 2006. *355*: 1780–1789.

89. Verhovsek M, Douketis JD, Yi Q, et al. Systematic review: D-dimer to predict recurrent disease after stopping anticoagulant therapy for unprovoked venous thromboembolism, *Ann Intern Med.* 2008. *149*(7): 481–490, W94.

90. Kyrle P, Minar E, Bialonczyk C, et al. The risk of recurrent venous thromboembolism in men and women, *N Engl J Med.* 2004. *350*: 2558.

91. Rodger MA, Kahn SR, Wells PS, et al. Identifying unprovoked thromboembolism patients at low risk for recurrence who can discontinue anticoagulant therapy, *Can Med Assoc J.* 2008. *179*(5): 417–426.

92. Beyth RJ, Quinn L, Landefeld CS. A multicomponent intervention to prevent major bleeding complications in older patients receiving warfarin: A randomized, controlled trial, *Ann Intern Med.* 2000. *133*: 687–695.

93. Hylek EM, Regan S, Go AS, et al. Clinical predictors of prolonged delay in return of the international normalized ratio to within the therapeutic range after excessive anticoagulation with warfarin, *Ann Intern Med.* 2001. *135*: 393–400.

94. Cannegieter SC, Rosendaal FR, Wintzen AR, et al. Optimal oral anticoagulant therapy in patients with mechanical heart valves, *N Engl J Med.* 1995. *333*: 11–17.

95. Fihn SD, McDonnell M, Martin D, et al. Risk factors for complications of chronic anticoagulation: A multicenter study: Warfarin Optimized Outpatient Follow-up Study Group, *Ann Intern Med.* 1993. *118*: 511–520.

96. Henderson MC, White RH. Anticoagulation in the elderly, *Curr Opin Pulm Med.* 2001. *7*: 365–370.

97. Palareti G, Legnani C, Lee A, et al. A comparison of the safety and efficacy of oral anticoagulation for the treatment of venous thromboembolic disease in patients with or without malignancy, *Thromb Haemost.* 2000. *84*: 805–810.

98. Ageno W, Gallus AS, Wittkowsky A, et al Oral anticoagulant therapy: Antithrombotic therapy and prevention of thrombosis, 9th ed: American College of Chest Physicians Evidence-based Clinical Practice Guidelines, *Chest.* 2012. *141*: e44S–e88S.

99. Crowther MA, Julian J, McCarty, et al. Treatment of warfarin-associated coagulopathy with oral vitamin K: A randomised controlled trial, *Lancet.* 2000. *356*: 1551–1553.

100. Nee R, Doppenschmidt D, Donovan DJ, Andrews TC. Intravenous versus subcutaneous vitamin K1 in reversing excessive anticoagulation, *Am J Cardiol.* 1999. *83*(2): 286–288: A6–A7.

101. Leissinger CA, Blatt WK, Hoots WK, Ewenstein B. Role of prothrombin complex concentrates in reversing warfarin anticoagulation: A review of the literature, *Am J Hematol.* 2008. *83*(2): 137–143.

102. Rosovsky RP, Crowther MA. What is the evidence for the off-label use of recombinant Factor VIIa (rVIIA) in the acute reversal of warfarin? ASH evidence-based review 2008, *Hematology. Am Soc Hematol Educ Program.* 2008. *2008*(1): 36–38.

103. Kovacs MJ, Kearon C, Rodger M, et al., Single-arm study of bridging therapy with low-molecular-weight heparin for patients at risk of arterial embolism who require temporary interruption of warfarin, *Circulation.* 2004. *110*: 1658–1663.

104. Spyropoulos AC, Turpie AG, Dunn AS, et al. Clinical outcomes with unfractionated heparin or low-molecular-weight heparin as bridging therapy in patients on long-term oral anticoagulants: The REGIMEN registry, *J Thromb Haemost.* 2006. *4*(6): 1246–1252.

105. Dunn AS, Turpie AGG. Perioperative management of patients receiving oral anticoagulants: A systematic review, *Arch Intern Med.* 2003. *163*: 901–908.

106. Garcia DA, Regan S, Henault LE, et al. Risk of thromboembolism with short-term interruption of warfarin therapy, *Arch Intern Med.* 2008. *168*(1): 63–69.

107. Bajkin BV, Popovic SL, Selakovic SD. Randomized, prospective trial comparing bridging therapy using low-molecular-weight heparin with maintenance of oral anticoagulation during extraction of teeth, *Oral Maxillofac Surg.* 2009. *67*(5): 990–995.

108. Ahmed I, Gertner E, Melson WB, et al. Continuing warfarin therapy is superior to interrupting warfarin with or without bridging anticoagulation therapy in patients undergoing pacemaker and defibrillator implantation, *Heart Rhythm.* 2010. *7*(6): 745–749.

109. Douketis JD, Spyropoulos AC, Spencer FA, et al. The perioperative management of antithrombotic therapy: American College of

Chest Physicians Evidence-Based Clinical Practice Guidelines (9th Edition), *Chest*. 2012. *141*(2): e326S–e350S.

110. Bates S, Greer IA, Middeldorp S, et al. VTE, thrombophilia, antithrombotic therapy and pregnancy: Antithrombotic therapy and prevention of thrombosis, 9th ed: American College of Chest Physicians Evidence-based Guidelines, *Chest*. 2012. *141*: e691S–e736S.

111. Greer IA, Nelson-Piercy C. Low-molecular-weight heparins for thromboprophylaxis and treatment of venous thromboembolism in pregnancy: A systematic review of safety and efficacy, *Blood*. 2005. *106*(2): 401–407.

112. Petila V, Kaaja R, Leinonen P, et al. Thromboprophylaxis with low molecular weight heparin (dalteparin) in pregnancy, *Thromb Res*. 1999. *96*: 275–282.

113. Rodger MA, Kahn SR, Cranney A, et al. Long-term dalteparin in pregnancy not associated with a decrease in bone mineral density: A substudy of a randomized controlled trial, *J Thromb Haemost*. 2007. *5*(8): 1600–1606.

114. Smith M, Norris L, Steer P, et al. Tinzaparin sodium for thrombosis treatment and prevention during pregnancy, *Am J Obstet Gynecol*. 2004. *190*: 495–500.

115. Crowther MA, Spitzer K, Julian J, et al. Pharmacokinetic profile of a low-molecular weight heparin (reviparin) in pregnant patients: A prospective cohort study, *Thromb Res*. 2000. *98*(2): 133–138.

116. Weitz JI, Hirsh J, Samama MM. New anticoagulant drugs: The Seventh ACCP Conference on Anticoagulant and Thrombolytic Therapy, *Chest*. 2004. *126*(3): 265S–286S

117. Büller HR, Davidson BL, Decousus H, et al. Fondaparinux or Enoxaparin for the initial treatment of symptomatic deep venous thrombosis: A randomized trial, *Ann Intern Med*. 2004. *140*(11): 867–873.

118. Büller HR, Davidson BL, Decousus H, et al. Subcutaneous fondaparinux versus intravenous unfractionated heparin in the initial treatment of pulmonary embolism, *N Engl J Med*. 2003. *349*(18): 1695–1702.

119. Weitz JI, Eikelboom JW, Samama MM. New antithrombotic drugs: Antithrombotic therapy and prevention of thrombosis, 9th ed.: American College of Chest Physicians Evidence-Based Clinical Practice Guidelines, *Chest*. 2012. *141*: e120S–e151S.

120. Eerenberg ES, van Es J, Sjipkens MK, et al. New anticoagulants: Moving on from scientific results to clinical implementation, *Ann Med*. 2011. *43*(8): 606–616.

121. Product monograph. Xarelto (rivaroxaban) tablets. http://www.bayer.ca

122. Mueck W, Lensing AWA, Agnelli G, et al. Population pharmacokinetics in patients treated with acute deep-vein thrombosis and exposure simulations in patients with atrial fibrillation, *Clin Pharmacokinet*. 2011. *50*: 6775–6786.

123. Hillarp A, Baghaei F, Fagerberg B, et al. Effects of the oral, direct factor Xa inhibitor rivaroxaban on commonly used coagulation assays, *J Thromb Haemost*. 2010. *9*(1): 133–139

124. Samama MM, Martinoli JL, LeFlem L, et al. Assessment of laboratory assays to measure rivaroxaban: An oral, direct factor Xa inhibitor, *Thromb Haemost*. 2010. *103*(4): 815–825.

125. Douketis JD. Pharmacologic properties of the new oral anticoagulants: A clinician-oriented review with a focus on perioperative management, *Curr Pharm Design*. 2010. *16*: 3436–3441.

126. Eerenberg ES, Kamphuisen PW, Sjipkens MK, et al. Reversal of rivaroxaban and dabigatran by prothrombin complex concentrate: A randomized, placebo controlled, crossover study in healthy subjects, *Circulation*. 2010. *124*(14): 1573–1579.

127. Product monograph. Eliquis (apixaban) tablets. www.bmscanada.ca.

128. Wong PC, Pinto DJ, Zhang D. Preclinical discovery of apixaban, a direct and orally bioavailable factor Xa inhibitor, *J Thromb Thrombolysis*. 2011. *31*(4): 478–492.

129. Raghavan N, Frost CE, Yu Z, et al. Apixaban metabolism and pharmacokinetics following oral administration, *Drug Metab Dispos*. 2009. *37*: 780–782.

130. Wang L, Zhang D, Raghaven N, et al. In vitro assessment of metabolic drug-drug interaction potential of apixaban through cytochrome P450 phenotyping, inhibition, and induction studies, *Drug Metab Dispos*. 2010. *38*(3): 448–458.

131. Becker RC, Yang H, Barrett Y, et al. Chromogenic laboratory assays to measure the factor Xa-inhibiting properties of apixaban, an oral, direct, and selective factor Xa inhibitor, *J Thromb Thrombolysis*. 2011. *32*(2): 183–187.

132. Product monograph. Pradax/Pradaxa (dabigatran etexilate) tablets. www.Boehringer-ingelheim.ca

133. Sorbera LA, Bozzo J, Castaner J. Dabigatran/Dabigatran etexilate, *Drug Future*. 2005. *30*(9): 877–885.

134. Strangier J, Rathgen K, Stahle H, et al. The pharmacokinetics, pharmacodynamics, and tolerability of dabigatran etexilate, a new oral direct thrombin inhibitor, in healthy subjects, *Br J Clin Pharmacol*. 2007. *64*(3): 292–303

135. Strangier J. Clinical pharmacokinetics and pharmacodynamics of the oral direct thrombin inhibitor dabigatran etexilate, *Clin Pharmacokinet*. 2008. *47*(5): 285–295.

136. Connolly SJ, Ezekowitz MD, Yusuf S, et al. Dabigatran versus warfarin in patients with atrial fibrillation, *N Engl J Med*. 2009. *361*: 1139–1151.

137. Schulman S, Eriksson BI, Goldhaber S, et al. Dabigatran or warfarin for extended maintenance therapy of venous thromboembolism, *J Thromb Haemost*. 2011. *9*(Suppl 2): 731–732. (Abstr. O-Thu-033).

138. Uchino K, Hernandez AV. Dabigatran association with a higher risk of acute coronary events: Meta-analysis of non-inferiority randomized controlled trials, *Arch Intern Med*. 2012. *172*(5): 397–402.

139. Hohnloser SH, Oldgren J, Yang S, et al. Myocardial ischemic events in patients with atrial fibrillation treated with dabigatran or warfarin in the RE-LY (Randomized evaluation of long-term anticoagulation therapy) trial, *Circulation*. 2012. *125*: 669–676.

140. van Ryn J, Stangier J, Haertter S, et al. Dabigatran etexilate: A novel, reversible, oral direct thrombin inhibitor: Interpretation of coagulation assays and reversal of anticoagulant activity, *Thromb Haemost*. 2010. *103*(6): 1116–1127.

141. Stangier J, Rathgen K, Stahle H, et al. Influence of renal impairment on the pharmacokinetics and pharmacodynamics of oral dabigatran etexilate: An open-label parallel-group, single-centre study, *Clin Pharmacokinet*. 2010. *49*(4): 259–268.

142. Lindahl TL, Baghaei F, Blixter IF, et al. Effects of the oral, direct thrombin inhibitor dabigatran on five common coagulation assays, *Thromb Haemost*. 2011. *105*(2): 371–378.

143. Eriksson BI, Borris LC, Friedman RJ, et al. Rivaroxaban versus enoxaparin for thromboprophylaxis after hip arthroplasty, *N Engl J Med*. 2008. *358*: 2765–2775.

144. Turpie AG, Lassen MR, Davidson BL, et al. Rivaroxaban versus enoxaparin for thromboprophylaxis after total knee arthroplasty (RECORD4): A randomized trial, *Lancet*. 2009. *373*(9676): 1673–1680.

145. Lassen MR, Ageno W, Borris LC, et al. Rivaroxaban versus enoxaparin for thromboprophylaxis after total knee arthroplasty, *N Engl J Med*. 2008. *358*(26): 2776–2786.

146. Eriksson BI, Friedman R. Dabigatran etexilate: Pivotal trials for venous thromboembolism prophylaxis after hip or knee arthroplasty, *Clin Appl Thromb Haemost*. 2009. *15*(Suppl 1): 25S–31S.

147. Lassen MR, Raskob GE, Gallus A, et al. Apixaban or enoxaparin for thromboprophylaxis after knee replacement, *N Engl J Med*. 2009. *361*(18): 594–604.

148. Lassen MR, Raskob GE, Gallus A, et al. Apixaban versus enoxaparin for thromboprophylaxis after knee replacement (ADVANCE-2): A randomized double-blind trial, *Lancet*. 2010. *375*(9717): 779–780.

149. Lassen MR, Gallus A, Raskob GE, et al. Apixaban versus enoxaparin for thromboprophylaxis after hip replacement, *N Engl J Med*. 2010. *363*(26): 1–12.

150. Connolly SJ, Ezekowitz MD, Yusuf S, et al. Dabigatran versus warfarin in patients with atrial fibrillation, *N Engl J Med.* 2009. *361*: 1139–1151.

151. Patel MR, Mahaffey KW, Garg J, et al. Rivaroxaban versus warfarin in nonvalvular atrial fibrillation, *N Engl J Med.* 2011. *365*: 883–891.

152. Granger CB, Alexander JH, McMurray JJV, et al. Apixaban versus warfarin in patients with atrial fibrillation, *N Engl J Med.* 2011. *365*(11): 981–992.

153. Schulman S, Kearon C, Kakkar AK, et al. Dabigatran versus warfarin in the treatment of acute venous thromboembolism, *N Engl J Med.* 2009. *361*(24): 2342–2352.

154. Schulman S, Eriksson BI, Goldhaber S, et al. Dabigatran or warfarin for extended maintenance therapy of venous thromboembolism, *J Thromb Haemost.* 2011. *9*(Suppl 2): 731–732 (Abstr. O-Thu-033).

155. Schulman S, Baanstra D, Eriksson BI, et al. Dabigatran vs. placebo for extended maintenance therapy of venous thromboembolism, *J Thromb Haemost.* 2011. *9*: 22 (Abstr. O-Mo-037).

156. Bauersachs R, Berkowitz SD, Brenner B, et al. Oral rivaroxaban for symptomatic venous thromboembolism, *N Engl J Med.* 2010. *363*: 2499–2510.

157. Buller HR, Prins MH, Lensing AWA, et al. Oral rivaroxaban for the treatment of symptomatic pulmonary embolism, *N Engl J Med.* 2012. *366*(14): 1287–1297.

158. Elsharawy M, Elzayat E. Early results of thrombolysis vs anticoagulation in ileofemoral venous thrombosis, *Eur J Vasc Endovasc Surg.* 2002. *24*(3): 209–214.

159. Jackson LS, Wang XJ, Dudrick SJ, et al. Catheter directed thrombolysis and\or thrombectomy with selective endovascular stenting as alternatives to systemic, anticoagulation for treatment of acute deep vein thrombosis, *Am J Surg.* 2005. *190*(6): 863–868.

159. Enden T, Haig Y, Lkow NE, et al. Long-term outcome after additional catheter-directed thrombolysis versus standard treatment for acute ileofemoral deep vein thrombosis (the CaVenT study): A randomised controlled trial, *Lancet.* 2012. *379*(9810): 31–38.

160. Wormald JR, Lane TR, Herbert PE, et al. Total preservation of patency and valve function after percutaneous pharmacomechanical thrombolysis using the Trellis-8 system for an acute, extensive deep vein thrombosis, *An R Coll Surg Engl.* 2012. *94*(2): e103–e105.

161. Comerota AJ, Gale SS. Techniques of contemporary ileofemoral and infrainguinal venous thrombectomy, *J Vasc Surg.* 2006. *43*(1): 185–191.

162. Meissner MH, Gloviczki P, Comerota AJ, et al. Early thrombus removal strategies for acute venous thrombosis: Clinical practice guidelines of the Society for Vascular Surgery and the American Venous Forum, *J Vasc Surg.* 2012. *55*(5): 1449–1462.

163. Decousus H, Leizorovicz A, Parent F, et al. A clinical trial of vena cava filters in the prevention of pulmonary embolism in patients with proximal deep-vein thrombosis, *N Engl J Med.* 1998. *338*(7): 409–415.

164. Mismetti P, Rivron-Guillot K, Quenet S, et al. A prospective long-term study of 220 patients with a retrievable vena cava filter for secondary prevention of venous thromboembolism, *Chest.* 2007. *131*(1): 223–229.

165. Young T, Tang H, Aukes J, et al. Vena caval filters for the prevention of pulmonary embolism, *Cochrane Database Syst Rev.* 2007. *4*: CD0006212.

166. Tschoe M, Kim HS, Brotman DJ, et al. Retrievable vena cava filters: A clinical review, *J Hosp Med.* 2009. *4*(7): 441–448.

167. Streiff MB. Vena cava filters: A comprehensive review, *Blood.* 2000. *95*(12): 3669–3677.

168. Fox MA, Kahn SR. Post-thrombotic syndrome in relation to vena cava filter placement: A systematic review, *J Vasc Interv Radiol.* 2008. *19*(7): 981–985.

41.

DIAGNOSIS AND MANAGEMENT OF HEPARIN-INDUCED THROMBOCYTOPENIA

Theodore E. Warkentin

INTRODUCTION

The Vein Book would be incomplete without a discussion of heparin-induced thrombocytopenia (HIT) for three reasons. First, deep venous thrombosis (DVT) is almost always initially treated with heparin, thus creating the potential for this immune-mediated adverse drug reaction. Second, venous thrombosis itself is the most common complication of HIT.[1,2] Third, the treatment of HIT-associated DVT with warfarin can precipitate severe venous limb ischemia (phlegmasia cerulea dolens), with potential for limb loss (venous limb gangrene).

DEFINITION OF HIT

HIT can be defined as any clinical event (or events) best explained by platelet-activating anti-platelet factor 4 (PF4)/heparin antibodies ("HIT antibodies") in a patient who is receiving, or who has recently received, heparin.[1] In most patients, this includes a large platelet count fall that usually exceeds 50%.[1-3] The clinical importance of HIT primarily stems from its strong association with thrombosis.

PATHOGENESIS

The key event in HIT pathogenesis is formation of platelet-activating antibodies of immunoglobulin G (IgG) class that recognize a "self" protein, PF4, bound to heparin. Multimolecular complexes of PF4, heparin, and IgG form on platelet surfaces, leading to platelet activation (via platelet Fc IgG receptors) and formation of procoagulant platelet-derived microparticles, thereby stimulating hypercoagulability (increased thrombin generation). Heparin molecules bind to PF4 in relation to their chain length, perhaps explaining why unfractionated heparin (UFH) is more likely to cause HIT than low molecular weight heparin (LMWH) or fondaparinux.[3,4] Once triggered, the prothrombotic risk of HIT persists (or even worsens) for several days, despite stopping heparin.[1,5]

CLINICAL PRESENTATION

THE "4 T'S"

Thrombocytopenia is common in heparin-treated patients, yet only a minority have HIT. A clinical scoring system, the "4 T's," helps predict which patients have HIT, based on assessment of: *T*hrombocytopenia, *T*iming, *T*hrombosis, and the absence of o*T*her explanation(s) (see Table 41.1).[1,2] Evaluation of this scoring system suggests that HIT antibodies are unlikely (<5%) when a low score (≤3) is obtained, but likely (50–80%) with a high score (≥6).[6] An intermediate score (4 or 5) usually indicates a clinical profile compatible with HIT but also with another plausible explanation, such as sepsis.

Most patients with HIT have moderate thrombocytopenia, with platelet count nadirs usually between 20 to 150×10^9/L (median nadir, 60×10^9/L); only 5 to 10% develop a platelet count fall to less than 20×10^9/L.[1,2] At least 90% of patients evince a 50% or greater platelet count fall; especially in postoperative patients (who usually exhibit thrombocytosis after postoperative day 5), even a large platelet count decline may not necessarily cause the platelet count to fall below 150×10^9/L.[3]

Typically, the platelet count begins to fall 5 to 10 days after starting heparin, although a more rapid platelet count fall can occur if HIT antibodies are already present because of a recent exposure to heparin.[7] This link between "rapid-onset HIT" and recent heparin use is explained by the unusual transience of HIT antibodies, which become undetectable a median of 50 to 80 days (depending on the assay performed) after an episode of HIT.[7] Indeed, the transience of HIT antibodies, together with the inability to regenerate HIT antibodies before day 5 following reexposure, provides

Table 41.1 CLINICAL SCORING SYSTEM FOR HIT: THE "4 T'S"

	POINTS (0, 1, OR 2 FOR EACH OF 4 CATEGORIES: MAXIMUM POSSIBLE SCORE = 8)		
	2	1	0
Thrombocytopenia	>50% platelet fall to nadir >20	30–50% platelet fall (or >50% fall resulting from surgical hemodilution); or nadir 10–19	<30% platelet fall; or nadir <10
Timing* of onset of platelet fall (or other sequelae of HIT)	days 5–10; or <day 1 with recent heparin (past 30 days)	>day 10 or timing unclear; or <day 1 with recent heparin (past 31–100 days)	<day 4 (no recent heparin)
Thrombosis or other sequelae	proven new thrombosis; skin necrosis; or anaphylactoid reaction after IV UFH bolus	progressive or recurrent thrombosis; erythematous skin lesions; suspected thrombosis (not proven)	None
OTher cause(s) of platelet fall	none evident	Possible	definite

Pretest probability score: 6–8= HIGH; 4–5 = INTERMEDIATE; 0–3 = LOW

*First day of immunizing heparin exposure considered day 0.

Reprinted, with modifications, from Reference 6 with permission.

a rationale for using intraoperative heparin anticoagulation during cardiac or vascular surgery in a patient with previous HIT, provided that platelet-activating antibodies are no longer detectable.[7,8]

Rarely, HIT begins several days after heparin already has been stopped ("delayed-onset HIT"); this syndrome is associated with strong positive tests for HIT antibodies.[9] Sera from these patients activate platelets in vitro without the need to add heparin.

Thrombosis is the most important complication of HIT and occurs in most patients.[1-5] Both venous and arterial thrombi can occur (see Table 41.2). The odds ratio for thrombosis ranges from 20 to 40.[2,10]

VENOUS THROMBOSIS AND HIT

Venous thrombosis is the most common complication of HIT, usually manifesting as unilateral or bilateral lower limb DVT.[1,2] Indeed, DVT occurs in about 50% of patients with HIT, with half of these (i.e., 25% overall) developing symptomatic pulmonary embolism. In one study, upper limb DVT occurred in 10% of HIT patients with use of a central venous catheter (CVC); compared with controls, both HIT and CVC use were strongly associated with upper limb DVT, illustrating that a localizing risk factor (vessel injury from the CVC) interacts with systemic hypercoagulability (HIT), thereby influencing the type and location of thrombosis.[11]

Table 41.2 THROMBOSIS AND OTHER SEQUELAE OF HIT

VENOUS THROMBOSIS	ARTERIAL THROMBOSIS	MISCELLANEOUS
DVT (50%): new, progressive, recurrent; lower limb (often bilateral); upper limb (at site of venous catheter); phlegmasia cerulea dolens	Aortic or iliofemoral thrombosis resulting in acute limb ischemia or infarction (5–10%) or spinal cord infarction (rare)	Heparin-induced skin lesions at injection sites (10–20%): erythematous plaques, skin necrosis
Coumarin-induced venous limb gangrene (5–10% of DVT treated with coumarin)	Acute thrombotic stroke (3–5%)	Coumarin-induced skin necrosis involving "central" sites (breast, abdomen, thigh, calf, etc.; rare)
PE (25%): with or without right-sided cardiac intra-atrial or intraventricular thrombi	Myocardial infarction (3–5%)	Acute anaphylactoid reactions post IV heparin bolus (25% of sensitized patients receiving IV bolus or SC LMWH injection):
	Cardiac intraventricular or intra-atrial thrombosis, in situ or via embolization of DVT (rare)	
Cerebral (dural) sinus thrombosis (rare)	Thrombosis involving miscellaneous arteries (rare): upper limb, renal, mesenteric, spinal, and others	Inflammatory: fever, chills, flushing
Splanchnic vein thrombosis: adrenal hemorrhagic infarction* (rare): bilateral (acute or chronic adrenal insufficiency) or unilateral; mesenteric or portal vein thrombosis	Embolization of thrombus from heart or proximal aorta can also contribute to microvascular ischemic syndromes	Cardiorespiratory: tachycardia, hypertension, dyspnea, cardiopulmonary arrest (rare)
		Gastrointestinal: nausea, vomiting, diarrhea
		Neurological: transient global amnesia, pounding headache
		Overt DIC (10–20%)

*secondary to adrenal vein thrombosis

Estimated frequencies of the various complications of HIT are given in parentheses. Rare indicates an estimated frequency <3% of HIT patients.

(Reprinted, with modifications from Reference 2)

PHLEGMASIA CERULEA DOLENS AND VENOUS LIMB GANGRENE

Venous limb ischemia (phlegmasia cerulea dolens, venous limb gangrene) can result if coumarins such as warfarin are used to treat DVT associated with HIT (see Figure 41.1).[2,12–15] This results from disturbed procoagulant-anticoagulant balance: HIT creates hypercoagulability (increased thrombin generation), and coumarin impairs synthesis of the vitamin K–dependent natural anticoagulant, protein C. A supratherapeutic international normalized ratio (INR), usually >3.5, is characteristic of venous limb ischemia, and represents a surrogate marker for severe protein C depletion (reflecting parallel reduction in factor VII). Rarely, overt (decompensated) disseminated intravascular coagulation (DIC) can explain microvascular thrombosis and limb ischemia in the absence of coumarin (see Figure 44.1).[2] Venous gangrene is a more common explanation for limb loss in HIT than the white clot syndrome (discussed subsequently).

ARTERIAL THROMBOSIS

Occlusion of large or medium-sized arteries by platelet- and leukocyte-rich "white clots" is the classic explanation for limb ischemia in HIT (see Figure 41.1).[2] The distal aorta and iliofemoral arteries are most frequently involved, leading to acute limb ischemia with absent pulses. The thrombi can form either in situ or as a result of embolization from a more proximal location, including the left ventricle or proximal aorta. Other arterial events that are relatively common in HIT include thrombotic stroke and myocardial infarction.

LIMB ISCHEMIA AND THROMBOCYTOPENIA

Table 41.3 lists several diagnostic considerations when a patient presents with the combination of thrombocytopenia and an ischemic limb.[16] Absence of pedal pulses suggests occlusion of large arteries by thromboemboli. Palpable (or Doppler-identifiable) pulses, especially in the setting of DVT, suggests venous limb ischemia, due to coumarin or severe DIC.

At least 5% of patients with HIT develop limb necrosis requiring amputation.[17] Sometimes, limb loss is iatrogenic (warfarin-related) and thus potentially preventable (see later). Timely thrombectomy can salvage limbs in some circumstances (see later).

MISCELLANEOUS COMPLICATIONS

Less than 10% of patients who develop HIT during subcutaneous (SC) injections of UFH or LMWH develop necrotizing skin lesions at the injection sites.[1,2] These patients appear to be at relatively high risk of developing arterial thrombosis.[2]

HIT can also present as an *acute systemic* (or *anaphylactoid*) *reaction*.[1,2,18] These follow intravenous (IV) bolus injection of heparin to a patient with circulating HIT antibodies. Symptoms and signs, which begin 5 to 30 min post injection, are listed in Table 41.2. Abrupt platelet count declines accompany these reactions.

Approximately 10 to 20% of patients with HIT show laboratory evidence of overt (decompensated) DIC, including elevated INR and/or activated partial thromboplastin time (APTT), reduced fibrinogen, red cell

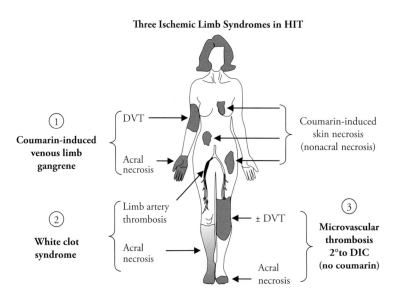

Three Ischemic Limb Syndromes in HIT

① **Coumarin-induced venous limb gangrene** — DVT, Acral necrosis

Coumarin-induced skin necrosis (nonacral necrosis)

② **White clot syndrome** — Limb artery thrombosis, Acral necrosis

± DVT

③ **Microvascular thrombosis 2° to DIC (no coumarin)** — Acral necrosis

Figure 41.1   Three ischemic limb syndromes in HIT. (1) Coumarin-induced venous limb gangrene is characterized by acral (distal extremity) necrosis in a limb with DVT. The INR is usually >3.5. (2) White clot syndrome is characterized by large artery occlusion by platelet-rich white clots. (3) Rarely, microvascular thrombosis secondary to DIC can explain acral limb necrosis even in the absence of coumarin therapy; affected limbs may or may not have associated DVT. For comparison, the classic form of coumarin-induced skin necrosis is shown, which usually involves nonacral sites, such as breast, abdomen, or thigh.   Reprinted, with modifications, from Reference 15, with permission.

Concurrence of limb ischemia/necrosis and thrombocytopenia suggests one of several hematologic emergencies.

(A) **HIT-associated arterial thrombosis.** Occlusion of large lower-limb arteries by platelet-rich "white clots" is characteristic of HIT. The major clue is an otherwise unexplained platelet count fall that begins 5 or more d after starting heparin. Urgent thromboembolectomy may be limb-sparing. Sensitive assays for HIT antibodies give strong positive results.

(B) **Adenocarcinoma-associated DIC.** Severe venous or arterial thrombosis can develop in patients with metastatic adenocarcinoma who have DIC, especially within hours after stopping heparin. A clinical clue is an otherwise unexplained rise in platelet count that occurred during initial heparin therapy.

(C) **Warfarin-induced phlegmasia cerulea dolens/venous limb gangrene.** Coumarin anticoagulants (e.g., warfarin) can lead to venous ischemia (phlegmasia cerulea dolens) or venous limb gangrene in patients with DIC caused by HIT or adenocarcinoma. Limb loss can occur even though the limb pulses are palpable.

(D) **Sepsis-associated macro- or microvascular thrombosis.** Acquired natural anticoagulant failure (e.g., antithrombin or protein C depletion) can complicate DIC associated with sepsis, leading to acral limb ischemia or necrosis.

(E) **Septic embolism.** Rarely, infective endocarditis or aneurysmal thrombosis leads to the constellation of thrombocytopenia associated with infection and acute limb ischemia.

(F) **Antiphospholipid syndrome.** Autoimmune thrombocytopenia and hypercoagulability can interact to produce acute limb ischemia and thrombocytopenia in a patient with antiphospholipid syndrome.

Reprinted, with modifications, from Reference 16 with permission.

---

fragments, or circulating nucleated red cells.[2] These patients can develop ischemic limb necrosis in spite of nonheparin anticoagulant therapy.[14,17,19] Indeed, HIT-associated DIC—by elevating APTT values—can result in suboptimal therapy by APTT-adjusted therapeutic agents ("APTT confounding").[17,19]

LABORATORY TESTING FOR HIT ANTIBODIES

Two types of assays detect HIT antibodies.[1,20] Most widely used are the commercial enzyme-immunoassays (EIAs) that test for antibodies reactive against PF4/polyanion complexes. In contrast, platelet activation assays exploit this pathologic feature of HIT. As a general rule, the stronger a positive test is, the greater the likelihood the patient has HIT.[21]

PLATELET ACTIVATION ASSAYS

The best platelet activation assays utilize "washed" platelets, for example, the platelet serotonin release assay (SRA). When performed by experienced labs, this assay is sensitive for clinically important HIT antibodies, with high specificity (usually >95%).[20] However, washed platelet activation assays are technically demanding and available in only a few reference centers.

PF4/POLYANION IMMUNOASSAYS

Solid-phase EIAs detect antibodies that react with PF4 complexed with heparin or other polyanions. IgG-specific EIAs have similar high sensitivity as polyspecific EIAs (that detect additionally IgA and IgM), but with greater diagnostic specificity (since only IgG antibodies cause HIT).

ICEBERG MODEL

Figure 41.2 shows the interrelationships among different HIT antibody assays, thrombocytopenia (i.e., HIT), and the subset with HIT-associated thrombosis (HIT-T).[4,20] Five features are illustrated: (1) washed platelet activation assays (e.g., SRA) and EIAs have similar high sensitivity for clinical HIT; (2) the SRA has greater diagnostic *specificity* for clinical HIT than the EIAs; (3) the IgG-specific EIA has greater diagnostic specificity than the polyspecific EIA-IgG/A/M; (4) only a subset of heparin-treated patients who form antibodies develop clinical HIT; and (5) increased risk of thrombosis is not observed in patients who develop antibodies in the absence of a significant platelet count fall.

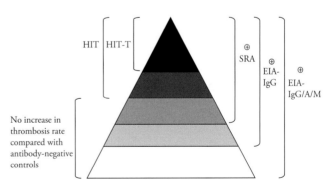

Figure 41.2 Iceberg model of HIT. This model depicts several features of HIT, including the hierarchy of sensitivity and specificity of three different types of assays: (i) platelet activation assay that utilizes washed platelets, for example, platelet SRA; (ii) PF4/heparin EIA that detects IgG class antibodies (EIA-IgG); and (iii) polyspecific EIA that detects antibodies of IgG, IgM, and/or IgA class (EIA-IgG/A/M). Clinical HIT indicates either of the top two levels of the iceberg, including the subset of patients with HIT complicated by thrombosis (HIT-T). The frequency of thrombosis among patients who do not develop thrombocytopenia is similar to that of antibody-negative controls.

TREATMENT

Section A of Table 41.4 lists six general principles of treatment.[1,8,17] If heparin is stopped in a patient with strongly suspected (or serologically confirmed) HIT, an appropriate nonheparin anticoagulant should be initiated. This is because 35 to 50% of patients with serologically confirmed HIT develop symptomatic thrombosis (including 5% thrombotic death rate) when heparin is stopped because of thrombocytopenia alone ("isolated" HIT).[1,5,8] Interestingly, antibody levels can decrease, and platelet counts can recover, even if heparin is continued in some patients with HIT.[22]

Given the high frequency of DVT, routine duplex ultrasonography is recommended.[16,17] Testing for HIT antibodies provides important corroborative (if strongly positive) or contrary (if negative or only weakly positive) information.[21] A negative test for HIT antibodies allows for resumption of heparin.

In the United States, two nonheparin anticoagulants, lepirudin (see later) and argatroban (see later), are approved for treatment of HIT. Fondaparinux, although not specifically approved for HIT, appears effective for this disorder,[17,23] and is increasingly utilized for this indication (see below).

CONTRAINDICATIONS: WARFARIN, PLATELET TRANSFUSIONS, VENA CAVA FILTERS

Warfarin

Warfarin is ineffective in acute HIT and predisposes to microvascular thrombosis.[12–15] Venous limb gangrene is a more common manifestation of *coumarin necrosis* in HIT than is "classic" skin necrosis. In patients with acute HIT, it is recommended that warfarin be postponed (or avoided

---

Table 41.4 **TREATMENT PRINCIPLES WHEN HIT IS STRONGLY SUSPECTED (OR CONFIRMED)**

A. General principles

1. Discontinue and avoid all heparin (including LMWH).

2. Give a nonheparin, alternative anticoagulant.

3. Postpone warfarin pending substantial platelet count recovery (give vitamin K if warfarin has already been started).

4. Test for HIT antibodies.

5. Investigate for lower limb DVT.

6. Avoid prophylactic platelet transfusions.

B. Nonheparin anticoagulant options during vascular surgery

Lepirudin

Intraoperative bolus*: 0.2–0.4 mg/kg IV (immediately before vascular clamping) followed by 0.05–0.10 mg/kg/h** (target APTT, 1.5–2.5 × baseline);

Intraoperative "flush" solution consisting of 0.1 mg/ml lepirudin (maximum, 250 ml administered during surgery);

Postoperative anticoagulation, ranging from 0.05 mg/kg/h (target APTT 1.5–2.0 × baseline APTT) or 15 mg bid SC in patients at relatively low risk for postoperative reocclusion (e.g., surgery involving aorta, iliac, femoral, or carotid arteries) to 0.10 mg/kg/h (target APTT 1.5–2.5 × baseline) for patients at relatively high risk of postoperative reocclusion (e.g., popliteal bypass).**

Argatroban

Intraoperative bolus*: 0.1 mg/kg bolus, followed by 0.5 to 2 μg/kg/min infusion (= 0.03 to 0.12 mg/kg/h) for intraoperative and postoperative anticoagulation (target APTT 1.5–3.0× baseline APTT).

Danaparoid

Intraoperative bolus*: 2,250 anti-Xa U for patient weighing 60–75 kg (bolus dose adjusted to 1,500 and 3,000 U for patients weighing <60 and >75 kg, respectively).

Intraoperative "flush" solution: 750 U in 250 ml normal saline (maximum, 250 ml if the intraoperative bolus has been given).

Postoperative anticoagulation, ranging from low (prophylactic dose), i.e., 750 U bid or tid SC or higher (therapeutic dose) usually 200 U/h (with target anti-Xa levels between 0.5 and 0.8 U/ml)

* Assumes patient has absent or low drug levels at start of surgery (otherwise bolus may not be required).

** In case of renal insufficiency, dosing must be decreased by up to 90%. As anesthesia results in decreased renal perfusion, the dose of lepirudin should be reduced by approximately 30% (with APTT adjustments) during surgery and in the early postoperative period even in a patient stably anticoagulated prior to surgery. The APTT should be monitored frequently during and following surgery.

Use of these agents for intraoperative anticoagulation represents "off-label" use.

bid, twice-daily; tid, thrice daily; U, units.

Section A is modified from Reference 29. Section B is modified from Reference 28, which also provides additional supporting literature.

completely) pending substantial resolution of thrombocytopenia (preferably, platelet count >150 × 10⁹/L), with subsequent gradual initiation of warfarin anticoagulation.[8]

Administration of vitamin K is advised when acute HIT is diagnosed after warfarin has already been started:[8,14] besides reducing risk of coumarin necrosis, this reduces risk of underdosing of lepirudin and argatroban, since warfarin prolongs the APTT used to monitor these anticoagulants.

Platelet Transfusions

Prophylactic platelet transfusions are not recommended, as petechiae and other evidence of impaired hemostasis usually are not seen in HIT; in theory, transfused platelets might contribute to increased thrombotic risk.

Vena Cava Filters

In my opinion, vena cava filters should be avoided, as their use in acute HIT often is complicated by massive lower limb venous thrombosis. Further, the presence of a filter might tempt physicians to avoid or minimize needed anticoagulation.

ALTERNATIVE NONHEPARIN ANTICOAGULANTS

Five alternative nonheparin anticoagulants have a rational basis for use in managing HIT.[17] Three (lepirudin, argatroban, bivalirudin) are direct thrombin inhibitors (DTIs), whereas two (danaparoid, fondaparinux) can be classified as indirect (antithrombin [AT]-dependent) inhibitors of activated factor X (Xa).

LEPIRUDIN (REFLUDAN)

Lepirudin is a recombinant hirudin that forms irreversible 1:1 complexes with thrombin.[17] (Hirudin is the thrombin inhibitor produced by the medicinal leech.) This 65-amino acid polypeptide (6,980 Da) exhibits exceptionally high affinity for thrombin (Ki = 0.0001 nmol/L) resulting from bivalent binding, as it recognizes both the fibrin(ogen) binding site and a region near the active (catalytic) site of thrombin. Its irreversible binding to thrombin could contribute to its efficacy. The half-life of lepirudin (about 80 min) increases greatly in renal insufficiency. As no antidote exists, major dose reduction is required for renally compromised patients.

Lepirudin is approved by the US Food and Drug Administration (FDA) for the treatment of HIT complicated by thrombosis. The approved dose (normal kidneys) is 0.4 mg/kg by IV bolus followed by an initial infusion rate at 0.15 mg/kg/h, adjusted for target APTT 1.5 to 2.5 times baseline. However, this protocol frequently results

in overdosing and bleeding, and therefore consensus conference guidelines[8] recommend much lower dosing, as follows: (1) no bolus; (2) initial infusion rate, 0.05 to 0.10 mg/kg/h (assumes normal renal function, otherwise dosing is much lower[8]); and (3) APTT monitoring at 4-h intervals until steady state is reached, and after any dose adjustment. An important problem arises when there is baseline APTT prolongation (e.g., severe HIT-associated DIC, preceding coumarin therapy, hepatic dysfunction, etc.): in this situation, APTT monitoring is not reliable, potentially contributing to adverse outcomes.[17,19]

Compared with historical controls, lepirudin treatment of serologically confirmed HIT complicated by thrombosis was associated with reduced thrombotic events, from approximately 25% to 7% (relative risk reduction [RRR], 0.72).[17] Lepirudin also appeared effective for treating isolated HIT.[8]

Lepirudin's foreign structure can trigger antihirudin antibodies that sometimes alter its pharmacokinetics, for example, drug accumulation resulting from impaired renal excretion of lepirudin-IgG complexes. Thus, daily APTT monitoring is required. Fatal anaphylaxis following IV bolus administration has been reported.

Recently (April 2012), the manufacturer discontinued lepirudin world-wide, although it may remain available in some jurisdictions through another manufacturer.

ARGATROBAN

Argatroban (Argatroban [US], Novastan [non-US]) is a synthetic, small-molecule DTI derived from arginine (527 Da). It reversibly binds to the active site pocket of thrombin alone and thus is a univalent DTI. The Ki of argatroban for human thrombin is 40 nmol/L, indicating lower affinity for thrombin than hirudin.[17] Its half-life is 40 to 50 min, and it undergoes hepatobiliary excretion. Argatroban is FDA-approved for the prophylaxis or treatment of thrombosis in patients with HIT.

Argatroban is not immunogenic, and anaphylaxis has not been reported. The usual dose is 2 μg/kg/min adjusted by APTT (usual target, 1.5–3 times baseline APTT), but lower starting doses are frequently given (0.5–1.2 μg/kg/min).[8] The starting dose should be reduced by 75% in a patient with significant liver dysfunction, or in a patient in the intensive care unit.

Compared with historical controls, argatroban treatment of clinically suspected HIT complicated by thrombosis was associated with reduced thrombotic events, from approximately 35% to 16% (RRR, 0.55). The lower RRR compared with lepirudin could reflect the shorter mean treatment duration of argatroban therapy in its clinical evaluation compared with lepirudin (7 vs. 14 d, respectively),[10] or perhaps differences in its fundamental mechanism of action (reversible vs. irreversible thrombin inhibition).

Prolongation of the INR by argatroban is considerably greater than with lepirudin,[24] which can complicate argatroban-warfarin overlap. Argatroban's greater effect on the INR results from its relatively low affinity for thrombin, and thus the need for greater molar concentrations (approximately twenty-fold) to double the APTT, compared with lepirudin. Plasma concentrations of argatroban ($\sim$1.0 μmol/L) are similar to the theoretical maximum amount of thrombin generated in the INR reaction.

BIVALIRUDIN

Bivalirudin (Angiomax) is a twenty-amino acid *hirulog* (analogue of hirudin) that unites a C-terminal segment of twelve amino acids (dodecapeptide) derived from hirudin to an active site-binding tetrapeptide sequence (d-Phe-Pro-Arg-Pro) at its N-terminus, bridged by four glycines (2,180 Da).[25] Indeed, bivalirudin connotes this bivalent binding to thrombin. Unlike hirudin, however, bivalirudin interaction with thrombin is transient, as plasma proteases cleave bivalirudin near its N-terminus. The affinity of bivalirudin for human thrombin (Ki = 2 nmol/L) is between that observed for lepirudin and argatroban; accordingly, its ability to prolong the INR is intermediate in comparison with these other two DTIs.[24] Bivalirudin has undergone off-label use in HIT, particularly in the setting of off-pump and on-pump (cardiopulmonary bypass) cardiac surgery.[25]

DANAPAROID (ORGARAN)

Danaparoid (Orgaran) is a "heparinoid" (mixture of anticoagulant glycosaminoglycans) that has both anti-Xa and antithrombin (anti-IIa) activity (anti-Xa/anti-IIa ratio = 22; 6,000 Da [mean]). It is available in Canada and Europe, but was withdrawn from the United States in 2002. It is effective for treatment and prevention of thrombosis in HIT, but its long half-life (25 h), lack of an antidote, and inability to inhibit clot-bound thrombin make it less than ideal for anticoagulation during vascular surgery.

FONDAPARINUX (ARIXTRA)

Fondaparinux (Arixtra), a synthetic indirect (AT-dependent) inhibitor of factor Xa, is modeled after the AT-binding pentasaccharide region of heparin (1,727 Da). Despite its small size (compared with natural heparin), anti-PF4/heparin antibodies are generated as often during fondaparinux therapy as with LMWH.[26] However, the antibodies formed do not cross-react with PF4/fondaparinux, suggesting that fondaparinux causes HIT even less often than LMWH, and probably is effective for treatment of HIT-associated thrombosis[17,23] (a situation for which LMWH is considered contraindicated[8]). Since fondaparinux is FDA-approved for prevention and treatment of venous thromboembolism (2.5 mg and 7.5 mg once daily by SC injection, respectively,

for average-sized adults), it is appropriate for many patients with a previous history of HIT, in which repeat use of heparin usually is avoided. As with danaparoid, the long half-life of fondaparinux (17 h), the lack of an antidote, and its inability to inhibit clot-bound thrombin make it less than ideal for anticoagulation during vascular surgery.

MANAGEMENT OF THE ISCHEMIC LIMB

EVALUATION OF LIMB ISCHEMIA

The clinician must determine whether there is large and medium-size artery thrombosis that could be amenable to surgical thromboembolectomy, or whether limb ischemia reflects microvascular thrombosis, thus indicating a medical rather than surgical emergency (see Figure 41.1). Often, microvascular thrombosis is associated with proximal DVT in the same limb, but can also be associated with arterial thrombosis particularly in the setting of overt DIC.

Arterial Thromboembolectomy

The vascular surgeon who manages a patient with limb-threatening ischemia due to artery occlusion in HIT faces the dilemma of how to anticoagulate such a patient during potentially limb-salvaging thromboembolectomy, as UFH is at least relatively contraindicated. However, for patients with acute (or recent) HIT requiring thromboembolectomy, it is unknown whether nonheparin anticoagulation achieves better outcomes over intraoperative anticoagulation with heparin.[27] A further issue is that in the emergency setting of thromboembolectomy for critical limb ischemia, there may not be sufficient time to obtain HIT antibody test results, consult a hematologist, or even organize alternative anticoagulation.

Section B of Table 41.4 lists various nonheparin options for intraoperative anticoagulation.[28] However, experience during vascular surgery with any of these approaches is minimal, and so risk-benefit considerations of any operative intervention must be judged individually. Whether monitoring is best performed using APTT, activated clotting time (ACT), or ecarin clotting time (ECT) is unknown.

Venous Limb Ischemia

Medical Management

Severe venous limb ischemia is a medical emergency, as effective anticoagulation may prevent its progression. Vitamin K (e.g., 10 mg IV over 30–60 min) is recommended for the patient who has received warfarin, or who has an elevated INR, since vitamin K antagonism or deficiency can explain venous limb ischemia.[12–15] The syndrome of phlegmasia cerulea dolens can be prodromal for venous gangrene, and prompt institution of effective anticoagulation could avoid critical limb ischemia.[12] Sometimes systemic or catheter-direct thrombolysis is given, but a caveat is that fibrin(ogen) degradation products produced by thrombolysis will bind and protect thrombin from its physiologic inhibitors, potentially worsening consumptive coagulopathy. Thus, in my opinion, at least moderate-dose anticoagulation should be given to a patient who is receiving thrombolysis (e.g., lepirudin, 0.05–0.10 mg/kg/h or danaparoid 100–200 U/h after an initial danaparoid bolus).

Surgical Management

A surgical role for severe venous limb ischemia is less certain. Fasciotomy is sometimes performed in patients with suspected compartment syndrome, but this may delay or interrupt much-needed aggressive anticoagulation. Further, it is uncertain to what extent compartment syndromes contribute to limb ischemia in patients with HIT-associated DVT and associated microvascular thrombosis.

Preoperative and Postoperative Anticoagulation

A patient with HIT-associated thrombosis who requires intraoperative anticoagulation with a nonheparin anticoagulant may already be receiving this agent during the immediate preoperative period, thus obviating the need for a full intraoperative dose. There is also the dilemma of whether to continue the anticoagulant immediately postoperatively, or whether to suspend infusion until postoperative hemostasis appears secure. However, the prothrombotic nature of acute HIT suggests that continuing anticoagulation even during the immediate postoperative period (at least in low-to-moderate doses) can be appropriate.

REFERENCES

1. Warkentin TE. Heparin-induced thrombocytopenia: Pathogenesis and management, *Br J Haematol.* 2003. *121*: 535–555.
2. Warkentin TE. Clinical picture of heparin-induced thrombocytopenia. In: Warkentin TE, Greinacher A, eds. *Heparin-induced thrombocytopenia*, 5e. Boca Raton, FL: CRC Press. 2013: 24–76.
3. Warkentin TE, Roberts RS, Hirsh J, Kelton JG. An improved definition of immune heparin-induced thrombocytopenia in postoperative orthopedic patients, *Arch Intern Med.* 2003. *163*: 2518–2524.
4. Linkins LA, Lee DH. Frequency of heparin-induced thrombocytopenia. In: Warkentin TE, Greinacher A, eds. *Heparin-induced thrombocytopenia*, 5e. Boca Raton, FL: CRC Press. 2013: 110–150.
5. Warkentin TE, Kelton JG. A 14-year study of heparin-induced thrombocytopenia, *Am J Med.* 1996. *101*: 502–507.
6. Lo GK, Juhl D, Warkentin TE, Sigouin CS, Eichler P, Greinacher A. Evaluation of pretest clinical score (4 T's) for the diagnosis of heparin-induced thrombocytopenia in two clinical settings, *J Thromb Haemost.* 2006. *4*: 759–765.
7. Warkentin TE, Kelton JG. Temporal aspects of heparin-induced thrombocytopenia, *N Engl J Med.* 2001. *344*: 1286–1292.
8. Linkins LA, Dans AL, Moores LK, Bona R, Davidson BL, Schulman S, et al. Treatment and prevention of heparin-induced thrombocytopenia: Antithrombotic Therapy and Prevention of Thrombosis, 9th ed: American College of Chest Physicians Evidence-Based Clinical Practice Guidelines, *Chest.* 2012. *141*(Suppl 2): e495S–e530S.
9. Warkentin TE, Kelton JG. Delayed-onset heparin-induced thrombocytopenia and thrombosis, *Ann Intern Med.* 2001. *135*: 502–506.
10. Warkentin TE. Management of heparin-induced thrombocytopenia: A critical comparison of lepirudin and argatroban, *Thromb Res.* 2003. *110*: 73–82.
11. Hong AP, Cook DJ, Sigouin CS, Warkentin TE. Central venous catheters and upper-extremity deep-vein thrombosis complicating immune heparin-induced thrombocytopenia, *Blood.* 2003. *101*: 3049–3051.
12. Warkentin TE, Elavathil LJ, Hayward CPM, Johnston MA, Russett JI, Kelton JG. The pathogenesis of venous limb gangrene associated with heparin-induced thrombocytopenia, *Ann Intern Med.* 1997. *127*: 804–812.
13. Smythe MA, Warkentin TE, Stephens JL, Zakalik D, Mattson JC. Venous limb gangrene during overlapping therapy with warfarin and a direct thrombin inhibitor for immune heparin-induced thrombocytopenia, *Am J Hematol.* 2002. *71*: 50–52.
14. Warkentin TE. Should vitamin K be administered when HIT is diagnosed after administration of coumarin?, *J Thromb Haemost.* 2006. *4*: 894–896.
15. Warkentin TE. Heparin-induced thrombocytopenia: IgG-mediated platelet activation, platelet microparticle generation, and altered procoagulant/anticoagulant balance in the pathogenesis of thrombosis and venous limb gangrene complicating heparin-induced thrombocytopenia, *Transfus Med Rev.* 1996. *10*: 249–258.
16. Warkentin TE. Heparin-induced thrombocytopenia. In: Hoffman R, Benz EJ Jr, Silberstein LE, Heslop HE, Weitz JI, Anastasi J, eds. *Hematology: Basic principles and practice,* 6e. Philadelphia: Churchill Livingstone Elsevier. 2013: 1913–1924.
17. Warkentin TE. Agents for the treatment of heparin-induced thrombocytopenia, *Hematol Oncol Clin North Am.* 2010. *24*: 755–775.
18. Warkentin TE, Greinacher A. Heparin-induced anaphylactic and anaphylactoid reactions: Two distinct but overlapping syndromes, *Expert Opin Drug Saf.* 2009. *8*: 129–144.
19. Greinacher A, Warkentin TE. The direct thrombin inhibitor hirudin, *Thromb Haemost.* 2008. *99*: 819–829.
20. Warkentin TE, Sheppard JI. Testing for heparin-induced thrombocytopenia antibodies, *Transfus Med Rev.* 2006. *20*: 259–272.
21. Warkentin TE, Sheppard JI, Moore JC, Sigouin CS, Kelton JG. Quantitative interpretation of optical density measurements using PF4-dependent enzyme-immunoassays, *J Thromb Haemost.* 2008. *6*: 1304–1312.
22. Warkentin TE, Sheppard JI, Moore JC, Cook RJ, Kelton JG. Studies of the immune response in heparin-induced thrombocytopenia, *Blood.* 2009. *113*: 4963–4969.
23. Warkentin TE, Pai M, Sheppard JI, Schulman S, Spyropoulos AC, Eikelboom JW. Fondaparinux treatment of acute heparin-induced thrombocytopenia confirmed by the serotonin-release assay: A 30-month, 16-patient case series. *J Thromb Haemost.* 2011. *9*: 2389–2396.
24. Warkentin TE, Greinacher A, Craven S, Dewar L, Sheppard JI, Ofosu FA. Differences in the clinically effective molar concentrations of four direct thrombin inhibitors explain their variable prothrombin time prolongation, *Thromb Haemost.* 2005. *94*: 958–964.
25. Warkentin TE, Greinacher A, Koster A. Bivalirudin, *Thromb Haemost.* 2008. *99*: 830–839.
26. Warkentin TE, Cook RJ, Marder VJ, et al. Anti-platelet factor 4/heparin antibodies in orthopedic surgery patients receiving antithrombotic prophylaxis with fondaparinux or enoxaparin, *Blood.* 2005. *106*: 3791–3796.
27. Warkentin TE, Pai M, Cook RJ. Intraoperative anticoagulation and limb amputations in patients with immune heparin-induced thrombocytopenia who require vascular surgery, *J Thromb Haemost.* 2012. *10*: 148–150.
28. Warkentin TE. Heparin-induced thrombocytopenia and vascular surgery, *Acta Chir Belgica.* 2004. *104*: 257–265.
29. Warkentin TE, Greinacher A. Appendix 4: Six treatment principles of HIT. In: Warkentin TE, Greinacher A, eds. *Heparin-induced thrombocytopenia*, 5e. Boca Raton, FL: CRC Press. 2013: 625.

42.

OPERATIVE VENOUS THROMBECTOMY

Anthony J. Comerota and Steven S. Gale

INTRODUCTION

Contemporary venous thrombectomy has the potential of offering patients with extensive iliofemoral and/or infrainguinal deep vein thrombosis (DVT) an opportunity for rapid resolution with significant reduction in postthrombotic morbidity. Early experience with venous thrombectomy was enthusiastically received because of reports of excellent patency without severe postthrombotic sequelae.

Mahorner et al.[1] and Haller and Abrams[2] reported excellent patency rates in patients operated on early for iliofemoral venous thrombosis. Haller and Abrams reported an 85% patency rate with 81% of survivors having normal legs without postthrombotic swelling. However, a subsequent follow-up report indicated higher rates of rethrombosis with failure to prevent postthrombotic sequelae, despite a patent deep venous system, presumably due to valvular incompetence.[3] This damaging report was a 5-year follow-up of patients originally described by Haller and Abrams. They reported that 94% of patients returning for follow-up had significant edema and skin changes, which required elastic stockings and leg elevation. Patients who underwent follow-up phlebography were found to have incompetent valves, although this represented only approximately 25% of the patients initially treated. Lansing and Davis[3] brought attention to the fact that two of the three postoperative deaths (in the thirty-four patients initially operated) were from pulmonary embolism (PE) and that there was a 30% wound complication rate, an average transfusion requirement of 1,000 ml, and a mean hospital stay of 12 d.

Critics of operative venous thrombectomy frequently fail to mention that the early technique was unlike modern thrombectomy procedures, with patients undergoing cut-downs on their iliac veins, femoral veins, and vena cava, often with flush and irrigation procedures performed to clear the venous system of thrombus, whereas venous thrombectomy today is performed with balloon catheters, and autotransfusion devices are available to minimize the need for blood transfusion. Completion phlebograms were essentially nonexistent with no effort to either identify or correct underlying venous pathology. Arteriovenous fistulae were not constructed, and it is unclear to what degree patients were anticoagulated either during the procedure or postoperatively.

The report by Lansing and Davis suffered from a selection bias, since it is likely that the patients with the most severe postthrombotic sequelae were returning for follow-up and therefore were the most heavily represented in their series. Furthermore, the patients reported represented only 50% of those initially operated on, with phlebographic examination in far fewer. Another damaging report was that of Karp and Wylie,[4] who reported uniform rethrombosis following iliofemoral venous thrombectomy. Although the patients' clinical symptoms appeared to be improved, the predischarge phlebographic documentation of rethrombosis led to further disinterest in venous thrombectomy.

Subsequent reports of successful thrombectomy from European centers,[5–12] with success rates reported as high as 88% without mortality, were for the most part ignored by surgeons in the United States. Moreover, until 2008, guideline authors overlooked a multicenter randomized trial evaluating contemporary venous thrombectomy versus standard anticoagulation.[13–15] Patients underwent systematic follow-up with routine venous imaging and physiologic measurements. Peer-reviewed reporting occurred at 6 months,[13] 5 years,[14] and 10 years[15] of follow-up. Patients randomized to venous thrombectomy demonstrated improved patency ($P < 0.05$), lower venous pressures ($P < 0.05$), less leg swelling ($P < 0.05$), and fewer postthrombotic symptoms ($P < 0.05$) compared with anticoagulation.

Fortunately, a number of vascular centers have persisted in using thrombectomy,[12,16] and with the ongoing experience and refinement of technique,[17] the results have markedly improved. Most notable among these technical improvements are the use of a venous thrombectomy catheter (large balloon), fluoroscopic-guided thrombectomy with completion intraoperative phlebography, correction of an underlying venous stenosis, construction of an arteriovenous fistula (AVF), and immediate and prolonged therapeutic anticoagulation, often catheter-directed.

RESULTS OF OPERATIVE VENOUS THROMBECTOMY

Although the early mortality rate in Haller and Abrams series was 9%, with two of the three fatalities attributed to PE, by the mid-1980s a progressive reduction in operative mortality was observed. Eklof and Juhan[18] reported their large experience in 230 patients undergoing venous thrombectomy for iliofemoral venous thrombosis. They reported no fatal PE and only one operative death. It is apparent that the application of venous thrombectomy now can be based on its effectiveness relative to competitive forms of therapy in reducing early morbidity and the late sequelae of iliofemoral venous thrombosis, rather than on the concern that the procedure will fail or be accompanied by complications.

Successful venous thrombectomy significantly reduces early morbidity in patients with phlegmasia cerulea dolens and phlegmasia alba dolens. The patients' pain and edema quickly subside and the discoloration resolves. The definition of benefit, however, may be masked by the additional cost of the operation, the need for blood transfusion, incisional discomfort, and wound complications. Interestingly, even if thrombectomy is not complete or is followed by some degree of rethrombosis, the limb rarely returns to its former morbid state if elevation and anticoagulation are continued. In our experience, thrombectomy has failed only when our own treatment guidelines were not observed. Although several patients may not have benefited, no patient has been made clinically worse, and we have yet to observe a symptomatic PE following the procedure.

The long-term benefits of venous thrombectomy relate to its ability to achieve proximal patency and maintain distal valve competence. Both are influenced by initial technical success and the avoidance of recurrent thrombosis. Initial success in achieving patency is, in turn, influenced by timely intervention and attention to technical detail. Pooled data from a number of contemporary reports on iliofemoral venous thrombectomy (Tables 42.1, 42.2) have indicated that the early and long-term patency for the iliofemoral venous segment is in the 75–80% range compared with 30% patency in patients treated with anticoagulation alone,[19] and femoral-popliteal venous valve function is preserved in the majority of patients.

TECHNIQUE

The incremental goals that we believe are important for successful venous thrombectomy are summarized in Table 42.3. During the past two decades, the technique of venous thrombectomy has been refined and improved. Most of the principles of a successful procedure follow those established for patients undergoing arterial reconstruction for acute arterial occlusion. A number of important technical modifications have evolved, however, beginning with the accurate preoperative definition of the extent of thrombus (both proximally and distally) and whether the thrombus has embolized to the pulmonary vascular bed. The proximal extent of thrombus can be clearly defined by contralateral iliocavagraphy. It is especially important

Table 42.1 **VENOUS THROMBECTOMY WITH ARTERIOVENOUS FISTULA: LONG-TERM ILIAC VEIN PATENCY**

AUTHOR/YEAR (REFERENCE NO.)	NO.	FOLLOW-UP (MO)	PATENT ILIAC VEIN (%)
Plate et al. 1984 (13)	31	6	76
Piquet et al. 1985 (5)	57	39	80
Einarsson et al. 1986 (6)	58	10	61
Vollmar 1986 (7)	93	53	82
Juhan et al. 1999 (8)	150	102	84
Torngren et al. 1988 (9)	54	19	54
Rasmussen et al. 1990 (10)	24	20	88
Eklof et al. 1996 (12)	77	48	75
Neglen et al. 1991 (11)	34	24	88
Meissner et al. 1996 (25)	27	12	89
Pillny et al. 2003 (26)	97	70	90
Hartung et al. 2008 (27)	29	63	86
Holper et al. 2009 (28)	25	68	84
TOTAL	756	55 mo (mean)	80% (mean)

Adapted from Comerota AJ, Gale SS. Surgical venous thrombectomy for iliofemoral deep vein thrombosis. In: Greenhalgh RM, ed. *Towards vascular and endovascular consensus*. London: BIBA Publishing. 2005. Used with permission.

Table 42.2 VENOUS THROMBECTOMY WITH ARTERIOVENOUS FISTULA: LONG-TERM VALVE COMPETENCE OF FEMOROPOPLITEAL VENOUS SEGMENT

AUTHOR/YEAR (REFERENCE NO.)	NO.	FOLLOW-UP (MO)	FEMORAL-POPLITEAL VALVE COMPETENCE
Plate et al. 1984 (13)	31	6	52
Einarsson et al. 1986 (6)	53	10	42
Ganger et al. 1989 (29)	17	91	82
Neglen et al. 1991(11)	37	24	56
Kniemeyer et al. 1993 (30)	37	55	80
Juhan et al. 1999 (8)	150	60	80
Meissner et al. 1996 (25)	27	60	30
TOTAL	352	45 mo (mean)	63% (mean)

From Comerota AJ, Gale SS. Surgical venous thrombectomy for iliofemoral deep vein thrombosis. In: Greenhalgh RM, ed. *Towards vascular and endovascular consensus*. London: BIBA Publishing. 2005. Used with permission.

to determine whether thrombus has extended into the vena cava. Magnetic resonance venography (MRV) with gadolinium or spiral computerized tomography (CT) scan with contrast may obviate the invasive procedure in some patients. Our preference is spiral CT scan with contrast of the head, chest, abdomen, and pelvis. Extending the imaging not only localizes the proximal extent of thrombus, but also screens for other pathology.

During the operation, complete thrombus removal is ensured by completion phlebography. Correction of an underlying venous stenosis with balloon angioplasty and stenting (if needed) is critical to obtain unobstructed venous drainage into the vena cava. Residual iliac vein obstruction produces venous hypertension at best and often leads to recurrent venous thrombosis. Therefore, it must be identified and corrected. A properly constructed AVF increases venous velocity through the previously thrombosed iliofemoral venous system without increasing venous pressure, thereby decreasing the risk of rethrombosis. Prolonged therapeutic anticoagulation is important to prevent recurrence.

The more recent modifications, which include balloon catheter thrombectomy of the vena cava during suprarenal caval balloon occlusion for nonocclusive caval clot, infrainguinal venous thrombectomy followed by early and continued postoperative anticoagulation through a catheter remaining in the posterior tibial vein, and construction of an AVF, are likely to further improve outcome. The sequential details of the contemporary venous thrombectomy are described in the following sections.

Table 42.3 **TECHNIQUE OF CONTEMPORARY VENOUS THROMBECTOMY**

1. Identify etiology of extensive venous thromboembolic process
   a. Complete thrombophilia evaluation
   b. Rapid CT scan of head, chest, abdomen, and pelvis
2. Define full extent of thrombus
   a. Venous duplex examination
   b. Contralateral iliocavagram, MRV, or spiral CT
3. Prevent pulmonary embolism (numerous techniques)
   a. Anticoagulation
   b. Vena cava filter (if nonocclusive caval clot)
   c. Balloon occlusion of vena cava during thrombectomy
   d. Positive end-expiratory pressure during thrombectomy
4. Perform a complete thrombectomy
   a. Iliofemoral (vena cava) thrombectomy
   b. Infrainguinal venous thrombectomy (if required)
5. Ensure unobstructed venous inflow to and outflow from thrombectomized iliofemoral venous system
   a. Infrainguinal venous thrombectomy (if required)
   b. Correct iliac vein stenosis (stent)
6. Prevent recurrent thrombosis
   a. Arteriovenous fistula
   b. Continuous therapeutic anticoagulation
   c. Catheter-directed postoperative anticoagulation (if infrainguinal venous thrombectomy is required)
   d. Extended oral anticoagulation

MRV, magnetic resonance venography; CT, computerized tomography

PREOPERATIVE PROCEDURES

1. Evaluate the patient for an underlying thrombophilia. Since the majority of patients with DVT do not develop this degree of extensive thrombosis, the likelihood of identifying an underlying thrombophilia is high. If the patient is already anticoagulated, blood is sent for antiphospholipid antibody, Factor V Leiden, prothrombin gene mutation, and homocysteine tests. These can be reliably performed in patients who are already being treated with heparin. The

results of the hypercoagulable evaluation are important for appropriate recommendations regarding duration of anticoagulation. A blood sample is also sent for type and cross-match.

2. Delineate the full extent of thrombus. It is always important to know whether clot is involving the vena cava. A contralateral iliocavagram frequently is performed to assess the vena cava (Figure 42.1). Additionally, a rapid spiral CT scan with contrast of the head and chest examines for PE as well as brain and thoracic pathology. The subsequent abdominal and pelvic CT scans during the same contrast infusion can identify the proximal extent of thrombus and any intra-abdominal or pelvic pathology that may be etiologically associated with the DVT (Figure 42.2). We have found PE in approximately 50% of our patients. We have also found renal cell carcinoma with tumor thrombus extending into the vena cava, adrenal tumors, retroperitoneal lymphoma, hepatic metastases from unknown primaries, and iliac vein aneurysms. Each of these is critically important for proper patient management and would have been overlooked had the CT scan not been performed.

3. Therapeutic anticoagulation with unfractionated heparin (UFH) or low molecular weight heparin (LMWH) is initiated after the blood samples are drawn for the thrombophilia evaluation. UFH is used during the procedure and early postoperative period. Although LMWH is as effective as UFH, intravenous UFH offers better temporal control of the degree of anticoagulation.

4. Vena caval filtration is not routinely required. An exception may be those patients with nonocclusive thrombus extending into the vena cava (Figure 42.1). The recently introduced optional (nonpermanent) vena cava filters have been used with plans for early retrieval. Patients with caval thrombus also have been managed with balloon occlusion of the proximal vena cava at the time of balloon catheter thrombectomy. The protective vena caval balloon is positioned during preoperative iliocavagraphy from the contralateral femoral vein using fluoroscopic guidance. After positioning, the balloon remains deflated until the time of thrombus extraction (Figure 42.3).

5. The operating room is prepared for fluoroscopy. An autotransfusion device is made available during the procedure.

OPERATIVE DETAILS

6. General anesthesia is recommended for the majority of patients.

7. A longitudinal inguinal incision is made with exposure and control of the common femoral vein, femoral vein, saphenofemoral junction, and profunda femoris vein (Figure 42.4A).

8. A longitudinal venotomy is made in the common femoral vein at about the level of the saphenofemoral junction. The precise location of the venotomy depends on the extent and location of the thrombus. Since the common femoral vein is dilated, closure of the longitudinal venotomy with

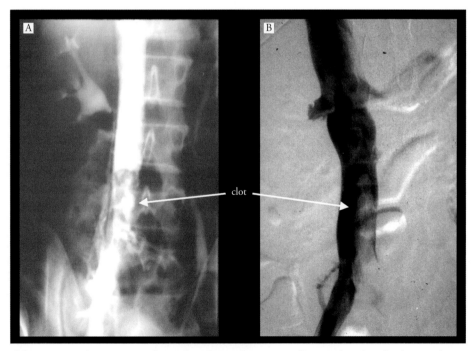

Figure 42.1 Contralateral iliocavagrams showing nonocclusive thrombus in the vena cava illustrate the value of imaging to detect proximal extent of thrombus. From: Comerota AJ, Gale SS. Surgical venous thrombectomy for iliofemoral deep vein thrombosis. In: Greenhalgh RM, ed. *Towards vascular and endovascular consensus*. London: BIBA Publishing. 2005. Used with permission.

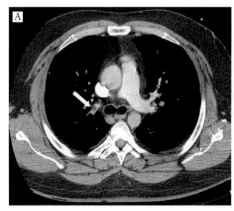
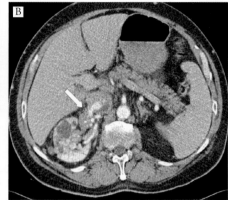

Figure 42.2 Asymptomatic PE (arrow, A) and renal cell carcinoma (arrow, B) identified with CT scan of chest as part of the evaluation of patients with iliofemoral DVT. From: Comerota AJ, Gale SS. Surgical venous thrombectomy for iliofemoral deep vein thrombosis. In: Greenhalgh RM, ed. *Towards vascular and endovascular consensus*. London: BIBA Publishing. 2005. Used with permission.

fine monofilament suture can be achieved without compromising vein lumen.

9. The infrainguinal venous thrombectomy is performed first. The leg is elevated and compressed from the toes proximally with a tightly wrapped rubber bandage. The foot is dorsiflexed and the leg squeezed and milked to remove the clot from below.

10. If infrainguinal clot persists, a cut-down on the medial portion of the lower leg is performed to expose the posterior tibial vein in order to accomplish a balloon catheter infrainguinal venous thrombectomy (Figure 42.4B). A #3 or #4 balloon catheter is passed proximally from below to exit from the common femoral venotomy (Figure 42.5A). The stem of a plastic IV catheter (12–14

gauge) is slid halfway onto the balloon catheter coming up from below and another (#4) balloon catheter is placed into the opposite end of the plastic sheath. Pressure is applied to the syringes attached to the two catheters by a single operating surgeon; this secures the balloons inside the sheath. The #4 balloon catheter is guided distally through the venous valves and clotted veins (Figure 42.5B) to the level of the posterior tibial venotomy (Figure 42.5C). The infrainguinal venous thrombectomy is then performed with a #4 or #5 balloon catheter, if necessary (Figure 42.5, D and E), repeating catheter passage as required until no further thrombus is extracted.

11. Following the infrainguinal balloon catheter thrombectomy, the infrainguinal venous system is vigorously

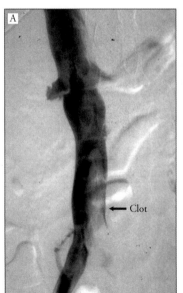
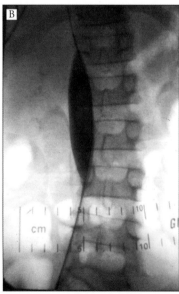
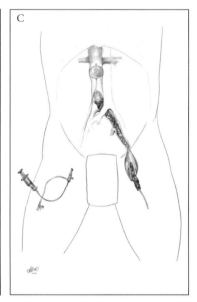

Figure 42.3 Preoperative iliocavagram shows nonocclusive thrombus extending from the left iliofemoral venous system into the vena cava (A). A suprarenal balloon catheter was placed from the contralateral femoral vein and inserted under fluoroscopy. The balloon is inflated at the time of thrombectomy (B). Schematic of iliocaval thrombectomy performed with the double balloon catheter technique, protecting the patient from pulmonary embolism (C). From Reference 17. Used with permission.

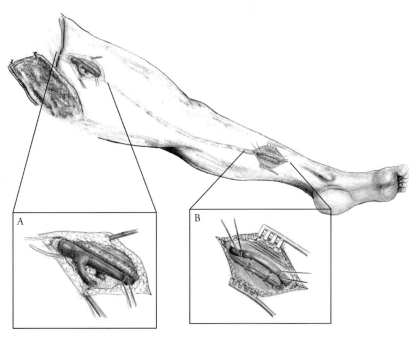

Figure 44.4 Exposure of the common femoral, femoral, and profunda femoris veins (A). Exposure of the posterior tibial vein (B). From: Comerota AJ, Gale SS. Contemporary venous thrombectomy. In: Fischer JE, Bland KI, eds. *Mastery of surgery*, 5e. Philadelphia, PA: Lippincott Williams & Wilkins. 2006. Used with permission.

flushed with a heparin-saline solution to hydraulically force residual thrombus (which can be considerable) from the deep venous system by placing a #14–#16 red rubber catheter into the proximal posterior tibial vein and flushing with a bulb syringe (Figure 42.6). After flushing, a vascular clamp is applied below the femoral venotomy, and the infrainguinal venous system is then filled with a dilute plasminogen activator solution using approximately 4–6 mg of rt-PA in 200 cc of saline. The plasminogen activator solution remains in the infrainguinal veins for the remainder of the procedure. If the infrainguinal venous thrombectomy is not successful due to chronic thrombus in the femoral vein, the femoral vein is ligated and divided below the profunda. Patency of the profunda is ensured by direct thrombectomy, if required.

12. The proximal thrombectomy is performed by passing a #8 or #10 venous thrombectomy catheter partway into the iliac vein for several passes to remove thrombus before advancing the catheter into the vena cava. The proximal thrombectomy is performed under fluoroscopy using a contrast-saline solution to expand the balloon. This is especially important if a vena cava filter is present, there is clot in the vena cava, or resistance to catheter passage is encountered. The anesthesiologist should apply positive end-expiratory pressure during the iliocaval thrombectomy to further reduce the risk of PE. If there is clot in the vena cava, the caval thrombectomy can be performed with a protective balloon catheter inflated above the thrombus and the thrombectomy performed under fluoroscopy (Figure 42.3).

13. After completion of the iliofemoral thrombectomy, the iliofemoral venous system is examined with intraoperative phlebography/fluoroscopy to ensure unobstructed venous drainage into and through the vena cava (Figure 42.7). Any underlying iliac vein stenosis is corrected with balloon angioplasty using a stent if venous recoil occurs. If a stent is used, a diameter of 12 mm or greater is recommended.

14. After closing the venotomy with fine monofilament suture, an end-side AVF is constructed using the end of the proximal saphenous vein or a large proximal branch of the saphenous vein anastomosed to the side of the superficial femoral artery (Figure 42.8A). The anastomosis should be limited to 3.5–4.0 mm in diameter. Frequently the proximal saphenous vein requires thrombectomy to restore patency prior to the AVF.

15. A piece of polytetrafluoroethylene (PTFE) or a silastic band is placed around the saphenous AVF and a large permanent monofilament suture (#0) looped and clipped, leaving approximately 2 cm in the subcutaneous tissue (Figure 42.8A). This will guide future dissection in the event that operative closure of the AVF becomes necessary; however, most do not.

16. Common femoral vein pressures are measured before and after the AVF is opened. Pressures should not change. If the venous pressure increases when the AVF is opened, the iliac veins should be reevaluated for residual stenosis or obstruction, and the proximal lesion corrected. If the pressure remains elevated, the AVF is constricted to decrease flow and normalize pressure.

17. If there appears to be notable serous fluid in the wound, a search for transected lymphatics is performed and they are ligated or coagulated. A #7 Jackson-Pratt drain (or other similar closed suction drain) is placed in the wound to evacuate hematoma or serous fluid that may accumulate postoperatively. The drain exits through a separate puncture

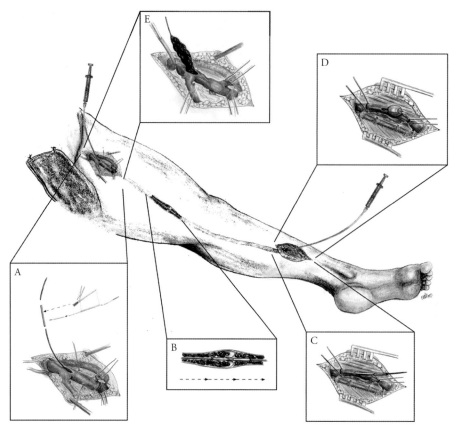

Figure 42.5 Technique of infrainguinal balloon catheter venous thrombectomy begins with passage of a #3 or #4 balloon catheter from the posterior tibial vein proximally, exiting the femoral venotomy. A silastic IV sheath is placed halfway onto the catheter and another #4 balloon catheter inserted into the other end of the sheath (A). The balloons are inflated to fix the catheter tips inside of the sheath with pressure applied by a single individual guiding them distally through the clotted veins and venous valves (B). Catheters and sheath exit the posterior tibial venotomy (C). The thrombectomy catheter balloon is gently inflated as the catheter is pulled proximally (D) to exit the femoral venotomy, extracting thrombus (E).   From Reference 17. Used with permission.

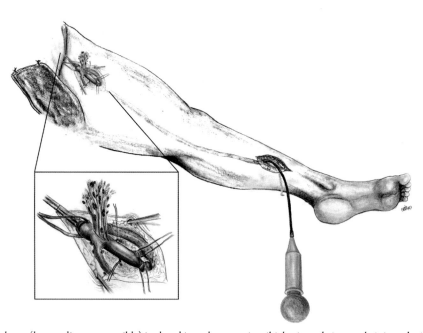

Figure 42.6 A red rubber catheter (largest diameter possible) is placed into the posterior tibial vein and vigorously injected with a heparin-saline solution using a bulb syringe to flush residual thrombus. After flushing, the femoral vein is clamped and the leg veins injected with 150–200 cc of a dilute UK or rt-PA solution.   From Reference 17. Used with permission.

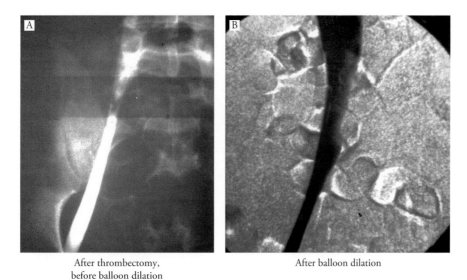

After thrombectomy,
before balloon dilation

After balloon dilation

Figure 42.7   After thrombectomy, the right common iliac vein shows residual stenosis (A). Following iliac vein venoplasty, the stenosis is corrected, restoring unobstructed venous drainage into the vena cava (B).   From: Comerota AJ, Gale SS. Surgical venous thrombectomy for iliofemoral deep vein thrombosis. In: Greenhalgh RM, ed. *Towards vascular and endovascular consensus.* London: BIBA Publishing. 2005. Used with permission.

site adjacent to the incision. The wound is closed with multilayered running absorbable sutures to achieve a hemostatic and lymphostatic wound closure.

18. The distal posterior tibial vein is ligated. An infusion catheter (typically a pediatric feeding tube) is brought into the wound via a separate stab incision in the skin and inserted and fixed in the proximal posterior tibial vein (Figure 42.8B). This catheter is used for postoperative heparin anticoagulation and a follow-up (predischarge) phlebogram. This ensures maximal heparin concentration into the affected venous segment. A 2-0 monofilament suture is looped around the posterior tibial vein (and catheter) and

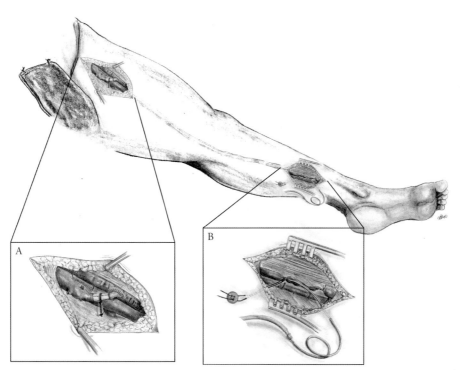

Figure 42.8   The venotomy is closed with fine monofilament suture, and a 3.5- to 4.0-mm AVF is constructed sewing the transected end of the saphenous vein to the side of the superficial femoral artery. A piece of PTFE (5-mm graft) or similar wrap is placed around the saphenous AVF, looped with #0 monofilament suture and the ends clipped, leaving approximately 2–2½ cm in the subcutaneous tissue to guide surgical closure of the AVF, should it be necessary (A). The distal posterior tibial vein is ligated. An infusion catheter (pediatric NG-tube) is brought into the wound through a separate stab wound in the skin and inserted and fixed in the proximal posterior tibial vein. The proximal posterior tibial vein and catheter is looped with #0 monofilament suture and fixed to the skin through a sterile button, which is used to snugly occlude the posterior tibial vein at the time of catheter removal (B).   From Reference 17. Used with permission.

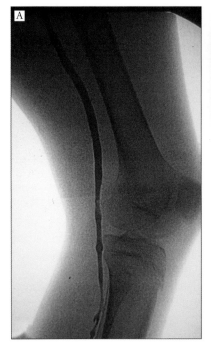
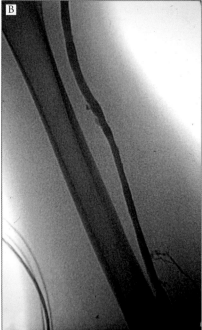

Figure 42.9 An ascending phlebogram evaluates venous patency prior to catheter removal, after the patient is therapeutic on warfarin. From: Comerota AJ, Gale SS. Contemporary venous thrombectomy. In: Fischer JE, Bland KI, eds. *Mastery of surgery*, 5e. Philadelphia, PA: Lippincott Williams & Wilkins. 2006. Used with permission.

both ends exit the skin. Both ends of the suture are passed through the holes of a sterile button, which is secured snugly to the skin when the catheter is removed. This obliterates the proximal posterior tibial vein and eliminates the risk of bleeding following catheter removal. Prior to catheter removal, an ascending phlebogram is performed through the catheter to once again examine the veins phlebographically (Figure 42.9).

POSTOPERATIVE DETAILS

19. After wound closure, antibiotic ointment and sterile dressings are placed on the wounds. The patient's leg is wrapped with sterile gauze and multilayered elastic bandages from the base of the toes to the groin. The bandages are snugly applied, with the posterior tibial vein catheter exiting between the layers of the bandage on the lower leg.

20. Full anticoagulation is continued postoperatively with UFH through the catheter in the posterior tibial vein. The heparin solution and pump are attached to an IV pole with wheels and the patient is allowed (encouraged) to ambulate. Oral anticoagulation is begun when the patient is awake and resumes oral intake. The heparin infusion is continued for a minimum of 4–5 d and the INR reaches 2–3.

21. Intermittent pneumatic compression garments are used on both legs during the postoperative period when the patient is not ambulating.

22. Prior to removing the posterior tibial vein catheter, a predischarge ascending phlebogram is obtained to evaluate patency of the femoropopliteal and iliofemoral venous segments. In the presence of an AVF, there may be significant

washout of contrast in the common femoral vein, thereby mitigating good visualization of the iliac venous segments. Any significant stenosis in the iliofemoral venous segment should be treated to maintain unobstructed venous drainage into the vena cava.

23. Oral anticoagulation is continued for an extended period of time, at least 1 year in all patients and indefinitely in many.

24. Upon discharge the patient is prescribed 30–40 mmHg ankle gradient compression stockings and instructed to wear the stockings from the time he/she awakens in the morning until bedtime. Compression stockings further reduce postthrombotic sequelae.[20, 21]

DISCUSSION

The 2008 American College of Chest Physicians (ACCP) Evidence-based Clinical Practice Guidelines (8th ed.) recommends that patients with iliofemoral DVT should be considered for a management strategy designed to remove thrombus from the iliofemoral system in order to reduce postthrombotic sequelae (Grade 2B).[22] Many patients are now treated as outpatients for acute DVT. However, when common femoral vein thrombosis with occlusion is identified by venous duplex, we would recommend that the patient be hospitalized and the strategy that is summarized in Figure 42.10 adopted. If the patient is not a candidate for catheter-directed thrombolysis, the recommendation for venous thrombectomy (Grade 2C) should be followed.

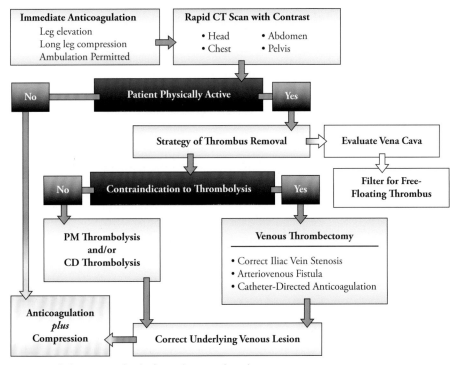

Management of Iliofemoral DVT

Figure 42.10 Algorithm: Recommended treatment for iliofemoral venous thrombosis. From: Comerota AJ, Gale SS. Contemporary venous thrombectomy. In: Fischer JE, Bland KI, eds. *Mastery of surgery*, 5e. Philadelphia, PA: Lippincott Williams & Wilkins. 2006. Used with permission.

Successful thrombus removal results in improved quality of life and fewer postthrombotic sequelae.[13–15,23] A randomized trial of catheter-directed thrombolysis versus anticoagulation has shown better patency and preserved valve function in those treated with thrombolytic therapy.[24] Patients who have iliofemoral DVT and contraindications to lytic therapy should be considered for venous thrombectomy if they present within 10 d of the onset of their DVT.

Aggressive anticoagulation combined with leg compression[20,21] is the preferred treatment for patients who have a contraindication to thrombolysis, are poor operative candidates, have a prolonged duration of venous thrombosis, or are critically ill or bedridden.

Contemporary venous thrombectomy has substantially improved the early and long-term results of patients with extensive DVT compared to the initial reports. The major technical differences between the initial and contemporary procedures are listed in Table 42.4. Recent reports of those performing venous thrombectomy and the long-term results of a large Scandinavian randomized trial confirm significant benefit compared to anticoagulation alone. Therefore, vascular surgeons should include contemporary venous thrombectomy as part of their routine operative armamentarium.

Table 42.4 **VENOUS THROMBECTOMY: COMPARISON OF OLD AND CONTEMPORARY TECHNIQUES**

TECHNIQUE	OLD	CONTEMPORARY
Pretreatment phlebography/ CT scan	Occasionally	Always
Venous thrombectomy catheter	No	Yes
Operative fluoroscopy/ phlebography	No	Yes
Correct iliac vein stenosis (stent)	No	Yes
Arteriovenous fistula	No	Yes
Infrainguinal thrombectomy	No	Yes
Full post-op anticoagulation	Occasionally	Yes
Catheter-directed anticoagulation	No	Yes
IPC post op	No	Yes

IPC, intermittent pneumatic compression

Adapted from Comerota AJ, Gale SS. Surgical venous thrombectomy for iliofemoral deep vein thrombosis. In: Greenhalgh RM, ed. *Towards vascular and endovascular consensus*. London: BIBA Publishing. 2005. Used with permission.

REFERENCES

1. Mahorner H, Castleberry JW, Coleman WO. Attempts to restore function in major veins which are the site of massive thrombosis, *Ann Surg.* 1957. *146*(3): 510–522.
2. Haller JA, Abrams BL. Use of thrombectomy in the treatment of acute iliofemoral venous thrombosis in forty-five patients, *Ann Surg.* 1963. *158*: 561–569.
3. Lansing AM, Davis WM. Five-year follow-up study of iliofemoral venous thrombectomy, *Ann Surg.* 1968. *168*(4): 620–628.
4. Karp RB, Wylie EJ. Recurrent thrombosis after iliofemoral venous thrombectomy, *Surg Forum.* 1966. *17*: 147.

5. Piquet P. Traitement chirurgical des thromboses iliocaves: Exigences et resultats. In: Kieffer E, ed. *Chirurgie de la veine cave inferieure et de ses branches*. Paris: Expansion Scientifique Francaise. 1985. 210–216.

6. Einarsson E, Albrechtsson U, Eklof B. Thrombectomy and temporary AV-fistula in iliofemoral vein thrombosis: Technical considerations and early results, *Int Angiol*. 1986. 5(2): 65–72.

7. Vollmar JF. Robert May memorial lecture: Advances in reconstructive venous surgery, *Int Angiol*. 1986. 5(3): 117–129.

8. Juhan C, Alimi Y, Di Mauro P, Hartung O. Surgical venous thrombectomy, *Cardiovasc Surg*. 1999. 7(6): 586–590.

9. Torngren S, Swedenborg J. Thrombectomy and temporary arterio-venous fistula for ilio-femoral venous thrombosis, *Int Angiol*. 1988. 7(1): 14–18.

10. Rasmussen A, Mogensen K, Nissen FH, Wadt J, Skibsted L. Acute iliofemoral venous thrombosis: 26 cases treated with thrombectomy, temporary arteriovenous fistula, and anticoagulants, *Ugeskr Laeger*. 1990. 152(40): 2928–2930.

11. Neglen P, al-Hassan HK, Endrys J, Nazzal MM, Christenson JT, Eklof B. Iliofemoral venous thrombectomy followed by percutaneous closure of the temporary arteriovenous fistula, *Surgery*. 1991. 110(3): 493–499.

12. Eklof B, Kistner RL. Is there a role for thrombectomy in iliofemoral venous thrombosis?, *Semin Vasc Surg*. 1996. 9(1): 34–45.

13. Plate G, Einarsson E, Ohlin P, Jensen R, Qvarfordt P, Eklof B. Thrombectomy with temporary arteriovenous fistula: The treatment of choice in acute iliofemoral venous thrombosis, *J Vasc Surg*. 1984. 1(6): 867–876.

14. Plate G, Akesson H, Einarsson E, Ohlin P, Eklof B. Long-term results of venous thrombectomy combined with a temporary arterio-venous fistula, *Eur J Vasc Surg*. 1990. 4(5): 483–489.

15. Plate G, Eklof B, Norgren L, Ohlin P, Dahlstrom JA. Venous thrombectomy for iliofemoral vein thrombosis: 10-year results of a prospective randomised study, *Eur J Vasc Endovasc Surg*. 1997. 14(5): 367–374.

16. Comerota AJ, Aldridge SC, Cohen G, Ball DS, Pliskin M, White JV. A strategy of aggressive regional therapy for acute iliofemoral venous thrombosis with contemporary venous thrombectomy or catheter-directed thrombolysis, *J Vasc Surg*. 1994. 20(2): 244–254.

17. Comerota AJ, Gale SS. Technique of contemporary iliofemoral and infrainguinal venous thrombectomy, *J Vasc Surg*. 2006. 43(1): 185–191.

18. Eklof B, Juhan C. Revival of thrombectomy in the management of acute iliofemoral venous thrombosis, *Contemp Surg*. 1992. 40: 21.

19. Akesson H, Brudin L, Dahlstrom JA, Eklof B, Ohlin P, Plate G. Venous function assessed during a 5 year period after acute ilio-femoral venous thrombosis treated with anticoagulation, *Eur J Vasc Surg*. 1990. 4(1): 43–48.

20. Brandjes DP, Buller HR, Heijboer H, et al. Randomised trial of effect of compression stockings in patients with symptomatic proximal-vein thrombosis, *Lancet*. 1997. 349(9054): 759–762.

21. Prandoni P, Lensing AW, Prins MH, et al. Below-knee elastic compression stockings to prevent the post-thrombotic syndrome: A randomized, controlled trial, *Ann Intern Med*. 2004. 141(4): 249–256.

22. Kearon C, Kahn SR, Agnelli G, Goldhaber SZ, Raskob G, Comerota AJ. Antithrombotic therapy for venous thromboembolic disease: ACCP evidence-based clinical practice guidelines (8th ed), *Chest*. 2008. 133(6): 454S–545S.

23. Comerota AJ, Throm RC, Mathias SD, Haughton S, Mewissen M. Catheter-directed thrombolysis for iliofemoral deep venous thrombosis improves health-related quality of life, *J Vasc Surg*. 2000. 32(1): 130–137.

24. Elsharawy M, Elzayat E. Early results of thrombolysis vs anticoagulation in iliofemoral venous thrombosis: A randomised clinical trial, *Eur J Vasc Endovasc Surg*. 2002. 24(3): 209–214.

25. Meissner AJ, Huszcza S. Surgical strategy for management of deep venous thrombosis of the lower extremities, *World J Surg*. 1996. 20(9): 1149–1155.

26. Pillny M, Sandmann W, Luther B, et al. Deep venous thrombosis during pregnancy and after delivery: Indications for and results of thrombectomy, *J Vasc Surg*. 2003. 37(3): 528–532.

27. Hartung O, Alimi YS, Di Mauro P, Portier F, Juhan C. Endovascular treatment of iliocaval occlusion caused by retroperitoneal fibrosis: Late results in two cases, *J Vasc Surg*. 2002. 36(4): 849–852.

28. Holper P, Kotelis D, Attigah N, Hyhlik-Durr A, Bockler D. Longterm results after surgical thrombectomy and simultaneous stenting for symptomatic iliofemoral venous thrombosis, *Eur J Vasc Endovasc Surg*. 2010. 39(3): 349–355.

29. Ganger KH, Nachbur BH, Ris HB, Zurbrugg H. Surgical thrombectomy versus conservative treatment for deep venous thrombosis: Functional comparison of long-term results, *Eur J Vasc Surg*. 1989. 3(6): 529–538.

30. Kniemeyer HW, Sandmann W, Schwindt C, Grabitz K, Torsello G, Stuhmeier K. Thrombectomy with arteriovenous fistula for embolizing deep venous thrombosis: An alternative therapy for prevention of recurrent pulmonary embolism, *Clin Investig*. 1993. 72(1): 40–45.

43.

PERMANENT VENA CAVA FILTERS

INDICATIONS, FILTER TYPES, AND RESULTS

Ali F. AbuRahma and Patrick A. Stone

INTRODUCTION

The incidence of pulmonary embolism (PE) is estimated to be around 355,000 patients per year and results in as many as 240,000 deaths per year in the United States.[1] The standard treatment for PE remains therapeutic anticoagulation. However, 5 to 8% of patients receiving therapeutic anticoagulation for PE experience a second PE episode.[2,3] Complications of anticoagulation also occur in up to 26% of patients.[2,3] There are many instances in which anticoagulation is either contraindicated or patients experience a complication of anticoagulation necessitating its discontinuation. In these situations, inferior vena cava (IVC) filter insertion is indicated to prevent PE.

Since the introduction of the first percutaneous Greenfield filter in 1984,[4] several lower profile percutaneously inserted caval filters have been developed; and presently, ten devices are approved by the US Food and Drug Administration.

THE IDEAL CAVAL FILTER

Several ideal caval filter characteristics have been recognized.[5] These characteristics include: (1) biocompatible, nonthrombogenic, with infinite implant lifetime performance; (2) secure fixation within the IVC; (3) high filtering efficiency with no impedance of flow; (4) small caliber delivery system with ease of percutaneous insertion with a simple and controlled release mechanism amenable to repositioning; (5) low access site thrombosis; (6) low cost; (7) retrievability; (8) magnetic resonance imaging (MRI) compatibility. Many of these features have been achieved in some of the newer IVC devices; however, the ideal device has yet to be developed. Long-term performance characteristic of caval filters is particularly significant in patients being considered for prophylactic IVC filter insertion.

INDICATIONS AND CONTRAINDICATIONS FOR CAVAL FILTER INSERTION

Although the data on the benefit versus the risk of caval filters are limited, the use of these filters has increased dramatically. Stein et al.[6] reported that the use of caval filters in the United States between 1979 and 1999 increased 2,000%. The number of patients who had caval filters increased from 2,000 in 1979 to 49,000 in 1999. Forty-five percent of caval filter insertions were in patients with deep vein thrombosis (DVT) alone in 1999, 36% were in patients with PE, and 19% were in patients who were presumably at high risk, but did not have DVT or PE listed as a discharge code.[6,7]

Table 43.1 summarizes the various absolute and relative indications for IVC filter insertion. This table includes the established indications for caval filter placement and also summarizes indications that may be debatable or controversial.[8,9]

Overall, patients with complications of anticoagulation or contraindications to anticoagulation should be managed with caval filter insertion alone. In certain cases, both caval filtration and anticoagulation may be used to protect patients, for example, patients with chronic PE who are being considered for pulmonary embolectomy or patients with severe cardiopulmonary compromise that places them at greater risk if any additional embolic insults occur.

Relative indications for caval filters included the presence of iliofemoral thrombosis with a free-floating tail ≥5 cm long. Although this indication has been questioned by a prospective trial,[10] thrombus with a free-floating tail ≥5 cm long may still be appropriately treated with caval filters. Other such indications are septic PE, chronic PE in patients with cor pulmonale, and high-risk patients including those with significant cardiopulmonary disease, occlusion of more than 50% of the pulmonary bed, or both, who could not tolerate any recurrent thromboembolism.

Table 43.1 **INDICATIONS FOR IVC FILTER INSERTION**

A. Absolute Indications

  1. Recurrent thromboembolic disease despite anticoagulation therapy

  2. Significant complication of anticoagulation therapy that forced therapy to be discontinued

  3. Uncontrolled anticoagulation: sub- or supratherapeutic despite patient compliance

  4. Recurrent PE in a patient with an IVC filter in place

  5. Contraindication to anticoagulation:

       Bleeding complication of anticoagulation

       Recent bleeding

       Recent major trauma or surgery

       Hemorrhagic stroke

       Heparin-induced thrombocytopenia or thrombocytopenia (<50,000/mm^3)

       Central nervous system neoplasm, aneurysms, or vascular malformation

       Guaiac-positive stools

  6. In conjunction with pulmonary embolectomy

B. Relative Indications

  1. Large, free-floating iliofemoral thrombus

  2. Propagating iliofemoral thrombus despite adequate anticoagulation

  3. Thromboembolic disease with limited cardiopulmonary reserve

  4. Chronic thromboembolic disease (undergoing pulmonary embolectomy)

  5. Poor compliance with medications

  6. Septic PE

  7. Severe ataxia; at risk for falls on anticoagulation therapy

  8. DVT thrombolysis

  9. Renal-cell cancer with renal vein or IVC involvement

  10. Prophylactic in high risk patients: massive trauma, pelvic or lower extremity fractures, head injury

Several authorities have suggested that the indications for filter insertions be made more liberal to include patients who have sustained massive trauma and remain at high risk of thromboembolism, but do not actually have the disease.[11–13] Others have advocated the use of filters in patients with malignancy who are at risk for PE or who have thromboembolism.[14–17] The routine use of caval filtration for DVT instead of anticoagulation in high-risk older surgical patients and in pregnant patients with DVT or PE have also been advocated.[18]

There has been a change in vena cava filter placement in some centers over the past decade. Yunus et al. reviewed their institution's experience and found a six-fold increase in the number of IVC filters placed when comparing 1995 with 2005.[19] With a decreasing profile of filters, a trend toward more liberal indications for placement by their center by increased number of filters placed for infrapopliteal DVT or for a prophylactic indication.

A significant change was also demonstrated by the specialty of the physician inserting the IVC filter. While interventional radiologists continued to place 50% of the filters, the number of filters deployed by vascular/trauma surgeons increased to 24%, and cardiologists decreased to 29%.[19]

The only known absolute contraindications to IVC filter insertion are complete thrombosis of the IVC and inability to gain access to the IVC. Replacement of IVC filters in younger patients (adolescent age) should also be avoided because of the lack of performance data lasting several decades. These patients would likely have such devices implanted for extended periods of time.

PROPHYLACTIC CAVAL FILTER INSERTION IN TRAUMA PATIENTS

Patients with multiple trauma have been considered for prophylactic caval filters. The usual prophylactic measures that are useful in the prevention of thromboembolic disease in surgical or medical patients, often fail in multiple trauma patients. Prophylaxis is often started too late in these trauma patients and there is frequent venous stasis and/or associated venous injury along with hypercoagulable states. Venous compression devices and venous surveillance ultrasonography cannot be applied in many of these patients because of external fixation devices, the extent of edema, or the application of casts.

Although several reports have advocated the use of caval filters in high-risk trauma patients, others have cautioned against routine prophylactic caval filter placement. In one large series, prophylactic caval filters would not have benefited 95% of high-risk patients without a DVT and would not have prevented any deaths.[20] Most investigators have attempted to identify trauma patients at particularly high risk for thromboembolism and recommended prophylactic caval filter insertion.[21,22] These high-risk patients (e.g., brain or spinal cord injury, pelvic, and multiple long bone fractures) have been demonstrated to have a fifty-fold increase in thromboembolic complications compared with other trauma patients. Most studies have demonstrated favorable outcomes with caval filters in such patients, however others have failed to show this benefit.[12,21–24]

Wojcik et al.[25] reported on a series of 105 blunt trauma patients who were treated with permanent caval filters for treatment of DVT and prophylaxis, with a mean follow-up of 29 months. There was no PE in the patients in whom filters were placed, and no patients experienced any clinically significant complications related to caval filter insertions. They also reported minimal migration of only one filter and one caval occlusion (0.95%). However, eleven patients (10.4%) experienced symptoms of leg swelling after hospital discharge, and twenty-eight of the sixty-four patients with prophylactically placed caval filters had a DVT after filter placement.

Rodriguez et al.[13] also reported on their experience of Greenfield filter insertions in trauma patients within 48 h, with a PE-related mortality decrease from 17 to 2.5%, and only two of forty patients developed significant venous stasis of the lower extremities.

Leon et al.[26] reported on the prophylactic use of IVC filters in seventy-four patients undergoing high-risk spinal surgery. Criteria for usage were (1) history of thromboembolism, (2) diagnosed thrombophilia, (3) malignancy, (4) bed-ridden for over 2 weeks prior to surgery, (5) staged procedures or multiple levels, (6) combined anterior/posterior approaches, (7) expected need for significant iliocaval manipulation during exposure, and (8) single-stage anesthetic time over an 8-h period. Seventy patients had at least two risk factors. Patients were evaluated for filter complications, DVT, and PE. At a mean follow-up of 11 months, one patient developed PE. Twenty-seven limbs in twenty-three patients developed DVT. Five limbs had isolated calf DVT, and twenty-two had proximal vein involvement. Insertion site DVT accounted for nearly one-third of the DVTs. Six patients died from unrelated complications. They concluded that despite the high incidence of DVT following high-risk spinal surgery, prophylactic caval filter placement appears to protect patients from PE.[26]

With the advances in the use of retrievable filters, the indication of prophylactic caval filters in trauma patients may be justified.

PROPHYLACTIC CAVAL INSERTION IN PATIENTS WITH MALIGNANCY

Patients with malignancies have hypercoagulable states and experience frequent thromboembolic events.[14,27] Some studies suggest that despite adequate anticoagulation, thromboembolism can occur in such patients to a greater degree than in other patients. The associated comorbidities of patients with malignancies undergoing cancer therapy frequently places them at greater risk for bleeding complications from anticoagulation. The use of caval filters in these patients has been applied with conflicting results. In a recent report, the American College of Chest Physicians Consensus Committee on PE discouraged the routine use of IVC filters in cancer-associated DVT/PE and recommended the use of anticoagulation therapy until a randomized controlled study comparing the two modalities becomes available.[20] The use of filters has also been criticized in these patients because of the high cost and high mortality rate experienced in these patients in many IVC filter studies.[14]

CAVAL FILTER INSERTION IN SEPTIC PATIENTS

The FDA guidelines for intravascular filters state that filters should not be implanted in patients with a risk of septic embolism.[28] Therefore, in septic patients who have a contraindication to anticoagulation, the physician must choose between placing the caval filter in contradiction to FDA guidelines and leaving the patient at increased risk of PE. However, this has been challenged recently. A review of a registry of 2,600 patients in whom Greenfield filters were inserted over a 15-year period suggests that filter placement may be a safe method of PE prophylaxis in septic patients.[29] In reviewing 175 patients in this study with a diagnosis of sepsis at the time of caval filter placement, they noted an initial 33% mortality rate in this group, however the mortality leveled out over time, suggesting the cause of death is related not to caval filter insertion but rather to the process of sepsis itself. No filters were removed from any patients, and the recurrent PE rate was 1.7%. Thus, it appears that caval filter placement in septic patients receiving appropriate antibiotics, especially patients with contraindications to anticoagulation, may benefit from caval interruption. It should be noted that the employed filters in this study are made of titanium and stainless steel, both of which are inert materials.

CAVAL FILTER INSERTION DURING PREGNANCY

The choice of therapy for DVT of the lower extremity during pregnancy has been widely debated. Warfarin passes through the placenta to the fetus and may cause fetal complications and/or death. Heparin, in contrast, does not cross the placenta, but its long-term use may be impractical and may increase the risk of bleeding, osteoporosis, and neurological complications.

AbuRahma et al.[18] analyzed eighteen pregnant patients who had Greenfield filters inserted for DVT of the lower extremity and/or PE. The DVT diagnosis was made using duplex imaging. Conventional full-dose intravenous heparin was initiated until the filter was inserted, followed by subcutaneous heparin until labor, and continued for 6 weeks postpartum in thirteen patients who were breast-feeding. Warfarin was given postpartum in the other five patients. The indications for Greenfield insertion included three patients with PE while on anticoagulation, two with significant bleeding secondary to anticoagulation, four for free-floating iliofemoral DVT, two for heparin-induced thrombocytopenia, and seven with iliofemoropopliteal DVT occurring 1–3 weeks prior to labor, for prophylactic reasons. The mean fluoroscopy time during filter insertion was less than two minutes. There was no fetal or maternal morbidity or mortality. In long-term follow-up (mean: 78 months), no PE or filter-related complications were encountered.

THE RESULTS OF IVC FILTER TRIALS

The available data suggest that the risk of caval filter placement for prevention of recurrent PE is justified in the face of contraindications and failure of anticoagulation. Since caval filters are considered the standard of care in such instances, controlled trials for these indications may be unethical.[30]

Well-designed randomized prospective trials to determine the clinical role for caval filters are mostly lacking,[30] although numerous case studies documenting the outcomes of widely used caval filters have been published. The large randomized study (Prevention du Risque d'Embolie Pulmonaire par Interruption Cave Study Group [PREPIC]) assessing the value of caval filters compared with standard anticoagulation therapy was published in 1998.[31] This study included 400 patients with proximal lower extremity DVT who were at risk for PE; 200 patients were randomized to a filter group (four different filters were used: the titanium Greenfield, Bird's Nest, Vena Tech, and Cardil), and 200 were randomized to a nonfilter group. Both groups received standard anticoagulation. The rate of recurrent venous thromboembolism (recurrent PE and/or DVT), death, and major bleeding were analyzed at 12 days and 2 years. This study concluded that the beneficial effect of an IVC filter in PE prevention (1.1% versus 4.8% at day 12, p = 0.03) was outweighed by an excess of recurrent DVT (20.8% versus 11.6% at 2 years, p = 0.02), without a decrease in overall mortality.

This conclusion stimulated intense criticism for multiple reasons. First, the study was originally planned to include 800 patients (44 sites), but because of difficulty in enrollment, this study was stopped after only 400 patients had enrolled. Second, the statistical power for comparing PE incidences at 2 years was extremely low because of a limited number of data points, which did not allow meaningful assessment of delayed PE rates. Third, although the overall mortality rates were similar, there were no deaths caused by PE in the filter group, whereas 80% of the deaths in the nonfilter group were related to PE. Fourth, the study did not include a group of patients who received IVC filters without concomitant anticoagulation, which accounts for the majority of patients in clinical practice. Fifth, a higher rate of recurrent DVT did not outweigh the benefit of a decreased PE rate and reduced PE-related deaths because of greater gravity of recurrent PE in comparison with recurrent DVT.

In 2000, White et al.[32] reported the results of a population-based study of the effectiveness of caval filters among patients with venous thromboembolism and concluded that insertion of filters was not associated with a significant reduction in the incidence of rehospitalization for PE.[32] This study evaluated hospital discharge data from California hospitals from 1991 to 1995 and was designed to determine the cumulative incidence at 1 year of rehospitalization for PE or venous thrombosis among patients with thromboembolism treated with caval filters, compared with the incidence in a control population with thromboembolism not treated with filters. There were 3,622 patients treated with filters, and 64,333 control patients were admitted with a diagnosis of venous thromboembolism. Patients initially admitted with PE were significantly more likely to be readmitted for PE than patients with an initial episode of venous thrombosis only, among patients with caval filters (relative risk of 6.72) and control patients (relative risk of 5.3). Risk-adjusted proportional hazards models showed no significant difference between patients treated with filters and control patients in the relative hazard for readmission for PE. This study was limited because the patients treated with filters had significantly more comorbidities, a higher frequency of previous PE, and a lack of information regarding anticoagulation therapy. The authors concluded that patients with caval filters were at increased risk of caval occlusion because of accumulation of thrombus at the level of the filter, which was felt to be caused by clot accumulation during the time of recurrent thromboembolism.

In 2000, Athanasoulis et al.[33] reported a retrospective study with several different caval filters over a 26-year period. A total of 1,765 filters were implanted in 1,731 patients. A review of hospital records revealed a prevalence of PE after filter placement of 5.6%, with fatal PE occurring in 3.7% of patients. Major complications occurred in 0.3% of procedures and IVC thrombosis occurred after filter placement in 2.7%. They concluded that caval filters provided protection from life-threatening PE with minimal morbidity and few complications.

TECHNICAL CONSIDERATIONS FOR IVC FILTER INSERTION

Caval filter insertion is usually performed under fluoroscopy, either in the operating room with C-arm fluoroscopy or in the radiology or endovascular suite, where better imaging can be obtained. A preoperative venacavogram should be obtained prior to filter insertion. The insertion of all currently available IVC filters requires venous access using the Seldinger technique. The introducer sheath is placed over a dilator, which is advanced over 0.035- to 0.038-inch guide wire. The filter is inserted into the sheath after the dilator and guide wire have been removed, placed in the proper position, usually below the level of the renal vein using an imaging technique, and deployed by unsheathing technique. In the majority of cases, the ideal level of placement is L2 or L3; however placement in the suprarenal IVC or superior vena cava may be indicated in some situations. The entrance site is usually the femoral vein (preferably, the right femoral) or the internal jugular vein.

The radiographic diameter of the IVC should be measured, with correction for magnification, which can be as much as 25%. A very large cava (above 30 mm in diameter) may be found in patients with right-sided heart failure. It may be safer to introduce separate filters into each iliac vein in these patients. Thrombus within the cava should not be allowed to contact the filter to prevent the propagation of thrombus through the filter. If thrombus does extend to the level of the renal vein, or the distal IVC is thrombosed, the filter should be placed at the level of T12 (suprarenal). After removal of the carrier system and the guide wire, a follow-up abdominal radiograph is obtained to confirm the position of the filter.

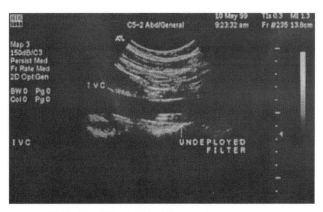

Figure 43.1 Undeployed filter within delivery catheter. (From Reference 36)

IVC FILTER PLACEMENT AT THE BEDSIDE USING DUPLEX ULTRASONOGRAPHIC TECHNIQUE

This technique has been very helpful in patients in the intensive care unit.[34–36] Bedside placement of IVC filters has several advantages, including minimizing the risk of contamination of central lines and dislodgement of intravenous catheters during transfer from the ICU to the operating room or angiography suite. Many of these critically ill patients are on mechanical ventilation with continuous monitoring and/or on vasopressor support, which makes their move to other areas of the hospital rather difficult and hazardous. Many of these patients also have unstable pelvic fractures or spinal injuries. These patients can have their IVC filters inserted using a movable fluoroscopy unit.

Recently, the use of transcutaneous duplex ultrasonography to visualize the IVC for placement of filters has been adapted in several centers.[34–36] This technique has several advantages, including the ability of performing the procedure at the bedside, avoiding the use of contrast material with its potential nephrotoxicity and ionizing radiation. The femoral veins, iliac veins, and the IVC can usually be visualized using duplex technology. Similarly, the internal jugular vein can be used as an access for the filter.

The patient is generally placed in the supine position for abdominal ultrasound examination. It is advisable for these patients to be NPO (for "nil per os," or "nothing by mouth") or to have their tube feedings discontinued for several hours to facilitate visualization of the IVC. The vascular technologist is generally positioned opposite to the operating surgeon. Once the IVC is identified and the renal veins are located, a long J guide wire is inserted into the venous access and can be visualized crossing the IVC. The delivery system, including the filter, is passed over the guide wire and can be visualized using the duplex ultrasound. Once the delivery system is properly positioned, the IVC filter can be deployed under direct vision. After inserting the IVC filter, the delivery system is then removed. A plain abdominal X-ray is then obtained to confirm the proper filter position (Figures 43.1, 43.2, and 43.3).

Conners et al.[36] reported on 284 patients (out of 325 patients) who underwent duplex ultrasound-guided IVC filter placement. Poor IVC visualization, IVC thrombosis, and unsuitable anatomy prevented duplex ultrasound-guided filter placement in forty-one patients (12%). There were no procedure-related deaths or septic complications. Technical complications occurred in twelve patients (4%). Filter misplacement occurred in six patients (2%), access thrombosis in one (<1%), migration in one (<1%), bleeding in one (<1%), and IVC occlusion in three (1%). Pulmonary emboli after IVC filter placement occurred in one patient with a misplaced filter. Average hospital charges related to duplex ultrasound-guided filter placement were $2,388 less than the fluoroscopic placement charges.

Others have reported on the use of intravascular ultrasound for bedside insertion of IVC filters.[35,37–39]

OTHER IMAGING MODALITIES FOR IVC FILTER INSERTION

IVC filters have been traditionally inserted using conventional fluoroscopy, and more recently, transabdominal duplex ultrasound or intravascular ultrasound. Recently, other authorities have evaluated the role of other modalities in evaluating the IVC for filter placement. Holtzman et al.[40] reported on the successful use of CO_2 cavagrams in

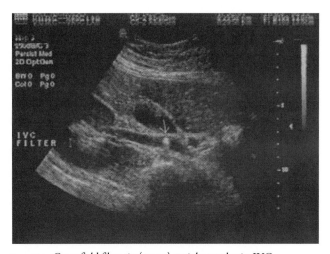

Figure 43.2 Greenfield filter tip (arrow) at right renal vein-IVC junction. (From Reference 36)

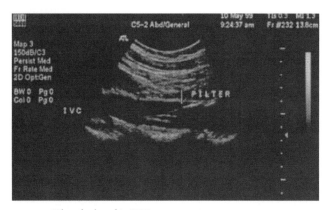

Figure 43.3   Filter deployed in IVC.   (From Reference 36)

twenty-five adult trauma patients requiring IVC filter placement, and Brown et al.[41] conducted a prospective study comparing gadolinium, CO_2, and iodinated contrast material for planning IVC filter placement in forty patients. They concluded that CO_2 and gadolinium had limitations when compared with iodinated contrast material. Gadolinium provided superior consistency in identifying relevant landmarks for filter placement. CO_2 demonstrated significantly greater mean correlative error than gadolinium at initial and repeat readings.[41]

USE OF SUBCLAVIAN VEIN FOR INFERIOR VENA CAVA FILTER INSERTION

With the increasing use of central venous catheters and difficulty in venous access in some patient populations, alternatives to the traditional jugular and femoral vein approaches have been investigated.

Certain patient populations can pose challenges to using the standard routes of IVC deployment. Trauma injuries can create difficulties in jugular access secondary to cervical immobilization, as well as limited exposure to access to femoral vessels secondary to lower extremity immobilization or fractures. Femoral vessel access may likewise be compromised in patients with iliofemoral DVT. In addition, some patients requiring IVC filters may also require long-term central venous catheter placement. Combined placement of both a vena cava filter and a subclavian long-term central catheter in these patients can provide a single expeditious procedure, especially if other access sites are compromised.

Davison et al.[42] reported successful placement of the TrapEase filter in five patients by using the antecubital vein. Ricco et al.[43] reported successful placement of LGM vena cava filters using the subclavian vein approach in eight patients.

In 2004, we reported the results of 135 patients with TrapEase IVC filter placement over a 2-year period.[44] In a majority of cases, the choice of subclavian vein approach was based primarily on surgeon preference. Other circumstances for subclavian vein deployment included cervical immobilization secondary to trauma, desire for concomitant placement of a subclavian long-term central venous access catheter, and patient body habitus limiting exposure to the internal jugular vein. There were 135 filters placed during this 2-year period. The internal jugular vein approach was used in fifty-six patients, the femoral vein approach in thirty-nine patients, and the subclavian vein approach in forty patients. Thirty-nine of the forty TrapEase filter placements using the subclavian vein were successful; twenty-six were deployed through the right subclavian vein, and fourteen through the left subclavian vein. The single failed subclavian deployment was due to the inability to pass the guide wire adequately into the IVC after successful cannulation of the right subclavian vein. No insertion complications were encountered. We concluded that the subclavian vein provides an alternative site for access for the TrapEase IVC filter.

SUPRARENAL IVC FILTER PLACEMENT

In certain clinical circumstances, suprarenal caval filter insertion is needed because it is impossible or inadvisable to place an IVC filter in the usual infrarenal location. Indications of these filters include: (1) patients with renal vein thrombosis, (2) infrarenal vena caval thrombosis, (3) requirement for IVC filtration in the presence of ovarian vein thrombosis in the postpartum state or the presence of a large patent left ovarian vein (pregnancy or childbearing age), (4) the presence of thrombus propagating proximal to a filter below the renal veins, (5) extensive IVC thrombosis extending to or above the renal veins, including tumor thrombus from hepatic or renal tumors, (6) malposition or migration of a prior filter above the renal veins, and (7) recurrent PE following infrarenal IVC filter placement, preferably after an upper extremity emboli source has been ruled out.

Several studies have concluded that suprarenal IVC filter insertion is both safe and effective with clear indications for filter placement.[45–47] A higher rate of caudal migration was noted compared to infrarenal caval filters. The optimum choice for suprarenal IVC filters is, perhaps, either a titanium Greenfield filter or a wire-guided stainless steel Greenfield filter.

Kalva et al.[48] reported a 20-year experience of patients who had implants of suprarenal IVC filters. In their series of seventy patients only one patient had a documented PE during follow-up. Additionally, thirty patients had follow-up computed tomography (CT) of the abdomen at just over 1-year mean, and demonstrated thrombus in the filter in three patients, penetration of the IVC in two and fracture in one additional patient.

SUPERIOR VENA CAVA FILTER INSERTION

Several authorities have reported their experience in small case series, with placement of filters in the superior vena cava (SVC).[49-53] These authorities felt that superior vena cava filters were beneficial in certain clinical indications, however others reported SVC thrombosis secondary to SVC filters.[53] Several studies have suggested that PE is not a rare complication of upper extremity DVT, however it is believed that catheter-related upper extremity DVT can expose patients to a greater risk of PE. Indications for these filters would include contraindications to thrombolytic and anticoagulation therapy. The stainless steel Greenfield filter is generally believed to be an ideal choice for SVC filtration because of its short length, alternating hook design, and being over the wire, allowing tracking and precise positioning. Guide wire entrapment may be more prone to occur with SVC filter placement.

FILTER PLACEMENT IN OVERSIZED IVCs

Oversized IVCs are generally defined as IVCs more than 28 mm in diameter. The Bird's Nest filter is the device approved by the FDA for use in an oversized IVC. If this device is not available, insertion of bilateral common iliac vein filters is acceptable. It has also been noted that the titanium Greenfield filter and the new stainless steel Greenfield filter with alternating hooks may not be subject to the same 28-mm-diameter IVC size limitation as the original Greenfield filter, with significantly better fixation in 34-mm-diameter IVCs. This is due to a wider base and redesigned hook pattern.

AVAILABLE CAVAL FILTER DEVICES

STAINLESS STEEL GREENFIELD FILTERS

This filter is the "gold standard" to which all current and future filters should be compared. It is stainless steel, cone-shaped, and 4.6 cm in length from the apex to the base. It consists of six legs that affix to the wall of the vena cava with small recurved hooks.[54] The legs are 2 mm apart at the apex and 6 mm apart at the base when it is expanded in the vena cava (Figure 43.4). Due to its high patency rate, this filter has been placed above the renal veins in patients with thrombosis to the level of the renal veins. It has also been placed in the SVC in rare circumstances. The filter was originally designed for placement by operative technique by way of the internal jugular or femoral veins.

The largest clinical experience was reported by Greenfield and Michna; 469 patients were followed for 12 years,[55] with a long-term patency rate of 98%. The study also showed a failure to insert the filter in 0.6% of patients, misplacement of the filter in 2.5%, tilt of the filter in 1.7%, proximal migration in 0%, venous stasis in 5%, and a recurrent PE rate in 4%. Other studies confirm and support these findings.[56,57]

Similar results have been obtained in other follow-up series, with long-term patency rates in excess of 95%. The 20-year experience demonstrated the same low rate of recurrent PE and high rate of caval patency as seen in earlier reports.[58] The results of suprarenal filter placement are very comparable, with a 100% long-term patency rate in the twenty-two patients studied in the series of sixty-nine filters placed at this level since 1976.[59,60]

TITANIUM GREENFIELD FILTERS

The titanium Greenfield filter (Boston Scientific, MA; Figure 43.4) is made of titanium alloy. Its cone shape is similar to that of the stainless steel Greenfield filter, but it is 8 mm wider at the base and 0.5 cm taller. It weighs 0.25 g, as opposed to 0.56 g for the stainless steel Greenfield filter, and it can be compressed to a diameter of 0.144 inch.[54]

A recurved hook design with an 80-degree angle will serve as a barrier to penetration beyond the axis of the limb and should limit both upward and downward vectors of force that might induce migration.[60] The mechanical properties of the titanium Greenfield filter have been tested extensively, and it shows a remarkable resistance to flexion fatigue and induced corrosion. The titanium Greenfield filter requires a 12 Fr carrier system and an introducer sheath of 14 Fr. This reduction in size of the overall system has led to a reduction in insertion site venous thrombosis. Placement of the titanium Greenfield filter requires a guide wire inserted percutaneously or by way of cutdown in the right jugular or femoral vein over which a dilator system and attached 14-Fr sheath are passed. When the dilator and sheath are in the IVC at the desired level, the dilator is removed. The titanium Greenfield filter carrier system is then placed through the sheath with fluoroscopic guidance. Both the sheath and carrier are retracted as a unit to release the filter. The carrier and sheath are removed and gentle pressure is applied to the insertion site to promote hemostasis. This design reduces premature misfire, which would place the filter in the sheath rather than in the patient. A new control handle that allows no manipulation other than retraction of the carrier for discharge of the filter decreases the risk of premature discharge. The filter is also preloaded into the carrier system, which decreases the concern of crossed limbs.

The behavior of the titanium Greenfield filter seems comparable to the stainless steel Greenfield filter with increased corrosion resistance and tolerance to flexion stress. In addition, because of its decreased carrier size, both entry and positioning have been facilitated, and bleeding during percutaneous filter insertion has been eliminated.

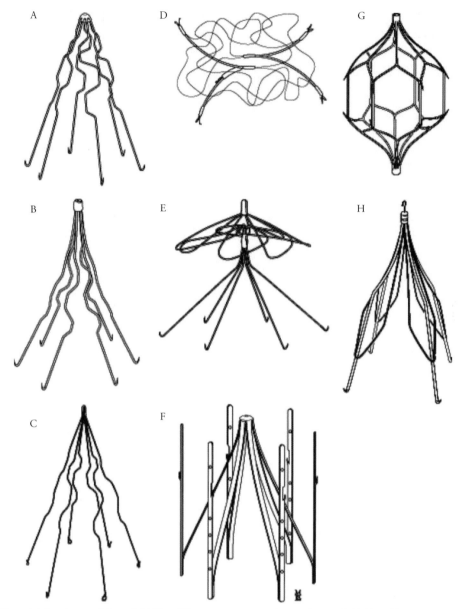

Figure 43.4 Vena cava filters: (a) Stainless steel Greenfield filter, (b) percutaneous stainless steel Greenfield filter, (c) titanium Greenfield filter, (d) Bird's Nest filter, (e) Simon Nitinol filter, (f) Vena Tech filter, (g) Nitinol TrapEase filter, (h) Gunther Tulip filter. (With permission from Hann CL, Streiff MB. The role of vena caval filters in the management of venous thromboembolism. *Blood Reviews*. 2005. 19: 179–202, published by Elsevier).

Experience with this filter has accumulated since the device was approved by the FDA in 1991. The initial prospective multicenter trial showed that filter insertion was successful in 181 out of 186 patients (97%): placement of the remainder was precluded only because of unfavorable anatomy.[61] Initial follow-up data, obtained from all participating centers at 30 d, showed minimal filter movement in 11%; with no significant proximal migration. There was evidence of penetration of the wall of the IVC in only one case (0.8%), with no clinical sequelae. In another clinical study of the titanium Greenfield filter, the follow-up period was extended to at least 12 months. The late patency rate was 99%, with recurrent PE in 3.7% of 176 patients who were enrolled in this study.[62]

STAINLESS STEEL OVER-THE-WIRE GREENFIELD FILTER

This is a 12-Fr stainless steel filter (Boston Scientific, MA) that is used as an alternative device for percutaneous placement (Figure 43.4). This device allows for over-the-wire delivery and a flexible carrier system to facilitate safe delivery. It is the tallest of the Greenfield filters, at 4.9 cm, with a resting base diameter of 3.2 cm, between those of the titanium Greenfield filter (3.8 cm) and the original Greenfield filter (3.0 cm). Two of the six hooks of this filter are angled distally (Figure 43.4), which facilitates secure fixation within the vena cava. The device is manufactured from the same material as the original stainless steel Greenfield filter, but the wires exit from the apex at a different angle, which facilitates delivery via a 12-Fr system. The results of clinical trials of this filter have demonstrated comparable results to the 24-Fr and titanium filters with respect to efficacy (95%) and patency (95%).[63]

BIRD'S NEST FILTER

The use of the Bird's Nest filter (Cook, Bloomington, IN) was first reported in 1984,[64] and a large series of 568 patients was reported in 1988.[65] The device consists of four stainless steel wires 25 cm long and 0.18 in diameter. The wires are preshaped into a criss-crossing, nonmatching array of bends intended to provide multiple barriers to thromboemboli (Figure 43.4). The end of each wire is attached to a strut that ends in a hook for fixation to the wall of the vena cava.[64,65] One strut is z-shaped so that a pusher wire can be attached for insertion. The filter was redesigned in 1986 using a stiffer 0.46 mm wire to improve fixation. Modification of the filter resulted in as increase in the preload system from 8-Fr to a 12-Fr size. During insertion of the filter, the pusher is used to set the first group of hooks into the caval wall. The wires are then extruded with the goal of closely packing the formed loops into a 7-cm segment of the infrarenal vena cava. The second group of hooks are then pushed into the wall of the cava, and the pusher is removed by unscrewing it from the filter. The theoretical advantages of this filter include: (1) the ability to trap small emboli; (2) the ability to accommodate cavae as large as 40 mm in diameter; (3) the possibility that wires may be able to occlude nearby collaterals; (4) avoidance of the need for intraluminal centering because of the configuration of the device; and (5) the lack of radically oriented struts, thereby limiting the tendency toward caval wall penetration. Only 37 of 481 patients with the filter in place for more than six months were available for follow-up. Seven patients (19%) had occlusion of the vena cava; three symptomatic patients had pulmonary angiography for recurrent thromboembolism that was confirmed in one (3%), and proximal migration was seen in five patients resulting in one death secondary to the filter being embedded in a massive PE. These results occurred before strut modification. In a study of the new modified strut, there were three cases of filter migration in thirty-two placements;[66] two were identified within 24 h of placement and were corrected by angiographic manipulation, and one was not detected until six months after placement, and it was embedded in the right atrium and ventricle and could not be repositioned.

More recently, Nicholson et al.[67] reported on the long-term clinical follow-up of the Bird's Nest filters in a small group of patients. Seventy-eight consecutive patients with filters placed between 1989 and 1994 were recalled for clinical assessment and imaging studies. Recurrent PE occurred in 1.3% of patients, and IVC occlusion in 4.7%. There was no filter migration. Wire prolapse was visualized

in 70% by abdominal plain film. CT also showed asymptomatic penetration of the IVC wall in 85.3% of the patients studied. Aortic penetration was also reported, resulting in a clinically significant aortic pseudoaneurysm from penetration of one of the filter struts, which required repair.[68] The rate of IVC occlusion associated with the Bird's Nest device appears to be similar to other caval devices, although estimates range from 0% to 19%.[64,69]

SIMON NITINOL FILTER

The Nitinol filter (Bard, Covington, GA), first described in 1977, is made of a nickel-titanium alloy and is a pliable straight wire when cool, but transforms rapidly into a previously imprinted, rigid shape when warmed. The filter is a 28-mm dome shape with eight overlapping loops, below which the wires are shaped into a cone with six diverging legs with terminal hooks, used to affix it to the vena cava wall (Figure 43.4).[70] The filter wire is advanced rapidly with a feeder pump using iced, normal saline infused through a 9-Fr delivery catheter. When it is discharged from the storage tube, it expands instantly, assumes the appropriate shape, and is locked into place (Figure 43.4).

Of 103 patients undergoing placement at seventeen centers, only forty-four were available for follow-up.[70] There were three cases of recurrent PE, seven cases of confirmed vena cava occlusion, and two suspected cases based on clinical examination. In a more recent study of 224 patients, 65 patients (29%) completed a 6-month follow-up.[71] Four percent of patients developed recurrent PE, one of which was fatal; 19.6% had caval occlusion; and three deaths were associated with massive caval thrombosis. It is currently believed that the Nitinol filter may be thrombogenic.[71]

In 1998, Poletti et al.[72] reported on the long-term performance of Simon Nitinol filters in 114 consecutive patients with an average follow-up of 27 months. They prospectively evaluated thirty-eight of these patients, and the remaining patients were retrospectively evaluated from follow-up clinical data. Five patients (4.4.%) had recurrent PE and 5.3% had documented DVT, with thrombosis at the exit site noted in 3.5%. Filter migration was not found in this series, but IVC thrombosis was noted in 3.5%. The Nitinol filter was found to have penetrated the IVC wall in 95% of patients, and was found to be in contact with adjacent organs in 76%; however all of these were asymptomatic. Sixty-three percent of the filters were eccentrically positioned within the vena cava, and 16% were found to have partial disruption that did not appear to affect filter function. In 2001, Wolfe et al.[73] reported a recurrent PE rate of 7.7% with evidence of IVC penetration in all 117 patients they analyzed. Strut fracture was noted in 2.9% of patients, and 19% had eccentrically oriented filters. There were no cases of IVC thrombosis in their study.

VENA TECH FILTER

The Vena Tech filter (B. Braun, Boulogne, France) was first introduced in France in 1986. It is a cone-shaped filter with stabilizing struts added to each limb that are designed for percutaneous use. The filter is made of phynox and is a stamped, six-prong device with hooked stabilizers with sharp ends intended to center and affix the device (Figure 43.4).[74,75] The filter uses a 12-Fr catheter system, usually inserted through the right internal jugular vein over a guide wire.

The early experience from France shows 100 attempts at insertion, resulting in 98 filter discharges. Eighty-two filters were in the correct position, eight showed a tilt of 15 degrees or greater, and eight had opened incompletely, with three of these associated with a tilt.[74] A more recent report showed a 2% recurrent embolism rate, a 23% rate of insertion site venous thrombosis, a 92% IVC patency rate at six months, a 14% migration rate, and a 6% rate of incomplete opening of the filter.[75] Breakage of the stabilizer struts has also been reported. This filter was designed to prevent tilt, but continues to show a high incidence of tilting.

Long-term studies of this device by Crochet et al.[76,77] have demonstrated that there has been a 73% incidence of filter occlusion over time.

VENA TECH LOW PROFILE FILTER

The Vena Tech low profile filter (Vena Tech LP) has a release wire design contained within a 6-Fr introducer sheath, which allows placement of the filter through alternative venous access sites. This filter is 43 mm in height and 40 mm in diameter in its unconstrained state. This filter was approved in 2001 by the FDA for placement in IVCs that were 28 mm or less in diameter, but can be used for a cava as large as 35 mm.[78]

GUNTHER TULIP FILTER

The Gunther Tulip filter (Cook, Inc.) is a low-profile filter that uses the same funnel-shaped design as the Greenfield filter (Figure 43.4). This filter was introduced in 1992 for use in Europe and has been available in the United States since 2001. The filter is constructed from elgiloy, and an MRI-compatible material. It consists of four main struts, each 0.45 mm in diameter, configured as a cross. Each strut has an elongated wire loop that extends inferiorly three-fourths of the length from the apex to the hooked end of the four main cross struts. The four main struts contain 1-mm-long hooks at the inferior end for caval fixation. The filter is 30 mm in diameter and 45 mm long in its fully expanded state. The filter can be placed using 8.5-Fr introducer sheaths via the femoral or jugular vein.

This filter is FDA-approved for permanent implantation. Although the Gunther Tulip filter is used as a

retrievable filter in Europe, it has not received FDA approval for this application. Several Canadian medical centers have reported successful retrieval of this filter using an endovascular approach within 12 to 14 d after insertion. Recent reports state that the filter can actually be repositioned every seven days; which potentially increases the likelihood that it can be removed.[79]

Millward et al.[80] reported the results of placement of Gunther Tulip filters in ninety patients from eight hospitals. Filter retrieval was attempted in fifty-two patients with fifty-three filters, and was successful in fifty-two filters. The duration of filter implantation was 2 to 25 d, with a mean implantation time of 9 d. In thirty-nine patients in whom the filter was not retrieved (a mean follow-up of 85 days), two filter occlusions (5%) were noted. No other complication of filter placement were noted.

G2 FILTER

The G2 filter jugular/subclavian system (Bard, Figure 43.5) consists of a filter and delivery system. It can be delivered via the femoral and jugular/subclavian approaches, and a separate delivery system is available for each approach. It consists of twelve shape-memory nitinol wires emanating from a central nitinol sleeve. These twelve wires form two levels of filtration of emboli: the legs provide the lower level of filtration, and the arms provide the upper level of filtration. The delivery system consists of a 10-Fr introducer sheath and dilator, the G2 filter, and a delivery device. The filter is packaged preloaded within the delivery device, and it is designed to act as a permanent filter.

When clinically indicated, the G2 filter may be percutaneously removed after implantation using the recovery cone removal system. It is intended to be used in an IVC with a diameter of ≤28 mm. The system consists of a dilator and introducer set and a delivery device. The dilator accepts a

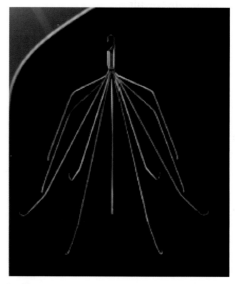

Figure 43.5   G2 filter.

0.038-inch guide wire and allows for an 800-psi maximum pressure contrast power injection. The 10-Fr introducer sheath contains a radiopaque tip and hemostasis valve with a side port for saline infusion and a delivery mechanism to deploy the G2 filter. The delivery device contains a spline cap that mechanically separates the filter hooks from one another in a unique pattern to prevent leg entanglement. Once the introducer sheath is in position, the delivery device is advanced through the introducer sheath until the introducer and delivery hubs snap together. The safety clip is then removed. The introducer hub is pulled back over the pusher wire handle to unsheath and release the filter, allowing it to recover to its predetermined shape. Nonclinical testing has demonstrated that the G2 filter is MRI conditional. It can be scanned safely under specific conditions. The jugular or subclavian delivery system should not be used for the femoral approach, as this will result in improper filter orientation within the IVC.

A clinical study involving 100 patients was conducted to assess the safety of removal of the G2 filter. Sixty-one patients underwent a filter retrieval procedure, and fifty-eight were successful. Of the forty-two patients who did not have their filter retrieved, six died of unrelated causes, three withdrew, two were lost to follow-up, and thirty-one failed to meet retrieval eligibility criteria (within 6 months after filter placement). The time to retrieval in the fifty-eight patients with successful filter retrievals ranged from five to 300 d, with a mean of 140 d.[81,82]

TRAPEASE FILTER

The TrapEase caval filter (Cordis, Figure 43.4), approved by the FDA in 2002, is a symmetric double-basket caval filter constructed from nickel-titanium (nitinol) material. It is a small profile filter that is inserted through a 6-Fr introducer. It has a unique biconvex symmetric filter that allows a single filter to be placed from either direction. This filter has six struts that frame the filter in a diamond or trapezoidal configuration and ends in two superior and inferior baskets created by six struts converging at the apex of the filter. Proximal and distal hooks are fixed at the straight struts that parallel the wall of the cava. The superior basket is conical and oriented in the conventional concave position. The inferior basket is oriented in a mirror position with the apex pointing inferiorly (Figure 43.4). The hook is placed at one apex of the filter for manipulation and possible retrieval of the filter. The filter can be inserted through the femoral, jugular, subclavian, or antecubital vein.[42,44] The deployed filter measures 50–62 mm in length and is approved for vena cavas <30 mm in diameter and it is MRI compatible.

Rousseau et al.[83] reported the results of a small French multicenter prospective trial to evaluate the TrapEase IVC filter. A total of sixty-five patients were enrolled in twelve centers throughout Europe and Canada. They reported a 95.4% technical success rate in filter placement, with a

clinical success rate of 100% at 6 months (with no symptomatic PE). There was no filter migration, filter fracture, vessel wall penetration, or insertion site thrombosis during this short follow-up period, however two patients had early IVC thrombosis within 30 d.

Schutzer et al.[84] reported the results of a retrospective study of 189 consecutively inserted infrarenal TrapEase filters at a single institution over a 22-month period. The technical success rate was 100%, with a symptomatic caval thrombosis rate of 1.5%, one case of symptomatic PE, and one case of intracardiac migration.[85]

Kalva et al.[86] reviewed the clinical and imaging data of 751 patients who had TrapEase IVC filters placed during a 4-year period. Indications for filter placement were: contraindications to anticoagulation (61%), complications of anticoagulation (6%), failure of anticoagulation (5%), and prophylaxis (28%). Filters were placed in the infrarenal (n = 738) or suprarenal (n = 13) position through a femoral (n = 729) or jugular vein (n = 22) approach. Follow-up CT scans of the chest and abdomen were evaluated for recurrent PE and filter-related complications, respectively.

During a mean 295-day clinical follow-up, 7.5% of patients developed symptoms of PE, and one (0.1%) death was attributed to PE. Chest CT performed for various clinical indications in 219 patients at a mean of 192 days showed PE in 15 patients (6.8%; 2/3 were symptomatic, but none were fatal). Follow-up abdominal CTs at a mean of 189 days showed fracture of filter components in 3.0%, thrombus within the filter in 25%, thrombus extending beyond the filter in 1.5%, near total caval occlusion in 0.7%, and no cases of migration. They concluded that the TrapEase vena cava filter is effective in the prevention of PE, with minimal complications.

COMPARISON OF VARIOUS PERMANENT IVC FILTER DEVICES

Table 43.2 summarizes various commonly used caval filters. As noted in this table, the majority of filters are comparable in regard to their effectiveness in preventing recurrent PE, with some variations in regard to the incidence of IVC thrombosis and DVT. They also vary somewhat on the rates of migration.

Usoh et al.,[87] in a prospective randomized study, compared the outcome of the Greenfield filter with the TrapEase filter. One hundred and fifty-six patients were enrolled over a 2-year period, prior to the study's premature termination. During the mean 12- month follow-up (range, 0–39 months), symptomatic IVC iliac vein thrombosis developed in five patients (6.9%) in the TrapEase group, compared to none in the Greenfield group (p = 0.019). No access-site thrombosis, filter migration, misplacement, or IVC perforation occurred. Recurrent PE was suspected in one of the five patients with IVC iliac vein thrombosis. The

Table 43.2 COMPARISON OF VARIOUS IVC FILTERS

FILTER (REF)	CARRIER	TYPE OF EVALUATION	NO.	F.U. (MOS.)	RECURRENT PE	IVC THROMBOSIS	DVT	MIGRATION RATE (%)	MISPLACEMENT RATE (%)
Stainless steel Greenfield (61)	24 F	Meta-analysis	3184	18 (1–60)	2.6% (0–9%)	3.6% (0–18%)	5.9% (0–18%)	35%; >3 mm	4%
Titanium Greenfield (61)	12 F	Meta-analysis	511	5.8 (0–81)	3.1% (0–3.8%)	6.5% (1–31%)	22.7% (0–36%)	11%; >9 mm	0.5%
Stainless steel over-the-wire Greenfield (94)	12 F	Case series	599	26	2.6%	1.7%	7.3%	—	—
Bird's nest (61)	12 F	Meta-analysis	1426	14.2 (0–60)	2.9% (0–4.2%)	3.9% (0–15%)	6% (0–20%)	9%	—
Simon nitinol (61)	7 F	Meta-analysis	319	16.9 (0–62)	3.8% (0–5.3%)	7.7% (4–18%)	8.9% (8–11%)	1.2%	—
Vena Tech (61)	12 F	Meta-analysis	1050	12 (0–81)	3.4% (0–8%)	11.2% (0–28%)	32% (0–32%)	14%; >10 mm	—
Vena Tech Low Profile	6 F	—	30	2.3	0%	0%	10.3%	—	—
Gunther tulip (95)	8.5 F	Clinical trial	83	4.5 (0–36)	3.6%	9.6%	—	—	—
TrapEase (96)	6 F	Clinical trial	189	(0–24)	0%	1.5%	—	—	—

—, none or not reported

overall mortality rate was 42.3% (sixty-six patients), and the 30-d mortality rate was 13.5% (twenty-one patients: ten TrapEase and eleven Greenfield). They concluded that a higher rate of symptomatic IVC iliac vein thrombosis was associated with TrapEase filter placement.

Corriere et al.[88] conducted a comparative analysis of consecutive patients undergoing placement of retrievable versus permanent IVC filters to analyze the incidence of IVC thrombosis during a 4-year period at one institution. A total of 189 IVC filter cases (165 permanent and 24 retrievable) were examined. Over a median follow-up of 8.5 months, no significant hemorrhage, no IVC filter migration, and four cases of vena cava thrombosis were observed. Vena cava thrombosis was observed more frequently with retrievable IVC filters, compared to permanent IVC filters (12.5% versus 0.6%; $p = 0.007$). All observed vena cava thromboses were associated with severe clinical symptoms and occurred in patients who received opposed biconical IVC filter designs (TrapEase and OptEase). Although causative factors remain unclear, filter design and resultant flow dynamics may play an important role, because all episodes of vena cava thrombosis occurred in patients with a single-filter design.

Fox and Kahn[89] conducted a systematic review to assess the frequency of symptoms and signs of postthrombotic syndrome in relation to IVC filter placement. They also assessed whether the initial indication for IVC filter placement—prevention of PE in a patient without known venous thrombosis (i.e., primary prevention) versus prevention of PE in patients with known venous thrombosis (i.e., secondary prevention)—or concurrent use of anticoagulation or compression stockings influenced this rate. Eleven articles describing 1,552 patients met the criteria for review. At a mean follow-up of 4.5 years, the weighted pooled incidence of edema was 43%, and that of chronic skin changes (including venous ulcers) was 12%. Among patients who had IVC filter insertion for secondary prevention, 52% had edema and 14% had skin changes at follow-up, compared with 20% and 8%, respectively, in patients who received an IVC filter for primary prevention. One study reported no difference in the frequency of symptoms and signs of postthrombotic syndrome according to whether anticoagulation was initiated in addition to filter placement.

Nazzal et al.,[90] in a retrospective review of 400 IVC filter implants, predominately permanent filters (80% TrapEase and Greenfield); demonstrated a significant difference in filter complications based on filter type. Migration and or tilt were seen more frequently with Bard filters, compared to other filters individually ($p < 0.004$, 11.8% versus 0.55% as a group), and IVC thrombosis was significantly more common with the TrapEase filter. Specifically, in patients with either hypercoagulable or malignant conditions, 25% of patients developed IVC thrombosis with the TrapEase filter, compared to none in its absence.

Additional complications related to permanent IVC filters include penetration and perforation of the IVC into the gastrointestinal tract. A systematic review of the literature reported symptomatic duodenal perforations in twenty-one patients. The most common presentation was abdominal pain, with most presenting over 2 years after implant. The most common IVC filter was the Greenfield filter in 7/19 of known filter type. Management varied from the trimming of the legs of the filter with intestinal repair to complete extraction of filter and caval repair.[91]

FOLLOW-UP AFTER IVC FILTERS

There is no specific protocol for late follow-up of patients receiving IVC filters, especially when the patient is asymptomatic. It is generally believed that a simple physical examination in conjunction with a plain abdominal X-ray can detect the majority of complications of IVC filters. CT scanning and duplex ultrasonography are helpful in assessing any abnormalities. Venography should be reserved for patients in whom these modalities are not helpful.

In a prospective observational study of patients with permanent IVC filters,[92] patients without a contraindication for anticoagulation were evaluated with duplex examination of the IVC lower extremity veins at least once per year. Patients with IVC thrombus were managed with a more intensive anticoagulation regimen by specified protocol. Despite anticoagulation, new PEs were diagnosed in 5% of patients, new DVTs in 20%, IVC thrombus in 30%, and a major bleeding episode occurred in 7%. With these prospective ultrasound-based findings despite anticoagulation, it raises concerns for long-term implantation, even in patients who can receive anticoagulation.

COMMENTS/CONCLUSIONS

Many different and ingenious caval filters are currently available on the market for clinical use; however, the perfect filter has not been developed. It appears likely that caval filters do reduce the incidence of PE, but may result in IVC thrombosis and a higher incidence of recurrent lower extremity DVT than is seen with anticoagulation alone. Prospective randomized trials comparing the efficacy of filters and various filter devices are presently lacking. Each of these filters has its own advantages and disadvantages, therefore the physician must select a filter that is suitable to his patient and the one with which he or she is familiar. Because of concerns over the long-term performance characteristics of caval filters, it is best to adhere to strict indications for filter insertion.

Recently, Berczi et al.[93] investigated the long-term retrievability of IVC filters and whether we should abandon permanent devices, and they concluded that there is still a definite role for permanent filters, which have a far longer clinical practice history—and this is the Achilles heel of the retrievable filters. Follow-up (preferably prospective) is necessary for all retrievable filters, regardless of whether or not they are retrieved. Until these data become available, we should restrict ourselves to the present indications for permanent filters. If long-term follow-up data on a larger number of cases confirm that retrievable filters are as safe and effective as permanent filters, use of retrievable filters is likely to expand.

REFERENCES

1. Bick RL. Hereditary and acquired thrombophilia: Preface, *Semin Thromb Hemost*. 1999. *25*: 251–253.

2. Stein PD, Henry JW, Relyea B. Untreated patients with pulmonary embolism: Outcome, clinical, and laboratory assessment, *Chest*. 1995. *107*: 931–935.

3. Douketis JD, Keaton C, Bates S, et al. Risk of fatal pulmonary embolism in patients with treated venous thromboembolism, *JAMA*. 1998. *279*: 458–462.

4. Tadavarthy SM, Castaneda-Zuniga W, Salomonowitz E, et al. Kimray-Greenfield vena cava filter: Percutaneous introduction, *Radiology*. 1984. *151*: 525–526.

5. Grassi CJ. Inferior vena caval filters: Analysis of five currently available devices, *Am J Roentgenol*. 1991. *156*: 813–821.

6. Stein PD, Kayali F, Olson RE. Twenty-one-year trends in the use of inferior vena cava filters, *Arch Intern Med*. 2004. *164*: 1541–1545.

7. Anderson RC, Busey HI. Retrievable and permanent inferior vena cava filters: Selected considerations, *Pharmacotherapy*. 2006. *26*: 1595–1600.

8. Quirke TE, Ritota PC, Swan KG. Inferior vena caval filter use in US trauma centers: A practitioner survey, *J Trauma*. 1997. *43*: 333–337.

9. American College of Chest Physicians' Consensus Committee on Pulmonary Embolism. Opinions regarding the diagnosis and management of venous thromboembolic disease, *Chest*. 1998. *113*: 499–504.

10. Pacouret G, Alison D, Pottier JM, et al. Free-floating thrombus and embolic risk in patients with angiographically confirmed proximal deep venous thrombosis: A prospective study, *Arch Intern Med*. 1997. *157*: 305–308.

11. Rogers FB, Shackford SR, Wilson J, et al. Prophylactic vena cava filter insertion in severely injured trauma patients: Indications and preliminary results, *J Trauma*. 1993. *35*: 637–641.

12. Khansarinia S, Dennis JW, Veldenz HC, et al. Prophylactic Greenfield filter placement in selected high-risk trauma patients, *J Vasc Surg*. 1995. *22*: 231–235.

13. Rodriguez JL, Lopez JM, Proctor MC, et al. Early placement of prophylactic vena caval filters in injured patients at high risk for pulmonary embolism, *J Trauma*. 1996. *40*: 797–802.

14. Rosen MP, Porter DH, Kim D. Reassessment of vena caval filter use in patients with cancer, *J Vasc Interv Radiol*. 1994. *5*: 501–506.

15. Losef SV, Barth KH. Outcome of patients with advanced neoplastic disease receiving vena caval filters, *J Vasc Interv Radiol*. 1995. *6*: 273–277.

16. Fink JA, Jones BT. The Greenfield filter as the primary means of therapy in venous thromboembolic disease, *Surg Gynecol Obstet*. 1991. *172*: 253–256.

17. Cohen JR, Tenenbaum N, Citron M. Greenfield filter as primary therapy for deep venous thrombosis and/or pulmonary embolism in patients with cancer, *Surgery*. 1991. *109*: 12–15.

18. AbuRahma AF, Mullins DA. Endovascular caval interruption in pregnant patients with deep vein thrombosis of the lower extremity, *J Vasc Surg*. 2001. *33*: 375–378.

19. Yunus TE, Tariq N, Callahan RE, et al. Changes in inferior vena cave filter placement over the past decade at a larger community-based academic health center, *J Vasc Surg*. 2008. *47*: 157–165.

20. Spain DA, Richardson JD, Polk HC Jr, et al. Venous thromboembolism in the high-risk trauma patient: Do risks justify aggressive screening and prophylaxis?, *J Trauma*. 1997. *42*: 463–469.

21. Shackford SR, Davis JW, Hollingsworth-Fridlung P, Brewer NS, Hoyt DB, Mackersie RC. Venous thromboembolism in patients with major trauma, *Am J Surg*. 1990. *159*: 365–369.

22. Pasquale M, Fabian TC, EAST Ad Hoc Committee on Practice Management Guideline Development. Practice management guidelines for trauma from the Eastern Association of Trauma, *J Trauma*. 1998. *44*: 941–956.

23. Rogers FB, Strindberg G, Shackford SR, et al. Five-year follow-up of prophylactic vena cava filters in high-risk trauma patients, *Arch Surg*. 1998. *133*: 406–412.

24. McMurty AL, Owings JT, Anderson JT, et al. Increased use of prophylactic vena cava filters in trauma patients failed to decrease overall incidence of pulmonary embolism, *J Am Coll Surg*. 1999. *189*: 314–320.

25. Wojcik R, Cipolle MD, Feren I, et al. Long-term follow-up of trauma patients with a vena cava filter, *J Trauma*. 2000. *49*: 839–843.

26. Leon L, Rodriguez H, Tawk RG, Ondra SL, Labropoulos N, Morasch MD. The prophylactic use of inferior vena cava filters in patients undergoing high-risk spinal surgery, *Ann Vasc Surg*. 2005. *19*: 442–447.

27. Falanga A, Donati MB. Pathogenesis of thrombosis in patients with malignancy, *Intl J Hematol*. 2001. *73*: 137–144.

28. US Food and Drug Administration, Center for Devices and Radiological Help: Guidance for Cardiovascular Intravascular Filter 510(K) Submissions. Document issued on November 26, 1999. Online at: www.fda.gov/MedicalDevices/DeviceRegulationandGuidance/GuidanceDocuments/ucm073776.htm

29. Greenfield LJ, Proctor MC. Vena caval filter use in patients with sepsis: Results in 175 patients, *Arch Surg*. 2003. *138*: 1245–1248.

30. Becker DM, Philbrick JT, Selby JB. Inferior vena cava filters: Indications, safety, effectiveness, *Arch Intern Med*. 1992. *152*: 1985–1994.

31. Decousus H, Leizorovicz A, Parent F, et al. A clinical trial of vena caval filters in the prevention of pulmonary embolism in patients with proximal deep-vein thrombosis: Prevention du Risque d'Embolie Pulmonaire par Interruption Cave Study Group, *N Engl J Med*. 1998. *338*: 409–415.

32. White RH, Zhou H, Kim J, Romano PS. A population-based study of the effectiveness of inferior vena cava filter use among patients with venous thromboembolism, *Arch Intern Med*. 2000. *160*: 2033–2041.

33. Athanasoulis CA, Kaufman JA, Halpern EF, Waltman AC, Geller SC, Fan CM. Inferior vena caval filters: review of a 26-year single-center clinical experience, *Radiology*. 2000. *216*: 54–66.

34. Nunn CR, Neuzil D, Naslund T, et al. Cost-effective method for bedside insertion of vena caval filters in trauma patients, *J Trauma*. 1997. *43*: 752–758.

35. Matsumura JS, Morasch MD. Filter placement by ultrasound technique at the bedside, *Seminars Vasc Surg*. 2000. *13*: 199–203.

36. Conners MS, Becker S, Guzman RJ, et al. Duplex scan-directed placement of inferior vena cava filters: A five-year institutional experience, *J Vasc Surg*. 2002. *35*: 286–291.

37. Corriere MA, Passman MA, Guzman RJ, Dattilo JB, Naslund TC. Comparison of bedside transabdominal duplex ultrasound versus contrast venography for inferior vena cava filter placement: What is the best imaging modality, *Ann Vasc Surg*. 2005. *19*: 229–234.

38. Oppat WF, Chiou AC, Matsumura JS. Intravascular ultrasound-guided vena cava filter placement, *J Endovasc Surg*. 1999. *6*: 285–287.

39. Garrett JV, Passman MA, Guzman RJ, Dattilo JB, Naslund TC. Expanding options for bedside placement of inferior vena cava filters

with intravascular ultrasound when transabdominal duplex ultrasound imaging is inadequate, *Ann Vasc Surg.* 2004. *18*: 329–334.

40. Holtzman RB, Lottenberg L, Bass T, Saridakis A, Bennett VJ, Carrillo EH. Comparison of carbon dioxide and iodinated contrast for cavography prior to inferior vena cava filter placement, *Am J Surg.* 2003. *185*: 364–368.

41. Brown DB, Pappas JA, Vedantham S, Pilgram TK, Olsen RV, Duncan JR. Gadolinium, carbon dioxide, and iodinated contrast material for planning inferior vena cava filter placement: A prospective trial, *J Vasc Interv Radiol.* 2003. *14*: 1017–1022.

42. Davison BD, Grassi CJ. TrapEase inferior vena cava filter placed via the basilic arm vein: A new antecubital access, *J Vasc Interv Radiol.* 2002. *13*: 107–109.

43. Ricco J, Dubreuil F, Renaud P, et al. The LGM Vena-Tech caval filter: Results of multicenter study, *Ann Vasc Surg.* 1995. *9*(Suppl): S89–S100.

44. Stone PA, AbuRahma AF, Hass SM, et al. TrapEase inferior vena cava filter placement: Use of subclavian vein, *Vasc Endovasc Surg.* 2004. *38*: 505–509.

45. Greenfield LJ, Proctor MC. Supra-renal filter placement, *J Vasc Surg.* 1998. *28*: 432–438.

46. David W, Gross WS, Colaiuta E, Gonda R, Osher D, Lanuti S. Pulmonary embolus after vena cava filter placement, *Am Surg.* 1999. *65*: 341–346.

47. Streiff MB. Vena caval filters: A comprehensive review, *Blood.* 2000. *95*: 3669–3677.

48. Kalva SP, Chalpoutake C, Wicky S, Greenfield AJ, Waltman AC, Athanasoulis CA. Suprarenal inferior vena cava filters: A 20 year single center experience, *J Vasc Interv Radiol.* 2008. *19*(7): 1041–1047.

49. Hoffman MJ, Greenfield LJ. Central venous septic thrombosis managed by superior vena cava Greenfield filter and venous thrombectomy: A case report, *J Vasc Surg.* 1986. *4*: 606–611.

50. Pais SO, Orchis DF, Mirvis SE. Superior vena caval placement of Kimray-Greenfield filter, *Radiology.* 1987. *165*: 385–386.

51. Owen EWJ, Schoettle GPJ, Harrington OB. Placement of a Greenfield filter in the superior vena cava, *Ann Thorac Surg.* 1992. *53*: 896–897.

52. Ascher E, Hinforani A, Tsemekhin B, Yorkovich W, Gunduz Y. Lessons learned from a 6-year clinical experience with superior vena cava Greenfield filters, *J Vasc Surg.* 2000. *32*: 881–887.

53. Lidagoster MI, Widman WE, Chevinski AH. Superior vena caval occlusion after filter insertion, *J Vasc Surg.* 1994. *20*: 158–159.

54. Greenfield LJ. Vena cava interruption: Devices and results. In: Bergan JJ, Yao JST, eds. *Venous disorders.* Philadelphia, PA: WB Saunders. 1991. 556.

55. Greenfield LJ, Michna BA. Twelve-year clinical experience with the Greenfield vena cava filter, *Surgery.* 1988. *104*: 706–712.

56. Gomez GA, Cutler BS, Wheeler HB. Transvenous interruption of the inferior vena cava, *Surgery.* 1983. *93*: 612–619.

57. Chimochowski GE, Evans RH, Zarins CK, et al. Greenfield filter versus Mobin-Uddin umbrella: The continuing quest for the ideal method of vena caval interruption, *J Thorac Cardiovasc Surg.* 1980. *79*: 358–365.

58. Greenfield LJ, Proctor MC. Twenty-year clinical experience with the Greenfield filter, *Cardiovasc Surg.* 1995. *3*: 199–205.

59. Greenfield LJ, Cho KJ, Proctor MC, et al. Late results of suprarenal Greenfield vena cava filter placement, *Arch Surg.* 1992. *127*: 969–973.

60. Greenfield LJ, Whitehill TA. New developments in caval interruption: Current indications and new techniques for filter placement. In: Veith FJ, ed. *Current critical problems in vascular surgery.* St. Louis, MO: Quality Medical. 1992. Vol. 4, 113–121.

61. Greenfield LJ, Cho KH, Proctor M, et al. Results of a multicenter study of the modified hook-titanium Greenfield filter, *J Vasc Surg.* 1991. *14*: 253–257.

62. Greenfield LJ, Proctor MC, Cho KH, et al. Extended evaluation of the titanium Greenfield vena caval filter, *J Vasc Surg.* 1994. *20*: 458–464.

63. Cho KJ, Greenfield LJ, Proctor MC, et al. Evaluation of a new percutaneous stainless steel Greenfield filter, *J Vasc Interv Radiol.* 1997. *8*: 181–187.

64. Roehm JOF Jr, Gianturco C, Barth MH, et al. Percutaneous transcatheter filter for the inferior vena cava: A new device for treatment of patients with pulmonary embolism, *Radiology.* 1984. *150*: 255–257.

65. Roehm JOF Jr, Johnsrude IS, Barth MH, et al. The bird's nest inferior vena cava filter: Progress report, *Radiology.* 1988. *168*: 745–749.

66. McCowan TC, Ferris EJ, Keifsteck JE, et al. Retrieval of dislodged bird's nest inferior vena caval filters, *J Vasc Intervent Radiol.* 1988. *3*: 179–183.

67. Nicholson AA, Ettles DF, Paddon AJ, Dyet JF. Long-term follow-up of the bird's nest IVC filter, *Clin Radiol.* 1999. *54*: 759–764.

68. Campbell JJ, Calcagno D. Aortic pseudoaneurysm from aortic penetration with a bird's nest vena cava filter, *J Vasc Surg.* 2003. *38*: 596–599.

69. Lord RS, Benn I. Early and late results after bird's nest filter placement in the inferior vena cava: Clinical and duplex ultrasound follow up, *Aust NZJ Surg.* 1994. *64*: 106–114.

70. Simm M, Athanasoulis CA, Kim D, et al. Simon nitinol inferior vena cava filter: Initial clinical experience, *Radiology.* 1989. *172*: 99–103.

71. Dorfman GS. Percutaneous inferior vena caval filters, *Radiology.* 1990. *174*: 987–992.

72. Poletti PA, Becker CD, Prina L, et al. Long-term results of the Simon nitinol inferior vena cava filter, *Eur Radiol.* 1998. *8*: 289–294.

73. Wolfe F, Thurnher S, Lammer J. Simon nitinol vena cava filters: Effectiveness and complications, *Rofo Fortschr Geb Rontgenstr Neuen Bildgeb Verfahr.* 2001. *173*: 924–930.

74. Ricco JB, Crochet D, Sebilotte P, et al. Percutaneous transvenous caval interruption with the "LGM" filter: Early results of a multicenter trial, *Ann Vasc Surg.* 1988. *3*: 242–247.

75. Murphy TP, Dorfman GS, Yedlicka JW, et al. LGM vena cava filter: Objective evaluation of early results, *J Vasc Interv Radiol.* 1991. *2*: 107–115.

76. Crochet DP, Stora O, Ferry D, et al. Vena Tech-LGM filter: Long-term results of a prospective study, *Radiology.* 1993. *188*: 857–860.

77. Crochet DP, Brunel P, Trogrlic S, et al. Long-term follow-up of Vena Tech-LGM filter: Predictors and frequency of caval occlusion, *J Interv Radiol.* 1999. *10*: 137–142.

78. Kinney TB. Update on inferior vena cava filters, *J Vasc Interv Radiol.* 2003. *14*: 425–440.

79. Tay KH, Martin ML, Webb JG, Machan LS. Repeated Gunther Tulip inferior vena cava filter repositioning to prolong implantation time, *J Vasc Intervent Radiol.* 2002. *13*: 509–512.

80. Millward SF, Oliva VL, Bell SD, et al. Gunther Tulip retrievable vena cava filter: Results from the Registry of the Canadian Interventional Radiology Association, *J Vasc Interv Radiol.* 2001. *12*: 1053–1058.

81. Grande WJ, Trerotola SO, Reilly PM, et al. Experience with the recovery filter as a retrievable inferior vena cava filter, *J Vasc Interv Radiol.* 2005. *16*: 1189–1193.

82. Asch MR. Initial experience in humans with a new retrievable inferior vena cava filter, *Radiology.* 2002. *225*: 835–844.

83. Rousseau H, Perreault P, Otal P, et al. The 6-F nitinol TrapEase inferior vena cava filter: Results of a prospective multicenter trial, *J Vasc Interv Radiol.* 2001. *12*: 299–304.

84. Schutzer R, Ascher E, Hingorani A, et al. Preliminary results of the new 6F TrapEase inferior vena cava filter, *Ann Vasc Surg.* 2003. *17*: 103–106.

85. Porcellini M, Stassano P, Musumeci A, Bracale G. Intracardiac migration of nitinol TrapEase vena cava filter and paradoxical embolism, *Eur J Cardiothorac Surg.* 2002. *22*: 460–461.

86. Kalva SP, Wicky S, Waltman AC, Athanasoulis CA. TrapEase vena cava filter: Experience in 751 patients, *J Endovasc Ther.* 2006. *13*: 365–372.

87. Usoh F, Hingorani A, Ascher E, et al. Prospective randomized study comparing the clinical outcomes between inferior vena cava Greenfield and TrapEase filters, *J Vasc Surg.* 2010. *52*: 394–399.

88. Corriere MA, Suave KJ, Ayerdi J, et al. Vena cava filters and inferior vena cava thrombosis, *J Vasc Surg.* 2007. *45*: 789–794.

89. Fox MA, Kahn SR. Postthrombotic syndrome in relation to vena cava filter placement: A systematic review, *J Vasc Interv Radiol.* 2008. *19*: 981–985.

90. Nazzal M, Chan E, Nazzal M, et al. Complications related to inferior vena cava filters: A single-center experience, *Ann Vasc Surg.* 2010. *24*(4): 480–486.

91. Malgor RD, Labropoulos N. A systematic review of symptomatic duodenal perforation by inferior vena cava filters, *J Vasc Surg.* 2012. *55*: 856–861.

92. Jajduk B, Tomkowski WZ, Malek G, Davidson BL. Vena Cava filter occlusion and venous thromboembolism risk in persistently antico-agulated patients, *Chest.* 2010. *137*(4): 877–882.

93. Berczi V, Bottomley JR, Thomas SM, Taneja S, Gaines PA, Cleveland TJ. Long-term retrievability of IVC filters: Should we abandon permanent devices?, *Cardiovasc Intervent Radiol.* 2007. *30*: 820–827.

94. Greenfield LJ, Proctor MC. The percutaneous Greenfield filter: Outcomes and practice patterns, *J Vasc Surg.* 2000. *32*: 888–893.

95. Neuerburg JM, Funther RW, Vorwerk D et al. Results of a multicenter study of the retrievable Tulip vena cava filter: Early clinical experience, *Cardiovasc Intervent Radiol.* 1997. *20*: 10–16.

96. Porcellini M, Stassano P, Musumeci A, Bracale G. Intracardiac migration of nitinol TrapEase vena cava filter and paradoxical embolism, *Eur J Cardiothorac Surg.* 2002. *22*: 460–461.

44.

COMPLICATIONS OF VENA CAVA FILTERS

Teresa L. Carman and Linda M. Graham

BACKGROUND

Venous thromboembolism (VTE) is optimally treated by anticoagulation. When anticoagulation must be withheld, inferior vena cava (IVC) interruption affords protection against major embolic events. IVC interruption has progressed from cava ligation, plication, or caval clips to percutaneously placed devices. Complications associated with surgical caval interruption and first-generation IVC filters have driven the modification and design of devices to minimize endothelial cell interaction, use smaller deployment hardware, use alloys compatible with magnetic resonance imaging (MRI) and computed tomography (CT) imaging, and have decreased thrombogenicity. Currently available devices include permanent filters that once deployed remain in place indefinitely and optionally retrievable filters that may be left in place permanently or may be removed within weeks to months depending on the device. Optionally retrievable filters have modifications to the caval attachment sites and/or hooks at one end to facilitate removal. This is appealing because absolute contraindications to systemic anticoagulation may be short-lived, and the long-term outcomes of IVC filters may not be as benign as once thought. So optionally retrievable filters are designed to provide the efficacy of a permanent filter and yet minimize the complications of a long-term indwelling vascular device. There are no unique indications or recommendations that have been made regarding optionally retrievable IVC filters.[1] The decision regarding the use of a permanent or optionally retrievable filter must be made individually for each patient.

Table 44.1 outlines the current absolute and relative indications for IVC filter placement. Contraindications to anticoagulation, complications of anticoagulation, or thromboembolism (pulmonary embolism [PE] or recurrent/propagation of deep venous thrombosis [DVT]) despite adequate anticoagulation are considered indications for filter placement.[2] These accepted indications are frequently expanded to include a number of relative indications. In addition, in some centers IVC filters are used for primary prophylaxis against pulmonary embolism.[3,4] With

these indications in mind it is important to recognize that an IVC filter does not treat VTE but protects that patient from the most serious adverse event, massive, fatal pulmonary embolism. Anticoagulation should be initiated despite the presence of a filter when deemed safe.[2] However, there are no recommendations regarding the duration of anticoagulation in this setting.

There has been a trend toward increasing IVC filter use for both VTE management and for primary prophylaxis. In a recent population based study of 9,665 IVC filters the authors demonstrated a 40% increase in filter placement; 1,446 filters were placed in 1991 with an increased to 2,447 filters in 1995. Sixty percent (5,621/9,665) of the filters were deployed in patients without a primary diagnosis of VTE (i.e., used for primary or secondary VTE prophylaxis).[5] During a 21-year period data from the National Hospital Discharge Survey (NHDS) database demonstrated an increase in filter placement from 2,000 in 1979 to 49,000 in 1999. In 1999, 45% of filters were placed in patients with DVT, 36% in patients with PE, and 19% of IVC filters were placed in patients without a coded diagnosis for VTE.[6] Registries of patients treated for VTE have demonstrated IVC filter insertion rates of 2% in Spain compared with 14% in a US study.[7,8] In the US study, 33% of IVC filters were inserted for primary prophylaxis in patients with DVT, and 17% were placed for indications other than the three absolute indications for IVC filter placement.[8]

The robust use of IVC filters for prophylaxis and for relative indications is concerning, given the lack of comparative data or prospective, randomized trials regarding IVC filter use. Most of the literature regarding the use and complications of IVC filters is derived from case series, retrospective studies, or prospective trials enrolling patients with a single filter type.[9] In addition, as more filters are approved there is little long-term data for most devices.

Several comprehensive reviews of IVC filters and filter complications have been published detailing the design, deployment, and complications of both the permanent and optionally retrievable filters.[10–13] The use and complications

Table 44.1 INDICATIONS FOR INFERIOR VENA CAVA (IVC) FILTER PLACEMENT

Absolute indications
• Contraindication to anticoagulation either permanent or temporary
• Complications of anticoagulation that prevent further therapy
• Recurrent pulmonary embolism or iliofemoral deep vein thrombosis despite adequate anticoagulation

Relative indications
• Difficulty managing anticoagulation or poor compliance
• Inability to manage anticoagulation despite patient compliance
• Massive pulmonary embolism
• Poor cardiopulmonary reserve
• Increased risk for complications of anticoagulation
• Recurrent pulmonary embolism despite an IVC filter
• Prior to pulmonary thromboendarterectomy for chronic thromboembolic disease
• Prior to thrombolysis
• Free floating proximal deep venous thrombosis
• Iliocaval thrombus

Prophylactic indications (when mechanical or pharmacologic prophylaxis is suboptimal)
• Trauma patients with multiple fractures, pelvic injury, spinal cord or head trauma
• Surgical patient with high risk for VTE including neurosurgery, orthopedic, or bariatric
• Medical patient with a high risk for VTE

Table 44.2 COMPLICATIONS RELATED TO INFERIOR VENA CAVA FILTERS

Venous thromboembolism
Recurrent deep venous thrombosis
Thrombus propagation
Recurrent pulmonary embolism
Inferior vena cava thrombosis
Insertion site complications
Insertion site thrombosis
Hematoma/hemorrhage
Arteriovenous fistula
Infection
Deployment complications
Tilting
Malposition in the incorrect vein/vessel
Failure to fully deploy
Device complications
Strut fracture
Strut embolism
IVC perforation or strut extrusion
Guide wire entrapment
Migration (proximally or distally)
Filter embolism

complications are uncommon. Four (0.16%) filter-related deaths were noted in one review.[14]

of the stainless steel Greenfield filter and its modified designs have been best studied and characterized. Considerably less literature is published regarding the most recently approved filters. One can only assume that these filters will have the same success and complication rates as the devices that have a longer history of use. Certainly IVC filters appear to prevent major pulmonary embolism in patients with DVT, however, complications related to IVC filter use are not negligible. Complications may include VTE, deployment and positioning issues, insertion site complications, and migration after placement. Table 44.2 lists complications related to permanent or optionally retrievable IVC filters. There are no large case series or comparable studies examining the true rates of complications by filter-type. It is also important to note that radiographic follow-up after filter placement is not standardized and there are no guidelines for identifying patients who should undergo additional radiographic imaging after filter placement. Many complications, such as minor degrees of filter migration, limited penetration through the caval wall or even compromise of the structural integrity of the filter, may be clinically silent. Major complications related to IVC filters, such as migration or significant caval perforation, are relatively rare. Life-threatening

THROMBOTIC COMPLICATIONS

Thrombotic complications related to IVC filters including recurrent DVT (propagation of an existing thrombus into additional venous segments or involvement of new venous segments including the contralateral limb), PE, IVC or filter thrombosis, and insertion site thrombosis are well documented, however, they have not been thoroughly studied. There are no prospective comparative studies of IVC filters so it is difficult to determine whether the risk of recurrent venous thrombosis relates to the presence of a filter or if specific design issues are related to thrombogenesis. Since it is unlikely that comparative studies of specific devices will be performed, however, further study of filter design and thrombogenicity may help clarify factors contributing to these events.

DVT

A comprehensive review of IVC filters by Streiff in 2000 reported on complications from the then available filters including the stainless steel Greenfield (SSG), titanium Greenfield (TG), Bird's Nest (BN), Simon nitinol (SN), and Vena Tech (VT).[11] Most studies involved relatively few patients and were either retrospective reviews or prospective follow-up performed by chart review, questionnaires, or clinic visits as opposed to serial radiographic surveillance. In this review the SSG and the BN filters had the lowest rates of recurrent deep venous thrombosis, 5.9% and 6%, respectively.[11] The highest rates of DVT have been seen with the TG (22.7%), the VT (32%), and the TrapEase filters (45.7%).[11,12]

Both retrospective and prospective studies have demonstrated an increased incidence of recurrent DVT after IVC filter placement despite the use of anticoagulation.[15–17] The only prospective, randomized trial of IVC filter outcomes was performed by the PREPIC study group. Four hundred patients with proximal DVT at risk for PE were randomized to receive treatment with either anticoagulation alone or an IVC filter followed by anticoagulation. This trial used the Vena Tech and the Titanium Greenfield filters in 56% and 26.5% of patients, respectively, and there was no significant difference in the duration of anticoagulation between the two groups.[16] At both 2 and 8 years of follow-up, there was a significantly increased risk of recurrent DVT in patients with an IVC filter compared to patients without filters (Table 44.3).[15,16]

If recurrent deep venous thrombosis is suspected, patients should undergo further evaluation. Imaging with venous duplex ultrasound or venogram may help determine whether the patient has had proximal or distal propagation of existing thrombus or recurrent DVT in a new venous segment. In some cases determining the age or chronicity of the thrombus is difficult. In this setting further investigation with D-dimer or alternative imaging modalities may assist in making the determination.

Given the risk for recurrent VTE, anticoagulation should be initiated when possible even after an IVC filter has been placed. Guidelines have been published regarding current anticoagulation recommendations. It is unclear at this time whether the presence of an IVC filter should extend the duration of anticoagulation for a particular clinical situation.[2,18] Some practitioners advocate long-term anticoagulation in patients with vena caval filters, but this has not been well studied. For now, the duration of anticoagulation must be individualized for each patient.[2]

Table 44.3 **2-YEAR AND 8-YEAR RESULTS OF THE PREPIC TRIAL OF ANTICOAGULATION WITH OR WITHOUT AN INFERIOR VENA CAVA FILTER TO PREVENT PULMONARY EMBOLISM**

| | RECURRENT DVT | | SYMPTOMATIC PE | |
	2 Years	8 Years	2 Years	8 Years
Filter	20.8%	35.7%	3.4%	6.2%
No Filter	11.6%	27.5%	6.3%	15.1%
P	0.02	0.16	0.042	0.008

From References 15 and 16.

PE

IVC filter placement is one method of managing DVT and preventing PE in patients unable to be anticoagulated. However, despite IVC interruption, PE may occur. The origin of pulmonary emboli in this setting includes propagation of thrombus proximal to the IVC filter (Figure 44.1), small emboli that pass through the filter, emboli from unprotected venous beds including the upper extremity, or embolism through developed pelvic or abdominal veins or collaterals such as the azygous or ovarian vein. Cumulative rates of recurrent symptomatic PE in the PREPIC trial were 1.1%, 3.4%, and 6.2% at 12 d, 2-year, and 8-year follow-up, respectively. At 2 years there was no difference in the rate of symptomatic PE between the groups, however, by 8 years of follow-up there was a 63% decrease in the risk of recurrent PE in patients with an IVC filter compared to patients without (Table 44.3).

Two patients (1%) suffered fatal PE.[15,16] From the reviews by Streiff and Kinney, forty studies of the SSG filter demonstrated a composite rate of pulmonary embolism of 2.6%, with a range of 0–9%.[11,12] The composite rates for the other available filters were: TG 3.1% (range 0–3.8%), BN 2.9% (range 0–4.2%), SN 3.8% (range 0–5.3%), and VT 3.4% (range 0–8%). The rates of fatal pulmonary embolism were between 0.3% in the VT series up to 1.9% for the SN filter.[11,12] Athanasoulis et al. documented a fatal PE rate of 3.7% following filter insertion in a 26-year review of their

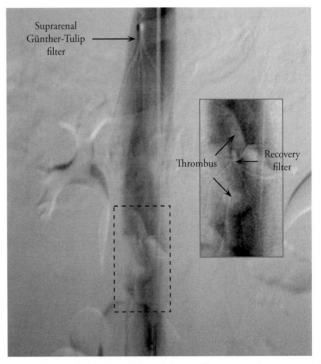

Figure 44.1 Thrombus both within and above a filter (inset) demonstrated by venogram in a patient who developed massive pulmonary embolism despite the presence of an infrarenal Recovery filter. A suprarenal Günther-Tulip filter was placed to protect against further embolism until anticoagulation could be initiated.

IVC filter experience.[19] So, the rates reported for recurrent symptomatic pulmonary embolism and fatal pulmonary embolism are not negligible. Studies have not addressed clinical conditions likely to predispose to this complication.

In a patient with suspected PE, PE protocol chest CT, pulmonary angiography, or ventilation/perfusion nuclear medicine lung scanning should be performed. If the diagnosis is confirmed, the source of the event should also be identified. IVC filter thrombosis can be investigated using contrast enhanced abdominal CT with venous phase imaging or contrast vena cavography. Duplex ultrasound of unprotected venous beds should also be performed to evaluate other potential sources of embolism.

IVC THROMBOSIS OR OCCLUSION

IVC thrombosis may result from innate thrombogenicity of the filter, trapped emboli within the filter, or propagation of thrombus through the venous system up to and including the filter (Figure 44.2). The PREPIC trial documented symptomatic IVC thrombosis in 13% of patients after 8-years of follow-up.[16] Other reports have documented IVC filter thrombosis rates of 0–31%. Once again the SSG and BN filters have documented the lowest rates of IVC thrombosis, 3.6% and 3.9% respectively. The highest rates of IVC thrombosis occurred with the VT filter, 11.2%.[10] In

initial studies, the TrapEase filter had a documented IVC filter thrombosis rate at 6 months of 3.1%.[20]

Early studies of optionally retrievable filters documented IVC thrombosis in up to 10% of patients with the Günther-Tulip filters.[21,22] In addition, thrombus trapped within the filter at attempted retrieval has been documented in 10% of Günther-Tulip and 22% of Recovery filters suggesting the filters may have performed well in preventing PE;[21] whether this could lead to eventual caval thrombosis if the filter is not removed is unknown. Longer follow-up is required to determine whether the rates of IVC thrombosis in optionally retrievable filters will remain constant or increase over time.

When IVC thrombosis is identified, or if the source of the pulmonary embolism is suspected or documented to be due to thrombosis proximal to the filter, management must be individualized. One option is placement of a more proximal vena caval filter, typically suprarenal placement (Figures 44.1 and 44.2). The major concern in this setting is the continued propagation of the thrombus with the potential for involvement of the renal veins. In the hands of a skilled interventionist, filter thrombosis can be managed by endovascular techniques (Figure 44.3). Mechanical and

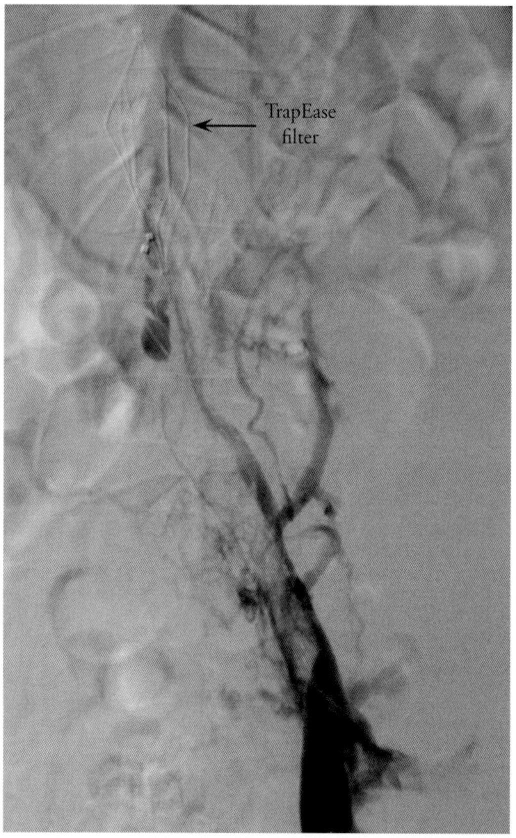

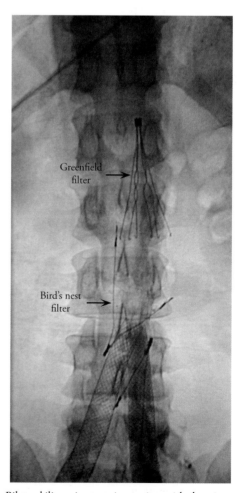

Figure 44.2 Chronic IVC and filter thrombosis demonstrated below a TrapEase filter with collateral drainage.

Figure 44.3 Bilateral iliac vein stents in a patient with chronic venous occlusion following Bird's Nest and Greenfield filter placement.

pharmacologic thrombolysis may be used to restore patency of the IVC filter.[23-25] Other endovascular techniques including balloon maceration of the thrombus or stent placement to collapse the filter and exclude it from the IVC have been reported.[23,26]

POSTTHROMBOTIC SYNDROME

After a DVT, clinical symptoms of the postthrombotic syndrome increase over time. At 8-year follow-up, postthrombotic symptoms are observed in approximate 70% of patients with DVT with or without IVC filter placement.[16] Fox and Kahn recently published a review of postthrombotic syndrome (PTS) related to IVC filter placement for either primary or secondary prophylaxis. They included 1,552 patients in 11 studies in their pooled analysis. Overall, 43% (647/1,507), 12% (176/1,470) and 3.4% (501/1,470) of patients suffered edema, trophic skin changes of PTS, or venous stasis ulcers following IVC filter placement.[27] Given the high rate of postthrombotic complications in patients with VTE, recurrent symptoms of discomfort, erythema, edema, and increased warmth are not uncommon and may lead to repeated investigation for recurrent DVT. Compression stockings are recommended following a DVT with or without IVC filter placement to decrease the development of PTS symptoms.

INSERTION SITE COMPLICATIONS

Insertion site complications after filter placement have perhaps the most varied manifestations. These complications occur in 4–11% of all filter insertions.[12] Some are site-dependent while others may be directly related to the device delivery system. Insertion site complications range from minor bleeding to major complications that may be the source of significant morbidity and even mortality. Death related to IVC filter insertion has been reported to occur in 0.12% of patients.[12]

Most of the complications are similar to other procedures in which central venous access is obtained; bleeding (major or minor), arteriovenous fistula, infections, vessel damage/rupture, and access site thrombosis. Some of the vascular complications at the access site are considered to be directly related to the profile of the delivery system. This has been a major reason for the development of new filters with a lower profile delivery system, which limits the size of the venipuncture and potentially decreases these complications. The internal jugular vein is often a preferred site of access, but due to its anatomic proximity to vital structures, complications related to access at this site may have devastating consequences. Stroke caused by inadvertent carotid puncture, pneumothorax, vocal cord paralysis caused by damage to the recurrent laryngeal nerve, arrhythmia, and air embolism have all been documented.

Insertion site DVT is likely the most common access site complication following IVC filter placement. With routine surveillance, insertion site thrombosis has been identified in 14–64% of patients. Since IVC filters may be inserted by femoral, jugular, or brachial routes, insertion site thrombosis may occur in an unprotected venous bed.[12] The newer low-profile delivery systems may decrease the risk for insertion site thrombosis, but to document the actual frequency of this complication, studies will need to incorporate routine surveillance of the insertion site into protocols.

DEPLOYMENT COMPLICATIONS

Deployment complications are largely dependent on the technical skill and the equipment used to place the filter as well as the filter type. These complications may be generalized into tilting or malposition, incorrect anatomical placement, or failure of the device to fully deploy at its intended site. An incorrectly deployed filter may not achieve the desired protection from pulmonary embolism and yet exposes the patient to all the complications of the procedure, the potential for migration, and possible thrombosis as previously discussed. In addition, the patient and the physician may derive a false sense of security from the filter placement, despite the suboptimal deployment. Thus, incorrect deployment of a filter has clinical implications as well as possible secondary complications.

MALPOSITIONING

Filter malposition or tilting theoretically may result in inadequate protection from pulmonary embolism. For permanent filters, this is traditionally managed with either observation or additional filter placement, typically in the suprarenal position. In a single-center study of 486 patients undergoing duplex ultrasound-guided (n = 435) or intravascular ultrasound (IVUS)-guided (n = 51) IVC filter insertion, by Corriere et al., twelve patients (2.4%) had inadequate positioning as determined by postoperative radiography.[28] Two of these patients had no further filter manipulation, three had a second filter placed under fluoroscopic guidance, and five patients had filters retrieved and repositioned under fluoroscopic guidance. All five patients undergoing retrieval and repositioning in this series had Greenfield filters, which are not traditionally regarded as retrievable. This manipulation was possible using endovascular techniques.[28] In another long-term study of Greenfield filters followed by abdominal radiography, Messmer et al. reported five patients (7%) in whom the filter was at an angle of more than 16 degrees from the vertical.[29] A change in filter angle may result from displacement of a strut into the right renal vein as well as from physiologic changes.[29] Retrievable filters are typically manipulated at the time of insertion to achieve minimal tilting. In the review by Stein et al., 12% (20/169) of Günther Tulip filters and 6% (2/32) Recovery filters were tilted.[21]

The effect of IVC filter tilt and asymmetry on filter function is considered controversial. Clinical concerns include reduced protection from emboli due to a larger space between the struts allowing transit of thrombi as well as a potential for increased thrombogenicity due to flow disturbances from the asymmetric filter struts along the vessel wall. A study conducted by Katsamouris et al. demonstrated when centered, the original Greenfield IVC filter allowed passage of small clots, and eccentric positioning (defined as >14°) allowed small and large clots to pass through the filter.[30] Another study by Greenfield and Proctor showed that alignment only assumed importance when the IVC is larger than 22 mm.[31] One clinical study evaluated recurrent PE and caval thrombosis in patients with titanium Greenfield IVC filters and included a subgroup analysis of patients with filter asymmetry, defined by strut pattern in the cava. Out of a total of 738 filters, asymmetry was found in 42 cases (5%). Recurrent PE was diagnosed in a total of 3 of 35 patients (8.6%) with asymmetric filters compared with 11 of 338 patients (3.3%) with symmetric IVC filters ($P = NS$).[32]

While it is difficult to know exactly how tilting or malpositioning affects the functioning of a given device in view of the lack of routine clinical follow-up, device modifications have been used to reduce this complication. The currently available Greenfield filters use a guide wire deployment system designed to promote midline deployment. Other devices have adopted a symmetrical filter design to optimize vertical deployment. Modifications such as a dual level filter design have also been used optimize centering and to provide more efficient thrombus trapping.

INADVERTENT DEPLOYMENT IN AN INCORRECT VESSEL

Filter deployment in the incorrect vessel or at an unplanned location in the appropriate vessel can occur. Misplaced filter deployment has been documented in the right atrium,[18] the innominate vein,[33] above the renal veins, juxtaposed to the renal veins or partially within a renal vein,[19] and in the iliac vein.[34] Forty-six IVC filters that were inadvertently placed in the suprarenal IVC, juxtarenal IVC, or renal vein were compared with infrarenal IVC filters.[19] No differences in filter efficacy were identified. PE after filter placement was identified in 7% of patients, but renal complications were not discussed.[19] Although a misplaced filter is an unusual complication and in most cases is tolerated without clinical effect, serious consequences may occur in some settings and the utmost care should be used to avoid inadvertent deployments.

Venous anomalies may lead to problems in filter deployment. Anomalous IVC or renal vein anatomy, megacava (>30 mm), small caliber cava, congenital absence of the vena cava, double cava, left-sided vena cava, caval thrombus, circumaortic renal veins, retroaortic veins, multiple renal veins, or congenital absence of the kidneys may affect deployment. In one study, anatomical variation or IVC thrombosis was documented in 9.6% of patients prior to deployment and warranted an adjustment in the deployment strategy in 4% of patients.[19] Imaging by venography/cavography using iodinated contrast, gadolinium, or occasionally carbon dioxide has traditionally been used prior to IVC filter placement. More recent reports have focused on using duplex ultrasound or IVUS, which may allow for bedside insertion in patients who are critically ill or if transportation is difficult due to extensive spine or orthopedic injuries.

FAILURE TO DEPLOY

The failure of vena caval filters to fully deploy is frequently discussed but rarely documented in the literature (Figure 44.4). While this complication may manifest as filter migration or even embolization, most cases are not clinically apparent. Partial deployment has usually been attributed to a malfunction of the filter itself that occurs on a case-by-case basis and is not necessarily design specific. In one study of Vena Tech filters, major complications of placement occurred in three patients, all when the right internal jugular vein was used for introduction. One filter was inadvertently placed in the right renal vein and two

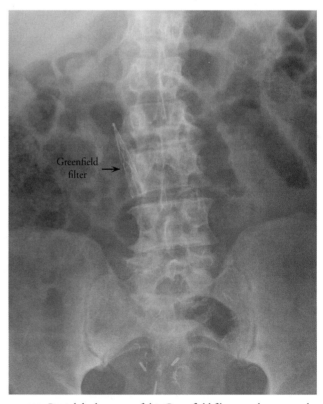

Figure 44.4 Partial deployment of this Greenfield filter was documented by abdominal radiograph.

filters failed to open fully.[35] Deployment complications with the Greenfield filter and modified designs have been documented in another series.[19] The TrapEase filter has not demonstrated failure to deploy, however, filter shortening and maldeployment have been documented.[20] In many cases the failure to fully open can be addressed at the time of filter placement with endovascular manipulation of underdeployed or partially deployed filters.

DEVICE COMPLICATIONS

Complications that are device and equipment specific provide an impetus for the development of new filter designs and delivery systems. Strut fracture due to compromise of the structural integrity of the filter has been documented for most filter designs.[19] To date there are no large series comparing strut fractures among different filter types. Because of the lack of routine imaging follow-up, the identification of a strut fracture is typically a serendipitous discovery during radiological imaging performed for other clinical indications. Clinical issues may arise when a fractured strut embolizes to the cardiopulmonary circulation or is extruded thru the IVC into adjacent structures. In some cases the fractured leg may be retrieved and in other cases this may be impractical.[36] The most vulnerable points for fracture are welded seams. To this extent filters such as the TrapEase or OptEase, which are laser cut in a unibody style, are less likely to have fracture complications.

Guide wire entrapment is another device-related complication that may occur at the time of filter placement or when a wire is passed thru the filter for central access. In one in vitro study, the TrapEase filter entrapped 3.0-mm and 1.5-mm J-tipped guide wires, whereas the Vena Tech LP (low profile) and Günther Tulip filters did not.[37] Another study described entrapment of both the 1.5-J and 3-J guide wires by the stainless steel Greenfield and Vena Tech LGM devices.[38] The 1.5-J guide wire became entrapped regardless of engagement pattern; while the 3-J became entrapped only when engaged in the hole in the apex of the SSG and VT filters. In a series of superior vena cava filters, 56% of patients had subsequent central access without complications.[39] In another series, one filter was dislodged during central line placement and repositioned into the innominate vein.[33] This complication may be avoidable if fluoroscopy is used during central access in patients with residing filters. Retrieval of an entrapped guide wire can be a technically challenging proposition, snares and other endovascular devices may be used for percutaneous retrieval.

MIGRATION

Filters are long-term intravascular devices that are subject to a number of external forces that may change their

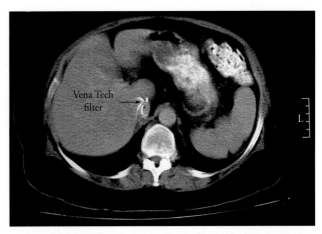

Figure 44.5   Vena Tech filter with migration to the level of the intrahepatic inferior vena cava demonstrated on CT scan.

position as well as dimensions over time.[40] These changes can result clinically in filter migration or penetration/extrusion through the vessel wall. Case series have documented migration in all filter types.[10] The Vena Tech filter appears to be most affected by this complication; up to 18% migrated in one study.[10] Migration may be cephalad or caudal; typically movement >20 mm is considered clinically significant. In one study of sixty-nine patients with a Greenfield IVC filter in place for 1–9 years evaluated with supine abdominal radiographs, the filter span diameter had increased by 3–11 mm in twenty-two (32%) patients, and had decreased by 3–18 mm in six patients (9%). Twenty patients (29%) had caudal migration of 3-18 mm, and four (6%) had cephalad migration.[29]

Proximal migration to clinically significant structures such as the intrahepatic IVC (Figure 44.5) or the right atrium may occur.[19] A number of case reports describe serious complications of embolization to the heart, including pericardial tamponade and intracardiac migration with life-threatening arrhythmias.[40,41,42] Retrieval of these filters has been attempted using endovascular techniques. However, because of the unusual location, retrieval may require extraordinary measures including surgical procedures with cardiopulmonary bypass or circulatory arrest. It is unclear what places a patient at risk for filter embolism. Occasionally, embolization is considered to have occurred because of a large thrombus burden entrapped within the filter.[22,40] Routine clinical follow-up and serial radiographic surveillance has not been advocated following IVC filter placement, so migration is usually identified serendipitously unless a serious clinical consequence occurs.

EXTRUSION

Most filters will have some change in dimension following placement.[30] Extrusion of the filter struts through the caval wall is a near universal phenomenon (Figure 44.6).[10,40,43]

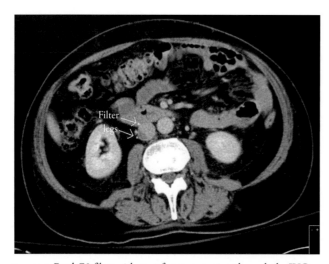

Figure 44.6 Bard G2 filter with strut foot penetration through the IVC wall (arrows).

In a study to determine the long-term clinical and radiographic outcome of patients who undergo insertion of a Bird's Nest filter, perforation of the caval wall was universal but not clinically symptomatic.[44] Strut extrusion typically does not assume clinical importance until there is involvement of adjacent structures and associated clinical complications.

There are a number of case reports in the literature detailing individual clinical experiences and unusual complications resulting from strut or even filter extrusion from the IVC. Reports of small bowel obstruction occurring as a result of volvulus occurring around an extruded filter strut,[45] a fragmented IVC filter penetrating the aorta and causing a small infrarenal aortic pseudoaneurysm,[46] hydronephrosis caused by transcaval penetration of a Bird's Nest filter,[47] laceration of a lumbar artery by a stainless steel Greenfield filter strut that resulted in a near fatal hemorrhage,[48] and upper gastrointestinal bleeding secondary to Bird's Nest inferior vena caval filter migration into the duodenum[49] to name a few. These are rare, usually reportable, complications of filter placement.

RETRIEVAL COMPLICATIONS

The optionally retrievable filters typically have FDA approval for both permanent and retrievable options. However, most of the optionally retrievable filters have little to no data available on their long-term performance when used as permanent filters. There are no unique indications for the use of optionally retrievable filters compared to permanent devices. In addition, there are no absolute indications for retrieval or removal of an IVC filter unless it is a source of morbidity.[1] When used as an optionally retrievable filter, two visits to the interventional suite are required; initially for placement and when indicated for removal. This creates a potential for increased numbers of complications not only related to the device or to venous access (Table 44.2) but also an entirely new category of complications related

to the explantation of devices. Retrieval complications may include injury to the IVC during retrieval, failure to retrieve, device fracture, and retained legs/hooks. Furthermore, explantation complications can be of a serious nature (e.g., caval perforation).

The FDA has recommended maximum dwell times before which the devices should be retrieved. However, studies have demonstrated safe retrieval with longer indwelling durations. Binkert et al.[50] have reported the retrieval of such type of filter at 317 days without complications on follow-up venogram. Repeated repositioning has been used to prolong the deployment of these devices.[51] While most retrievable IVC filters are placed in patients with a well-defined, short-term risk for VTE and contraindications to anticoagulation, the percentage of retrievable filters actually removed is less than 50%.[52] The most common reason stated for not retrieving a filter is due to caval or filter thrombus or continued contraindication to anticoagulation. All retrieved filters have strands of organized thrombus on the filter struts. The presence of small thrombi does not dictate the need to abort the retrieval, but larger thrombi preclude filter removal. Given the large numbers of these filters remaining in situ, data on the potential longer-term complications of these filters should be emerging.

Data on failed retrievals based on technical difficulties is sparse. Most limited case series of the various filter types report successful snaring and device retrieval with no caval injuries.[53,54] In one series, retrieval failure was related to device angulation within the vena cava that precluded safe capture.[53] Difficulties with retrieval may be encountered more frequently with longer dwell times, but data is lacking at present.

SPECIAL CONSIDERATIONS

There are identified patient populations in whom IVC filter use generates special consideration. These include trauma patients, children, pregnant women, and patients with septicemia. In the trauma population IVC filter placement has gained popularity as a mechanism of both primary and secondary prophylaxis. The body of literature regarding filter use in this setting is growing. On the other hand, very few studies focus on filter placement in children, during pregnancy, or in patients with septicemia.

In most clinical settings filters are deployed into the infrarenal IVC. However, placement in the suprarenal IVC or superior vena cava has also been used for specific clinical indications. Superior vena cava positioning has been employed to protect against embolism from upper extremity DVT.

TRAUMA

The use of IVC filters for primary prophylaxis in trauma patients has increased, especially when sequential compression or pharmacologic therapy is contraindicated, for example, in vertebral fracture or spinal cord injury, multiple lower extremity fractures, and closed head injury. The use of IVC filters for primary prophylaxis in this setting is open to controversy. Analysis of 450,375 patients registered in the American College of Surgeons National Trauma Data Bank identified a VTE (DVT, PE, or both) rate of 0.36%. The mortality rate in patients with PE was 18.7%. A total of 3,883 patients had IVC filters placed; 83% were prophylactic. This analysis also identified risk factors for VTE including: age ≥ 40 (OR 2.29); pelvic or lower extremity fracture (OR 2.93 and 3.16 respectively); spinal cord injury with paralysis (OR 3.39); head injury (OR 2.59); more than 3 d of ventilator dependency (OR 10.62); venous injury (OR 7.93); shock (OR 1.95); and major surgery (OR 4.32).[55] Yet data regarding IVC filter use in the trauma setting is based solely on case series reports and retrospective registry studies. Girard et al. reviewed sixteen series published before 1999 with a total of 1,112 trauma patients.[56] PE occurred following IVC filter placement in 0-3.9% of cases. Fatal PE was documented in a single patient in each of two studies. DVT was identified in 0–20.6% of patients. IVC thrombosis or occlusion occurred in 0–6.7% of cases. Insertion site thrombosis and procedural complications were identified in 0–5.7% and 0–4.6% of cases respectively.[56] The results do not support the general use of filters in all trauma patients, but since this review encompassed reports prior to 1999, the use of newer, low profile devices may demonstrate more favorable results. Furthermore, selected use of filters in high-risk subgroups of trauma patients may be appropriate.

Optionally retrievable filters have also been used in the trauma population. In recently published series, recurrent DVT was documented in 2.9% and 8.6%; and in one study, insertion site DVT was documented in 1.9%.[34,57] Filter retrieval was successful in 51% and 66% of patients. If the practice of permanent or optionally retrievable filter placement for primary prophylaxis in the trauma population is to be supported, further systematic study is should be encouraged.

CHILDREN

Thromboembolic events are less frequent in children than adults. When present, the options for therapy remain the same. The potential for growth and increased life-expectancy for children raises concerns regarding the use of IVC filters. One study has published results of IVC filter placement in fifteen children with clinical follow-up. No insertion complications, migration, or filter related mortality occurred. During follow-up, one patient demonstrated PTS symptoms and three patients had common femoral vein reflux, but no recurrent PE occurred.[58] In another study of eight patients; three patients died. The remaining five patients, followed up to 13 months, demonstrated no filter migration, IVC occlusion or thrombosis, or symptomatic PE.[59] Chaudry et al. published their experience with deployment in three children with successful retrieval in two.[60] From the limited

data available, IVC filter placement in children may serve as a useful management tool in patients with a contraindication to anticoagulation. Children do not appear to have an increased risk of complications compared with other study groups. However, if successful retrieval can be accomplished this may also decrease concerns for long-term complications.

SEPTICEMIA

Infectious complications of IVC filters appear as case reports,[61] but there is a paucity of data regarding this complication or the use of filters in septic patients. The single retrospective publication of IVC filter placement is patients with septicemia demonstrated no need for filter retrieval due to infectious complications.[62] Documented 30-d survival was 67%. Filter complications included caval occlusion (1%), recurrent nonfatal PE (1%), recurrent DVT (2.9%), and procedure/deployment complications in 8.6% of patients.[62] Rare case reports of IVC filter infection should not sway the decision to place an IVC filter when clinically indicated in patients with septicemia.

ATYPICAL FILTER LOCATION

Nontraditional locations for filter placement are used in various clinical circumstances. Filters may be place in iliac veins in patients with a mega cava (>40 mm). Suprarenal IVC filter placement may be indicated in patients with an anomalous IVC, thrombus or mass in the IVC that precludes infrarenal placement, or filter occlusion or thrombosis. Suprarenal placement has also been advocated in women who are pregnant or of child-bearing age, although there is very little literature to support this practice.[63] Concern surrounds suprarenal IVC filter placement due to the risk for IVC thrombosis or thrombus propagation and the potential for fatal renal vein thrombosis. This complication has been seen, however, it appears to be relatively rare.[59,63,64] From one survey of cancer patients with suprarenal IVC filter placement two of thirteen patients developed renal vein thrombosis.[64] Greenfield et al. reviewed data on 148 suprarenal IVC filters and compared outcomes to 1,932 infrarenal IVC filters placed during the same period.[65] Overall there was no statistically significant difference in the complication rates between the two filter groups. Recurrent PE was documented in 8% and 4% of suprarenal IVC and infrarenal IVC filters, respectively. Caval occlusion was found in 5% of patients. There were no renal complications.[65] While suprarenal IVC filter placement does not appear to be complicated by a preponderance of renal vein thrombosis, in patients with advanced malignancy, a single functioning kidney, chronic kidney disease, or previous renal vein thrombosis, suprarenal IVC filter placement should be avoided if possible.

In view of the very limited treatment options available, superior vena cava filters are sometimes used in patients with upper extremity DVT who have a contraindication to anticoagulation or experience PE despite adequate anticoagulation.[33,39] In one series, no filter migration, dislodgement, or fracture was identified in forty-one patients (median follow-up 12 weeks). No clinical symptoms of SVC syndrome were identified. Central venous catheters or Swan-Ganz catheters were subsequently placed in 56% of patients without complication. One patient had subsequent PE related to left lower extremity DVT.[39] Usoh et al. reviewed their experience in 154 patients with SVC filter placement.[33] Only fifty-eight patients survived longer than 60 d. In-hospital death was documented in 49% of patients unrelated to the SVC filter or VTE. In forty of the fifty-eight patients surviving more than 60 d, no migration was identified by follow-up radiographs. One filter was misplaced in the innominate vein and remained patent at 2 months of follow-up. No patients had clinical symptoms of PE or SVC thrombosis following filter placement. Three patients suffered SVC perforation and cardiac tamponade. One patient was noted to have an aortic perforation at the time of autopsy.[33] Upper extremity DVT is not free of typical thromboembolic complications. SVC filter placement may be an alternative form of management in this clinical setting. However, the relative increase in the use of indwelling catheters and transvenous devices such as pacemakers and defibrillators may make permanent deployment of a filter in this position less favorable. Optionally retrievable filters may have a role in this setting, but data is lacking at present.

CONCLUSION

IVC filter use is increasing. In many cases the deployment is for indications other than a contraindication or complication of anticoagulation. Device development and design has been directed toward decreasing the complications associated with IVC filters. Despite device improvements, complications related to IVC filters remain a significant clinical concern. Deployment should be used when clinically indicated; however, a focus on retrieval when possible may also be warranted. Further study of all of these considerations is warranted.

REFERENCES

1. Kaufman JA, Kinney TB, Streiff MB, et al. Guidelines for the use of retrievable and convertible vena cava filters: Report from the Society for Interventional Radiology multidisciplinary consensus conference, *J Vasc Interv Radiol.* 2006. *17*: 449–459.
2. Kearon C, Kahn SR, Agnelli G, Goldhaber S, Raskob GE, Comerota AJ. Antithrombotic therapy for venous thromboembolic disease: American College of Chest Physicians evidence based clinical practice guidelines (8th edition), *Chest.* 2008. *133*: 454S–545S.
3. Girard P, Tardy B, Decousus H. Inferior vena cava interruption: How and when?, *Annu Rev Med.* 2000. *51*: 1–15.
4. Crowther MA. Inferior vena cava filters in the management of venous thromboembolism, *Am J Med.* 2007. *120*(10 Suppl 2): S13–S17.
5. White RH, Zhou H, Kim J, Romano PS. A population-based study of the effectiveness of inferior vena cava filter use among patients with venous thromboembolism, *Arch Intern Med.* 2000. *160*: 2033–2041.
6. Stein PD, Kayali F, Olson RE. Twenty-one-year trends in the use of inferior vena cava filters, *Arch Intern Med.* 2004. *164*: 1541–1545.
7. Arcelus JI, Caprini JA, Monreal M, Suárez C, González-Farjardo J. The management and outcome of acute venous thromboembolism: A prospective registry including 4011 patients, *J Vasc Surg.* 2003. *38*: 916–922.
8. Jaff MR, Goldhaber SZ, Tapson VF. High utilization rate of vena cava filters in deep vein thrombosis, *Thromb Haemost.* 2005. *93*: 1117–1119.
9. Girard P, Stern J, Parent F. Medical literature and vena cava filters: So far so weak, *Chest.* 2002. *122*: 963–967.
10. Whitehill TA. Current vena cava filter devices and results, *Semin Vasc Surg.* 2000. *13*: 204–212.
11. Streiff MB. Vena caval filters: A comprehensive review, *Blood.* 2000. *95*: 3669–3677.
12. Kinney TB. Update on inferior vena cava filters, *J Vasc Interv Radiol.* 2003. *14*: 425–440.
13. Imberti D, Prisco D. Retrievable vena cava filters: Key considerations, *Thromb Res.* 2008. *122*: 442–449.
14. Becker DM, Philbrick JT, Selby JB. Inferior vena cava filters: Indications, safety, effectiveness, *Arch Intern Med.* 1992. *152*: 1985–1994.
15. Decousus H, Leizorovicz A, Parent F, et al. A critical trial of vena cava filters in the prevention of pulmonary embolism in patients with proximal deep-vein thrombosis, *N Engl J Med.* 1998. *338*: 409–415.
16. PREPIC Study Group. Eight-year follow-up of patients with permanent vena cava filters in the prevention of pulmonary embolism, *Circulation.* 2005. *112*: 416–422.
17. Billett HH, Jacobs LG, Madsen EM, Giannattasio ER, Mahesh S, Cohen HW. Efficacy of inferior vena cava filters in anticoagulated patients, *J Thromb Haemost.* 2007. 5: 1848–1853.
18. Gomes MPV, Kaplan KL, Deitcher SR. Patients with inferior vena caval filters should receive chronic thromboprophylaxis, *Med Clin N Am.* 2003. *87*: 1189–1203.
19. Athanasoulis CA, Kaufman JA, Halpern EF, Waltman AC, Geller SC, Fan C. Inferior vena caval filters: Review of a 26-year single-center clinical experience, *Radiology.* 2000. *216*: 54–66.
20. Rousseau H, Perreault P, Otal P, et al. The 6-F nitinol TrapEase inferior vena cava filter: Results of a prospective multicenter trial, *J Vasc Interv Radiol.* 2001. *12*: 299–304.
21. Stein PD, Alnas M, Skaf E, et al. Outcome and complications of retrievable inferior vena cava filters, *Am J Cardiol.* 2004. *94*: 1090–1093.
22. Ku GH, Billett HH. Long lives, short indications: The case for removable inferior vena cava filters, *Thromb Haemost.* 2005. *93*: 17–22.
23. Vedantham S, Vesely TM, Parti N, et al. Endovascular recanalization of the thrombosed filter-bearing inferior vena cava, *J Vasc Interv Radiol.* 2003. *14*: 893–903.
24. Angle JF, Matsumoto AH, Al Shammari M, Hagspiel KD, Spinosa DJ, Humphries JE. Transcatheter regional urokinase therapy in the management of inferior vena cava thrombosis, *J Vasc Interv Radiol.* 1998. 9: 917–925.
25. Poon WL, Luk SH, Yam KY, Lee ACW. Mechanical thrombectomy in inferior vena cava thrombosis after caval filter placement: A report of three cases, *Cardiovasc Intervent Radiol.* 2002. *25*: 440–443.
26. Joshi A, Carr J, Chrisman H, et al. Filter-related, thrombotic occlusion of the inferior vena cava treated with a Gianturco stent, *J Vasc Interv Radiol.* 2003. *14*: 381–385.
27. Fox MA, Kahn SR. Postthrombotic syndrome in relation to vena cava filter placement: A systematic review, *J Vasc Interv Radiol.* 2008. *19*: 981–985.

28. Corriere MA, Passman MA, Guzman RJ, Dattilo JB, Naslund TC. Retrieving "nonretrievable" inferior vena caval Greenfield filters: A therapeutic option for filter malpositioning, *Ann Vasc Surg.* 2004. *18*: 629–634.

29. Messmer JM, Greenfield LJ. Greenfield caval filters: Long-term radiographic follow-up study, *Radiology.* 1985. *156*: 613–618.

30. Katsamouris AA, Waltman AC, Delichatsios MA, Athanasoulis CA. Inferior vena cava filters: In vitro comparison of clot trapping and flow dynamics, *Radiology.* 1988. *166*: 361–366.

31. Greenfield LJ, Proctor MC. Experimental embolic capture by asymmetric Greenfield filters, *J Vasc Surg.* 1992. *16*: 436–443.

32. Greenfield LJ, Proctor MC, Cho KJ, Wakefield TW. Limb asymmetry in titanium Greenfield filters: Clinically significant?, *J Vasc Surg.* 1997. *26*: 770–775.

33. Usoh F, Hignorani A, Ascher E, et al. Long-term follow-up for superior vena cava filter placement, *Ann Vasc Surg.* 2009. *23*: 350–354.

34. Rosenthal D, Wellons ED, Lai KM, Bikk A. Retrievable inferior vena cava filters: Early clinical experience, *J Cardiovasc Surg.* 2005. *46*: 163–169.

35. Millward SF, Peterson RA, Moher D, et al. LGM (Vena Tech) vena caval filter: Experience at a single institution, *J Vasc Interv Radiol.* 1994. *5*: 351–356.

36. Hull JE, Robertson SW. Bard Recovery filter: Evaluation and management of vena cava limb perforation, fracture, and migration, *J Vasc Interv Radiol.* 2009. *20*: 52–60.

37. Stavropoulos SW, Itkin M, Trerotola SO. In vitro study of guide wire entrapment in currently available inferior vena cava filters, *J Vasc Interv Radiol.* 2003. *14*: 905–910.

38. Kaufman JA, Thomas JW, Geller SC, Rivitz SM, Waltman AC. Guide-wire entrapment by inferior vena caval filters: In vitro evaluation, *Radiology.* 1996. *198*: 71–76.

39. Spence LD, Gironta MG, Malde HM, Mickolick CT, Geisinger MA, Dolmatch BL. Acute upper extremity deep venous thrombosis: Safety and effectiveness of superior vena caval filters, *Radiology.* 1999. *210*: 53–58.

40. Proctor MC, Cho KJ, Greenfield LJ. In vivo evaluation of vena caval filters: Can function be linked to design characteristics?, *Cardiovasc Intervent Radiol.* 2000. *23*: 460–465.

41. Lahey SJ, Meyer LP, Karchmer AW, et al. Misplaced caval filter and subsequent pericardial tamponade, *Ann Thorac Surg.* 1991. *51*: 299–300; discussion 301.

42. Bach JR, Zaneuski R, Lee H. Cardiac arrhythmias from a malpositioned Greenfield filter in a traumatic quadriplegic, *Am J Phys Med Rehabil.* 1990. *69*: 251–253.

43. Hoekstra A, Hoogeveen Y, Elstrodt JM, Tiebosch AT. Vena cava filter behavior and endovascular response: An experimental in vivo study, *Cardiovasc Intervent Radiol.* 2003. *26*: 222–226.

44. Starok MS, Common AA. Follow-up after insertion of Bird's Nest inferior vena caval filters, *Can Assoc Radiol J.* 1996. *47*: 189–194.

45. Kupferschmid JP, Dickson CS, Townsend RN, Diamond DL. Small-bowel obstruction from an extruded Greenfield filter strut: An unusual late complication, *J Vasc Surg.* 1992. *16*: 113–115.

46. Putterman D, Niman D, Cohen G. Aortic pseudoaneurysm after penetration by a Simon nitinol inferior vena cava filter, *J Vasc Interv Radiol.* 2005. *16*: 535–538.

47. Stacey CS, Manhire AR, Rose DH, Bishop MC. Bird's nest filter causing symptomatic hydronephrosis following transmural penetration of the inferior vena cava, *Cardiovasc Intervent Radiol.* 2004. *27*: 61–63.

48. Woodward EB, Farber A, Wagner WH, et al. Delayed retroperitoneal arterial hemorrhage after inferior vena cava (IVC) filter insertion: Case report and literature review of caval perforations by IVC filters, *Ann Vasc Surg.* 2002. *16*: 193–196.

49. al Zahrani HA. Bird's nest inferior vena caval filter migration into the duodenum: A rare cause of upper gastrointestinal bleeding, *J Endovasc Surg.* 1995. *2*: 372–375.

50. Binkert CA, Bansal A, Gates JD. Inferior vena cava filter removal after 317-day implantation, *J Vasc Interv Radiol.* 2005. *16*: 395–398.

51. Tay KH, Martin ML, Fry PD, Webb JG, Machan LS. Repeated Gunther Tulip inferior vena cava filter repositioning to prolong implantation time, *J Vasc Interv Radiol.* 2002. *13*: 509–512.

52. Rectenwald JE. Vena cava filters: Uses and abuses, *Semin Vasc Surg.* 2005. *18*: 166–175.

53. Lam RC, Bush RL, Lin PH, Lumsden AB. Early technical and clinical results with retrievable inferior vena caval filters, *Vascular.* 2004. *12*: 233–237.

54. Millward SF, Bhargava A, Aquino J Jr, et al. Gunther Tulip filter: Preliminary clinical experience with retrieval, *J Vasc Interv Radiol.* 2000. *11*: 75–82.

55. Knudson MM, Ikossi DG, Khaw L, Morabito D, Speetzen LS. Thromboembolism after trauma: An analysis of 1602 episodes from the American College of Surgeons National Trauma Data Bank, *Ann Surg.* 2004. *240*: 490–498.

56. Girard TD, Philbrick JT, Angle JF, Becker DM. Prophylactic vena cava filters for trauma patients: A systematic review of the literature, *Thromb Res.* 2003. *112*: 261–267.

57. Hoff WS, Hoey BA, Wainwright GA, et al. Early experience with retrievable inferior vena cava filters in high-risk trauma patients, *J Am Coll Surg.* 2004. *199*: 869–874.

58. Cahn MD, Rohrer MJ, Martella MB, Cutler BS. Long-term follow-up of Greenfield inferior vena cava filter placement in children, *J Vasc Surg.* 2001. *34*: 820–825.

59. Reed RA, Teitelbaum GP, Stanley P, Mazer MJ, Tonkin ILD, Rollins NK. The use of inferior vena cava filters in pediatric patients for pulmonary embolus prophylaxis, *Cardiovasc Intervent Radiol.* 1996. *19*: 401–405.

60. Chaudry G, Padua HM, Alomari AI. The use of inferior vena cava filters in young children, *J Vasc Interv Radiol.* 2008. *19*: 1103–1106.

61. Lin M, Soo TB, Horn LC. Successful retrieval of an infected Günther Tulip IVC filter, *J Vasc Interv Radiol.* 2000. *11*: 1341–1343.

62. Greenfield LJ, Proctor MC. Vena caval filter use in patients with sepsis: Results in 175 patients, *Arch Surg.* 2003. *138*: 1245–1248.

63. Kalva SP, Chlapoutaki C, Wicky S, Greenfield AJ, Waltman AC, Athanasoulis CA. Suprarenal inferior vena cava filters: A 20-year single-center experience, *J Vasc Interv Radiol.* 2008. *19*: 1041–1047.

64. Marcy P, Magné N, Frenay M, Bruneton J. Renal failure secondary to thrombotic complications of suprarenal inferior vena cava filters in cancer patients, *Cardiovasc Intervent Radiol.* 2001. *24*: 257–259.

65. Greenfield LJ, Proctor MC. Suprarenal filter placement, *J Vasc Surg.* 1998. *28*: 432–438.

45.

TEMPORARY FILTERS AND PROPHYLACTIC INDICATIONS

Robert B. Rutherford, John C. McCallum, and Nikhil Kansal

Since the development of retrievable vena cava filters (RVCFs), their use for prophylactic indications has contributed to the trend of increasing inferior vena cava (IVC) filter use for patients at risk for venous thromboembolic disease. A preceding chapter has dealt with permanent filters, whose indications and results are relatively well established, but recently a number of temporary or retrievable filter devices have been introduced, and their use is also increasing. In certain respects two of these upward trends, in prophylactic indications and the use of RVCFs, are linked in that both are most commonly used in dealing with patients who have not had a pulmonary embolus (PE) but who are considered to be at high risk of this dreaded complication, yet only for a limited period of time. This chapter will appraise both of these burgeoning practices, and the available evidence regarding these remarkable shifts in the use of VCFs.

THE RATIONALE BEHIND THE USE OF TEMPORARY OR RETRIEVABLE VCFS

The preceding chapter dealt with the complications of vena cava filters, which, it will be seen, provide part of the justification for using temporary or retrievable filters (RVCFs). The justification for using RVCFs is based on two oft-related circumstances: (1) the risk of PE is limited in duration in a number of patient categories and (2) the complications associated with leaving a VCF in situ can be significant over time. The latter consideration is particularly pertinent in otherwise healthy younger patients with an extended longevity outlook who would be at risk of these problems for many years.

This was just a theoretical position until a randomized prospective trial suggested that this was indeed the case. The PREPIC trial (Prevention du Risque d'Embolie Pulmonaire par Interruption Cave) has been widely quoted as evidence to support the use of RVCFs. This trial randomized 400 patients with proximal deep venous thrombosis (DVT) and a variety of indications for VCF placement into no filter and filter groups, both receiving heparin (contraindication to anticoagulant [AC] therapy was not represented). The choice of filter used was optional and included Vena Tech LGM, Titanium Greenfield, Cardial, or Bird's Nest. After 12 days, there was a significant protection against PE by the filters (1.1% vs. 4.8%, p = 0.03) and a very suggestive advantage against fatal PE (0.0% vs. 2.0%, p = 0.12). At two years, the protection against PE (3.4% vs. 6.3%, p = 0.16) and fatal PE (0.5% vs. 2.5%, p = 0.21) appeared to persist, but statistical significance was lost because of diminishing numbers of patients. However, at two years, there was a significantly higher rate of DVT among the filter group (21% vs. 12%, p = 0.02). The conclusion was that although filters protected against PE, they carried a higher risk of later DVT. Whether this late DVT risk was related to the thrombogenicity of some of the filters used, and/or associated caval thrombosis due to disturbed flow or intimal changes is not known, and the results were not analyzed relative to filter type. Follow-up data at 5 and 8 years showed the same trends in terms of DVT, but statistical significance, though close, was lost (p = 0.06 at five years and p = 0.08 at eight years).

Some have used these late follow-up data to claim that there is not a long-term risk of DVT associated with leaving in VCFs, whereas others have countered that the trends are still clear but that, like many long-term studies, the loss of patients to follow-up undermines statistical significance. Nevertheless, this study added great impetus to the development of temporary, retrievable filters for prophylactic indications representing a limited duration of risk of PE.

Most recent data regarding outcomes from RVCF are derived largely from single-institution, observational case series. There is little randomized controlled data. A recent Cochran Review[1] found that the PREPIC trial and one other trial met consideration for inclusion and analysis in a review of randomized controlled trials looking at the effectiveness of vena cava filters in preventing pulmonary embolism. In the other trial, Fullen et al.[2] found that cava filters were effective in reducing PE relative to controls without filters in 129 patients, however the patient population was noted to have a high rate of atherosclerotic heart disease and heart failure, and no difference in mortality was noted.

With the exception of these studies, which compare permanent filters to no filter, these authors are not aware of a randomized controlled trial of RVCFs versus no filter, nor of RVCFs versus permanent filters.

CURRENTLY AVAILABLE RVCFS

It is not the purpose of this chapter to compare individual filters (Figure 45.1). Nevertheless, specific filters will be mentioned in the discussion that follows; therefore they should be identified here. Currently available RVCFs that have been approved by the FDA for use in the United States include the Günther Tulip (Cook), the Celect (Cook), the OptEase (Cordis), the Option (Rex Medical), the Meridian (Bard), and the Eclipse (Bard). Meridian and Eclipse are new marketing names for the second-generation Bard RVCF. Bard's RVCF was initially marketed as the "Recovery" filter, then significant changes were made it its design including increased numbers of struts, leading to the "G2" device. Subsequent names for this second-generation device include the "G2x," and both the "Meridian" and "Eclipse" products are based on the second-generation "G2" body, with minor changes (personal communication with the manufacturer).

PROBLEMS WITH CURRENT RVCFS

In spite of the impressive technological advances associated with the development of RVCFs, there are still a number of limiting factors that must be pointed out. Removal of many if not most of the current temporary filters becomes increasingly difficult with passage of time because of thrombus in the filter and/or adherence at points of endothelial contact. As a result many have simply been left in. Thrombus in a filter can be interpreted as good (a potential PE has been trapped) or bad (device thrombogenicity). This problem in retrieving temporary filters may have resulted in renaming them optional filters, meaning that they can be used as either temporary/retrievable filters or left in as permanent filters. This implies that it is quite permissible (i.e., no significant penalty) to leave them in. This name change may be a marketing ploy because, as of this writing, no good long-term outcome data on these new optional filters has been published to justify leaving them indefinitely (e.g., low rates of recurrent PE, filter migration, filter or caval thrombosis, distal DVT, etc.). Instead, a growing body of

literature suggests that complications persist over time and filters should be removed as soon as the indication for their placement has ceased to be applicable.

Since 2007, a number of retrospective studies have been published that report extending dwell times for RVCFs, periods of time that the filters can be left in place and still be successfully removed. Table 45.1 includes data for recent reports on successful retrieval rates of RVCFs, mean dwell times, as well as range of time in place. While several studies report filters being left in place for over a year, no case series reports an average dwell time over 200 days.[3] Filter tilt, incorporation of filter struts into the walls of the vena cava by endothelialization, and the presence of a significant amount of trapped thrombus have been reported as the major pathophysiologic processes that increase the difficulty of filter removal. As endovascular specialists have increased their experience with removing vena cava filters, their ability to remove what were previously thought to be technically irretrievable filters has improved. This is demonstrated in the technical success rates seen among attempted filter removals in Table 45.1, which range from 78–100%, despite increasing dwell times.

The reported experience with the greatest claim regarding safe dwell time before a RVCF is removed has been with the Günther Tulip, which demonstrated the feasibility of retrieval at 494 days, with a range of 3–494 days and a mean of 58.9 days, in a case series by Smouse et al.[3] They report technically successful removal in 248 of 275 attempts (90%) to remove filters, among 554 patients in whom retrievable filters were placed, thereby representing a 44% removal rate among all filters placed. They report that "unsuccessful attempts (n = 27) were attributed primarily to improper hook orientation (n = 10), or excessive tissue in-growth at the filter legs (n = 16)." They did not report accumulated thrombus as a major reason for inability to remove filters. They provide a breakdown of successful retrieval attempts over time via a Kaplan-Meier analysis, and report successful retrieval of greater than 99% at 4 weeks, greater than 94% at 12 weeks, greater than 67% at 26 weeks, and greater than 37% at 52 weeks.

The case series reporting the claim regarding the greatest safe average dwell time involved the Celect filter, the successor to the Günther Tulip. Lyon et al.[6] reported removal at an average of 179 days, with a range of 5–466 days among 95 patients, with a successful removal rate of 96.6% They reported 100% successful retrieval at 50 weeks, and 74% at 55 weeks, representing 9 patients with filters removed after 52 weeks.

With reports of filters left in place for several months at a time with predictable retrieval rates, the practice of repositioning filters, once thought to extend the dwell time while enabling retrievability, is moving into disuse. Neither Smouse et al. nor Lyon et al. repositioned filters, and still reported the longest dwell time of a filter to these authors' knowledge.[3,6] A review by Berczi et al.[14] concluded that "the

Table 45.1 CLASSICAL COMPLICATIONS AND DEVICE RETRIEVAL RATES PERCENTAGES COMPLETED

STUDY	TOTAL NUMBER OF FILTERS PLACED	STUDY TYPE	FILTER TYPE	FOLLOW-UP DURATION (MONTHS)	PE [NUMBER (%)]	DVT	IVC OCCLUSION/ THROMBOSIS (%)	SUCCESSFUL RETRIEVALS/ ATTEMPTED RETRIEVALS (%)	MEAN DURATION BETWEEN PLACEMENT AND SUCCESSFUL RETRIEVAL (RANGE) DAYS
Given et al.[4]	322	PO	GT	NR	1 (<1%)	NR	NR	188/205 (92%)	76.95 (1–309)
Johnson et al.[5]	100	PO	Option	6	8 (8%)	18 (18%)	3 (3%)	36/39 (92%)	67.1 (1–175)
Lyon et al.[6]	95	PO	Cel	12	1 (1%)	1 (1%)	0 (0%)	56/58 (97%)	179 (5–466)
Sangwaiya et al.[7]	73	RO	Cel	2	2 (2%)	1 (1%)	0 (0%)	14/15 (93%)	84 (5–381)
Cantwell et al.[8]	241	RO	Rec, G2	25	5 (2%)	0 (0%)	NR	127/133 (95%)	NR
9. Charles et al.[9]	140	RO	G2	NR	NR	NR	NR	26/26 (100%)	122 (11–260)
Smouse et al.[3]	554	PO	GT	NR	3 (<1%)	NR	NR	248/275 (90%)	59 (3–494)
Hammond et al.[10]	317	RO	GT, others	NR	2 (<1%)	NR	10 (3%)	100/128 (78%)	NR
Ziegler et al.[11]	150	PO	OptEase	6	0 (0%)	1 (<1%)	4	NR	NR
Onat et al.[12]	228	RO	OptEase	NR	6 (3%)	NR	1	115/124 (93%)	11 (4–23)
Oliva et al.[13]	27	PO	OptEase	1	0 (0%)	1 (4%)	0	21/21 (100%)	11.1 (5–14)

Key: PO, prospective observational; RO, retrospective observational; GT, Günther Tulip; Cel, Celect; Rec, Recovery; NR, not reported.

Table 45.1 represents recent data related to classical outcomes as measured for RVCFs.

In addition to these outcomes, the widespread use retrievable filters has highlighted additional concerns about complications including filter fracture, migration, tilt, malposition, and IVC perforation. The rates of these are reported in Table 45.2.

original implantation time of 10–14 days has been extended to more than 100 days as the mean implantation time" for many filters.

While these studies suggest that removal of an RVCF is technically possible at a longer period of time than previously thought, the proportion of patients in whom retrieval is attempted remains small. This is reportedly due in large part to ongoing contraindications to anticoagulation and the need for prevention of PE, as well as loss to follow-up. A recent study from the trauma literature by Rogers et al.[15] reported that a concerted effort involving phone contact, patients' family members, rehabilitation facilities, and social workers was able to achieve a 59% retrieval rate among filters that could have been removed.

In summary, successes with predictably removing RVCFs at greater than 100 days has expanded their application to the point where a retrievable filter is more likely to placed for a temporary indication than is a permanent filter. The longer dwell times with subsequent safe removal has moved the field away from a previous paradigm of serially repositioning the filter to promote retrievability.

PROPHYLACTIC INDICATIONS: CRITICAL APPRAISAL

The major and steady increases in the use of prophylactic indications over the last three or four decades, to the point where it clearly dominates over therapeutic indications, have a number of likely reasons, but because all the conditions for which VCFs are being applied were all present by the time effective permanent VCFs were available, in the late 1960s, it seems appropriate to question the justification for such a large increase, particularly since there does not appear to be good data-based evidence for most prophylactic indications. Some general statements can be made about prophylactic indications in some respects, but in other respects it is necessary to focus on individual categorical prophylactic indications to pinpoint key issues.

CHANGES IN REFERRAL PATTERNS AND SPECIALIST PERFORMING THE PROCEDURE

The placement of VCFs, in the period after well-designed permanent devices were developed and available, was performed through remote cut-down under general or local anesthesia with sedation, with what was then an acceptably low procedural morbidity and mortality, the latter usually being attributable to intercurrent disease rather than operative misadventures. What percutaneous placement of the newer low-profile devices offered was the avoidance of open surgery, empirically attractive to referring physicians. Although vascular surgeons continued to participate in these trends and introduce new technology and technical approaches, percutaneous placement increasingly opened the door to other interventionalists (e.g., an interventional radiologist, cardiologist, or other specialist with catheter skills). In addition, the referring physicians more often were those without a primary interest in the management of venous thrombo-embolish (VTE) and AC therapy (e.g., an oncologist, trauma surgeon, bariatric surgeon, orthopedic surgeon, neurosurgeon). This combination of less knowledgeable, less critical physician referrals and ready acceptance by service-oriented interventionalists may have played a major role in liberalizing the indications for prophylactic VCF use.

LACK OF ADEQUATE EVIDENCE ON WHICH TO BASE DECISIONS REGARDING VCF USE

These changing referring physician–interventionalist arrangements may have resulted in not only an apparent lack of critical appraisal of expanding indications but also a dearth of critical outcome assessments. In a Medline search of 568 references from 1975 to 2000 on VCFs, Girard et al.[16] found that 65% either were retrospective studies (33.3%) or case reports (31.7%), 12.9% were animal or in vitro experiments, and only 7.4% were prospective studies. Only 16 studies involved more than 100 cases, and there was only one randomized study. In contrast, 47.4% of 531 references on heparin in VTE were randomized prospective trials. This is a striking contrast and should serve as a challenge to those involved with VCF placement to come up with higher level data on which to base current practice.

RECENT OUTCOMES DATA FROM RVCFS

Fracture, migration, tilt, malposition, and IVC perforation have all been reported as complications of RVCF placement. Nicholson et al. reported a high prevalence of fracture and embolization with Bard "Recovery" (first generation) and "G2" (second generation) filters: 13 of 80 patients had a least one filter fracture (16%), and they reported five cases of fractured strut fragments embolizing to the heart, causing three patients to develop life-threatening sequelae.[17] Most of these events occurred with the first-generation RVCF, and were in part the impetus for the development of the second-generation filter. The risk of embolization and fracture has become evident with the passage of sufficient time to observe these rare risks. While other studies have cited significantly lower rates of embolization and fracture, these studies were not designed to detect such events and may underestimate them.

Filter tilt is reported in many of the studies listed in Table 45.2. Smousse et al.[3] report that 209 of 554 patients were observed to have some degree of filter tilt, however they do not report the degree of tilt nor the clinical significance

Table 45.2 FILTER FRACTURE, MIGRATION, TILT, MALPOSITION, AND IVC PERFORATION

STUDY	TOTAL NUMBER OF FILTERS PLACED	FILTER TYPE	MEAN FOLLOW-UP DURATION (MONTHS)	FILTER FRACTURE	FILTER MIGRATION	FILTER TILT (DEGREE)	FILTER MAL-POSITION	IVC PERFORATION
Nicholson et al.[17]	80	Rec	38 (average)	13	NR	NR	NR	NR
Smouse et al.[3]	554	GT	NR	NR	NR	209 (any)	NR	1
Hammond et al.[10]	516	GT, others	NR	1	NR	2 (any)	3	1
Oliva et al.[13]	27	OptEase	1	0	0	0	0	0
Ziegler et al.[11]	150	OptEase	5	3	1	8 (>15)	1	0
Onat et al.[12]	228	OptEase	NR	0	0	9 (NR)	NR	0
Johnson et al.[5]	100	Option	6	0	2	NR	NR	0
Lyon et al.[6]	95	Cel	12	0	0	40 (>5)	0	0
Sangwaiya et al.[7]	73	Cel	2	1	1	4 (>15)	NR	4
Cantwell et al.[8]	241	Rec, G2	25	9	41	36 (any), 11 (>15)	NR	0
Charles et al.[9]	140	G2	NR	0	1	5 (>15)	0	0
Given et al.[4]	322	GT	NR	1	1	NR	NR	2

Key: GT, Günther Tulip; Opt, Option; Cel, Celect; Rec, Recovery; Trap, TrapEase; NR, not reported.

of this finding. Among the authors cited in Table 45.2, there seems to be no consensus as to the degree of filter tilt that is clinically significant, only that it contributes to retrieval difficulty in some cases and is seen commonly.

In a statement issued via their website, the FDA reported that from 2005 to 2010, there were "921 device adverse event reports involving IVC filters, of which 328 involved device migration, 146 involved embolizations (detachment of device components), 70 involved perforation of the IVC, and 56 involved filter fracture."[18] The statement did not differentiate between permanent and retrievable filters, nor was there a quantification of the number of filters placed from which this number of complications stemmed. The FDA went on to recommend that retrievable filters be removed as soon as possible.

In summary, filter fracture, migration, tilt, malposition, and IVC perforation have all been reported as complications of RVCF placement and retrieval. The rates and clinical significance of these events are not clearly defined.

ISSUES WITH INDIVIDUAL PROPHYLACTIC INDICATIONS

Each prophylactic indication category deserves individual comment in terms of VCF use.

Multiple Trauma

Multiple long bone fractures, severe closed head injuries, vertebral spine injuries with and without cord injury, pelvic or acetabular fractures, associated major direct venous trauma, and essentially any other multiple system trauma predicted to require extended period of immobilization

are generally considered to be reasonable prophylactic indications for inserting a VCF, but each subgroup deserves clearer definition. Severe, multisystem trauma is associated with periods of hypercoagulability, and in some instances, involves direct or indirect venous trauma or endothelial damage. These types of trauma are known to be associated with a high risk of VTE, and AC therapy is usually contraindicated. Intermittent pneumatic compression (IPC) and/or duplex surveillance (DS) is another prophylactic measure to be considered, and IVC filter placement is appropriate only when this is not practical or deemed effective. It is important to note that these patients need protection only until they are ambulatory or AC therapy can be instituted.

Although the justification for temporary caval filtration relates to the limited duration of the need for protection, it is spurred by the fact that most trauma patients are young and their expected longevity is great relative to the duration of this need. Nevertheless, the duration of risk may be quite long in many of these types of trauma relative to the safe indwelling time of most current retrievable filters. In such cases, with predictably long immobilization (e.g., spinal fractures, pelvic fractures, multiple long bone fractures), it might be better to use a permanent filter, the one with the best long-term performance record.

VCFs have been reported to be effective for this category of prophylactic use. Langhan et al.[19] reported a 99.5% effectiveness but also reported a 12.8% rate of DVT after filter insertion, with an additional 10.3% in those followed later. However, only 47% returned for follow-up (a problem with trauma patients), and the filter was visualized in only 52% of those. On a survey questionnaire of the others, twenty-seven had leg swelling, fourteen had other extremity symptoms, nine had shortness of breath, seven had chest pain, and four had venous skin changes. It cannot be determined, from such a follow-up, how many of these reported problems could have reflected VTE. There were three non-fatal filter complications, but all twenty-seven deaths were attributed to the trauma, not the VCF. Clearly, the protection against PE was excellent but, much like the PREPIC trial,[1] there appears to be a penalty for this approach in the form of DVT.

Better follow up has been achieved as mentioned earlier by Rogers et al. through a program of "disciplined follow-up."[15] They reported that among 7,949 trauma admissions, 420 (5.2%) met criteria for filter placement, and among those 160 were available for removal and 94% were successfully removed (59%).

Rosenthal et al.[20] reported that for patients with multiple trauma, filters were successfully placed with 96.8% technical success. None of the nineteen deaths was reportedly from VCF placement, and there were complications in only 5.3%. One patient had a PE after filter removal. Follow-up in this study was short, and the incidence of DVT was not documented. In another evaluation of this approach from a trauma center, Duperier et al.[21] reported a low rate of insertion complications in 133 consecutive multiple trauma patients, but "DVT was observed in 30% of patients despite 92% being on prophylaxis"; 26% were de novo. In this experience, the filter was inserted an average of 6.8 +/- 0.6 (SE) days after trauma. In the previously cited experience of Langhan et al.,[19] the mean insertion day was 6. This delay in insertion of the VCF in earlier trauma experiences, before the practice of bedside filter insertion under ultrasound guidance, reinforces the potential value of this relatively recent capability.

The *American College of Chest Physicians Evidence Based Clinical Practice Guidelines* (8th edition)[22] enumerates many concerns regarding a lack of solid evidence to support prophylactic use of VCF in trauma patients. The authors observe that prospective studies have shown no difference in the rates of PE among patients with and without prophylactic filters, and that filters are associated with short- and long-term complications, and may delay initiation of proven effective thromboprophylaxis. However they recognize that there is an indication for patient with a proven proximal DVT and either an absolute contraindication to full-dose anticoagulation or planned major surgery in the near future. They go on to encourage practitioners to implement therapeutic anticoagulation as soon as the contraindication resolves.

One critical appraisal of the prophylactic use of VCFs in trauma patients has been recently been reported by Knudsen et al.[23] In an analysis of 1,602 episodes of VTE from the American College of Surgeons National Trauma Data Bank, the authors observed that 90% had at least one of nine accepted risk factors, and found the following factors correlated significantly with outcome: age (>40), lower extremity fracture, a high trauma score, head injury,

prolonged ventilator support (>3 days), venous injury, and major operative procedure. Eighty-six percent had prophylactic IVC filters placed, but 11% had no identifiable risk factors. They concluded that (1) patients who need VTE prophylaxis after trauma can be identified by risk factors, and (2) the use of prophylactic IVC filters in trauma patients should be reexamined.

Patients with Neurological Problems Resulting in Paralysis or Prolonged Immobilization

Paralyzed or otherwise immobilized patients are at high risk for VTE, but many can be managed by AC therapy. In those in whom anticoagulants are contraindicated, if the limbs are accessible (i.e., not injured or encumbered), IPC and DS can be used, and may be effective. There are, however, patients in whom AC therapy is contraindicated or in whom the limbs are not accessible for IPC or DS (e.g., closed head or acute cord injuries associated with long bone fractures) in which VCFs may be justified. Outside of this exemplary exception, other forms of prophylaxis probably should be used with some form of surveillance for DVT added.

Several articles attest to this generic advice. Maxwell et al.[24] studied 111 spinal cord–injured patients from a registry of 8,269 trauma admissions, and found that using these other means of prophylaxis, there was an overall incidence of DVT and PE of 9.0% and 1.8%, respectively, but with no deaths. Mean hospital stay was 23 days, and DS was performed an average of 2.3 +/- 2.1 times. The incidence of DVT and PE with low molecular weight (LMW) heparin alone was 11.1% and 2.8%, respectively, but when this was combined with DS, it was only 7.4% and 0%, respectively, so the latter combination was recommended. By comparison, in a subgroup with long bone fractures, the incidence of DVT was 37.5%. They concluded that IVC filters were needed only in spinal cord injury patients with associated long bone fractures, in those with detected DVT or its progression under surveillance, or when AC therapy was contraindicated.

Gorman et al.[25] noted that among a group of fifty-four spinal cord–injured patients who received prophylactic VCF, eleven experienced DVT during their hospitalization, relative to a comparison group of fifty-eight similar patients who did not receive filters, among whom only three developed DVTs. They went on to conclude that without other indications for prophylaxis with VCF, SCI alone should not precipitate prophylaxis with VCF.

This agrees with guidelines developed by a committee of neurosurgeons[26] who agreed that low-dose LMW heparin alone is insufficient and recommended rotating beds, IPC, and DS in addition, with VCF inserted only if DVT was detected. Thus, recent opinion appears to suggest that the role of VCFs in this category should be limited to those who develop DVT despite other forms of prophylaxis.

Patients with Advanced Malignancy

Patients with advanced malignancy have been shown to be at increased risk of VTE, and AC therapy may not be adequately protective. Prophylactic VCF use has been debated, but the trend now favors therapeutic use (i.e., only after VTE). Risk factors have been identified.[27] Univariate analysis and logistic regression models identified the following as significant risk factors for recurrent VTE: the appearance of new metastases, a history of DVT, and neutropenia as a result of chemotherapy. Other studies have identified stage of disease and type of malignancy as specific risk factors for VTE. The effectiveness of VCFs in preventing PE has not in itself been challenged, but use of this indication for VCF placement clearly must be balanced by patient prognosis as demonstrated by three sobering reports. Jarrett et al.[28] reported on 116 patients with VCFs placed for advanced malignant disease. Its effectiveness was suggested by the fact that two had recurrent DVT and three had PE after VCF, but it was the issue of patient survival that was challenged. Life table analysis showed survival to be 68% at 30 days, 49.4% at 3 months, and 26.8% at 1 year. Of those with stage IV disease, 46% died within 6 weeks and only 13.7% were alive at 1 year. Damascelli et al.[29] reported 106 patients with malignancy in whom RVCFs were placed and who were anticoagulated to a target international normalized ratio (INR) of 1.5–2.0. With a median follow-up of 217 days, they reported only three PEs, all of these occurring in patients who had already had a PE. However, they admit that "at the time of manuscript preparation, 44 of 106 patients were alive, 29 of them continuing with caval filtration combined with oral anticoagulation." Shunn et al.[30] reported 97.5% protection against PE in forty patients with advanced malignancy receiving VCFs, but also a high (20%) complication rate. In addition, 30% survived less than 30 days. It is difficult to justify the use of a RVCF in these patients. Their risk of thromboembolism is unlikely to decrease during their lifetime.

Major Surgery Associated with a High Risk of DVT

Certain categories of major surgery have a predicted high VTE risk, and yet the use of AC prophylaxis may be contraindicated or presumed ineffective. In such patients, VCF has been felt to be indicated. Some well-known examples of such VCF use include pelvic surgery, hip surgery, major surgery with history of DVT, major surgery with known or suspected hypercoagulable state, major venous reconstructions with VTE risk, and gastric bypass surgery for morbid obesity. As a general criticism, in many of these applications, the risk of VTE, the duration of risk, and the benefits of VCFs are poorly documented in the literature, and few studies involve valid comparisons with alternative methods of prophylaxis. Nevertheless, it is clear that individual high-risk patients can be identified, and when alternative methods of prophylaxis are either contraindicated or ineffective, VCF placement should be considered. As a general rule, in this subcategory, an RVCF should be used if the patient can be ambulatory or AC therapy can be instituted in about three weeks, otherwise a permanent filter may be preferable. Thus, although supporting data are scant, individual high-risk patients can be reasonably chosen on their own merits, and it is difficult to take exception with this practice.

Bariatric surgery has received much recent attention, and although the intervention itself has been challenged by many, some data and guidelines have emerged for prophylactic VCF use with this operation. Open gastric bypass for morbid obesity carries a 1 to 4% PE risk in spite of other methods of prophylaxis including IPC, LMW heparin, and a push for early ambulation. Using RVCFs, Gariulo[31] reported a reduced PE rate in open gastric bypass for patients with a BMI >55, but there was a 14% complication rate. Factors associated with a high risk of VTE have been identified[32] to include BMI >60, truncal obesity, venous stasis dermatitis, and hypoventilation/sleep apnea syndrome. Logically, one would add those with a history of VTE and a known or probable hypercoagulable state.

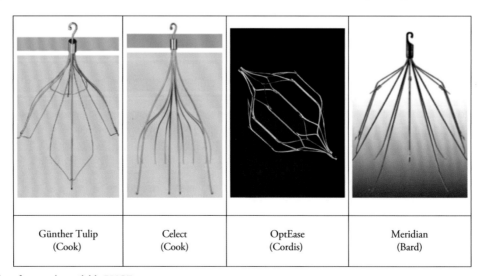

| Günther Tulip (Cook) | Celect (Cook) | OptEase (Cordis) | Meridian (Bard) |

Figure 45.1   Examples of currently available RVCF.

Similarly, Vaziri et al.[33] reported the use of prophylactic VCF placement in thirty patients with a history of VTE scheduled to undergo bariatric surgery. Patients underwent a combination of open and laparoscopic procedures, and in the patients deemed to be at high risk due to their history, prophylactic VCF were placed after induction of anesthesia and immediately prior to the bariatric procedure. At follow-up ultrasonography on approximately postoperative day 19, six patients (21%) were noted to have recurrent DVT. Twenty-seven of the thirty patients underwent follow-up venogram, and four patients (15%) were noted to have significant thrombus trapped by the VCF. No patients were discovered to have PE.

It has been said that this operation has a short, defined period of risk for VTE that is ideal for retrievable VCFs. On the other hand, VCF placement can be challenging in morbidly obese patients, especially the superobese (BMI >60). Duplex ultrasound guidance is impossible, but intravascular ultrasound can be used to advantage in placing a filter in these patients. In the face of great enthusiasm for this indication for prophylactic VCF use, the author would insert a word of caution: no prospective studies, comparing VCFs with alternative methods of VTE prophylaxis, have been carried out, and most of the published reports related to its use have dealt with open gastric bypass. It is quite conceivable that the laparoscopic approach, with its earlier ambulation, may significantly reduce the VTE risk. Whether this is sufficient to allow the adjunctive use of IPC and LMW heparin to be effective deserves investigation. In the meantime, the risk factors listed earlier should serve as guidelines for selective VCF use.

SUMMARY AND CONCLUSIONS

The current use of prophylactic indications for caval filter placement and the RCVFs that have been developed for this purpose have been reviewed. Based on this, some recommendations can be confidently made, but there is a clear need better information, clarifying higher level studies on which to base prophylactic indications. Also, there appears to be room for further improvements in RVCF design, or possibly the modification of an existing permanent filter with good long-term outcomes so that it can be retrieved if necessary. It may or may not be possible to design a truly optional filter, one that can be retrieved as needed or left in permanently without penalty. If not, the use of two types of filters will persist as the best strategy—the best RCVF and best permanent filter being chosen based on duration of patient risk with safe indwelling time in the former. Better supporting data are required to support either use. It is also apparent that, in respect to categories of prophylactic indications, current practice is not based on a high level of medical evidence and, in fact, the use of VCFs in some of these settings appears to be excessive and subjectively determined. It is hoped that prophylactic indications

within each subcategory will be refined in the future by indication-specific prospective analyses of critical outcome data compared with alternative methods of prophylaxis, and that these studies also will identify the factors significantly affecting outcome as a basis for more objective guidelines for application. The need for evidence-based medicine here is obvious. Industry-driven trials of single devices are not, in themselves, acceptable for this purpose and tend to promote excessive prophylactic use rather than control it. On the other hand, if one believes in the potential of new technology to bring about continuing improvements, industry can be expected to develop even better retrievable caval filters, those which ultimately could be proven safe and effective for prophylactic use in patients temporarily at high risk for VTE, specifically filters that can be retrieved or repositioned safely, without being compromised by entrapped clot or contact point endothelialization for longer periods of time relative to the risk of VTE. Until then, it is hoped that this critical appraisal of the prophylactic use of VCFs, and the current temporary filters that increasingly are linked to it, will help guide physicians engaged in this practice.

REFERENCES

1. Young T, Tang H, Hughes R. Vena caval filters for the prevention of pulmonary embolism. *Cochrane Database Syst Rev.* 2010. Feb 17;(2):CD006212.
2. Fullen WD, Miller EH, Steele WF, McDonough JJ. Prophylactic vena caval interruption in hip fractures. *J Trauma.* 1973. 13(5):403–410.
3. Smouse HB, Rosenthal D, Thuong VH, Knox MF, Dixon RG, Voorhees WD 3rd, McCann-Brown JA. Long-term retrieval success rate profile for the Günther Tulip vena cava filter. *J Vasc Interv Radiol.* 2009. 20(7): 871–877.
4. Given MF, McDonald BC, Brookfield P, et al. Retrievable Gunther Tulip inferior vena cava filter: experience in 317 patients. *J Med Imaging Radiat Oncol.* 2008. 52(5):452–457.
5. Johnson MS, Nemcek AA Jr, Benenati JF, et al. The safety and effectiveness of the retrievable option inferior vena cava filter: a United States prospective multicenter clinical study. *J Vasc Interv Radiol.* 2010. 21(8): 1173–1184.
6. Lyon SM, Riojas GE, Uberoi R, et al. Short- and long-term retrievability of the Celect vena cava filter: results from a multi-institutional registry. *J Vasc Interv Radiol.* 2009. 20(11): 1441–1448.
7. Sangwaiya MJ, Marentis TC, Walker TG, Stecker M, Wicky ST, Kalva SP. Safety and effectiveness of the celect inferior vena cava filter: preliminary results. *J Vasc Interv Radiol.* 2009. 20(9): 1188–1192.
8. Cantwell CP, Pennypacker J, Singh H, Scorza LB, Waybill PN, Lynch FC. Comparison of the recovery and G2 filter as retrievable inferior vena cava filters. *J Vasc Interv Radiol.* 2009. 20(9): 1193–1199.
9. Charles HW, Black M, Kovacs S, et al. G2 inferior vena cava filter: retrievability and safety. *J Vasc Interv Radiol.* 2009. 20(8):1046–1051.
10. Hammond CJ, Bakshi DR, Currie RJ, et al. Audit of the use of IVC filters in the UK: experience from three centres over 12 years. *Clin Radiol.* 2009. 64(5): 502–510.
11. Ziegler JW, Dietrich GJ, Cohen SA, Sterling K, Duncan J, Samotowka M. PROOF trial: protection from pulmonary embolism with the OptEase filter. *J Vasc Interv Radiol.* 2008. 19(8):1165–1170.
12. Onat L, Ganiyusufoglu AK, Mutlu A, Sirvanci M, Duran C, Ulusoy OL, Hamzaoglu A. OptEase and TrapEase vena cava filters: a single-center experience in 258 patients. *Cardiovasc Intervent Radiol.* 2009. 32(5): 992–997.

13. Oliva VL, Szatmari F, Giroux MF, Flemming BK, Cohen SA, Soulez G. The Jonas Study: Evaluation of the retrievability of the Cordis OptEase inferior vena cava filter, *J Vasc Interv Radiol.* 2005. *16*: 1439–1445.

14. Berczi V, Bottomley JR, Thomas SM, Taneja S, Gaines PA, Cleveland TJ. Long-term retrievability of IVC filters: should we abandon permanent devices? *Cardiovasc Intervent Radiol.* 2007. *30*(5): 820–827.

15. Rogers FB, Shackford SR, Miller JA, Wu D, Rogers A, Gambler A. Improved recovery of prophylactic inferior vena cava filters in trauma patients: the results of a dedicated filter registry and critical pathway for filter removal. *J Trauma Acute Care Surg.* 2012. *72*(2): 381–384.

16. Girard P, Stern JB, Parent F. Medical literature and vena cava filters: So far so weak. *Chest.* 2002. *122*: 963–967.

17. Nicholson W, Nicholson WJ, Tolerico P, et al. Prevalence of fracture and fragment embolization of Bard retrievable vena cava filters and clinical implications including cardiac perforation and tamponade. *Arch Intern Med.* 2010. *170*(20): 1827–1831.

18. Inferior Vena Cava (IVC) Filters: Initial Communication: Risk of Adverse Events with Long Term Use. FDA MedWatch. Posted 9 August 2010. Available at https://www.accessdata.fda.gov/scripts/medwatch/medwatch-online.htm. Accessed 20 February 2012.

19. Langhan EM, Miller RS, Casey WJ, et al. Prophylactic inferior vena cava filters in trauma patients at high risk: Follow-up examination and risk benefit assessment. *J Vasc Surg.* 1999. *30*: 484–490.

20. Rosenthal D, Wellons ED, Levitt AB, Shuler FW, Conner RE, Henderson VJ. Role of prophylactic temporary inferior vena cava filter placed at the ICU bedside under ultrasound guidance in patients with multiple trauma. *J Vasc Surg.* 2004. *40*: 958–964.

21. Duperier T, Mosenthal A, Swan KG, Kaul S. Acute complications associated with Greenfield filter insertions in high risk patients. *J Vasc Surg.* 2003. *37*: 976–983.

22. Greets WH, Bergqvist D, Pineo GF, et al. Prevention of Venous Thromboembolism: American College of Chest Physicians. Evidence-based clinical practice guidelines (8th edition), *Chest.* 2008. *133*: 381S–453S.

23. Knudsen MM, Ikossi DG, Khaw L, et al. Thromboembolism after trauma: an analysis of 1602 episodes from the American College of Surgeons National Trauma Data Bank. *Ann Surg.* 2004. *240*: 96–104.

24. Maxwell RA, Chavarria-Aguilar M, Cockerham WT, et al. Routine prophylactic vena cava filtration is not indicated after acute spinal cord injury. *J Trauma.* 2002. *52*(5): 902–906.

25. Gorman PH, Qadri SF, Rao-Patel A. Prophylactic inferior vena cava (IVC) filter placement may increase the relative risk of deep venous thrombosis after acute spinal cord injury, *J Trauma.* 2009. *66*: 707–712.

26. Deep venous thrombosis and thromboembolism in patients with spinal cord injuries. Neurosurgery. 2002. *50*(3 suppl): s73–s80.

27. Lin J, Proctor MC, Varma M. Factors associated with recurrent VTE in patients with malignant disease. *J Vasc Surg.* 2003. *37*: 976–983.

28. Jarrett BP, Dougherty MJ, Calligaro KD. Inferior vena cava filters in malignant disease. *J Vasc Surg.* 2002. *36*: 704–707.

29. Damascelli B, Ticha V, Patelli G, et al. Use of a retrievable vena cava filter with low-intensity anticoagulation for prevention of pulmonary embolism in patients with cancer: an observational study in 106 cases. *J Vasc Interv Radiol.* 2011. *22*(9):1312–1319.

30. Shunn CD, Shunn GB, Vona-Davis L, Waheed U. Inferior vena cava filter placement in late stage cancer. Presented at the 17th Annual Meeting of the American Venous Forum. San Diego, California. February 10, 2005.

31. Gariulo NJ. Patient selection for retrievable inferior vena cava filters. *Endovasc Today.* 2004. *3*: 42–44.

32. Sappala JA, Wood MH, Schuhknecht MP, et al. Fatal pulmonary emboli after bariatric operations for morbid obesity: A 24 year retrospective analysis. *Obes Surg.* 2003. *13*: 819–825.

33. Vaziri K, Bhanot P, Hungness ES, Morasch MD, Prystowsky JB, Nagle AP. Retrievable inferior vena cava filters in high-risk patients undergoing bariatric surgery. *Surg Endosc.* 2009. *23*(10):2203–2207.

46.

THROMBOLYTIC THERAPY FOR ACUTE VENOUS THROMBOSIS

Anthony J. Comerota and Santiago Chahwan

INTRODUCTION

Despite evidence demonstrating that patients with iliofemoral venous thrombosis suffer more severe postthrombotic sequelae than patients with infrainguinal deep venous thrombosis (DVT), the majority of physicians treat all patients with acute DVT with anticoagulation alone. A treatment approach that includes a strategy of thrombus removal and optimal anticoagulation is not adopted by most clinicians, even in patients with extensive venous thrombosis.

Unquestionably, there have been enormous advances in anticoagulation. Anticoagulants, such as low molecular weight heparins (LMWHs) and pentasaccharides, and other families of agents, such as the direct thrombin inhibitors, serve to limit progression of thrombosis and, with proper duration of therapy, prevent recurrences; however, they are not designed to clear thrombus from the deep venous system.

It appears that patients with iliofemoral DVT are a clinically relevant subset of patients with acute DVT who suffer severe postthrombotic morbidity.[1-3] O'Donnell and colleagues[1] were among the first to bring to our attention the high incidence of postthrombotic venous ulceration, the large number of recurrent hospitalizations, and the loss in financial productivity in these patients. Akesson et al.[2] showed that 95% of patients with iliofemoral DVT treated with anticoagulation alone had ambulatory venous hypertension at 5 years, and 90% suffered symptoms of chronic venous insufficiency. During this relatively short follow-up, 15% of patients already developed venous ulceration, and another 15% had debilitating symptoms of venous claudication. Delis et al.[3] demonstrated that venous claudication occurred in 40% of patients with iliofemoral DVT treated with anticoagulation when they were studied with exercise testing.

UNDERSTANDING POSTTHROMBOTIC VENOUS INSUFFICIENCY

Many physicians fail to recognize the difference in the pathophysiology of primary versus postthrombotic venous insufficiency. As a result, the value of thrombus removal in preventing postthrombotic morbidity in patients with acute DVT is underestimated. The pathophysiology of chronic venous insufficiency is ambulatory venous hypertension, which is defined as an elevated venous pressure during exercise. In individuals with a normal deep venous system, ambulatory venous pressures in the lower leg and foot should drop to less than 50% of the standing venous pressure. In patients with postthrombotic syndrome, the ambulatory venous pressure drops very little, and in those with persistent proximal venous occlusion, the ambulatory pressures may actually rise above standing pressure. This degree of ambulatory venous hypertension often leads to the debilitating symptoms of venous claudication.

The anatomic components contributing to ambulatory venous hypertension are venous valvular incompetence and luminal obstruction. It has been consistently shown that the most severe postthrombotic sequelae and the highest ambulatory venous pressures occur in patients with valvular incompetence accompanied by luminal venous obstruction.[4,5]

Venous obstruction is not synonymous with occlusion. Occlusion is complete obliteration, whereas obstruction (for the most part) is relative narrowing of the lumen. Although relative degrees of obstruction are reliably quantitated on the arterial side of the circulation, technology has not advanced to the point that allows this degree of accuracy on the venous side. Furthermore, physicians often cannot put venous obstruction into proper perspective pathophysiologically in terms of its contribution to postthrombotic discomfort or distal leg soft tissue damage. Our ability to identify and quantitate venous obstruction is so poor that there is widespread underappreciation regarding the importance of the contribution of obstruction to postthrombotic morbidity.

Unfortunately, physiologic testing on the venous side of the circulation has not kept pace with similar advances on the arterial side of the vascular tree. Vascular laboratories have traditionally (and paradoxically) tested the hemodynamics of venous obstruction with patients in the resting, supine position with their legs elevated, which is the standard position for measuring maximum venous outflow, the commonly accepted test for venous obstruction. However, the pathophysiology of chronic venous disease is defined in the upright, exercising patient, with increased arterial inflow stressing venous return. Phlebograms of postthrombotic recanalized veins frequently document patency, and noninvasive studies may indeed show normal maximal venous outflow values, giving the mistaken impression that venous obstruction contributes little to postthrombotic morbidity.

This is clearly illustrated by the patient represented in Figure 46.1, who had iliofemoral DVT 10 years earlier and was suffering with severe postthrombotic syndrome and a venous ulcer. Noninvasive testing demonstrated that the patient had valvular incompetence but a normal 3-s maximal venous outflow. An ascending phlebogram was interpreted as "the classic tree-barking appearance of chronic venous disease. There is no evidence of venous obstruction." The following day the patient underwent a classic Linton procedure, which included femoral vein ligation with division just below its junction with the profunda femoris vein. A cross-section of the divided femoral vein is shown in Figure 49.1, along with its corresponding level on the

ascending phlebogram. The vein shows multiple recanalization channels and substantial luminal obstruction. This severity of luminal obstruction becomes hemodynamically important in the exercising limb, in which substantial increases in arterial flow occur as a result of exercise. With exercise, venous outflow becomes restricted by the luminal obstruction, significantly contributing to ambulatory venous hypertension. Of course, the valves within these diseased veins are destroyed, and patients also have valvular incompetence.

It makes intuitive sense that eliminating the acute thrombus leading to the persistent venous obstruction would benefit patients over the long term, and indeed it does. Furthermore, thrombus extraction not only eliminates venous obstruction but also preserves valvular function.

BENEFITS OF THROMBUS REMOVAL

There is increasing evidence that thrombus removal or early thrombus resolution after acute DVT is associated with improved outcomes. Benefits of thrombus removal derive from data generated from experimental animal studies, findings from natural history studies of acute DVT treated with anticoagulation, venous thrombectomy data, and observations following systemic and catheter-directed thrombolysis.

Cho and colleagues[6] and Rhodes and associates[7] have used a canine experimental model of acute DVT to compare the results of thrombolysis versus placebo and mechanical thrombectomy. They demonstrated that thrombolysis with urokinase preserves endothelial function and valve competence, both immediately and at 4 weeks after therapy. There was less residual thrombus in veins treated with urokinase, thereby preserving the vein's structural integrity.

The aforementioned experimental observations translated into clinical outcome when the University of Washington investigators performed a natural history study of acute DVT treated with anticoagulation.[8-11] This NIH-supported effort resulted in observations indicating that persistent obstruction of proximal veins was associated with distal valve incompetence. The combination of venous obstruction and valve incompetence was associated with the most severe postthrombotic morbidity. Spontaneous clot lysis naturally restored venous patency. If spontaneous lysis occurred early (within 90 days), valve function was frequently preserved.

The initial trials of thrombolytic therapy for acute DVT involved systemic administration of the plasminogen activators. The cumulative results of these trials demonstrated that although 45% of patients had substantial or complete lysis, the majority did not.[12] Those whose clot was successfully lysed had a significant reduction in postthrombotic morbidity and preservation of venous valve

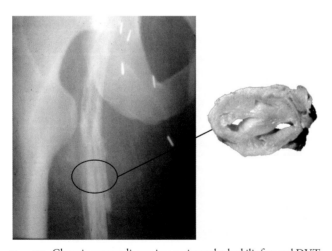

Figure 46.1 Chronic venous disease in a patient who had iliofemoral DVT 10 years earlier. The patient suffered with the postthrombotic syndrome leading to multiple hospitalizations due to venous ulcers. Ascending phlebography showed chronic venous disease with "no evidence of obstruction." An IPG was normal. A classic Linton procedure, which includes ligation of the femoral vein distal to its junction with the profunda, was performed, showing recanalization of the femoral vein with significant luminal obstruction.

function. Goldhaber et al.[13] reviewed the results from eight trials of systemic streptokinase treatment for acute DVT and found that moderate or significant thrombolysis was achieved almost three times more frequently among patients treated with thrombolytic therapy than among patients treated with anticoagulation alone. However, there was nearly a four-fold increased risk of major bleeding in those receiving thrombolytic therapy, thereby focusing the attention of clinicians on the hemorrhagic morbidity of lytics rather than their potential for long-term benefit.

The long-term efficacy of thrombus removal in patients with acute iliofemoral DVT was further substantiated by the Scandinavian investigators who performed a randomized trial of iliofemoral venous thrombectomy with an arteriovenous fistula (AVF) and anticoagulation versus anticoagulation alone.[14–16] Follow-up at 6 months, 5 years, and 10 years demonstrated clear benefit in patients randomized to venous thrombectomy. Early thrombus removal resulted in improved patency of the iliofemoral venous system, lower venous pressures, less edema, and fewer postthrombotic symptoms.

These observations, extending from the basic research laboratory through systemic thrombolysis and operative venous thrombectomy, support the concept that thrombus removal in patients with acute iliofemoral DVT results in significantly less postthrombotic morbidity. Unfortunately, the favorable results of contemporary venous thrombectomy have not led to much enthusiasm for the operative procedure in the United States. Additionally, physicians are unwilling to accept the higher risk of bleeding complications with lytic therapy; therefore, systemic thrombolysis for acute DVT is infrequently used and not recommended, which is appropriate in light of the improved results with catheter-directed lysis.

INTRATHROMBUS CATHETER-DIRECTED THROMBOLYSIS

RATIONALE

The mechanism by which thrombolysis results in clot dissolution is the activation of fibrin-bound plasminogen.[17] When circulating GLU-plasminogen binds to fibrin, it is modified to LYS-plasminogen, which has greater affinity for plasminogen activators. When delivered into the thrombus, a plasminogen activator efficiently activates LYS-plasminogen. The intrathrombus delivery protects the plasminogen activator from neutralization by circulating plasminogen activator inhibitors and also protects the resultant plasmin from neutralization by circulating alpha 2-antiplasmins.

Catheter-directed techniques that deliver the plasminogen activator into the thrombus theoretically can accelerate thrombolysis, which increases the likelihood of a successful outcome. By reducing the overall dose and duration of infusion of the plasminogen activator, it is reasonable that complications will be minimized.

RESULTS

Numerous reports have emerged supporting favorable outcomes of catheter-directed thrombolysis for acute DVT.[18–25] Three of the larger reports demonstrate approximately an 80% success rate (see Table 46.1). Initial success rates might have been higher had treatment been restricted to only patients with acute iliofemoral DVT. However, patients who had more distal and chronic venous thrombosis were included, resulting in a lower overall success rate. In these three studies, 422 patients were treated with remarkably consistent rates of success and complications.[18–20] Catheter-directed urokinase was used in each of these studies. Underlying iliac vein stenoses were treated with balloon angioplasty, stenting, or both to achieve unobstructed venous drainage into the vena cava and reduce the risk of recurrent thrombosis (see Figure 46.2).

Major bleeding occurred in 5 to 10% of cases, with the majority resulting from puncture site bleeding. Intracranial bleeding was rare, occurring in only three patients in the National Venous Registry.[19] This resulted in the death of one patient. Pulmonary embolism (PE) occurred in 1% of patients in the series reported by Bjarnason et al.[18] and the National Venous Registry, and fatal PE occurred in only one out of the 422 patients. Therefore, death as a result of catheter-directed thrombolysis was rare.

Since 2000, most patients treated with catheter-directed thrombolysis were managed with urokinase. Since urokinase was removed from the market, catheter-directed alteplase and reteplase have demonstrated similarly good results.[22–25]

An interesting new therapeutic approach was reported by Chang et al.[23] when they used intrathrombus bolus dosing of rtPA in twelve lower extremities of ten patients with acute DVT. They infused rtPA intrathrombus using the pulse-spray technique and no more than 50 mg per treatment. After the pulse-spray bolus, patients were returned to their rooms and brought back the following day for repeat venographic examination. Continuous infusion was not used. Patients had treatment repeated for up to four daily sessions. Results were excellent; eleven lower extremities had significant or complete lysis, and the remaining leg had 50 to 75% lysis. Although the average total dose of rtPA was 106 mg, bleeding complications were minor, and no patient had a decrease in hematocrit more than 2%. This technique is deserving of further study to evaluate whether others can obtain similarly good results.

A further analysis of the patients treated in the National Venous Registry[19] offers important clinical insight into catheter-directed thrombolysis for patients with acute DVT. Of the 287 patients treated in both academic and

Table 46.1 RESULTS OF CATHETER-DIRECTED THROMBOLYSIS WITH UROKINASE IN THREE CONTEMPORARY SERIES: EFFICACY AND COMPLICATIONS

	BJARNASON ET AL.[18] (N = 77)	MEWISSEN ET AL.[19] (N = 287)	COMEROTA ET AL.[20] (N = 58)
Efficacy			
Initial Success	79%	83%	84%
Iliac	63%	64%	78%
Femoral	40%	47%	–
Primary Patency at 1 yr	63%	64%	78%
Iliac	40%	47%	–
Femoral	54%	74%	89%
Iliac Stent: Patency at 1 yr	75%	53%	71%
+Stent			
–Stent			
Complications			
Major Bleed	5%	11%	9%
Intracranial Bleeding	0%	<1%	0%
Pulmonary Embolism	1%	1%	0%
Fatal Pulmonary Embolism Death	0%	0.2%	0%
Secondary to Lysis	0%	0.4%	0% (? 2%)*

*Death due to multiorgan system failure 30 d post lysis, though not related to lytic therapy.

community centers, 66% had acute DVT, 16% had chronic DVT, and 19% had an acute episode superimposed on a chronic condition. Seventy-one percent of the patients presented with iliofemoral DVT and 25% with femoropopliteal DVT. Catheter-directed thrombolysis with intrathrombus infusion of urokinase was the preferred approach. However, some patients were treated with urokinase infused into a foot vein, which was essentially systemic thrombolysis. Phlebographic evaluation showed that 31% of patients had complete lytic success and 52% had 50 to 99% lytic success. In 17% of patients, less than 50% of the thrombus was dissolved. When urokinase was not infused intrathrombus, success rates fell dramatically. In the subgroup of patients with acute, first-time iliofemoral DVT, 65% of the patients enjoyed complete clot lysis.

During follow-up, thrombosis-free survival was observed in 65% at 6 months and in 60% at 12 months. There was a significant correlation (P < 0.001) of thrombosis-free survival with the results of initial therapy. Seventy-eight percent of patients with complete clot resolution had patent veins at 1 year, compared with only 37% of those in whom less than 50% of the clot was dissolved. Interestingly, in the subgroup of patients with acute, first-time iliofemoral DVT who had successful thrombolysis, 96% of the veins remained patent at 1 year. In addition to sustained patency, early success directly correlated with valve function at 6 months. Sixty-two percent of patients with less than 50% thrombolysis had venous valvular incompetence, whereas 72% of patients who had complete lysis had normal valve function (P < 0.02).

The large database of the National Venous Registry offered an opportunity to objectively evaluate the long-term impact of catheter-directed thrombolysis on patients with iliofemoral DVT. Since the National Venous Registry collected data only on patients treated with thrombolytic therapy, a contemporary cohort of patients with iliofemoral DVT treated with anticoagulation in the same institutions was identified. All anticoagulated patients were candidates for lytic therapy but were treated with anticoagulation alone due to physician preference. A validated quality-of-life (QOL) questionnaire was used to query patients at 16 and 22 months post treatment. Of the ninety-eight patients studied, sixty-eight were treated with catheter-directed lysis and thirty treated with anticoagulation alone. Those treated with catheter-directed thrombolysis reported a significantly better QOL than those treated with anticoagulation alone. The QOL results were directly related to the initial success of thrombolysis. Patients who had a successful lytic outcome reported a significantly better Health Utilities Index, better physical functioning, less stigma of chronic venous disease, less health distress, and fewer overall postthrombotic symptoms. Patients in whom catheter-directed thrombolysis failed had similar outcomes to patients treated with anticoagulation alone. These efficacy data combined with the observed reduction in complications offer a sound argument for the management of patients with iliofemoral DVT with catheter-directed thrombolysis.

A small, randomized trial performed by Elsharawy et al.[26] demonstrated that catheter-directed thrombolysis versus anticoagulation alone offered significantly better outcomes at 6 months. Assuming patients are properly managed with anticoagulation, the 6-month observations should reflect their long-term outcome.

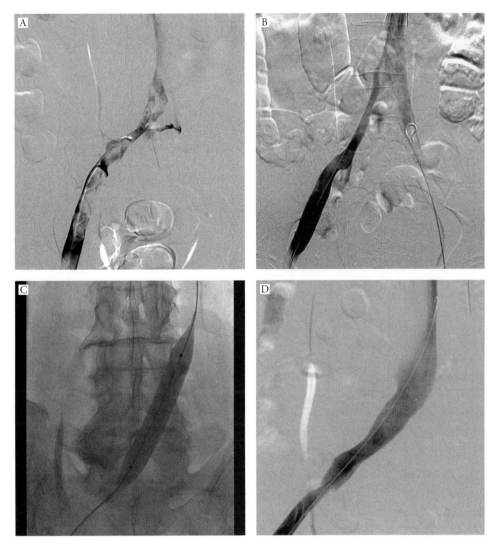

Figure 46.2 (A) Initial phlebogram (prone iliocavagram) of a patient with extensive iliofemoral DVT who presented with a swollen, painful left leg. Using ultrasound guidance, the catheter was positioned into the thrombus of the iliofemoral segment. A plasminogen activator (t-PA) was infused at 1 mg/h. (B) After 22 hours of catheter-directed t-PA infusion, the patient had a good phlebographic and clinical response. A stenosis of the left iliac vein was identified. (C) The stenosis was treated with balloon angioplasty, and a 16-mm Wallstent was deployed and dilated. (D) Final phlebogram showing unobstructed venous drainage into the vena cava.

We believe that the results available to date support a strategy of catheter-directed thrombolysis for acute iliofemoral DVT in patients who have no contraindication to thrombolytic therapy. If a contraindication to lytic therapy exists, a contemporary venous thrombectomy (Chapter 45) followed by long-term anticoagulation should be considered.

PATIENT EVALUATION AND TECHNIQUE OF CATHETER-DIRECTED THROMBOLYSIS

PATIENT EVALUATION

It is intuitive and clinically apparent that patients with iliofemoral DVT have a greater stimulus to thrombosis than the majority of patients with DVT and therefore warrant a search for an underlying etiology. Asymptomatic pulmonary emboli are present in at least 50%. It is important that the PE be recognized early, since up to 25% will subsequently become symptomatic, manifesting as pleuritic chest discomfort once the inflammatory pulmonary process reaches the pleural surface. If the PE is not recognized, the clinician often mistakenly assumes that the pleuritic symptoms are due to a new PE and failure of treatment. A spiral CT scan of the chest with contrast evaluates the pulmonary vasculature for PE and other thoracic pathology (see Figure 46.3A). The CT is extended to the abdomen and pelvis to identify the proximal extent of thrombus and to evaluate for abdominal or pelvic pathology (see Figure 46.3B). This has been an important addition to the evaluation of these patients, as we have found serious unsuspected pathology with surprising frequency. Renal cell carcinoma, adrenal

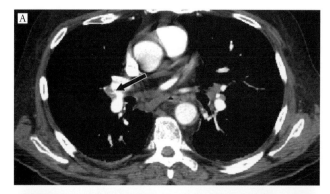

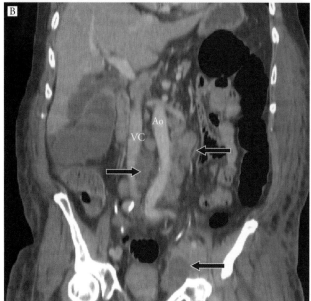

Figure 46.3 Initial CT scan of the chest, abdomen, and pelvis of a 65-year-old male with chronic low back pain who presented with left lower extremity phlegmasia cerulea dolens. The chest CT (A) shows an asymptomatic pulmonary embolus (arrow). The abdominal CT (B) shows extensive retroperitoneal and pelvic lymphadenopathy (arrows) compressing the distal vena cava and the left iliac system. All patients presenting with iliofemoral DVT by duplex ultrasound receive chest, abdominal, and pelvic CT scans as part of the initial workup.

tumors, retroperitoneal lymphoma, hepatic metastases, iliac vein aneurysms, and vena caval atresia all have been identified. A full hematologic evaluation for an underlying thrombophilia is also performed.

TECHNIQUE

There has been an evolution of catheter-directed thrombolytic techniques since around 2000. The preferred approach is through an ultrasound-guided popliteal vein puncture with antegrade passage of the infusion catheter. Through this approach physicians can incorporate adjunctive mechanical thrombectomy techniques.

If the popliteal vein is thrombosed, an additional catheter is placed through an ultrasound-guided tibial vein puncture. Using catheters that achieve long segments of thrombus infusion is advised.

There also has been an evolution in the dose and volume of plasminogen activator. Since the activation of fibrin-bound plasminogen is not dose dependent, exposure to the plasminogen activator is all that is required. The volume of the lytic solution has increased with a decrease in the concentration (dose) of plasminogen activator. It is now our preference to increase the volume of lytic infusion to 80 to 100 ml per hour. The larger volume is intended to saturate the thrombus, exposing more fibrin-bound plasminogen to the plasminogen activator. Phlebograms are obtained at 12-h intervals and are used to monitor the success of lysis and reposition catheters if necessary. Vena caval filters are not routinely used but are recommended for patients with free-floating thrombus in the vena cava. A retrievable filter can be used in the patient in whom only temporary protection is needed.

Following successful thrombolysis, the venous system is examined with completion phlebography. If a stenosis exists, which is frequently observed in the left common iliac vein where it is compressed by the right common iliac artery, the vein is dilated and stented if necessary. The addition of intravascular ultrasonography has improved the evaluation of iliac compression and the precision of stent deployment when these lesions are corrected. Residual areas of stenosis must be corrected for long-term success; otherwise, the patient faces a high risk of rethrombosis. If a stent is used, it should be sized appropriate to the normal diameter of the common iliac vein.

ADJUNCTIVE TECHNIQUES TO CATHETER-DIRECTED THROMBOLYSIS

Percutaneous mechanical thrombectomy techniques are discussed in detail in Chapter 46. There appears to be a higher incidence of embolic complications with mechanical thrombectomy. In a prospective evaluation of pulse-spray pharmacomechanical thrombolysis of clotted hemodialysis grafts,[27] it was found that PE (documented by ventilation perfusion scan) occurred in 18% of patients treated with a plasminogen activator pulse-spray solution versus 64% of patients treated with a heparinized saline pulse-spray solution (P = 0.04). Since clotted hemodialysis grafts are in direct communication with the venous circulation, they can be considered similar to proximal veins with acute DVT. Observations would likely be magnified when treating larger venous thromboses.

In an experimental model, Greenberg and associates[28] evaluated mechanical, pharmacomechanical, and pharmacologic thrombolysis. Their findings are consistent with anecdotal clinical observations as well as the results reported by Kinney and associates.[27] Greenberg et al. demonstrated that pulse-spray mechanical thrombectomy was associated with the largest number and greatest size of distal emboli. When urokinase was added to the solution, the embolic particles diminished in number and in size and increased the speed of lysis with reperfusion. Catheter-directed thrombolysis alone was associated with the slowest reperfusion but the fewest distal emboli. In general, mechanical thrombectomy alone most often is inadequate. Hemolytic complications of rheolytic mechanical thrombectomy are common and occasionally can result in anemia and renal dysfunction.

A new device recently released for segmental and controlled pharmacomechanical thrombolysis is the reengineered Trellis catheter (Bacchus Vascular, Santa Clara, CA), which is a hybrid catheter that isolates the thrombosed vein segment between two occluding balloons (see Figure 46.4). A lytic agent is infused into the thrombus between the occluding balloons. The intervening catheter shaft assumes a sine wave or spiral configuration and, when activated, spins at 15,000 rpm. After 10 to 15 min, the liquified thrombus and remaining fragments are aspirated. Phlebographic evaluation of the result is performed before moving on to treat additional thrombosed vein segments (see Figure 49.4). The advantages of such a device are its ability to incorporate mechanical and pharmacologic therapies, even in patients with a contraindication to thrombolytic therapy since the infusate is aspirated, and the rapidity with which treatment

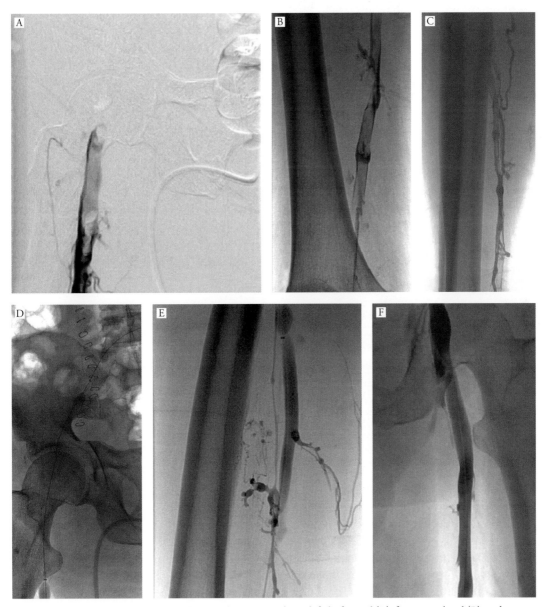

Figure 46.4 (A–C) Phlebogram of a patient 2 d after exploratory laparotomy shows left iliofemoral (A), femoropopliteal (B), and posterior tibial (C) DVT. The treatment goal was to lyse the extensive thrombus rapidly with minimal systemic exposure to the plasminogen activator. (D) This was accomplished using segmental pharmacomechanical thrombolysis with the hybrid Trellis peripheral infusion system (Bacchus Vascular, Santa Clara, CA) and ultrasound-accelerated thrombolysis of popliteal and tibial thrombus with the EKOS LysUS® System (EKOS Corp, Bothell, WA). The Trellis system achieves isolated thrombolysis between two occluding balloons by lytic infusion and mechanical drug dispersion with the intervening catheter rotating at 15,000 rpm. This mechanism of thrombolysis enables focused treatment of thrombus within the target vessel. (E, F) Phlebogram 30 min after using the Trellis system shows resolution of the thrombus in the iliac and femoral veins.

can be achieved. The rationales behind the design of this catheter are:

1. Rapidly resolve thrombus during a short course of treatment.

2. Limit or avoid exposure to thrombolytic therapy by aspirating liquified thrombus and infused lytic agent.

3. Prevent PE by proximal balloon occlusion.

A clinical trial designed to evaluate the success and complication rate of this technique is under way.

An interesting new adjunct to catheter-directed thrombolysis is the addition of the emission of ultrasound waves from the infusion catheter while delivering the plasminogen activator (see Figure 46.5). Several reports have emerged indicating that an infusion catheter with ultrasound transducers built into the infusion end of the catheter can be used to accelerate thrombolysis.[29–32] In vitro studies have demonstrated that ultrasound enhances the fibrinolytic activity of tissue plasminogen activator (t-PA).[33–35] The potential mechanism for augmented clot lysis has been extrapolated from in vitro studies showing that ultrasound produces clot fragmentation in the presence of t-PA, and consequently, more t-PA binds to fibrin-binding sites due to the larger available surface area.[36–38] The concept of a transducer-tipped catheter that delivers a fibrinolytic drug in combination with high frequency, low-intensity ultrasound has been well described. In vivo models[39] and clinical trials[40] are now under way to assess the potential value of ultrasound enhancement of thrombolysis for the management of acute DVT.

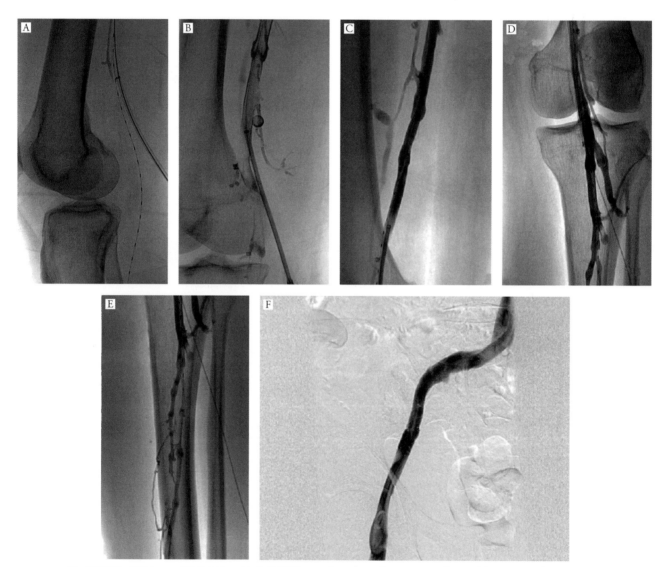

Figure 46.5   (A) The EKOS LysUS System (EKOS Corp, Bothell, WA) is an ultrasonic infusion system designed for controlled and selective infusion of thrombolytics into the thrombosed veins. Ultrasound waves accelerate thrombolysis, reducing treatment time. The catheter was advanced proximally from an ultrasound-guided posterior tibial vein puncture. (B) Phlebogram showing popliteal vein thrombus. (C–E) Post ultrasound lysis, dissolution of thrombus in the distal femoral vein (C), popliteal vein (D), and posterior tibial vein (E). (F) Angioplasty and stenting were performed on the left iliac vein, establishing normal venous drainage into the inferior vena cava.

The patient with phlegmasia cerulea dolens, summarized in Figure 46.4, illustrates the advantage of using segmental, pharmacomechanical thrombolysis and ultrasound-enhanced catheter-directed thrombolysis to shorten treatment duration and limit exposure to the thrombolytic agent, maximizing the chance of a successful outcome.

Thrombolysis is effective and has become safer with the direct intrathrombus infusion and adjunctive mechanical techniques. As technology continues to improve, lytic infusion times will shorten, more patients will be offered a treatment strategy that includes thrombus removal, and many patients will be spared their otherwise certain postthrombotic morbidity.

REFERENCES

1. O'Donnell TF Jr, Browse NL, Burnand KG, Thomas ML. The socioeconomic effects of an iliofemoral venous thrombosis, *J Surg Res.* 1977. *22*: 483–488.
2. Akesson H, Brudin L, Dahlstrom JA, Eklof B, Ohlin P, Plate G. Venous function assessed during a 5 year period after acute iliofemoral venous thrombosis treated with anticoagulation, *Eur J Vasc Surg.* 1990. *4*: 43–48.
3. Delis KT, Bountouroglou D, Mansfield AO. Venous claudication in iliofemoral thrombosis: Long-term effects on venous hemodynamics, clinical status, and quality of life, *Ann Surg.* 2004. *239*: 118–126.
4. Shull KC, Nicolaides AN, Fernandes é Fernandes J, et al. Significance of popliteal reflux in relation to ambulatory venous pressure and ulceration, *Arch Surg.* 1979. *114*: 1304–1306.
5. Johnson BF, Manzo RA, Bergelin RO, Strandness DE Jr. Relationship between changes in the deep venous system and the development of the postthrombotic syndrome after an acute episode of lower limb deep vein thrombosis: A one- to six-year follow-up, *J Vasc Surg.* 1995. *21*: 307–312.
6. Cho JS, Martelli E, Mozes G, Miller VM, Gloviczki P. Effects of thrombolysis and venous thrombectomy on valvular competence, thrombogenicity, venous wall morphology, and function, *J Vasc Surg.* 1998. *28*: 787–799.
7. Rhodes JM, Cho JS, Gloviczki P, Mozes G, Rolle R, Miller VM. Thrombolysis for experimental deep venous thrombosis maintains valvular competence and vasoreactivity, *J Vasc Surg.* 2000. *31*: 1193–1205.
8. Killewich LA, Bedford GR, Beach KW, Strandness DE Jr. Spontaneous lysis of deep venous thrombi: Rate and outcome, *J Vasc Surg.* 1989. *9*: 89–97.
9. Markel A, Manzo RA, Bergelin RO, Strandness DE Jr. Valvular reflux after deep vein thrombosis: Incidence and time of occurrence, *J Vasc Surg.* 1992. *15*: 377–382.
10. Meissner MH, Manzo RA, Bergelin RO, Markel A, Strandness DE Jr. Deep venous insufficiency: The relationship between lysis and subsequent reflux, *J Vasc Surg.* 1993. *18*: 596–605.
11. Caps MT, Manzo RA, Bergelin RO, Meissner MH, Strandness DE Jr. Venous valvular reflux in veins not involved at the time of acute deep vein thrombosis, *J Vasc Surg.* 1995. *22*: 524–531.
12. Comerota AJ, Aldridge SE. Thrombolytic therapy for acute deep vein thrombosis, *Semin Vasc Surg.* 1992. *5*: 76–84.
13. Goldhaber SZ, Buring JE, Lipnick RJ, Hennekens CH. Pooled analyses of randomized trials of streptokinase and heparin in phlebographically documented acute deep venous thrombosis, *Am J Med.* 1984. *76*: 393–397.
14. Plate G, Einarsson E, Ohlin P, Jensen R, Qvarfordt P, Eklof B. Thrombectomy with temporary arteriovenous fistula: The treatment of choice in acute iliofemoral venous thrombosis, *J Vasc Surg.* 1984. *1*: 867–876.
15. Plate G, Akesson H, Einarsson E, Ohlin P, Eklof B. Long-term results of venous thrombectomy combined with a temporary arterio-venous fistula, *Eur J Vasc Surg.* 1990. *4*: 483–489.
16. Plate G, Eklof B, Norgren L, Ohlin P, Dahlstrom JA. Venous thrombectomy for iliofemoral vein thrombosis: 10-year results of a prospective randomised study, *Eur J Vasc Endovasc Surg.* 1997. *14*: 367–374.
17. Alkjaersig N, Fletcher AP, Sherry S. The mechanism of clot dissolution by plasmin, *J Clin Invest.* 1959. *38*: 1086–1095.
18. Bjarnason H, Kruse JR, Asinger DA, et al. Iliofemoral deep venous thrombosis: Safety and efficacy outcome during 5 years of catheter-directed thrombolytic therapy, *J Vasc Interv Radiol.* 1997. *8*: 405–418.
19. Mewissen MW, Seabrook GR, Meissner MH, Cynamon J, Labropoulos N, Haughton SH. Catheter-directed thrombolysis for lower extremity deep venous thrombosis: Report of a national multicenter registry, *Radiology.* 1999. *211*: 39–49.
20. Comerota AJ, Kagan SA. Catheter-directed thrombolysis for the treatment of acute iliofemoral deep venous thrombosis, *Phlebology.* 2001. *15*: 149–155.
21. Verhaeghe R, Stockx L, Lacroix H, Vermylen J, Baert AL. Catheter-directed lysis of iliofemoral vein thrombosis with use of rtPA, *Eur Radiol.* 1997. *7*: 996–1001.
22. Shortell CK, Queiroz R, Johansson M, et al. Safety and efficacy of limited-dose tissue plasminogen activator in acute vascular occlusion, *J Vasc Surg.* 2001. *34*: 854–859.
23. Chang R, Cannon RO III, Chen CC, et al. Daily catheter-directed single dosing of t-PA in treatment of acute deep venous thrombosis of the lower extremity, *J Vasc Interv Radiol.* 2001. *12*: 247–252.
24. Castaneda F, Li R, Young K, Swischuk JL, Smouse B, Brady T. Catheter-directed thrombolysis in deep venous thrombosis with use of reteplase: Immediate results and complications from a pilot study, *J Vasc Interv Radiol.* 2002. *13*: 577–580.
25. Sillesen H, Just S, Jorgensen M, Baekgaard N. Catheter-directed thrombolysis for treatment of ilio-femoral deep venous thrombosis is durable, preserves venous valve function and may prevent chronic venous insufficiency, *Eur J Vasc Endovasc Surg.* 2005. *30*(5): 556–562.
26. Elsharawy M, Elzayat E. Early results of thrombolysis versus anticoagulation in iliofemoral venous thrombosis: A randomised clinical trial, *Eur J Vasc Endovasc Surg.* 2002. *24*: 209–214.
27. Kinney TB, Valji K, Rose SC, et al. Pulmonary embolism from PulseSpray pharmacomechanical thrombolysis of clotted hemodialysis grafts: Urokinase versus heparinized saline, *J Vasc Interv Radiol.* 2000. *11*: 1143–1152.
28. Greenberg RK, Ouriel K, Srivastava S, et al. Mechanical versus chemical thrombolysis: An in vitro differentiation of thrombolytic mechanisms, *J Vasc Interv Radiol.* 2000. *11*: 199–205.
29. Steffen W, Fishbein MC, Luo H, et al. High intensity, low frequency catheter-delivered ultrasound dissolution of occlusive coronary artery thrombi: An in vitro and in vivo study, *J Am Coll Cardiol.* 1994. *24*: 1571–1579.
30. Rosenschein U, Gaul G, Erbel R, et al. Percutaneous transluminal therapy of occluded saphenous vein grafts: Can the challenge be met with ultrasound thrombolysis?, *Circulation.* 1999. *99*: 26–29.
31. Tachibana K, Tachibana S. Ultrasound energy for enhancement of fibrinolysis and drug delivery: Special emphasis on the use of a transducer-tipped ultrasound system. In: Siegel RJ, ed. *Ultrasound angioplasty.* Boston: Kluwer. 1996. 121–133.
32. Tachibana K, Tachibana S. Prototype therapeutic ultrasound emitting catheter for accelerating thrombolysis, *J Ultrasound Med.* 1997. *16*: 529–535.
33. Trubestein G, Engel C, Etzel F, Sobbe A, Cremer H, Stumpff U. Thrombolysis by ultrasound, *Clin Sci Mol Med Suppl.* 1976. *3*: 697s–698s.
34. Ariani M, Fishbein MC, Chae JS, et al. Dissolution of peripheral arterial thrombi by ultrasound, *Circulation.* 1991. *84*: 1680–1688.
35. Rosenschein U, Bernstein JJ, DiSegni E, Kaplinsky E, Bernheim J, Rozenzsajn LA. Experimental ultrasonic angioplasty: Disruption of

atherosclerotic plaques and thrombi in vitro and arterial recanalization in vivo, *J Am Coll Cardiol*. 1990. *15*: 711–712.

36. Lauer CG, Burge R, Tang DB, Bass BG, Gomez ER, Alving BM. Effect of ultrasound on tissue-type plasminogen activator-induced thrombolysis, *Circulation*. 1992. *86*: 1257–1264.

37. Hong AS, Chae JS, Dubin SB, Lee S, Fishbein MC, Siegel RJ. Ultrasonic clot disruption: An in vitro study, *Am Heart J*. 1990. *120*: 418–422.

38. Drobinski G, Brisset D, Philippe F, et al. Effects of ultrasound energy on total peripheral artery occlusions: Initial angiographic and angioscopic results, *J Interv Cardiol*. 1993. *6*: 157–163.

39. Atar S, Luo H, Nagai T, Siegel RJ. Ultrasonic thrombolysis: Catheter-delivered and transcutaneous applications, *Eur J Ultrasound*. 1999. *9*: 39–54.

40. EKOS Corporation, Bothell, WA. Retrospective evaluation of thrombolysis with EKOS Lysus System.

47.

PERCUTANEOUS MECHANICAL THROMBECTOMY IN THE TREATMENT OF DVT

Colleen M. Johnson, Pritham P. Reddy, and Robert B. Mclafferty

INTRODUCTION

Deep venous thrombosis (DVT) is associated with significant morbidity and mortality. Symptomatic DVT affects 250,000 to 300,000 people per year in the United States and is responsible for approximately 300,000 hospital admissions per year.[1–4] Nearly 50,000 deaths each year are attributable to pulmonary embolism (PE) from DVT.[3] The costs for treatment of DVT are estimated between $1.2 and $2.4 billion per year.[5]

Once the diagnosis of DVT is established, the goals of therapy are: (1) prevention of PE, (2) prevention of thrombus propagation, (3) preservation of valvular function, and (4) prevention of postthrombotic syndrome (PTS). Traditionally, treatment involves unfractionated heparin (UH) or low molecular weight heparin (LMWH) as a bridge to oral anticoagulation. In addition to the prevention of PE and PTS, therapeutic anticoagulation aids in the prevention of clot propagation. Asbeutah et al. reported 5-year follow-up of fifty-one patients with fifty-four DVTs for PTS. Twenty-six limbs were noted to have proximal involvement. When treated with anticoagulation alone, 34% had thrombus resolution at 1 month. Sixty-five percent of limbs went on to develop reflux, and 54% progressed to chronic venous insufficiency within 1 year of diagnosis.[6]

Surgical thrombectomy is an open procedure whereby thrombus is manually extracted from a venotomy most commonly created in the femoral vein. Thrombus proximal to the inguinal ligament is removed using a balloon catheter and thrombus below is removed by compression of the limb with an esmarch wrap (Spectrum Laboratories, Rancho Dominguez, CA). Problems with this technique include denuding endothelium, damage to the valves, and incomplete thrombus removal. Although thrombectomy is advocated by some as the preferred method of treatment for DVT, the vast majority of patients continue to be treated with anticoagulation.

With the advent of thrombolytic drugs, some institutions have treated DVTs with intravenous administration.[7–9] Although thrombolysis theoretically satisfies all therapeutic goals, complete thrombus resolution occurs in only about 50% of patients with nonobstructive thrombus and 10% of those with obstructive thrombi.[10,11] Serious bleeding complications such as retroperitoneal hematoma and intracranial hemorrhage are markedly elevated in patients receiving systemic therapy when compared with patients treated with anticoagulation alone.[12–15]

Regional or catheter-directed thrombolysis (CDT) has been used with some success. Potential advantages include administration of the pharmacologic agent directly into the thrombus and less systemic side effects. AbuRahma et al. reported complete resolution of symptoms in 83% of patients undergoing CDT compared with 3% in the group receiving anticoagulation alone.[16] CDT also has proven advantageous in the prevention of recurrent DVT in a large majority of patients.[17] Unfortunately, bleeding complications continue to plague 4 to 6% of patients, and intracranial hemorrhage still occurs in a small minority of patients.[18,19] CDT usually requires 1 to 3 d of continuous therapy and represents a major disadvantage to prompt and safe treatment. Comerota et al. reported a 21% incidence of severe PTS in patients treated for DVT with heparin alone, compared to 5% in those treated with streptokinase.[20] CDT in the management of DVT also has been proven superior to anticoagulation alone when evaluating health-related quality of life.[21]

Percutaneous mechanical thrombectomy (PMT) refers to the technique whereby a catheter utilizing mechanical means can be used independently or coupled with pharmacologic thrombolysis in the treatment of DVT. Preliminary data show that treatment with PMT may provide quicker thrombus resolution than CDT alone.[21,22] With an increasing emphasis on minimal invasiveness, recent years have witnessed an endovascular revolution that has ushered in many different types of PMT catheters. Herein we provide a comprehensive review of the PMT catheters and descriptions of more common treatment techniques.

TECHNIQUE

In order to successfully perform PMT, several general premises must be considered. These include whether to place a temporary vena cava filter, determining optimal site for venous access, and how to traverse the thrombosis. Although the technique unique to each PMT catheter is highly variable, these general principles apply to most clinical scenarios in treating DVT. Following thrombus removal, subsequent interventions such as balloon angioplasty and/or stenting can be performed if necessary.

TEMPORARY INFERIOR VENA CAVA (IVC) FILTER PLACEMENT

The risk of fatal PE during thrombolytic therapy of iliac vein thrombus has been reported as high as 6%.[24] All PMT devices, including those that aspirate during treatment, generate small particles that can migrate to the pulmonary circulation. The placement of a retrievable IVC filter has become a valuable adjunct to PMT. There are many types of temporary IVC filters available with different time periods for retrieval (see Table 47.1). Additionally, each filter varies in the approach to deployment and retrieval. These important issues must be considered prior to PMT.

An in vitro model of early large-volume DVT demonstrated that in placing an IVC filter prior to PMT, 99% of particles larger than 500 μm were either macerated by the device or captured by the filter.[25] Trerotola et al. demonstrated a significant number of clinically significant segmental and subsegmental pulmonary emboli while evaluating the Arrow-Trerotola Percutaneous Thrombectomy Device (Arrow International, Reading, PA) in a canine model.[26] Further investigations determined that use of a temporary IVC filter reduced the number of pulmonary emboli as diagnosed by pulmonary angiography.[27]

In the majority of patients, placement of a retrievable IVC filter should be performed just prior to PMT. Generally, access to the deployment site should be void of

thrombus, and guide wire traversal should be observed with fluoroscopy for any deviation or difficulty that may indicate the presence of thrombus. A venogram should be obtained prior to deployment of the IVC filter to identify the renal veins and to further ensure the proposed deployment location is devoid of any thrombus. A low threshold to perform venography by selective catheterization should be considered if nonselective venography fails to show important venous tributaries.[28]

Depending on the results of PMT, the filter can be removed immediately or remain in place 1 to 3 weeks during the healing process. The IVC filter should remain in place if contraindications to anticoagulation arise, development of recurrent DVT, or increases in DVT risk occur.

VENOUS ACCESS

If possible, the same venous access for IVC filter placement should be used when selecting an access site to perform PMT. The ipsilateral common femoral vein is the optimal access site for thrombus confined to the iliocaval segments. In this clinical scenario, the IVC filter should be placed via the contralateral femoral vein. If the thrombosis is confined to a single lower extremity, possible access sites include either common femoral vein or the ipsilateral popliteal vein. The internal jugular vein can also be used to access DVT in the lower extremities.

Generally, access to lower extremity DVT from the external iliac vein to the superficial femoral vein is from the contralateral common femoral vein. Selective catheterization comes over the iliac vein bifurcation and the involved contralateral venous segments are accessed in a retrograde direction. If the thrombus burden is high or there is anticipated difficulty in performing a retrograde cannulation, antegrade access through the ipsilateral popliteal vein is preferred.

The antegrade approach through the ipsilateral popliteal vein to treat iliofemoral DVT remains the most common alternative to the contralateral approach. With the patient in the prone position, duplex ultrasound is required for needle guidance. A micropuncture kit that uses a 22-gauge needle and a 0.014-inch wire aids in providing a nontraumatic, safe access. Advantages of antegrade access through

Table 47.1 **RETRIEVABLE IVC FILTERS**

FILTER	INSERTION SITES			RETRIEVAL SITES		
	FEMORAL	JUGULAR	ANTECUBITAL	FEMORAL	JUGULAR	ANTECUBITAL
ALN (ALN Implants Chirurgicaux, Ghisonaccia, France)	X	X	X		X	
Recovery (Bard Peripheral Vascular, Tempe, AZ)	X	X	X	X	X	X
Günther Tulip (Cook Medical, Bloomington, IN)	X	X	X	X	X	
OptEase (Cordis Endovascular, Warren, NJ)	X	X			X	
SafeFlo (Rafael Medical, Caesarea, Israel)	X				X	

the popliteal vein include ease of traversing valves and minimal need for selective catheterization.

Other more remote sites such as the jugular and subclavian veins have been used to gain access to DVT. More commonly these access sites may be required for direct access to the confluence of the common iliac veins. Occasionally, common iliac vein stenosis in combination with thrombosis can be negotiated only via a retrograde approach from the brachiocephalic veins. Treating iliofemoral DVT may require dual access with the use of a snare to pull the wire from one access site to another, thereby providing for more stable access to treat with PMT. In the case of upper extremity DVT treatment, venous access generally is obtained at the ipsilateral basilic vein. This also requires ultrasound guidance and use of a micropuncture kit.

TRAVERSING THE THROMBUS

After defining the venous segment by venography as an entry point to the thrombus, stable access with a sheath or guiding catheter usually is required. A stiff hydrophilic guide wire (Boston Scientific; Natick, MA) allows optimal manipulation and guidance in gaining access into thrombus. As the wire is advanced, a catheter is advanced over the wire to maintain crossing and increase stability. Usually a straight catheter such as a 4-Fr. glidecath (Boston Scientific, Natick, MA) is used in combination with a stiff angled guide wire (Boston Scientific, Natick, MA). Alternatively, an angled catheter such as a Kumpe catheter (Cook; Bloomington, IN) can be used with a straight guide wire (Boston Scientific; Natick, MA). These combinations are particularly useful when traversing thrombus in a retrograde direction. Valve leaflets can be negotiated with slow directed movements under magnified fluoroscopy.

Another technique that can facilitate crossing thrombs is forming the guide wire into a long "J" configuration. This maneuver takes advantage of the stiff portion of the guide-wire while preventing trauma to the vein wall because the floppy tip is in a "J" shape. When pushing antegrade through older thrombus, this technique may prove useful. Emphasis should be placed on not forcing wires, catheters, and PMT systems into position. Careful continuous fluoroscopic imaging is mandatory when moving wires and catheters and observing their tracking path is vital to avoiding injury. A manifold hand injection system with the ability to withdraw contrast and dilute with saline is helpful in facilitating quick, periodic views to assure correct catheter position.

DEVICES

PMT catheters can be categorized a variety of ways. One important distinction is whether the catheter has complete or incomplete wall contact. Advantages of complete wall contact include more thorough thrombus dissolution. Potential disadvantages include endothelial and valvular damage. PMT catheters also can be categorized by their method of thrombus dissolution. These mechanical methods include rheolytic aspiration, rotational thrombectomy, and ultrasonic fragmentation. Rheolytic devices remove thrombus based on the Venturi effect. This adaptation of the Bernoulli effect states that fluid moving at high speeds generates low pressure zones. These low pressure zones create a partial vacuum, termed the Venturi effect. In rheolytic thrombectomy devices, high speed saline jets are directed into the thrombus creating low pressure zones near the catheter where the fragments are aspirated through the device via the vacuum effect. Theoretic advantages of rheolytic aspiration include less valvular damage and decreased endothelia damage.

The rotational devices are designed to spin at varying speeds within the thrombus causing fragmentation. This mechanism also can result in increased endothelial damage. Ultrasonic fragmentation occurs through the delivery of high-frequency, low-energy ultrasound. The ultrasound waves cause the aggregated fibrin strands to dissociate, resulting in both increased permeability of the thrombus and exposure of new plasminogen activator sites on the fibrin strands. Thrombolytic drugs are forced into the thrombus by the radial pressure generated by the ultrasound waves.

Finally, PMT catheters are designed to either aspirate fragmented thrombus or create a near liquefaction of thrombus that migrates into the venous circulation. Ultimately, the microemboli are propelled to the pulmonary circulation, where endogenous lysis takes place. The aspiration catheters can increase blood loss associated with the procedure, and, therefore, the operator must be vigilant in monitoring the aspirated volume. Clinically significant sequelae of pulmonary emboli from the nonaspiration catheters have not been reported after treatment for DVT. Table 47.2 includes the commercially available devices subsequently discussed in this chapter.

ANGIOJET
THROMBECTOMY SYSTEM

Indications for use approved by the US Food and Drug Administration (FDA) of the AngioJet thrombectomy system (ATS; Possis Medical, Minneapolis, MN) include treatment of peripheral arterial occlusions, thrombosed hemodialysis grafts, and DVT. This dual lumen catheter (see Figure 47.1) operates on the Bernoulli-Venturi principles. Saline or a thrombolytic drug are infused by the drive unit to generate approximately 10,000 psi of pressure within the catheter. The infusate is ejected from the catheter in retrograde-directed, pulsatile jets. The jets generate low pressure zones that allow for thrombus maceration and aspiration. An exhaust port near the tip of the catheter allows for aspiration thereby avoiding the potential for localized

Table 47.2 **PMT DEVICES**

DEVICE	METHOD OF THROMBUS REMOVAL	WALL CONTACT	ASPIRATION CATHETER	FDA APPROVED INDICATION
AKonya Eliminator	Mechanical	Mechanical	No	Thrombosed AVF and dialysis grafts
Arrow-Trerotola	Mechanical	Complete	Yes	Thrombosed AVF and dialysis grafts
AngioJet				
XMI	Rheolytic	Incomplete	Yes	Coronary or vein graft lesions >2 mm
XVG	Rheolytic	Incomplete	Yes	Thrombosed infrainguinal arteries >3 mm
Xpeedior 120	Rheolytic	Incomplete	Yes	Thrombosed infrainguinal arteries >3 mm
AVX	Rheolytic	Incomplete	Yes	Thrombosed dialysis grafts
XMI-RX+	Rheolytic	Incomplete	Yes	Thrombosed infrainguinal arteries >2 mm
DVX	Rheolytic	Incomplete	Yes	Thrombosed infrainguinal arteries >3 mm
Castaneda Over-the-Wire Brush	Mechanical	Complete	No	Thrombosed dialysis grafts
Helix Clot Buster Thrombectomy Device (Amplatz Device)	Mechanical	Incomplete	No	Thrombosed AVF and dialysis grafts
Lysus Infusion System	Ultrasonic	Incomplete	No	Selective infusion of medication into peripheral vessels
Oasis Thrombectomy System	Rheolytic	Complete	Yes	Thrombosed dialysis grafts
ProLumen	Mechanical	Incomplete		Thrombosed dialysis grafts
Thrombex PMT	Mechanical	Incomplete		Thrombosed dialysis grafts
Trellis Infusion System	Mechanical	Incomplete	Yes	
X-Sizer Catheter System	Mechanical		Yes	Thrombosed dialysis grafts

endothelial damage from a more eccentrically placed vortex. Ninety-nine percent of the particulate matter generated by the ATS is 0 to 12 μm in diameter.[29] A separate pump drive unit is necessary for the catheter to function with dual lumen tubing that delivers the infusate and collects the effluent. The system functions in an isovolumetric manner with 60 cc/min being infused and aspirated simultaneously.[30]

Multiple catheters have been designed for use in vessels of varying diameters and locations (see Table 47.3). Additionally, different types of tubing are available to allow for saline infusion or power pulsation. Power pulsation is designed to force standard pharmacologic thrombolytics into the thrombus. In contrast, traditional CDT uses *lacing*, whereby the drug seeps from the multiple side holes of an infusion catheter.

Sharafuddin et al. evaluated endothelial damage incurred after use of the ATS compared to the Fogarty balloon embolectomy in a canine model. The ATS-treated vessels had significantly more endothelial coverage than vessels treated with the Fogarty balloon.[31] Segments treated with the ATS showed no difference in endothelial coverage or valvular damage when histologically compared to untreated control segments.

Thrombus extraction rates using the ATS range from 52 to 95%.[22] This wide range of variability appears to be related to the adjunctive use of pharmacologic thrombolysis.[32] The ATS has been used in the treatment of symptomatic lower extremity DVT with success. Bush et al. reported the use of the ATS in the treatment of twenty-three limbs in twenty patients. Technical success was achieved in fifteen of the twenty-three treated limbs. The remaining limbs demonstrated varying degrees of thrombus removal. Seven of twelve patients being treated for iliofemoral DVT had prophylactic IVC filters placed. Marked clinical improvement within 24 h of therapy was noted in 74% of patients. Only three minor bleeding complications were noted, and no one required a blood transfusion.[33]

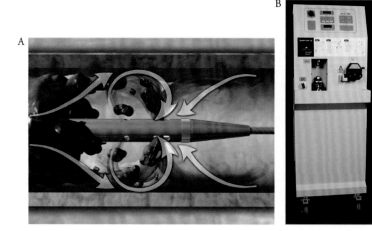

Figure 47.1 (A) Demonstration of the Bernoulli-Venturi effect as used by the Angiojet thrombectomy system. (B) The free-standing pump drive unit for the Angiojet thrombectomy system.

Table 47.3 ANGIOJET THROMBECTOMY SYSTEM CATHETERS

CATHETER	MIN. VESSEL DIAMETER	WORKING LENGTH	GUIDEWIRE COMPATIBILITY	SHEATH COMPATIBILITY
XMI-OTW	>2 mm	135 cm	0.014″	4 Fr.
XMI-RX+	>2 mm	135 cm	0.014″	4 Fr.
XVG	>3 mm	140 cm	0.014″	5 Fr.
Xpeedior	>3 mm	120 cm	0.035″	6 Fr.
DVX	>3 mm	90 cm	0.035″	6 Fr.

Kasirajan et al. reported similar results in seventeen patients treated with the ATS. Thrombus extraction rates were lower with only 24% having >90% thrombus removal. Adjunctive thrombolytic therapy was used in nine of thirteen that demonstrated less than 90% thrombus extraction. Eighty-two percent of patients had significant clinical improvement, and no complications were reported.[34]

The ATS also has been successfully used in the management of Paget-Schroetter's syndrome, PE, and mesenteric venous thrombosis.[35-37]

AKONYA ELIMINATOR

The Eliminator catheter (IDev Technologies, Houston, TX) is a nonmotor-driven thrombectomy device approved by the FDA for thrombectomy of dialysis grafts. The device uses a 6-Fr. adjustable basket that can accommodate vessels from 2 to 10 mm in diameter. The catheter has directional control that allows easy navigation of tortuous vessels. The catheter has no drive unit, and through manipulation in an axial direction or manual rotation, the thrombus can be stripped from the vein wall.

ARROW-TREROTOLA PERCUTANEOUS THROMBECTOMY DEVICE

The Arrow-Trerotola Percutaneous Thrombectomy Device (ATPTD) fragments thrombus using a self-expanding 9-mm fragmentation cage. The device comes as either an over-the-wire configuration or the original design whereby the cage is constrained by a sheath. The latter device must be positioned across the thrombus before withdrawing the sheath and releasing the fragmentation cage. In both devices, the cage rotates at 3,000 rpm and is pulled through the thrombus. The rotating cage strips and macerates thrombus from the vein wall creating a slurry that can be aspirated through the sheath. Two passes of the device usually provide optimal clot fragmentation.[38]

Damage to the veins after thrombectomy with the ATPTD was assessed in an experimental canine model. The device was passed five times in the antegrade direction through thrombosed lateral saphenous veins. The venous segments were assessed for endothelial loss, the presence of thrombus, and valvular damage. Compared to valves designated as controls in untreated thrombosed lateral saphenous

veins, valves in the experimental group treated with ATPTD had significantly less inflammatory cell infiltrates.[39]

Technical success rates are reported between 92 and 100% when treating thrombosed dialysis grafts.[38,40,41] Procedure times are markedly shortened when compared to pulse-spray thrombolysis.[38] Ninety-day patency rates range from 39 to 70%.[38,41] Preliminary work has begun to evaluate the ATPTD for treating DVT. Animal studies indicate promising local success rates, but segmental and subsegmental pulmonary emboli were demonstrated with concomitant increases in mean and systolic pulmonary arterial pressure. Increasing pCO_2 and acidosis were also observed.[42] The thrombus fragments produced by the device range in size from <1 mm to as high as 3 mm.[42] Truong et al. reported successful PMT using the ATPTD in a patient that presented with a subacute iliocaval thrombosis. A temporary Günther basket filter was placed prior to intervention. At 3 months, magnetic resonance imaging (MRI) demonstrated no recurrent thrombosis in the treated vessels.[43]

HELIX CLOT BUSTER

Previously marketed as the Amplatz Thrombectomy Device, the HELIX Clot Buster (ev3, Plymouth, MN) was the first device approved by the FDA for percutaneous treatment of thrombosed dialysis grafts. Basic components include an impeller mounted on a drive shaft that is powered by a compressed air turbine. Rotation of the impeller at 150,000 rpm creates a vortex at the distal tip of the catheter that draws in the thrombus and recirculates the particulate matter. Particles from this PMT catheter are less than 1,000 microns.[44] Success rates of the HELIX for treatment of thrombosed dialysis grafts range from 79 to 93%.[45,46] The blunt tip design of the HELIX make it difficult to navigate tortuous vessels.

Successful treatment of venous thrombosis has been reported in multiple vascular segments using the HELIX. Uflacker reported treatment of nine acute and subacute venous thromboses in the IVC and iliac veins (n = 3), SVC and subclavian veins (n = 3), portal vein and transjugular intrahepatic portosystemic shunt (TIPS) (n = 2), and an IVC to pulmonary artery Fontan conduit (n = 1). Thromboses had been present from 2 d to four weeks. Three patients had failed prior CDT with urokinase. PMT was successful in all CDT failures, but each required an adjunctive measure to ensure long-term patency. One patient being treated for an iliocaval thrombosis developed intraprocedural shortness of breath attributed to pulmonary embolism despite placement of an IVC filter.[47] Similarly, Smith et al. reported using the HELIX in patients with DVT who had relative or absolute contraindications to pharmacologic thrombolysis. Treatment of DVT was performed in the superior mesenteric vein, bilateral femoral veins, and the SVC and brachiocephalic veins.[48] Additionally, the HELIX has been used to treat major and minor pulmonary emboli.[49]

HYDROLYSER

This multilumen catheter (Cordis, Warren, NJ) is designed for over-the-wire use. It utilizes the Venturi effect to fragment thrombus (see Figure 47.2). Simultaneous infusion of thrombolytic drugs or saline is possible through an injection port. Aspiration takes place through a 6-mm elliptical exhaust port that is located 4 mm proximal to the distal tip of the catheter.

Disadvantages of the Hydrolyser (see Figure 47.3) can include possible fluid overload and hemolysis. Additionally, the guide wire may obstruct the exhaust port and decrease the amount of thrombus extracted. The eccentrically located exhaust port creates an imbalanced vortex. This may result in tenting of the vessel toward the low pressure region and increase the endothelial damage.[22]

The Hydrolyser was compared to the ATS in an in vitro model to determine the degree of embolization.[50] The catheters were also compared with and without the guide wires in place, as previous data has indicated decreased effectiveness when the guide wire remained. The Hydrolyser demonstrated greater thrombus resolution and less distal embolization when compared to the ATS. Thrombus destruction was improved for both catheters when the guide wire remained in the catheter.[51]

Successful cases of PMT using the Hydrolyser for the treatment of acute DVT and pulmonary embolism have been reported.[52-54] Henry et al. reported 83% technical success in a variety of patients with arterial, bypass graft, and venous thrombosis.[53] Thrombus less than 10 d old provided the optimal therapeutic window when using the Hydrolyser, and segments treated took less than 4 min on average.[53] Poon et al. reported on three women that had IVC thromboses treated with the Hydrolyser. None of these patients could receive heparin or thrombolytics due to neurosurgical problems. All patients were successfully treated with the Hydrolyser and had complete resolution of their lower extremity edema. Each patient had an IVC filter placed, and one patient required a second treatment with the Hydrolyser.[54]

LYSUS INFUSION CATHETER SYSTEM

The Lysus Infusion Catheter System (EKOS Corporation, Bothell, WA) uses high-frequency, low-powered ultrasound to lyse thrombus. After traversal of the thrombus with guide wire, a multiholed drug delivery catheter is advanced over the guide wire. The guide wire is removed and the ultrasound core is placed within the catheter. The ultrasound core contains many ultrasound transducers along its length, and a separate control system regulates the ultrasound output and temperature. The core is actively cooled by a saline infusion that exits the distal tip of the catheter during treatment. Thrombolytic drugs are infused via the multiholed delivery catheter and the radial force generated by the ultrasound propels the drug away from the catheter and deeper into the more permeable thrombus.

OASIS

The Oasis catheter (Boston Scientific, Natick, MA), originally marketed as the Shredding Embolectomy Thrombectomy catheter, is a triple-lumen catheter placed over a guide wire that allows for the infusion of saline and simultaneous aspiration of thrombus. In contrast to the ATS system, which requires a separate drive unit, the Oasis can be powered by a standard power injector. The presence of the dedicated wire lumen also avoids a reduction in suction through the exhaust lumen that can be observed with the ATS device.

In a canine DVT model, the Oasis catheter has an 80% procedural success rate. All vessels exhibited endothelial denudation that occasionally extended into the

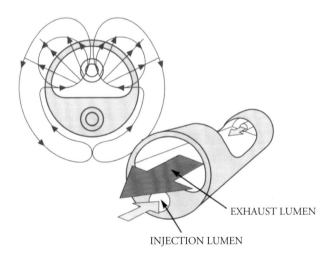

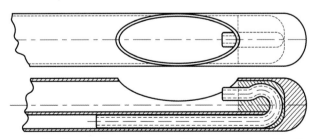

Figure 47.2 The Venturi effect as used in the Hydrolyser Catheter (Cordis Endovascular, Warren, NJ).

EXHAUST LUMEN

INJECTION LUMEN

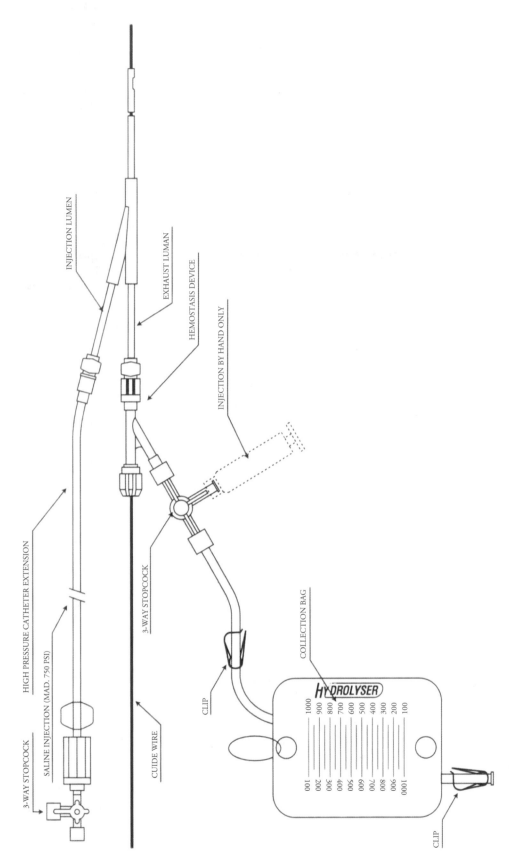

Figure 47.3 The Hydrolyser set-up.

internal elastic lamina, while no injury extended to the media. Significant pulmonary embolization was not observed.[55]

Technical success in the treatment of thrombosed dialysis grafts approaches 90%, and clinical success, defined as the ability to access the grafts for dialysis, ranges from 76 to 81%.[56,57] Takahashi et al. reported a single case of successful use of the Oasis thrombectomy device to treat a symptomatic mesenteric venous thrombosis in the portal and superior mesenteric veins.[58]

PROLUMEN

Approved for use in hemodialysis access, the ProLumen (Datascope, Montvale, NJ) is a self-contained thrombectomy catheter that requires no additional equipment. The device contains a 0.035-inch stainless steel S-wire with a radiopaque tip. With a 5.8-Fr outer diameter, the catheter has a handheld battery-operated drive unit that rotates the sigmoid shaped S-wire at approximately 4,000 rpm. The S-wire maintains contact with the graft wall to release adherent thrombus. No reports are published to date using the ProLumen for treatment of DVT.

TRELLIS-8 THROMBECTOMY SYSTEM

The Trellis-8 Thrombectomy System (Bacchus Vascular, Santa Clara, CA) combines CDT and PMT by isolating the thrombosed venous segment between proximal and distal occlusion balloons. After a thrombolytic drug is infused into this closed system, a sinusoidal wire mixes the lytic agent into the thrombus together. The balloon occlusion limits systemic exposure to the lytic agent and prevents pulmonary emboli. The slurry created in the treated segment is then aspirated to remove lysed clot and the residual active drug.

The Trellis-8 Thrombectomy System (see Figure 47.4) has been successful in treating both upper and lower

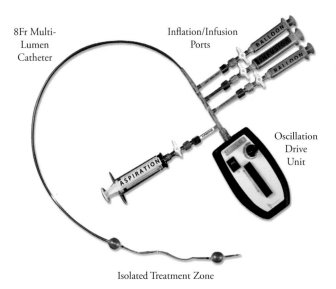

8Fr Multi-Lumen Catheter

Inflation/Infusion Ports

Oscillation Drive Unit

Isolated Treatment Zone

Figure 47.4 The Trellis-8 Thrombectomy System.

extremity venous thrombosis. Arko et al. reported use of the TTS to treat two patients with axillosubclavian vein thrombosis.[59] Ramaiah et al. used the TTS to treat an iliofemoral thrombosis. In both reports, use of the TTS resulted in shorter treatment times when compared with CDT alone, and decreased doses of the thrombolytic agent used. No bleeding complications were reported in any of the patients described. Neither patient described had a bleeding complication or PE reported.[59,60]

X-SIZER

The X-Sizer helical thrombectomy catheter (ev3, Plymouth, MN) is composed of a rotating helical cutter that is housed in an outer sheath. The device is attached to a vacuum source for the aspiration of particulate matter created during the procedure. The device has been evaluated in the coronary arterial circulation, but to date treatment of hemodialysis grafts, the peripheral arterial tree, and the venous system has not been reported.

DISCUSSION

An increasing number of patients with acute DVT are undergoing treatment with PMT. Advantages of PMT include immediate improvement of symptoms, decreased treatment times and complications when compared to CDT alone, and a possible reduction in the incidence and severity of PTS. Although many PMT catheters are commercially available, only the Trellis-8 Thrombectomy System and the ATS lytic power pulse system are approved by the FDA for treatment of acute DVT.

Some PMT catheters, such as those just mentioned, are designed to allow for the concomitant infusion of thrombolytic agents in order to more thoroughly remove thrombus. The combination of PMT and pharmacologic thrombolysis can drastically reduce the treatment times compared to CDT alone. Arko et al. reported complete thrombus removal in two patients using the Trellis-8 Thrombectomy System with Alteplase (Genentech, South San Francisco, CA) for upper extremity DVT. These two patients were treated at a single setting and received 5 mg of Alteplase over 10 min.[59]

When evaluating these devices in the treatment of thrombosed hemodialysis access, the ATS, ATPTD, and Oasis were found to have equivalent technical success rates when compared to pulse-spray thrombolysis.[28,56,61] The procedure times were significantly shorter in the groups that underwent PMT.[38,56] Complications such as bleeding requiring transfusion, PE, and arterial embolization were less in the PMT arm, but statistical significance was not reached due to the small number of patients.[38]

PMT most often allows patients to be treated in a single setting, thereby avoiding multiple trips to the angiography suite. Ramaiah et al. reported a single case of a patient that developed increased thrombus burden while on heparin. After failure following 36 h of CDT with reteplase (Centocor, Horsham, PA), PMT using the Trellis-8 Thrombectomy System was successful with complete clot lysis in 45 minutes.[60] Similar results have been reported in the treatment of upper extremity DVT when using the Trellis-8 Thrombectomy System.[59]

Bleeding complications may be less when compared to CDT. In seventeen patients treated with PMT for lower extremity DVT, Kasirajan et al. observed no hemorrhagic or access site complications.[34] Bush et al. reported two patients that developed access site hematomas and one that developed a retroperitoneal hematoma out of twenty patients treated for DVT with the ATS. None required surgical intervention or transfusion.[33]

The discovery of an underlying venous stenosis can occur after PMT. Thirty-eight to 95% of patients have been shown to have a lesion that is treated with percutaneous angioplasty or primary stenting. Importance should be placed on opening these stenoses so as to avoid outflow obstruction. Reducing outflow obstruction helps prevent recurrent DVT and further reduces the severity of PTS.

Many authors have described the use of various PMT catheters in the treatment of DVT. To date no prospective randomized in vivo trial has been performed comparing PMT to other various methods of DVT treatment. In an in vitro model, Müller-Hülsbeck et al. compared the ATS without a guide wire, with a 0.016-inch guide wire, and with a 0.035-inch guide wire to the Hydrolyser, Oasis, and Amplatz Thrombectomy. Interestingly, the ATS had significantly less thrombus removal using the 0.016-inch guide wire compared to other configurations. No significant difference was found among the other catheters. The highest percentage of embolism was noted with the ATS.[50]

Delomez et al. reported use of the Amplatz Thrombectomy Device in eighteen patients with symptomatic lower extremity DVT. Successful recanalization was reported in 83% of patients. A permanent IVC filter was placed in one patient and a temporary filter placed in another. No pulmonary emboli were reported.[62] The time thrombus was present prior to treatment ranged from 4 to 240 d. The age of DVT that can still be optimally treated with PMT has not been determined. Generally 2 weeks represents a common window used by many practicioners.[47,62–64] Thrombi older than this begin to have a denser fibrin network and are more resistant to PMT. Moreover, older thrombi are associated with an increased incidence of distal embolization.[63]

PMT can also be used alone or in conjunction with thrombolytic therapy. In one study comparing multiple thrombectomy devices and lytic agents, Vendatham et al. reported improved results when coupling the two modalities compared to using either independently.[23] This retrospective review analyzed twenty patients who underwent twenty-two procedures. Due to the retrospective nature of the study, the methods of CDT and the timing and use of PMT could not

be controlled. Vendatham reported an 82% procedural success when both modalities were combined. Major bleeding requiring transfusion occurred in three patients. Reduced doses and thrombolytic infusion times were observed in those undergoing adjunctive PMT. Based on his findings, he concluded that PMT has an important role in the endoluminal therapy for DVT.[23] Siablis et al. compared the ATS with CDT for the treatment of massive pulmonary embolism. He found significant decrease in the mean urokinase dose and duration of therapy in the ATS group.[36]

Many clinical scenarios exist in daily practice in which pharmacologic therapy with either thrombolytic agents or anticoagulation are contraindicated. Although an IVC filter can be placed for prophylaxis against PE, serious short- and long-term sequelae can still threaten the limb. Aside from the short-term decrease in quality of life from edema and pain, the long-term sequelae of PTS are devastating. Multiple reports illustrate resolution of edema, pain, and disability with the use of PMT alone.[33,34,48] Other advantages include minimizing bleeding complications and shorter hospital stays. The benefits of immediate improvement of leg edema following the use of PMT are underestimated. Although PMT is not indicated in some scenarios (e.g., patients with very poor prognosis and DVT), a majority of patients may prove to benefit. More prospective studies are needed to help determine who will benefit most. As technology continues to change rapidly, past studies can be difficult to interpret. Future research must also take into account quality-of-life measures in the short and long term.

Potential disadvantages of PMT are related to the individual catheter designs. Common to the catheters that utilize the Venturi effect is the potential for fluid overload resulting in congestive heart failure and pulmonary edema. The ATS, Hydrolyser, Oasis, and ATD are all designed to function in an isovolumetric manner. Müller-Hülsbeck et al. evaluated all four PMT devices in an in vitro model, and found that none functioned isovolumetrically. The ratio of infused saline to aspirated fluid improved for the ATS when the guide wire was left in place. The Oasis was noted to have the greatest discrepancy between infused saline and aspirated fluid.[50]

Another potential disadvantage of all PMT catheters is hemolysis. Qian et al. found no significant differences regarding the hemolytic effect when comparing the Helix thrombectomy catheter and the ATD.[65] Gandini et al. evaluated plasma free hemoglobin (PFH) levels and hematocrit in eight patients treated for iliocaval thrombosis with the ATD, and found no significant abnormality in either parameter in any patient after treatment.[66] Uflacker reported a significant increase in PFH in thirteen patients treated with the ATD. The PFH levels returned to normal within 24 h.[47] In preclinical evaluations, treatment with the ATS resulted in a transient increase in PFH and a concomitant decrease in the hematocrit.[31] In eighteen patients treated with the ATS for DVT, Delomez et al. reported no postoperative anemia. One patient developed a transient increase in haptoglobin without clinical sequelae.[62] However, Danetz et al. reported two patients with chronic renal insufficiency who developed pancreatitis after using the ATS.[67] The degree of hemolysis is directly proportional to the length of PMT. In patients with chronic renal insufficiency, minimizing the treatment time and careful attention to the hydration status may ameliorate the occurrence of posttreatment pancreatitis. Use of the ATPTD has not resulted in clinically significant elevation of the PFH after treatment of thrombosed hemodialysis grafts.[38]

Based on these observations, patients with renal and hepatic insufficiency should proceed with caution when considering PMT. The increased PFH can result in intranephronal cast formation resulting in acute renal failure. The increased PFH also increases heme catabolism, which enhances the formation of tetrapyrrol unconjugated bilirubin. The unconjugated bilirubin is metabolized and excreted by the liver. Those with abnormal liver function may not tolerate the increased PFH.[47] Although these considerations are paramount, no case of renal failure or fulminant hepatic failure has been reported after PMT.

CONCLUSION

PMT offers many benefits in short-term therapy for DVT. Faster thrombus removal, smaller doses of thrombolytic agents, and shorter treatment times translate into improved symptom relief, decreased complications, and more efficient patient care. Additionally, more rapid thrombus resolution potentially can preserve valvular function and decrease the incidence and severity of PTS. PMT should be considered as first-line therapy for patients presenting with DVT. Advanced endovascular skills, as well as being well versed in possible complications of PMT, are required to provide safe and effective patient care.

REFERENCES

1. Anderson FA, Wheeler HB, Goldberg RJ, et al. A population-based perspective of the hospital incidence and case fatalities of deep vein thrombosis and pulmonary embolism: The Worcester DVT study, *Arch Intern Med.* 1991. *151*: 933–938.
2. Sharafuddin MJ, Sun S, Hoballah JJ, et al. Endovascular management of venous thrombotic occlusive disease of the lower extremities, *J Vasc Interv Radiol.* 2003. *14*: 405–423.
3. Bravo SM, Reinhart RD, Meyerovitz MF. Percutaneous venous interventions, *Vasc Med.* 1998. *3*: 61–66.
4. Wakefield TW, Greenfield LJ. Diagnostic approaches and surgical treatment of venous thrombosis and pulmonary embolism, *Hematol Oncol Clin North Am.* 1993. *7*: 1251–1267.
5. Carson J, Kelle M, Duff A, et al. The clinical course of pulmonary embolism, *N Engl J Med.* 1992. *326*: 1240–1245.
6. Asbeutah AM, Riha AZ, Cameron JD, McGrath BP. Five-year outcome study of deep venous thrombosis in the lower limbs, *J Vasc Surg.* 2004. *40*: 1184–1190.
7. D'Angelo A, Mannucci PM. Outcome of treatment of deep-vein thrombosis with urokinase: Relationship to dosage, duration of therapy, age of the thrombus and laboratory changes, *Thromb Haemost.* 1984. *51*: 236–239.
8. Marder VJ, Brenner B, Totterman S, et al. Comparison of dosage schedules of rt-PA in the treatment of proximal deep vein thrombosis, *J Lab Clin Med.* 1992. *119*: 485–495.
9. Schweizer J, Kirch W, Koch R, et al. Short- and long-term results after thrombolytic treatment of deep venous thrombosis, *J Am Coll Cardiol* 2000. *36*: 1336–1343.
10. Meyerovitz MF, Polak JF, Goldhaber SZ. Short-term response to thrombolytic therapy in deep venous thrombosis: Predictive value of venographic appearance, *Radiology.* 1992. *184*: 345–348.
11. Ott P, Eldrup E, Oxholm P, et al. Streptokinase therapy in the routine management of deep venous thrombosis in the lower extremities: A retrospective study of phlebographic results and therapeutic complications, *Acta Med Scand.* 1986. *219*: 295–300.
12. Eichlisberger R, Fruachiger B, Widmer MT, et al. Late sequelae of deep venous thrombosis: A 13-year follow-up of 223 patients, *Vasa.* 1994. *23*: 234–243.
13. Goldhaber SZ, Buring JE, Lipnick RJ, et al. Pooled analyses of randomized trials of streptokinase and heparin in phlebographically documented acute deep venous thrombosis, *Am J Med.* 1984. *76*: 393–397.
14. Bounameux H, Banga JD, Bluhmki E, et al. Double-blinded, randomized comparison of systemic continuous infusion of 0.25 versus 0.50 mg/kg/24 h of ateplase over 3 to 7 days for treatment of deep venous thrombosis in heparinized patients: Results of the European Thrombolysis with rt-PA in Venous Thrombosis (ETTT) trial, *Thromb Haemost.* 1992. *67*: 306–309.
15. Francis CW, Totterman S. Magnetic resonance imaging of deep vein thrombi correlates with response to thrombolytic therapy, *Thromb Haemost.* 1995. *73*: 386–391.
16. AbuRhama AF, Perkins SE, Wulu JT, et al. Iliofemoral deep venous thrombosis: Conventional therapy versus lysis and percutaneous transluminal angioplasty and stenting, *Ann Surg.* 2001. *233*: 752–760.
17. Sharma GVRK, Folland ED, McIntyre KM, et al. Long term benefit of thrombolytic therapy in patients with pulmonary embolism, *Vasc Med.* 2000. 5: 91–95.
18. Castaneda F, Li R, Young K, et al. Catheter-directed thrombolysis in deep venous thrombosis with use of reteplase: Immediate results and complications from a pilot study, *J Vasc Interv Radiol.* 2002. *13*: 577–580.
19. Meissner MH. Thrombolytic therapy for acute deep vein thrombosis and the venous registry, *Rev Cardiovasc Med.* 2002. 3(Suppl): S53–S60.
20. Comerota AJ, Aldridge SA, Cohen G, et al. A strategy of aggressive regional therapy for acute iliofemoral thrombosis with contemporary venous thrombectomy or catheter-directed thrombolysis, *J Vasc Surg.* 1994. *20*: 244–254.
21. Comerota AJ. Quality-of-life improvement using thrombolytic therapy for iliofemoral deep vein thrombosis, *Rev Cardiovasc Med.* 2002. 3: S61–S67.
22. Kasirajan K, Haskal ZJ, Ouriel K. The use of mechanical thrombectomy devices in the management of acute peripheral arterial occlusive disease, *J Vasc Interv Radiol.* 2001. *12*: 405–411.
23. Vendantham S, Vesely TM, Parti N, et al. Lower extremity venous thrombolysis with adjunctive mechanical thrombectomy, *J Vasc Interv Radiol.* 2002. *13*: 1001–1008.
24. Grimm W, Schwieder G, Wagner T. Fatal pulmonary embolism in venous thrombosis of the leg and pelvis during lysis therapy, *Dtsch Med Wschr.* 1990. *115*: 1183–1187.
25. Wildberger JE, Haage P, Bovelander J, et al. Percutaneous venous thrombectomy using the Arrow-Trerotola percutaneous thrombolytic device (PTD) with temporary caval filtration: In vitro investigations, *Cardiovasc Intervent Radiol.* 2005. *28*: 221–227.

26. Trerotola SO, McLennan G, Davidson D, et al. Preclinical in vivo testing of the Arrow-Trerotola percutaneous thrombolytic device for venous thrombosis, *J Vasc Interv Radiol*. 2001. *12*: 95–103.

27. Trerotola SO, McLennan G, Eclavea AC, et al. Mechanical thrombolysis of venous thrombosis in an animal model with use of temporary caval filtration, *J Vasc Interv Radiol*. 2001. *12*: 1075–1085.

28. Danetz JS, McLafferty RB, Ayerdi J, et al. Selective venography versus nonselective venography before vena cava filter placement: Evidence for more, not less, *J Vasc Surg*. 2003. *28*: 928–934.

29. Stahr P, Rupprecht HJ, Voigtlander T, et al. A new thrombectomy catheter device (AngioJet) for the disruption of thrombi: An in vitro study, *Catheter Cardiovasc Interv*. 1999. *47*: 381–389.

30. Bush RL, Lin PH, Lumsden AB. Mechanical thrombectomy in deep venous thrombosis, *J Invas Cardiol*. 2004. *16*: 16S–22S.

31. Sharafuddin MJ, Hicks ME, Jennson ML, et al. Rheolytic thrombectomy with the Angioget F105 catheter: Preclinical evaluation of safety, *J Vasc Interv Radiol*. 1997. *8*: 939–945.

32. Silva JA, Ramee SR, Collins TJ, et al. Rheolytic thrombectomy in the treatment of acute limb-threatening ischemia: Immediate results and six-month follow-up of the multicenter AngioJet registry, *Cathet Cardiovasc Diagn*. 1998. *45*: 386–393.

33. Bush RL, Lin PH, Bates JT, et al. Pharmacomechanical thrombectomy for treatment of symptomatic lower extremity deep venous thrombosis: Safety and feasibility study, *J Vasc Surg*. 2004. *40*: 965–970.

34. Kasirajan K, Gray B, Ouriel K. Percutaneous AngioJet thrombectomy in the management of extensive deep venous thrombosis, *J Vasc Interv Radiol*. 2001. *12*: 179–185.

35. Schneider DB, Curry TK, Eichler CM, et al. Percutaneous mechanical thrombectomy for the management of venous thoracic outlet syndrome, *J Endovasc Ther*. 2003. *10*: 336–340.

36. Siablis D, Karnabatidis D, Katsanos K, et al. AngioJet rheolytic thrombectomy versus local intrapulmonary thrombolysis in massive pulmonary embolism: A retrospective data analysis, *J Endovasc Ther*. 2005. *12*: 206–214.

37. Ruy R, Lin TC, Kumpe D, et al. Percutaneous mesenteric venous thrombectomy and thrombolysis: Successful treatment followed by liver transplantation, *Liver Transpl Surg*. 1998. *4*: 222–225.

38. Trerotola SO, Vesely TM, Lund GB, et al. Treatment of thrombosed hemodialysis access grafts: Arrow-Trerotola percutaneous thrombolytic device versus pulse-spray thrombolysis, *Radiology*. 1998. *206*: 403–414.

39. McLennan G, Trerotola SO, Davidson D, et al. The effects of a mechanical thrombolytic device on normal canine vein valves, *J Vasc Interv Radiol*. 2001. *12*: 89–94.

40. Lazzaro CR, Treretola SO, Shah H, et al. Modified use of the Arrow-Trerotola percutaneous thrombolytic device for the treatment of thrombosed hemodialysis access grafts, *J Vasc Interv Radiol*. 1999. *10*: 1025–1031.

41. Roček M, Peregrin JH, Laštovička J, et al. Mechanical thrombolysis of thrombosed hemodialysis native fistulas with use of the Arrow-Trerotola percutaneous thrombolytic device: Our preliminary experience, *J Vasc Interv Radiol*. 2000. *11*: 1153–1158.

42. Trerotola SO, McLennan G, Davidson D, et al. Preclinical in vivo testing of the Arrow-Trerotola percutaneous thrombolytic device for venous thrombosis, *J Vasc Interv Radiol*. 2001. *12*: 1295–1103.

43. Truong TH, Spuentrup E, Staatz G, et al. Mechanical thrombectomy of iliocaval thrombosis using a protective expandable sheath, *Cardiovasc Intervent Radiol*. 2004. *27*: 254–258.

44. Yasui K, Qian Z, Nazarian GK, et al. Recirculation-type Amplatz clot macerator: Determination of particle size and distribution, *J Vasc Interv Radiol*. 1993. *4*: 275–278.

45. Sofocleous CT, Cooper SG, Schur I, et al. Retrospective comparison of the Amplatz thrombectomy device with modified pulse-spray pharmacomechanical thrombolysis in the treatment of thrombosed hemodialysis access grafts, *Radiology*. 1999. *213*: 561–567.

46. Uflacker R, Rajagopalan PR, Selby JB, et al. Thrombosed dialysis access grafts: Randomized comparison of the Amplatz thrombectomy device and surgical thromboembolectomy, *Eur Radiol*. 2004. *14*: 2009–2014.

47. Uflacker R. Mechanical thrombectomy in acute and subacute thrombosis with use of the Amplatz device: Arterial and venous applications, *J Vasc Interv Radiol*. 1997. *8*: 923–932.

48. Smith GJ, Molan MP, Brooks DM. Mechanical thrombectomy in acute venous thrombosis using an Amplatz thrombectomy device, *Australas Radiol*. 1999. *43*: 456–460.

49. Müller-Hülsbeck S, Brossmann J, Jahnke T, et al. Mechanical thrombectomy of major and massive pulmonary embolism with use of the Amplatz thrombectomy device, *Invest Radiol*. 2001. *36*: 317–322.

50. Müller-Hülsbeck S, Grimm J, Leidt J, et al. Comparison of in vitro effectiveness of mechanical thrombectomy devices, *J Vasc Interv Radiol*. 2001. *12*: 1185–1191.

51. Bucker A, Schmitz-Rode T, Vorwerk D, et al. Comparative in vitro study of two percutaneous hydrodynamic thrombectomy systems, *J Vasc Interv Radiol*. 1996. *7*: 445–449.

52. Fava M, Loyola S, Huete I. Massive pulmonary embolism: Treatment with the hydrolyser thrombectomy catheter, *J Vasc Interv Radiol*. 2000. *11*: 1159–1164.

53. Henry M, Amor M, Henry I, et al. The hydrolyser thrombectomy catheter: A single-center experience, *J Endovasc Surg*. 1998. *5*: 24–31.

54. Poon WL, Luk SH, Yam KY, et al. Mechanical thrombectomy in inferior vena cava thrombosis after caval filter placement: A report of three cases, *Cardiovasc Intervent Radiol*. 2002. *25*: 440–443.

55. Qian Z, Wholey M, Ferral H, et al. Recanalization of thrombosed superficial femoral arteries with a hydraulic thrombectomy catheter in a canine model, *Am J Roentgenol*. 1999. *173*: 1557–1563.

56. Barth KH, Gosnell MR, Palestrant AM, et al. Hydrodynamic thrombectomy system versus pulse-spray thrombolysis for thrombosed hemodialysis grafts: A multicenter prospective randomized comparison, *Radiology*. 2000. *217*: 678–684.

57. Sahni V, Kaniyur S, Malhotra A, et al. Mechanical thrombectomy of occluded hemodialysis native fistulas and grafts using a hydrodynamic thrombectomy catheter: Preliminary experience, *Cardiovasc Intervent Radiol*. 2005. *28*(6): 714–721.

58. Takahashi N, Kuroki K, Yanaga K. Percutaneous transhepatic mechanical thrombectomy for acute mesenteric venous thrombosis, *J Endovasc Ther*. 2005. *12*: 508–511.

59. Arko FR, Cipriano P, Lee E, et al. Treatment of axillosubclavian vein thrombosis: A novel technique for rapid removal of clot using low-dose thrombolysis, *J Endovasc Ther*. 2003. *10*: 733–738.

60. Ramaiah V, Del Santo PB, Rodriguez-Lopez JA, et al. Trellis thrombectomy system for the treatment of iliofemoral deep venous thrombosis, *J Endovasc Ther*. 2003. *10*: 585–589.

61. Sofocleous CT, Cooper SG, Schur I, et al. Retrospective comparison of the Amplatz thrombectomy device with modified pulse-spray pharmacomechanical thrombolysis in the treatment of thrombosed hemodialysis access grafts, *Radiology*. 1999. *213*: 561–567.

62. Delomez M, Beregi JP, Willoteaux S, et al. Mechanical thrombectomy in patients with deep venous thrombosis, *Cardiovasc Interv Radiol*. 2001. *24*: 42–48.

63. Coleman CC, Krenzel C, Dietz CA, et al. Mechanical thrombectomy: Results of early experience, *Radiology*. 1993. *189*: 803–805.

64. Bjarnason H, Kruse JR, Asinger DA, et al. Iliofemoral deep venous thrombosis: Safety and efficacy outcome during five years of catheter-directed thrombolytic therapy, *J Vasc Interv Radiol*. 1997. *8*: 405–418.

65. Qian Z, Kvamme P, Ragheed D, et al. Comparison of a new recirculation thrombectomy catheter with other devices of the same type: In vitro and in vivo evaluations, *Invest Radiol*. 2001. *37*: 503–511.

66. Gandini R, Maspes F, Sodani G, et al. Percutaneous iliocaval thrombectomy with the Amplatz device: Preliminary results, *Eur Radiol*. 1999. *9*: 951–958.

67. Danetz JS, McLafferty RB, Ayerdi J, et al. Pancreatitis caused by rheolytic thrombolysis: An unexpected complication, *J Vasc Interv Radiol*. 2004. *15*: 857–860.

48.

DIAGNOSIS AND MANAGEMENT OF PRIMARY AXILLOSUBCLAVIAN VENOUS THROMBOSIS

Niren Angle

BACKGROUND AND HISTORY

Venous thrombosis resulting from compression of the axillosubclavian vein at the thoracic outlet is a condition that, in contrast to most vascular disorders, afflicts young, otherwise healthy, and frequently quite physically active individuals. It is the venous manifestation of thoracic outlet compression, otherwise known by its eponym—Paget-Schroetter syndrome. Sometime around the 1950s, the term "thoracic outlet syndrome" (TOS) crept into the parlance of the medical and surgical literature, and was first used to describe both the arterial and neurogenic conditions, recognizing the not-infrequent overlap between the vascular and the neurologic manifestations of compression at the thoracic outlet. As Machleder has written, "neurovascular compression at the thoracic outlet is perhaps best developed in the context of the historical evolution of etiologic concepts, and the unique anatomic characteristics that underlie the varied clinical manifestations."[1]

The first two cases of spontaneous or effort-related axillosubclavian vein thrombosis were published independently over 100 years ago by Paget in England[2] and Von Schroetter in Germany.[3] In 1949, E. S. R. Hughes analyzed 320 cases of spontaneous upper extremity venous thrombosis in the medical literature and in recognition of the fact that this represented a unique disorder, named it the Paget-Schroetter syndrome.[4] At that time, surgical thrombectomy was the mainstay of therapy, with the goal being to restore venous patency, and was attended by high early rethrombosis rates. Until the 1980s, this remained the mainstay of therapy, at which time the availability of catheter-directed thrombolysis introduced a significant improvement in the treatment of this condition.

A significant amount of natural history data of this condition is available, which attests to the fact that untreated patients with Paget-Schroetter syndrome develop varying degrees of disability as a result of the chronic venous hypertension accompanied many times with recurrent episodes of venous thrombosis. Tilney et al. reported a 74% incidence of related disability,[5] whereas Linblad from Sweden reported it in the range of 25%.[6] In addition, there is a finite incidence of pulmonary thromboembolism as well.[7] Upper extremity venous thrombosis accounts for approximately 2% of deep venous thrombosis. In sum, Paget-Schroetter syndrome represents a condition that afflicts a young, active, and productive segment of the population, and if not aggressively treated, will result in significant disability that affects the function and productivity of this group of people.

THE ANATOMY OF THE THORACIC OUTLET

The superior opening of the bony thorax is now considered to be the thoracic outlet, sometimes termed the "superior thoracic aperture." The anatomic features of the thoracic outlet are descriptive in their own right in terms of explaining the varied clinical manifestations that encompass the thoracic outlet syndromes, namely the arterial, venous, and neurogenic TOS subtypes.

In a review in 1986, the neurologist W. S. Fields wrote:

All shoulder girdle compression syndromes have one common feature, namely, compression of the brachial plexus, the subclavian artery, and subclavian vein, usually between the first rib and the clavicle. With elevation of the upper limb, there is a scissorlike approximation of the clavicle superiorly and the first rib inferiorly. Grouping the various conditions under the single heading of thoracic outlet syndrome has resulted in more correct diagnosis and improved therapy.[8]

The anatomic feature underlying compression in the thoracic outlet is the presence of four spaces through which the neurovascular structures must traverse in their path from the neck to the axilla. These four spaces are the superior thoracic aperture, the interscalene triangle, the costoclavicular passage, and the subcoracoid space.[9] Of these, the interscalene triangle is a space bordered by the anterior scalene muscle anteriorly, the middle scalene muscle posteriorly, and the first rib inferiorly. The subclavian vein can also be compressed by first rib anomalies or by abnormal muscular insertions.[1,10] The costoclavicular space is most commonly the area where the subclavian vein is compressed in Paget-Schroetter syndrome; this is a space made up of the subclavius muscle anteriorly, the clavicle anteriorly, the first rib posteriorly, and the scapula and subscapularis muscle posterolaterally.

The inciting cause of Paget-Schroetter syndrome now is recognized to be compression and constriction at the costoclavicular portion of the axillosubclavian vein, the critical stenosis of which results in thrombus formation, extending distally from that junction into the axillary and often the brachial veins. The thrombosis always occurs in the area of chronic compression and resultant narrowing at the thoracic outlet. The vein is compressed between a hypertrophied anterior scalene muscle and subclavius tendon and the first rib. One may also occasionally see a large exostosis at the costoclavicular junction.

PRESENTATION

The male-to-female ratio is approximately 2:1, commonly in the third decade, although Urschel et al. have published their large experience with male:female ratios being roughly equal.[11] Patients typically will provide a recent history of strenuous or repetitive upper arm activity prior to the onset of symptoms. The typical patient is one who is either a competitive athlete or one whose profession requires repetitive upper arm exertion. This is primarily a condition of the young/middle-aged active person, and as such, the condition is quite disabling. The typical patient may be a student that swims, plays tennis competitively, lifts weights, or alternatively, a fireman, professional athlete, or a worker that performs heavy and repetitive lifting.

In a group of fifty consecutive patients at UCLA treated for Paget-Schroetter syndrome, Machleder described thirty-one men with a mean age of 24 (range 14–50 years) and nineteen women with a mean age of 38 (range 23–51 years).[12] All but one of the men had been engaged in vigorous physical activity at the time of the onset of symptoms, and ten of these were student athletes. Eleven women were engaged in sedentary occupations, and eight were involved in activities involving upper extremity exertion.

The patient will typically notice severe and uniform swelling of the upper extremity rather suddenly. Usually, there is a slight rubor or more commonly, some cyanosis. Collateral veins around the shoulder and chest on the affected side start becoming prominent within a few days. If these symptoms are ignored or the patient is not definitively treated, over days the symptoms of heaviness, aching, tightness, and arm swelling may improve and may resolve. These symptoms may be mild or not noticeable at rest after adequate time has gone by but the observant patient will notice that with mild activity involving the upper arm, swelling, heaviness, fatigue, and sweating are easily evident. It is these symptoms and outcomes that one attempts to prevent by prompt treatment and decompression of the thoracic outlet.

It is important to remember that the physical exam findings are dependent on the time from symptom onset to examination. In the patient with a recent onset (i.e., hours to days), one will expect to see edema, tightness, cyanosis, and symptoms of heaviness and aching, and rarely pain and tenderness. If many days to weeks have elapsed, the patient at rest may show little of these signs. In this case, if one exercises the patient by having them do push-ups in a warm room, one may note more duskiness and prominence of collateral veins. With continued exercise, the patient may complain of pain, particularly in the supraclavicular, pectoral, or axillary regions. Upon cessation of exercise, these signs and symptoms resolve rapidly.

DIAGNOSIS

The diagnosis of spontaneous or effort thrombosis of the axillosubclavian vein is not a subtle endeavor. The symptoms as just described are the sine qua non of this condition, and these symptoms in the right patient must be considered due to axillosubclavian thrombosis until proven otherwise.

Imaging is the next step. However, if acute thrombosis is suspected, prompt anticoagulation with heparin is indicated. More often than not though, by the time the patient presents to a physician who can make the correct diagnosis, the elapsed time is more on the order of days rather than hours. Even in this situation, the patient should be anticoagulated with heparin.

The definitive study to confirm the clinical suspicion and facilitate treatment is a contrast venogram. Noninvasive studies such as duplex ultrasound, in my opinion, have little to offer in this situation. There are a limited number of published reports on the sensitivity and specificity of ultrasonography in comparison with contrast venography.[13,14] The reported sensitivity and specificity rates vary from 78 to 100% and 82 to 100%, respectively. No studies specifically have addressed interobserver and intraobserver variability, but it is a widely known fact that ultrasonography is operator dependent in daily practice and that some patients may be more difficult to investigate, such as those with very extensive edema or obesity.

The proximal axillosubclavian vein is difficult to image directly with ultrasound except in the case of a slender individual. Magnetic resonance venography (MRV) is better at imaging the axillosubclavian vein and for this diagnosis, but once again, access into the venous system is going to be necessary for the first step of treatment. In the presence of clinical suspicion (i.e., a sudden onset of swelling, aching, heaviness), cyanosis and pain in one arm is venous thrombosis until proven otherwise. I would submit that even with a negative duplex, unless the vein was clearly imaged throughout its course, the chances of a false negative duplex ultrasound should make contrast venography the definitive study that allows for diagnosis and treatment.

In addition to being the gold standard, contrast venography is a seamless road to the next step of therapy, namely, catheter-directed thrombolysis of the clotted vein. Prior to the advent of and the demonstrated safety and efficacy of catheter-directed thrombolysis, the treatment of these patients primarily would be surgical thrombectomy with its associated high rethrombosis rates or warfarin anticoagulation.

In a recent paper from the United Kingdom, the authors reviewed their experience with Paget-Schroetter syndrome in four district hospitals.[15] The majority of these patients were treated by nonsurgeons and were treated with warfarin anticoagulation. This treatment strategy was rewarded with a 33% rate of persisting disability—in the authors' estimation, an unacceptably high rate in this era. These results are not dissimilar to the outcomes noted before the use of thrombolysis and thoracic outlet decompression.

VENOGRAPHY

Diagnostic venography is performed by accessing the antecubital veins on the affected side. The patient is supine and the venogram is performed ideally with the arm at the patient's side and with the arm at right angles to the chest wall. Figures 48.1 and 48.2 demonstrate the venograms of

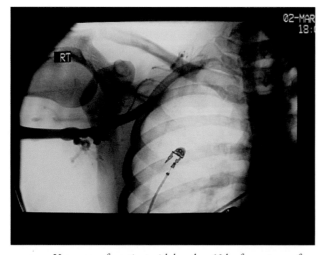

Figure 48.1   Venogram of a patient with less than 12 h of symptoms of arm swelling, aching, and heaviness. The venogram shows abrupt cutoff of contrast with no visible collateral venous channels, suggesting an acute thrombosis of the axillosubclavian vein.

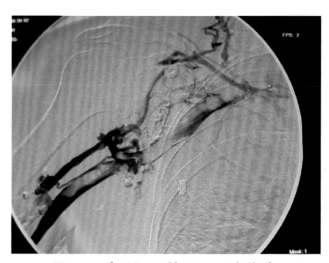

Figure 48.2   Venogram of an 18-year-old swimmer with 6 h of onset of acute arm swelling, pain, and dusky discoloration, which reveals extensive thrombosis of the axillary and subclavian veins.

patients with acute axillosubclavian vein thrombosis. By contrast, Figure 48.2 shows a venogram with long-standing venous thrombosis of the axillosubclavian vein. Note the extensive collateralization around the shoulder joint.

TREATMENT

THROMBOLYSIS

The contrast venogram confirms the diagnosis of Paget-Schroetter syndrome and allows for immediate treatment. Once the thrombosis is confirmed, an infusion catheter can be positioned into the vein and thrombolytic therapy can be initiated. The thrombolytic agent of choice in the 1990s used to be urokinase, but, due to the withdrawal of urokinase from the market in the late 1990s, new experience was gained with the use of alternative agents such as tissue plasminogen activator (tPA) and reteplase (Retevase). Urokinase has since been reintroduced into the market, but all these agents have proven to be safe and efficacious. Urokinase can be administered at doses of 125,000 U to 250,000 U/h. tPA is administered at an initial dose of anywhere from 0.5 to 3 mg/h and reteplase is administered at doses of 0.5 to 1 U/h. Typically, the period of lytic therapy is less than 24 h, but if the clot is of a longer duration, then longer infusion times are necessary.

Lytic therapy allows for complete clot lysis with minimal trauma to the venous endothelium compared to surgical thrombectomy. Upon completion of lysis, one may see a stricture of the vein due to extrinsic compression in the thoracic outlet. The temptation to perform a balloon angioplasty at this time must be strongly resisted. The reason is that until and unless the thoracic outlet is decompressed and the causative compression relieved, balloon angioplasty is destined to fail. Similarly, placement of a venous stent at this time is also to be strongly condemned, as it is doomed to failure. Urschel et al. reported on a series of patients with Paget-Schroetter syndrome treated at outside hospitals with lysis and intravenous stent placement without operative decompression of the thoracic outlet.[16] Out of twenty-two patients treated thus, twenty-two patients reoccluded their vein from 1 d to 6 weeks after stent placement. This is an illustration of a treatment that is not only *not* successful, but is to be condemned in light of the fact that patients treated optimally have such a good outcome following lysis and first rib resection.

TREATMENT FOLLOWING THROMBOLYSIS

Following successful thrombolysis, one is faced with either a patient with a patent axillosubclavian vein with luminal narrowing due to extrinsic compression or stricture due to long-standing extrinsic narrowing, or a patient with a widely patent axillosubclavian vein with no stenosis or with stenosis only in the stressed, arm abducted position. Certainly, if there is evidence of venous stenosis after thrombolysis, it is prima facie evidence of the fact that compression of the axillosubclavian vein is due to thoracic outlet compression and accordingly, operative decompression of the thoracic outlet should be performed. If the axillosubclavian vein following thrombolysis appears to be patent without any evidence of stenosis in the neutral position, the vein should be studied in the stressed position. The provocative maneuvers employed can be any or all of the following:

- Abduction and external rotation
- Arm overhead
- Arm pulled down to the side

If vein compression with any or all of these maneuvers is noted, we would recommend first rib resection with subtotal scalenectomy. If no vein compression is noted with any of these maneuvers, then the decision becomes a little more difficult. Although it is perfectly defensible to anticoagulate the patients for 3 to 6 months, first rib resection still should be considered since it is still the most likely cause of spontaneous thrombosis of the axillosubclavian vein in an otherwise normal healthy patient.

TIMING OF OPERATIVE THERAPY

Thrombolysis results in recanalization of the vein and relief of arm swelling, aching, heaviness, and other symptoms. Until a few years ago, the maxim was that following lytic therapy, the patient should be anticoagulated for 4 to 6 weeks

with warfarin, and after this time had passed, a transaxillary first rib resection would be performed. This algorithm was based more on a theoretical consideration of the perivenous inflammation rather than any data suggesting that early rib resection was hazardous. This algorithm was challenged by a number of groups performing early first rib resection with equal safety, and the added benefit of avoiding prolonged warfarin use in these young patients. We reported on the safety of such an approach wherein following thrombolysis, we performed a transaxillary first rib resection on the same admission with no difference in complications or efficacy.[17]

Accordingly, we would now recommend that the patient presenting with acute axillosubclavian vein thrombosis should have a venogram, then lytic therapy, followed by transaxillary first rib resection on the same admission. This approach results in quick and definitive therapy. Recognizing that in a subset of patients (approximately 30%) there will be a residual venous stricture despite decompression of the thoracic outlet due to long-standing extrinsic compression, it is our practice to perform a venogram on all patients approximately 2 weeks following first rib resection. If a significant stenosis is identified at that time, a percutaneous transluminal angioplasty (PTA) is performed. These lesions respond very nicely to PTA alone, and we have not found the use of a stent in this situation necessary. Figure 48.3 demonstrates the venogram of one such patient that had thrombolysis, then transaxillary first rib resection, followed by PTA of a venous stenosis 2 weeks following first rib resection.

OPERATION

In 1966, Roos reported a series of fifteen patients treated by removal of the first rib from a transaxillary approach.[18] This was a major milestone, as the dramatic superiority of this technique was widely recognized and quickly accepted. The transaxillary first rib resection is the standard operation

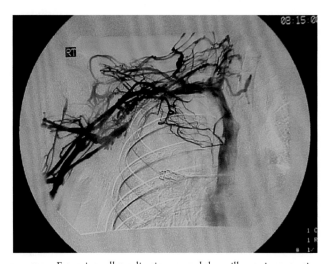

Figure 48.3   Extensive collateralization around the axillary vein suggesting a more long-standing thrombosis of the axillosubclavian vein.

for removal of the first thoracic rib. Alternative approaches to the removal of the first rib involve an infraclavicular approach to the anterior first rib and/or a supraclavicular approach to removal of the entire first rib. Some authors have found that there is a higher incidence of brachial plexus injuries with the supraclavicular approach compared to the transaxillary approach.

The transaxillary first rib resection has become the gold standard since its description by Roos in 1966. It provides a rapid and direct approach to the first rib and the incision is discreet and cosmetically appealing. The limitations are that it tends to be an operation in which visualization can be limited due to the fact that one is operating in a cavity with limited visualization, particularly for more than one person. However, with experience, this operation can be done quite easily and with excellent results.

The exact details of the operation can be obtained in a variety of good atlases and will be only briefly described here. The patient is placed in a true lateral position with a pad placed under the other axilla to prevent injury to the brachial plexus. The affected arm is prepped into the field so that it is mobile, and the assistant elevates the stockinette-clad arm by means of a double wrist lock. The arm elevation/retraction is done on an intermittent basis to prevent arm ischemia and brachial plexus injury.

The incision is made transversely at the lower margin of the axilla between the latissimus dorsi and the pectoralis major. This incision is deepened through the subcutaneous tissues and one reaches the cul de sac of fascia that separates the axilla from the thoracic outlet. The view from this incision is such that one sees anteriorly the subclavian vein separated from the subclavian artery by the anterior scalene muscle, with the brachial plexus posterior to the subclavian artery. The anterior scalene is divided sharply and anteriorly. The subclavius muscle and tendon that commonly compress the vein are also divided. The first rib is divided with a bone cutter and the cut edges smoothed appropriately. One can get an excellent view and a complete resection of the first rib through the transaxillary approach. The operation typically takes less than 2 h, and the patient recovery is excellent. Operative details can be obtained by reading the description of Roos[19] as well as the atlas authored by Valentine and Wind.[9]

INTERMITTENT COMPRESSION OF THE AXILLOSUBCLAVIAN VEIN

Thoracic outlet compression can also manifest with intermittent signs and symptoms of arm swelling, aching, pain, and heaviness that resolve within minutes of onset of symptoms. This phenomenon is termed "McLeery's syndrome" and represents a variant of venous thoracic outlet syndrome. All the clinical and anatomic features of Paget-Schroetter syndrome are present, and it is only distinguished by the

fact that the vein has not proceeded to thrombosis. The treatment for this condition should be the same, namely, first rib resection for decompression of the thoracic outlet. Following first rib resection, the patient should undergo venography to ensure that there is no underlying venous stenosis and if there is, PTA of the vein should be performed.

THE ISSUE OF THE CONTRALATERAL VEIN

In the UCLA series, 61% of patients studied with bilateral venography had thrombosis of compression of the contralateral vein.[12] This is the impetus for the recommendation that the patient presenting with symptoms on one side should undergo venography of the contralateral side. Out of forty-one patients studied, twenty patients demonstrated compression and stricture of the contralateral vein, that is, "the unaffected side," in the neutral position and another five patients had evidence of hemodynamically significant compression in the stress position. For this reason, the patient presenting with venous TOS symptoms on one side should have the other side studied and electively repaired by undergoing first rib resection with subtotal scalenectomy.

RESULTS OF TREATMENT

Elman recently published the results of a review of the literature to ascertain the outcomes of patients with upper extremity deep venous thrombosis. The frequency of post-thrombotic syndrome (PTS) after upper extremity deep venous thrombosis ranged from 7 to 46%, and residual thrombosis and axillosubclavian vein thrombosis appeared to be associated with an increased risk of PTS.[20] In addition, quality of life was impaired in patients with upper extremity PTS, especially after venous thrombosis of the upper arm. For this reason, dissolution of venous clot and decompression of the thoracic outlet must be viewed as an imperative.

The results of first rib resection in the context of the algorithm just discussed are excellent. Urschel's series represents one of the largest experiences of 486 patients treated with expeditious lysis and transaxillary first rib resection.[22] Early lysis and decompression is safe in expert hands, effective, and of minimal morbidity. Transaxillary rib resection early after Paget-Schroetter syndrome must be considered the gold standard of therapy. In Machleder's series, fifty consecutive patients were entered into a sequential treatment program for spontaneous axillosubclavian vein thrombosis.[21] Forty-three had initial thrombolytic or anticoagulant treatment followed by longer-term warfarin treatment. This paper preceded the evolution of the treatment algorithm wherein first rib resection was performed right away on the same admission following thrombolysis. Thirty-six (72%) underwent surgical correction of the underlying structural abnormality, and nine patients had postoperative balloon angioplasty. Ninety-three percent of patients with a patent vein and 64% of those with an occluded vein were essentially free of symptoms. After surgical correction there were no episodes of recurrent thrombosis in a mean follow-up period of 3.1 years. Urschel reported a large series of patients with thoracic outlet syndrome, a subset of whom were patients with venous TOS or Paget-Schroetter syndrome.[21] Long-term results indicated that 205 extremities had good results (the patient returned to work without symptoms). Twenty-four patients had fair results (intermittent swelling but able to work), and eleven patients had poor results (chronic swelling). Seven of the poor results occurred in the thirty-five patients seen initially more than 3 months after the thrombotic episode. No patient had phlegmasia cerulea dolens. There were no deaths. These results were in marked contrast to those of thirty-five patients treated with only anticoagulants: ten good results, sixteen fair results, and nine poor results. Urschel's data provides the exclamation point for a series of reports from other institutions that attest to the good outcomes following this method of diagnosis and treatment.

CONCLUSION

In our opinion, conservative, read nonoperative, management for this patient population represents suboptimal treatment, and operative decompression results in better clinical results, better quality of life, and definitive treatment with very low recurrence rates. This illustrates the reason why prompt lysis and first rib resection should be considered the treatment of choice for Paget–Schroetter syndrome.

Paget–Schroetter syndrome is a disabling condition that tends to afflict the young and active and results in considerable long-term compromise of quality of life and disabling symptoms if appropriate and definitive treatment as described earlier is not undertaken. Prompt thrombolysis followed by first rib resection is the treatment of choice for patients with venous TOS that present with thrombosis or with McLeery's syndrome. The transaxillary first rib resection as described by Roos is the gold standard, but anterior approach via a supraclavicular and/or infraclavicular approach also can be used. PTA of the vein should not be undertaken unless the thoracic outlet is surgically decompressed. Venous stents are virtually never necessary, as PTA alone in our experience results in long-term venous patency as attested to by the earlier results. A majority of patients will have venous compression in the thoracic outlet on the contralateral side. Prophylactic first rib resection is recommended for the contralateral side on an elective basis. The evolution of the treatment of Paget-Schroetter syndrome has evolved over the last 2 decades and as it stands, prompt

thrombolysis and early first rib resection (same hospital admission) is associated with very good results and represents the optimal therapy for this condition.

REFERENCES

1. Kashyap VS, Ahn SS, Machleder HI. Thoracic outlet neurovascular compression: Approaches to anatomic decompression and their limitations, *Sem Vasc Surg*. 1998. *11*: 116–122.
2. Paget J. *Clinical lectures and essays*. London: Longmans Green. 1985.
3. Schroetter V. L. *Erkrankungen der Fegasse*. Vienna: Holder. 1884.
4. ESRH. Venous obstruction in the upper extremity (Paget-Schroetter's syndrome), *Int Abstr Surg*. 1949. *88*: 89–127.
5. Tilney ML, Griffiths HJ, Edwards EA. Natural history of major venous thrombosis of the upper extremity, *Arch Surg*. 1970. *101*(6): 792–796.
6. Lindblad B, Bornmyr S, Kullendorff B, Bergqvist D. Venous haemodynamics of the upper extremity after subclavian vein thrombosis, *Vasa*. 1990. *19*(3): 218–222.
7. Harley DP, White RA, Nelson RJ, Mehringer CM. Pulmonary embolism secondary to venous thrombosis of the arm, *Am J Surg*. 1984. *147*(2): 221–224.
8. Fields WS, Lemak NA, Ben-Menachem Y. Thoracic outlet syndrome: Review and reference to stroke in a major league pitcher, *Am J Roentgenol*. 1986. *146*(4): 809–814.
9. Valentine RJ, Wind GG. *Anatomic exposures in vascular surgery*, 2e. 2003. Philadelphia: Lippincott Williams & Wilkins. 577.
10. McCarthy MJ, Varty K, London NJM, Bell PR. Experience of supraclavicular exploration and decompression for treatment of thoracic outlet syndromes, *Ann Vasc Surg*. 1999. *13*: 268–274.
11. Urschel HC Jr, Razzuk MA. Neurovascular compression in the thoracic outlet: Changing management over 50 years, *Ann Surg*. 1998. *228*(4): 609–617.
12. Machleder H. *Vascular disorders of the upper extremity*, 3e. 1998. Armonk, New York: Futura. 515.
13. Baarslag HJ, Koopman MM, Reekers JA, van Beek EJ. Diagnosis and management of deep vein thrombosis of the upper extremity: A review, *Eur Radiol*. 2004. *14*(7): 1263–1274.
14. Gaitini D, Kaftori JK, Pery M, Engel A. High-resolution real-time ultrasonography: Diagnosis and follow-up of jugular and subclavian vein thrombosis, *J Ultrasound Med*. 1988. *7*(11): 621–627.
15. Fassiadis N, Roidl M, South M. Are we managing primary upper limb deep venous thrombosis aggressively enough in the district?, *Int Angiol*. 2005. *24*(3): 255–257.
16. Urschel HC Jr, Patel AN. Paget-Schroetter syndrome therapy: Failure of intravenous stents, *Ann Thorac Surg*. 2003. *75*(6): 1693–1696; discussion 1696.
17. Angle N, Gelabert HA, Farooq MM, et al. Safety and efficacy of early surgical decompression of the thoracic outlet for Paget-Schroetter syndrome, *Ann Vasc Surg*. 2001. *15*(1): 37–42.
18. Roos DB. Transaxillary approach for first rib resection to relieve thoracic outlet syndrome, *Ann Surg*. 1966. *163*(3): 354–358.
19. Roos DB, Owens JC. Thoracic outlet syndrome, *Arch Surg*. 1966. *93*(1): 71–74.
20. Elman EE, Kahn SR. The postthrombotic syndrome after upper extremity deep venous thrombosis in adults: A systematic review, *Thromb Res*. 2005. *117*(6): 609–614.
21. Machleder HI. Evaluation of a new treatment strategy for Paget-Schroetter syndrome: Spontaneous thrombosis of the axillary subclavian vein, *J Vasc Surg*. 1993. *17*(2): 305–315; discussion 316–317.
22. Urschel HC Jr, Patel AN. Surgery remains the most effective treatment for Paget-Schroetter syndrome: 50 years' experience. *Ann Thor Surg*. 2008. *84*(1): 254–260.

49.

SUBCLAVIAN VEIN OBSTRUCTION

TECHNIQUES FOR REPAIR AND BYPASS

Richard J. Sanders

Subclavian vein obstruction, also called venous thoracic outlet syndrome (venous TOS) can be partial or complete. Partial obstruction is due to stenosis; complete obstruction is usually due to thrombosis.

ETIOLOGY

The two categories of causes are primary and secondary. *Primary* subclavian vein obstruction is due to congenital narrowing of the vein at the point where the vein enters the mediastinum just proximal to being joined by the jugular vein. This point lies on the inner aspect of the first rib and is bounded medially by the costoclavicular ligament and superiorly by the subclavius tendon (see Figure 49.1).[1] In most people with narrowing at this point, it may only be demonstrable when the arm is elevated; it appears normal with the arm at the side. As many as 20% of the population have been demonstrated by dynamic venography to have significant narrowing in this area.[2] Fortunately, only a small fraction of these people ever become symptomatic. It is postulated that those who become symptomatic do so because of repetitive movement with the arm in elevated positions causing chronic irritation and fibrosis of the intima in the critical area. Thus, stenosis may be the first pathologic step, which may or may not be followed by thrombosis. Primary subclavian vein thrombosis is also called effort thrombosis, idiopathic thrombosis, or Paget-Schroetter syndrome. The cause of primary subclavian vein obstruction is always *extrinsic* to the vein.

Secondary subclavian vein obstruction is due to known causes such as tumor, coagulopathy, or iatrogenic factors like catheters or wires. Subclavian vein catheters are by far the most common cause of subclavian vein obstruction and thrombosis. For some unknown reason, thrombosis from such catheters seldom causes severe enough symptoms to require treatment other than anticoagulation. With the exception of tumors, the causes of secondary subclavian vein obstruction are always *intrinsic*.

SIGNS AND SYMPTOMS

Swelling of the entire arm is the primary symptom. Swelling limited to the fingers and hand can occur with neurogenic thoracic outlet syndrome and is not indicative of venous obstruction unless the whole arm is involved. Other symptoms are cyanosis, a feeling of fullness, aching, or pain. Some patients have mild paresthesia. Physical examination confirms the swelling and cyanosis. The only other significant finding is dilated subcutaneous veins over the shoulder and upper chest wall of the affected side.

DIAGNOSIS

The two diagnostic tools in use today are duplex scanning and venography. Venous pressure measurements also can be used, but these are cumbersome and unreliable unless there is obvious arm swelling. Duplex scanning requires an experienced technician because the clavicle lies directly over the critical part of the subclavian vein. Though duplex scanning is fairly reliable for total occlusion of the vein, accurate diagnosis of stenosis without thrombosis is difficult. Venography remains the gold standard for evaluating the subclavian vein. A venogram with the arm at rest is usually enough to make the diagnosis of total occlusion, but subclavian vein stenosis may be demonstrable only with dynamic positioning, elevating the arm to 90 degrees and 180 degrees.

TREATMENT

The approach to managing subclavian vein obstruction is three-fold:

1. Remove the thrombus. For recent thrombus, thrombolysis or thrombus extraction with appropriate devices is always the first step. If unsuccessful, surgical thrombectomy can be considered.

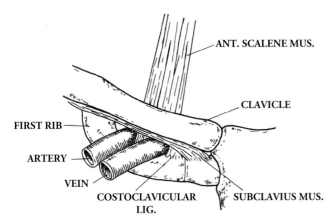

Figure 49.1   Anatomy of the costoclavicular space. The subclavian vein can easily contact the costoclavicular ligament, subclavius muscle, clavicle, first rib, or anterior scalene muscle.   Reprinted with permission from Sanders RJ. Subclavian vein obstruction. In: Bergan JJ, Yao ST, ed. *Venous Disorders*. Philadelphia: WB Saunders; 1991: 256.

2. Remove the extrinsic cause. First rib resection with venolysis is the primary procedure for treating the underlying cause. This should follow removal of the thrombus when dealing with thrombosis, but this is the only treatment needed for nonthrombotic subclavian vein obstruction. Adequate venolysis can be achieved through transaxillary or infraclavicular approaches. In most patients, the supraclavicular route does not provide adequate exposure to divide all the ligaments and totally free the vein. In reports where the supraclavicular route has been tried, the majority of patients also required an additional infraclavicular incision to complete the operation.[3–6] Thus, unless the supraclavicular route is needed to treat neurogenic TOS, venous decompression is best performed through the other approaches.

3. Remove the intrinsic obstruction. Treatment of the intrinsic venous obstruction should be considered only after the first two steps have been completed. In the large majority of patients with subclavian vein obstruction, symptoms will be completely or almost completely relieved once the thrombus has been removed and the subclavian vein decompressed by rib resection and venolysis. Thus, no further treatment is needed. Only in patients who continue to have significant swelling and pain is venous reconstruction indicated.

There are three approaches to relieving intrinsic subclavian vein obstruction:

- Balloon angioplasty
- Endovenectomy with vein patch
- Subclavian vein bypass

BALLOON ANGIOPLASTY

Percutaneous balloon angioplasty (PTA) is usually successful in treating stenosis when performed after the subclavian vein has been decompressed by resection of the first rib

and the attached ligaments. Prior to first rib resection, the extrinsic pressure around the vein prevents its expansion, making PTA ineffective. Studies of PTA performed prior to rib resection have revealed not only uniform failure but in several patients, rethrombosis was precipitated by the attempt.[7]

More than one center has followed a protocol of routine balloon angioplasty in those patients with residual stenosis either immediately after rib resection in the operating room suite, or within a few days of rib resection in the angio suite.[5,8] The results have been successful in over 90% of the patients. This certainly raises the question of whether or not this should be used in all patients with residual stenosis following surgical decompression. However, in our experience, we have not found it necessary to use PTA routinely on all postoperative stenoses, although we do use it on tight stenoses with collaterals as seen on resting venograms. Patients with stenosis of less than 80 to 90% have been followed and if symptoms of swelling and aching persist, PTA is performed. This protocol has been quite successful as seldom have patients with residual postoperative stenosis been symptomatic and required additional treatment.

ENDOVENECTOMY WITH VEIN PATCH

If thrombolysis has been incomplete and residual thrombus or tight stenosis remains, two approaches may be employed. Either proceed with first rib resection and venolysis, followed by PTA, or consider opening the vein, performing surgical thrombectomy, endovenectomy, and closing the venotomy with a vein patch graft. The same technique also has been applied to total occlusion of less than 2 cm.[9] Unfortunately, in some patients adequate proximal venous control cannot be obtained without opening the mediastinum. A median sternotomy down to the first interspace and then a transverse incision into the interspace will free enough of the manubrium to elevate the clavicle and provide excellent exposure for the procedure.[10] Although we have had 100% success with this technique in eleven patients, it is an extensive procedure requiring several weeks to completely recover from the operation. It makes sense to try PTA first if at all possible. Endovenectomy can be performed a day or two later if PTA fails. Endovenectomy is performed via a 12- to 14-cm infraclavicular incision, splitting the pectoralis major fibers between sternal and clavicular heads, and mobilizing the subclavian vein. If the first rib is still present, it is now excised, dividing the anterior end at the costal cartilage then removing as much additional cartilage and manubrium as needed to expose the subclavian vein as far medial as possible. The subclavian vein is palpated to locate the proximal end of the thickened vein. If the proximal vascular clamp can be applied on thin, soft vein, no further exposure is needed. If the proximal vein cannot be reached because of the overhanging sternum, the

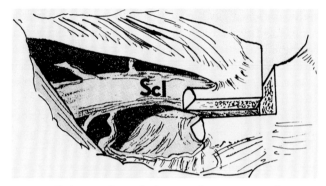

Figure 49.2 Technique of sternal splinting to first interspace with transverse extension laterally to free the clavicle with a small piece of sternum attached. This provides excellent exposure of subclavian-innominate junction. Repair is with two or three sutures of heavy Dacron or wire. Reprinted with permission from Molina JE. A new surgical approach to the innominate and subclavian vein, *J Vasc Surg*. 1998. *27*: 576–581.

trap door sternal flap of Molina through the first interspace is created to expose the subclavian-innominate junction (see Figure 49.2). Following distal and proximal control, the patient is heparinized and a venotomy performed over the thickened venous segment. Thrombectomy is performed first, removing all organized clot proximal and distal to the venotomy with embolectomy forceps. Thickened, organized clot that is firmly adherent to the intima cannot be removed with embolectomy forceps. This often has the appearance of a tumor inside the vein. This must be excised

sharply with scissors or a knife, leaving a small rim of clot remaining against venous intima. It is impossible to find a smooth plane of dissection in the vein wall as is done with arterial endarterectomy. When this is attempted in a vein, the adventitia usually is perforated. It is best to simply leave a 1- to 2-mm thickness of organized clot against the vein wall (see Figure 49.3). A saphenous vein patch is used to close the venotomy. In most patients, we have left a few centimeters of the saphenous vein graft unopened, in continuity with the distal tip of the patch. The end of this vein is then sewn to the side of the axillary artery to create a temporary arteriovenous fistula (AVF) that will flow directly over the endovenectomy segment. This is done to prevent postoperative thrombosis of the repair, which tends to occur in low-pressure systems when a fresh, rough surface has been left in the vein.[11] The fistula can be closed 2 to 3 months later. Because it can be very difficult to find the AVF at this time, we place a 2-0 or 3-0 Prolene suture loosely around the AVF to aid closing it (going through the same skin incision). Placing the suture doubly around the AVF allows it to be pulled up and tied so that the vein itself does not require dissection. Because the ends of the suture are usually difficult to find, leaving the ends of the suture long and bringing them up into the subcutaneous tissue over a button will make them easier to find. An alternative to this is to create a temporary AVF in the ipsilateral arm. In dialysis patients who already have a functioning AVF in the ipsilateral arm, another AVF is unnecessary.

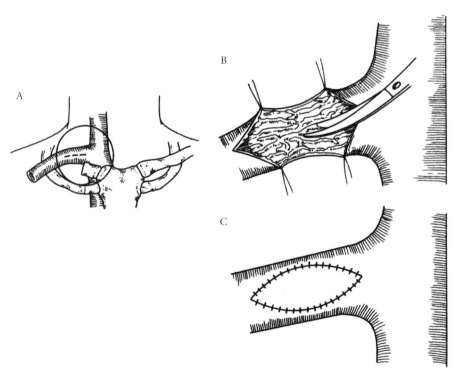

Figure 49.3 Technique of endovenectomy of the subclavian-innominate junction and patch graft with autogenous vein. Reprinted with permission from Sanders RJ. Management of subclavian vein obstruction. In Bergan JJ, Kistner RL, eds. Atlas of venous surgery. Philadelphia, PA: WB Saunders; 1992: 267.

SUBCLAVIAN VEIN BYPASS INDICATIONS

When subclavian vein thrombosis cannot be resolved, total occlusion becomes a chronic problem. Treatment is indicated only for significant symptoms of swelling and pain. Patients whose veins cannot be opened by thrombolytic therapy should be anticoagulated for several months and followed. Many patients will recanalize without additional treatment. Among those who remain occluded, the majority will enjoy symptomatic improvement over the next six to 12 months by the development of adequate collaterals. In one study of 95 patients treated only with anticoagulants, 60% were totally asymptomatic or had minimal symptoms, 27% had symptoms only with moderate exercise, and only 13% were symptomatic at rest.[11]

CHOICE OF BYPASS

Venography is necessary to determine the type of bypass to perform. For occlusions limited to 5 to 6 cm, with good inflow, axillojugular vein transposition is our procedure of choice. This procedure is limited to short occlusions. For longer occlusions, the jugular vein will not reach the more distal axillary vein and some type of graft must be used. Aortic homografts are our first choice. This procedure is limited to short occlusions. For longer occlusions, the jugular vein will not reach the more distal axillary vein and some type of graft must be used.

Aortic homografts,[10] saphenous vein spiral[13] or panel grafts, prosthetic materials, and even transposition of the contralateral cephalic vein sewn to the brachial or axillary vein[14] all have been successful. Because subclavian vein bypass is seldom needed there is no large database to help one choose the best graft material. In dialysis patients who already have a functioning AVF, the easiest bypass is with a prosthesis from the axillary to the internal jugular vein.

Although this is prosthetic material, the AVF will usually maintain high enough pressure and flow to prevent thrombosis.[14]

TECHNIQUE OF JUGULOAXILLARY VEIN BYPASS

The technique is described in Figure 49.4. An infraclavicular incision 2 to 3 cm below the midclavicle is used.

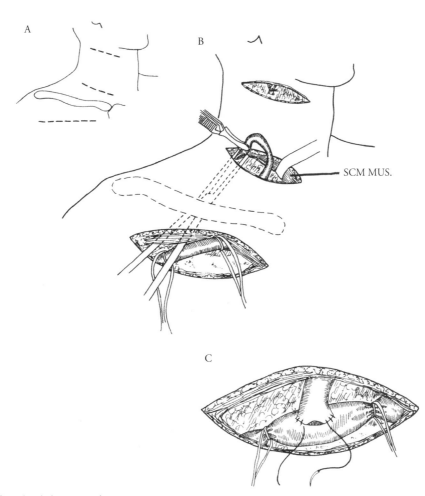

Figure 49.4 Technique of jugulosubclavian vein bypass. Reprinted with permission from Sanders RJ. Subclavian vein obstruction. In: Bergan JJ, Yao ST, ed. *Venous Disorders*. Philadelphia: WB Saunders; 1991: 256.

The pectoralis major is split between clavicular and sternal heads. The pectoralis minor tendon is divided and the axillary and subclavian veins mobilized and surrounded with vessel loops. Two transverse incisions are made in the neck to dissect the internal jugular vein. The first is 2 cm above the clavicle, 5 to 6 cm long, and directly over the sternocleidomastoid muscle. The sternal and clavicular heads of this muscle are split, and the internal jugular vein dissected circumferentially and surrounded with a Penrose drain. The vein is totally freed as far as possible both proximally and distally by dividing all bands. A second incision, 4 to 5 cm long, is made below the mandible. Through this incision the cephalic portion of jugular vein is freed proximally to the base of the skull and distally to meet the freed portion of vein in the tunnel between the two incisions.

A tunnel is created behind the clavicle between the subclavian vein and the supraclavicular incision. The subclavius muscle is divided and a kidney pedicle clamp passed between the two incisions. The tunnel is dilated bluntly so that the jugular vein can pass easily through it without compression in the tunnel. The jugular vein is marked with a stitch on its anterior wall for orientation. The vein is clamped and divided close to the base of the skull. The cephalic end is suture ligated. The distal end is carefully passed down the jugular tunnel, brought out through the lower neck incision, and freed as far as possible below the clavicle up to the subclavian vein junction. The vein is then passed though the tunnel beneath the clavicle. The patient is heparinized and a longitudinal venotomy is performed, excising a narrow rim of the vein wall. Passing a 12- to 14-French catheter through the vein prior to performing the anastomosis is a good way to check that the subclavian vein is unobstructed and not kinked in its path to the innominate vein. An end-to-side anastomosis is performed with 6-0 Prolene. Some surgeons have elected an end-to-end anastomosis; either is effective.

Because venous repairs are subject to thrombosis due to low flow pressures,[11] a temporary AVF is created between the axillary vein and axillary artery, provided there is adequate room on the axillary vein distal to the anastomosis. We have used ringed or spiral reinforced 6-mm PTFE for the AVF. This is placed in a loop that comes up into the subcutaneous tissue to make it easier to find when the temporary AVF is taken down. We usually remove the AVF in about 3 months.[16] An alternative AVF can be created in the arm or antecubital space if creating it between axillary vessels appears too difficult.

REFERENCES

1. Sanders RJ. Subclavian vein obstruction. In: Bergan JJ, Yao ST, ed. *Venous Disorders*. Philadelphia: WB Saunders; 1991: 256.
2. Dunant JH. Subclavian vein obstruction in thoracic outlet syndrome, *Inter Angio*. 1984. *3*: 157–159.
3. Thompson RW, Schneider PA, Nelken NA, Skioldebrand CG, Stoney RJ. Circumferential venolysis and paraclavicular thoracic outlet decompression for effort thrombosis of the subclavian vein, *J Vasc Surg*. 1992. *16*: 723–732.
4. Azakie A, McElhinney DB, Thompson RW, Raven RB, Messina LM, Stoney RJ. Surgical management of subclavian-vein effort thrombosis as a result of thoracic outlet compression, *J Vasc Surg*. 1998. *28*: 777–786.
5. Schneider DB, Dimuzio PJ, Martin ND, et al. Combination treatment of venous thoracic outlet syndrome: Open surgical decompression and intraoperative angioplasty, *J Vasc Surg*. 2004. *40*: 599–603.
6. Melby SJ, Vedantham S, Narra VR, et al. Comprehensive surgical management of the competitive athlete with effort thrombosis of the subclavian vein (Paget-Schroetter syndrome), *J Vasc Surg*. 2008. *47*: 809–820.
7. Machleder HI. Evaluation of a new treatment strategy for Paget-Schroetter syndrome: Spontaneous thrombosis of the axillary-subclavian vein, *J Vasc Surg*. 1993. *17*: 305–317.
8. Kreienberg PB, Chang BB, Darling C III, et al. Long-term results in patients treated with thrombolysis, thoracic inlet decompression, and subclavian vein stenting for Paget-Schroetter syndrome, *J Vasc Surg*. 2001. *33*: S100–S105.
9. Molina JE. Need for emergency treatment in subclavian vein effort thrombosis, *J Am Coll Surgeons*. 1995. *181*: 414–420.
10. Molina JE. A new surgical approach to the innominate and subclavian vein, *J Vasc Surg*. 1998. *27*: 576–581.
11. Johnson V, Eiseman B. Evaluation of arteriovenous shunt to maintain patency of venous autograft, *Am J Surg*. 1969. *118*: 915–920.
12. Gloviczki P, Kazmier FJ, Hollier LH. Axillary subclavian venous occlusion: The morbidity of a nonlethal disease, *J Vasc Surg*. 1986. *4*: 333–337.
13. Doty DB, Baker W. Bypass of superior vena cava with spiral vein graft, *Ann Thorac Surg*. 1976. *22*: 490–493.
14. Hashmonai M, Schramek A, Farbstein J. Cephalic vein cross-over bypass for subclavian vein thrombosis: A case report, *Surgery*. 1976. *80*: 563–564.
15. Sanders RJ, Cooper MA. Surgical management of subclavian vein obstruction, including six cases of subclavian vein bypass, *Surgery*. 1995. *118*: 856–863.
16. Sanders RJ, Rosales C, Pearce WH. Creation and closure of temporary arteriovenous fistulas for venous reconstruction or thrombectomy: Description of technique, *J Vasc Surg*. 1987. *6*: 504–505.
17. Sanders RJ. Subclavian vein obstruction. In: Bergan JJ, Kistner RL, eds. *Atlas of venous surgery*. Philadelphia: WB Saunders. 1991.
18. Sanders RJ, Haug CE. *Thoracic outlet syndrome: A common sequela of neck injuries*. Philadelphia: JB Lippincott. 1991.

50.

SUPERFICIAL THROMBOPHLEBITIS

RECOMMENDATIONS FOR DIAGNOSIS AND MANAGEMENT

Joann M. Lohr

Superficial thrombophlebitis is a relatively common inflammatory process that affects the superficial veins. This may include the upper extremity, lower extremity, trunk, chest wall or penis, and has been described in various locations. The symptoms include pain, reddening of the skin, and swelling of the surrounding tissue.

The predisposing risk factors for superficial vein thrombophlebitis (SVTP) and superficial venous thromboembolism (SVT) are similar and include immobilization, varicose veins, postoperative time period, trauma, pregnancy, postpartum, active malignancy, use of oral contraceptives and hormone replacement therapy, obesity, chemotherapy, and prolonged immobilization. Treatment is aimed at reducing the local symptoms, especially pain, and preventing the development of more serious complications, especially thrombus propagation or embolization.

The incidence of SVT increases with age, in the third decade it is 0.05 per 1,000 per year in males and 0.31 per 1,000 per year in females. In the eighth decade it is 1.8 per 1,000 per year in males and 2.2 per 1,000 per year in females. It has a female proportion of 55–70% with a mean age of 60 years.[1]

Virchow's Triad is well established. It includes changes in blood flow, changes in vessel walls, and changes in the characteristics of the blood flow, all of which come into play with the development of SVT.

PATHOPHYSIOLOGY

Local inflammatory mediators are altered with development of SVT. This includes the prostaglandins, leukotrienes, metabolites of arachidonic acid, nitric oxide, swelling of the endothelial cells, and polymorphonuclear leukocyte infiltration of the tunica media resulting in vessel wall injury and potentiation of the thrombotic process.[2,3]

Predisposing factors include varicose veins; inherited thrombophilias including Factor V Leiden, prothrombin (2102A) gene mutations, deficiencies of antithrombin, heparin cofactor, protein C or S deficiencies, lupus anticoagulant antibodies, and anticardiolipin antibodies; and abnormal fibrinolytic activity.

Characteristic patient populations and triggering risk factors include female proportion 55–70% with a mean age of 60 years, obesity 20%, pregnancy, oral contraceptives, hormonal replacement, history of deep vein thrombosis (DVT), long-haul flights, prolonged immobilization, recent surgery, trauma, or sclerotherapy.[4]

A red, hot, tender, palpable cord along a superficial vein is the most common physical examination finding. When looking at risk factors, clinical findings, venous duplex ultrasound findings and treatment in all of the patients, Gorty and colleagues found the most common risk factor was the presence of varicose veins followed by a history of SVT, previous DVT, recent surgery, leg trauma, cancer, hormone use, (either oral contraceptive or replacement), or hypercoagulable state. Pain was by far the most common symptom.[5]

Superficial vein thrombophlebitis appears in two distinct forms. One is varicose vein thrombophlebitis, representing the vast majority of cases. It is characterized by a large thrombus in a varicose vein and a modest inflammatory process localized in the surrounding vessel but not in its wall. The other rarer form of SVTP affects a nonvaricosed vein. Abundant intima proliferation and media fibrosis with nonimportant thrombosis are the hallmarks of this form, which may be associated with a systemic disease. Although SVTP is perceived as trivial and benign, the coexistence of mostly distal DVT with propagation to the popliteal or femoral and even pulmonary emboli (PE) have been reported. The prevalence of these complications varies widely from 6–53% for coexistence of DVT to 2.6–15% for propagation, and 0–33% for asymptomatic PE. Risk factors for these complications are those known to be associated with DVT.[6]

NATURAL HISTORY

Patients with a SVTP of the leg have a ten-fold increased risk of developing DVT during the subsequent 6 months when compared with an age- and sex-matched group without SVTP. The absolute risk of DVT, however is just 2.7%.[7] Swelling of a leg within 6 months after a SVTP should prompt diagnostic testing for DVT.[7]

Treatment with low molecular weight heparin (LMWH) or nonsteroidal anti-inflammatory drugs (NSAIDs) during the 10 d following SVTP decreases the risk of the developing DVT by about 15% and 9% respectively.[7]

Independent predictive factors for complications were SVT of recent onset (odds ratio [OR], 3.01; 95% confidence interval [CI], 1.44–6.27), severe chronic venous insufficiency (OR, 2.75; CI, 1.10–6.89), male gender (OR, 2.17; CI, 1.28–36.8), and a history of venous thromboembolism (VTE) (OR, 2.07; CI, 1.06–4.04). Only severe chronic venous insufficiency was an independent risk factor and predictor of the development of DVT or PE (OR, 4.50; CI, 1.30–15.61).[8] Knowledge of the predictive factors may be useful in determining the appropriate treatment in patients with SVTP.[8]

Vascular surgeons have given little attention to superficial thrombophlebitis involving the lesser saphenous vein. Dr. Ascher and The New York Group in 2003 reported that lesser saphenous vein thrombosis more often is associated with DVT (65.6%) than previously believed. While most lesser saphenous vein thrombophlebitis will improve in 18 months, that associated with DVT will resolve sooner. Whether anticoagulation accounted for this difference remains to be demonstrated.[9]

The risk of development of subsequent DVT following SVT is really not fully appreciated. The mechanisms, time relations, and risks factors for DVT arising on earlier SVT are still unclear. Most patients will have complete resolution of symptoms at 3 weeks. At that time, thrombus disappeared completely in 26% of cases. Thrombus regression was similar to venous blood flow outflow direction—proximal to femoral area. Thrombus propagation has been observed following regression of local symptoms of SVT.[10]

The William Beaumont Group in 1996 identified 263 patients with isolated SVT. Eleven percent of these patients had documented progression to deep involvement. The most common site of deep vein involvement was progression of the disease from the great saphenous in the thigh to the common femoral vein with the majority of these being nonocclusive and up to two-thirds having a free-floating component. Other sites of extension were the above-knee saphenous vein through thigh perforators to occlude the femoral vein in the thigh, as well as extension of the below-knee saphenous vein into the popliteal vein or extension of the below-knee thrombi into the tibioperoneal veins with calf perforators. This group recommended proximal vein thrombosis be treated with anticoagulation or at least

followed with sequential duplex scanning so that definitive therapy may be initiated if progression was noted. Most distal SVT should be followed carefully clinically and repeat duplex scan performed if progression is noted or patient symptoms worsen.[11]

DIAGNOSIS

The diagnosis of SVT is made in a clinical setting, but ultrasonography is useful to eliminate the diagnostic or concomitant DVT. For SVT of the lower limb varicose veins represent the principal cause, but underlying conditions (i.e., autoimmune diseases, malignancy, or thrombophilia) must be sought in cases of idiopathic, migrant, or recurrent DVT and in the absence of varicose veins. Concomitant DVT and PE can occur in approximately 15% and 5% respectively. A 1-month prophylactic dose of low-molecular weight heparin plus elastic stockings could be an appropriate strategy in most cases.[12]

In all cases of clinical SVT a duplex examination of both the superficial and deep venous symptoms is necessary in order to provide a complete diagnosis. The treatment of SVT depends on the situation and the size of the thrombi. In case of associated DVT, the most important treatment is of the DVT. The use of heparin or LMWH (therapeutic doses) is proved for patients with coexisting DVT, and is thought to be appropriate for ascending SVT as well. Superficial vein thrombosis must be considered a risk factor for the development of DVT, and patients should be treated from this point of view. Biologic analysis and complete check-up are mandatory in cases of varicose thrombosis in young patients and in cases of recurrence.[13]

Duplex ultrasound is somewhat controversial but it can be used to confirm the diagnosis of thrombus and identify the popliteal and saphenofemoral functions. It can also rule out contiguous and noncontiguous DVT. Superficial vein thrombosis and concomitant DVT have been reported in a wide spectrum from 2.6 to 65.6%.[14]

The differential diagnosis includes the clinical setting, cellulitis, panniculitis, erythema nodosum, insect bites, and lymphangitis. In at least one case, a ruptured infected superficial femoral artery aneurysm has been misdiagnosed as an SVT.[15]

The main histopathologic differential diagnosis of superficial and venous thrombophlebitis is cutaneous polyarteritis nodosa. Biopsy and complementary techniques as well as clinical signs and symptoms will usually allow the diagnosis to be made. Superficial vein thrombosis is usually characterized by an autoresolving vasculitis of medium-sized veins of the upper subcutaneous tissue or the deep dermis that clinically manifests as a tender or painful palpable cord-like structure. Superficial vein thrombosis for the most part involves the lower extremity, but special locations including the anterior chest wall or the penis, characterize specific clinical forms including Mondor's disease.[16]

Thrombophlebitis migrans is a footprint for Buerger's disease and has been discussed in a descriptive study from northeast Iran.[17] Congenital malformations and venous abnormalities may also present as migratory SVT or unusual presentations of DVT.[18]

Mondor's disease was originally described in 1939 as a superficial venous thrombophlebitis of the thoracoepigastric veins in women. This term has also been applied to the superficial dorsal vein of the penis. This may actually be underreported as patients may be reluctant to seek medical care, especially if they associate their condition with deviant behavior. Injection of illegal substances in subcutaneous veins may also cause thrombosis. Extrinsic venous compression may also result in occlusion and this may occur with infection, sexual devices, and neoplastic diseases as well as a tool belt worn around the waist causing venous pooling and vessel trauma. A careful history is critically important in evaluating the patients.[19]

Other unusual cases of superficial thrombophlebitis have been reported in association with sickle cell episodes.[20]

Thrombophilias may also present as recurrent SVTs or SVTs of unusual locations.[21]

Laparoscopy and laparoscopic procedures may have an increased risk for the development of thrombosis due to increased abdominal pressure and negative Trendelenburg positioning. In patients with varicose veins and a history of thromboembolism, laparoscopy-associated risk factors for the development of thromboembolic complications may be aggravated. These patients with varicose veins and a history of venous thromboembolism need to be considered carefully for prolonged laparoscopic and robotic procedures.[22] Primary care practitioners may be confronted with this complication more often because, due to legislative regulations, patients are discharged earlier from the hospital after laparoscopic interventions.[22]

Several studies have shown an increased incidence of inherited thrombophilias, in particular the presence of Factor V Leiden and/or hyperhomocysteinemia in patients affected by SVT. Acquired molecular prothrombotic conditions associated with SVT are mainly represented by the antiphospholipid syndrome or acquired activated protein C resistance. Few studies have focused on the association of molecular prothrombotic conditions in oncological patients affected by SVT.[23]

From a pathologic point of view, it is important to distinguish SVT localized at the lower or upper extremity or also unusual sites of thrombosis. Moreover, it is also important to differentiate SVT of large venous vessels from SVT of small venous vessels because of the possibility of embolization. Another relevant problem is related to the possibility of detection of small thrombus because of the presence of a short peripheral venous catheter placed for the administration of drugs, fluids, antibiotics, parenteral nutrition, chemotherapy, and blood derivatives. Nursing surveillance and catheter maintenance at the site of IV access is critical to decrease the risk of infectious SVT.[23]

Trousseau described spontaneous, recurrent superficial migratory thrombophlebitis associated with occult cancers, and this was later correlated with disseminated microangiopathy (platelet-rich clots in small blood vessels). This is often associated with mucinous adenocarcinomas, which secrete abnormally glycosylated mucins and mucin fragments into the bloodstream. Since carcinoma mucins can have binding sites for selectins, the hypothesis is that selectin-mucin interactions might trigger this syndrome. When highly purified, tissue-factor-free carcinoma mucin preparations were intravenously injected into mice, platelet-rich microthrombi were rapidly generated. This pathology was markedly diminished in P- or L-selectin-deficient mice. Heparin (an antithrombin-potentiating agent that can also block P- and L-selectin recognition of ligands) ameliorated this platelet aggregation, but had no additional effects on P- or L-selectin-deficient mice. Inhibition of endogenous thrombin by recombinant hirudin also did not block platelet aggregation. Mucins generated plate aggregation in vitro in hirudinized whole blood, but not in platelet-rich leukocyte-free plasma nor in whole blood from L-selectin-deficient mice. Thus, Trousseau syndrome is likely triggered by the interactions of circulating carcinoma mucins with leukocytes L-selectin and platelet P-selectin without requiring accompanying thrombin generation. Wahrenbrock and colleagues' data may also explain why heparin ameliorates Trousseau syndrome, while vitamin K antagonists that merely depress thrombin production do not.[24]

One of the problems with migratory thrombophlebitis is that patients may have advanced disease prior to presentation. The exact workup of patients with SVT for occult malignancy is unsettled at this time.

Superficial vein thrombosis is commonly encountered in pregnancy. It is critical the obstetrician recognize the potential for complications and embolic events and that Doppler ultrasound be utilized to rule out potential deep venous extension in these patents. While thromboembolism remains a leading cause of maternal death, the potential dangers of symptomatic thrombophlebitis should not be overlooked.[25]

Mondor's disease or "wire-like" changes most commonly presents in middle-aged women and is idiopathic. It may be related to strenuous exercise or trauma and it has been associated with breast cancer. It may also be seen however in pregnant women and it may also be mistaken for scleroderma.[26]

Thrombophilias may play a minor role in the etiology of SVT associated with pregnancy.[27] A careful obstetrical and gynecological history is important and is critical to maintain a high index of suspicion.

Primary hypercoagulable states are those conditions associated with an increased risk of thrombosis caused by a specific measurable defect in the proteins of coagulation and/or fibrinolytic systems. These disorders are frequently inherited and include deficiencies with antithrombin III, heparin cofactor 2, protein C, protein S, abnormal fibrinolytic activity, dysfibrinogenemia, and Hageman trait. Patients with lupus anticoagulant and anticardiolipin antibody syndrome with thrombotic episodes are also considered to have a primary hypercoagulable state.[28]

A high suspicion of underlying thrombophilia needs to be considered in patients who have SVT in unusual sites or in patients who have SVT with no varicose vein involvement.[29-31]

High Factor VIII concentration is an independent risk factor for SVT.[31]

The lower threshold for testing for hypercoagulable disorders should be maintaining patients with recurrent recalcitrant or unusual patterns of SVT thrombosis.[32]

In addition, elevated body mass index (BMI ≥ 28 kg/m^2) has also been associated with increased risk of SVT.[33,34]

Association of eosinophilia with SVT is a rare situation that can reveal neoplasia, malignancy blood disorders, or vasculitis, but SVT has recently been described with the hypereosinophilic syndrome.[35]

Thrombophlebitis may be a complication of the incompetent greater saphenous vein and usually has a benign outcome when this occurs (see Figure 50.1). However, a free-floating thrombus tip in the femoral vein is a challenge to treat, and surgical ligation may be needed to prevent the risk of embolization when ascending SVT extends to the femoral vein with a free-floating thrombus tip (see Figure 50.2). Use of color duplex sonography is important in differentiating this and establishing the diagnosis.[36,37]

Dr. Lowell S. Kabnick and colleagues presented endovenous heat induced thrombus (EHIT) following endovenous vein obliteration at the American Venous Forum in 2006. They tried to categorize this process as producing a non-normal SVT as the thrombus after endovenous procedures is hyperechoic whereas a de novo thrombus is hypoechoic.

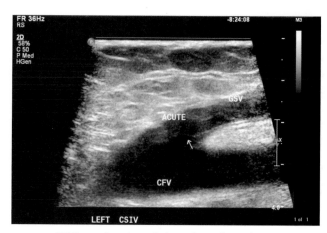

Figure 50.2   SVT extending through the sapheno-femoral junction into the common femoral vein.

They classified their patients' thrombi into four categories. A Class I venous thrombus is superficial and extends just to the deep junction. It is located at the saphenofemoral junction or saphenopopliteal junction and does not extend into the deep system. For this class, no treatment was needed. A Class II nonocclusive venous thrombus with a less than 50% extension into the deep system and a cross-sectional diameter of less than 50% was thought to need follow-up and possible antiplatelet agents. A Class III venous thrombus has a cross-sectional extension into the deep system, is nonocclusive but greater than 50%. Finally, a Class IV venous thrombus completely occludes the common femoral vein and should be treated as DVT.[38]

Upper extremity SVT is most frequently associated with iatrogenic conditions using intravenous catheters, drugs, chemotherapy, and heroin. Suppurative thrombophlebitis is an infection of the vein wall. It is usually associated with intravenous catheter placement and accounts for approximately 10% of all nosocomial infections. It is more common in patients with burns or cancer or those receiving steroids. The skin flora, especially *Staphylococcus aureus*, are the most common pathogens. Suppurative thrombophlebitis should be suspected when the patient is having phlebitis or presents with a fever greater than 102°F. The diagnosis of suppurative thrombophlebitis is usually straightforward. It can be made by the demonstration of pus coming from the wound of the removed intravenous device or aspiration of pus percutaneously from the involved vein. Treatment of superficial suppurative thrombophlebitis consists mainly of venotomy of the affected vessel and systemic antimicrobial therapy.[39,40]

Septic thrombophlebitis in the superficial veins is a potentially devastating complication. Local inflammatory changes are present in less than half of the patients with sepsis and may not manifest until several days after the catheter has been removed. A high index of suspicion is necessary to reach a timely diagnosis and proceed with definitive surgical therapy. In the setting of persistent sepsis without an identifiable source, the diagnosis of septic thrombophlebitis

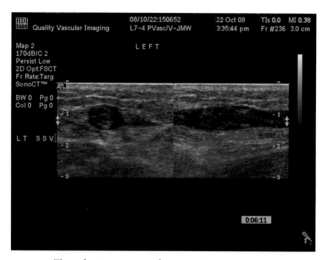

Figure 50.1   Thrombus in greater saphenous vein.

should be considered and the evidence of its presence actively sought.[40]

Fungi are increasingly recognized as microorganisms causing superficial suppurative thrombophlebitis and are again managed by aggressive surgical therapy and antifungal agents.[41]

Clinically silent DVT is much more common in patients without varicose veins. A clinical marker for complications of SVT is the occurrence of SVT in a patient who does not have varicose veins. This should prompt a search for underlying associated diseases.[42]

A substantial number of patients with SVT exhibit venous thromboembolism at presentation; however, some do not develop this complication until the subsequent 3 months. Risk factors for complications at 3 months were male sex, history of DVT or PE, previous cancer, and absence of varicose veins. These findings should prompt consideration of alternative therapy and prolonged treatment for patients in these high risk groups.[43]

Gorty, Milio, and colleagues reported that SVT in a normal vein with extension occurred in 20.8 to 23.7% of their patient populations with thrombus propagation.[44,45]

Superficial venous thrombosis occurs in 125,000 new cases per year in the United States. A "healthy vein" is involved in 25% of these cases with propagation reported to occur in 2.6 to 15% of cases and 5% to have PE. The mortality rate for SVT is 0–1% and the mortality rate for DVT is 5%.[4]

The course of SVT is usually benign with septic complications occurring more commonly with upper extremity thrombi and more commonly iatrogenic. The DVT that occurs has been associated in 5.6 to 36% of cases. This may be contiguous in 50–70% or noncontiguous. With a noncontiguous pattern, a hypercoagulable state should be considered. Patients with concomitant DVT have symptomatic PEs reported in 0.5 to 4%. Physicians who systematically perform lung scans on patients should know that PEs may be present in up to 33% of patients.[4]

The lower extremities account for 60–80% of SVTs for the most part involving the great saphenous vein; 10–20% involved the short saphenous vein. Other veins are involved 10–20% of the time and 5–10% of cases are bilateral. Upper extremity and neck SVTs are more commonly iatrogenic. The anterior thoracic or thoracoabdominal wall veins or veins of the penis or groin may also be involved.[4]

TREATMENT

Anticoagulants have been shown to decrease the incidence of new SVT and DVT.[45]

Considering patients with SVT and varicose veins, Factor V Leiden in the nonspreading group is present in 6.7%. In patients with complications it may be found in 35.7%. Prothrombin mutation is present in 4.4% of SVT patients without complications and is found in 7.9% of patients with spreading SVT. The methylenetetrahydrofolate reductase (MTHFR), a C677T mutation, is found in 6.7% of patients with nonspreading SVT and 21.4% of patients with spreading complications.[45]

If you compare this same study looking at patients with SVT involving normal veins, Factor V Leiden is found in 26.3% of patients with nonspreading situation and 60% in patients with spreading. Prothrombin mutation is found in 7.9% of nonspreading and 20% of those with ascending complication. The MTHFR C677T mutation is found in 40% of those with spreading or present in only 23.7% of patients with nonspreading.[45]

Knowledge and correct identification of all veins routinely imaged in the upper extremities and lower extremities is critical to the proper management of SVT and DVT. Unfortunately, in Ziehler and colleagues' survey only 12% of physicians were able to correctly identify all of the veins routinely imaged in either upper extremity or lower extremity duplex venous scans.[46]

At the Good Samaritan Hospital John J. Cranley Vascular Laboratory, thrombus location is reported as superficial or deep, and also according to the location by zones to allow sequential comparison and comparison between technologists. (See Figures 50.3 and 50.4.)

Ascending phlebitis closer than 5 cm to the deep venous system has been treated surgically. However, there is no consensus in the literature as to how to treat ascending thrombophlebitis. The surgical procedure can be performed under local anesthesia, and is safe and efficient.[47]

Varicose vein thrombectomy, when performed concurrently, gives patients better postoperative pain control.

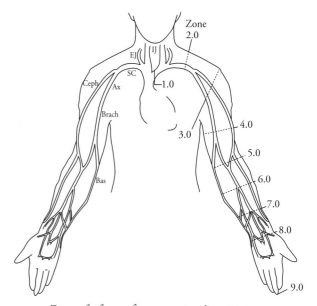

Figure 50.3   Zones of reference for upper extremity venous scanning: midline = 1.0, acromion = 3.0, elbow = 5.0, wrist = 8.0, and fingertips = 9.0.   From Lohr et al. *J Vasc Surg* 1991;14:618–23.

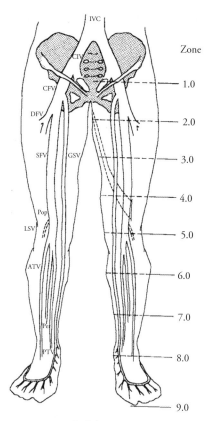

Figure 50.4   In an average-sized adult, one zone equals a length of approximately 10 cm on the extremity. Zone 1 is defined as the intersection of the femoral vessels with the inguinal ligament. Zone 5 is an imaginary line passing from midpatella to the popliteal crease. Zone 8 corresponds to a line from midmedial malleolus to the midlateral malleolus. Zone 9 corresponds to the tips of the toes. With use of the above landmarks, the thigh and calf are subdivided into four and three equal zones, respectively.   From Lohr et al. *Am J Surg* 1995;170:86–90.

Duplex scanning affords 100% accuracy in both determining the presence of thrombosis and its extent.[48]

Treatment of superficial thrombophlebitis may be provided by a variety of measures. These include local anti-inflammatory applications including gels, creams, and sprays, local incision and expression of clots, microthrombectomy, and ligation of connecting points, compression bandaging and stockings, immediate mobilization and walking exercises, analgesias and anti-inflammatory drugs, surgery with high ligation and completed varicose vein excision, anticoagulation with unfractionated heparin, LMWH in prophylactic or therapeutic doses, and oral anticoagulants.[49]

Treatment with a therapeutic or prophylactic dose of LMWH or an NSAID reduces the incidence of SVT extension or recurrence but not the VTE. More randomized control trials are needed before any evidence-based recommendations on the treatment of SVT for the prevention of VTE can be given.[50]

In a comparison of high and low doses of LMWH for the treatment of SVT of the legs, a double-blind

randomized control trial suggested therapeutic doses of LMWH administered for one month in patients with SVT of the great saphenous vein did not improve results obtained when compared with prophylactic doses administered for the same period. The patients were followed for three months.[51]

The recent CHEST guidelines stated that peripheral vein infusion thrombophlebitis is estimated to occur in 25–35% of hospitalized patients with peripheral IV catheters. No control trials have evaluated systemic anticoagulants for the treatment of infusion thrombophlebitis.[52]

The CHEST guidelines suggest oral diclofenac or another NSAID as a Grade 2B recommendation. Topical diclofenac gel, Grade 2B, or heparin gel, Grade 2B, are recommended for resolution of symptoms for up to 2 weeks. We recommend against the use of systemic anticoagulation in this population as a Grade 1C recommendation.[52] Superficial venous thrombosis has been less studied than DVT; however it is more common. Treatment of superficial thrombophlebitis has been the subject of a recent Cochrane meta-analysis.[53]

The CHEST guidelines recommend that patients with spontaneous SVTP be treated with prophylactics or intermediate doses of LMWH or unfractionated heparin as a Grade 2B for at least 4 weeks. They suggest an alternative of 4 weeks of LMWH or unfractionated heparin and a vitamin K agonist with a target INR of 2.5 with a range of 2 to 5 that can be overlapped with 5 d of LMWH or unfractionated heparin and continued for 4 weeks. This is a Grade 2C recommendation. They suggest oral NSAIDs not be given in addition to anticoagulants. Anticoagulation is a 2B recommendation, and they recommend medical treatment with anticoagulants over surgical treatment as a Grade 1B recommendation. It is thought likely that less extensive SVT (i.e., where the affected venous segment is short in length or further from the saphenofemoral junction) does not require treatment with anticoagulation at all. It is reasonable to use oral or topical NSAIDs for symptoms and control of these cases.[52]

The optimal duration of treatment for SVT as well as the best regimen is unclear. General questions about the treatment of SVT remain unresolved. Large and adequately designed randomized control trials are needed to assess the actual role of NSAIDs and LMWH to ascertain whether these drugs are actually comparable, and whether used in combination they may be more effective and as safe compared with a single treatment. Another important issue is to clarify the optimal duration of SVT treatment. Current available data suggest that LMWH given for a week is probably too short to prevent VTE in the long term. A prolongation of LMWH or NSAID treatment for at least a month might be considered. Whether a topical treatment might add some benefit if given in combination with LMWH or NSAIDs remains unclear. Finally, whether treatment needs to be adapted based on location and the etiology of superficial thrombophlebitis warrants further investigation.[53]

The goal of treatment for SVT is to improve local symptoms while preventing the development of complications such as VTE and PE. Topical treatment alone does not seem a reasonable approach to treat these patients. The most effective approach to treat SVT may be represented by LMWH which has been shown to prevent VTE events and extension and/or recurrence of SVT. In addition, the administration of LMWH does not seem to carry a high risk of bleeding, although these data are very preliminary.[53-55]

It is advisable to repeat duplex scanning to determine whether propagation of thrombus exists as an adjuvant in those patients who are not actively treated.[56]

The three main local actions of heparin on the skin can be defined as (1) the anticoagulant action; (2) the microcirculatory-modulatory action determining important control of the microcirculation in case of excessive vasoconstriction or vasodilatation; and (3) the "facilitatory action" on skin permeability, allowing other drugs to diffuse better and faster into the skin producing a better therapeutic effect. Observation suggests important clinical applications for local liposomal heparin action.[57,58]

Exercise may reduce pain as well as decrease the possibility of deep vein extension. Bed rest should be avoided in patients with SVT. DVT prophylaxis should be established in patients with reduced mobility. Antibiotics usually do not have a place in superficial vein thrombophlebitis unless there are documented episodes of infection.[59]

Extended thrombus prophylaxis may be indicated in patients with a history of venous thrombosis and genetic mutations due to the enhanced risk of recurrence. Patient groups with thrombophilias might benefit from extended oral anticoagulation or vitamin supplementation if clinically warranted.[60]

There are no good data on the use of pentasaccharide for use of prophylaxis or treatment.[61]

The incidence of deep and superficial thromboembolism and symptoms was significantly reduced by day 12 in all active treatment groups treated with LMWH. No episodes of death or major hemorrhage occurred in this study.[62]

When high-dose and low-dose unfractionated heparin were evaluated in patients with acute SVT of the thigh, unmonitored high doses of unfractionated heparin were more effective than prophylactic doses for the prevention of thromboembolic complications and did not enhance the risk of bleeding complications.[63]

Local treatment with Essaven Gel in comparison with placebo showed a decrease in the analogue symptomatic score and in the skin temperature in the placebo group that was due to skin manipulation and massage while the SVT treated group had improved symptoms and decreased skin temperature faster. This would suggest an effective symptomatic improvement with Essaven Gel.[64]

The Belgian Thrombosis Guidelines Group recommends immediate mobilization in elastic compression for all patients with SVT.[65]

Dr. Jason Lee and Dr. Maziyar Kalani from Stanford in California suggested that in patients with refractory SVT surgical intervention such as phlebectomy, sclerotherapy, saphenofemoral junction ligation, or saphenous vein stripping are all potentially acceptable treatments.[66]

Researchers at the University of Michigan in 2001 also suggested that ligation of above-knee superficial thrombophlebitis that does not involve the deep system may be a suitable alternative.[67]

A combination of LMWH and an anti-inflammatory agent is more effective than LMWH alone as a standard treatment for SVT with improved symptom resolution and reduction of pain and tenderness.[68]

The Cincinnati group has previously demonstrated that ligation is a safe alternative and may be combined with compression in outpatient treatment with LMWH in the management of SVT.[37]

The use of duplex ultrasound can safely identify patients who need ligation.[69]

The exact results and treatment recommendations need to be individualized and further trials are needed. An article in the *New England Journal of Medicine* suggested a cost-benefit analysis needs to be done to evaluate the pricing of medications and other interventions in consideration of the range of patients being treated to identify patients in whom treatments may be most beneficial and cost-effective, but rapidly expanding those to others may be less clear and must be considered carefully. Dr. Goldman suggests phase 3.5 trials to document the cost, the effect on quality of life, and the cost-effectiveness of new interventions so as to reach a consensus regarding their worthiness.[70]

Goldman suggests that the exact treatment for SVT needs to be individualized with special care given to the presentation, the pattern of disease, and the potential complications. If only tributaries are involved local heat, nonsteroidal anti-inflammatories, graduated compression, frequent ambulation, and elevation may be appropriate. Anticoagulation is needed if there is concomitant DVT, if the SVT is not responding to therapy, if there is involvement of the great saphenous vein at the saphenofemoral junction or of the small saphenous and the saphenopopliteal junction, if there are known underlying hypercoagulable states, or if patients have had frequent recurrences. When a healthy vein is involved, the treatment workup should include evaluation for underlying diseases and thrombophilias, a careful duplex evaluation to evaluate for propagation, and a hypercoagulable workup. Surgical intervention is potentially indicated for patients with a very symptomatic SVT in varicose veins and reflux in the great saphenous vein. Timing of surgical treatment is controversial. Ultimately the treatment of SVT needs to be decided on an individual patient basis.[70]

REFERENCES

1. Coon WW. Tecumseh Community Health Study, *Circulation.* 1973. *48*: 839–846.
2. Lewis GHG, Heckle JF. Infusion thrombophlebitis, *Br J Anaesth.* 1985. *57*: 220–233.
3. Guildyal SK, Pande RC, Mirsa TR. Histopathology and bacteriology of post-infusion phlebitis, *Inter Surg.* 1975. *60*: 341–344.
4. Decousus H, Epinat M, Cuillot K, Boissier C, Tardy B. Superficial vein thrombosis: Risk factors, diagnosis, and treatment, *Curr Opin Pulm Med.* 2003. *9*: 393–397.
5. Gorty S, Palton-Adkins J, DaLanno M, Starr J, Dean S, Satiana B. Superficial venous thrombosis of the lower extremities: Analysis of risk factors and recurrence and role of anticoagulation, *Vasc Medicine.* 2004. *9*: 1–6.
6. Blattler W, Schwarzenbach B, Largiader J. Superficial vein thrombophlebitis-serious concern or much ado about little?, *VASA.* 2008. *37*: 31–38.
7. Van Weert H, Dolan G, Wichers I, de Vries C, ter Riet G, Buller H. Spontaneous superficial venous thrombophlebitis: Does it increase risk for thromboembolism?, *J Fam Practice.* 2006. *55*: 52–57.
8. Quenet S, Laport S, Decousus H, Leizorovicz A, Epinat M, Mismetti P. Factors predictive of venous thrombotic complications in patients with isolated superficial vein thrombosis, *J Vasc Surg.* 2003. *38*: 944–949.
9. Ascher E, Hanson JN, Salles-Cunha S, Hingorani A. Lesser saphenous vein thrombophlebitis: Its natural history and implications for management, *Vas Endovasc Surg.* 2003. *37*: 421–427.
10. Gorski G, Norszczyk W, Kostewicz W, et al. Progress of local symptoms of superficial vein thrombosis vs. duplex findings, *VASA.* 2004. *33*: 219–225.
11. Chengelis DL, Bendick PJ, Glover JL, Brown OW, Ranval TJ. Progression of superficial venous thrombosis to deep vein thrombosis, *J Vasc Surg.* 1996. *24*: 745–749.
12. Decousus H, Epinat M, Duillot K, Quenet S, Boissier C, Tardy B. Superficial vein thrombosis: Risk factors, diagnosis, and treatment, *Curr Opin Pulm Med.* 2003. *9*: 393–397.
13. Guex JJ. Thrombotic complications of varicose veins: A literature review of the role of superficial venous thrombosis, *Dermatol Surg.* 1996. *22*: 378–382.
14. Marchiori A, Mosena L, Prandoni P. Superficial vein thrombosis: Risk factors, diagnosis, and treatment, *Semin Thromb Hemost.* 2006. *32*: 737–743.
15. Coppin T, Lebrun E, Barroy JP. Rupture of infected superficial femoral artery aneurysm: A case report, *Acta Chir Belg.* 2002. *102*: 276–278.
16. Rodriguez-Peralto JL, Carrillo R, Rosales B, Rodriguez-Gil Y. Superficial thrombophlebitis, *Semin Cutan Med Surg.* 2007. *26*: 71–76.
17. Fazeli B, Modagheh H, Ravra H, Kazemzadeh G. Thrombophlebitis: Migrans as a footprint of Buerger's disease: A protective-descriptive study in north-east of Iran, *Clin Rheumatol.* 2008. *27*: 55–57.
18. Evanchuk DM, Von Gehr A, Zehnder JL. Superficial venous thrombosis associated with congenital absence of the inferior vena cava and previous episode of deep venous thrombosis, *Am J Hematol.* 2008. *83*: 250–252.
19. Griger DT, Angel TE, Grisier DB. Penile Mondor's disease in a 22-year-old man, *J Am Osteopath Assoc.* 2001. *101*: 235.
20. Nachmann MM, Jaffe JS, Ginsberg PC, Horrow MM, Harkaway RC. Sickle cell episode manifesting as superficial thrombophlebitis of the penis, *J Am Osteopath Assoc.* 2003. *103*: 102.
21. Boehlen F. Superficial thrombophlebitis of the chest wall associated with anticardiolipin antibodies: Antiphospholipid syndrome or Mondor's disease?, *Lupus.* 2004. *13*: 70–71.
22. Holzheimer RG. Laparoscopic procedure as a risk factor of deep venous thrombosis, superficial ascending thrombophlebitis, and pulmonary embolism: Case report and review of the literature, *Eur J Med Res.* 2004. *9*: 417–422.
23. Micco PD. Superficial vein thrombosis in malignancy: An underestimated problem, *Exp Oncol.* 2008. *30*: 4–5.
24. Wahrenbrock M, Borsig L, Le D, Varki N, Varki A. Selectin-mucin interactions as a probable molecular explanation for the association of Trousseau syndrome with mucinous adenocarcinomas, *J Clin Invest.* 2003. *112*: 853–862.
25. Kupelian AS, Huda MSB. Pregnancy, thrombophlebitis, and thromboembolism: What every obstetrician should know, *Arch Gynecol Obstet.* 2007. *275*: 215–217.
26. Duff P. Mondor disease in pregnancy, *Obstet Gynecol.* 1981. *58*: 117.
27. McCall MD, Ramsey JE, Talt RC, et al. Superficial vein thrombosis: Incidence in association with pregnancy and prevalence of thrombophilia defects, *Thromb Haemost.* 1998. *79*: 741–742.
28. Samlaska CP, James WD. Superficial thrombophlebitis: I. Primary hypercoagulable states, *J Am Acad Dermatol.* 1990. *22*: 975–989.
29. Pereira de Godoy JM, Fernades Goday M, Batigalia F, Braile DM. The association of Mondor's disease with protein S deficiency: Case report and review of literature, *J Thromb Thrombolys.* 2002. *13*: 187–189.
30. Pereira de Godoy JM, Braile DM. Protein S deficiency in repetitive superficial thrombophlebitis, *Clin Appl Thromb-Hem.* 203. *9*: 61–62.
31. Schonauer V, Kyrle PA, Weltermann A, et al. Superficial thrombophlebitis and risk for recurrent venous thromboembolism, *J Vasc Surg.* 2003. *37*: 834–838.
32. Leon LR, Labropoulos N. Superficial vein thrombosis and hypercoagulable states: The evidence, *Persp Vasc Surg Endovasc Ther.* 2005. *17*: 43–46.
33. De Moerloose P, Wutschert R, Heinzmann M, Perneger T, Reber G, Bounameaux H. Superficial vein thrombosis of lower limbs: Influence of factor V Leiden, factor II G20210A and overweight, *Thromb Haemost.* 1998. *80*: 239–241.
34. Martinell I, Cattaneo M, Tailoi E, de Stefano V, Chusolo P, Mannucci PM. Genetic risk factors for superficial vein thrombosis, *Thromb Heamost.* 1999. *82*: 1215–1217.
35. Terrier B, Piette AM, Kerob D, et al. Superficial venous thrombophlebitis as the initial manifestation of hypereosinophilic syndrome, *Arch Dermatol.* 2006. *142*: 1606–1610.
36. Raulin S, Raulin C, Greve B. Free-floating thrombus in the femoral vein: A challenge in phlebologic diagnostics, *Eur J Dermatol.* 2001. *11*: 564–568.
37. Lohr JM, McDevitt DT, Lutter KS, et al. Operative management of greater saphenous thrombophlebitis involving the saphenofemoral junction, *Am J Surg.* 1992. *164*: 269–275.
38. Kabnick LS, Ombrellino M, Agis H, et al. *Endovenous heat induced thrombus (EHIT) following endovenous vein obliteration: To treat or not to treat? A new perioperative thrombolic classification.* Presented at the 18th Annual Meeting of the American Venous Forum, Miami, Florida, February 23, 2006.
39. Villani C, Johnson DH, Cunha BA. Bilateral suppurative thrombophlebitis due to *Staphylococcus aureus, Heart Lung.* 1995. *24*: 342–344.
40. Katz SC, Pachter L, Cuschman JG, et al. Superficial septic thrombophlebitis, *J Trauma.* 2005. *59*: 750–753.
41. Murray CK, Beckius ML, McAllister K. Fusarium proliferatum superficial suppurative thrombophlebitis, *Mil Med.* 2003. *168*: 426–427.
42. Jerkic Z, Karic A, Karic A. Clinically silent deep vein thrombosis in patients with superficial thrombophlebitis and varicose veins at legs, *Med Arh.* 2009. *63*: 284–287.
43. Decousus H, Quéré I, Presles E, et al. Superficial venous thrombosis and venous thromboembolism, *Ann Intern Med.* 2010. *152*: 218–224.
44. Gorty S, Patton-Adkins P, DaLanno M, Staar J, Dean S, Satiana B. Superficial venous thrombosis of the lower extremities: Analysis of risk factors, and recurrence and role of anticoagulation, *Vasc Med.* 2004. *9*: 1–6.
45. Milio G, Siragusa S, Minà C, et al. Superficial venous thrombosis: Prevalence of common genetic risk factors and their role on spreading to deep veins, *Thromb Res.* 2008. *123*: 194–199.

46. Zierler BK, Meissner MH, Cain K, Strandness DE. A survey of physicians' knowledge and management of venous thromboembolism, *Vas Endovasc Surg.* 2002. *36*: 367–375.

47. Rohrbach N, Mouton WG, Naef M, Otten KT, Zehnder T, Wagner HE. Morbidity in superficial thrombophlebitis and its potential surgical prevention, *Swiss Surg.* 2003. *9*: 15–17.

48. Murgia AP, Cisno GC, Manfredini R, Liboni A, Zamboni P. Surgical management of ascending saphenous thrombophlebitis, *Int Angiol.* 1999. *18*: 343–347.

49. De Maeseneer MGR. Superficial thrombophlebitis of the lower limb: Practical recommendations for diagnosis and treatment, *Acta Chir Belg.* 2005. *105*: 145–147.

50. Wichers IM, Di Nisio M, Miller HR, Middeldorp S. Treatment of superficial vein thrombosis to prevent deep vein thrombosis and pulmonary embolism: A systematic review, *Haematolgica.* 2005. *90*: 672–677.

51. Vesalio Investigators Group. High vs. low doses of low-molecular-weight heparin for the treatment of superficial vein thrombosis of the legs: A double-blind, randomized trail, *J Thromb Haemost.* 2005. *3*: 1152–1157.

52. Kearon C, Kahn SR, Agnelli G, Goldhaber S, Raskob GE, Comerota AJ. Antithrombotic therapy for venous thromboembolic disease, *Chest.* 2008. *133*: 454S–545S.

53. De Nisio M, Wishers IM, Middledorp S. Treatment for superficial thrombophlebitis of the leg (review). *The Cochrane Library* 2010; 6.

54. Decousus H, Leizorovicz A. Superficial thrombophlebitis of the legs: Still a lot to learn, *J Thromb Haemost.* 2005. *3*: 1149–1151.

55. Bounameaux H, Righini M, Gal GL. Superficial thrombophlebitis of the legs: Still a lot to learn: A rebuttal, *J Thromb Haemost.* 2006. *4*: 289.

56. Hill SL, Hancock DH, Webb TL. Thrombophlebitis of the great saphenous vein: Recommendations for treatment, *Phlebology.* 2008. *23*: 35–39.

57. Cesarone MR, Belcaro G, Corsi M, et al. Local heparin, superficial vein thrombosis. *Angiology.* 2007. *58*(Suppl 1): 36S–40S.

58. Katzenschlager R, Ugurlouglu A, Sipos G, et al. Efficacy and tolerability of liposomal heparin spray-gel as an add-on treatment in the management of superficial venous thrombosis, *Angiology.* 2007. *58*(Suppl 1): 27S–35S.

59. Cesarone MR, Belcaro G, Agus G, et al. Management of superficial vein thrombosis and thrombophlebitis: Status and expert opinion document, *Angiology.* 2007. *59*(Suppl 1): 7S–15S.

60. Kyrle PA, Eichinger S. The risk of recurrent venous thromboembolism: The Austrian study on recurrent venous thromboembolism, *Wiener Klinische Wochenschrift.* 2003. *115*: 471–474.

61. Kalodiki E, Nicolaides N. Superficial thrombophlebitis and low-molecular-weight heparins, *Angiology.* 2002. *53*: 659–663.

62. Decousus H. A pilot randomized double-blind comparison of a low-molecular weight heparin, a non-steroidal anti-inflammatory agent, and placebo in the treatment of superficial vein thrombosis, *Arch Intern Med.* 2003. *163*: 1657–1663.

63. Marchiori A, Verlato F, Sabbion P, et al. High versus low doses of unfractionated heparin for the treatment of superficial thrombophlebitis of the leg: A prospective, uncontrolled, randomized study, *Haemotolgica.* 2002. *87*: 523–527.

64. De Sanctis MT, Cesarone MR, Incandela L, Belcaro G, Griffin M. Treatment of superficial vein thrombosis with standardized application of Essaven Gel, *Angiology.* 2001. *52*(Suppl 3): S57–S62.

65. De Maeseneer MG, Thrombosis Guidelines Group of the Belgian Society and Haemostasis and Belgian Working Group on Angiology. Superficial thrombophlebitis of the lower limb: Practical recommendation for diagnosis and treatment, *Acta Chir Belg.* 2005. *105*: 145–147.

66. Lee JT, Kalani MA. Treating superficial venous thrombophlebitis, *J Natl Compr Canc Netw.* 2008. *6*: 760–765.

67. Sullivan V, Denk PM, Sonnad SS, Eagleton MJ, Wakefield TW. Ligation versus anticoagulation: Treatment of above-knee superficial thrombophlebitis not involving the deep venous system, *J Am Coll Surg.* 2001. *193*: 556–562.

68. Uncu H. A comparison of low-molecular-weight heparin and combined therapy of low-molecular-weight heparin with an anti-inflammatory agent in the treatment of superficial vein thrombosis, *Phlebology.* 2009. *24*: 56–60.

69. Beatty J, Fitridge R, Benveniste G, Greenstein D. Acute superficial venous thrombophlebitis: Does emergency surgery have a role?, *Int Angiol.* 2002. *21*: 93–95.

70. Goldman L, Ginsberg J. Superficial phlebitis and phase 3.5 trials, *N Engl J Med.* 2010. *363*: 1278–1280.

PART IV

CHRONIC VENOUS INSUFFICIENCY

51.

THE PRIMARY CAUSE OF CHRONIC VENOUS INSUFFICIENCY

Michel Perrin and Oscar Maleti

BACKGROUND

DEFINITION

Primary venous insufficiency (PVI) is chronic venous dysfunction whose cause is neither congenital or secondary (postthrombotic). Restricting our attention to chronic venous insufficiency, that is, CEAP classes C_3–C_6 as defined in the VEIN-TERM consensus conference,[1] we will discuss only patients that present edema or chronic skin or subcutaneous lesions including healed and active ulcers, and we will limit our focus to the primary cause of these problems. Nevertheless it must be mentioned that edema is confusing, as transient edema does not have the same severity grade as permanent edema.

HISTORY

For a long time C_3–C_6 classes were supposed to be secondary (postthrombotic), but now we know, thanks to ultrasound investigations, that primary etiology is common in patients classified C_3–C_6.

One of the major merits of the CEAP classification has been to take in account the etiology, information that was missing in previous classifications.

In the updated CEAP, another credit has been added, the use of the advanced CEAP. In the advanced CEAP all the signs listed in the C classes must be reported.[2] For example, a patient presenting with varices, edema, pigmentation, and active ulcer will be classified $C_{2,3,4a,6}$. In the problem that we are dealing with in this chapter the descriptor etiology will always be primary, the descriptor anatomy will inform what venous system is abnormal: superficial, deep, perforator and their possible combinations; lastly the descriptor physiopathology will provide information on the physiologic anomaly that was identified in the eighteen veins or groups of veins listed in the descriptor anatomy. For example, using advanced CEAP, a patient presenting reflux in the great saphenous vein above and below the knee, the small saphenous vein, and the calf perforators, and an obstruction of the common iliac vein will be classified $A_{s,p,d}$, $P_{r2,3,4,18,o7}$.

If we return to the patient described above in terms of clinical and etiologic descriptors and if we add the anatomical and physiopathological descriptors, he will be classified $C_{2,3,4,6}$, E_p, $A_{s,p,d}$, $P_{r2,3,4,18,o7}$. Until now, the advanced CEAP has been used in few epidemiological studies.[3] In this chapter, its use allows precise identification of not only the etiology but also the underlying anatomical and physiopathological anomalies of venous ulcer.

EPIDEMIOLOGIC STUDIES

Only recent epidemiologic studies will be analyzed. Some studies report the prevalence of C_3–C_6 in the general adult population.[4–8] This information is displayed in Table 51.1, but in these studies no data were provided concerning relationships between etiology and clinical class.

COHORT STUDIES

Until now precise information on the etiology, anatomic or physiopathologic abnormalities have been only available in C_5–C_6 patients.

Analyzing 182 legs presenting chronic venous ulcers (C_5–C_6) examined by duplex color sonography (DCS), Magnusson identified a primary etiology in 127 (69.8%) and secondary in 55 (30.2%).[8] Among the primary patients, sixty-two (49%) had only superficial insufficiency, forty-five (35%) a combination of deep and superficial reflux, fourteen (11%) had deep reflux alone (half of them in this subgroup had previously undergone saphenous vein surgery), and six (5%) had no identifiable reflux.

Mac Daniel used DCS examination and air plethysmography (APG) in examining ninety-nine ulcerated legs (C_6).

Table 51.1 PREVALENCE OF CVI PATIENTS

STUDY FIRST AUTHOR (REF NO.)	POPULATION STUDIED (NUMBER) AGE	CLASSIFICATION USED TO IDENTIFY CLINICAL STATUS	PREVALENCE
San Diego Population study Criqui (2)	Cross-sectional study University Employees active or retired (2,211) ?	CEAP	Edema 5.8% Trophic changes 6.2%
Edinburgh Vein Study* Evans (3)	Cross-sectional population study Edinburgh Residents (1,566) 16–84	Widmer clinical classes CVI 2 = C4 in the CEAP CVI 3 = C5–6 in the CEAP	M = 2.3% F = 1.3%
Polish study Jawien (4)	Cross-sectional population study Polish adults rural (21%) and urban area seeking medical help regardless of the cause (40,095) ?	CEAP	Edema 10% Trophic changes 5.1%
Bonn Study Pannier (5)	Cross-sectional population study Bonn and rural respondents (3,072) 18–64	CEAP	Edema 10% Trophic changes 2.5 %

* In the Edinburgh Vein Study ankle flare was used to qualify CVI 1, but as this sign is not listed in the CEAP classification, prevalence numbers might be distorted. Conversely edema is not listed in the Widmer classification.

Sixty-four percent of the patients had a primary etiology and 36% secondary.[9]

In another series of 111 C_5–C_6 legs, fifty-seven (51%) had superficial incompetence alone.[10] In the group with deep incompetence six legs (5%) had isolated deep venous incompetence and forty-two legs (44%) had mixed superficial and deep venous reflux. Knowing that only twenty legs were listed as suspected (fourteen) or proven (6) deep vein thrombosis, it is obvious that etiology was primary in most legs.

Tassiopoulos reviewed thirteen studies reported between 1980 and 1998 which used DCS to assess 1,249 limbs with chronic venous ulceration.[11] The incidence of previous DVT was 32% (95%; confidence interval [CI] 27–36) in 405 limbs where this information was documented. Ninety-two percent of the 1,249 limbs assessed demonstrated venous reflux with isolated superficial venous reflux present in 45% and combined deep and superficial reflux in 43% of the limbs.

A large English survey gives the pattern of venous reflux in 496 limbs (C_5–C_6)[12] (see Table 51.2).

Nevertheless there is another series in which results concerning the patterns of reflux are more instructive. One hundred and twenty seven C_4–C_6 legs were compared with 274 C_{0s}–C_3. The most obvious difference between the two groups was the presence of an axial deep reflux in the C_4–C_6 group (odds ratio [OR], 2.7; CI 1.56–4.57; see Figure 51.1).[13]

In contrast, presence of axial reflux in superficial veins did not increase prevalence of skin changes (OR 0.73; CI 0.44–1.2). The authors concluded that continuous axial deep venous reflux is a major contributor to increased prevalence of skin changes or ulcer with chronic venous disease compared with segmental deep venous reflux above or

Table 51.2 PATTERN OF VENOUS REFLUX IN 496 LIMBS WITH CHRONIC VENOUS ULCERATION

PATTERNS OF REFLUX	NUMBER OF LIMBS	PERCENTAGE
Isolated SVR	230	46.4
SVR+ IPVs	28	5.6
SVR+ sDVR	54	10.9
SVR+ sDVR+ IPVs	9	1.8
SVR+ f-l DVR	88	17.7
SVR+ f-l DVR + IPVs	21	4.2
Isolated f-l DVR	49	10
Isolated sDVR	7	1.4
Isolated IPVs	2	0.4
f-l DVR + IPVs	7	1.4
sDVR+ IPVs	1	0.2

Abbreviations: SVR=superficial venous reflux; IPVs=incompetent calf perforating veins; sDVR= segmental deep venous reflux was defined as deep venous incompetence in the presence of at least one competent deep vein valve above or below the refluxing segment knowing that three venous segments were investigated, the femoral, the below-knee popliteal, and the gastrocnemius veins; f-l DVR= full-length deep venous reflux.

(Adapted from Reference 10)

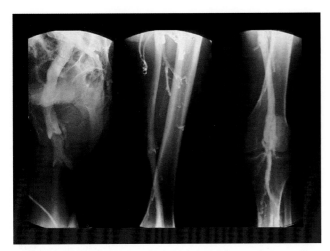

Figure 51.1   Descending venography. Deep axial reflux grade 4 according to Kistner.

below the knee. Information on etiology was reported on the whole group: E_p 302 legs (75%), E_s 99 legs (25%), but not per class.

In the very well documented series of ninety-eight limbs graded C_6, sixty-six extremities (67%) were primary.[3] Superficial reflux with or without involvement of other systems was seen in eighty-four extremities (86%), incompetent perforators were identified in seventy-nine limbs (81%), and seventy-two legs (73%) had deep reflux with or without involvement of other systems.

In the deep reflux subgroup, twenty-two extremities out of seventy-two had a reflux grade 3 and 4 according to Kistner classification[14] (grade 3 = 7; grade 4 = 15). Since the VEIN-TERM consensus conference, grades 3 and 4 are termed "axial reflux."[2] It is worth noting that all patients with a reflux grade 4 had a combination of superficial and/or perforator insufficiency (ten superficial+ perforator, four isolated superficial, one isolated perforator). Nevertheless six legs had no axial superficial reflux.

From all these studies it is clearly established at present that in patients classified C_4–C_6 primary etiology is at least as frequent as secondary etiology. This statement leads to practical management.

MANAGEMENT OF C_4–C_6 PATIENTS

For some authors,[5] only patients who have chronic and permanent changes in the skin and subcutaneous tissues of the lower leg are referred to clinically as having chronic venous insufficiency (CVI), but in the updated CEAP, C3 patients have been included in CVI.[2]

As CVI is an expression of severity in chronic venous disease, management guidelines for CVI patients need to be stated both in terms of investigations and treatment.

INVESTIGATIONS

Besides clinical examination, all C_3–C_6 patients must be investigated on level II as defined in the revision of the CEAP, which means mandatory DCS.[2] In most cases, that allows documentation using the advanced CEAP classification. In other words, the physical signs, absence or presence of symptoms, etiology, and anatomic and physiopathologic abnormalities are usually clearly identified. It is essential to know in every anatomical system, superficial, deep, and perforator, what veins are obstructed or refluxing and what etiology is identified: primary, secondary, or congenital.

In patients with CVI we recommend complementing the CEAP classification by using the updated venous severity scoring system,[15] as we know that in patients with C_3–C_6 the two other scoring systems, venous segmental disease score (VSDS) and the venous disability score (VDS), might be useful, although not validated.[16] When there is a discrepancy between symptoms, C class and DCS findings complementary investigations are needed, such as venography, venous helical CT scan, magnetic resonance imaging, intravascular ultrasound (IVUS), and so forth, according to the venous disease type.

To quantify the global CVI severity investigations such as ambulatory venous pressure and air plethysmography are useful.

TREATMENT
Methods of Treatment

The various treatment methods will be not described in this chapter, as they are detailed in other chapters of the book. Grossly they can be divided in two groups: conservative and invasive or mini-invasive. The first includes compression, drugs, and physiotherapy; the second includes open surgery and endovenous procedures in the three venous systems, knowing that ablation (chemical or thermal) is only used in superficial and perforator veins.

The main difference between conservative and nonconservative treatments is very important to keep in mind. Conservative treatment is usually prescribed regardless of the etiology, anatomy, and physiopathology of the CVI.

On the contrary operative treatments are selective, taking into account etiology, anatomic lesions, and physiopathologic disorders. Superficial venous reflux can be treated by open surgery and endovascular ablation, and the different techniques can be combined.

For treating perforator insufficiency all techniques can be used: sclerotherapy, thermal ablation, ligation by open surgery, and subfascial endoscopic perforator surgery (SEPS).

Deep venous surgery is supposed to treat obstruction or reflux. In primary etiology, obstruction was supposed to be infrequent compared to reflux, but according to Raju and Neglen, primary iliac vein obstruction prevalence is underestimated and underdiagnosed.[17]

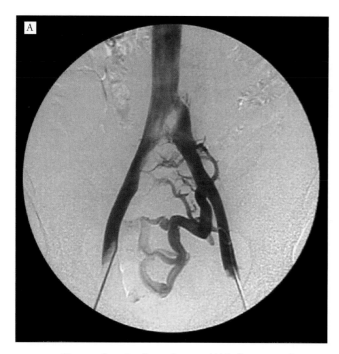

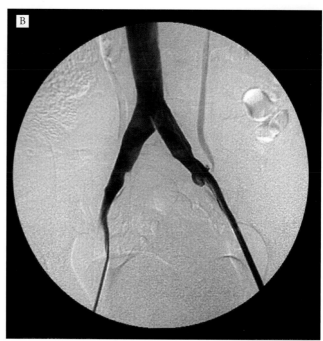

Figure 51.2   Venography using femoral access: (A) Left common iliac vein compression and reflux in left internal iliac vein. (B) Same patient after stenting. Reflux is no longer identified.

For treating primary deep iliocaval obstruction, ballooning and stenting is the method of choice (see Figure 51.2 A B), whereas valvuloplasty is the most used procedure for treating primary deep vein reflux (Figure 51.3).[17,18]

Treatment Results

As the information concerning the outcome of the various treatments is provided elsewhere in this volume, we will focus on patients C_3–C_6 with PVI.

Surprisingly few studies give precise information both on the clinical class and etiology in CVI except for classes C_5–C_6 Only controlled randomized trials (RCTs) with few exceptions will be analyzed here.

Elastic Compression

First of all it must be underlined that long-term compliance with compression is difficult to estimate (between 30 to 60%), but is not influenced by the severity of the venous disease.[19]

Efficacy of compression according to the clinical class:

C_3. Compression reduces edema, but in all the studies both etiology and physiopathologic disorders are not stated. There is no RCT comparing compression to operative treatment.

C_{4a} (eczema, pigmentation). There is no RCT comparing compression to operative treatment.

C_{4b} (lipodermatosclerosis, atrophie blanche). One RCT has shown that stockings improve lipodermatosclerosis, but C_{4b} etiology is not detailed in this study.[20]

C_5–C_6 (healed ulcer, active ulcer). Many RCTs comparing different bandages are available, but the results according to the etiology are not documented.

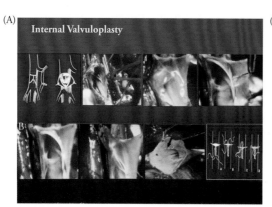

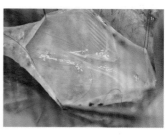

Figure 51.3   Internal valvuloplasty. The floppy incompetent deep valve is repaired. At the end of the procedure the free borders of the valve are in contact.

In two trials compression is compared to surgery. In the first trial, seventy-five venous leg ulcers (VLUs)[21]—fifty-one of primary etiology (forty-seven isolated superficial venous insufficiency and fourteen with a combination of superficial and deep vein reflux), thirteen postthrombotic, and one congenital—were randomized between minimally invasive surgical hemodynamic correction of reflux (CHIVA is the French acronym for this method) and compression. Healing was shorter in the CHIVA group ($P < 0.02$). At a mean follow-up of 3 years, recurrence rate was lower in the CHIVA group ($P < 0.05$) and investigation parameters such as quality of life (QoL) were improved in the CHIVA group. But primary and secondary etiology were not evaluated separately, the extent of the reflux was not documented, and the number of patients was small.

In the ESCHAR study, 500 consecutive patients with VLUs presenting superficial venous reflux and mixed superficial and deep reflux were randomized in two groups receiving either compression alone or in combination with superficial venous surgery.[22,23] Deep venous reflux was assessed in three locations: common femoral or femoral veins, above-knee popliteal vein, and below-knee popliteal vein. When one or two of the three studied deep segments were refluxing, deep reflux was denominated segmental deep; when the three segments were involved, it was classified as total deep.

Primary end points were 24-week healing rates and 4-year recurrence rates. Results were analyzed on an intention-to treat basis. Overall healing rates were similar in both groups.

The rate of ulcer recurrence at 4 years was 56% for the compression group and 31% for the compression plus surgery group ($P < 0.01$).

At 4 years for patients with isolated superficial venous reflux, VLU recurrence rates were 51% for the compression group and 27% for the compression plus surgery group ($P < 0.01$)—At 3 years for patients who had superficial + segmental deep reflux, VLU recurrence rates were 52% for the compression group and 24% for the compression plus surgery group ($P = 0.04$)—At 3 years for patients who had superficial + axial deep reflux, VLU recurrence rates were 46% for the compression group and 32% for the compression plus surgery group ($P = 0.33$).

These results are in accordance with Adam's article.[24] In a series of thirty-nine patients with VLUs in which superficial and segmental deep reflux were combined, segmental deep reflux resolved in nineteen of thirty-nine (49%) and ulcer healing occurred in thirty of thirty-nine (77%) limbs at 12 months after isolated superficial venous surgery.

Chemical Ablation in Presence of Superficial Reflux
There is no RCT comparing chemical ablation with other treatment in PVI restricted to C_3–C_6 patients, but several articles report good outcomes in venous ulcer after foam sclerotherapy, however, etiology and presence or absence of combined deep reflux are not always specified.[25,26]

Two prospective studies are available, the first one included twenty-eight C6 limbs treated by ultrasound-guided foam sclerotherapy as an adjunct for compression. Of chronic VLUs, 96% healed within 3 months, and only two healed VLUs (7%) had recurred at 12 months.[27]

Another study with long-term follow-up is available. C_6 patients were followed during a 45- to 68-month period after HL and ultrasound-guided foam sclerotherapy. At 4-year follow-up, the ulcer recurrence rate was around 30% in the present study, a value comparable with that in the ESCHAR study[23] (estimated recurrence rate 31%) in which patients were treated by conventional surgery plus compression.[28]

Open Surgery in Presence of Superficial Reflux
In the three RCTs comparing surgery + compression with compression alone in C_5–C_6 patients only superficial venous surgery was performed.[21–23] In the first one[21] it was the CHIVA technique, that is high ligation + disconnection of the tributaries from the saphenous trunk. In the second,[22,23] the procedures were isolated saphenofemoral junction or saphenopopliteal disconnection, or combination of high ligation, tributary stab avulsion, and saphenous trunk stripping (only for the great saphenous vein).

There are no RCTs for C_3–C_4 patients comparing surgery with other treatment.

Thermal Ablation in Presence of Superficial Reflux
There are many observational studies and RCTs comparing open surgery with thermal ablation, but the outcome is not reported according to the C class excepted in two.

In one, 560 C_6 patients presenting saphenous and perforator reflux were treated by endovenous laser ablation (EVLA) or classical surgery. The authors concluded that EVLA healed most leg ulcers with primary CVI and reduced the recurrence of ulcers within the first 3 years after treatment, but the treatment protocol is not clear.[29]

In another observational study, in 88 limbs with recalcitrant VLUs, treated in a dedicated wound center by compression over 5 weeks and showing no improvement, incompetent superficial and perforator veins were treated by endovenous ablation. Following successful ablation, the healing rate for healed ulcers improved significantly ($P > 0.05$). After a minimum observation period of 6 months 76.3% of patients healed in 142 +/− 14 days. Twelve patients with twenty-six ulcers did not heal.[30]

Perforator Surgery
Although SEPS has been largely used for treating C_5–C_6 patients whatever the etiology, there are no RCTs comparing results of superficial surgery with superficial surgery + SEPS. In the North American Subfascial Endoscopic Surgery Perforator study[31] (146 patients) SEPS was combined with superficial venous surgery in 103 patients (71%). Patients with primary valvular incompetence had 1-year

(limbs at risk 41) and 2-year (limbs at risk 25) recurrence rates of 15% and 20%, respectively, compared with 47% after 2 years in those of secondary etiology.

Deep Venous Surgery for Reflux

There are no RCTs comparing conservative treatment with surgery for correcting deep venous reflux. Outcomes of this surgery remain difficult to judge, as in PVI superficial, perforator, and deep reflux are frequently combined.

Nevertheless in many series treated by deep venous reconstructive surgery, conservative treatment, or/and superficial surgery, perforator ligation had been used previously and was unsuccessful.

The results of valvuloplasty, which is the procedure of choice for correcting primary deep reflux, are summarized in Table 51.3.

In our series the ulcer recurrence-free survival was 75% at 5 years (44 limbs) for PVI (C_5–C_6) and among the twenty-four limbs with PVI (C_4) no ulcer occurred after deep venous reconstructive surgery.[32]

Grossly deep valvuloplasty with or without previous or concomitant superficial venous surgery and perforator ligation is credited at 5 years with 70% good clinical (no ulcer recurrence) and hemodynamic results: competence of the valve(s) repaired.[18]

It is worth noting that in all series treated by valve repair, the deep reflux was an axial reflux.

Endovenous Treatment for Obstruction

Again there is no RCT comparing conservative treatment to ballooning and stenting, but most of the patients treated operatively were previously not improved or stabilized by conservative treatment. In a series of 334 limbs combining primary reflux and iliac vein compression (nonthrombotic iliac vein lesion: NIVL) 183 were C_3, 69 C_4, 6 C_5, and 39 C_6.[17] All were treated by dilatation and stenting. Outcome was appreciated separately in limbs with isolated

Table 51.3 **VALVULOPLASTY RESULTS**

AUTHOR YEAR	SURGICAL TECHNIQUE	NUMBER OF LIMBS (NUMBER OF VALVES REPAIRED)	ETIOLOGY PVI/TOTAL	FOLLOW-UP MONTHS (MEAN)	ULCER RECURRENCE OR NON HEALED ULCER (%)	HEMODYNAMIC RESULTS COMPETENT AVP □ VALVE (%) VRT ■	
Masuda 1994 (37)	I	32	27/32	48–252 (127)	(28)	24/31 (77)*	□ ↗ 81% (av) ■ ↗ 50% (av)
Raju 1996 (38)	I	68 (71)	/	12–144	16/68 (26)	30/71 (42)	/
Raju 1996 (38)	TMEV	47 (111)	/	12–70	14/47 (30)	72/111	/
Sottiurai 1996 (39)	I	143	/	9–168 (81)	9/42 (21)	107/143 (75)	/
Perrin 2000 (32)	I	85 (94)	65/85	12–96 (58)	10/35 (29)	72/94 (77)	■ Normalized 63% (av)
Raju 2000 (40)	TCEV	141 (179)	98/141	1–42	(37)	(59)	□ ↗ 15% (av) ■ Normalized 100%
Tripathi 2004 (41)	I TMEV	90 (144) 12 (19)	118	(24)	(32) (50)	(79.8) (31.5)	//
Rosales 2006 (42)	TMEV	17 (40)	17/17	3–122 (60)	3/7 (43)	(52)	□ ↗ 50% (av)
Wang 2006 (43)	TMEV	(40)	40/40	(36)	/	(91)	■ ↗ 50% (av)
Lehtola 2008 (44)	I TMEV I+TMEV	12 7 1	5/12 3/7 0/1	24–78 (54)	/	(55)	/

ABBREVIATIONS

I = Internal Valvuloplasty

PVI = Primary Venous Insufficiency

TMEV = Transmural External Valvuloplasty

TCEV = Transcommissural External Valvuloplasty

□ AVP = Ambulatory Venous Pressure

■ VRT = Venous Refill Time

av = average

↗ = Improved

* No reflux or less than 1s

compression and compression and reflux, knowing that reflux was not treated. The cumulative results observed at 2.5 years after stent placement in the NIVL subsets with reflux and without reflux respectively were complete relief of swelling for 47% and 53%, complete stasis ulcer healing for 67% and 76%.

INDICATIONS

According to the reported results recommendations according to Guyatt's grading can be given.[33]

ISOLATED SUPERFICIAL INSUFFICIENCY

In presence of isolated superficial insufficiency operative treatment is strongly recommended (Grade 1 B). As there are now no RCTs comparing long-term outcome of the various operative treatments (open surgery or chemical or thermal ablation) the choice of the procedure to be used is not clear. In the presence of major reflux at a very dilated saphenofemoral or saphenopopliteal junction, particularly when the terminal valve is incompetent, high ligation (HL) remains legitimate combined with trunk saphenous stripping and stab avulsion of the incompetent tributaries.

Endovenous ablation does not include HL, and postoperatively a nonrefluxing patent saphenous stump is usually identified at the saphenofemoral junction. What the long-term results should be in the patients who had an incompetent terminal valve with a massive reflux preoperatively, we don't know. When terminal valve is competent endovenous ablation must be considered.

ASSOCIATION OF SUPERFICIAL AND CALF PERFORATOR VEINS INSUFFICIENCY

There is no consensus agreement in this situation. As a first step isolated superficial venous surgery looks reasonable (recommendation 1C). If persistent incompetent perforators are identified after operative treatment and when the patient is not improved, namely recurrent ulcer or progressive lipodermatosclerosis, they should be treated by surgery (SEPS) or endovenous procedure (recommendation 1B).

COMBINATION OF SUPERFICIAL VENOUS INSUFFICIENCY WITH OR WITHOUT PERFORATOR INSUFFICIENCY AND DEEP VENOUS REFLUX

Presence of a deep segmental deep venous reconstructive surgery is seldom considered, and the patient management is the same as stipulated in the paragraphs above.

In presence of axial deep reflux, phlebologists and some vascular surgeons model their attitude to the one adopted when a segmental reflux is identified. Compression is prescribed after control of superficial and perforator incompetence.

But for others, including our teams, in patients graded C5–C6 deep venous reconstructive surgery must be considered after failure of operative superficial reflux treatment in absence of contraindication, namely ineffective calf pump (recommendation grade 1A).

Valvuloplasty (single, multilevel, multisystem) is the most suitable technique, internal is preferred by most surgeons, knowing this procedure has provided better outcome than external valvuloplasty[18] (see Figure 51.3).

ISOLATED PRIMARY DEEP VEIN REFLUX

This presentation is not common, but C_5–C_6 or C_{4b} class findings in young patients who are reluctant to wear compression for all their lifetime and with extended deep reflux are candidates for valve reconstruction[18] (recommendation grade 1A).

PRIMARY ILIOCAVAL AND FEMORAL OBSTRUCTION COMBINED WITH SUPERFICIAL REFLUX

There is a consensus in patients presenting CVI to treat first obstruction by stenting, but a single-stage combination of percutaneous venous stenting and superficial ablation in patients with severe chronic venous disease is safe.[34]

PRIMARY OBSTRUCTION COMBINED WITH DEEP REFLUX

Indications for treating primary iliocaval compression remain debated, primarily because obstruction identification and its severity are not easy to determine. According to Neglen, only IVUS is reliable.[35] In symptomatic patients with CVI, most authors recommend ballooning and stenting (recommendation grade 1A).[36] But if the patient is not improved, valvuloplasty must be considered in patients presenting persistent axial reflux.[18]

POSTOPERATIVE COMPRESSION

This problem is not resolved. There is no rule stating how long a patient must wear elastic compression after any kind of surgery. One must rely on clinical features, other investigations, or both. When there is no more edema or skin or subcutaneous change, or when DCS and photoplethysmography parameters become normal or subnormal, compression should be discarded.

GUIDELINES FOR PROSPECTIVE STUDIES

First of all an epidemiologic survey in the general population is desirable in order to know the prevalence and incidence of PVI in CVI patients and the respective numbers in the different classes (C_3, C_{4a}, C_{4b}, C_5, and C_6). Besides it would be essential to obtain full information in each group on the different anomalies according to the anatomical location: isolated superficial, perforator, and deep vein insufficiency and their various combinations.

Concerning treatment the following studies should be recommended:

In patients with isolated superficial reflux, RCT comparing chemical ablation with open surgery and thermal ablation. Many studies have been published but only one with a middle term follow-up.

In patients combining superficial and perforator reflux RCT with two arms is needed: one arm where patients will be treated by superficial venous surgery, the other by a combination of superficial surgery and perforator operative treatment.

In patients with deep anomalies RCTs would be difficult to put in place, as the number of patients is small and their anatomic and physiopathologic patterns are mixed.

CONCLUSIONS

Primary venous insufficiency is at least as frequent as secondary in CVI.

As a result, all patients with CVI should be investigated with DCS to fulfill all the headings of the advanced CEAP classification, but most importantly to identify superficial venous insufficiency. Once identified, this isolated anomaly is easily correctible by operative treatment.

When combined with perforator incompetence, there is no consensus for treating them in combination as the first step.

Primary deep vein reflux when axial, needs complementary investigations. Valvuloplasty must be considered in the absence of contraindications, particularly in patients not improved by conservative and/or superficial vein treatment with or without perforator surgery.

Primary deep vein obstruction seems to be underdiagnosed in patients when there is a discrepancy between symptoms, C class, and DCS findings.

REFERENCES

1. Eklof B, Perrin M, Delis K, Rutherford R, VEIN-TERM Transatlantic Interdisciplinary Faculty. Updated terminology of chronic venous disorders: The VEIN-TERM Transatlantic Interdisciplinary consensus document, *J Vasc Surg.* 2009. *49*: 498–501.
2. Eklöf B, Bergan JJ, Carpentier PH, et al. For the American Venous Forum's International Ad Hoc Committee for Revision of the CEAP Classification: Revision of the CEAP classification for chronic venous disorders: A consensus statement, *J Vasc Surg.* 2004. *40*: 1248–1252.
3. Danielsson G, Eklof B, Grandinetti A, Kistner RL, Masuda EM, Sato DT. Reflux from thigh to calf, the major pathology in chronic venous ulcer disease: Surgery indicated in the majority of patients, *Vasc Endovascular Surg.* 2004. *39*: 209–218.
4. Criqui MH, Jamosmos M, Fronek A, et al. Chronic venous disease in an ethnically diverse population, the San Diego population study, *Am J Epidemiol.* 2003. *158*: 448–456.
5. Evans CJ, Fowkes FGR, Ruckley CV, Lee AJ. Prevalence of varicose veins and chronic venous insufficiency in men and women in the general population: Edinburgh vein study, *J Epidemiol Community Health.* 1999. *53*: 149–153.
6. Jawien A, Grzela T, Ochwat A. Prevalence of chronic venous insufficiency in men and women in Poland: Multicentre cross-sectional study in 40,095 patients, *Phlebology.* 2003. *18*: 110–122.
7. Pannier-Fischer F, Rabe E. Epidemiology of chronic venous diseases, *Hautarzt.* 2003. *54*: 1037–1044.
8. Magnusson MB, Nelzén O, Sivertsson R. A colour Doppler ultrasound study of venous reflux in patients with chronic leg ulcers, *Eur J Vasc Endovasc Surg.* 2001. *21*: 353–360.
9. Mac Daniel HB, Marston WA, Farber MA, et al. Recurrence of chronic venous ulcers on the basis of clinical, etiologic, anatomic and physiopathologic criteria and air plethysmography, *J Vasc Surg.* 2002. *35*: 723–728.
10. Grabs AJ, Wakely MC, Nyamekye I, Ghauri ASK, Poskitt KR. Colour duplex ultrasonography in the rational management of chronic venous leg ulcers, *Br J Surg.* 1996. *83*: 1380–1382.
11. Tassiopoulos AK, Golts E, Labropoulos N. Current concepts in chronic venous ulceration, *Eur J Vasc Endovasc Surg.* 2000. *20*: 27–32.
12. Adam DJ, Naik J, Harstone T, London NJM. The diagnosis and management of 689 chronic leg ulcers in a single visit assessment clinic, *Eur J Vasc Endovasc Surg.* 2003. *25*: 462.
13. Danielsson G, Arfvidssson B, Eklof B, Lurie F, Kistner RL. Deep axial reflux, an important contributor to skin changes or ulcer in chronic venous disease, *J Vasc Surg.* 2003. *38*: 1336–1341.
14. Kistner RL, Ferris RG, Randhawa G, Kamida CB. A method of performing descending venography, *J Vasc Surg.* 1986. *4*: 464–468.
15. Vasquez MA, Rabe E, McLafferty RB, et al. Revision of the venous clinical severity score: Venous outcomes consensus statement: Special communication of the American Venous Forum Ad Hoc Outcomes Working Group, *J Vasc Surg.* 2010. *52*: 1387–1396.
16. Rutherford RB, Padberg FT, Comerota AJ, Kistner RL, Meissner MH, Moneta GL. Venous severity scoring: An adjunct to venous outcome assessment, *J Vasc Surg.* 2000. *31*: 1307–1312.
17. Raju S, Neglen P. High prevalence of nonthrombotic iliac vein lesions in chronic venous disease: A permissive role in pathogenicity, *J Vasc Surg.* 2006. *44*: 136–144.
18. Maleti O, Perrin M. Reconstructive surgery for deep vein reflux in the lower limbs: Techniques, results, and indication, *Eur J Vasc Endovasc Surg.* 2011. *41*: 837–848.
19. Raju S, Hollis K, Neglen P. Use of compression stockings in chronic venous disease: Patient compliance and efficacy, *Ann Vasc Surg.* 2007. *21*(6): 790–795.
20. Vandongen YK, Stacey MC. Graduated compression elastic stockings reduce lipodermatosclerosis and ulcer recurrence, *Phlebology.* 2000. *15*: 33–37.

21. Zamboni P, Cisno C, Marchetti P, et al. Minimally invasive surgical management of primary venous ulcers vs compression treatment: A randomized clinical trial, *Eur J Vasc Endovasc Surg*. 2003. *25*: 313–318.

22. Barwell J, Davies C, Deacon J, et al. Comparison of surgery and compression with compression alone in chronic venous ulceration (ESCHAR study): Randomised controlled trial, *Lancet*. 2004. *363*: 1854–1859.

23. Gohel MS, Barwell JR, Taylor M, et al. Long term results of compression plus surgery in chronic venous ulceration (ESCHAR): Randomized controlled trial, *Br Med J*. 2007. *335*: 83–88.

24. Adam DJ, Bello M, Harstone T, London NJM. Role of superficial venous surgery in patients with combined superficial and segmental deep venous reflux, *Eur J Vasc Endovasc Surg*. 2003. *25*: 469–472.

25. Cabrera J, Redondo P, Becerra A, et al. Ultrasound-guided Polidocanol microfoam in the management of venous leg ulcers, *Arch Dermatol*. 2004. *140*: 667–673.

26. Bergan J, Pascarella L, Mekenas L. Venous disorders: Treatment with sclerosant foam, *J Cardiovasc Surg*. 2006. *47*: 9–18.

27. Darvall KAL, Bate GR, Adam DJ, Silverman SH, Bradbury AW. Ultrasound-guided foam sclerotherapy for the treatment of chronic venous ulceration: A preliminary study. *Eur J Vasc Endovasc Surg*. 2009. *38*: 764–769.

28. Figueiredo M, de Araujo SP, Figueiredo MF. Late follow-up of saphenofemoral junction ligation combined with ultrasound-guided foam sclerotherapy in patients with venous ulcers. *Ann Vasc Surg*. 2012. *26*: 977–981.

29. Magi G, Agus GB, Antonelli P, Nardoianni V, Sereni O, Bavera PM. Long-term results of endovenous laser treatment of saphenous and perforator reflux in cases of venous leg ulcers, *Acta Phlebol*. 2009. *10*: 17–22.

30. Harlander-Locke M, Lawrence P, Alktaifi A, Jimenez JC, Rigberg D, DeRubertis B. The impact of ablation of incompetent superficial and perforator veins on ulcer healing rates, *J Vasc Surg*. 2012. *55*: 458–464.

31. Gloviczki P, Bergan JJ, Rhodes JM, Canton LG, et al. Mid-term results of endoscopic interruption for chronic venous insufficiency: Lessons learned from the North American Subfascial Endoscopic Perforator Surgery Registry, *J Vasc Surg*. 1999. *29*: 489–502.

32. Perrin M. Reconstructive surgery for deep venous reflux: A report on 144 cases, *Cardiovasc Surg*. 2000. *8*: 246–255.

33. Guyatt G, Gutterman D, Baumann MH, et al. Grading strength of recommendations and quality of evidence in clinical guidelines: Report from an American College of Chest Physicians Task Force, *Chest*. 2006. *129*: 174–181.

34. Neglén P, Hollis KC, Raju S. Combined saphenous ablation and iliac stent placement for complex severe chronic venous disease. *J Vasc Surg*. 2006. *44*: 828–833.

35. Neglen P, Raju S. Intravascular ultrasound scan evaluation of the obstructed vein, *J Vasc Surg*. 2002. *35*: 694–700.

36. Neglen P, Hollis KC, Olivier J, Raju S. Stenting of the venous outflow in chronic venous disease: Long-term stent-related outcome, clinical and hemodynamic results, *J Vasc Surg*. 2007. *46*: 979–990.

37. Masuda EM, Kistner RL. Long-term results of venous valve reconstruction: A 4 to 21 year follow-up, *J Vasc Surg*. 1994. *19*: 391–403.

38. Raju S, Fredericks RK, Neglen PN, et al. Durability of venous valve reconstruction techniques for "primary" and post-thrombotic reflux, *J Vasc Surg*. 1996. *23*: 357–367.

39. Sottiurai VS. Results of deep vein reconstruction, *Vasc Surg*. 1997. *31*: 276–278.

40. Raju S, Berry MA, Neglén P. Transcommissural valvuloplasty: technique and results, *J Vasc Surg*. 2000. *32*: 969–976.

41. Tripathi R, Sieunarine K, Abbas M, et al. Deep venous valve reconstruction for nonhealing leg ulcers: Techniques and results, *ANZ J Surg*. 2004. *74*: 34–39.

42. Rosales A, Slagsvold CE, Kroese AJ, et al. External venous valve plasty (EVVP) in patients with primary chronic venous insufficiency (PCVI), *Eur J Vasc Endovasc Surg*. 2006. *32*: 570–576.

43. Wang SM, Hu ZJ, Li SQ, Huang XL, Ye CS. Effect of external valvuloplasty of the deep vein in the treatment of chronic venous insufficiency of the lower extremity, *J Vasc Surg*. 2006. *44*: 1296–1300.

44. Lehtola A, Oinonen A, Sugano N, et al. Deep venous reconstructions: long-term outcome in patients with primary or post-thrombotic deep venous incompetence, *Eur J Vasc Endovasc Surg*. 2008. *35*: 487–493.

52.

CONVENTIONAL SURGERY FOR CHRONIC VENOUS INSUFFICIENCY

William Marston

INTRODUCTION

Successful treatment of patients with symptomatic chronic venous insufficiency (CVI) requires a detailed analysis of the anatomic and physiologic correlates of venous dysfunction. Using this information the physician may determine whether correction of the source of CVI is possible and if so, which procedures may be useful to do so. With the proliferation of minimally invasive procedures in the last decade, conventional surgical correction of venous insufficiency is performed less frequently. However these procedures remain useful in some instances as the primary procedure of choice. Regardless of whether a surgical, endovenous, injection-based, or other procedure is performed, the goal is the same: Correction of abnormal venous reflux or obstruction resulting in CVI. Hemodynamic testing may be performed before and after a procedure is performed to document objective improvement and predict long-term success.

Patients with CVI require treatment for limb swelling, skin changes, and ulceration, as well as the pain and disability associated with these objective signs. Although cosmetic considerations should not be ignored, the primary concern in CEAP classes 3–6 is to effectively obliterate abnormal reflux and minimize recurrence for long-term symptom resolution.

In this chapter, diagnostic evaluation and indications for intervention in these patients will be discussed. The options for surgical management of various anatomic types of venous insufficiency will be reviewed and contrasted to nonsurgical techniques.

PRESENTATION OF PATIENTS WITH CVI

A commonly held perception is that less severe CVI (CEAP clinical classes 2–3) is typically a sequela of superficial venous reflux while more severe CVI (CEAP classes 4–6) is associated with deep venous reflux. For this reason, the majority of patients treated with venous leg ulcers never are referred to a venous specialist for consideration of a corrective procedure. Several authors have defined the anatomy of reflux in patients with advanced CVI, and isolated saphenous or saphenous and perforator reflux is not uncommon, occurring in 20–35% of patients in various series. Also, as outlined by Drs. Neglen, Raju, and Kistner in other chapters, many patients with deep venous insufficiency causing severe CVI may be improved with surgical or endovenous procedures, reducing symptoms and the incidence of recurrent ulcers.

For these reasons, all patients with advanced CVI with or without limb ulceration who are candidates for corrective procedures should be studied with diagnostic studies to determine the anatomy and physiology of their individual case. Referral to a venous specialist familiar with surgical and nonsurgical options will allow the optimal method of correction to be selected.

DIAGNOSTIC TESTING FOR PATIENTS WITH CVI

The rational treatment of patients with chronic venous insufficiency (CVI) and its sequelae requires the use of non-invasive studies performed by experienced vascular technologists to identify dysfunction in the patient's venous system. Information on both the anatomic sites of venous dysfunction and its hemodynamic importance are required to allow treatment plans to be formulated and optimal results to be achieved. Selecting surgical therapy without a knowledge of which vein segments are abnormal is essentially blind surgery and cannot result in optimal results.

DUPLEX ULTRASOUND

Imaging techniques using ultrasound combined with Doppler interrogation of the venous system have been validated as sensitive methods of diagnosis of deep venous thrombosis. Important information for patients with CVI that would be detected with this technique includes the presence or absence of venous obstruction or other changes typical of previous deep venous thrombosis (DVT). This information will help to determine whether the patient's CVI is due to obstruction, reflux, or both (pathophysiology). The presence of outflow obstruction in the iliac veins and/or IVC can often be detected looking at flow patterns, phasicity, and respiratory variation in the common femoral vein. In addition to an examination of the deep and superficial systems, the perforator veins are carefully examined for evidence of incompetence.

Secondly, venous reflux in the deep and superficial venous systems is evaluated with the patient in the standing position using duplex ultrasound and either manual compression or a rapid inflation/deflation system to elicit reflux. Systematic interrogation of the common femoral, superficial femoral, popliteal, greater saphenous, and lesser saphenous veins is conducted, allowing an anatomic map of venous reflux in the limb to be constructed.

Using this information, the clinician can determine the etiology, anatomy, and pathophysiology of CVI for the patient. For example, the patient that has superficial and perforator disease may be differentiated from the patient with superficial and deep reflux, allowing alternate treatment plans to be selected. Although duplex evaluation provides detailed information on the anatomy of venous disease, it cannot define the importance of anatomic abnormalities in the venous function of the limb.

PHOTOPLETHYSMOGRAPHY

Plethysmography is defined as the determination of changes in volume, and various techniques of plethysmography have been evaluated in the noninvasive examination of the venous system. A representative photoplethysmography (PPG) tracing is reproduced in Figure 52.1 and illustrates the primary measure obtained, the refill or recovery time (VRT), which represents the time required for the PPG tracing to return to 90% of baseline after cessation of calf contraction. PPG does not produce a quantitative measure, but the refill time has been found to correlate closely with ambulatory venous pressure (AVP) measurements. The use of an above-knee tourniquet inflated to 50 mm Hg has been described to differentiate the contribution of the deep and superficial venous systems to venous reflux.

Limbs affected with CVI typically have a much shorter VRT than normal limbs. As such, PPG can provide a relatively simple measure of whether venous insufficiency is present or not. However, the technique can vary depending on the site of photosensor placement and the small sample area obtained.

PPG measurements have not been proven to be a strong discriminator of the severity of CVI. Nicolaides and Miles reported that normal limbs were well identified by a PPG refill time of greater than 18 seconds with their protocol. Abnormal limbs with CVI consistently had a refill time of <18 seconds. However, in the abnormal group, PPG refill time could not differentiate between degrees of CVI, with similar PPG refill times obtained in patients with AVP measurements ranging from 45 to 100 mm Hg. Therefore, PPG is a poor test for assessing the results of venous corrective surgical procedures.

AIR PLETHYSMOGRAPHY

Air plethysmography (APG) uses a technique to improve on the shortcomings of PPG and other types of plethysmography that have limited sampling areas. It employs a low-pressure air-filled cuff measuring 30 to 40 cm in length that is applied to the lower leg, allowing quantitative evaluation of volume changes of the entire lower leg from knee to ankle. The technique is described in Chapter 5. In 1988, Christopoulos et al. described the use of APG for evaluation of normal limbs and those affected with CVI. A venous filling index (VFI) < 2 ml/s was associated with clinically normal limbs, and increasing levels of VFI were associated with more severe symptoms (Table 52.1).[1] The VFI is believed to provide a reasonable approximation of the global function of the lower extremity venous system in resisting reflux in the standing position.

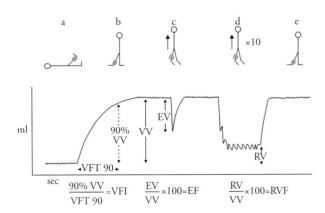

Figure 52.1 APG values measured.

Table 52.1 PREVALENCE OF THE SEQUELAE OF VENOUS DISEASE IN RELATION TO VFI IN 134 LIMBS WITH VENOUS DISEASE STUDIED WITH AIR PLETHYSMOGRAPHY

VFI, ML/S	SWELLING (%)	SKIN CHANGES (%)	ULCERATION (%)
<3	0	0	0
3–5	12	19	0
5–10	46	61	46
>10	76	76	58

(From Reference 17)

The ejection fraction (EF) and residual volume fraction (RVF) are measures of the efficacy of the calf muscle to pump blood out of the leg. The RVF was found to correlate closely with AVP throughout the range of AVP measurements, with lower RVF values representing better calf pump function (normal RVF defined as <35%).

In an evaluation of 186 limbs, Criado et al. assessed the ability of APG parameters to predict the clinical severity of CVI. They reported that, of the APG parameters measured, VFI was the best predictor of the clinical severity of CVI with an 80% sensitivity and 99% positive predictive value for detecting abnormal reflux.[2] EF measurements were unable to differentiate between classes of CVI, and RVF measurements, though able to differentiate, were less useful than the VFI. Further work with APG measurements has demonstrated that the postoperative VFI can predict the long-term symptomatic outcome for patients after venous surgical procedures. Ninety-four percent of patients in whom the VFI corrected to <2 ml/s after surgery were asymptomatic at a mean follow-up time of 44 months (Figure 52.2).[3]

In summary, APG, by sampling a large portion of the calf area, provides a better measure than PPG of the global venous function of the limb. It provides a quantitative analysis that appears to be useful in the selection and follow-up of patients undergoing venous reconstructive or ablative surgery.

INDICATIONS FOR INTERVENTION

The indications for intervention in patients with CVI are variable and depend on the severity of symptoms, options for correction, and the functional and medical status of the patient. Patients in CEAP clinical class 3 and 4 suffering symptoms of swelling and skin changes may be managed with compression stockings and skin lubricants with general improvement. However, compliance with compression stocking use is generally believed to be poor in the long term. Patients who are candidates for a corrective procedure will typically choose intervention, particularly younger, more active patients. In clinical classes 5 and 6, the primary

indication for intervention is to reduce the risk of recurrent ulceration. Patients with active ulcers can expect ulcer healing in 10–12 weeks on average using various high compression bandaging systems.[4] Unfortunately, patients with larger ulcers and those of long duration heal more slowly in most cases. It is not clear whether intervention with correction of CVI will accelerate healing in these cases, but it is reasonable to perform corrective procedures if possible prior to ulcer healing.

Anatomically, any combination of superficial, perforator, and/or deep venous disease may result in severe CVI. Marston et al. reported that 29% of limbs with CVI and leg ulceration displayed superficial or superficial and perforator disease on standing reflux examination (Table 52.2).[4] Small saphenous reflux may also be sufficient to cause leg ulceration with no other abnormalities, typically resulting in ulceration near the lateral malleolus. The contribution of incompetent perforators to global venous insufficiency remains controversial and will be discussed in detail below, but it is clear that some leg ulcers are associated with large incompetent perforators that should be ligated.

A significant percentage of patients with severe CVI are found to have abnormal venous function in multiple systems. Over 27% percent displayed both deep and superficial reflux in a study of 138 limbs with leg ulceration (Table 52.2). It is not always clear whether these patients will experience an improvement in the severity of symptoms if their superficial or superficial and perforator abnormalities are corrected. This issue will be discussed in detail below.

Hemodynamic evaluation using APG is very useful in the management of patients with multisystem venous insufficiency. Patients with deep and superficial reflux may be initially treated with superficial stripping or ablation, and the APG can be repeated to determine the degree of improvement without addressing the deep venous reflux. As noted above, postoperative normalization of the VFI is associated with minimal symptoms at late follow-up. Therefore, a patient who has improvement in the VFI with correction of only one anatomic component of their venous reflux can be followed conservatively, while a patient with a persistent hemodynamic abnormality with a poor VFI can be considered for further intervention. Ulcer recurrence can also be predicted based on the VFI. McDaniel et al reported that a

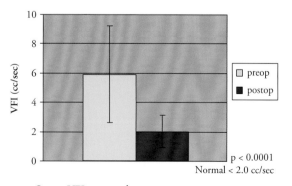

Figure 52.2   Owens VFI post-op data.

Table 52.2 ANATOMIC DISTRIBUTION OF VENOUS REFLUX IN 138 LIMBS WITH CEAP CLINICAL CLASS 6 CVI.

ANATOMIC SITE	INCIDENCE
Deep alone	43.5%
Deep and superficial	21.0%
Deep, perforator, and superficial	6.5%
Superficial alone	18.1%
Superficial and perforator	10.9%

postintervention VFI > 4 was associated with a significantly increased incidence of recurrent limb ulceration. Therefore, patients who are treated conservatively with venous leg ulcers resulting in healing may be considered for intervention to correct venous insufficiency based on the risk of recurrence predicted by APG evaluation.

CONVENTIONAL SURGICAL PROCEDURES FOR CORRECTION OF CVI

SUPERFICIAL VENOUS REFLUX— GREAT SAPHENOUS VEIN

Traditional surgical techniques for removal of the great saphenous vein (GSV) have typically employed ligation of the vein at the saphenofemoral junction (SFJ) and removal of the vein between the groin and knee or groin and ankle using a stripping technique. The goal of high ligation is to identify and divide all venous branches communicating with the SFJ to minimize the potential for recurrent reflux pathways resulting in recurrent symptoms. Unfortunately it appears that many patients developing recurrent venous insufficiency do so because of neovascular generation of new venous communications reestablishing the SFJ, or dilation of preexisting venous tributaries. At this point it is theorized that the surgical procedure itself is the primary stimulus for neovascularization, and there is hope that endovenous techniques may prove to be associated with a lower incidence of recurrent venous insufficiency after intervention.

Numerous methods have been described for removal of the saphenous veins after high ligation. The current trend is toward minimizing the invasiveness of surgical intervention, and numerous alternatives to surgical stripping have been introduced. However, it should be noted that stripping procedures themselves have undergone a significant evolution. Using minimal incisions, tumescent local anesthesia, ultrasound guidance, and careful dissection, the GSV can be removed through two small incisions with relatively little bruising or postoperative discomfort in the majority of cases. In Chapter 23, saphenous stripping techniques are reviewed in detail. Key advances have included the use of detailed preoperative venous mapping to plan surgery and the use of intraoperative ultrasound to locate the SFJ and precisely place incisions.

The following issues in superficial venous surgery will be discussed in detail below:

- Saphenofemoral ligation alone or ligation and saphenous stripping
- Saphenous stripping to the ankle or to the knee
- Small saphenous reflux
- Need for concomitant varicosity ablation

Saphenofemoral Ligation Alone or Ligation and Saphenous Stripping

It has long been debated whether high ligation alone or with varicosity ablation is sufficient for the treatment of superficial venous reflux. Proponents argue that preservation of the saphenous vein is preferable to allow later use as a conduit and that the rate of recurrent symptoms without stripping is acceptable. Hammarsten et al. reported a random allocation of forty-two patients to high ligation with varicosity avulsion or high ligation with saphenous stripping and varicosity avulsion.[5] At a mean follow-up of 52 months there was no difference in the rate of recurrent symptomatic varicose veins (VV) between the two treatment groups (12% in those with stripping and 11% in those without). Venous Doppler evaluation of the residual saphenous vein revealed that 78% would be suitable for use as an arterial conduit.

Proponents of high ligation with GSV stripping have noted the increased incidence of recurrent reflux in the saphenous vein after high ligation alone and maintain that optimal results require routine saphenous stripping. Investigators looking at the residual GSV after high ligation without stripping have identified frequent residual reflux in the GSV. McMullin et al. reported residual reflux in twenty-four of fifty-two cases (46%) after SFJ ligation and found that those with persistent reflux did not correct VRTs measured by PPG.[6] de Haan et al. measured reflux duration and velocities at several levels in the GSV before and after high ligation in twenty-nine limbs.[7] While nearly all (97%) had reflux in the proximal saphenous vein abolished, 52% demonstrated persistent saphenous reflux at the knee.

The Gloucestershire Vascular Group reported 5-year follow-up of 110 limbs randomized to high ligation alone compared with ligation plus stripping.[8] Although patient satisfaction was similar in the two groups, significantly fewer patients in the stripping group required reoperation for recurrent saphenous reflux with symptomatic varicosities (6%) compared to the high ligation–only group (20.8%). Regardless of the type of intervention, VV recurrence appears to depend on the length of follow-up. In Fischer's definitive report of the long-term follow-up of limbs treated with high ligation and stripping, 47% of patients followed for an average of 34 years developed clinically evident varicosity recurrence.[9] The primary benefit of stripping appears to be a reduction in the number of limbs requiring reoperation. It has been suggested that this relates to the improved hemodynamic outcome in limbs treated with stripping, resulting in a lower incidence of persistent pain and swelling that would require reoperation.

Balancing the improved hemodynamic result with saphenous stripping has been the occurrence of increased complications with this procedure. While there is an increased incidence of bruising and hematoma in the thigh with stripping, this can be minimized by the use of tumescent anesthesia and other techniques as noted above. The most significant complication attributed to saphenous stripping involves injury to the saphenous nerve. Fully described below, there is a significant incidence of saphenous nerve deficit after stripping, which is reduced when stripping stops at the level of the knee. Overall, few patients appear to have long-term deficits from this injury.

In summary, high ligation and varicosity ablation is likely to be an acceptable procedure for less severe classes of CVI where the reduced recovery time and reduced potential for bruising and nerve injuries is more important. Although some patients develop recurrent reflux, several authors have reported that sequential sclerotherapy of saphenous branches is able to eliminate recurrent reflux when it develops.

However, in more severe classes of CVI, the primary aim is to correct the hemodynamic abnormality resulting in symptoms. For many patients, the need for repeat procedures to maintain control of saphenous reflux is undesirable. The high incidence of residual saphenous reflux and significant frequency of reoperation when stripping is not performed argue in favor of high ligation and stripping as the preferred surgical operation for CVI with symptoms due to GSV reflux.

Saphenous Stripping to the Ankle or to the Knee

If GSV stripping is chosen as a component of a procedure for the treatment of CVI, the surgeon must determine the length of vein to remove. In most cases, the vein refluxes both at the SFJ and throughout its course. Traditionally, many surgeons have elected to strip the entire vein from groin to ankle. The saphenous vein is easily identified at the ankle, and retrograde passage of the stripper is generally unobstructed. However, the saphenous nerve is in close proximity to the vein beginning just below the knee in many patients and may be susceptible to injury during stripping procedures. For these reasons, some surgeons have recommended limiting stripping at a point just below the knee.

To determine whether a limited GSV stripping to the knee would be sufficient to yield improvement in venous hemodynamics, Nishibe et al. studied 110 limbs before and after removal of the above knee segment of GSV using duplex ultrasound APG.[10] They found that venous hemodynamics as measured by APG were markedly improved after limited GSV stripping. The majority of patients experienced correction of the abnormal preoperative VFI (4.0 ± 0.35 ml/s) to the normal range (1.4 ± 0.15, p < 0.001). The incidence of apparent saphenous nerve injury on assessment at 2–3 weeks after surgery was 4.5%, with most of these patients reporting numbness, mild to moderate pain, or sensitivity to touch in the affected areas.

Holme and colleagues conducted a prospective randomized study in which 163 patients were randomized to high ligation and stripping of the GSV to the ankle (Group A)

compared to high ligation and stripping to the knee (Group B).[11] Three months after surgery, 94% of patients in Group A reported good or excellent relief of symptoms compared to 97% of patients in Group B (p = NS). Evidence of saphenous injury was identified in 39% of limbs in Group A compared to 7% in Group B (p < 0.001). In a subsequent report, the same authors reported long-term follow-up of the same patient cohort. Three years after randomization, 29% of limbs in group A were reported to display symptoms of permanent saphenous nerve injury compared to only 5% in Group B (p < 0.01). At 5 years of follow-up, recurrent varices were seen in 10% of patients in each group.

In a detailed study of the incidence and clinical impact of saphenous nerve injury, Morrison and Dalsing evaluated 127 limbs treated with saphenous stripping to the ankle at a mean follow-up of 4.5 years.[12] Overall, 40% of patients reported symptoms of saphenous nerve injury at some point after operation. At last follow-up 17% reported the symptoms were persistent, but only 2.3% reported that the symptoms negatively affected their quality of life.

Although the symptoms of saphenous nerve injury may rarely be severe, minor complaints are frequent. It appears that the hemodynamic results of stripping to the knee are similar to total saphenous stripping in most cases. Therefore, most authors have recommended stripping to the knee as the treatment of choice for axial GSV reflux.

Small Saphenous Reflux

Often overlooked is the possibility that severe CVI may be due solely to reflux in the small saphenous vein (SSV). Labropolous et al. studied 226 limbs with reflux isolated to the SSV, comprising approximately 10% of their patients with CVI.[13] Symptoms were present in 61% of patients, but only 18.5% were severe enough to be classified as CEAP clinical class 4–6. In a report of twenty limbs with isolated lateral perimalleolar ulcers, Bass and colleagues found isolated SSV reflux at the saphenopopliteal junction (SPJ) in 15 (75%).[14] After SSV ligation at the junction, all ulcers healed within 12 weeks. Lin et al. found that SSV incompetence was frequently associated with severe CVI and is less commonly corrected surgically than GSV insufficiency.[15] They recommended that SSV examination and correction should assume greater importance in the management of symptomatic CVI. In general, SSVs with sufficient reflux to cause severe CVI are large, dilated veins with numerous varicose tributaries. Hemodynamic evaluation with plethysmography is often useful to determine whether isolated SSV reflux is hemodynamically significant. Patients with SSV reflux are unlikely to have significant symptoms without an abnormal venous filling index.

Prior to intervention for patients with SSV incompetence, the anatomy of the vein must be carefully determined. The variable course of the SSV has been well documented, and the vein may terminate at numerous points into the popliteal vein, the femoral vein, the vein of Giacomini, or elsewhere. The presence of a large persistent superficial vein in the lateral thigh that does not join the deep system should alert the clinician to the possibility of a variant of Klippel-Trenaunay syndrome with hypoplastic deep veins.

Preoperative or intraoperative mapping of the SSV with ultrasound will assist with operative planning and identification of the SPJ. The SSV may give off several branches just distal to the SPJ, and it is believed to be beneficial to ligate these branches to minimize residual collateral reflux. Similar to GSV surgery, controversy has existed concerning the need for stripping of a portion of the SSV. Although no randomized trials have compared sahpenopoliteal ligation to ligation with SSV stripping, most authors have recommended stripping a portion of the SSV. Stripping should generally not involve the lower third of the calf, given the increased risk of injury to the sural nerve.

Need for Concomitant Varicosity Ablation

Correction of saphenous and perforator insufficiency will improve hemodynamics with reduction in symptom severity. However, to many patients, the primary sign of their "vein problem" is the visible varicosities, and most prefer varicosity removal or ablation whenever necessary. In conventional surgical treatment, this typically has been performed at the time of saphenous stripping, taking advantage of the anesthetic and eliminating the need for subsequent procedures. Some practitioners prefer to perform saphenous stripping alone, noting that many varicosities will improve after this procedure, never requiring removal. Since the introduction of endovenous ablative techniques, more patients are treated initially with endovenous ablation without varicosity ablation. In many limbs, residual varicosities contract and fade in the absence of continued venous hypertension so that no further ablative procedures are required. Ambulatory phlebectomy or sclerotherapy may be performed after endovenous ablation for limbs with residual varicosities as needed at the patient's request.

Patients with more severe CVI typically have large varicosities, which may be less likely to resolve without removal. The author's practice has been to recommend elimination of these varicosities at the time of saphenous correction. If incompetent perforating veins (IPVs) are present in the calf, they typically communicate with the posterior arch vein rather than the GSV. Varicosity ablation may be important to eliminate outflow pathways for IPVs as described below. There is little evidence that hemodynamic or symptomatic improvement depends on varicosity removal in most patients, so this decision must be individualized based on the status of the varicosities and the patient's wishes.

A variety of techniques have been described to address prominent varicosities. The standard technique for surgical removal has involved surgical incisions overlying prominent

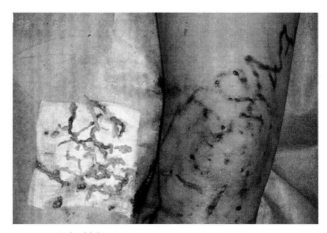

Figure 52.3   Stab phlebectomy.

varicosities and avulsion, followed by limb compression to minimize bleeding and hematoma formation. Over the years, this procedure has been performed through smaller and smaller incisions to its current technique using fine instruments specifically designed to fish out varicosities through microincisions (Figure 52.3). Cosmetic results have improved markedly using this technique, which is fully described in Chapter 26.

Although varicosities can be reliably ablated with this technique, it may be a tedious, time-consuming method in patients with extensive varicosities. For this reason, Spitz developed an alternative method for varicosity removal utilizing a powered phlebectomy device allowing large areas of varicose veins to be rapidly removed through two small incisions (Trivex, Smith and Nephew, Inc., Andover MA). The technique is fully described in Chapter 27. In a randomized study, the results of powered phlebectomy were compared to surgical varicosity removal. Powered phlebectomy was found to significantly reduce the number of required incisions and a trend toward shorter operative time was noted. No difference was found in the incidence of bruising, cellulites, pain, or recovery time. Cosmetic results were perceived by the patients to be equivalent, and no difference in varicosity recurrence was found 6 and 12 months after surgery. The authors concluded that the results of powered phlebectomy were equal to standard phlebectomy, with the potential to shorten surgical time particularly in patients with more extensive varicosities.

Residual varicosities may also be treated with sclerotherapy using a variety of sclerosants as discussed in Chapters 18–21.

RESULTS OF CONVENTIONAL SAPHENOUS SURGERY

Numerous studies have reported on short- and long-term results after saphenous surgery, including symptom relief, varicosity resolution, recurrent varicosities, need for reoperation, and quality-of-life improvement. Bergan reported on the results of 702 limbs undergoing conventional surgical procedures in an outpatient setting.[16] The most common complication was ecchymosis in the medial thigh, none severe enough to require further treatment. Less frequent complications included numbness in the saphenous nerve distribution (6.5%) and lymphocele along the saphenous tract (2.5%). There were no reported cases of DVT in this series. Hospitalization was required in only three patients.

The hemodynamic improvement in patients undergoing saphenous surgery has been well documented. Using APG, correction of saphenous reflux has been demonstrated to result in marked improvement in venous filling index, ejection fraction, and residual volume fraction.[3] Patient satisfaction with the procedure is generally high, but not universally so. Mackay et al. reported on 155 patients who were treated with high ligation and GSV stripping assessed by a questionnaire.[17] Nearly two-thirds of patients reported a perceived postoperative complication within the first 2 weeks after surgery, most relating to bruising, pain, and numbness. Six months after surgery, 80% of patients were satisfied with the outcome, with the most common reason for dissatisfaction being residual varicosities.

Chronic venous disease has been reported to negatively affect patient quality of life as assessed by a variety of outcome measures. Using various methodology, investigators have reported that saphenous vein surgery significantly improves quality of life both initially following surgery, and at midterm follow-up several years later.

For patients with CEAP clinical class 5 and 6 disease, Barwell et al. performed a randomized study comparing the efficacy of saphenous stripping plus compression compared with compression alone for healing and prevention of venous leg ulcers.[18] Termed the ESCHAR study, 500 patients with isolated superficial reflux (60%) or combined superficial and deep venous disease (40%) were enrolled. Demographic factors were similar in the two groups. Ulcer healing was no different with 65% healed in each group by life table analysis at 24 weeks after randomization. Significantly fewer patients in the surgery group experienced recurrent ulceration in 15% at 1 year and 24% at 3 years compared to 34% at 1 year and 52% at 3 years for the group treated with compression alone.

In summary, saphenous stripping procedures have a proven ability to correct venous hemodynamic dysfunction due to abnormal reflux resulting in reduced patient symptoms and improved quality of life in the majority of patients. Though not able to speed healing for venous leg ulcers, the rate of recurrent ulceration is significantly reduced compared to treatment without surgical correction. Complications of surgery are most often minor and self-limited, but an occasional patient may develop nagging discomfort from saphenous neuralgia, and the rare incidence of DVT cannot be ignored.

ALTERNATIVES TO CONVENTIONAL SAPHENOUS SURGERY

Numerous alternatives to conventional saphenous surgery have been promoted to effectively eliminate saphenous reflux without the need for surgical incisions or saphenous removal. These include:

- Hemodynamic correction of varicose veins (CHIVA)

- External banding to restore saphenous competence

- Endovenous ablation

  - Radiofrequency
  - Laser

- Sclerotherapy

  - Ultrasound guided
  - Foam

When considering the optimal management of patients with more severe CVI, the primary goal is to abolish axial reflux and prevent its recurrence. In these patients, recanalization or reopening of the previously treated saphenous vein usually results in recurrence of the preintervention symptoms, including pain, swelling, worsening skin changes, and possibly ulceration. Most patients who have suffered leg ulcers related to CVI, if given a choice, will choose an intervention that is most likely to minimize the risk of ulcer recurrence. None of the alternatives to saphenous stripping have been studied in a randomized trial to prove benefit in reducing venous ulcer recurrence. As a surrogate we can assume that if the GSV or SSV remains closed with no reflux throughout the length from groin to knee, the patient should experience a benefit similar to high ligation and stripping procedures.

Saphenous banding procedures to attempt to reestablish competence of the sentinel valve at the SFJ using either external banding materials, or endovenous radiofrequency have met with variable results. Despite encouraging reports of success in some studies, others have generated disappointing results with high recurrence rates, such that these techniques are not widely used currently.

Sclerotherapy using ultrasound guidance has been described as a means for occluding the GSV or SSV, thereby correcting reflux. Initial attempts employed liquid sclerosants, and though many saphenous veins were successfully treated, recanalization rates were high in many studies (18.8%—23.8%). More recently, foam sclerotherapy has been studied for occlusion of the GSV, with several studies finding improved results compared to liquid sclerotherapy.[19] In a randomized study, 88 patients were treated with either sclerosing foam or sclerosing liquid via direct puncture of the GSV under duplex guidance.[19] Three weeks after treatment repeat examination with duplex ultrasound revealed that only 40% of patients treated in the liquid sclerotherapy group had eliminated reflux throughout the GSV compared to 84% in the foam sclerotherapy group. From these studies, it appears that the recurrence rate for liquid sclerotherapy is unacceptably high for treatment of the GSV. Using a foam sclerosant will significantly increase success rates, but they may still be inferior to high ligation and stripping.

Of the listed alternatives to saphenous ligation and stripping procedures, endovenous ablation has been the most widely studied, including randomized comparisons to stripping. Early studies with both techniques have demonstrated initial saphenous closure rates of over 90%. Long-term data reporting the incidence of saphenous recanalization are now emerging, with acceptable 3- to 5-year results. In the EVOLVeS study, radiofrequency ablation (RFA) was compared with ligation and stripping in eighty-six limbs including quality-of-life measures and follow-up ultrasound examinations at routine intervals. Initial success rates at elimination of saphenous reflux were 100% in the stripping group and 95% in the RFA group.[20] Time to return to normal activities and return to work were significantly less in the RFA group. Quality of life surveys revealed a significantly better global score and a significantly better pain score for RFA 1 week post procedure, but these differences progressively decreased over time. At 2 years of follow-up, two patients in the RFA group had developed recanalization of an initially closed saphenous vein (4%), but global quality-of-life scores still favored RFA. One patient in the RFA group and four treated with ligation and stripping were found to have evidence of neovascularization on ultrasound examination. Recurrent VV occurred in 14% of RFA limbs and 21% of stripped limbs (p = NS).

In another randomized study comparing RFA to saphenous stripping in eighty-eight patients, similar results were reported as patient satisfaction, quality-of-life improvement, and analgesic requirements all significantly favored RFA early after surgery.[21]

Clearly, further long-term study is required to define the optimal use of endovenous procedures. However, in amenable patients, these techniques appear to be viable alternatives to surgical stripping. Long-term recurrence rates must be carefully studied, but the possibility that endovenous ablation will produce less neovascular regeneration at the SFJ is intriguing and will certainly be followed closely.

COMBINED DEEP AND SUPERFICIAL VENOUS INSUFFICIENCY

Treatment of patients with symptomatic CVI and isolated superficial venous insufficiency is usually recommended given the reproducible improvement with correction of saphenous reflux and the low-risk procedures available for this patient group. In patients with CEAP class 4–6 disease, superficial insufficiency is often identified in combination with deep disease. As noted above, 27% of limbs studied with active or healed ulcers were reported as having combined reflux. In this situation the clinician must determine whether symptom improvement is likely from treatment of superficial reflux alone, or if the patient is more likely to require deep venous reconstruction.

Several authors have reported that when superficial reflux in the GSV or SSV is present, the more proximal deep vein segment will occasionally reflux solely due to the superficial vein incompetence. Correction of the superficial reflux reliably results in resolution of the deep vein segment reflux. In this situation GSV incompetence would be seen along with reflux in the common femoral vein, but the femoral and popliteal veins would be competent. With SSV reflux, popliteal reflux would be noted cranial to the SPJ, but not caudal to the junction. With these patterns of reflux, superficial ablative procedures are recommended using the same criteria used for superficial incompetence alone.

Treatment of limbs demonstrating true deep venous insufficiency, defined as reflux in the femoral and popliteal veins, combined with superficial reflux is controversial. Walsh and Sales reported resolution of deep venous reflux after GSV stripping in over 90% of cases, but Scriven reported that deep venous reflux usually did not correct.[22] Puggioni et al. recently reported a study of thirty-eight limbs with combined deep and superficial reflux studied with duplex ultrasound before and after saphenous stripping.[22] Deep venous reflux was corrected in one-third of patients, and femoral vein reflux corrected more frequently when only segmental reflux was present in that vein rather than axial reflux throughout the deep venous system. Puggioni et al. note that the majority of limbs reported by Walsh and Sales demonstrated segmental reflux that may be more likely to correct with superficial surgery than axial reflux.

Padberg and colleagues reported a hemodynamic follow-up of eleven limbs with deep and superficial disease treated with superficial stripping and perforator ligation in some cases.[23] Although only 27% of limbs studied postoperatively were found to have correction of deep venous reflux, significant improvement in both clinical symptom scores and the venous filling index were demonstrated. Marston et al. reviewed the clinical and hemodynamic results of forty patients with both femoropopliteal and superficial reflux treated with endovenous ablation of the GSV and/or SSV.[24] They found that the amount of clinical improvement depended on the maximal reflux velocity (MRV) in the deep venous system. When MRV in the popliteal or femoral vein was less than 10 cm/s, limbs had significantly better outcomes than limbs with MRV > 10 cm/s as measured by both VFI (p = 0.01) and venous clinical severity score (VCSS) (p = 0.03).

In summary, it is reasonable to consider superficial ablative intervention in patients with combined deep and superficial insufficiency. Those with proximal or segmental reflux of lower velocity are more likely to benefit than patients with full axial or higher velocity reflux in the deep venous system.

THE SIGNIFICANCE OF PERFORATOR REFLUX IN CVI

The incidence of perforator incompetence increases as the clinical severity of CVI worsens. The majority of limbs in CEAP clinical classes 5 and 6 have been reported to contain perforators with incompetence on duplex imaging. For this reason, some clinicians believe that incompetent perforators should be corrected whenever they are diagnosed. Unfortunately it is difficult to clearly determine the hemodynamic significance of incompetent perforators because they are usually seen in limbs that also display superficial and/or deep system incompetence. There clearly are cases where incompetent perforators are seen in a limb previously treated with saphenous stripping with persistent symptoms of CVI. In these patients, perforator interruption is necessary. But it is unclear whether perforators should routinely undergo ligation in severe CVI at the time of saphenous ablation.

CONVENTIONAL SURGICAL LIGATION OF IPVS

When the surgeon believes that IPVs are associated with clinical symptoms, elimination of perforator reflux can be performed using a variety of techniques. Open surgical ligation, mini-incision ligation, subfascial endoscopic ligation, and percutaneous ablation can all be considered. Until the last decade, only open surgical perforator ligation was performed, usually using the Linton procedure. As originally described by Linton, the procedure involves a medial lower limb incision placed over the site of the clinically significant IPVs. Dissection proceeds down to the level of the fascia, where the perforators are located and ligated with suture ligatures (Figure 52.4). The use of skin flaps was advocated to help reduce the potential for skin breakdown at the incision site postoperatively.

Though the Linton procedure was effective at eliminating perforator reflux, it has been associated with a high incidence of complications, mostly occurring at the incision site in the area of hyperpigmented, scarred skin typical

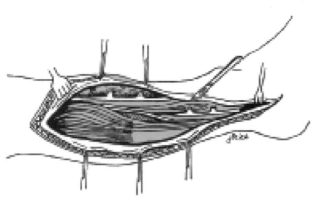

Figure 52.4 Linton procedure.

of advanced CVI. In a report of thirty-seven limbs treated with the Linton procedure, Stuart et al. reported that calf wound complications occurred in seven patients (19%), and the average hospital time was 9 d.[25] Recurrent ulceration was reported in 7–22% of treated limbs at varying lengths of follow-up after the Linton procedure.

For these reasons, alternate methods were developed to ligate IPVs while eliminating the need for surgical incisions in the area of diseased skin expected to be at risk for compromised wound healing. The most widely performed alternative to the Linton procedure employs endoscopy to facilitate subfascial perforator ligation (SEPS) through a small remote incision just below the knee. See Chapter 53 for a full description of this technique. The primary benefits of this technique have been reported to include more rapid recovery and fewer perioperative complications with equivalent hemodynamic results in comparison to the Linton procedure. In a prospective comparison of the Linton procedure to SEPS, Pierik et al. randomized thirty-nine patients to open or endoscopic perforator ligation.[26] 1997 In the open group, 53% of patients developed postoperative wound infection compared to 0% in the SEPS group (p < 0.001). Ulcer healing rates and recurrence rates were similar in the two groups.

Other alternate options have been reported for treatment of refluxing perforators. Perforator ligation has been reported using a mini-incisional technique minimizing wound complications. Results have been reasonably good, but experience is limited. Initial reports of the use of endoluminal techniques have suggested that percutaneous ablation of perforator veins is feasible. Larger prospective studies are needed to determine the efficacy of these less invasive methods.

A more fundamental question concerns the indications for perforator ligation. This remains controversial with proponents arguing that perforators are frequently present in severe CVI and should be ligated whenever present. Skeptics argue that perforators are usually present in combination with superficial and/or deep venous incompetence and the relative contribution of the incompetent perforator to venous insufficiency is less important. Iafrati et al. reported on the treatment of fifty-one limbs with perforator reflux and leg ulcers using SEPS.[27] Venous disability scores improved significantly after the procedure, and 74% of limb ulcers healed within 6 months. The recurrent ulceration rate was low at 13%. Excellent results were obtained, but thirty-five of the fifty-one limbs were treated concomitantly with saphenous or varicose vein removal. Of note, SEPS performed without saphenous surgery was associated with delayed ulcer healing.

Tawes et al. reported a large retrospective multicenter experience using SEPS in over 800 limbs with CVI.[28] The majority of patients (532) were in CEAP clinical class 5 or 6. Concomitant GSV removal was performed in 55% of cases. Reported results were excellent, with 92% of limb ulcers healing at 4–14 weeks after SEPS. Recurrent ulceration occurred in only 4% at a mean follow-up of 15 months. From this review, the authors concluded that until definitive level I evidence is available, SEPS is advocated as optimal therapy for patients with CVI and incompetent perforator veins.

Mendes et al. studied a common subset of patients with IPVs, those with concomitant saphenous reflux and IPVs.[29] Twenty-four limbs were studied before and after surgery with duplex ultrasound and APG. In all limbs, saphenous stripping was performed, with powered phlebectomy added in patients with prominent varicosities. No SEPS or other specific treatment for the IPVs was performed. After surgery, 71% of the limbs no longer contained IPVs. Hemodynamic improvement on APG occurred in all limbs, with the VFI improving from 6.0 ± 2.9 preoperatively to 2.2 ± 1.3 after surgery (p < 0.001). They concluded that either the varicosity ablation performed an extrafascial perforator ligation by removing the outflow tract for the IPVs, or the IPVs were of relatively little hemodynamic importance in comparison to saphenous reflux in this patient group.

It is not clear whether IPVs found in limbs coexisting with deep venous reflux should be ligated, particularly in the absence of corrective surgery for the deep venous system. In the North American SEPS Registry report, there was an increased incidence of leg ulcer recurrence in patients with deep venous insufficiency after SEPS. No prospective randomized studies have been performed to further evaluate these important questions.

It is obvious that the treatment of limbs found to contain IPVs remains controversial in many situations. Perhaps the primary problem in this debate is the lack of a comprehensive definition of perforator incompetence based on their potential to cause venous hemodynamic dysfunction. Delis and colleagues previously suggested that all perforators demonstrating outward flow are not equal, proposing that the volume of outward flow in 1 s after compression release (based on perforator size and velocity of reflux) may be used to define classes of perforator reflux.[30] They proposed that the early hemodynamic function of the IPV determines its clinical impact on the leg, rather than the duration of reflux. The maximum diameter of IPVs may also be important in determining the hemodynamic impact of IPVs. Further research on diagnosis and management of IPVs is required to allow optimal treatment of IPVs.

CONCLUSION

In patients with severe CVI, the primary goal is elimination of abnormal venous reflux resulting in venous hypertension. Rational treatment of this diverse group of patients requires detailed anatomic and hemodynamic assessment with duplex and plethysmography. Postprocedure reassessment can reveal the results of therapy and direct further management. Standard surgical techniques for correction of superficial and perforator incompetence are being replaced by less invasive methods that appear in early and mid-term studies to have comparable symptomatic and hemodynamic results. Long-term study will be required to evaluate the critical areas of neovascularization and symptom recurrence after these alternative methods.

REFERENCES

1. Christopoulos D, Nicolaides AN, Szendro G. Venous reflux: Quantitation and correlation with the clinical severity of chronic venous disease, *Br J Surg.* 1988. *75*: 352.
2. Criado E, Farber MA, Marston WA, Danniel PF, Burnham CB, Keagy BA. The role of air plethysmography in the diagnosis of chronic venous insufficiency, *J Vasc Surg.* 1998. *27*: 660–670.
3. Owens LV, Farber MA, Young ML. The value of air plethysmography in predicting clinical outcome after surgical treatment of chronic venous insufficiency, *J Vasc Surg.* 2000. *32*: 961–968.
4. Marston WA, Carlin RE, Passman MA, et al. Healing rates and cost efficacy of outpatient compression treatment for leg ulcers associated with venous insufficiency, *J Vasc Surg.* 1999. *30*: 491–498.
5. Hammarsten J, Pedersen P, Cederlund CG, Campanello M. Long saphenous vein saving surgery for varicose veins. A long-term follow-up. *Eur J Vasc Surg.* 1990. *4*(4): 361–364.
6. McMullin GM, Coleridge Smith PD, Scurr JH. Objective assessment of high ligation without stripping the long saphenous vein, *Br J Surg.* 1991. *78*: 1139–1142.
7. De Haan RJ, Legemate DA, van Gurp JM, Leeuwenberg A. Quantitative measurements of venous reflux by duplex scanning of the incompetent long saphenous vein before and after high ligation at the saphenofemoral junction, *Eur J Surg.* 1999. *165*: 861–864.
8. Dwerryhouse S, Davies B, Harradine K, Earnshaw JJ. Stripping the long saphenous vein reduces the rate of reoperation for recurrent varicose veins: Five-year results of a randomized trial, *J Vasc Surg.* 1999. *29*: 589–592.
9. Fischer R, Linde N, Duff C, Jeanneret C, Chandler JG, Seeber P. Late recurrent saphenofemoral junction reflux after ligation and stripping of the greater saphenous vein, *J Vasc Surg.* 2001. *34*: 236–240.
10. Nishibe T, Nishibe M, Kudo F, Flores J, Miyazaki K, Yasuda K. Stripping operation with preservation of the calf saphenous veins for primary varicose veins: Hemodynamic evaluation, *Cardiovasc Surg.* 2003. *11*: 341–345.
11. Holme JB, Skajaa K, Holme K. Incidence of lesions of the saphenous nerve after partial or complete stripping of the long saphenous vein, *Acta Chir Scand.* 1990. *156*: 145–148.
12. Morrison C, Dalsing MC. Signs and symptoms of saphenous nerve injury after greater saphenous vein stripping: Prevalence, severity, and relevance for modern practice, *J Vasc Surg.* 2003. *38*: 886–890.
13. Labropoulos N, Giannoukas AD, Delis K, et al. The impact of isolated lesser saphenous vein system incompetence on clinical signs and symptoms of chronic venous disease, *J Vasc Surg.* 2000. *32*: 954–960.
14. Bass A, Chayen D, Weinmann EE, Ziss M. Lateral venous ulcer and short saphenous vein insufficiency, *J Vasc Surg.* 1997. *25*: 654–657.
15. Lin JC, Iafrati MD, O'Donnell TF Jr, Estes JM, Mackey WC. Correlation of duplex ultrasound scanning-derived valve closure time and clinical classification in patients with small saphenous vein reflux: Is lesser saphenous vein truly lesser?, *J Vasc Surg.* 2004. *39*: 1053–1058.
16. Bergan JJ. Surgical management of primary and recurrent varicose veins. In Gloviczki P, Yao JST, eds. *Handbook of venous*

disorders: *Guidelines of the American Venous Forum*, 2e. New York: Arnold. 2001. 289–302.

17. Mackay DC, Summerton DJ, Walker AJ. The early morbidity of varicose vein surgery, *JR Nav Med Serv.* 1995. *81*: 42–46.

18. Barwell JR, Davies CE, Deacon J, et al. Comparison of surgery and compression with compression alone in chronic venous ulceration (ESCHAR study): Randomized controlled trial, *Lancet.* 2004. *363*: 1854–1859.

19. Hamel-Desnos C, Desnos P, Wollmann JC, Ouvry P, Mako S, Allaert FA. Evaluation of the efficacy of Polidocanol in the form of foam compared with liquid form in sclerotherapy of the greater saphenous vein: Initial results, *Dermatol Surg.* 2003. *29*: 1170–1175.

20. Lurie F, Creton D, Eklof B, et al. Prospective randomized study of endovenous radiofrequency obliteration (closure procedure) versus ligation and stripping in a selected population (EVOLVeS Study), *J Vasc Surg.* 2003. *38*: 207–214.

21. Subramonia S, Lees T. Randomized clinical trial of radiofrequency ablation or conventional high ligation and stripping for saphenous varicose veins, *Br J Surg.* 2010. *97*(3): 328–336.

22. Puggioni A, Lurie F, Kistner RL, Eklof B. How often is deep venous reflux eliminated after saphenous vein ablation, *J Vasc Surg.* 2003. *38*: 517–521.

23. Padberg FT Jr, Pappas PJ, Araki CT, Thompson PN, Hobson RW 2nd. Hemodynamic and clinical improvement after superficial vein ablation in primary combined venous insufficiency with ulceration, *J Vasc Surg.* 1996. *24*: 711–718.

24. Marston WA, Brabham VW, Mendes R, Berndt D, Weiner M, Keagy BA. The importance of deep venous reflux velocity as a determinant of outcome in patients with combined superficial and deep venous reflux treated with endovenous saphenous ablation, *J Vasc Surg.* 2008. *48*: 400–406.

25. Stuart WP, Asam DJ, Bradbury AW, Ruckley CV. Subfascial endoscopic perforator surgery is associated with significantly less morbidity and shorter hospital stay than open operation (Linton's procedure), *Br J Surg.* 1997. *84*: 1364–1365.

26. Pierik EGJM, van Urk H, Hop WCJ, Wittens CHA. Endoscopic versus open subfascial division of incompetent perforating veins in the treatment of venous leg ulceration: A randomized trial, *J Vasc Surg.* 1997. *26*: 1049–1054.

27. Iafrati MD, Pare GJ, O'Donnell TF, Estes J. Is the nihilistic approach to surgical reduction of superficial and perforator vein incompetence for venous ulcer justified?, *J Vasc Surg.* 2002. *36*: 1167–1174.

28. Tawes RL, Barron ML, Coello AA, Joyce DH, Kolvenbach R. Optimal therapy for advanced chronic venous insufficiency, *J Vasc Surg.* 2003. *37*: 545–551.

29. Mendes RR, Marston WA, Farber MA, Keagy BA. Treatment of superficial and perforator venous incompetence without deep venous insufficiency: Is routine perforator ligation necessary?, *J Vasc Surg.* 2003. *38*: 891–895.

30. Delis KT, Husmann M, Kalodiki E, Wolfe JH, Nicolaides AN. In situ hemodynamics of perforating veins in chronic venous insufficiency, *J Vasc Surg.* 2001. *33*: 773–782.

53.

SUBFASCIAL ENDOSCOPIC PERFORATOR VEIN SURGERY(SEPS) FOR CHRONIC VENOUS INSUFFICIENCY

Peter Gloviczki, Manju Kalra, and Alessandra Puggioni

Surgical interruption of incompetent perforating veins was first suggested by Linton in 1938[1] to treat patients with venous ulcers. The rationale for ligating incompetent perforators was to decrease ambulatory venous hypertension in patients with advanced venous disease by decreasing abnormal transmission of pressure from the deep to the superficial veins. Linton's original operation, that required a long skin incision, resulted in a high rate of wound complications. Subsequently proposed operations using shorter skin incisions were either incomplete or, similar to Linton's operation, resulted in frequent wound complications. Subfascial endoscopic perforator vein surgery (SEPS) was developed to replace the open techniques and it became instantly popular because of the minimally invasive nature of the procedure combined with a lesser rate of wound complications. SEPS has been an effective, minimally invasive technique to interrupt incompetent medial perforating veins of the leg.[2–25]

SURGICAL TECHNIQUE

SEPS was first performed in Germany by Hauer in 1985, who used a simple one-port endoscopic instrument to interrupt perforating veins.[2] Two main techniques for SEPS have been developed.

The first has been a perfection of the original technique of Hauer, by Fischer,[3,5,14] with further development by Bergan and colleagues,[9,11,18] and Wittens and Pierik.[7,13,20,25] It uses a single scope with channels for both the camera and working instruments (see Figure 53.1). Improvement in instrumentation for this technique resulted in using carbon dioxide insufflation through the single working channel to inflate and enlarge the subfascial space.

The second technique of SEPS uses instrumentation from laparoscopic surgery, and it was introduced by

O'Donnell.[23] Carbon dioxide insufflation was added to this technique simultaneously by Conrad in Australia[6] and by our group at the Mayo Clinic.[8,15,21] The two-port technique employs one port for the camera and a separate port for instrumentation, thereby making it easier to work in the subfascial space. The 5-mm port is placed more posterior, halfway between the main port and the ankle. First the limb is exsanguinated with an Esmarque bandage and a thigh tourniquet is inflated to 300 mmHg to provide a bloodless field. A 10-mm endoscopic port next is placed in the medial aspect of the calf 10 cm distal to the tibial tuberosity, proximal to the diseased skin (see Figure 53.2). A balloon dissector is used to widen the subfascial space and facilitate access after port placement. The distal 5-mm port is placed halfway between the first port and the ankle (about 10–12 cm apart), under direct visualization with the camera. Carbon dioxide is insufflated into the subfascial space and pressure is maintained around 30 mmHg to improve visualization and access to the perforators. Using laparoscopic scissors inserted through the second port, the remaining loose connective tissue between the calf muscles and the superficial fascia is sharply divided.

The subfascial space is then explored from the medial border of the tibia to the posterior midline, down to the level of the ankle, and up to the level of the 10-mm port. All direct and indirect perforators encountered are occluded and divided with a harmonic scalpel or electrocautery, or the vein is cut with scissors between clips. A paratibial fasciotomy next is made by incising the fascia of the posterior deep compartment, close to the tibia, to avoid injury to the posterior tibial vessels and the tibial nerve. The posterior tibial perforators (Cockett II and Cockett III) are frequently located within an intermuscular septum, or frankly, in the deep posterior compartment, behind the paratibial fascia (see Figure 53.3). This has to be incised before identification and division of the perforators can be

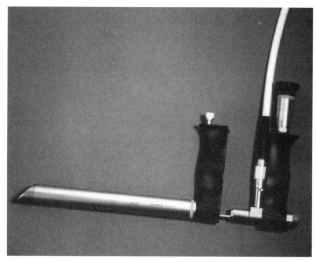

Figure 53.1   Olympus endoscope for the subfascial perforating vein interruption. The scope can be used with or without carbon dioxide insufflation. It has an 85-degree angle field of view, and the outer sheath is either 16 or 22 mm in diameter. The working channel is 6 × 8.5 mm, with a working length of 20 cm.[39]

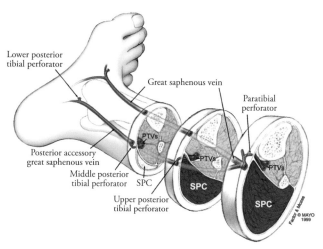

Figure 53.3   The anatomy of the medial perforating veins of the leg. PTVs = posterior tibial veins, SPC = superficial posterior compartment [40]

accomplished. The medial insertion of the soleus muscle on the tibia may also have to be exposed to visualize proximal paratibial perforators. The paratibial fasciotomy can aid in distal exposure, but reaching retromalleolar Cockett I perforator endoscopically is usually not possible, and if incompetent, may require a separate small incision over it to gain direct exposure.

After completion of the endoscopic portion of the procedure the instruments and ports are removed, the CO_2 is manually expressed from the limb. Twenty ml of 0.5% marcain solution is instilled into the subfascial space for postoperative pain control. The tourniquet can be left inflated during the time stab avulsion of varicosities is performed on the foot, ankle, or calf. After deflating the tourniquet,

laser or radiofrequency ablation or, occasionally, high ligation and stripping of the great or small saphenous vein, if incompetent, is performed. All stab wounds and the area surrounding the saphenous vein is infiltrated with tumescent diluted anesthetic solution. The port sites are closed in two layers with dissolvable sutures, the stab wounds are closed with paper tapes, and the limb is wrapped with an elastic bandage. A single dose of low molecular weight heparin is given subcutaneously during the procedure to decrease the risk of perioperative deep vein thrombosis. Elevation is maintained at 30 degrees postoperatively for 3 h, after which ambulation is permitted. SEPS is an outpatient procedure, and patients are discharged the same day or within 24 hours following overnight observation. In the long term they are instructed to use a firm compression (30 to 40 mmHg) elastic garment.

RESULTS OF SEPS

Experience with SEPS continues to grow, and results from several centers are summarized in Table 53.1. The safety and efficacy of SEPS has been established in the North American SEPS Registry[17,24] and in nonrandomized case series.[2–16,18–23] In a randomized trial SEPS had a lower wound complication rate (0%) than traditional open surgical techniques (53%) at 21 months after surgery.[25]

The North American SEPS (NASEPS) registry compiled data from 146 patients, 101 of whom had active ulcers (C6) at the time of operation (see Figures 53.4 and 53.5).[17,24] Wound complication rate was 6%, and one deep venous thrombosis occurred at 2 months after surgery. The midterm (24 months) results of the NASEPS registry demonstrated an 88% cumulative ulcer healing rate at 1 year. The median time to ulcer healing was 54 days. Cumulative rate of ulcer recurrence was significant: 16% at 1 year, 28% at 2 years,

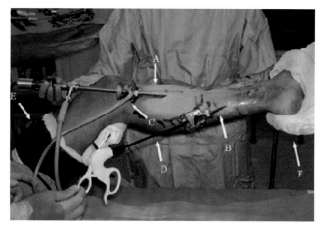

Figure 53.2   Two-port technique of SEPS. One 10-mm port (A) for the camera and a 5-mm port (B) for instrumentation are inserted. Carbon dioxide is insufflated into the subfascial space (C), and pressure is maintained around 30 mmHg. All perforators encountered are divided with the harmonic scalpel (D). Note the thigh tourniquet (E) and the leg holder (F) to facilitate the operation.[38]

Table 53.1 PUBLISHED RESULTS OF SUBFASCIAL ENDOSCOPIC PERFORATOR VEIN SURGERY (SEPS)*

FIRST AUTHOR, YEAR	LIMBS (NO.)	LIMBS WITH HISTORY OF ULCER (NO.)**	LIMBS WITH ACTIVE ULCER (NO.)	SAPHENOUS ABLATION (%)	WOUND DEHISCENCE/ SEROMA (NO.)	HEMATOMA (NO.)	PARESTHESIA (NO.)	INFECTION/ CELLULITIS/ THROMBOPHLEBITIS (NO.)	ULCER HEALING %	LIMBS WITH ULCER RECURRENCE (NO.) φ	MEAN FOLLOW-UP (MONTHS)
Jugenheimer and Junginger[4] 1992	103	NR	17	NR	3	6	10	0	94	0	27
Pierik et al.[29] 1995	40	40	16	10	0	0	0	3	100	1	46
Bergan et al.[9] 1996	31	25	15	100	2	2	0	6	93	0	NR
Rhodes et al.[30] 1998	31	25	12	77	3	2	2	2	100	1	11
Glowiczki et al.[17] 1999	146	122	101	60	0	0	10	5	84	26	24
Lee et al.[31] 2001	36	19	NR	92	0	0	2	4	89	2	14
Sybrandy et al.[20] 2001	20	20	20	70	0	0	0	0	85	2	46
Baron et al.[32] 2001	45	45	37	40	0	0	0	0	89	0	10
Iafrati et al.[33] 2002	51	51	29	55	1	2	0	0	74	7	38
Ciostek et al.[34] 2002	146	74	36	90	0	0	19	5	86	11	56
Kalra et al.[21] 2002	103	76	42	72	5	5	4	14	90	21	39
Bianchi et al.[35] 2003	74	74	58	77	0	3	0	9	91	4	44

*From Reference 38, with permission

**CEAP Classes 5 and 6

φ Disease Class 6

φ Recurrence calculated for Class 5 and 6

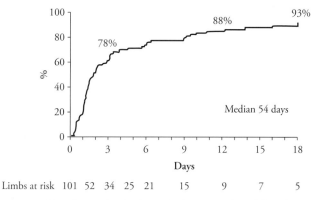

Limbs at risk 101 52 34 25 21 15 9 7 5

Figure 53.4   Cumulative ulcer healing in 101 patients after subfascial endoscopic perforator vein surgery. The 90-day, 1-year, and 1.5-year healing rates are indicated. The standard error is less than 10% at all time points.[24]

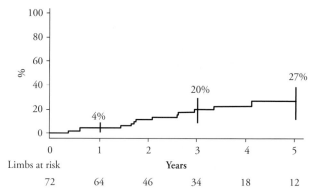

Limbs at risk   72   64   46   34   18   12

Figure 53.6   Cumulative ulcer recurrence in seventy-two patients in the Mayo Clinic series after subfascial endoscopic perforator vein surgery (SEPS). The 1-, 3-, and 5-year recurrence rates are indicated. All class 5 limbs at the time of SEPS and class 6 limbs that subsequently healed are included. The start point (day 0) for time to recurrence in class 6 patients was the date of initial ulcer healing. The standard error is less than 10% at all time points.[21]

but still compared favorably with results of nonoperative management. Higher rate of ulcer healing was observed in those who underwent SEPS with saphenous vein stripping, compared with limbs that underwent SEPS alone: 3- and 12-month cumulative ulcer healing rates of 76% and 100% versus 45% and 83% (*P* < 0.01), respectively.

In a prospective study Nelzen et al. reported on results of 149 SEPS procedures in 138 patients.[19] Forty-five percent of limbs had venous ulceration (C6–thirty-six limbs, C5–thirty-one limbs) and deep venous insufficiency was present in 7% of limbs. During a median follow-up of 32 months, thirty-two of thirty-six ulcers healed, more than half (19/36) within 1 month. Three ulcers recurred, one of which subsequently healed during follow-up. At a median follow-up of 7 months following surgery, 91% of patients were satisfied with the results of the operation.

Our results at Mayo Clinic were reported by Kalra et al.[21] One hundred and three consecutive SEPS procedures were performed over a 7-year period. Venous ulceration affected 74% of limbs (C6–forty-two limbs, C5–thirty-four limbs),

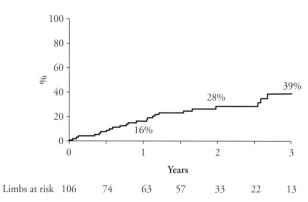

Limbs at risk   106   74   63   57   33   22   13

Figure 53.5   Cumulative ulcer recurrence in 106 patients of the North American Registry after subfascial endoscopic perforator vein surgery (SEPS). The 1-, 2-, and 3-year recurrence rates are indicated. All class 5 limbs at the time of SEPS and class 6 limbs that subsequently healed are included. The start point (day 0) for time to recurrence in class 6 patients was the date of initial ulcer healing. The standard error is less than 10% at all time points.[24]

and deep venous incompetence was present in 89% of limbs. On life-table analysis 30-, 60-, and 90-d cumulative ulcer healing rates were 41%, 71%, and 80% with a median time to ulcer healing of 35 d. These results compare favorably with the 65% ulcer healing rates at 6 months, reported in the ESCHAR study that randomized patients to conservative management versus superficial venous surgery.[26] Mean follow-up in the SEPS study at Mayo was 3.25 years and 1-, 3-, and 4-year cumulative ulcer recurrence rates were 4%, 20%, and 27% (see Figure 53.6).

In the most recent report from the Mayo Clinic, Puggioni et al. demonstrated excellent healing rates after SEPS in patients without previous deep vein thrombosis.[27] Eighty-eight SEPS procedures were performed in eighty-one patients with active (n = 50) or healed (n = 38) ulcers. Median follow-up was 35 months. Forty-four ulcers healed, for a crude ulcer healing rate of 88%. Median time to ulcer healing was 35 days, 90-d and 1-year cumulative ulcer healing rates were 79% and 88%. All six ulcers that did not heal by the time of last follow-up had previous deep vein thrombosis. Ulcer healing in postthrombotic limbs at 1 year was 73% versus 100% in primary valvular incompetence (p = 0.02). Not surprisingly, healing rates were higher in those patients who had SEPS with superficial ablation versus those who had SEPS alone. Also, limbs with femoropopliteal reflux have decreased healing rates. SEPS with or without ablation of the incompetent superficial system was effective in decreasing ulcer recurrence as well. Eighteen ulcers recurred during follow-up, for an overall crude ulcer recurrence rate of 18/82 (22%). Freedom from ulcer recurrence at 1, 2, and 3 years were 96%, 90%, and 74%. Patients with primary valvular incompetence did very well, with freedom from ulcer recurrence at the same time intervals of 98%, 94%, and 85%, versus rates in postthrombotic syndrome of 90%, 78%, and 50% (p = 0.06). Factors associated with ulcer recurrence were active smoking and a previous deep venous thrombosis.

Hemodynamic improvement after SEPS was previously reported by Rhodes and colleagues used strain-gauge plethysmography to quantitate calf muscle pump function and venous incompetence before and after SEPS.[15] The authors observed significant improvement in both calf muscle pump function and venous incompetence in thirty-one limbs studied within 6 months after SEPS. Twenty-four of the thirty-one limbs underwent saphenous stripping in addition to SEPS. Normalization of venous incompetence occurred in up to 50% of limbs studied, and this improvement was associated with a favorable clinical outcome. Although limbs undergoing SEPS alone had significant clinical benefits, the hemodynamic improvements did not reach statistical significance. This is likely related to both the small number of patients and the predominance of postthrombotic syndrome in this subgroup.

Patients with primary valvular incompetence have better clinical outcome and also significantly better hemodynamic improvement compared with those with postthrombotic limbs. Proebstle et al., using light reflection rheography before and 8 weeks following SEPS, showed significant improvement in limbs with primary valvular incompetence.[16] Using foot volumetry, Stacey and coworkers demonstrated that perforator vein ligation with ablation of saphenous reflux improved calf muscle pump function in limbs with primary valvular incompetence, although the relative expelled volume did not return to normal.[28] However, no hemodynamic benefit was found in postthrombotic limbs.

Although the role of SEPS in postthrombotic syndrome remains controversial, most patients still show marked symptomatic improvement in disability (pain and swelling), when assessed with the venous clinical scores.[21] Also, recurrent ulcers are usually smaller, more superficial, and single more often than multiple, and heal again easily with conservative management.

In a meta-analysis of twenty published studies on SEPS, Tenbrook et al. analyzed the benefits and risks of surgical treatment in 1,140 limbs with advanced chronic venous insufficiency.[36] After SEPS, with or without superficial venous ablation, ulcers in 88% of limbs healed. The recurrence rate in 611 limbs was 13% at a mean time of 21 months (see Figure 53.7). Risk factors for no healing and recurrent ulcers included new or recurrent incompetent perforator veins, postthrombotic syndrome, deep vein obstruction and ulcers larger than 2 cm in diameter. Surgical complications included wound infection (6%), hematoma (9%), neuralgia (7%), and deep venous thrombosis (1%). Randomized controlled trials are still needed to define the role of SEPS in the treatment of venous ulcer disease. Unpublished data of the Dutch randomized trial indicate benefits of SEPS in patients with large medial ulcers, in those with recurrent ulcers, and in patients who undergo the SEPS procedure in expert venous centers.[37]

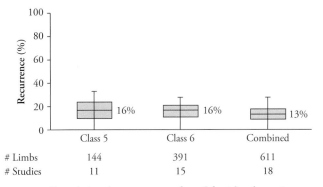

	Class 5	Class 6	Combined
# Limbs	144	391	611
# Studies	11	15	18

Figure 53.7 Cumulative ulcer recurrence after subfascial endoscopic perforator surgery (SEPS) in a meta-analysis of 611 limbs with C5 and C6 disease. *Horizontal lines*, point estimates; *boxes*, 95% confidence intervals; *error bars*, ranges for individual studies that contributed to each estimate; *class 5*, recurrence in limbs with class 5 disease at SEPS; *class 6*, recurrence in limbs with class 6 disease at SEPS in which ulcers subsequently healed; *combined*, recurrence in limbs with class 5 and class 6 disease. Number of limbs and studies in class 5 and class 6 disease do not total those in the combined group, because not all studies reported data separately for limbs with class 5 and class 6 disease.[36]

CONCLUSIONS

Initial exuberance with SEPS focused much needed attention to chronic venous disease and the underlying venous anatomy and pathophysiology. Limitations of perforator ablations alone in treating patients with ulcers were also soon recognized. Without doubt, SEPS should be combined with ablation of the incompetent superficial system, performed either as staged or as combined procedures. Results have been excellent on both ulcer healing and recurrence in primary valvular incompetence without associated femoropopliteal reflux, but long-term ulcer healing could not be achieved in half of the operated patients with postthrombotic syndrome. Incompetent perforators are but one of the contributing factors to ambulatory venous hypertension, and in patients with postthrombotic syndrome and deep vein occlusion they likely are important outflow channels that should be preserved to assure the collateral venous circulation. Introduction of less invasive techniques for perforator ablation, such as ultrasound-guided sclerotherapy or radiofrequency ablation may diminish the role of SEPS in the future, but results should be compared and analyzed before we diminish the use of a safe and effective endoscopic technique for ablation of the perforating veins.

REFERENCES

1. Linton RR. The operative treatment of varicose veins and ulcers, based upon a classification of these lesions, *Ann Surg.* 1938. *107*: 582–593.
2. Hauer G. Endoscopic subfascial discussion of perforating veins: Preliminary report [German], *Vasa.* 1985. *14*(1): 59–61.
3. Fischer R. Surgical treatment of varicose veins: Endoscopic treatment of incompetent Cockett veins, *Phlebologie.* 1989.

4. Jugenheimer M, Junginger T. Endoscopic subfascial sectioning of incompetent perforating veins in treatment of primary varicosis, *World J Surg.* 1992. *16*(5): 971–975.

5. Fischer R, Sattler G, Vanderpuye R. The current status of endoscopic treatment of perforators (in French), *Phlebologie.* 1993. *46*: 701–707.

6. Conrad P. Endoscopic exploration of the subfascial space of the lower leg with perforator vein using laparoscopic equipment: A preliminary report, *Phlebology.* 1994. *9*: 154–157.

7. Wittens CH, Pierik RG, van Urk H. The surgical treatment of incompetent perforating veins [Review] [63 refs], *Euro J Vasc Endovasc Surg.* 1995. *9*(1): 19–23.

8. Gloviczki P, Cambria RA, Rhee RY, Canton LG, McKusick MA. Surgical technique and preliminary results of endoscopic subfascial division of perforating veins, *J Vasc Surg.* 1996. *23*(3): 517–523.

9. Bergan JJ, Murray J, Greason K. Subfascial endoscopic perforator vein surgery: A preliminary report, *Ann Vasc Surg.* 1996. *10*(3): 211–219.

10. Padberg FT Jr, Pappas PJ, Araki CT, Back TL, Hobson RW. Hemodynamic and clinical improvement after superficial vein ablation in primary combined venous insufficiency with ulceration [see comments], *J Vasc Surg.* 1996. *24*(5): 711–718.

11. Sparks SR, Ballard JL, Bergan JJ, Killeen JD. Early benefits of subfascial endoscopic perforator surgery (SEPS) in healing venous ulcers, *Ann Vasc Surg.* 1997. *11*(4): 367–373.

12. Stuart WP, Adam DJ, Bradbury AW, Ruckley CV. Subfascial endoscopic perforator surgery is associated with significantly less morbidity and shorter hospital stay than open operation (Linton's procedure) [see comments], *Br J Surg.* 1997. *84*(10): 1364–1365.

13. Pierik EG, van Urk H, Wittens CH. Efficacy of subfascial endoscopy in eradicating perforating veins of the lower leg and its relation with venous ulcer healing, *J Vasc Surg.* 1997. *26*(2): 255–259.

14. Fischer R, Schwahn-Schreiber C, Sattler G. Conclusions of a consensus conference on subfascial endoscopy of perforating veins in the medial lower leg, *Vasc Surg.* 1998. *32*: 339–347.

15. Rhodes JM, Gloviczki P, Canton LG, Heaser TV, Rooke T. Endoscopic perforator vein division with ablation of superficial reflux improves venous hemodynamics, *J Vasc Surg.* 1998. *28*: 839–847.

16. Proebstle TM, Weisel G, Paepcke U, Gass S, Weber L. Light reflection rheography and clinical course of patients with advanced venous disease before and after endoscopic subfascial division of perforating veins, *Dermatol Surg.* 1998. *24*: 771–776.

17. Gloviczki P, Bergan JJ, Menawat SS, et al. Safety, feasibility, and early efficacy of subfascial perforator surgery: A preliminary report from the North American Registry, *J Vasc Surg.* 1997. *25*(1): 94–105.

18. Murray JD, Bergan JJ, Riffenburgh RH. Development of open-scope subfascial perforating vein surgery: Lessons learned from the first 67 patients, *Ann Vasc Surg.* 1999. *13*: 372–377.

19. Nelzen O. Prospective study of safety, patient satisfaction, and leg ulcer healing following saphenous and subfascial endoscopic perforator surgery, *Br J Surg.* 2000. *87*: 86–91.

20. Sybrandy JE, van Gent WB, Pierik EG, Wittens CH. Endoscopic versus open subfascial division of incompetent perforating veins in the treatment of venous leg ulceration: Long-term follow-up, *J Vasc Surg.* 2001. *33*: 1028–1032.

21. Kalra M, Gloviczki P, Noel A, et al. Subfascial endoscopic perforator vein surgery in patients with postthrombotic syndrome: Is it justified?, *Vasc Endovasc Surg.* 2002. *36*: 41–50.

22. Illig KAS, Shortell CK, Ouriel K, Greenberg RK, Waldman D, Green RM. Photoplethysmography and calf muscle pump function after subfascial endoscopic perforator ligation, *J Vasc Surg.* 1999. *30*(6): 1067–1076.

23. O'Donnell TF. Surgical treatment of incompetent communicating veins. In: Bergan JJ, Kistner RL, eds. *Atlas of venous surgery.* Philadelphia: W.B. Saunders. 2000. 111–124.

24. Gloviczki P, Bergan JJ, Rhodes JM, Canton LG, Harmsen S, Ilstrup DM. Mid-term results of endoscopic perforator vein interruption for chronic venous insufficiency: Lessons learned from the North American subfascial endoscopic perforator surgery registry: The North American Study Group, *J Vasc Surg.* 1999. *29*(3): 489–502.

25. Pierik EG, van Urk H, Hop WC, Wittens CH. Endoscopic versus open subfascial division of incompetent perforating veins in the treatment of venous leg ulceration: A randomized trial, *J Vasc Surg.* 1997. *26* 1049–1054.

26. Barwell JR, Davies CE, Deacon J, et al. Comparison of surgery and compression with compression alone in chronic venous ulcer (ESCHAR Study): Randomized control trial, *Lancet.* 2004. *363*: 1854–1859.

27. Puggioni A, Kalra M, Noel A, Hoskin T, Gloviczki P. *Ulcer healing and recurrence after subfascial endoscopic perforator surgery (SEPS).* Presented at the 17th Annual Meeting of the American Venous Forum, San Diego, California, March, 2005.

28. Stacey MC, Burnand KG, Layer GT, Pattison M. Calf pump function in patients with healed venous ulcers is not improved by surgery to the communicating veins or by elastic stockings, *Br J Surg.* 1988. *75*: 436–439.

29. Pierik EGJM, Wittens CHA, van Urk H. Subfascial endoscopic ligation in the treatment of incompetent perforator veins, *Eur J Vasc Endovasc Surg.* 1995. *5*: 38–41.

30. Rhodes JM, Gloviczki P, Canton LG, Rooke T, Lewis BD, Lindsey JR. Factors affecting clinical outcome following endoscopic perforator vein ablation, *Am J Surg.* 1998. *176*: 162–167.

31. Lee DW, Chan AC, Lam YH, et al. Early clinical outcomes after subfascial endoscopic perforator surgery (SEPS) and saphenous vein surgery in chronic venous insufficiency, *Surg Endosc.* 2001. *15*: 737–740.

32. Baron HC, Saber AA, Wayne M. Endoscopic subfascial surgery for incompetent perforator veins in patients with active venous ulceration, *Surg Endosc.* 2001. *15*: 38–40.

33. Iafrati MD, Pare GJ, O'Donnell TF, Estes J. Is the nihilistic approach to surgical reduction of superficial and perforator vein incompetence for venous ulcer justified?, *J Vasc Surg.* 2002. *36*: 1167–1174.

34. Ciostek P, Myrcha P, Noszczyk W. Ten years experience with subfascial endoscopic perforator vein surgery, *Ann Vasc Surg.* 2002. *16*: 480–487.

35. Bianchi C, Ballard JL, Abou-Zamzam AM, Teruya TH. Subfascial endoscopic perforator vein surgery combined with saphenous vein ablation: Results and critical analysis, *J Vasc Surg.* 2003. *38*: 67–71.

36. Tenbrook JA Jr, Iafrati MD, O'Donnell TF Jr, et al. Systematic review of outcomes after surgical management of venous disease incorporating subfascial endoscopic perforator surgery, *J Vasc Surg.* 2004. *39*: 583–589.

37. Wittens CH, van Gent BW, Hop WC, Sybrandy JE. *The Dutch Subfascial Endoscopic Perforating Vein Surgery (SEPS) Trial: A randomized multicenter trial comparing ambulatory compression therapy versus surgery in patients with venous leg ulcers.* Presented at the Annual Meeting of the Society for Vascular Surgery, Chicago, Illinois, 2003, and at the Annual Meeting of the American Venous Forum, San Diego, California, 2005.

38. Puggioni A, Kalra M, Gloviczki P. Superficial vein surgery and SEPS for chronic venous insufficiency, *Semin Vasc Surg.* 2005. *18*(1): 41–48.

39. Bergan JJ, Ballard JL, Sparks S. Subfascial endoscopic perforator surgery: The open technique. In: Gloviczki P, Bergan JJ, eds. *Atlas of endoscopic perforator vein surgery.* London: Springer-Verlag. 1998. 141–149.

40. Mozes G, Carmichael SW, Gloviczki P. Development and anatomy of the venous system. In: Gloviczki P, Yao JST, eds. *Handbook of venous disorders*, 2e. London: Arnold. 2001. 11–24.

54.

ULTRASOUND-GUIDED SCLEROTHERAPY OF PERFORATING VEINS IN CHRONIC INSUFFICIENCY

Fedor Lurie, Alessandra Puggioni, and Robert L. Kistner

Correction of clinically important hemodynamic abnormalities, such as reflux and obstruction, is the major treatment objective in patients with chronic venous disease. Achieving this goal theoretically should convert the patient into being asymptomatic, eliminate or reverse existing signs, and prevent progression to more advanced stages of venous disease. Practical challenges that face the surgeon who will treat a patient with chronic venous disease include selection of which vein to treat and which technique to employ.

Recent development of new treatment options for reflux in the superficial venous system have established a new standard: patients can be treated in the office without a need for general anesthesia, can ambulate immediately after treatment, have insignificant postoperative pain, and have almost no negative impact on quality of life immediately after treatment. At the time when venous stripping was the only choice for patients with saphenous insufficiency, surgical interruption of perforating veins either by subfascial endoscopic surgery (SEPS) or through small incisions was considered minimally invasive. In a new clinical environment, invasiveness and wound complication risk of these surgical techniques exceeds that of treatment of saphenous veins.

This chapter presents a review of a nonsurgical treatment option for incompetent perforating veins, ultrasound-guided sclerotherapy, which combines the precision of surgical approach with minimal invasiveness of an injection.

HISTORICAL PERSPECTIVE

The first description of the perforating veins of the lower extremities is attributed to J. C. Von Loder, a German anatomist who worked at the end of the eighteenth century.[1] But it was not until the work of John Homans that the role of incompetent perforators was postulated, followed by development of surgical treatment.[2] After the precise definition of principles for perforator control was formulated in the 1930s by Robert R. Linton of Boston, and detailed investigations were performed by Frank Cockett of London, their modifications of perforator ligation became a universally accepted component of treatment of chronic venous disease. In the 1970s, DePalma and Edwards independently introduced a minimally invasive approach to perforator treatment addressing the problem of wound complications after subfascial ligation of incompetent perforators. Popularization of endoscopy in surgery inspired development of SEPS.[3,4] Incidence of wound complications was significantly decreased with SEPS, but the presence of other complications, such as deep venous thrombosis (DVT; less than 1%), superficial thrombophlebitis (3%), and saphenous neuralgia (7%),[5,6] as well as the technical complexity of the SEPS procedure and its high cost, stimulated interest in alternative techniques.

Compression sclerotherapy of incompetent perforating veins was introduced by Fegan in the 1950s.[7] He first hypothesized that, in order for this technique to be effective, patients must continuously wear postoperative compressive bandages. In one of his late publications, in 1979,[8] he reported:

The success of injection compression sclerotherapy depends on the facts: (1) that in the majority of patients with varicose veins and, in almost all those with symptoms incompetent perforating veins are present; and (2) that if these incompetent perforating veins are permanently occluded the superficial veins, no longer subjected to an abnormal blood flow, are capable of regaining their normal tone and diameter and the valves in them regain their competence. The aim of the injection technique is to prevent abnormal pressures and retrograde flow from the deep to the superficial venous system.

With growing popularity of sclerotherapy different techniques have been developed.[9] Results, however, were often unsatisfactory. In 1981 Cockett summarized main causes of failure in perforator injection as (1) inability to accurately locate the perforator, (2) potential damage by extravascular injection of sclerosant, (3) potential damage to posterior tibial artery, and (4) potential damage to deep veins causing DVT.[10]

Advances in ultrasound imaging in the 1980s and 1990s provided the technical basis for ultrasound-guided procedures. At the same time, reliable identification of perforating veins not only became possible but also was integrated into standard diagnostic protocols.[11] Together with new sclerosing agents, which can be effectively used in significantly lower concentrations with less damage to extravascular tissues, these advances helped to overcome the deficiencies of conventional sclerotherapy of perforating veins. By the late 1990s ultrasound-guided sclerotherapy (USGS) became popular in European countries and made its way to the United States.[12–15]

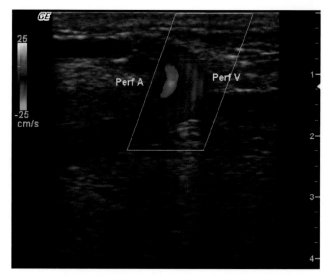

Figure 54.1   Perforating vessels. The perforating artery (Perf A) is located next to the perforating vein (Perf V) at the fascial opening.

BASIC CONSIDERATIONS

To perform echosclerotherapy of lower extremity perforating veins, a thorough knowledge of their anatomy and physiopathology is necessary. Perforator veins connect the superficial to the deep venous system and to the venous sinuses within the leg muscles. These veins usually contain a series of bicuspid valves, located in their subfascial segment, which prevent transmission of high pressure from the deep venous system into the superficial veins. The distribution of medial perforating veins connecting the superficial and deep systems in the calf and thigh is relatively constant. However, the number and anatomy of the numerous perforators to the muscular venous sinuses is unpredictable. Perforating veins are accompanied by perforating arteries supplying the skin and, sometimes, by cutaneous nerve branches and lymphatic vessels. Perforating arteries are usually smaller in diameter and located superior to the accompanied vein.[16] The presence of these arteries can often be confirmed by duplex scan[17] (see Figure 54.1).

The coexistence of perforating veins and arteries in the lower extremities was described first by Robert Linton, who established that "communicating" pedicles have venous and arterial components. He also described how these vessels run along the intermuscular fascial planes and noted that "the arteries are so small that it is not necessary to preserve them." Identification of the perforating arteries, although not always possible, becomes desirable when ultrasound-guided sclerotherapy of perforating veins is performed. Accidental injection of sclerosing agent into the arterial bed may possibly cause complications such as skin necrosis, and can be prevented by visual control, or by performing injections at a distance from the fascial opening where the perforating artery and vein are not in such close proximity to each other. The role of perforator arteries in pathogenesis of venous ulcers and sanogenesis after treatment is yet to be studied. As they provide blood supply to skin areas affected by venous disease, preservation of these vascular structures during treatment may be desirable. Our observations indicate that blood flow in perforating arteries increases after USGS.[17] If this hyperemia can be shown to be beneficial in ulcer healing, selective oblation of perforator veins by USGS could be more desirable than surgical interruption when both veins and arteries are interrupted. The same logic may be applied to perforating cutaneous nerves.

Perforator vein incompetence usually is associated with deep and/or superficial venous incompetence, but, if left untreated, can persist after successful treatment of saphenous reflux. Strong association of perforator incompetence with skin changes and ulceration has been well established, however, incompetent perforators are often present in less advanced stages of the disease, when their role in disease progression and/or recurrence of varicose veins is less obvious. Following the cases of persistent perforator veins after correction of other sources of reflux at Straub Clinic revealed association of patients' symptoms with isolated incompetent perforators, and relief of these symptoms after successful USGS. These findings and variations in anatomy support identification of not only perforator veins in areas of skin changes but also all those potentially clinically important as a treatment target.

Incompetent perforating veins 4 to 7 mm in diameter can be treated with this technique. Smaller veins seldom are incompetent, and larger veins require larger volumes of sclerosant, which potentially increases the risk of complications.

CLINICAL CONSIDERATIONS

Indications for USGS are not different from indications to surgical interruption of perforating veins. Cases of symptomatic chronic venous disease from C2 to C6 clinical class

(CEAP) that have demonstrable incompetent perforating veins at duplex ultrasound constitute the majority of indications. In primary disease, USGS can be performed at the time of initial treatment of saphenous reflux, or as a separate stage. In secondary (postthrombotic) disease, careful consideration should be given to the pathophysiologic role of incompetent perforators in each individual extremity. Incompetent perforators can constitute a major outflow track around an obstructed segment in some cases and be a contributor to skin ulceration in others.

USGS does not require anesthesia and can be performed in the office as well as in the operating room.

Patients with known allergic reactions to sclerotherapy agents, or who are pregnant or lactating should be excluded. The presence of severe arterial occlusive disease or active vasculitis is also a contraindication as inadvertent intraarterial injection potentially can result in limb loss.

SCLEROSING AGENTS

Sodium tetradecyl sulfate (Sotradecol) and sodium morrhuate are the agents frequently used for therapy of incompetent perforating veins. Polidocanol (Aethoxysklerol) is another valid drug for this purpose still awaiting FDA approval in the United States.

The mechanism of action of all these drugs is based on their detergent properties. Immediately after injection the endothelial cells in contact with the drug undergo swelling and disruption. This irreversible trauma causes localized thrombosis, vasospasm, and then vein fibrosis and reabsorption. Larger veins should be treated with increased concentrations rather than larger volumes, since the latter may cause escape of the drug into the deep veins and potentially into the systemic venous circulation.

Recent development of foam sclerotherapy opens new opportunities for treatment of perforating veins. In addition to different sclerosing agents and their concentrations, the use of foam introduces variability in type of gas, gas-to-liquid ratio, time between processing and use, size of the bubbles, and methods of preparation. This variability complicates analysis of results and development of guidelines. Until the standardization of sclerosing foams is developed, foam sclerotherapy continues to be based on the experience and preferences of a treating physician.

PREOPERATIVE DUPLEX

Duplex ultrasound scan plays the most important role in evaluation of the patient before USGS. Complete examination of deep and superficial venous systems including testing for obstruction and valvular incompetence is necessary in every case. Perforating veins should be identified by scanning all aspects of the calf and by following the course of the great saphenous vein (GSV), the vein of Giacomini,

or any incompetent nonsaphenous vein of the thigh. It is preferable to examine patients in a standing position, as the increased hydrostatic pressure makes perforating veins easier to visualize and evaluate. Incompetence of a perforating vein can be determined by registering of reversed flow (directed to the superficial veins) longer than 0.4 seconds, or by the size of the vein at the fascial opening exceeding 3.5 mm, or by the presence of both criteria.[11,18]

In addition to identification of incompetent perforator veins, ultrasound provides information on which veins are connected by these perforators, and thus allocates each perforator to a defined place in the hemodynamic map of the venous system of the affected extremity. At the time of duplex scan, incompetent perforating veins located in the areas of skin changes and ulcers, those connected with corona phlebectatica, or clusters of varicose veins, and those associated with symptoms should be separated from perforators found in asymptomatic limbs, and from those with a questionable hemodynamic role in the disease process. This information is crucial for development of a surgical plan and for a decision on how to treat each of the incompetent perforators.

TECHNIQUE

The procedure can be performed under general or local anesthesia during saphenous and varicose vein ablation, or as an isolated procedure in the outpatient clinic setting. When performed as a stand-alone procedure, no sedation or local anesthesia is required.

The procedure room is warmed to a comfortable temperature in order to avoid venous constriction, and the patient is positioned in the supine or prone position, depending on the location of veins to be treated. The skin is prepped with iodine solution, and a sterile latex cover is applied to the ultrasound probe. This must be oriented longitudinally, and after the target vein is identified, a 25-gauge needle connected to a 3-cc syringe is inserted into the skin close to the ultrasound transducer. The needle tip has to be oriented toward the perforating vein, along the sagittal plane of the probe. The target for the injection is the segment of perforating vein above the fascia (see Figure 54.2A). A small amount of venous blood is withdrawn in the syringe to confirm the correct position of the needle, and 1 to 2 cc of 1% sodium tetradecyl sulfate, or 5% sodium morrhuate is injected under duplex vision. The sclerosing agent can be easily seen by B-mode ultrasound imaging, thus monitoring each injection with ultrasound provides vital information regarding the precision of injection and volume of sclerosant needed to be injected to close the perforator, but not to cause damage of deep veins. Pain during injection, among other causes, can indicate that a perforating artery has been punctured, and therefore injection should be stopped to avoid serious complications.

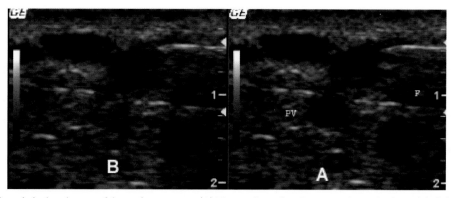

Figure 54.2 Ultrasound-guided sclerotherapy of the perforating vein. (A) The needle is placed in a vein above the fascia (F). (B) After an injection the perforating vein (PV) is filled with an echogenic material and has no flow.

The needle is withdrawn and compression applied for a few minutes. The vein is reimaged, and sclerotherapy is considered successful if no residual flow is observed in the treated perforator (see Figure 54.2A).

Larger veins can be treated by foam sclerotherapy. With this technique conventional sclerosing agent and air are mixed in order to form fine bubbles. The principle behind this method is that by displacing blood from the treated vein and increasing the contact time between the sclerosant and the vein more effective treatment can be achieved.

POSTOPERATIVE CARE

External compression is important for effective sclerotherapy. Even after a successful injection, inadequate compression of the treated area may allow blood flow through a damaged, thrombogenic endothelium, and so thrombophlebitis may develop at that site. Furthermore, adequate compression may improve the calf muscle pump, thus preventing propagation of thrombus into the deep veins. Recurrences may be due to inadequate initial or subsequent continuous compression until a fibrous occlusion occurs. Elastic bandages are applied to the extremity and maintained for 1 to 2 weeks and replaced by class II-III knee-high compression stockings thereafter. Patients with heavy elastic bandages should be warned to remove them should pain occur, before ischemia has caused any damage. Patients are encouraged to ambulate in order to prevent venous stasis that may lead to deep venous thrombosis.

RESULTS

Although available reports on results of USGS consistently demonstrate benefits of this treatment modality, their conclusions should be taken with caution.[12–13,15,19–22]

Important differences between USGS and surgical interruption of perforating veins should be considered when clinical results of perforating vein treatment are analyzed.

The true minimally invasive nature of USGS translates into minimal impact on patients' immediate posttreatment activity and quality of life. Early unrestricted ambulation can be a contributing factor for the treatment outcome.

Any surgical procedure, including SEPS, results in inflammation followed by scar formation in the area of the treated perforator. The impact of these processes on an extremity with CVI has not been defined, but presents theoretical possibilities either for prevention of development or recurrent perforators. On the one hand, postoperative scars may act as a mechanical barrier against reconnection of the deep and superficial systems, but on the other hand, postoperative inflammation might promote neovascularization, thus recurrence of perforators. In the case of USGS, the vein remains in place, therefore its recanalization is possible. Availability of information on objective documentation of immediate treatment success, and differentiation between reopening of treated perforator and development of new vessels can significantly impact interpretation of published data.

Utilization of different sclerosing agents in a variety of concentrations with differences in effects on the vein and surrounding tissue contributes to the complexity of interpretation of reported results.

Waiting for a higher level of evidence on USGS success, and for more precise definitions of outcome measures, one can rely only on clinical experience of groups and individuals performing a high volume of these procedures. The Straub clinic group performed over 3,000 injections of incompetent perforators in the early 2000s.[15,19–21] Immediate successful obliteration of the treated veins at the time of injection was obtained in 98% of cases. Skin complications with superficial skin necrosis occurred in six patients. Recurrence, defined as the presence of flow in a previously sclerosed perforating vein at duplex follow-up, was present in 23% of cases with a mean follow-up of 17 months. Venous clinical severity scores decreased on average from 11.95 pretreatment to 6.5 posttreatment (p < 0.05). Likewise, venous disability scores dropped from 1.86 pretreatment to 0.81 posttreatment (p < 0.05). Perforator recurrence was more common in limbs with ulcerations. Except for the rare occurrence of skin necrosis, cosmetic results were excellent, often with partial reversal of preexisting skin changes, and relief of symptoms.

COMPLICATIONS

Sclerotherapy of perforating veins is associated with minimal discomfort and pain and thus does not require local or general anesthesia. Occurrence of immediate or delayed pain at the site of injection or in a larger calf region should alert the operator against extravascular injection in the soft tissue or in a nearby artery. Intraarterial injection is extremely painful, whereas extravasation in the subcutaneous tissue may remain asymptomatic, unless the sclerosant solution had been mixed with normal saline, or a high concentration of sclerosant had been used. As a result of extravasation, superficial skin necrosis may occur. In our experience superficial skin necrosis occurred in less than 2% of patients, and usually resolved with minimal sequelae in a matter of weeks. A more serious complication is intraarterial injection, as this produces a diffuse endotheliitis blocking the arterioles, which may lead to tissue ischemia and gangrene. Should this complication occur, injection of procaine around the injected artery, local cooling, systemic heparinization, and infusion with low molecular weight dextran are recommended.

As discussed previously, a potential complication of inadequate compression is thrombophlebitis, because residual flow within a damaged vein predisposes to thrombosis of the vein and eventual recanalization. DVT, also rare, is probably due to injection of large volumes of sclerosant. Again, if sclerosing agents are injected in small amounts, only the intima, not the blood, should be affected. These agents are inactivated rapidly by the blood and are, paradoxically, hemolytic and not thrombotic. Another important point to stress is that patients must be encouraged to walk immediately after treatment and must continue this every day to prevent stagnant blood from collecting in the damaged veins.

It would be prudent to avoid injecting limbs of patients with known congenital or acquired prothrombotic state (bedridden, neoplastic, early postthrombosis).

Another possible, although rare, serious complication is anaphylactic shock. While performing injection sclerotherapy, all the necessary equipment to handle this situation must be readily available (oxygen, epinephrine, and steroids) as this could be a life-threatening event. We have not observed this complication during perforating vein sclerotherapy.

CONCLUSION

Ultrasound-guided sclerotherapy is a minimally invasive, alternative technique for the treatment of incompetent calf perforating veins. If a rigorous technique and careful precautions are undertaken, minimal complication rates and satisfactory clinical results can be achieved. After sclerotherapy, patients can resume their routine activities and return to work, and this is without doubt one of the most appealing aspects of this method. We believe that the adoption of this technique in experienced hands potentially could represent the standard method of treating incompetent perforators, as it is associated with minimal discomfort for the patient, acceptable recurrence rates, and is easily repeatable. These results are encouraging, but future research should define precise indications, optimal techniques, and measures for clinical and hemodynamic success for this procedure.

REFERENCES

1. Caggiati E, Mendoza M. The discovery of perforating veins, *Ann Vasc Surg*. 2004. *18*(4): 502–503.
2. Homans J. The operative treatment of varicose veins and ulcers, based upon a classification of these lesions, *Surg Gynecol Obstet*. 1916. *22*: 143–158.
3. Hauer G, Barkun J, Wisser I, Deiler S. Endoscopic subfascial discission of perforating veins, *Surg Endosc*. 1988. *2*(1): 5–12.
4. Gloviczki P, Cambria RA, Rhee RY, Canton LG, McKusick MA. Surgical technique and preliminary results of endoscopic subfascial division of perforating veins, *J Vasc Surg*. 1996. *23*(3): 517–523.
5. Rhodes JM, Gloviczki P, Canton LG, Rooke T, Lewis BD, Lindsey JR. Factors affecting clinical outcome following endoscopic perforator vein ablation, *Am J Surg*. 1998. *176*(2): 162–167.
6. Gloviczki P, Bergan JJ, Rhodes JM, Canton LG, Harmsen S, Ilstrup DM. Midterm results of endoscopic perforator vein interruption for chronic venous Insufficiency: Lessons learned from the North American subfascial endoscopic perforator surgery registry: The North American Study Group, *J Vasc Surg*. 1999. *29*(3): 489–502.
7. Fegan WG. Continuous compression technique for injecting veins, *Lancet*. 1963. *2*: 109–112.
8. Fegan WG. The treatment of varicose veins by injection sclerotherapy, *Edizioni Minerva Medica*. 1979.
9. Goor W. Sclerotherapy of incompetent perforating veins. In: May R, Partsch H, Staubesand J, eds. *Perforating veins*. Munich, Germany: Urban & Schwarzenberg. 1981.
10. Cockett F. Techniques of operations on perforating veins. In: May R, Partsch H, Staubesand J, eds. *Perforating veins*. Munich, Germany: Urban & Schwarzenberg. 1981.
11. Labropoulos N, Tiongson J, Pryor L, et al. Definition of venous reflux in lower extremity veins, *J Vasc Surg*. 2003. *38*(4): 793–798.
12. Guex JJ. Ultrasound guided sclerotherapy (USGS) for perforating veins (PV), *Hawaii Med J*. 2000. *59*: 261–262.
13. Thibault PK, Lewis WA. Recurrent varicose veins: Part 2: Injection of incompetent perforating veins using ultrasound guidance, *J Derm Surg Onc*. 1992. *18*: 895–900.
14. Schadeck M. Sclerotherapie des perforantes jambieres, *Phlebologie*. 1997. *50*(4): 683–688.
15. Puggioni A, Lurie F, Masuda E, Eklof B, Kistner R. *Ultrasound-guided sclerotherapy of incompetent perforators: Technique and duplex follow-up*. Pacific Vascular Symposium on Venous Disease, Kona, Hawaii, November, 2002.
16. Ghali S, Bowman N, Khan U. The distal medial perforators of the lower leg and their accompanying veins, *Br J Plast Surg*. 2005. *58*(8): 1086–1089.
17. Lurie F, Kessler D, Puggioni A, Masuda E. Blood flow in perforating arteries can change after oblation of incompetent perforating veins: Preliminary ultrasound observations: 6th European American Congress on Venous Diseases, Prague, Czech Republic, May 2005, *Praktika flebologie*. 2005. *14*(2): 55–56.

18. Sandri JL, Barros FS, Pontes S, Jacques C, Salles-Cunha SX. Diameter-reflux relationship in perforating veins of patients with varicose veins, *J Vasc Surg.* 1999. *30*(5): 867–875.

19. Masuda EM, Kessler DM, Puggioni A, Lurie F, Kistner RL, Eklof B. The effect of ultrasound-guided sclerotherapy of incompetent perforator veins on venous clinical severity and disability scores, *J Vasc Surg.* 2006. *43*(3): 551–556.

20. Puggioni A, Lurie F, Masuda E, Kistner R, Eklof B. *Ambulatory treatment of chronic venous disease with ultrasound guided sclerotherapy of perforating veins.* Society for Clinical Vascular Surgery, 31st Symposium, Miami, Florida, March, 2003.

21. Eklof B, Kessler D, Kistner R, et al. *Can duplex-guided sclerotherapy replace SEPS in the treatment of incompetent perforating veins?* Veith Symposium, New York, New York, November 20–23, 2003.

22. de Waard MM, der Kinderen DJ. Duplex ultrasonography-guided foam sclerotherapy of incompetent perforator veins in a patient with bilateral venous leg ulcers, *Dermatol Surg.* 2005. *31*(5): 580–583.

55.

PERFORATING VEINS

John J. Bergan, Luigi Pascarella and Nisha Bunke-Paquette

INTRODUCTION

The development of ankle hyperpigmentation, edema, atrophie blanche, and incipient ulceration, the cutaneous trophic changes of chronic venous insufficiency (CVI), is linked to a complex microangiopathy.[1] This, on a macro-vascular level is linked to ambulatory venous hypertension, which is enhanced by superficial and deep reflux. Also, it is linked to a lesser extent to venous obstruction. Thus it appears that venous hypertension is the fundamental pathogenic factor that leads to CVI.[2]

VALVE REMODELING PRODUCES DISTAL VENOUS HYPERTENSION

Our observations on ultrasound-proven, refluxing saphenous veins have shown that the endothelium of their venous valves and vein walls contain an infiltration of monocytes and an associated increased expression of intercellular adhesion molecules (ICAM-1). There is a statistically significant spatial correlation between CD68-positive monocytes and ICAM-1 in the various tissue areas of the valves and the vein walls.[3] The leukocytes and the expression of adhesion molecules are concentrated more on the proximal venous wall and valve cusp than on the distal wall and leaflet. This suggests a cause and effect relationship with venous hypertension.

The altered hemodynamics that accompany the venous hypertension change the plasma sheer stress, which, in turn, stimulates leukocyte pseudopod projection and adhesion of the leukocytes to the endothelium. It is a reduction, not an increase, in shear stress that leads to adhesion of the white cells on the endothelium.[4] Adhesion of the cells is followed by migration through the endothelium and interstitial macrophage infiltration.

The microscopic alterations, linked to venous hypertension described earlier are accompanied by gross tissue changes, which result in valve incompetency. Observations of these changes in primary venous insufficiency reveal dilation of the valvular annulus, atrophy of the cusp, and fibrotic remodeling of the valve and its annulus. Some have proposed that hemodynamic mechanical injury increases tissue damage to the annulus and cusps.[5] Others suggest that activated leukocytes release transforming growth factor-β_1 (TGF-β_1) gene expression, which alters environmental protein production.[6] This might explain the gross observations seen in affected valves.

VENOUS STASIS: AN INAPPROPRIATE TERM

Although the term "chronic venous insufficiency" (CVI) is in common usage and is becoming increasingly visible, the older term, "venous stasis" remains dominant. This is a tribute to John Homans of Harvard, who introduced the concept that venous stasis was the ultimate cause of venous ulceration.

Homans believed that there was a causal relation between venous ulcerations of the legs and blood stasis in patients with severe chronic venous insufficiency.[7] Blood stasis, as proposed by Homans, was determined by a shortage of oxygen content in the skin, and it was this that led to a condition of tissue hypoxia, necrosis, and ulceration.[7] Many observations in the last quarter century have demonstrated that shortage of oxygen is not the main cause of venous ulcers.

It has been hypothesized that presence of cutaneous arteriovenous fistulas might cause a deprivation of oxygen by shunting oxygenated blood away from skin already hypoxic from stasis. Such arteriovenous connections are easily demonstrated[8] by arteriography and microdissection in limbs with severe CVI but are not thought to contribute to the skin changes.[9] Coleridge Smith and others have shown that the content of oxygen in the skin and in varicose veins of limbs with venous ulcers is not decreased.[10] In fact, oxygen content in varicose veins is increased.[11] In addition, the oxygen diffusion defects suspected by histological findings of pericapillary fibrin cuffs have been refuted. Studies such as clearance of Xenon133 through liposclerotic skin have shown no significant oxygen barrier.[12]

PREULCERATIVE CUTANEOUS CHANGES

Inflammation dominates the early skin changes that precede venous ulceration. Increased leukocyte activation and an increased expression of soluble adhesion molecules have been demonstrated. There is a perivascular infiltration of the papillary plexus capillaries. Granulation tissue composed of lymphocytes, plasma cells, macrophages, histiocytes, and fibroblasts invades the subepithelial layer. This granulation tissue is responsible for the deposition of collagen fibers.[13] Collagen fibers appear to have completely lost their normal orientation in the cutaneous tissue. These lesions account for the inflammatory and postinflammatory process of tissue fibrosclerosis: lipodermatosclerosis.

When skin at the border of CVI is compared to normal skin in the same individual, the strong expression of ICAM-1 is seen in addition to a dense infiltration by T lymphocytes and macrophages. In some instances, the tissue also is infiltrated by an increased number of mast cells.[14] This is the typical picture of a chronic inflammatory reaction with an upregulation of endothelial adhesion molecules and dermal infiltration by T lymphocytes and macrophages in the skin of patients with CVI.

THE PERFORATING VEINS

Incompetent perforating veins are strongly associated with superficial venous reflux, and it is still controversial whether incompetent perforating veins are the primary cause of skin changes of chronic venous insufficiency or whether the incompetent perforating veins and skin changes are the result of superficial reflux. The cause of valvular dysfunction in perforating veins is not yet fully understood (see Figure 55.1).

Despite the classic studies of Linton[15] and Cockett,[16] it is still not known what the exact role of incompetent perforating veins is in the development of venous ulceration. Our observations suggest that venous hypertension is closely associated with valve damage and remodeling, which produces subsequent valve incompetence.[17] Therefore, it is useful to relate these findings to the valves in perforating veins.

It is well known that muscle contraction produces muscular compartment pressures in the range of 100 mm mercury and higher.[18] Such pressures exerted over time could initiate the cascade of molecular events, which eventuate in valvular incompetence. This valve incompetence would then produce the cutaneous "blow out" described as "spherical dilatations on veins under the skin" by Dodd and Cockett.[19] Failure of perforating vein valves due to their remodeling caused by repetitive compartment pressure elevation induced by normal exercise would lead to the skin changes described earlier.

A NEW HYPOTHESIS

A useful hypothesis is that venous hypertension, caused by superficial reflux and calf compartment pressure, is transmitted to unsupported venules of the skin. It is this sum of gravitational and hemodynamic pressure that stimulates the skin changes of chronic venous insufficiency. If this is true, a large component of ankle venous hypertension emanates from normal calf exercise with calf compartment pressures transmitted directly through the incompetent perforating vein valves to the skin (see Figure 55.2).

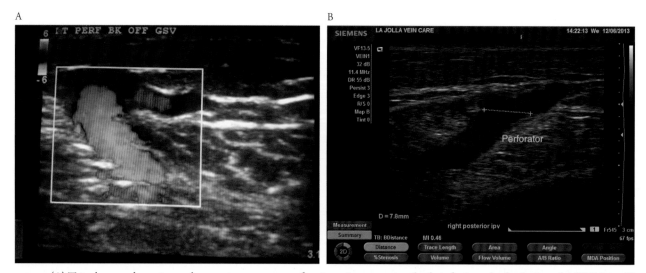

Figure 55.1   (A) This ultrasound scan image shows an incompetent perforating vein penetrating the deep fascia and refluxing into the GSV. It is calf muscle contraction that provides the pressure that is transmitted through a failed valve and elongates and dilates the superficial vein. (B) The IPV in this image is dilated and measures 7.8 mm in diameter.

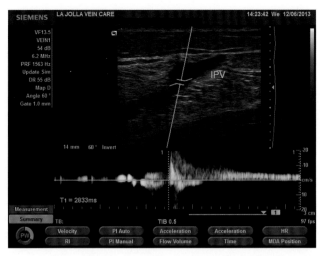

Figure 55.2 This perforating vein is shown penetrating the deep fascia. Its outward flow is demonstrated best by compression of distal soft tissues.

Indirect evidence of the importance of perforator veins in venous ulceration comes from surgical experience in dividing perforating veins in treatment of CVI.[20] A shorter ulcer healing time and improved hemodynamics have been found in limbs subjected to perforating vein surgery.[21]

De Palma showed in a crossover study that failure of conservative care, mainly consisting of compression, could be reversed by intervention with division of perforating veins.[22] This report, much like others,[23] is confused by the fact that 70% of the limbs had simultaneous stripping of the long saphenous vein at the time of perforator vein interruption. In fact, the sum of these two maneuvers did reduce venous hypertensive microangiopathy.

As ancient theories of causation of CVI gradually have been disproven as indicated earlier, it is no longer thought that venous blood stasis or ischemia due to arteriovenous fistulas, fibrin cuff development, or leukocyte trappings are important. Instead, a more logical explanation of the skin changes of chronic venous insufficiency is credible (see Table 55.1).

In development of the severe changes of CVI, first, venous hypertension and superficial venous valve failure are linked.[21] Sequential venous valve failure may be centrifugal or centripital. This allows venous hypertension to be transmitted to the ankle by superficial reflux. Next, perforating vein valves fail through the same mechanisms of venous hypertension-induced valve remodeling. Or, perforating veins acting as part of the private reflux recirculation can enlarge to the point of valvular incompetence[22] (see Figure 55.3).

Subsequent to perforating vein valve failure, subcutaneous changes of inflammation are produced by the inflammatory process,[14] and these lead to the clinical manifestations of chronic venous insufficiency.

As suggested previously, therapy of CVI supports this hypothesis. Compression treatment reduces ambulatory venous pressure and is effective in healing venous leg ulcers.[24] Superficial vein surgery reduces ambulatory venous pressure, allows healing of venous leg ulcer, and reduces the effects of CVI.[25] Perforator vein interruption by the Linton or endoscopic techniques reduces ambulatory venous pressure and ameliorates the chronic changes of CVI.[26,27]

Table 55.1 HYPOTHESES EXPLAINING GENESIS OF ADVANCED CHRONIC VENOUS INSUFFICIENCY

1. Superficial vein valve incompetence* raises distal venous pressure.
2. Perforating vein valve incompetence** raises distal venous pressure.
3. Additive effects of superficial and perforator incompetence produce profound distal venous hypertension.
4. Venous hypertension produces venulectasia, edema, leukocyte-endothelial interaction, and the inflammatory response.
5. Inflammation produces hyperpigmentation, fibrosis, and ulceration.

*Due to gravitational reflux induced valve remodeling.

**Due to muscle compartment pressure induced valve remodeling.

EXIT AND REENTRY PERFORATING VEINS

There are two fundamental facts that confuse understanding of perforating veins. The first relates to flow direction. Some perforating veins produce abnormal outflow from deep circulation to superficial circulation. This is demonstrated in Figure 55.1. This can be termed "perforating vein reflux." Other perforating veins demonstrate normal flow from the superficial system to the deep system. This is shown in the diagram of Figure 55.3 and the duplex scan shown in Figure 55.4. In situations of superficial venous incompetence and reflux, these can be called reentry perforating veins. It was Hach who understood this best, as he described the private circulation of reflux in superficial veins reentering to the deep system and the deep system in turn refluxing into the superficial veins.[24] It is most likely that it is the reentry perforating veins that disappear after adequately performed superficial venous stripping.

Another confusing factor in relating perforating veins to venous ulceration is the fact that venous ulceration is not directly related to severity of hemodynamic changes.[25] The lower limbs in a patient with bilaterally severe varicose veins might appear to be identical and might have identical hemodynamic measurements, but one limb might have all the stigmata of CVI and the other might have none. This is readily explained by the fact that skin changes are not caused by the venous hypertension or other hemodynamic changes but instead are dependent on leukocyte activation and the subsequent molecular changes that follow. In the absence of leukocyte activation, skin changes do not occur.

However, it may very well be that perforating vein outflow or reflux as detected by color flow Doppler duplex on

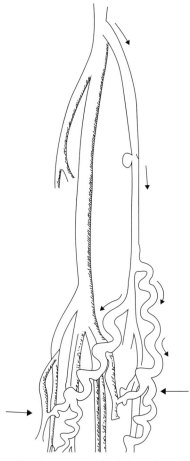

Figure 55.3 Normal perforating vein blood flow is from the superficial to the deep venous system. When saphenous vein reflux and varicose veins are present, the direction of flow is normal, but the perforating veins that allow reentry of reflux flow may enlarge and become incompetent as shown in this diagram. *(From Reference 27, with permission.)*

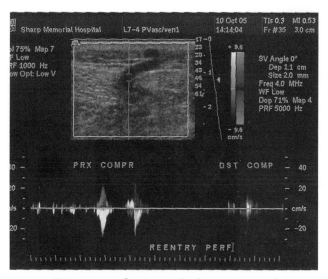

Figure 55.4 This reentry perforating vein has become tortuous because of increased flow. Distal compression causes its inward directed flow to stop. This resumes after distal compression release.

release of distal compression creates the hypertension in the subcutaneous venular network that elongates and dilates the capillaries, enlarges the intercellular junctions, produces edema, and triggers the inflammatory reaction that causes the skin changes.

If this is proven to be true, observations on the efficacy of measures to reduce cutaneous hypertension such as effective compression, superficial venous reflux ablation by foam sclerotherapy,[26] and perforator vein interruption will rest on a firm foundation. Even effective pharmacological intervention to moderate leukocyte activation is foreseeable.

CONCLUSIONS

Perforating veins and severe CVI are linked, and descriptions of molecular events associated with venous hypertension explain the relationship. These validate current medical and surgical therapy and point the way toward more effective and less cumbersome treatments in the future.

REFERENCES

1. Carpentier PH. Leukocytes in chronic venous insufficiency [in French], *J Mal Vasc*. 1998. *23*: 274–276.
2. Haenen JH, Janssen MCH, van Langen H, et al. The postthrombotic syndrome in relation to venous hemodynamics as measured by means of duplex scanning and strain-gauge plethysmography, *J Vasc Surg*. 1999. *29*: 1071–1076.
3. Takase S, Bergan JJ, Schmid-Schönbein GW. Expression of adhesion molecules and cytokines on saphenous veins in chronic venous insufficiency, *Ann Vasc Surg*. 2000. *14*: 427–435.
4. Moazzam F, DeLano FA, Zweifach BW, et al. The leukocyte response to fluid stress, *Proc Natl Acad Sci USA*. 1997. *94*: 5338–5343.
5. Corcos L, DeAnna D, Dini M, et al. Proximal long saphenous vein valves in primary venous insufficiency, *J Mal Vasc*. 2000. *25*: 27–36.
6. Hahn J, Junger M, Friedrich B, et al. Cutaneous inflammation limited to the region of the ulcer in chronic venous insufficiency, *VASA*. 1997. *26*: 277–281.
7. Homans J. The etiology and treatment of varicose ulcer of the leg, *Surg Gynecol Obstet*. 1917. *24*: 300–311.
8. Brewer AC. Arteriovenous shunts, *Br Med J*. 1950. *2*: 270–273.
9. Schalin, L. Arteriovenous communication to varicose veins in the lower extremities studied by dynamic angiography, *Acta Chir Scand*. 1980. *146*: 397–406.
10. Shami SK, Sarin S, Cheatle TR, Scurr JH, Coleridge Smith PD. Venous ulcers and the superficial venous system, *J Vasc Surg*. 1993. *17*: 487–490.
11. Blalock, A. Oxygen content of blood in patients with varicose veins, *Arch Surg*. 1929. *19*: 898–904.
12. Coleridge Smith PD. Pathogenesis of varicose veins and the chronic venous insufficiency syndrome. In: Goldman MP, Weiss RA, Bergan JJ, eds. *Varicose veins and telangiectasias: Diagnosis and management*. St. Louis, MO: Quality Medical. 1998.
13. Pappas PJ, You R, Rameshwar P, et al. Dermal tissue fibrosis in patients with chronic venous insufficiency is associated with increased transforming growth factor-β1 gene expression and protein production, *J Vasc Surg*. 1999. *30*: 1129–1145.
14. Scott HJ, Coleridge Smith PD, Scurr JH. Histological study of white blood cells and their association with lipodermatosclerosis and venous ulceration, *Br J Surg*. 1991. *78*: 210–211.

15. Linton RR. The postthrombotic ulceration of the lower extremity: Its etiology and surgical treatment, *Ann Surg.* 1953. *138*: 415–432.
16. Cockett FB. The pathology and treatment of venous ulcers of the leg, *Br J Surg.* 1955. *43*: 260–278.
17. Schmid-Schönbein GW, Takase S, Bergan JJ. New advances in the understanding of the pathophysiology of chronic venous insufficiency, *Angiology.* 2001. *52*(Suppl 1): S27–S34.
18. Arnoldi CC. Physiology and pathophysiology of the venous pump of the calf. In: Eklöf B, Gjöres JE, Thulesius O, Bergqvist D, eds. *Controversies in the management of venous disorders.* London: Butterworths. 1989. 11.
19. Dodd H, Cockett FB. *The pathology and surgery of the veins of the lower limb.* Edinburgh and London; E&S Livingstone. 1956. 344.
20. Gloviczki P, Bergan JJ, Rhodes JM, et al. Mid-term results of endoscopic perforator vein interruption for chronic venous insufficiency: Lessons learned from the North American subfascial endoscopic perforator surgery registry, *J Vasc Surg.* 1999. *29.* 489–502.
21. Rhodes JM, Gloviczki P, Canton L, et al. Endoscopic perforator vein division with ablation of superficial reflux improves venous hemodynamics, *J Vasc Surg.* 1998. *28*: 839–847.
22. DePalma RG, Kowallek DL. Venous ulceration: A crossover study from nonoperative to operative treatment, *J Vasc Surg.* 1996. *24*: 788–792.
23. Tawes RL, Barron ML, Coello AA, Joyce DH, Kolvenbach R. Optimal therapy for advanced chronic venous insufficiency, *J Vasc Surg.* 2003. *37*: 545–551.
24. Hach W. Die rezirkulationskreise der primren varicose, *Phlebologie.* 1991. *20*: 81–84.
25. Nicolaides AN, Hussein MK, Szendro G, et al. The relation of venous ulceration with ambulatory venous pressure measurements, *J Vasc Surg.* 1993. *17*: 414–419.
26. Bergan JJ, Pascarella L. Severe CVI: Primary treatment with sclerofoam, *Sem Vasc Surg.* 2005. *18*: 49–57.
27. Tibbs DJ. *Varicose veins and related disorders.* Oxford: Butterworth-Heineman. 1992.

56.

ENDOVASCULAR MANAGEMENT OF
ILIOCAVAL THROMBOSIS

Patricia E. Thorpe and Francisco J. Osse

INTRODUCTION

The term "endovenous" entered our vocabulary in the early 1990s to describe the percutaneous procedures performed to treat successive patients presenting with acute lower extremity deep vein thrombosis (DVT) superimposed on varying stages of chronic venous occlusive disease. Rarely did we see a case of "first episode" DVT. Gradually, the procedures evolved to include staged endovascular reconstruction of extensive, purely chronic axial vein occlusion in very symptomatic patients. During this time, the term "endovascular" had been touted, around the globe, as the new frontier in vascular surgery. Techniques developed between 1950 and 1975 by Seldinger, Amplatz, Dotter, Gruntzig, Judkins, and others, were "borrowed" and incorporated into innovative, percutaneous methods of treating aortic aneurysm and carotid disease. But, over the years, minimally invasive treatment of iliocaval obstruction has not become part of the repertoire of most vascular surgeons or interventional radiologists. This is a reflection of many factors. First, consider that peripheral vascular arterial disease is so prevalent that there are hardly enough physicians to care for the growing number of patients. Although chronic venous disease is the most common problem in vascular medicine, venous occlusive disease is technically challenging, often involving multiple segments, damaged valves, and difficult terrain to navigate. Few specialized tools have been developed, and those are mainly for addressing acute thrombosis. Furthermore, residents and fellows training in fragmented programs have trouble getting enough training in specialized areas of endovascular surgery. With limited time and energy, most focus on gaining experience with arterial disease. Catheter skills are essential in performing endovenous procedures. Venous cases can be more time-consuming than arterial procedures, and reimbursement is often less than for faster arterial interventions. It is nonetheless as gratifying to successfully treat chronic venous obstruction and relieve the heaviness and pain of venous hypertension as it is to open an occluded iliac artery and relieve claudication. So here we will begin with a chapter on the endovenous management of iliocaval thrombosis.

CLINICAL HISTORY AND EVALUATION

It is not a surprise that the clinical manifestations of iliocaval occlusion comprise a wide spectrum of signs and symptoms of venous hypertension. The recruitment of collateral pathways may be adequate as well as occult; some thrombosed individuals can remain symptom-free. Symptomatic individuals may present with variable lower extremity edema and a variety of complaints related to venous hypertension. There are three common clinical presentations among patients with chronic venous obstruction; (1) asymptomatic, (2) acutely symptomatic with underlying pathology, and (3) chronically symptomatic.[1] The clinical presentation reflects the venous pathology. Asymptomatic patients may have transient signs or symptoms that are not disabling. For example, asymptomatic patients may have limb, vulvar, or abdominal varices indicating venous hypertension, focal phlebitis within a varix or mild edema, intermittent groin pain, and a tiny ulcer (Figure 56.1). However, all of these signs and symptoms can increase in intensity and frequency if the venous flow pattern is further compromised. For example, superficial vein removal for varicosities, in a patient with iliofemoral occlusion, can lead to severe venous stasis and skin changes (Figure 56.2).

Acute caval thrombosis commonly presents with unilateral or bilateral lower limb edema, unexplained recent weight gain, and not infrequently, back pain. The lack of collateral flow causes lower limb edema, discoloration, and discomfort. The back pain reflects venous congestion in the sacral plexus. Patients have no difficulty recognizing the seriousness of their condition, even though it may have

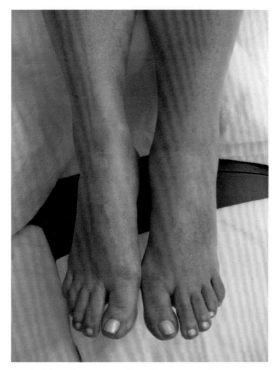

Figure 56.1   Left leg edema or nonthrombotic venous hypertension related to left iliac compression. Lymphedema can be a component.

Chronic inferior vena cava (IVC) occlusion can result in either bilateral or unilateral lower extremity edema. Prominent collateral veins can be seen on the lower anterior abdominal wall and in the perineal or pubic region (Figures 56.5, 56.6). Bilateral varicose veins may be present. Advanced skin changes including hyperpigmentation, lipodermatosclerosis and ulceration can develop. Venous stasis changes may lead to below-the-knee amputation years before the venous obstruction is identified. Patients with iliocaval occlusion often report that leg elevation does little to alleviate edema. This suggests a component of phlebolymphedema, perhaps secondary to venous obstruction.[2] Prolonged sitting can cause a vague inguinal ache. Exertion may cause venous claudication. Patients frequently report shortness of breath, even without any history of pulmonary embolus or respiratory ailments. Lower back discomfort or hematuria can be presenting signs. As a rule, patients with long-standing venous insufficiency, secondary to venous obstruction, are seen by primary care physicians long before they are referred to vascular specialists. Patients commonly report being told "there is not much we can do for you other than compression." Treatment of post-thrombotic syndrome commonly means compression stockings. Patients may have a remote history of iliofemoral DVT but no suspicion of central venous obstruction, since no one ever evaluated this area. Alternatively, they may have a prior diagnosis of iliocaval occlusion, or have been told that the IVC is absent following phlebography or if cross-sectional imaging. The chronically thrombosed cava becomes isodense with surrounding soft tissue, and large collaterals seen using computed tomography (CT) and magnetic resonance imagery (MRI) may be interpreted as lymphadenopathy and thereby prompt a search for malignancy.

developed gradually. Early on, symptoms can mimic sciatica and spinal, bowel, or bladder problems. However. when a critical mass of thrombus finally interrupts deep venous flow, venous hypertension progresses rapidly (Figures 56.3, 56.4).

Chronic iliocaval occlusion is often more difficult to diagnose, since collaterals and recanalization alter the hemodynamics which dictate the severity of the venous hypertension.

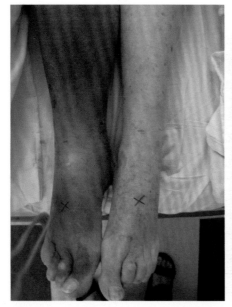
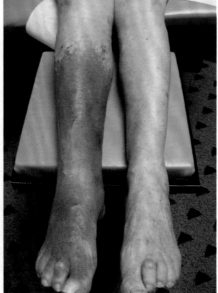

Figure 56.2   The right leg shows all the signs of advanced skin changes of chronic venous hypertension. The circumferential hyperpigmentation and lipodermatosclerosis became worse, and ulcers developed, after the patient underwent saphenous vein stripping for varicosities seven years before this photo. Her remote history of iliofemoral DVT went undiscovered until she presented with acute DVT following the stripping surgery. She responded to thrombolysis and iliac stenting, Her right leg improved, and the pain decreased significantly, which greatly enhanced her quality of life.

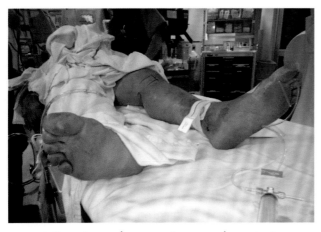

Figure 56.3 Cyanosis secondary to massive venous obstruction in a patient (Figure 56.4) with chronic bilateral iliocaval occlusion and acute left iliofemoral thrombosis.

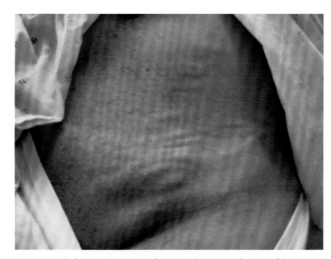

Figure 56.5 Abdominal varices indicating chronic occlusion of the inferior vena cava in a 45-year-old man with bilateral stasis ulcers.

IMAGING ILIOCAVAL DISEASE

The evaluation of obstructive venous disease utilizes multiple imaging modalities. We begin with duplex ultrasound (DU). The exam includes looking at the inflow and outflow of the limb. This means the exam includes below-the-knee veins as well as the iliac segments above the inguinal ligament. Wave-form analysis and velocity measurements are important when suspecting proximal obstruction. Specifically look for high velocities in the left common iliac segment, which can indicate a focal compression by the right iliac artery. Large collaterals adjacent to the common iliac might be present. However, they will show nonphasic flow. Nonphasic flow is seen in collaterals and axial veins distal to an obstructing lesion. A normal pattern returns

after stenting (Figure 56.7). Patients must be monitored for restenosis at 6-month intervals for the first 1–2 years post-op or if they become symptomatic. Many patients have a "normal" duplex exam even when they have restenosis. We find objective measurements are helpful. Labropoulos et al. established criteria for defining significant venous stenosis with DU.[3] Following baseline DU, patients underwent phlebography and intravascular pull-back pressure measurements before treatment of an identified stenosis. The data showed that a pressure gradient greater than or equal to 3.0 mmHg correlates with a greater than 50% stenosis. A peak velocity ratio of 2.5 correlated with a pressure gradient of 3.0 mmHg. These criteria pertain best to focal stenoses. In long-segment 12-mm stents, we find that diffuse intrastent hyperplasia will decrease the velocity. Therefore,

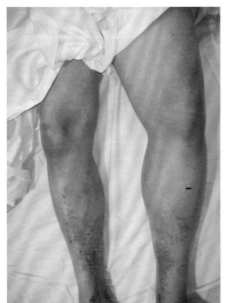

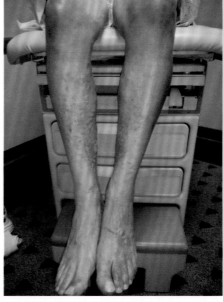

Figure 56.4 The initial thrombosis is this patient occurred after an aortobifemoral bypass 20 years prior to his presentation with hematuria and acute lower extremity edema that was clearly greater on the left. The image on the left shows his legs at 1 month follow-up after iliocaval reconstruction.

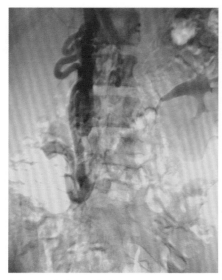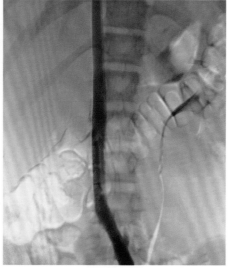

Figure 56.6   Venograms of the IVC before and after thrombolysis and stenting. This 17-year-old patient presented with acute left leg thrombosis. He has a single kidney and a pattern of chronic caval obstruction that was unknown prior to the DVT. His initial treatment was in 1997, and he remains patent with one subsequent intervention for focal caval and iliac in stent restenosis in 2007.

we use serial velocity measurements to screen for restenosis since visualization is unreliable.

Contrast phlebography provides the clearest understanding of obstructive disease. real-time digital phlebography

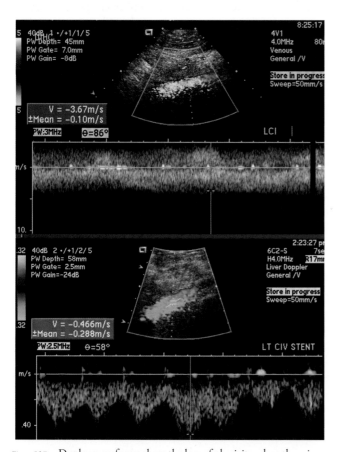

Figure 56.7   Duplex waveforms show the loss of phasicity when there is a proximal iliac obstruction. Following stent placement, the waveform is phasic, and the peak systolic velocity is similar to the other limb, which serves as a control.

shows rate of contrast clearance and contrast density patterns that can be helpful. A wide left common iliac segment indicates compression.

Demonstration of collaterals pathopneumonic for obstruction is clearly seen in patients with iliocaval obstruction. Magnetic resonance venography (MRV) and computed tomographic venography (CTV) reconstructions can demonstrate left vein iliac compression with multiple views (Figures 56.8, 56.9). However, both gadolinium and CO_2 have been shown to be less effective contrast agents than iodinated contrast in the venous system.[3] Thin-slice CT, widely used for diagnosis of pulmonary embolus, is not always sensitive for distal DVT.[4] The 64-slice CTV can produce impressive images of the lower extremities when contrast is injected distally via pedal intravenous access. We recommend that cross-sectional imaging and duplex be combined with phlebography if intervention is planned. Imaging of iliac compression is best done with intravascular ultrasound (IVUS). A decrease in cross-sectional area can be calculated, and the tightness of the anterior-posterior diameter relative to the transverse diameter indicates a hemodynamically significant lesion. We recommend documentation of the lesion with IVUS pre and post stenting.

TREATMENT OPTIONS

SYMPTOMATIC IVC OCCLUSION

Symptomatic IVC occlusion, whether acute or chronic, responds poorly to conservative therapy. Medical treatment with anticoagulation alone will do little to alleviate the multisegmental occlusion of large axial veins. Despite heparin,

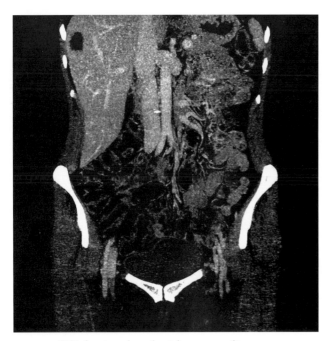

Figure 56.8   CTA showing where the right common iliac artery crosses the left common iliac vein.

warfarin, and autolysis, the risk of pulmonary embolus is high, and the threat of phlegmasia exists. Over time, the IVC syndrome may develop, leading to discomfort and disability. Historically, surgical intervention was reserved for severe cases and clinical results were mixed due to the morbidity of such high-risk surgery. In 2001, Jost et al. reported overall 3-year primary and secondary patency rates of 54% and 62% in patients undergoing surgical reconstruction for nonmalignant obstruction from 1985 to 1999.[5] In view of these limitations, endovascular repair of acute and

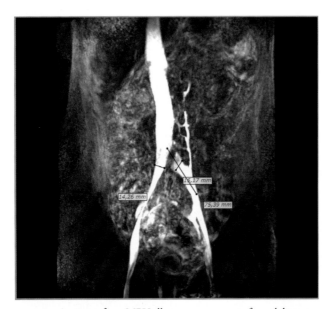

Figure 56.9   An image from MRV allows measurement of vessel diameters and shows the left common iliac vein compression and ascending lumbar collateral.

chronic IVC and combination iliocaval obstruction has evolved over the past 25 years. Early stainless steel stents were effective in strutting caval lesions, and they were associated with significant restenosis.[6,7] As early as April 1993, we began placing self-expanding metallic stents in chronically occluded iliac veins and the IVC. We have followed hundreds of patients over the years to track the long-term clinical outcomes and perform reinterventions to maintain patency.[8] Published reports since 2000 have shown endovenous reconstruction to be a safe, effective, and durable treatment option.[9-22] Following two decades of clinical experience, absent any large randomized trials, the minimally invasive, percutaneous approach has been declared an acceptable, if not preferred, treatment for symptomatic iliocaval obstruction or stenosis.[20] The 2008 guidelines published by the American College of Chest Physicians (ACCP) recommend phamacomechanical thrombolysis in preference to catheter-directed thrombolysis alone in the treatment of selected cases of acute DVT.[23]

NONTHROMBOTIC LEFT COMMON ILIAC OBSTRUCTION: MAY-THURNER

The prevalence of left iliac vein compression may be higher than concluded from autopsy studies in the 1940s. Originally described by Cockett and Thomas, the anatomical lesion was thought to be hemodynamically significant in approximately 30% of the population.[24,25] Two German pathologists, May and Thurner first described their iliac compression findings in 1957. Their names are associated with the clinical syndrome that reflects the mechanical risk factor for left leg thrombosis. Nonthrombotic manifestation of unilateral venous hypertension, due to common iliac vein narrowing, is now considered by some as an indication for stent placement,[17] The presence and persistence of such a lesion helps explain the high rethrombosis rate after balloon thrombectomy or early catheter-directed thrombolysis. Removal of acute iliofemoral thrombus without correction of the underlying lesion will almost invariably result in rethrombosis. Investigation with IVUS provides valuable information about the appearance and function of the common iliac vein near the bifurcation. Although in most patients duplex can identify the presence of collaterals or a focal shift in velocity (at the area of right iliac artery compression of the vein), direct visualization and measurement with IVUS are ideal. In the absence of thrombosis, a high-grade lesion is characterized by anteroposterior (AP) diameter of less than 3.0 mm, pressure gradient of ≥ 3.0 mmHg, distal stasis, and visible collateral veins. Such lesions merit consideration of stenting to prevent thrombosis in the future.

Neglen reported that a single anatomical lesion was identified in the proximal left common iliac vein in 36% of the 255 patients included in their study.[17] A smaller group,

8%, had a compressive lesion near the internal iliac bifurcation. In 46% of the patients, a combination of proximal and distal lesion was observed. Whereas the proximal lesion is more common on the left, there is an equal incidence of the distal narrowing. The cause of the distal lesions is extrinsic compression from the iliac artery, but relatively little fibrosis occurs at this level compared to the proximal lesions. The arterial compression and proximity of the spine can result in intrinsic vein wall thickening in the proximal left iliac. Bilateral common iliac compression is found in approximately 2% of the population. Whereas IVUS measurements and images are definitive, the phlebographic image is often misinterpreted as normal. The wider transverse diameter, and lighter contrast density, in the common iliac segment are consistent with AP narrowing of the vein. But, if collaterals are not seen, and the characteristic impression of the right iliac artery is not identified, the diagnosis can be missed with phlebography. Collaterals that are visualized with valsalva may not be apparent with normal respiration in a supine position.

ACUTE THROMBOTIC OBSTRUCTION

Catheter-directed thrombolysis, mechanical thrombectomy, and combination therapy have evolved over the past two decades. For the most part, patients presenting with phlegmasia cerulean dolens are referred for catheter-directed thrombolysis in centers where interventionalists are available. Patients not responding to standard heparin and warfarin therapy may also be referred for catheter-directed lysis. However, the majority of DVT patients treated in the emergency room are discharged with low molecular weight heparin and are no longer routinely hospitalized for bed rest. A multidisciplinary, multicenter clinical trial, under the auspices of the NIH, was initiated in 2007 to investigate the benefits of early endovascular thrombus removal (with thrombolysis and mechanical thrombectomy and adjunctive use of stents) compared with standard anticoagulation therapy.[27] Prevention of postthrombotic syndrome is a primary goal of early endovascular intervention. The objective of the study is the acquisition of Level I data, comparing anticoagulation alone with thrombus removal plus anticoagulation. The strategy of early thrombus removal reduces the likelihood of pulmonary embolus as well as postthrombotic syndrome.

Early observations of the natural history of DVT and subsequent evaluations following lysis revealed several findings. Distal valvular incompetence can develop in patients with persistent proximal obstruction, even if distal veins are not affected by the DVT.[28,29] Persistent residual thrombus is associated with a higher incidence of recurrent DVT.[30] Finally, the combination of obstruction and reflux leads to more severe postthrombotic syndrome than either condition alone.[29]

CHRONIC THROMBOTIC OBSTRUCTION: MAY-THURNER + THROMBOSIS

Prior to 2000, reports detailing the use of thrombolytic therapy and stents for use in venous thrombosis focused on patients with acute thrombosis, in whom about 50% have an underlying iliac lesion or May-Thurner compression.[31] Very often, the acute clinical presentation is deceptive, since the "critical mass" of thrombus that causes the clinical symptoms is composed of newer thrombus superimposed on a substrate of subacute or even chronic thrombus.

Endovascular stenting of chronic iliac occlusions, after removal of acute thrombus, has become familiar to interventionalists treating venous obstruction. Balloon angioplasty proved to be inadequate in treating iliac lesions.[32,33] We frequently use catheter-directed thrombolysis, with tissue plasminogen activator, to soften occlusive thrombus and facilitate guide-wire passage through apparently impossible occlusions. Venography and IVUS demonstrate the occlusive, echo-dense thrombus that obliterates the lumen (Figures 56.10, 56.11). The initial venograms will show very little of the residual caval and iliac segments. Following overnight thrombolysis, using a bilateral popliteal approach, the venogram will reveal additional venous anatomy. The procedure progresses very methodically in caval reconstructions. Serial angioplasty precedes simultaneous deployment of kissing self-expanding stents (Figures 56.12, 56.13). The long-term patency of large-caliber (12- to 16-mm) self-expanding stents placed in the common iliac segment is acceptable and compares

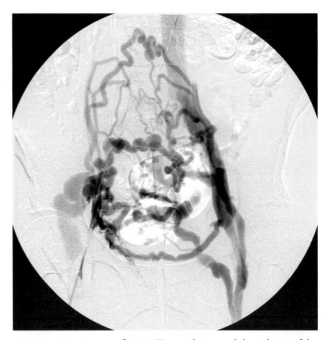

Figure 56.10 A venogram of a May-Thurner lesion and thromboses of the iliac veins. The image is taken with the patient prone on the angio table. Note the retroperitoneal and transpelvic collaterals.

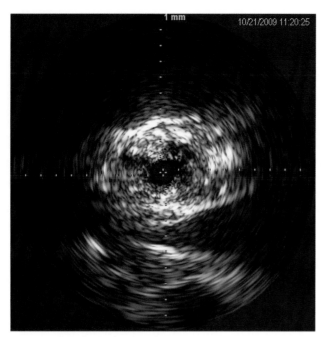

Figure 56.11   Intravascular ultrasound (IVUS) Volcano Eagle Eye 6F catheter image of a severe and chronic iliac occlusion where the residual lumen has been obliterated. It is usually necessary to used thrombolytic therapy to facilitate wire traversal of such lesions.

favorably to surgical thrombectomy, alone, and bypass surgery.[33] Neglen and Raju reported early experience with cannulation of totally occluded segments and technical success of stenting as 98% and 97%, respectively, in the treatment of ninety-four consecutive patients with suspected iliac vein obstruction.[12] In this series, the reported primary, assisted primary, and secondary patency rates at 1 year were 82%, 91%, and 92%, respectively.

The clinical impact of correcting the deep venous obstructive lesions in symptomatic patients can be measured in terms of quality of life as pain and swelling diminish when the venous hypertension is reduced by restoration of axial flow. In 2002, Raju et al. reported on the clinical impact of the venous stents in managing chronic venous insufficiency.[12] This was the first mention in the literature of the effect of stenting on the healing of venous stasis ulcers. Stasis dermatitis and ulceration was present in 69/304 (23%) limbs treated with stenting with or without saphenous ablation. They reported that the cumulative recurrence-free ulcer healing rate was 63% at 24 months. Furthermore, the rate of healing was not influenced by concomitant treatment of saphenous reflux. The reduction of pain and swelling after intervention were both statistically significant (P < 0.001).

IVC occlusion, in combination with iliac obstruction, can lead to severe venous hypertension when collateral circulation is inadequate. The IVC syndrome can include lower extremity swelling, stasis dermatitis and ulceration, varicosities, and loss of sensation and strength in the legs. Pain can be felt in the lower back, pelvis, or inguinal region in addition to the discomfort and heaviness in one or both limbs. It is most common to discover caval obstruction confined to the infrarenal cava. In patients in whom we have suspected an early thrombosis in infancy, the entire IVC was discovered to be very narrow, as if minimally recanalized following thrombosis.

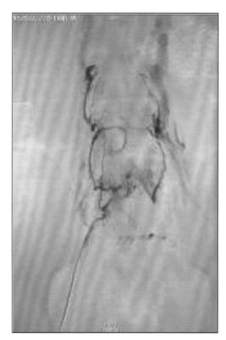
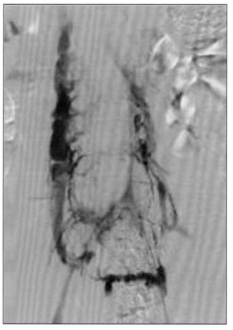

Figure 56.12   These images show the baseline cavagram and the result of overnight thrombolysis. Additional anatomy is revealed by infusing a thrombolytic agent for 12–18 hours via multi–side hole catheters advanced from a popliteal approach. In the second image, note the filling defects and the tram-track sign revealing the residual thrombus.

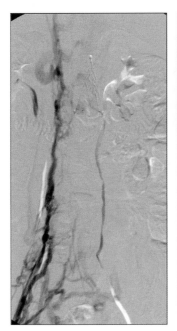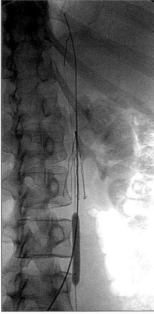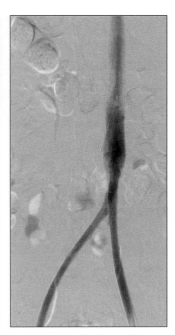

Figure 56.13   Three images showing the sequence of a baseline cavagram followed by stages of the reconstruction. Following bilateral popliteal catheter placement for thrombolysis, eventually a wire can be passed into the suprarenal cava. In this case, both wires pass through a previously occluded caval filter. Initial caval dilatation starts with small-diameter balloons and progresses to kissing 10- to 12- mm balloons. The third image shows the double barrel stents traversing the filter.

FOCAL ISSUES FOR ENDOVASCULAR THERAPY

A. IVUS: IVUS is an important tool in endovenous therapy. It has application in two main areas: (1) assessing the nonthrombosed common iliac segment and (2) in the follow-up examination of with signs and symptoms of restenosis. In the first instance, IVUS has proven to be the best way to image and evaluate the iliac stenosis in the May-Thurner syndrome.[11] Whereas the phlebogram will generally demonstrate widening of the transverse diameter of the common iliac segment, and decrease in the intensity of contrast, IVUS will clearly reveal the severity of the AP narrowing causing high venous resistance (Figures 56.14, 56.15). The presence of collaterals has previously thought to be necessary for diagnosis of a hemodynamically significant iliac lesion. Information from IVUS has shown that not all significant narrowings are accompanied by collaterals, which can be demonstrated phlebographically in the supine position.

B. RESTENOSIS: Restenosis is important issue in stenting. Untreated restenosis can lead to rethrombosis. Whereas early rethrombosis (<30 days) is usually due to inadequate anticoagulation or inflow and outflow issues, late loss of patency is most often due to intimal hyperplasia and subsequent thrombosis. When patients present with recurrent symptoms of limb edema or discomfort, the intensity is generally much less than the initial clinical presentation. The routine duplex exam will generally show patency of the stents. The wave form will remain phasic. Intimal hyperplasia, or in-stent restenosis, is best imaged

with IVUS. Before we had access to IVUS, we would redilate stents in patients with recurrent pain or edema. The symptoms and signs resolved. As little as 30–35% luminal decrease by intimal hyperplasia can cause recurrence

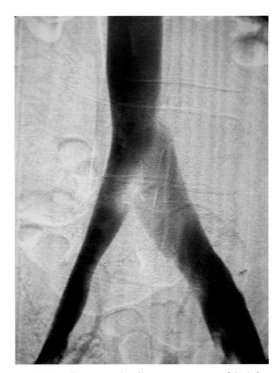

Figure 56.14   An excellent example of how compression of the left common iliac vein results in widening of the transverse diameter and narrowing of the anteroposterior lumen. On the venogram, this causes decrease in the intensity of contrast. This is the classic appearance of a May-Thurner compression on venography.

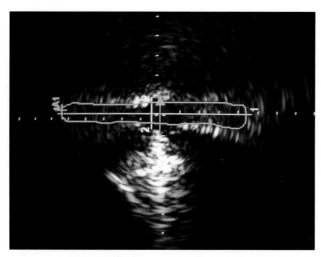

Figure 56.15   IVUS image the iliac compression seen in Figure 56.14. The AP diameter is "pancaked," and the echogenic rim indicates fibrotic thickening of the vein wall. This slit-like appearance shows why the contrast is less dense and why the flow velocity increases at the May-Thurner lesion.

of symptoms. In 2004, Neglen and Raju reported their observations of restenosis in venous stents and concluded that risk factors included a history of venous thrombosis, a positive test for thrombophilia, and longer stent systems extending below the inguinal ligament.[34] Gender and side had no significance. After 42 months of observation in 324 limbs treated with stenting, 23% had no sign of luminal narrowing on phlebography, 61% showed greater than 20% narrowing, and 15% showed greater than 50% narrowing. The value of identifying restenosis is in maintaining long-term patency of the stents. Their study showed that reintervention optimizes long-term patency. At 3 years, primary, primary assisted, and secondary patency were 75%, 90%, and 93%, respectively.

C. ANTICOAGULATION: Once flow is reestablished with stents, anticoagulation is important in patients with thrombophilia and those with significant residual distal thrombus and vein wall irregularity from previous DVT. Both conditions are risk factors for recurrent DVT despite good iliac flow. However, in patients with normal distal veins, the presence of a single or double iliac stent does not require long-term anticoagulation, per se. The use of anticoagulation and antiplatelet agents varies among clinicians. Low molecular weight heparin is used to bridge subtherapeutic international normalized ratio (INR) levels, particularly in patients who must travel more than 2 hours to return home. Plavix, 75 mg/d, is started prior to stenting and continued for 30 d. Patients not on warfarin also take 80 mg aspirin. It should be noted that rethrombosis of a metallic stent is a matter of urgency. In our experience, it is much more difficult, and sometimes not possible, to reopen chronic in-stent thrombosis. Unlike organized thrombus in native veins, the old thrombus in occluded stents is very hard to traverse.

D. STENTS: Self-expanding metallic stents are used in venous stenting. The 12- to 14-mm Wallstent (Boston Scientific, Natick, MA) has been used more than other stents because of the good long-term patency rates, the visibility under fluoroscopy, and the ability to reposition. Stent migration is rare, but can occur with any stent if it is undersized and the vein expands. Tandem Wallstents will not interlock as the SmartStent (Cordis, New Brunswick, NJ) will. The foreshortening of the Wallstent requires experience, and there are time when a stent that does not foreshorten is ideal. A single, high-grade focal stenosis requires a sufficiently long stent to prevent the stent from slipping (like a watermelon seed) to either side. In our experience, long-term success of these interventions is also related to establishing continuity of flow within the deep system of the entire lower extremity. Poor inflow from the tibiopopliteal segments, or the femoral may compromise long term patency as much as poor-outflow caused by under-stenting the iliac compression. Stents must extend into the IVC to completely treat the iliac compression. Otherwise, the compression persists and the stent can thrombose (Figure 56.16).

Pitfalls include the following situations. Visualizing the IVC with contrast alone can give a false estimate of the vein diameter. Above the thrombotic occlusion or stenosis, a normal vein may not expand with contrast injection due to low volume. Placement of an undersized stent can result in migration (Figure 56.17). A very tight, focal lesion should be treated with a longer stent. Trying to match the length of the lesion too closely can result in the stent slipping above or below the lesion during deployment (Figure 56.18). Adequate apposition to the vein wall, above or below the lesion, will prevent this problem. The ends of the self-expanding stents can be sharp. Adequate overlap of 15–20 mm at the interface

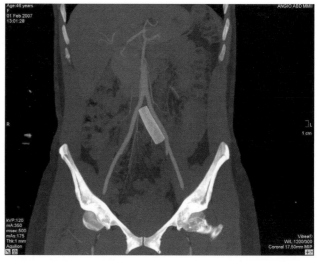

Figure 56.16   CT showing stent position too low in the iliac vein. It is below the right iliac artery, which can still compress the vein. Stents must be extended into the IVC by 1–2 centimeters. Failure to do so can result in early thrombosis of the stent.

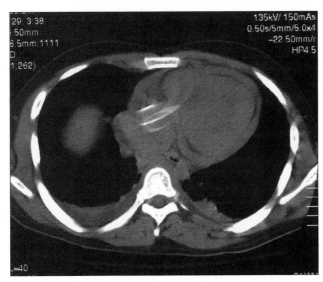

Figure 56.17   CT image of a stent that migrated to the right atrium. The stent was placed in the suprarenal IVC on the preceding day. Before IVUS, the diameter of the IVC could be underestimated with low-volume contrast imaging. The stent migrated to the heart and caused a tapenade. The percutaneous removal required a 16-Fr sheath in the jugular vein, a 20-mm goose-neck snare, a femoral catheter, a multidisciplinary team and determination. The 22-year-old patient made a full recovery.

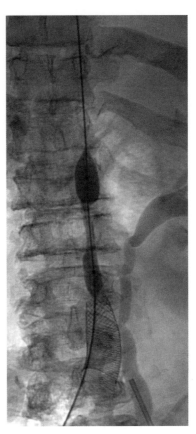

Figure 56.18   Deployment of a self-expanding stent in a very tight lesion can result in "watermelon seed" slippage, as seen in this image. Short tight lesions require longer stents to prevent this complication.

of stents during tandem deployment is important to prevent a bare area. This gap can be a site for restenosis. More importantly, it prevents possible perforation of the vein wall (Figure 56.19). In all instances, one must be prepared to address the complication. Snares can be use to retrieve a stent, and covered stents can be used to prevent exsanguination.

E. OCCLUDED VENOUS STENTS: Reopening a chronically occluded venous stent can be very difficult. It is much harder than reestablishing flow in a chronically occluded native vessel. If a stent thromboses, immediate intervention is recommended. Lysis of acute thrombus can restore patency. Chronic thrombus can be traversed, but there is no good way to debulk organized thrombus within the stent lumen. A pilot lumen may be achieved with rotational atherectomy using the JetStream 3 (Pathway Medical Technologies, Kirkland, WA) This will permit placement of the wire for dilatation. Cutting balloons and angioplasty may expand the channel, but we lack endovascular tools to "clean out" the stent. Placement of a new stent, within the lumen, may provide adequate flow. It is, however, hard to expand the inner stent when there is a circumferential layer of organized thrombus. There is a high risk of rethrombosis with a narrow lumen. Most of the iliac stent failures have been due to failure to place the stent high enough in the cava. The double barrel or kissing stent configuration requires extension of the two stents well above the bifurcation to maintain patency. Also, simultaneous balloon dilatation is recommended to avoid compressing a stent (Figure 56.20).

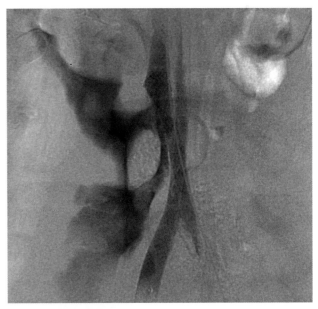

Figure 56.19   Dramatic contrast image of an iatrogenic caval tear and retroperitoneal extravasation. The two stents are not sufficiently overlapped. Care is taken not to oversize dilating balloons and to perform kissing balloon technique in the parallel caval stents. An uneven force was applied to the cava and stents and resulted in this perforation, which was treated effectively with a covered stent.

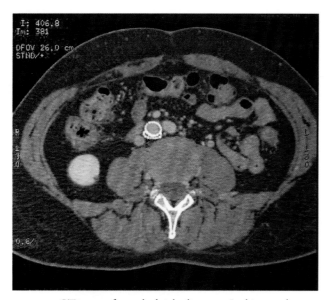

Figure 56.20   CT image of a crushed right iliac stent. In this case, the kissing Nitinol stents should have been extended higher into the cava to prevent this asymmetry. Furthermore, upon rethrombosis, the stent system should have been revised immediately.

F. DISTAL THROMBUS: The presence of acute and chronic tibiopopliteal thrombus can threaten the long-term patency of proximal reconstructions. We firmly believe that treatment of the entire limb is key to technical and clinical success. Complete understanding of the calf veins and popliteal inflow is important. Duplex and pedal phlebography are used to provide this information. In the event of thrombotic obstruction, flow-directed delivery of a thrombolytic agent can reduce calf and popliteal thrombus (Figures 56.21, 56.22). The saphenous vein is intermittently compressed against the malleolus and/or condyle, to redirect venous flow into the deep veins. The dedicated tourniquets, designed for this purpose, effectively promote thrombolysis of thrombus in the calf and popliteal segments (Tiger Surgical, Inc., Portland, OR).

G. IVC FILTERS: It is not generally thought to be necessary to place a caval filter while performing catheter-directed thrombolysis. The incidence of PE has been remarkably low, as the thrombus does not fragment without undue manipulation. However, mechanical thrombectomy for removal of acute thrombus poses the risk of embolism. In this case, temporary filters have been placed and subsequently removed. Occluded IVC filters can be safely and effectively bypassed. We have passed single and kissing Wallstents through and alongside all types of occluded filters without complication (Figures 56.6, 56.13, 56.23). Once the exchange guide wire has traversed this area of occlusion, serial balloon dilation will expand the tissue and allow stent deployment. Mechanical thrombectomy and thrombolysis can be effectively and safely used to restore flow in acutely thrombosed IVC bearing filters.[35] In our iliocaval series, successful recanalization of chronically occluded filters has also been performed with remarkable long-term patency.[8] Raju and Neglen encountered twenty-five patients with occluded IVC filters. Their results

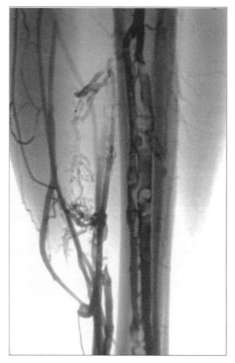
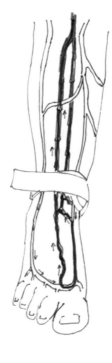

Figure 56.21   Contrast venogram shows acute tibial thrombus prior to flow-directed thrombolysis. The diagram shows placement of the DVT tourniquet, which was specifically designed for lytic infusions. Compression of the saphenous vein against the malleolus promotes flow into the deep venous system. In this manner, effective delivery of the thrombolytic drug can dissolve acute thrombus.

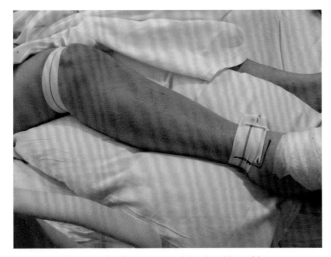

Figure 56.22　Photograph of a patient with both ankle and knee tourniquets in place for flow-directed lysis. A disc is positioned fluoroscopically to strategically compress the superficial vein against the bone.

also demonstrate the feasibility and low morbidity of stenting through a thrombosed filter.[37] Stent complications are quite rare, but they can happen.

H. ILIAC STENTS AND PREGNANCY: Young women undergoing stent procedures during child-bearing age were understandably concerned about whether or not an iliac stent would be an issue with pregnancy. On the contrary, treating a DVT or preventing thrombosis by stenting a May-Thurner compression mitigates against thrombosis during pregnancy and after delivery. Anticoagulation is managed by a hematologist or high-risk pregnancy specialist. In our experience, four women have delivered seven healthy children without complication. Hartung reported

that eight pregnancies occurred in six patients in whom a self-expanding stent had been previously placed for iliac compression. The recommendation to sleep on the right side and continue lovenox throughout the conception period and pregnancy parallel our experience.[40]

CLINICAL EXPERIENCE

In 2006, Raju reported a series of 120/4,217 (2.8%) patients with obstructive lesions of the IVC identified among patients with chronic venous insufficiency examined between 1997 and 2005.[1] The majority of the lesions were infrarenal (82%), 14% (14/97) were suprarenal but below the diaphragm, and four cases extended into the superior aspect of the intrahepatic IVC. In 93% of cases, lesion involved the common iliac segment, but in 7%, the lesion was limited to the IVC. Most of the IVC lesions 85/99 (86%) were stenotic (>60%) and not occlusive. There were fourteen occlusions in which seven of the attempted recanalizations were not successful. The CEAP clinical classification for the stented limbs included C3 (37%), C4 (26%), C5 (7%), and C6 (19%). The seven limbs with unhealed ulcers were found to have residual untreated reflux, which was predominantly in axial veins. There were nineteen limbs with active ulcers that underwent stenting. In twelve limbs (63%) the ulcers healed and remained healed at 24 months. Reflux was present in seventeen, involving both deep and superficial systems. Only two of these limbs underwent concurrent endovascular treatment of saphenous reflux. Although the other limbs had identified reflux, correction of the obstruction, alone, allowed healing of the ulcer. Stented patients experienced significant clinical improvement. After

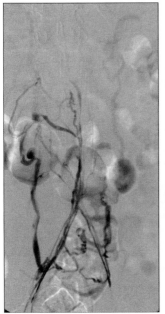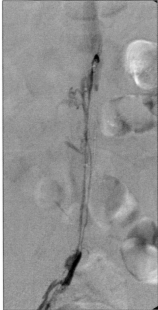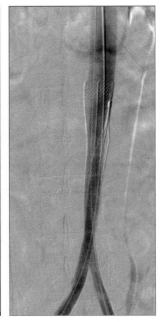

Figure 56.23　Three-image sequence showing baseline cavagram and subsequent reconstruction in a patient with IVC occlusion. Note the double barrel stents are extended parallel to the occluded filter.

3.5 years, the reduction in pain and swelling was 74% and 51%, respectively. At 24 months, cumulative primary and primary assisted patency were 58% and 82%, respectively. This is a valuable series, and the authors are to be commended for extensive experience and thoughtful review. Ninety percent of patients had symptomatic CVI, while 10% were essentially asymptomatic, including the four patients who had no idea there was a venous lesion prior to presenting with acute thrombosis distal to the IVC. Basically, the utilization of a complete venous investigation, including pelvic duplex, pressure testing, and transfemoral venography with IVUS uncovers a lot more venous pathology than anyone ever estimated. Whereas this degree of diagnostic investigation is not available in many institutions, the authors leave little doubt that venous obstruction is more prevalent than previously thought.

Thrombolytic therapy was not used except in treating acute DVT. Whereas we use catheter-directed thrombolysis to open and soften chronic thrombotic occlusions, the Raju and Neglen perform their procedures without thrombolysis. For the most part, thrombolysis was not required to pass a wire. However, lytic therapy may have facilitated difficult (unsuccessful) recanalization and diminished the incidence of residual stenoses that compressed stents and resulted in reintervention. Most of the lesions in this series were stenotic and, therefore, did require the opening of a primary channel. The authors make several technical points that I have similarly emphasized. First, complete stenting of diseased segments promotes reestablished continuity of deep venous flow, which is imperative to stent patency. Understenting should be discouraged in view of the observation that tributary flow passes through Wallstent interstices and traversing the inguinal ligament with overlapping, self-expanding metallic stents is well tolerated. Moreover, neither the initial venographic appearance, the extent of the lesion, nor the duration of the symptoms is a predictor of success or failure of guide-wire passage through a venous obstruction. Some chronic lesions are almost impossible and some are very easy. There must be genetic issues we do not yet recognize.

SUMMARY

Endovenous therapy represents a significant component in the treatment of chronic venous insufficiency due to thrombosis. The clinical options for treatment of residual obstruction, following DVT, now favor reconstruction of the native axial veins with self-expanding metallic stents. The evolution of the tools and techniques is ongoing, as the majority of the procedures have been adapted from arterial interventions. Because the venous system is characterized by lower pressure and lower flow state, compared with the arterial system, manipulations within veins are thrombogenic, and good technique is essential.

Appreciating that stents represent a form of bypass and, therefore, require good inflow as well as outflow to remain patent is fundamental. Often, this is not obvious to the inexperienced physician, who underestimates the role of residual thrombus in distal veins or the importance of a stent extending into the IVC by one centimeter. Chronic venous insufficiency is that "something old" that seems to be a renaissance topic in the midst of new pharmaceutical discoveries and the emerging field of endovenous surgery. Hopefully, continued innovation, multidisciplinary efforts, and clinical evidence will all support our efforts to better prevent DVT, to treat acute DVT in a timely manner, and, overall, reduce the incidence of postthrombotic venous insufficiency.

REFERENCES

1. Raju S, Hollis K, Neglén P. Obstructive lesions of the inferior vena cava: Clinical features and endovenous treatment, *J Vasc Surg*. 2006. *44*: 820–827.
2. Raju S, Owen SJ, Neglen P. Reversal of abnormal lymphoscintigraphy after placement of venous stents for correction of associated venous obstruction, *J Vasc Surg*. 2001. *34*: 779–784.
3. Brown DB, Pappas JA, Vedantham S, Pilgram TK, Olsen RV, Duncan JR. Gadolinium, carbon dioxide, and iodinated contrast material for planning inferior vena cava filter placement: A prospective trial. *J Vasc Interv Radiol*. 2003. *14*(8): 1017–1022.
4. David A, Peterson BA, Ella A, et al. Computed tomographic venography is specific but not sensitive for diagnosis of acute lower extremity deep venous thrombosis in patients with suspected pulmonary embolus, *J Vasc Surg*. 2001. *34*: 798–804.
5. Jost CJ, Gloviczki P, Cherry KJ Jr, et al. Surgical reconstruction of iliofemoral veins and the inferior vena cava for nonmalignant occlusive disease, *J Vasc Surg*. 2001. *2*: 320–328.
6. Zollikofer CL, Antonucci F, Stuckmann G, Mattias P, Salomonowitz EK. Historical overview on the development and characteristics of stents and future outlooks, *Cardiovasc Intervent Radiol*. 1992. *5*: 272–278.
7. Irving JD, Dondelinger RF, Reidy JF, et al. Gianturco self-expanding stents: Clinical experience in the vena cava and large veins, *Cardiovasc Intervent Radiol*. 1992. *5*: 328–333.
8. Thorpe P, Osse F, Dang H. Endovascular reconstruction for chronic iliac vein and inferior vena cava obstruction. In: Gloviczki P, Yao J, eds. *Handbook of venous disorders*, 2e. London: Arnold. 2001. 347–361.
9. O'Sullivan GJ, Semba CP, Bittner CA, et al. Endovascular management of iliac vein compression (May-Thurner) syndrome, *J Vasc Interv Radiol*. 2000. *11*: 823–836.
10. Razavi MK, Hansch EC, Kee ST, Sze DY, Semba CP, Dake MD. Chronically occluded inferior venae cavae: Endovascular treatment, *Radiology*. 2000. *1*: 133–138.
11. Neglén P, Raju S. Intravascular ultrasound scan evaluation of the obstructed vein, *J Vasc Surg*. 2002. *35*: 694–700.
12. Raju S, Owen SJ, Neglen P. The clinical impact of iliac venous stents in the management of chronic venous insufficiency, *J Vasc Surg*. 2002. *35*: 8–15.
13. Vedantham S, Vesely TM, Sicard GA, et al. Pharmacomechanical thrombolysis and early stent placement for iliofemoral deep vein thrombosis, *J Vasc Interv Radiol*. 2004. *15*: 565–574.
14. Allie DE, Hebert CJ, Lirtzman MD, et al. Novel simultaneous combination chemical thrombolysis/rheolytic thrombectomy therapy for acute critical limb ischemia: The power-pulse spray technique, *Catheter Cardio Inte*. 2004. *63*(4): 512–222.

15. Robbins MR, Assi Z, Comerota AJ. Endovascular stenting to treat chronic long-segment inferior vena cava occlusion, *J Vasc Surg.* 2005. *41*: 136–140.

16. te Riele WW, Overtoom TT, Van Den Berg JC, van de Pavoordt ED, de Vries JP. Endovascular recanalization of chronic long-segment occlusions of the inferior vena cava: Midterm results, *J Endovasc Ther.* 2006. *13*(2): 249–253.

17. Raju S, Neglen P. High prevalence of nonthrombotic iliac vein lesions in chronic venous disease: A permissive role in pathogenicity, *J Vasc Surg.* 2006. *44*: 136–144.

18. Neglén P, Hollis KC, Olivier J, Raju S. Stenting of the venous out-flow in chronic venous disease: Long-term stent-related outcome, clinical, and hemodynamic result, *J Vasc Surg.* 2007. *46*: 979–990.

19. Hilleman DE, Razavi MK. Clinical and economic evaluation of the trellis-8 infusion catheter for deep vein thrombosis, *J Vasc Interv Radiol.* 2008. *19*: 377–383.

20. Neglén P, Tackett TP Jr, Raju S. Venous stenting across the inguinal ligament, *J Vasc Surg.* 2008. *48*: 1255–1261.

21. Trabal J, Comerota A, LaPorte F, Kazanjian S, DiSalle R, Sepanski, D. The quantitative benefit of isolated, segmental, pharmacome-chanical thrombolysis (ISPMT) for iliofemoral venous thrombosis, *J Vasc Surg.* 2008. *48*: 1532–1537.

22. Raju S, Neglén P. Percutaneous recanalization of total occlusions of the iliac vein, *J Vasc Surg.* 2009. *50*: 360–368.

23. Hartung O, Loundou AD, Barthelemy P, Arnoux D, Boufi M, Alimi YS. Endovascular management of chronic disabling ilio-caval obstructive lesions: Long-term results, *Eur J Vasc Endovasc Surg.* 2009. *38*(1): 118–124.

24. Cockett FB, Thomas ML. The iliac compression syndrome, *Br J Surg.* 1965. *52*: 816–821.

25. Cockett FB, Thomas ML, Negus D. Iliac vein compression: Its rela-tion to iliofemoral thrombosis and the post-thrombotic syndrome, *Br Med J.* 1967. *2*: 14–19.

26. Labropoulos N, Borge M, Pierce K, Pappas PJ. Criteria for defining significant central vein stenosis with duplex ultrasound, *J Vasc Surg.* 2007. *46*: 101–107.

27. Comerota AJ. The ATTRACT trial: Rationale for early intervention for iliofemoral DVT, *Perspt Vasc Surg Endovasc Ther.* 2009. *4*: 221–224.

28. Killewich LA, Bedford GR, Beach KW, Strandness DE Jr. Spontaneous lysis of deep venous thrombi: Rate and outcome, *J Vasc Surg.* 1989. *9*: 89–97.

29. Johnson BF, Manzo RA, Bergelin RO, Strandness DE Jr. Relationship between changes in the deep venous system and the development of the postthrombotic syndrome after an acute episode of lower limb deep vein thrombosis: A one- to six-year follow-up, *J Vasc Surg.* 1995. *21*: 307–312.

30. Prandoni P. Risk factors of recurrent venous thromboemboli: The role of residual vein thrombosis, *Pathophysiol Haemost Thromb.* 2003. *33*: 351–353.

31. Markel A, Manzo RA, Bergelin RO, Strandness DE Jr. Valvular reflux after deep vein thrombosis: Incidence and time of occurrence, *J Vasc Surg.* 1992. *15*: 377–382.

32. Mewissen MW, Seabrook GR, Meissner MH, Cynamon J, Labropoulos N, Haughton SH. Catheter-directed thrombolysis for lower extremity deep venous thrombosis: Report of a national mul-ticenter registry [erratum appears in *Radiology.* 1999. *213*(3): 930], *Radiology.* 1999. *211*(1): 39–49.

33. Nazarian GK, Austin WR, Wegryn SA, et al. Venous recanalization by metallic stents after failure of balloon angioplasty or surgery: Four-year experience, *Cardiovasc Intervent Radiol.* 1996. *19*(4): 227–233.

34. Neglen P, Raju S. In-stent recurrent stenosis in stents placed in the lower extremity venous outflow tract, *J Vasc Surg.* 2004. *39*(1): 181–187.

35. Peter Neglén, MD, PhD, Rikki Darcey, BS, Jake Olivier, PhD, Seshadri Raju, MD. Bilateral stenting at the iliocaval confluence *J Vasc Surg* 2010;*51*:1457–1466.

36. Neglén P, Oglesbee MD, Raju S. Stenting of chronically obstructed inferior vena cava filters, *J Vasc Surg.* 2010. *51*(3): 794.

37. Bjarnason H, Kruse JR, Asinger DA, et al. Iliofemoral deep venous thrombosis: Safety and efficacy outcome during 5 years of catheter-directed thrombolytic therapy *J Vasc Interv Radiol.* 1997 *8*(3): 405–418.

38. Comerota AJ, Gravett MH. Iliofemoral venous thrombo-sis: A review, *J Vasc Surg.* 2007. *46*: 1065–1076.

39. Hartung O, Barthelemy P, Arnoux D, Boufi M, Alimi YS. Management of pregnancy in women with previous left ilio-caval stenting, *J Vasc Surg.* 2009. *50*: 355–359.

57.

POPLITEAL VEIN ENTRAPMENT

Seshadri Raju

opliteal vein entrapment is a rare clinical entity. *Anatomic* popliteal vein compression, however, can be demonstrated by imaging techniques in 27 to 42% of asymptomatic individuals with a 34% incidence of bilaterality.[1,2] In the frequency of the anatomic lesion and the rarity of the clinical expression, the entity perhaps resembles thoracic outlet syndrome. Compression of the popliteal vein is infrequently (±10%) associated with companion arterial compression, even though the very first case reported by Rich and Hughes in 1967 was.[3] Clinical features are often indistinguishable from other forms of chronic venous disease (CVD) and easily applicable diagnostic testing is lacking. Diagnosis currently depends on awareness of the entity and elimination of other causes of chronic venous insufficiency. Invasive monitoring of dynamic popliteal venous pressure with ankle maneuvers in suspected cases may be specific.[2]

INCIDENCE

The estimated incidence is less than 4% of all cases of CVD, probably much less. Sporadic case reports[4–15] and two series[2,16] can be found in the literature.

CLINICAL FEATURES

Contrary to expectations, the disease is not confined to the young; there appears to be no age or sex predilection.[2] Like other forms of CVD, common symptoms and signs are swelling, pain, and stasis skin changes including ulceration. Limb swelling extending above the knee joint probably rules out the condition as the primary pathology. Venous claudication may be present in some but not all. Cutaneous hyperpigmentation may extend more proximally beyond the gaiter area in some patients. Isolated popliteal valve reflux when symptomatic should arouse clinical suspicion of entrapment, as the former by itself is seldom symptomatic. Entrapment may result in popliteal vein thrombosis.[17]

INVESTIGATIONS

Popliteal vein compression on ascending venography is sensitive, but not specific. Popliteal vein compression should be demonstrated on active plantar flexion; passive dorsiflexion may also reproduce the lesion in some (see Figure 57.1). The site of compression is variable (high popliteal 11%, mid popliteal 39%, low popliteal 18%, and diffuse 32%), thus suggesting varied compressive mechanisms.

Like venography, duplex with ankle maneuvers can also demonstrate popliteal vein compression without any inference to causality of symptoms.[1] Associated popliteal artery compression with ankle maneuvers is present in about half of the limbs without clinical features of arterial insufficiency. Demonstration of arterial compression does not signify functionally significant associated venous compression.

Magnetic resonance imaging[18,19] may display abnormal features of the gastrocnemius muscle, which is frequently a part of the compressive mechanism, and it can help rule out other causes of compression such as the Baker's cyst.[9,14]

Abnormalities on ambulatory venous pressure measurement (pedal vein) and outflow fraction by occlusive plethysmography may be suggestive, but these tests are neither sensitive nor specific.[2] Similar comments apply to ejection fraction and residual volume measurements with air plethysmography (APG).

Dynamic popliteal vein pressure measurements (see Figure 57.2) with ankle maneuvers appear to be diagnostic and useful in assessing outcome after entrapment release.[2]

PATHOLOGY

The most frequent compressive mechanism is the gastrocnemius muscle due to abnormalities in the origin of the medial head (see Table 57.1). Postnatal extension of the medial head of the gastrocnemius muscle from the medial femoral condyle to involve portions of the adjacent femoral shaft is a normal event; excessive migration appears to result

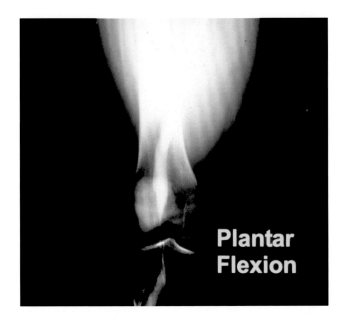

Figure 57.1 Popliteal vein compression with ankle maneuvers: mid popliteal (left). Discrete lesions at high and low popliteal locations as well as diffuse lesions (not shown) also occur.

Table 57.1 PATHOLOGICAL FEATURES IN THIRTY CASES OF ENTRAPMENT UNDERGOING RELEASE

COMPRESSIVE ENTRAPMENT MECHANISM	NUMBER
Gastrocnemius medial head anomalous origin	18*
Additional third head of gastrocnemius	1
Gastrocnemius lateral head origin from medial Condyle	5
Soleus sling	3
Thick perivenous fascia	13†
Abnormal course of vascular bundle lateral to the Lateral head	2
Unknown	1
PATHOLOGICAL CHANGES IN THE POPLITEAL VEIN	**NUMBER**
Sclerosis	13
Prestenotic Dilatation	1
Poststenotic Dilatation	4**
Postthrombotic Changes	2

*One case associated with atrophic lateral head.
**Two saccular aneurysms.
†Associated with other entrapment mechanisms.
(From Reference 2, with permission)

in compression of the vein. Compression by other muscles such as the lateral head of the gastrocnemius or the soleal sling are relatively rare. Compression of the vein by the tibial nerve may occur rarely.

The compressed vein segment often becomes sclerosed and stenotic. Both prestenotic and poststenotic dilatations occur, occasionally large enough to be classified as aneurysms. A thick perivenous fascia attached to the gastrocnemius muscle is an integral part of the compressive mechanism, which may explain the varied location of vein compression noted on venography. The entrapment mechanism likely involves prolonged spasm of the vein initiated by external compression by adjacent muscle. Elevation of the popliteal vein pressure persists long after cessation of active muscle contraction (see Figure 57.3). Entrapment may eventually lead to popliteal valve reflux[2] and perforator incompetence.[20] Unlike in popliteal artery entrapment,

anatomic course variations of the popliteal vein are relatively rare.

SURGICAL TREATMENT

The posterior approach[20] or the medial approach[2] to the popliteal fossa may be used. The posterior approach is preferable if anatomic course variations of the popliteal vasculature are suspected.

The medial head of the gastrocnemius is taken down from the bone with particular attention to the muscle extension beyond the condyle. This extension may be large enough to be described as a third head.[11] As recurrences with reattachment of the muscle can occur, resection of the medial head may be preferable to simple detachment of the muscle from its origin. Other compressive elements

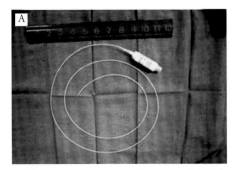 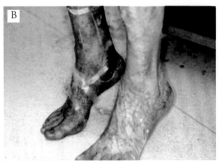

Figure 57.2 Calf exercise with percutaneously inserted Millar Probes. (A) The 2-Fr catheters have tip-mounted pressure transducers. (B) The catheter tip is positioned in the popliteal vein under fluoroscopy.

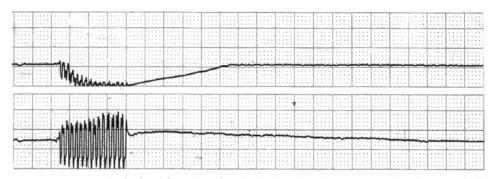

Figure 57.3 Simultaneous pressure tracings in the dorsal foot vein and popliteal vein with calf exercise. Note elevation in popliteal pressure and decrease in foot venous pressure after exercise. Popliteal pressure elevation persists for 100 seconds after cessation of exercise before slowly declining to baseline. (From Reference 2, with permission).

when present should be lysed as well. The vein should be cleared of its perivenous sheath and tributaries over a generous 10-cm length centered on the compressive point. Aneurysmal and stenotic segments should be resected and the vein repaired without any hint of tension, using a saphenous graft if necessary. The popliteal valve should be repaired if refluxive, particularly when skin changes are present. Axillary vein transfer may be required if primary valve reconstruction is not possible.[2] Perioperative antithrombotic prophylaxis including use of low molecular weight heparin, meticulous hemostasis, and closed drainage are necessary to achieve clean primary healing without local complications that may predispose to recurrence.

CLINICAL RESULTS

Excellent clinical results with relief of pain, swelling, and stasis skin changes have been reported particularly

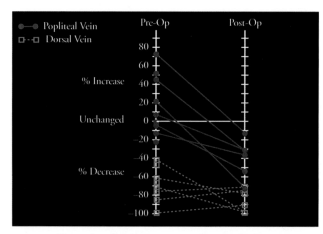

Figure 57.4 Elevated popliteal vein pressure after exercise decreases after entrapment lysis. Dorsal vein pressure (post exercise) shows little change. (From Reference 2, with permission).

when the diagnosis is firmly established on the basis of dynamic popliteal vein pressure measurements (see Figure 57.4).[2]

REFERENCES

1. Leon M, Volteas N, Labropoulos N, et al. Popliteal vein entrapment in the normal population, *Eur J Vasc Surg.* 1992. *6*(6): 623–627.
2. Raju S, Neglen P. Popliteal vein entrapment: A benign venographic feature or a pathologic entity? *J Vasc Surg.* 2000. *31*(4): 631–641.
3. Rich NM, Hughes CW. Popliteal artery and vein entrapment, *Am J Surg.* 1967. *113*(5): 696–698.
4. Edmondson HT, Crowe JA Jr. Popliteal arterial and venous entrapment, *Am Surg.* 1972. *38*(12): 657–659.
5. Connell J. Popliteal vein entrapment, *Br J Surg.* 1978. *65*(5): 351.
6. Mastaglia FL, Venerys J, Stokes BA, Vaughan R. Compression of the tibial nerve by the tendinous arch of origin of the soleus muscle, *Clin Exp Neurol.* 1981. *18*: 81–85.
7. Koplic S, Maskovic J, Radonic V. [Musculotendinous pressure on the arteries of the knee observed in a patient with obstructive entrapment syndrome of the popliteal artery and vein]. *Acta Chir Iugosl.* 1982. *29* Suppl 2: 189–193.
8. Zelli GP, Mattei E. [Unusual phlebopathy of the lower limbs. Considerations on a case of congenital compression (entrapment) of the popliteal vein]. *Ann Ital Chir.* 1982. *54*(3): 245–252.
9. Zygmunt S, Keller K, Lidgren L. Baker cyst causing nerve entrapment, *Scand J Rheumatol.* 1982. *11*(4): 239–240.
10. van Berge Henegouwen DP, Salzmann P, Lindner F. [Entrapment and cystic degeneration of the adventitia as a cause of occlusion of the popliteal artery], *Chirurg.* 1986. *57*(12): 797–800.
11. Iwai T, Sato S, Yamada T, et al. Popliteal vein entrapment caused by the third head of the gastrocnemius muscle, *Br J Surg.* 1987. *74*(11): 1006–1008.
12. Van Damme H, Ballaux JM, Dereume JP. Femoro-popliteal venous graft entrapment, *J Cardiovasc Surg* (Torino). 1988; *29*(1): 50–55.
13. Nelson MC, Teitelbaum GP, Matsumoto AH, Stull MA. Isolated popliteal vein entrapment, *Cardiovasc Intervent Radiol.* 1989–1990. *12*(6): 301–303.
14. Rettori R, Boespflug O. [Popliteal vein entrapment, popliteal cyst, desmoid tumor and fabella syndrome], *J Mal Vasc.* 1990. *15*(2): 182–187.

15. Sieunarine K, Prendergast FJ, Paton R, Goodman MA, Ibach EG. Entrapment of popliteal artery and vein, *Aust N Z J Surg*. 1990. *60*(7): 533–537.

16. di Marzo L, Cavallaro A, Sciacca V, Mingoli A, Tamburelli A. Surgical treatment of popliteal artery entrapment syndrome: A ten-year experience, *Eur J Vasc Surg*. 1991. *5*(1): 59–64.

17. Gerkin TM, Beebe HG, Williams DM, Bloom JR, Wakefield TW. Popliteal vein entrapment presenting as deep venous thrombosis and chronic venous insufficiency, *J Vasc Surg*. 1993. *18*(5): 760–766.

18. Fermand M, Houlle D, Cormier JM, Vitoux JF, Lignieres G. Popliteal vein entrapment shown by MR imaging, *AJR Am J Roentgenol*. 1990. *155*(2): 424–425.

19. Di Cesare E, Marsili L, Marino G, et al. Stress MR imaging for evaluation of popliteal artery entrapment, *J Magn Reson Imaging*. 1994. *4*(4): 617–622.

20. Di Marzo L, Cisternino S, Sapienza P, et al. [Entrapment syndrome of the popliteal vein: results of the surgical treatment], *Ann Ital Chir*. 1996. *67*(4): 515–519; discussion 519–520.

58.

VALVULOPLASTY IN PRIMARY VENOUS INSUFFICIENCY

DEVELOPMENT, PERFORMANCE, AND LONG-TERM RESULTS

Robert L. Kistner, Elna Masuda, and Fedor Lurie

Widespread interest in the occurrence of deep vein reflux, its clinical effects, the technique of direct valve repair, and the long-term results of valve repair followed the demonstration in 1968 that direct surgical repair of the femoral venous valve was feasible. This chapter will review the background on which the first repair was based and highlights that have evolved in this field since the first repair was reported in 1968.

THE FIRST VALVE REPAIR

The first valve repair[1] was the result of curiosity in a clinical case of swelling, pain, and work disability in a patient who suffered left leg deep venous thrombosis (DVT) following a high voltage electrical burn.

Two years following the injury this patient was unable to return to work due to swelling and pain in the extremity. An ascending venogram revealed the unexpected finding of patency of the entire deep venous system with traces of postthrombotic scarring in the popliteal vein and the lower thigh portion of the femoral vein. Since this finding did not offer an adequate explanation of the patient's symptoms (swelling above the knee), it was reasoned that the problem was due mainly to reflux rather than obstruction, and this led to the concept of descending venography to determine the valvular status in this extremity. The descending venogram showed full axial reflux of contrast from the common femoral vein (CFV) down through the popliteal vein and into the calf. It also showed a well-formed but incompetent valve at the upper end of the femoral vein (formerly termed the superficial femoral vein). Other valves were identified in the distal femoral vein. Evidence of postthrombotic scarring in the popliteal and superficial femoral veins was noted.

With the diagnosis of axial reflux as the cause of the patient's symptoms, it was elected to treat the patient after the teachings of Robert Linton[2] by controlling greater saphenous and perforator reflux, followed by control of the deep vein reflux by interrupting the upper end of the femoral vein just distal to the origin of the deep femoral vein in the groin. The patient previously had the saphenous vein stripped. The perforators of the calf were interrupted 3 d prior to exploration of the femoral vein, and the femoral vein was approached as a separate procedure.

Prior to surgery on the femoral vein, the finding of a normal-appearing valve in the upper femoral vein on the venogram resulted in the decision to explore the valve to see if it might be repairable prior to ligation of the femoral vein. When this exploration at surgery revealed a morphologically normal vein and valve structure with the single finding of elongation of the valve cusp, it was elected to attempt repair of this defect by shortening the leading edge of the two cusps. When this was done the valve appeared normal and it resulted in a totally competent valve upon closure of the vein. It was decided to accept this newly competent femoral valve as replacement for the originally intended ligation of the femoral vein. The patient was managed with full heparinization for the first postoperative week, then switched to Coumadin.

The clinical result was dramatic relief of his symptoms from the first postoperative day when he spontaneously remarked that his leg felt relieved of its congestion. He remained free of unilateral symptoms in this extremity for the remaining 13 years of his life.

This successful surgical repair of an incompetent femoral vein valve in 1968 led to a series of seventeen repairs that were the substance of the first national report of the procedure in 1975.[3] This series consisted of advanced venous insufficiency cases evaluated with ascending and descending venography to identify instances where severe clinical venous insufficiency was associated with axial deep vein reflux rather than deep obstruction.

BACKGROUND KNOWLEDGE OF NONTHROMBOTIC REFLUX DEEP VEIN DISEASE

Except for the publications of Gunnar Bauer in the 1940s,[4] clinically important deep vein reflux disease had been attributed to postthrombotic disease. Bauer was a brilliant investigator surgeon who worked in a small hospital in Mariestad, Sweden, in the mid-1900s. He experimented with venography in patients suspected of having venous disease and devised a method of performing descending venography, described in 1948. These venograms were performed with a needle in the CFV and with the patient in the 45-degree erect position. Static films were obtained to document findings. Bauer was the first to report nonthrombotic cases with high-grade axial reflux in the deep veins, and to associate these cases with advanced stages of clinical venous insufficiency. He treated these cases with popliteal vein ligation and reported early clinical success, but later follow-up of some of these cases by his peers in Sweden discredited the long-term value of popliteal vein ligation.

Bauer's descending venography resulted in activity in other sites around the world, as reflected by reports that appeared in the early 1950s.[5,6] Confusion arose from these reports when it was found that deep reflux was associated with symptoms in some cases, whereas other cases were asymptomatic. As a result of this confusion with descending venography and the report that popliteal vein ligation was a questionable procedure, this entity, which Bauer called "idiopathic nonthrombotic reflux," apparently lost credibility as an important cause of venous insufficiency in the 1950s and lay dormant until venous valve repair surfaced in 1975.

The description of the reflux entity that Bauer termed "idiopathic nonthrombotic venous insufficiency"[4] is identical to the present-day primary venous insufficiency. This entity is fundamentally different from postthrombotic disease since there is no element of gross inflammation or scarring of the vein or valve, or intraluminal obstruction with wall thickening as found in the postthrombotic cases.

TREATMENT OF DEEP VEIN REFLUX PRIOR TO 1968

There was great interest in the aggressive management of the chronic venous disease (CVD) leg prior to 1960, which is well summarized in the papers of Robert Linton of Boston from 1938 to 1953.[2,7] Linton refers to the epic work of Homans,[8] who drew attention to the importance of the perforator veins and concentrated on the excision of the diseased skin and scar tissue in the lower leg. Homans's understanding of the pathophysiology of CVD is amazing in view of the fact that he had no imaging studies to visualize the leg veins and depended entirely on clinical acumen to divine the relationship between the skin changes of CVD and the venous system. He came to understand that these changes were related to deep vein disease, which was attributed to postthrombotic changes in the veins through clinical examination alone. Linton embraced and amplified this thinking and devised a multipronged surgical effort to control venous hypertension by removing the saphenous vein, radically eliminating perforator veins in the calf, ligating the superficial femoral vein, and removing a large segment of deep fascia in the posterior calf to facilitate lymph drainage of the extremity. During the 1950s he was an intense advocate of aggressive surgical treatment for advanced venous insufficiency, essentially all of which he attributed to postthrombotic venous disease. His papers emphasize the importance of reflux in the genesis of postthrombotic sequelae as he describes the progression of the originally obstructive thrombosis to a refluxive postthrombotic state after recanalization of the thrombosed channels has occurred. Although his papers cite the work of Gunnar Bauer, there is little or no mention of ascending or descending venography or of nonthrombotic venous reflux disease in Linton's diagnostic workup of the postphlebitic patients.

EARLY INFLUENCE OF VALVULOPLASTY ON THE STUDY OF VENOUS DISEASE

The realization that there is an entity of primary reflux disease as a cause of axial reflux separate from postthrombotic reflux stimulated investigation into the frequency of the two conditions, their diagnostic criteria, and the implications their identification would have on management.

Among the questions that stimulated the interest of investigators were the need to know the frequency with which axial primary deep vein reflux occurred, the amount of damage it could contribute to the extremity, and the near- and long-term results of its repair. With the ability to repair reflux in the superficial, perforator, and deep veins, the concept of total repair of reflux was possible, and the question of which conditions would warrant this more aggressive treatment required investigation. For the first time, thorough knowledge of the pathophysiology in each segment of the venous tree had become of practical import because each could be repaired. This ultimately became a strong stimulus to revise the diagnosis of venous insufficiency into an objective image-driven study of the entire deep venous tree.

Some specific questions that stimulated new studies included:

1. What is the pathology of the repairable venous valve? Is it a postthrombotic valve with minimal damage? Is it a degenerative change in the noninflamed valve? Is it similar to the valve changes in saphenous varicose veins?

2. How often do deep veins develop incompetent valves?

3. Have they been repaired previously?

4. Can they be repaired reliably? How long will a repair last?

5. What are the clinical manifestations of nonthrombotic (pure) deep vein reflux?

These and many other questions led to investigations of advanced venous insufficiency cases that had to be done by venography since noninvasive ultrasound visualization of the veins was not available until the 1980s. Ascending venography was a known and developed test but descending venography was not. Since the early works of Bauer in devising descending venography had lost favor, and attention had been focused on postthrombotic deep vein disease, new studies with this technique were needed. In the interim, the improvement of fluoroscopic control with dynamic video recording and audio recording of descending venography permitted more definitive descending venograms than were heretofore available. These studies[9,10] resulted in confirmation of the early writings of Gunnar Bauer in which the two causes of deep vein reflux were described. The most important contribution of this newer technology was the ability to trace the dynamic retrograde flow of contrast in refluxing veins and compare this to the normal totally competent systems with well-defined valve outlines. As time progressed, it became possible to distinguish the postthrombotic diseased valves from the primary valves with a correlation to surgical findings in the range of 90% accuracy.

These reflux studies revealed that the clinical manifestations of CVD reflected by skin complications in the distal lower leg were similar whether the cause was postthrombotic reflux/obstruction or primary reflux, thereby establishing that the clinical appearance alone is not sufficient to differentiate between these two etiologies. This established with certainty that imaging of the veins in advanced CVD is critical to the accurate diagnosis of the disease process. The importance of differentiating these causes is emphasized because surgical repair techniques and the potential for long-term success are different for the two entities.

Surgical exploration of postthrombotic cases confirmed that these valves were scarred or completely destroyed in most cases and did not respond well to surgical repair, whereas the valves in primary cases were well-preserved, morphologically normal valves that could be reliably repaired.

The new surgical treatment of primary valve reflux was direct repair of the valve; however, the surgical treatment of postthrombotic reflux required valve substitution techniques rather than valve repair. Taheri's description[11] (see Figure 58.1) of transplantation of segments of arm veins that contain competent valves into the refluxing segments of the leg where valve destruction had occurred, and the alternative technique of vein transposition[12] (see Figure 58.1), which provided a substitute competent proximal valve in the outflow tract, were devised for use when there were no repairable primary valves available. These procedures were needed for the postthrombotic limb, but also find useful application in the primary limb when there are no repairable valves.

The question of how many valves are needed to provide clinical compensation to the extremity raised many doubts about repair of a single valve to correct severe venous insufficiency. The teleologic observation that the human has many more valves in the calf veins than in the proximal thigh suggested valves below the popliteal were more important than valves in the thigh, and predicted failure of proximal valve repair. The clinical observation of repaired primary valve cases did not confirm this rationale and has supported a different concept that a single valve interposed into an axial refluxing venous division at the thigh level will be adequate to reverse the clinical syndrome of deep reflux. This was based on the original reasoning that reflux from the heart to the calf, termed axial reflux, results in sequelae that can be ameliorated by

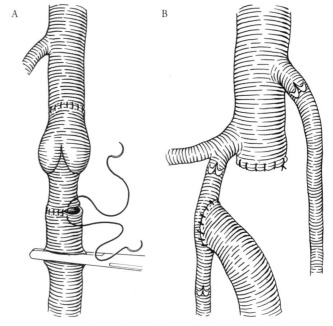

Figure 58.1 Valve substitution techniques: (A) Technique for valve substitution utilizing a harvested vein valve from the upper extremity. The substitute vein was placed end to end in the refluxing vein after the valve had been checked for competency. (B) Technique of valve substitution utilizing transposition of a refluxing vein to an adjacent vein by end-to-side anastomosis when the recipient vein had a competent proximal and distal valve. The proximal divided end of the transposed vein was oversewn to prevent a potential thrombotic pocket from developing postoperatively.

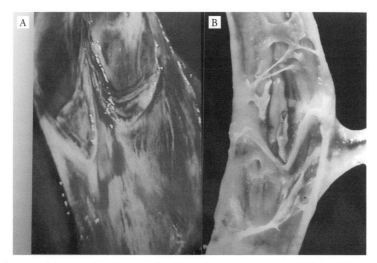

Figure 58.2 (A) Photograph of a valve with primary venous insufficiency to demonstrate the intima of the vein is healthy and free of scars, and the cusp is smooth, thin, and glistening but lies in folds due to elongation of the proximal margin, which presents as sagging edges in the opened vein. (B) Photograph of a severely distorted, scarred valve site following postthrombotic changes. This essentially unrecognizable valve site represents a far-advanced stage of the postthrombotic spectrum and demonstrates a dramatic difference from the primary valve.

decreasing the incompetent column essentially in half when a single competent valve is placed at the femoral-popliteal level.

When more than one (axial) anatomic division of the veins in the extremity is affected by incompetence, an additional valve is needed for the second division. The axial divisions are several: the usual common femoral–femoropopliteal–tibial route; the common femoral–profunda-popliteal–tibial route; the common femoral-saphenopopliteal-tibial route, including perforators; being the main three divisions. If the system contains large collaterals, other routes of atypical axial reflux can develop and need to be identified in individual cases. Eriksson[13] pointed out the importance of different routes of axial reflux when he reported failure in the case of repair of a single competent valve in the femoral vein that was attributed to residual incompetence in the adjacent refluxing profunda-popliteal axial segment. The dilemma of how many valves are needed can be solved by placing one valve in each refluxing axial tract, or by placing a single valve distal to all the refluxing segments, for example, placing a popliteal valve to protect the calf from reflux in both the femoral and the profunda outflow tracts. This location found favor in treatment of postthrombotic disease by O'Donnell[14] and Nash[15] with good results.

There have been advocates of providing more than one competent valve per axial segment, but none has proven that this is necessary. It makes common sense to repair a second valve if one is readily available, but the necessity of repairing a remote valve just to provide a second competent valve in a given axial route has not been widely followed.

PATHOLOGIC CHANGES OF FEMOROPOPLITEAL VALVES

The difference between the incompetent valves of the primary reflux cases and the valves of the postthrombotic cases is clear in both gross and microscopic study of these valves. The original description of the gross findings in the morphologically normal valve of primary disease[1] has stood the test of time. These valves are smooth and glistening and delicate, free of synechiae or scars, and surrounded by a normal endothelium in the surrounding vein wall. The abnormality in the primary incompetent deep vein valve is that the free margin of the valve is elongated and the valve cusp lies in folds with sagging margins when exposed at surgery (see Figure 58.2). The endothelial lining of the vein and the consistency of the valve and the vein wall are normal. This is in stark contrast to the grossly deformed valve site of some cases of postthrombotic disease, where the valves are literally destroyed by deforming scars and synechiae and are totally unrepairable (see Figure 58.2) and there is thickening of the wall of the vein.

Within the spectrum of valves exposed at surgery there are some valves that have features of both primary and secondary disease, such as a thin valve with smooth endothelium that also has one or more discrete synechiae, or scars, that deform the valve. Since pathologic material is rarely available to study the microscopic aspect of these valves, it may not be clear in a given case whether the valve pathology is truly primary or secondary or has elements of both. Some have reported long-term success with repairing scarred valves,[16] whereas the Straub experience has been that most of the valves with scarring develop late recurrence following an initial successful repair.

The microscopic difference in the vein wall between primary and secondary valve disease is striking. The microscopic pathology of the primary case involves increase of collagen, decrease of muscularis with entrapment of the muscularis by collagen bundles, and fragmentation of elastica. This set of conditions would correlate well with loss of tone in the vein wall and lead to dysfunction of the

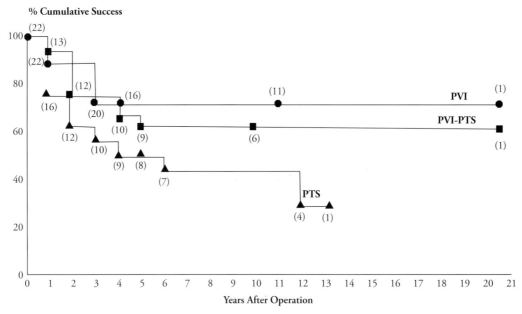

% Cumulative Success

Figure 58.3   Life table of results of primary internal repairs (PVI) compared to results after repair for mixed primary and postthrombotic disease (PVI-PTS) and results after repair for pure postthrombotic disease (PTS). Clinical criteria for repair were similar for all three groups. Criteria for appearing in this table were that the procedure had been performed 4–21 years prior to this report. The clinical results were superior but comparable for pure primary and mixed primary-secondary groups, but less effective in pure postthrombotic cases.[19]

attached venous valve without actually affecting the valve cusp.[17] The typical postthrombotic changes of inflammatory cells, hemosiderin deposits, and neovascularization are absent. A confounding factor in postthrombotic cases is that changes of both primary and secondary disease may be present, a finding we interpret to represent inflammatory secondary changes superimposed on primary degenerative wall changes.

In addition to cases of pure primary insufficiency and of secondary insufficiency, there is a large group of cases with advanced venous insufficiency who have had thrombophlebitis in the calf and popliteal veins, even extending into the lower femoral vein, who also have a refluxing valve in the proximal femoral vein that has all the features of a primary refluxing valve. In these limbs, repair of the proximal valve by valvuloplasty technique yields clinical results and durability of repair that mimics the results of pure primary reflux (see Figure 58.3). This phenomenon of separate areas of postthrombotic disease and primary disease in the same extremity occurred in the first valve treated by open repair in 1968. Caps has reported finding proximal incompetent valves in his studies of postthrombotic veins where the proximal valve was distant from the site of thrombosis[18] and reasoned this proximal incompetent valve to be a result of the thrombotic process but lacked prior valve studies to substantiate this. Our interpretation has favored the theory that these thin pliant repairable proximal valves are incompetent due to primary disease and were not clinically recognizable until the distal postthrombotic disease caused axial reflux, rather than attributing them to the phlebitic process. In either case, this finding of repairable proximal thigh

valves in extremities with more distal thrombotic disease is important because up to one third of the repairable valve cases in our series[19] fell into this category.

DISTRIBUTION OF PRIMARY INCOMPETENT VALVES

Primary incompetent veins and valves may occur in segmental or axial distribution. Axial reflux occurs most frequently in the saphenous veins, and often is limited to the saphenous veins in primary disease. The presence of axial reflux in the deep veins is significant in the more serious cases of primary reflux, which present with extensive aching, swelling, and disability.

This distribution of reflux is different from that of postthrombotic disease, where isolated reflux is often found in the deep veins but rarely in the saphenous veins. It is common to find the saphenous vein enlarged and still competent in late postthrombotic disease, but this would be extremely rare in primary disease. Volume flow studies often indicate the competent great saphenous vein is the major outflow tract in the postthrombotic extremity when the femoral and profunda veins have prominent elements of obstruction.

In a series of ninety-eight cases of venous ulcers[20] in which the distribution of reflux was studied, the deep veins showed reflux in 73% of cases, perforators in 80%, and saphenous veins in 86%. The etiologies in these cases were 67% primary and 33% postthrombotic disease. It is cogent that the deep veins demonstrated axial incompetence in one-third of primary cases and in two-thirds of secondary cases, and the great saphenous veins demonstrated axial incompetence in two-thirds of primary and one-third of postthrombotic cases. Even in these far-advanced cases of CVD the preponderance of deep vein reflux in postthrombotic disease contrasts with the preponderance of superficial reflux in the primary cases.

The source of the reflux and wall dilation in primary disease remains controversial between the top-down valvular theory and the contrasting theory that the basic problem begins with degeneration of the vein wall and involves the valves secondarily. Clinical evidence that the initial weakness occurs in the vein wall in primary disease has been presented,[21] and theoretical support for the primacy of wall changes can be deduced from the histologic changes in the vein wall described in the earlier section that described the pathologic changes of femoropopliteal valves. It is entirely possible that the wall changes result in dysfunction of the valve. Regardless of the initial event, elements of both wall weakness and valvular reflux clearly coexist as the degenerative process of primary disease matures.

The development of primary disease as a progressive phenomenon is well supported by the Bochum investigations,[22] in which young students were followed serially in 4-year increments during primary and secondary school and demonstrated progressive reflux in the saphenous and perforator veins, with minimal involvement of the deep veins. This is consistent with the observation that large numbers of early primary cases with varicose veins have no reflux in the deep veins, but progressive involvement beyond the saphenous and into the perforator veins and later into the deep veins is found in patients with more severe degrees of clinical disease as skin changes and ulceration becomes manifest. This contrasts sharply with the natural history of postthrombotic disease, which nearly always begins in the deep veins and spares the superficial veins.

SURGICAL CONSIDERATIONS ARISING FROM DEEP VEIN REFLUX PATTERNS

The axial reflux patterns of primary deep venous disease must be thoroughly diagnosed prior to planning deep vein valve repair. Primary cases often present with a single axial reflux tract that courses from the CFV through the femoral vein of the thigh to the popliteal and into the calf veins. In this case, a single valve repair in the femoral vein has been shown to be all that is needed to restore clinical compensation to the venous return. These cases usually have little or no communication between the distal profunda veins and the popliteal vein and seldom have other collaterals. The lack of collaterals is due to the lack of an obstructive element in the development of primary disease, in contrast to postthrombotic deep vein disease.

When the deep femoral vein is incompetent in addition to the femoral vein itself, attention needs to be directed to the distal communications between the profunda veins and the popliteal vein, usually via large connecting branches at the adductor canal (profunda-popliteal connecting veins). If there is significant distal reflux by the CFV deep femoral-popliteal route, a separate valve is needed for this tract. The choice when reflux occurs by both femoral and deep femoral tracts is either to provide one competent valve at the popliteal level, or two valves, one in the femoral and the other in the profunda veins. In postthrombotic disease the profunda-popliteal branches provide a collateral route of return flow when the femoral vein itself becomes occluded by the thrombotic process, and it persists when there are elements of relative obstruction in the scarred and recanalized femoral vein outflow tract.

CLINICAL CONTRIBUTIONS TO THE EXPERIENCE OF DEEP VEIN VALVE REPAIR

Following the report of repair of primary venous valve reflux in 1975,[3] a succession of clinical investigators initiated their own case series and developed innovative technical approaches to valve repair and valve substitution, generating diverse clinical results that resulted in new knowledge about lower extremity reflux disease. Interval reports from the Straub Clinic experience appeared in 1975,[3] 1979,[23] and 1982,[24] describing results of reconstruction in an enlarging group that initially consisted of primary valve repairs and subsequently included postthrombotic cases; this effort culminated in a 4- to 21-year follow-up report of the long-term results of these repairs in 1994.[19]

In 1982 and beyond, widespread reports from other sources presented new developments that have continued until the present. Among the initial publications are a large series of reconstructions for both primary and postthrombotic disease from the University of Mississippi,[25,26] a smaller series of valve repairs from Sweden[27] with description of the importance of the profunda vein reflux,[13] reports of the Northwestern University experience with transposition procedures,[28,29] report of valve repairs from Boston,[30] and multiple reports of valve substitution procedures beginning with Taheri in 1982[11] and 1986,[31] O'Donnell in Boston 1987,[32] and Nash in Australia 1988.[15] Lane (Australia) in 1988[33] described an external appliance to correct saphenous and femoral vein primary reflux.

Important contributions in the 1990 decade include a new variant in the technique of internal primary valve repair by Sottiurai followed by the initial reports of his series of deep vein reconstructions that has become one of the largest in the world,[34] and description of an angioscopic technique for valve repair by Gloviczki of the Mayo Clinic in 1991[35] supported by confirmatory series from Boston[36] and Japan.[37] DePalma described a type of cross-over study,[38] in which cases with unsuccessful nonsurgical management for advanced venous disease were converted to a surgical approach in 1996 and were followed for comparative control of the venous insufficiency state. In 2001, a well-designed study from Russia reported by Makarova[39] provided a glimpse into the natural history of primary disease and the potential effect deep surgical repair may have on this progression. The trap door technique of valve repair was reported by Tripathi in 2001,[40] followed by another large series of medical failure cases that were treated with this surgical repair and followed for 2 years.[41]

In 1990, a technique for external suture repair of the refluxing valve appeared.[42] The concept of controlling reflux from the outer side of the intact vein by suture or external appliance was found to be appealing because it is simpler, quicker, and safer than internal repair via venotomy. Many variations of the external approach have been developed, and enthusiastic reports continue to appear, some of which find results comparable with the open, internal repair. Important reports of enthusiasm for the external approach continue to flow from widely divergent sources, including Asia, Australia, Europe, and the United States, and speak to the desirability of a simple approach to deep vein reflux.

The fundamental difference between the internal and the external repairs is that the internal repair provides anatomically precise correction of the elongated leading edge of the valve cusp, and the external repair acts by altering the vein from the outside in one fashion or another and is not a precise correction of the valve cusp abnormality. Some believe the external repair can be performed in a manner to achieve the correction of the elongated valve cusp, but the evidence that this truly occurs lacks precision. Theoretical support for the concept of narrowing the base of the valve and deepening the valve pocket with the external repair is imaginable; and if the long-term results can be proven comparable or better than the internal repair, this would become the procedure of choice. At this time, though, the better results continue to follow open repair in the hands of those who are facile with both approaches. The overall statistics for long-term (>4 years) competence of the repaired valves lie in the range of 65 to 85% for internal repairs (see Table 58.1) compared to ranges of 50 to 65% for external repairs. In spite of this difference, situations when the external repair may be a better choice occur when technical or risk factors render the internal repair a more risky procedure than the surgeon may wish to undertake even though the internal repair carries a higher long-term competence rate.

INFLUENCE EXERTED BY THESE MULTIPLE REPORTS

As these reports developed, new knowledge emerged about CVD that was discovered through an intimate relationship

Table 58.1 **RESULTS OF INTERNAL VALVULOPLASTY**

AUTHOR	YEAR	# LIMBS	FU MOS	GOOD RESULTS	COMPETENT VALVE
Eriksson[44]	1990	27	6–108	70%	70% @ 4 yrs
Masuda[19]	1994	32	48–252	77%	77% @ 4–15 yrs
Lurie[45]	1997	49	36–108	–	85% @ 5 yrs
Perrin[46]	1997	75	24–96	–	85% @ >1 yr
Raju[47]	1996	68	12–144	76%	76% @ 2–10 yrs
Sottiurai[48]	1997	143	9–168	75%	75% @ >7 yrs
Tripathi[41]	2004	90	24	67%	79% @ 2 yrs

between improved diagnostics coupled with direct knowledge of the venous pathology derived from open surgery on the veins themselves. Points such as the following emerged:

1. Identical clinical presentations can develop from pure primary reflux to those seen in the reflux-obstructive changes of postthrombotic disease. This meant that definitive diagnosis (sufficient for surgical treatment) would have to be done by objective imaging techniques.

2. The practical importance of differentiating primary from secondary deep vein disease was established to permit deep venous surgical correction.

3. Global testing (venous pressures and much of plethysmography) has been replaced for practical value by more specific ultrasound imaging.

4. Results of treatment protocols began to be evaluated by noninvasive techniques, of which imaging has been the most specific.

5. Multiple approaches to repair of deep vein reflux in both primary and postthrombotic disease emerged from around the world.

6. The need for definitive diagnosis of the cause and distribution of segmental vein disease played an important role in stimulating the later development of the CEAP classification of chronic venous disease in 1994.[43]

INFLUENCE OF DEEP REPAIR ON MANAGEMENT OF CVD

With the definitive workup of all the vein segments mandated by the ability to repair reflux throughout the extremity in patients with advanced disease, clinical correlations between disease states and pathologic findings assumed increasing importance. Correction of axial superficial and deep reflux in all the patients who are symptomatic was not found reasonable because there are mildly symptomatic and even asymptomatic patients who have significant deep reflux in whom development of long-term serious sequelae has not been proven.

The initial aggressive surgical approach of repairing the deep system in those with advanced (C4–C6) disease who had not responded to medical therapy, the so-called total surgical repair of reflux in advanced cases, led to the criticism that many cases could probably be controlled for a significant period of time with lesser procedures limited to saphenous and perforator veins even though deep vein reflux persisted. This has been found to be true and resulted in a more conservative surgical approach that reserves deep vein reconstruction to cases that demonstrate failure of both medical and conventional saphenous and perforator surgery. Most of the series that have been reported since the early 1990s have reportedly followed this concept,[19,41,44-48] but the absence of criteria for adequate medical therapy, as well as provisions of satisfactory surgical treatment of saphenous and perforator veins, have resulted in the likelihood of considerable variability in case selection between the reports in the literature. Suffice it to say that the surgical selection of patients for deep repair has been largely restricted to resistant cases with serious manifestations of CVD who have not responded to initial efforts to control their problem by simpler methods up to the time of surgery.

For the surgeon and clinician, the clinical experience of the effect of placing a competent valve in the extremity of a patient with advanced primary disease is dramatic. Time and again the patient will recognize an immediate sense that the extremity is more comfortable. If an ulcer is present, a period of accelerated healing follows the successful repair. Improvement of C4 changes in the extremity become dramatic over the next several weeks to months. Over the course of months to years, the far-advanced changes of leathery dark skin may improve to soft skin and subcutaneous tissue with near-normal texture and turgor. The dark color of late-stage pigmentation can lighten considerably, although it rarely disappears entirely. Swelling will entirely disappear in some cases, but others retain an enlarged extremity that may or may not swell on a daily basis. For those who observe these favorable events after correction of deep vein reflux, there is no doubt about the import of deep vein reflux on the deranged physiology of advanced venous insufficiency. This phenomenon of clinical improvement after elimination of deep reflux is not new, having been mentioned by Homans, Linton, Bauer, and others after interruption of refluxing femoral or popliteal veins, which produced more temporary relief of symptoms.

A concept was advanced that repair of superficial reflux resulted in a decrease or disappearance of deep vein reflux in a high proportion of cases.[49] This concept supports the realization that axial deep reflux at times is a reflection of the interdependence of the superficial and deep segments of venous return. One study focused on the effect of ablation of superficial reflux in the presence of deep segmental versus axial reflux and concluded that the abolition of deep reflux by superficial ablation is unlikely when actual valvular deformity is present.[50] The knowledge that deep reflux may be decreased or eliminated by saphenous and perforator surgery reinforces the concept of initial repair in these veins prior to deep repair.

SURGICAL CONSIDERATIONS IN REPAIR OF PRIMARY DEEP VEIN REFLUX DISEASE

Practical questions that face the surgeon who will repair the deep vein reflux in primary disease include which vein to repair, the exact site of repair, and which surgical technique to employ.

PREOPERATIVE EVALUATION

Good surgical results begin with accurate diagnosis of the venous problem. The goal of the preoperative evaluation for deep vein reconstruction is to identify sites of both reflux and obstruction in all the venous segments from the inferior vena cava to the calf. This task is readily achieved with the aid of expert duplex scanning and venographic techniques.

It is incumbent on the surgeon who undertakes deep vein reconstruction to have expert scanning available to guide his choices at all stages of diagnosis and follow-up. The minimal requirements of the ultrasonographer should include experience in identification of reflux and obstruction in all the venous segments, ability to identify hemodynamically important tributaries of major veins and collateral flow routes, and most important, the capacity to individualize the scanning protocol to identify the anatomically and physiologically unique variations that occur in advanced venous disease. Since the knowledge of flow routes in CVD is still evolving, the ultrasonographer should have sufficient background to contribute to this progress as an essential member of the venous team.

With the advent of improving technology and technique in duplex scanning, the need for venography has been materially lessened over time for pure diagnostic purposes, but ascending and descending venography continue to be very helpful in planning deep vein surgical procedures.

Ascending venography provides a map of the physiologically preferred route of venous return from the foot when it is done in the erect position without tourniquets. When it shows deep return via the tibial, popliteal, and femoral vein without filling collaterals, one can deduce there is no important deep vein obstructive disease. Conversely, when it shows collateral patterns it is incumbent on the surgeon to search out and understand where the obstructive elements are located in the normal deep vein return vessels to produce these collaterals. In this way, both gross and subtle degrees of obstructive changes can be ferreted out and subtle elements of postthrombotic change can be detected. When collaterals are being studied, liberal use of tourniquets at the ankle, upper calf, and lower thigh may demonstrate filling of partially obstructed veins that had been bypassed by the ascending contrast because these veins presented higher resistance to outflow than the collateral routes.

Descending venography provides a map of the location of deep vein valves and a measure of their competence when performed with adherence to the details of the reported technique for detecting valve function.[10] It is best done with the treating surgeon in direct consultation with the radiologist at the time of the procedure in order to achieve optimal understanding of the morphology and the relative degree of competence and operability of the individual valves. This test should always include audio and video recording in order to be able to interpret the data on the film at future times. Catheter techniques allow for selective study of the femoral, profunda, saphenous, popliteal, and tibial veins. The X-ray table should move from the Trendelenburg to the erect position mechanically to take advantage of the effects of gravity on the venous flow in the standing position, and to be able to empty residual contrast from the veins by sharp Trendelenburg positioning.

The information gained from venography should be compared to the duplex scan data because they provide complementary information in most instances and, when there are differences between the studies, repetition of the scanning after venography will often provide clarification of important, even crucial, details.

PHYSIOLOGIC NONINVASIVE TESTING

The use of pressures and plethysmography in evaluation of the patient for surgery can be helpful in confirming that there is significant venous disease, but is seldom helpful in determining critical details of the preoperative workup. These tests are global in nature, especially the venous pressure test, and for this reason it can be used on a highly selective basis. Plethysmography provides more detail and is more practical than venous pressure, especially the VFI (venous filling index), which provides a measure of the reflux in the veins when the extremity is inverted. It has been related to the severity of venous insufficiency, and certain centers use this test as an important part of their estimation of severity of reflux in CVD and in reconstruction.[51]

PREOPERATIVE PLANNING: CHOICE OF SURGICAL TECHNIQUE AND PLACEMENT OF THE COMPETENT VALVE

In planning the surgical approach, the surgeon must decide which valve(s) to repair and which technique to use for the repair. The choice of the valve is dictated by the imaging studies, which show the axial refluxing segments and the location of the valves within these segments. There is no good evidence that repair of a valve above the femoral or profunda level is physiologically effective, but abundant evidence exists to support the finding that repair below the common femoral level is effective. The first point to ascertain is whether the reflux is limited to one or more axial distributions (femoral-popliteal-tibial vs. profunda-popliteal-tibial

vs. saphenous) from the groin to the calf because each of these routes of reflux requires at least one competent valve. When more than one valve in a segment is readily available for repair, it is opportune to repair the additional valve. When there is reflux in both femoral and profunda veins, placement of a single valve in the popliteal vein will control both routes of reflux; otherwise, at least one valve for each of the refluxing segments should be provided.

The choices for technique of repair are multiple. The first choice is whether to plan an internal or external repair. The internal repairs are the most reliable and durable, but external repairs are simpler and safer because the vein does not have to be opened. In the good-risk patient with a valve that appears favorable for the internal approach, it would be a logical choice to plan an internal repair. If it is a less favorable case by reason of surgical risk or anatomical exposure, as in an obese subject or an anatomically difficult position of the valve, the external repair may be preferable.

The internal repair can be done by any of several techniques, as discussed earlier. Since the follow-up statistics for valve competence are similar between the transvalvular[19] (see Figure 58.4), supravalvular,[47] and T-incision exposures,[48] the choice of technique is a matter of the surgeon's preference. If the surgeon has the technical facility, the angioscopic technique[35] is reasonable.

The external repair[52] (see Figure 58.5) of the deep valve has been well received by many surgeons. The significant advantages are that external repair is a simpler operation with less risk of complications because it does not require opening the vein and carries a very low likelihood of postoperative thrombosis, especially in the nonpostthrombotic patient. Heparin is not needed, which minimizes the chance for significant wound hematoma. The problem with the external repairs is that the long-term results are not as good as the internal repair in most reports. The expectation for long-term competence with external repair has been about 50% in the author's Straub Clinic experience compared to more than 70% competence with internal repair. Other centers have found the external repair results to be more comparable with but still not equal to the internal repair.[48,53] The use of external repair can be valuable when the repair is made difficult due to a deeply placed valve with limited exposure, or in the repair of a second valve to supplement an internal repair.[42] There are sizable reports of external circumferential suture repairs from Chinese,[54] Japanese,[55] and Italian[56] authors.

At this time, the summary statement for choice of surgical approach is that the internal repair provides an exact anatomical correction of the primary defect of elongation of the valve cusp, has produced the best results, and remains the procedure of choice for long-term results. When there are circumstances such as the need for a limited procedure or a difficult exposure, one of the exterior techniques may become the better alternative. In the primary case where there are no repairable valves, one of the valve

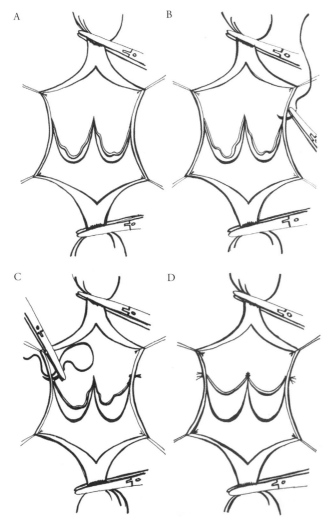

Figure 58.4 Original transvalvular technique of internal valve repair. (A) Diagrammatic appearance of sagging valve cusps as seen in the opened vein prerepair. (B) Technique of shortening the leading edge of the valve cusp for 2–3 mm distance with interrupted 7–0 monofilament suture introduced at the level of the commissure passing from outside to inside the vein, through the cusp near its leading edge, then returned to the level of the commissure and passing from inside to outside of the vein. (C) Introducing further similarly placed sutures, which will be done at both sides of the opened vein and in the center of the vein, where both valves meet. (D) Appearance of valve cusps after shortening the cusps to an appropriate length. This may require four to ten such sutures.

substitution techniques of transposition or transplantation of a valve-bearing arm segment can be used.

Regardless of technique, the principle is well demonstrated that restoration of competence to the lower extremity affected by primary axial reflux disease can effectively reverse advanced CVD even when this has been refractory to best medical therapy and to repair of saphenous and perforator reflux. The durability of the internal repair has been established, as cited in Table 58.1. Even in the absence of Grade I evidence based on prospective randomized trials, the collective clinical benefits of surgical reversal of extensive reflux are clear in the literature.

PUBLISHED RESULTS OF PRIMARY DEEP VEIN VALVE REPAIR

There are abundant data in the individual case series that advanced CVD resistant to more conventional measures of medical management and saphenous-perforator repair provides relief of pain, swelling, and disability, and is followed by a marked improvement in the recurrence rate of ulceration and debilitating skin changes.[19,32,38,41,44–46] These reports consistently demonstrate that resistant cases of advanced CVD due to primary reflux experience clinical relief of recurrent ulceration and skin changes in the range of 65 to 80% for periods that exceed 4- to 8-year follow-up (see Table 58.1). The results for clinical relief following repair of postthrombotic reflux and obstruction (in the range of 40–65%) are less favorable than the primary reports but represent significant salvage rates in cases that are otherwise committed to progressive disability and discomfort. This is understandable since postthrombotic disease is a more destructive and complicated problem because it reflects postinflammatory destruction of the vein wall and lumen and encompasses elements of obstruction in addition to the reflux, whereas primary disease is noninflammatory and degenerative in nature, and is restricted to the effects of reflux without morphologic obstruction.

The first presentation of truly long-term results (4–21 years) in 1994[19] provided initial data that cases with open repair of primary refluxing valves had a 73% chance of very long-term (>10 years) recurrence-free clinical improvement in the case of pure primary reflux, and 66% when the problem consisted of distal postthrombotic disease and proximal femoral vein primary valve disease. In all these cases the limb remained free of recurrence of the C4–C6 skin changes that constituted the indication for the operation. Similar results over 4 to 8 years, and beyond, have been presented by multiple other surgical series[19,45–48] that provide reproducibility for the original report. At least 30% of cases have voluntarily discarded elastic support against medical advice in several of these series and still remained free of recurrence over the long term. This result has never been reported with medical management and speaks to the critical importance of correction of deep vein reflux.

There has not been a randomized prospective trial of medical treatment versus superficial surgery (saphenous and perforator repair) versus deep surgery. The wide variation in pathologic findings of advanced CVD cases would make it difficult to accumulate exactly similar cases. Lacking this, the collected data of multiple, individual, carefully conducted studies with similar results provides impressive repeatable evidence (Level C) for validity to this approach to advanced primary venous reflux disease.

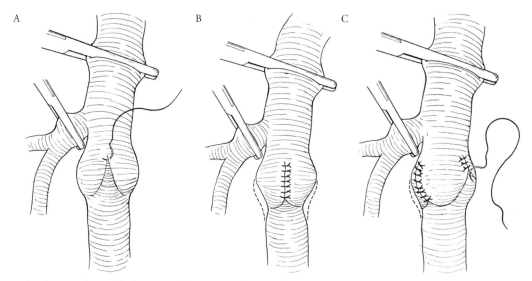

Figure 58.5   Original technique of external valve repair. (A) Interrupted sutures begin at the upper level of the commissure where the valve cusps originate. The suture passes into the vein from the outside to the inside to engage the valve cusps and is tied outside of the vein. (B) A series of similarly placed sutures passing down the valve secure the progressively decussating margin of the valve insertions until the base of the valve is reached. (C) Similarly placed sutures are then placed along the margins of the cusps on the opposite side of the vein.

PERSPECTIVE ON THE VALUE OF SURGICAL REPAIR IN DEEP VEIN VALVES

Caution is advised when comparing reports of nonsurgical treatment of deep reflux to those of deep surgical repair. There is a cogent difference between the cases in the surgical versus those in the nonsurgical reports of management for advanced CVD because the nonsurgical group has little definitive workup including a lack of detail about primary versus secondary disease and the extent of reflux or obstruction in the venous segments. In many instances the medically treated series are a mixture of first-time ulcers and recalcitrant ulcers, and the end point is the first healing of the ulcer. Data about recurrence of disease often are lacking. These reports lack the specificity of the reports of surgical deep repairs, all of which have been extensively evaluated to determine the etiology and the entire distribution of disease throughout the extremity and the recurrence rates are carefully traced. Since the surgical cases are nearly all resistant cases that have failed both medical management and surgical repair of superficial and perforator incompetence, the recurrence rate of ulcer and skin complications in these cases would be expected to be high and soon unless some correction had been done or some dramatic change in their way of life had occurred.

COMPLICATIONS OF DEEP VENOUS VALVE REPAIR

The complications of deep vein repair are primarily wound hematoma and DVT. Since the operation is performed under preoperative heparin and the heparin usually is continued postoperatively, there is increased opportunity for a wound hematoma to develop. If large enough, a wound hematoma can compromise an otherwise successful repair through local pressure and thrombosis of the venous segment. The frequency of this can be minimized by limiting the heparin dose to 400 to 800 units of heparin per hour for the first 2 postoperative days and by draining the wound with continuous wound suction with early surgical wound reexploration if bleeding is found in the first postoperative days.

Postoperative DVT is infrequent following open surgery for primary disease (incidence unknown, approximately 1–3%), but more frequent when the disease is postthrombotic or the patient is hypercoagulable. Since the potential for thrombosis is present, heparin has been recommended preoperatively and for the first 4 to 7 postoperative days until the patient is ambulatory and the wound is healing well without hematoma. If there is an element of postthrombotic disease in the patient, or other reason for hypercoagulability, heparin can be followed by Coumadin anticoagulation for weeks or indefinitely.

If the external repair is elected, the chance for DVT is virtually eliminated in the absence of hypercoagulability. When the underlying problem is mixed primary and postthrombotic disease it is wise to use aggressive heparin to prevent postoperative thrombosis that could result in transforming an original primary venous problem to a postthrombotic problem.

Postoperative thigh swelling is seen in some cases, probably due to lymphatic disruption from the surgical dissection. This will generally clear in about 6 weeks. Transfusions are rarely needed for this kind of surgery. Infections are unusual because it is a clean operation.

CONCLUSION

Surgical repair of deep vein valves for primary disease has been widely evaluated and found to have reproducible favorable results without recurrence in 65 to 80% of cases successfully operated on with internal repair. The repair can be performed in many different ways with the best long-term results achieved by open surgery, but with higher risk for complications after the open techniques than after the external techniques. Its use can be recommended in resistant CVD cases in which a repairable valve is identified.

In addition to pure primary disease, repairable valves can be found in the high thigh veins in a number of cases with distal deep vein thrombophlebitis when the more proximal valve(s) has been spared inflammatory involvement.

REFERENCES

1. Kistner RL. Surgical repair of a venous valve, *Straub Clinic Proc.* 1968. *34*: 41–43.
2. Linton RR. Modern concepts in the treatment of the postphlebitic syndrome with ulcerations of the lower extremity, *Angiology.* 1952. *3*: 431–439.
3. Kistner RL. Surgical repair of the incompetent femoral vein valve, *Arch Surg.* 1975. *110*: 1336–1342.
4. Bauer G. The etiology of leg ulcers and their treatment by resection of the popliteal vein, *J Int Chir.* 1948. 8: 937–967.
5. Lockhart-Mummery HE, Smitham JH. Varicose ulcer: A study of the deep veins with special reference to retrograde venography, *Br J Surg.* 1951. 38: 284–295.
6. Luke JC. The deep vein valves: A venographic study in normal and postphlebitic states, *Surgery.* 1951. *29*: 381–386.
7. Linton RR, Kelley JK. The postphlebitic ulcer: Surgical treatment with special reference to the communicating veins of the lower leg, *Am Heart J.* 1939. 17: 27–39.
8. Homans J. The etiology and treatment of varicose ulcer of the leg, *Surg Gynecol Obstet.* 1917. 24: 300–311.
9. Herman RJ, Neiman HL, Yao JST, et al. Descending venography: A method of evaluating lower extremity venous valvular function, *Radiology.* 1980. *137*: 63–69.
10. Kamida CB, Kistner RL. Descending phlebography: The Straub technique. In: Bergan JJ, Kistner RL, eds. *Atlas of venous surgery.* Philadelphia: W.B. Saunders Company. 1992. 105–109.
11. Taheri SA, Lazar L, Elias SM, et al. Surgical treatment of postphlebitic syndrome with vein valve transplant, *Am J Surg.* 1982. *144*: 221–224.
12. Kistner RL. Transvenous repair of the incompetent femoral vein valve. In: Bergan JJ, Yao JST, eds. *Venous problems.* Chicago: Year Book Medical Publishers. 1978. 493–513.
13. Eriksson I, Almgren B. Influence of the profunda femoris vein on venous hemodynamics of the limb. Experience from thirty-one deep vein valve reconstructions, *J Vasc Surg.* 1986. 4: 390–395.
14. O'Donnell TF. Popliteal vein valve transplantation for deep venous valvular reflux: Rationale, method and long-term clinical, hemodynamic and anatomic results. In: Bergan JJ, Yao JST, eds. *Venous disorders.* Philadelphia: W.B. Saunders Co. 1991. 273–295.
15. Nash T. Long-term results of vein valve transplants placed in the popliteal vein for intractable postphlebitic venous ulcers and preulcer skin changes, *J Cardiovasc Surg.* 1988. *29*: 712–716.
16. Raju S, Fredericks RK, Hudson CA, et al. Venous valve station changes in "primary" and post-thrombotic reflux: An analysis of 149 cases, *Ann Vasc Surg.* 2000. *14*: 193–199.
17. Rose SS, Ahmed A. Some thoughts on the aetiology of varicose veins, *J Cardiovasc Surg.* 1986. *27*: 534–533.
18. Caps MT, Manzo RA, Bergelin RO, et al. Venous valvular reflux in veins not involved at the time of acute deep vein thrombosis, *J Vasc Surg.* 1995. *22*: 524–531.
19. Masuda EM, Kistner RL. Long-term results of venous valve reconstruction: A 4 to 21year follow-up, *J Vasc Surg.* 1994. *19*: 391–403.
20. Danielsson G, Arfvidsson B, Eklof B, et al. Reflux from thigh to calf, the major pathology in chronic venous ulcer disease: Surgery indicated in the majority of patients. *Vasc Endovascular Surg.* 2004. *38*: 209–219.
21. Labropoulos N, Giannoukas AD, Delis K, et al. Where does venous reflux start? *J Vasc Surg.* 1997. *26*: 736–742.
22. Schultz-Ehrenburg U, Weindorf N, Matthes U, et al. An epidemiologic study of the pathogenesis of varices. The Bochum Study I-III, *Phlebologie.* 1992. *45*: 497–500.
23. Kistner RL, Sparkuhl MD. Surgery in acute and chronic venous disease, *Surgery.* 1979. 85: 31–43.
24. Ferris EB, Kistner RL. Femoral vein reconstruction in the management of chronic venous insufficiency: A 14-year experience, *Arch Surg.* 1982. *117*: 1571–1579.
25. Raju S. Venous insufficiency of the lower limb and stasis ulceration: Changing concepts in management, *Ann Surg.* 1983. *197*: 688–697.
26. Raju S, Fredericks R. Valve reconstruction procedures for nonobstructive venous insufficiency: Rationale, technique, and results in 107 procedures with two to eight-year follow-up, *J Vasc Surg.* 1988. 7: 01–310.
27. Eriksson I, Almgren B, Nordgren L. Late results after venous valve repair, *Int Angiol.* 1985. 4: 413–417.
28. Queral LA, Whitehouse WM, Flinn WR, et al. Surgical correction of chronic deep venous insufficiency by valvular transposition, *Surgery.* 1980. *87*: 688–695.
29. Johnson ND, Queral LA, Flinn WR, et al. Late objective assessment of venous valve surgery, *Arch Surg.* 1981. *116*: 1461–1466.
30. Huse JB, Nabseth DC, Bush HL Jr, et al. Direct venous surgery for venous valvular insufficiency of the lower extremity, *Arch Surg.* 1983. *118*: 719–723.
31. Taheri SA, Elias SM, Yacobucci GN, et al. Indications and results of vein valve transplant, *J Cardiovasc Surg.* 1986. *27*: 163–168.
32. O'Donnell TF, Mackey WC, Shepard AD, et al. Clinical, hemodynamic, and anatomic follow-up of direct venous reconstruction, *Arch Surg.* 1987. *122*: 474–482.
33. Jessup G, Lane RJ. Repair of incompetent venous valves: A new technique, *J Vasc Surg.* 1988. 8: 569–575.
34. Sottiurai VS. Technique in direct venous valvuloplasty, *J Vasc Surg.* 1988. 8: 646–648.
35. Gloviczki P, Merrell SW, Bower TC. Femoral vein valve repair under direct vision without venotomy: A modified technique using angioscopy, *J Vasc Surg.* 1991. *14*: 645–648.
36. Welch HJ, McLaughlin RL, O'Donnell TF Jr. Femoral vein valvuloplasty: Intraoperative angioscopic evaluation and hemodynamic improvement, *J Vasc Surg.* 1992. *16*: 694–700.
37. Hoshino S. Endoscopic valvuloplasty, *Vasc Surg.* 1997. *31*: 276.
38. DePalma RG, Kowallek DL. Venous ulceration: A crossover study from nonoperative to operative treatment, *J Vasc Surg.* 1996. *24*: 788–792.
39. Makarova NP, Lurie F, Hmelniker SM. Does surgical correction of the superficial femoral vein valve change the course of varicose disease? *J Vasc Surg.* 2001. *33*: 361–368.
40. Tripathi R, Ktenidis K. Trapdoor internal valvuloplasty—A new technique for primary deep vein valvular incompetence, *Eur J Vasc Endovasc Surg.* 2001. *22*: 86–89.
41. Tripathi R, Sieunarine K, Abbas M, et al. Deep venous valve reconstruction for nonhealing leg ulcers: Techniques and results, *ANZ J Surg.* 2004. *74*: 34–39.
42. Kistner RL. Surgical technique of external valve repair, *The Straub Foundation Proceedings.* 1990. *55*: 15–16.

43. Porter JM, Moneta GL. Reporting standards in venous disease: An update. International consensus committee on chronic venous disease, *J Vasc Surg.* 1995. *21*: 635–645.

44. Eriksson I. Reconstructive surgery for deep vein valve incompetence in the lower limb, *Eur J Vasc Surg.* 1990. *4*: 211–218.

45. Lurie F. Results of deep-vein reconstruction, *Vasc Surg.* 1997. *31*: 275–276.

46. Perrin MR. Results of deep vein reconstruction, *Vasc Surg.* 1997. *31*: 273–275.

47. Raju S, Fredericks RK, Neglen PN, et al. Durability of venous valve reconstruction techniques for "primary" and post-thrombotic reflux, *J Vasc Surg.* 1996. *23*: 357–367.

48. Sottiurai VS. Results of deep vein reconstruction, *Vasc Surg.* 1997. *31*: 276–278.

49. Walsh JC, Bergan JJ, Beeman S, et al. Femoral venous reflux abolished by greater saphenous vein stripping, *Ann Vasc Surg.* 1994. *8*: 566–570.

50. Puggioni A, Lurie F, Kistner RL, et al. How often is deep venous reflux eliminated after saphenous vein ablation? *J Vasc Surg.* 2003. *38*: 517–521.

51. McDaniel HB, Marston WA, Farber MA, et al. Recurrence of chronic venous ulcers on the basis of clinical, etiologic, anatomic, and pathophysiologic criteria and air plethysmography, *J Vasc Surg.* 2002. *35*: 723–728.

52. Kistner RL. External valve repair. In: Bergan JJ, Kistner RL, eds. *Atlas of venous surgery.* Philadelphia: W.B. Saunders Co. 1992. 131–133.

53. Raju S, Berry MA, Neglen P. Transcommissural valvuloplasty: Technique and results, *J Vasc Surg.* 2000. *32*: 969–976.

54. Wang S, Li X, Wu Z, et al. External valvuloplasty technique in deep venous valve insufficiency of the lower limbs, *Chin Med J.* 1999. *112*: 717–719.

55. Abe Y, Ueyama T, Endo M, et al. Long-term results after femoral vein valve repair for chronic venous insufficiency, *Zentralbl Chir.* 2002. *127*: 744–747.

56. Guarnera G, Furguiele S, Mascellari L, et al. External banding valvuloplasty of the superficial femoral vein in the treatment of recurrent varicose veins, *Int Angiol.* 1998. *17*: 268–271.

59.

PROSTHETIC VENOUS VALVES

Michael C. Dalsing

INTRODUCTION

The need for a prosthetic venous valve in the treatment of chronic deep venous valvular incompetence (CDVVI) or insufficiency becomes evident only after other options have failed or simply are not practical. The typical patient has end-stage chronic deep venous insufficiency afflicted with acute and/or recurrent venous ulceration resistant to standard medical therapy, has exhausted all superficial/perforator surgery that might be helpful, and has no autogenous venous valve available to use in the correction of the deep venous disease. In some cases, less advanced cases are considered for intervention because of severe lifestyle limiting concerns. These patients generally have postthrombotic disease that often renders the deep veins thickened and scarred yet recanalized resulting in unrelenting reflux while standing. The stiff, thickened, noncompliant vein makes intervention more difficult than in the case of primary insufficiency. These, our most challenging patients with venous disease, often are the most symptomatic and therefore any attempt to remedy the condition may result in a less impressive outcome than in other patient cohorts.

For the current discussion, the term "prosthetic" means dealing with the production or use of artificial body parts and the term "artificial" means not arising from natural growth. Therefore, a prosthetic venous valve is any venous valve substitute not originally arising from the recipient as a de novo venous valve. This eliminates consideration of autotransplantation, or valve transposition procedures. All other options are considered and generally fall into two categories: *Scaffold seeks incorporation as self after implantation* or *Scaffolds identified as self prior to implantation*. The quest for a minimally invasive venous valve implant will also be addressed, as it lends itself to some prosthetic valves and is certainly a desirable approach in the view of most patients.

DATA

SCAFFOLD SEEKS INCORPORATION AS SELF AFTER IMPLANTATION

Over the last few decades, several potential off-the-shelf implantable valves have been tested as a substitute for the autogenous venous valve. The valves may be allografts, xenografts, or synthetic in design.

Animal Studied/Poor Results

Transplantation of a fresh vein containing a valve from one canine to another without concern for rejection issues has been attempted. Of fourteen fresh allografts tested, using 24 hours of initial anticoagulation to boost patency, only 7% were patent and none competent over a 4-week study period.[1] Glutaraldehyde-preserved allografts, even when supported by a continuously functioning distal arteriovenous fistula (dAVF), would remain patent (80%) but rarely competent (25%) in the dog during a 7-week study.[2]

Xenograft transplantation initially was investigated using human umbilical vein that could be frozen, cleaned, fitted over an aluminum mandrel, and finally fixed with glutaraldehyde to sculpture a bicuspid valve for implantation.[3] The recipient was canine, and all ten transplants failed in 3 days both in terms of patency and competency. This experiment was unique in that the valve structure itself was not made in nature.

Completely synthetic designs also have been investigated. Using the same aluminum rod design to fashion a bicuspid valve with umbilical vein, liquid pellethane was made into a valve. All ten canine implanted valves thrombosed in 8 days.[3]

Animal Studied/Some Potential

Platinum or pyrite-carbon covered titanium center-hinged bileaflet valves have been implanted into the femoral vein

499

of three dogs.[4] Initial results demonstrated 100% patency and competency at approximately 3 months.[4] At 2 years, the valves demonstrated extensive neointimal hyperplastic ingrowth, which rendered the valves nonfunctional.[5] Although a long-term negative study in the canine model, these results do hold some promise that modification could extend the life of the valve sufficiently to be clinically useful.

Decellularization of venous valved allografts could provide a transplant devoid of the immunologic impact of donor cells. An early clinical experience with a cryopreserved decellularized allograft when used as a conduit for an arteriovenous fistula (AVF) appeared promising and incited very little antigenic response as determined by PRA (panel reactive antibody) levels.[6] This material, when used as a heart valve, demonstrated a similar lack of antigenic response and acceptable valve function.[7] However, a decallularized external jugular vein containing valve allograft when implanted into the venous system of a recipient sheep and without supportive anticoagulation demonstrated a 100% (four of four tested) occlusion rate at 6 weeks.[8] Although the only animal study using a decellularized venous valve allograft in the venous system had a negative conclusion, some clinical data using this material in other settings would suggest the need for further study.

Allografts of lyophilized vein containing a valve have been mechanically tested following rehydration with valve response much as one would observe in a native valve.[9] The valve cusps could withstand at least 350 mmHg retrograde pressure without rupture or insufficiency, and the valve closure time was an acceptable 0.31 ± 0.03 seconds. This allograft is totally untested as a potential venous valve substitute; there are no animal or clinical trials reported.

Fully Studied/Unsuccessful

The only allograft valve to reach clinical study involved standard allogenic crossmatching and cryopreservation as the storage process. Dog eurythrocyte antigen (DEA)-matched and cryopreserved veins containing valve allografts have been transplanted into recipient dogs with preestablished lower limb venous insufficiency. Following ligation of a high-flow dAVF that had functioned for 3 to 6 weeks, all four transplants remained patent and competent for 3 more weeks, at which time the animals were sacrificed for histologic evaluation.[10] The histology appeared very promising with what appeared to be endothelial cells present on the luminal surface and devoid of thrombus in the cusp sinuses (see Figure 59.1). From this study sprang the initial multicenter feasibility evaluation, which unfortunately suggested that a low-grade rejection phenomenon might be affecting the function of the valve transplants.[11] The primary patency rate was 67%

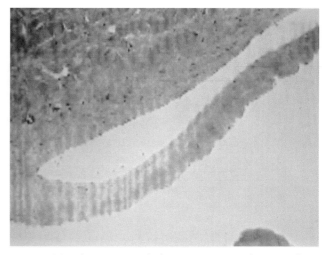

Figure 59.1   This photomicrograph shows a cryopreserved venous valve after removal from an animal model of CDVVI. Note the cellular lining of the valve cusp and minimal thickening.

and primary competency rate 56% at 6 months. A 2-year clinical study evaluating twenty-seven cryovalves reported a disappointing 27% patency and competency rate.[12] The cryopreserved valve allograft used in this study has failed early and in midterm clinical trial is no longer considered a viable substitute for the native valve in the treatment of CDVVI.

Glutaraldehyde-preserved bovine tissues have been used with success in cardiac surgery, and the technology exists to construct glutaraldehyde-preserved bovine venous valves of appropriate size for use in the lower leg of humans. Furthermore, the possibility of valve transplantation via a percutaneous route has been demonstrated to be feasible experimentally.[13] A percutaneously placed glutaraldehyde-preserved bovine venous segment with a contained valve demonstrated acceptable early results in the swine model.[14] At 2 weeks, the xenograft was patent and competent in the three surviving animals. This and other unpublished data were sufficiently compelling to begin clinical trials, but early clinical thrombosis with this particular experimental design was discouraging. A streamlined design was constructed (personal communication) but the new design may not have solved the clinical problem since the company that investigated this valve is no longer in existence.

Clinically Unavailable/Unstudied

Most recently, a bioprosthetic, bicuspid square stent-based venous valve has been developed and percutaneously placed in the external jugular vein of sheep in a feasibility study.[15] The valve is made of processed small intestinal submucosa (SIS; essentially collagen with growth factors remaining) stretched between a square metal frame with a slit cut in the middle of the SIS sheet to form the valve opening. The valve appears to be relatively resistant to thrombosis and does become repopulated with recipient endothelial cells following implantation.[15,16] When percutaneously deployed in the sheep external jugular vein, it demonstrated an 88% patency and competency rate, but tilting led to occlusion or valve insufficiency in three experimental animals.[15] This observation led to a design change to prevent misalignment within the vein wall and six of eight valves were competent at 5 weeks of study.[17] The company sponsoring the study of this valve (Cook, Inc., Bloomington, Indiana) confirms that the device is in research and development with some early clinical studies performed outside the United States. A third design change has taken place to improve venous hemodynamics around the valve cusps and thereby to prevent cusp thickening (see Figure 59.2).

Clinically Available/Unstudied

A cryopreserved superficial femoral vein containing valve allograft (cryovalve) remains available from the CryoLife company (CryoLife, Inc., Kennesaw, Georgia). It will maintain valve competency to 125 mmHg of tested retrograde valve pressure. It may require primary valvuplasty postthaw for optimal competency at the time of implant.[12] Without modification, it does not perform adequately to be recommended for the long-term treatment of patients with CDVVI but, if one could potentially modify the apparent rejection issues faced by the valve substitute, it might be useful.[11,12] The immunosuppression would have to be minimal and well tolerated and must not risk systemic infection, as the standard patient with a venous ulcer is not systemically infected but certainly does possess a port for potential infection. Cytotoxic T-cells to foreign endothelium may be the primary cause of rejection such that azathioprine or cyclosporine A would be potential immunosuppressive agents to consider. There are no clinical trials available investigating such a modified protocol for the use of the cryovalve in the treatment of CDVVI.

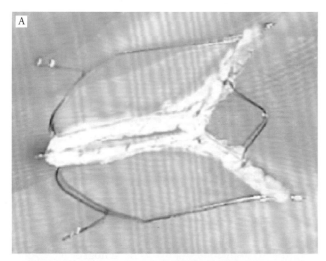

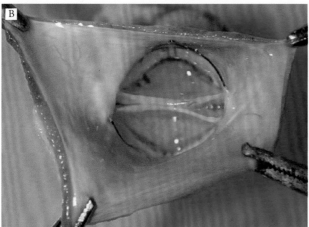

Figure 59.2   (A) This is the newest redesign of the SIS or Portland venous valve aimed at preventing tilting and to provide for a longer cusp, which is suggested to be a more hemodynamic structure. It was photographed from the side. (B) This is a SIS valve cusp photographed from the top to demonstrate the valve opening more clearly and to show its delicate structure. (With permission: Dr. Susan Pavenik).

SCAFFOLDS IDENTIFIED AS SELF PRIOR TO IMPLANTATION

Animal Studied/Some Potential

A venous valve can be made from a length of vein in the fashion of Eiseman and Malette. The basic technique involves an intussusception of the vein into itself with an appropriate bicuspid valve made by two sutures placed at 180 degrees from each other to hold the inner vein wall in the correct position.[18,19] The base tissue is autogenous vein, but the valve structure would be artificial because the vein tissue used is not a natural valve cusp. In the experimental studies, only operative heparinization was administered, and no long-term anticoagulation was provided to the animals. Short-term patency was excellent, with 90 to 100% of valves competent at physiologic pressures. The valve was certainly thicker than the native valve on gross and histologic study (see Figure 59.3).[18] However, when used in a chronic lower limb deep venous insufficiency canine model and transplanted to the femoral vein, the 90% venous refill time was modestly improved but not the venous filling time, which suggested that the valve was not as hemodynamically responsive as a native valve.[18] A modification of this valve involved thinning the adventitia and a part of the media to result in a thinner valve cusp after intussusception, and it has been investigated experimentally in the canine model.[20] The valve opened rapidly with minimal pressure (<3 cm of water) and closed at a pressure of 3 to 5 cm of water. Furthermore, it could withstand physiologic pressure without reflux. In the absence of prolonged anticoagulation, a thin layer of thrombus formed along the cusp wall resulting in valve incompetence. These studies suggested that such valves constructed of autogenous vein could function as a substitute of the native valve with the caution that these

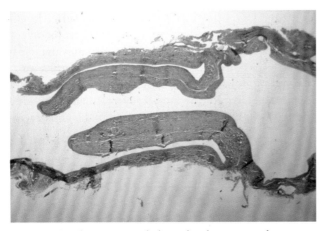

Figure 59.3 This photomicrograph shows that the invaginated vein valve design (Eiseman/Mallete design) results in a thicker valve than a normal venous valve even several weeks following implantation in a canine model.

valves may be more prone to thrombosis and possibly less responsive in a hemodynamic sense than a native valve. No clinical trials have blossomed from these experimental studies possibly because a significant length of vein is required for its construction, and patients with CDVVI often have little to spare.

Repopulating a decellularized external vein containing valve allograft with donor smooth muscle cells and endothelial cells would make for a transplant quite similar to an autogenous valve. One author has studied this approach in a sheep model with quite excellent results. The seeded allograft was transplanted into the external jugular vein of the sheep that provided the cells for seeding. Without the use of anticoagulation, nine of twelve seeded allograft transplants (75%) were patent and competent at 12 weeks. One transplant had occluded, and two others had valves frozen in the extracellular matrix of neointimal ingrowth.[8] The technique seems promising and did perform much better than the allograft without seeding (100% failure in 6 weeks). These grafts did not fare as well as the eight autografts, which demonstrated a 100% patency and competency rate at 6 weeks. There have been no clinical trials to date, but these early experimental data are promising.

Clinically Available/Under Study

The following clinical studies involve the use of autogenous venous tissue but not de novo venous valves. It is my personal feeling that some of these approaches sprang from an intraoperative clinical need for a valve in a situation where preoperative investigations had suggested the presence of an autogenous valve but in reality there was none. The solution worked so well that the investigators found it a viable option in other patients devoid of the standard options.

Dr. Raju and associates have a small series of patients who received de novo valve reconstruction procedures.[21] These procedures involve the use of saphenous vein, a tributary of the saphenous vein, or the axillary vein for a donor vein tissue. Semilunar cusps are fashioned out of donor vein after trimming adventitia and part of the media, and the tissue is sutured into the recipient vein with the nonendothelial surface directed toward the lumen to decrease the risk of thrombosis.[21] Little experience has been gained with this method outside of the good clinical results reported in Dr. Raju's small series.

Another attempt to use autogenous vein as a valve substitute has been reported by Plagnol et al.[22] This approach invaginates a stump of the great saphenous vein into the femoral vein to fashion a bicuspid valve. Both experimental and clinical results have been reported.[22] They report nineteen of twenty reconstructions to be patent and competent at a mean of 10 months. One valve demonstrated reflux because of insufficient valve size at the time of reconstruction. The invagination of an adventitial surface into the venous lumen is of some concern, not substantiated in this one report.

A vascular surgeon from Italy has reported a series of bicuspid or monocusp venous valves made from dissecting the intimal/medial wall of the thickened postphlebitic vein to form cusps. The initial seven cases were reported in 2002 with acceptable preliminary results such that continued study was deemed appropriate.[23] A more robust report was given at the recent American Venous Forum meeting in February of 2005.[24] Eighteen venous valves were constructed in sixteen patients with recurrent or nonhealing venous ulcers to treat chronic deep venous insufficiency due to the postthrombotic process. The patients were anticoagulated for 6 months. Early thrombosis below the valve occurred in two patients and there was one late occlusion just after beginning oral contraceptive therapy. Therefore, 83.3% of treated segments remained primarily patent with significantly improved duplex and air plethysmographic results at a mean 22 months of follow-up. This technique certainly seems promising if others can duplicate these impressive results.

THE MINIMALLY INVASIVE QUEST: LESSONS LEARNED AND POTENTIALS

Our initial experience with a Z-type stent having a vein containing valve lining the entire lumen of the metal exoskeleton demonstrated that the addition of metal barbs to aid in securing the implant to the vein wall added trauma and security of position, but not necessarily patency.[13] Slight oversizing of the device appeared to be the best design for a stable positioning and for function. The configuration of the Z-stent allows for a moderate expansion in the area of the valve (see Figure 59.4), hopefully providing an area for valve sinus function, which appears important to proper valve cleansing and is considered essential for long-term

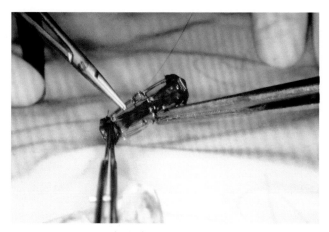

Figure 59.4 Our own method of attaching a vein containing valve to a self-expanding Z-stent overlaps the vein over the ends of the metal exoskeleton thus eliminating exposed metal as a potential site for thrombosis. Also note that the Z-stent expands somewhat more widely in its midsection (due to the restrictive nature of the attached vein circumference) to allow for sinus expansion if needed; however, scarring may prevent this motion over time.

function.[25] Rejection issues were not of concern because the tissue was an autogenous valve. No metal was exposed, as the vein overlapped the ends of the metal stent prior to implant. However, the presence of the metal exoskeleton could lead to scarring (noted in the study) and resulting compliance problems over time.

Using a self-expanding stent (Wallstent, Schneider, Inc., USA) with an autograft valve-bearing segment of vein secured within, and utilizing overexpansion to hold the device in place, a 1-week animal study (n = 5) demonstrated residual nonocclusive thrombus attached to the exposed stent struts on the downstream end of the valve/stent in all animals.[26] The animals were anticoagulated for 1 week post implantation. The valve and vein were normal in appearance and function, suggesting that the exposed metal was of concern as a site of thrombus formation. At 6 weeks, all valves (n = 6) were patent, and five were competent by manual strip test. These valve/stents were now fully incorporated without thrombus. The one incompetent valve appeared to have been recanalized with multiple small channels present, suggesting that the threat of thrombus is present until full incorporation, making it desirable to minimize clot formation as much as possible. Overall, the findings would suggest that the less exposed metal the better. The histologic images show that the vein wall is thickened with metal struts present within it. This would suggest that some compliant mismatch may develop, though it was not yet demonstrated during this 6-week study. However, the early animal results are promising. No clinical paper has been published with this valve/stent design to date.

A balloon expandable stent arrangement, with a more challenging glutaraldehyde-preserved xenograft valve mounted within, performed quite poorly, with all six inferior vena cava implants occluded at 2 months and with collateral circulation present.[27] One cannot be sure whether the presence of xenograft material, the bulk of metal present, or possibly the trauma of balloon expansion either to the recipient vein wall or the donor valve were factors in the poor results. Likely each factor contributed to some degree, and this particular valve/stent arrangement is unlikely to be the focus of investigation in the near future.

Percutaneous valve designs reaching clinical trials have demonstrated another observation of importance: less is better. As mentioned earlier, the glutaraldehyde-preserved xenograft that had reached clinical trial was being continually redesigned to decrease the bulk of xenograft present and to streamline the device. The optimal design was never reached. The current Portland (or SIS) valve uses a minimal metallic exoskeleton, compared with the previously mentioned investigations, with promising results.[15] A design change to aid in proper centering of the valve resulted in an increase in the exposed metal components, but still with good animal experimental results.[17] A finding of cusp thickening necessitated a lengthening of the valve cusps for improved hemodynamics. It remains to be seen whether the addition of more xenograft material will be an asset or a liability, as others have found with the presence of increasing foreign material.

The field of endovascular treatment for CDVVI is in its infancy. All that can be stated to date is that the concept is quite intriguing but much work is yet required even for a cursory understanding of the many facets involved with this approach.

CONCLUSIONS

A valve made of autogenous vein and surgically positioned into the lower leg venous system is currently the only artificial venous valve available with at least preliminary data to support its utility in the treatment of patients with end-stage CDVVI. There are potential nonautogenous off-the-shelf venous valve substitutes that are used in research and development but that lack clinical studies to support the transition to standard surgical use. All nonautogenous artificial venous valves to reach full clinical investigation have failed in early or midterm analysis. The quest for a percutaneous option is just beginning to be investigated, but early studies suggest that minimizing nonautogenous tissue and exposed metallic components is best.

No option presented in this review can substitute for a good autogenous venous valve in the treatment of chronic deep venous valvular incompetence. However, the quest continues for those unfortunate individuals who require surgery but have no current option available to them.

REFERENCES

1. McLachlin AD, Carroll SE, Meads GE, et al. Valve replacement in dogs, *Ann Surg*. 1965. *162*: 446–452.
2. Kaya M, Grogan JB, Lentz D, et al. Glutaraldehyde-preserved venous valve transplantation in the dog, *J Surg Res*. 1988. *45*: 294–297.
3. Hill R, Schmidt S, Evancho M, et al. Development of a prosthetic venous valve, *J Biomed Mater Res*. 1985. *19*: 827–832.
4. Taheri SA, Rigan D, Wels P, et al. Experimental prosthetic vein valve, *Am J Surg*. 1988. *156*: 111–114.
5. Taheri SA, Schultz RO. Experimental prosthetic vein valve. Long-term results, *Angiology*. 1995. *46*: 299–303.
6. Madden R, Lipkowitz G, Benedetto B, et al. Decellularized cadaver vein allografts used for hemodialysis access do not cause allosensitization or preclude kidney transplantation, *Am J Kidney Dis*. 2002. *40*: 1240–1243.
7. Elkins RC, Dawson PE, Goldstein S, et al. Decellularized human valve allograft, *Ann Thorac Surg*. 2001. *71*: S428–S432.
8. Teebken OE, Puschman C, Aper T, et al. Tissue-engineered bioprosthetic venous valve: A long-term study in sheep, *Eur J Vasc Endovasc Surg*. 2003. *25*: 305–312.
9. Reeves TR, Cezeaux JL, Sackman JE, et al. Mechanical characteristics of lyophilized human saphenous vein valves, *J Vasc Surg*. 1997. *26*: 823–828.
10. Burkhart HM, Fath SW, Dalsing MC, et al. Experimental repair of venous valvular insufficiency using a cryopreserved venous valve allograft aided by a distal arteriovenous fistula, *J Vasc Surg*. 1997. *26*: 817–822.
11. Dalsing MC, Raju S, Wakefield TW, Taheri S. A multicenter, phase I evaluation of cryopreserved venous valve allografts for the treatment of chronic deep venous insufficiency, *J Vasc Surg*. 1999. *30*: 854–866.
12. Neglén P, Raju S. Venous reflux repair with cryopreserved vein valves, *J Vasc Surg*. 2003. *37*: 552–557.
13. Dalsing MC, Sawchuk AP, Lalka SG, Cikrit DF. An early experience with endovascular venous valve transplantation, *J Vasc Surg*. 1996. *24*: 903–905.
14. Gomez-Jorge J, Venbrux AC, Magee C. Percutaneous deployment of a valved bovine jugular vein in the swine venous system: A potential treatment for venous insufficiency, *J Vasc Interv Radiol*. 2000. *11*: 931–936.
15. Pavcnik D, Uchida BT, Timmermans HA, et al. Percutaneous bioprosthetic venous valve: A long-term study in sheep, *J Vasc Surg*. 2002. *35*: 598–602.
16. Brountzos E, Pavcnik D, Timmersmans HA, et al. Remodeling of suspended small intestinal submucosa venous valve: An experimental study in sheep to assess the host cells' origin, *J Vasc Interv Radiol*. 2003. *14*: 349–356.
17. Pavcnik D, Kaufman J, Uchida B, et al. Second-generation percutaneous bioprosthetic valve: A short-term study in sheep, *J Vasc Surg*. 2004. *40*: 1223–1227.
18. Dalsing MC, Lalka SG, Unthank JL, et al. Venous valvular insufficiency: Influence of a single venous valve (native and experimental), *J Vasc Surg*. 1991. *14*: 576–587.
19. Wilson NM, Rutt DL, Browse NL. In situ venous valve construction, *Br J Surg*. 1991. *78*: 595–600.
20. Rosenbloom MS, Schuler JJ, Bishara RA, et al. Early experimental experience with a surgically created, totally autogenous venous valve: A preliminary report, *J Vasc Surg*. 1988. *7*: 642–646.
21. Raju S, Hardy JD. Technical options in venous valve reconstruction, *Am J Surg*. 1997. *173*: 301–307.
22. Plagnol P, Ciostek P, Grimaud JP, Prokopowicz SC. Autogenous valve reconstruction technique for post-thrombotic reflux, *Ann Vasc Surg*. 1999. *13*: 339–342.
23. Maleti O. Venous valvular reconstruction in postthrombotic syndrome. A new technique, *J Malad Vasc*, October 2002. *27*(4): 218–221.
24. Lugle M, Maleti O. *Neovalve construction in postthrombotic syndrome*. Presented at American Venous Forum, 17th Annual Meeting. February 9–13, 2005. San Diego, CA.
25. Lurie F, Kistner RL, Eklof B, Kessler D. Mechanism of venous valve closure and role of the valve in circulation: A new concept, *J Vasc Surg*. 2003. *38*: 955–961.
26. Ofenloch JC, Chen C, Hughes JD, Lumsden AB. Endoscopic venous valve transplantation with a valve-stent device, *Ann Vasc Surg*. 1997. *11*: 62–67.
27. Boudjemline Y, Bonnet D, Sidi D, Bonhoeffer P. Is percutaneous implantation of a bovine venous valve in the inferior vena cava a reliable technique to treat chronic venous insufficiency syndrome? *Medical Science Monitor*. 2004. *10*:BR 61–66.

60.

POSTTHROMBOTIC SYNDROME

CLINICAL FEATURES, PATHOLOGY, AND TREATMENT

Seshadri Raju

ostthrombotic syndrome (PTS) is a frequent sequel to deep venous thrombosis (DVT). PTS may take years and even decades to evolve fully. Recurrent DVT that may occur years after the initial event is a known risk factor for the development of PTS.[1] After a bout of DVT, only one-third of patients are asymptomatic over the long term; the other two-thirds have PTS, and half of these cases are severe.[2] The direct and indirect costs of this disease, which affects all adult age groups, are estimated to be substantial, arousing the interest of public health planners.

CLINICAL FEATURES

Major symptoms are orthostatic limb pain, swelling, and stasis skin changes including ulceration. Recurrent thrombophlebitis and recurrent cellulitis, the latter related to underlying tissue edema, are less well known features. Symptoms are present in varying combinations and severity in individual patients. A detailed comprehensive history-taking with leading questions is essential for proper assessment. For example, previous DVT or severe trauma to the limb may not be volunteered because the remote event years ago had been forgotten or not considered relevant to current complaints. The orthostatic nature of limb pain or the presence of nocturnal leg cramps and restless legs may not be revealed unless specifically solicited. Onset of limb pain when erect, and pain relief with leg elevation, walking, or use of stockings are characteristic of venous pain in postthrombotic syndrome. In some patients, leg elevation on a pillow at night is necessary to gain relief.

Limb swelling may be described by the patient as "severe" because it is painful, even though only mild pitting is evident on examination. Some patients may not even be aware of limb edema evident to the examiner because it is pain-free. Pain is absent in about 20% of patients. In about 10% of patients pain may be the only symptom with no other signs, and the diagnosis of PTS may be missed altogether because the limb looks "normal." Claudication type of symptoms with difficulty in climbing stairs is present in about 15% of patients. Exercise arterial pressure measurements will be normal in these individuals. The pain component is not adequately represented in the CEAP classification. Pain measurement using a visual analogue scale[3] is recommended. Type and frequency of analgesic use for pain relief is also a good gauge of pain.

Limb swelling increases as the day progresses; time of onset of leg swelling during the day is a rough indication of its severity. When limb measurements are used for assessment, they should be carried out at the same time of day for follow-up. The CEAP classification[4] and Venous Severity Scoring[5] are readily usable templates for proper clinical evaluation. Measures of quality of life (QOL) provide a view of outcome from the patient's perspective. The degree of disability and social constraint imposed by this disease can be surprising. The brevity of the CIVIQ[6] form renders it suitable for routine use.

DIFFERENTIAL DIAGNOSIS

A clinical diagnosis of postthrombotic syndrome can be made if characteristic clinical features and a clear history of prior deep venous thrombosis are present. Absence of a clear history does not rule out postthrombotic syndrome; about 30% of DVT are estimated to be silent. In others, DVT following trauma or surgery is simply missed as symptoms are submerged by expected postoperative pain—a common occurrence following orthopedic procedures on the hip or knee or for treatment of fractures. Differentiating "primary" disease from PTS may not be easy, as resolution of previous thrombosis may be so complete that no venographic residue remains and clinical presentation can be virtually identical.

PATHOLOGY

Our current view of PTS pathology is strongly influenced by the work of Strandness and colleagues.[7-10] Before these studies, postthrombotic clinical syndrome had been viewed as primarily related to the development of reflux. In a remarkable series of landmark papers, these authors showed that the dominant pathology was a combination of obstruction and reflux even though isolated obstruction and reflux occurred in some patients. The location and progression of postthrombotic reflux followed using serial duplex sonography was unexpected and intriguing. Reflux occurred not only in segments involved by thrombus but also in remote segments. Reflux occurred and progressed over time not only in deep venous segments distal to the thrombotic segment but also in proximal segments; in the distal segments, dilatation of the valve station due to cephalad obstruction was *not* found to be the cause of reflux. The fact that reflux occurs and progresses over time in superficial as well as deep valves proximal to the obstructed segment suggests a different (cytokines?), as yet poorly understood, mechanism.

Some patients present with femoral valve reflux and thrombosis in the distal femoral popliteal segment or even the calf. This clinical profile could be due to reflux-stasis induced distal thrombosis. Repair of the valve reflux can abate recurrent thrombosis. A similar type of clinical presentation can also result from evolution of de novo reflux above the thrombotic segment as described by Strandness and colleagues. Perivenous and mural fibrosis is a feature of these valves, with constriction and foreshortening of the valve station (Figure 60.1).[11] The valve cusps are redundant and reflexive, apparently as a result of restriction. The valve cusps can be repaired in the same way as the "primary" valve, using direct repair techniques.

INVESTIGATIONS

A comprehensive set of investigations are necessary for proper management of postthrombotic patients.

DUPLEX SONOGRAPHY

Duplex sonography is a qualitative tool; several duplex-derived parameters have been evaluated for quantification of reflux but a clinically usable metric has not been found. One such parameter in popular use, valve closure time (VCT), in fact correlates poorly with clinical severity. Peak reflux velocity has a better correlation, but not to a degree that is clinically usable.[12] An abnormal value for either parameter in the clinical setting therefore indicates the presence of reflux but not its severity. At present, relatively crude indices such as multisegment

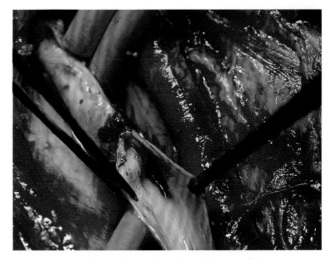

Figure 60.1   A possible mechanism for the production of valve redundancy and reflux in postthrombotic valve stations. Valve station fibrosis may lead to luminal constriction resulting in "secondary" valve leaflet redundancy and reflux. Foreshortening of the valve station may lead to widening of the commissural valve angle, contributing further to development of reflux.   (By permission, *Annals of Surgery*)

score (number of refluxive segments) or the presence of "axial" reflux are the best measures available to gauge severity. Iliac vein outflow obstruction, an important contributor to PTS,[13] is frequently impervious to duplex sonography.

VENOGRAPHY

Unlike duplex sonography, ascending venography provides a composite view of venous pathology. This is useful in secondary disease. Postthrombotic changes, segmental occlusions, and collateral patterns are readily apparent. The profunda femoris vein is the major natural collateral pathway in femoral stenoses and occlusions. This has an embryologic basis, as the profunda femoris is the early axial vein receding to the mature pattern later in embryologic development. A putative profunda-popliteal connection apparently exists as a high resistance embryologic residue; profunda collateral flow can be observed in venograms as early as a few hours after onset of acute DVT. In chronic femoral vein occlusions, the profunda enlarges to the same caliber as the normal femoral vein (Figure 60.2). This pattern of complete "axial" transformation of the profunda femoris vein[14] occurs in about 15% of postthrombotic limbs. Reflux may result from enlargement of the profunda valve station and may be severe with symptoms. Lesser degrees of profunda enlargement can be found in other cases, in which the femoral vein is not totally occluded but is stenotic.

Because the direction of collateral flow in the profunda is the same as natural flow direction in the vessel, it is very efficient. Once fully developed, the profunda fully compensates for the loss of femoral flow with little residual

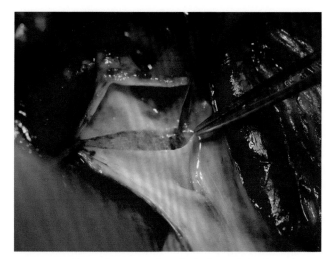

Figure 60.2   Axial transformation of profunda femoral vein through a large profunda-popliteal connection. The femoral vein is largely occluded with the distal end seen as a stump.   (By permission, *Surgery*)

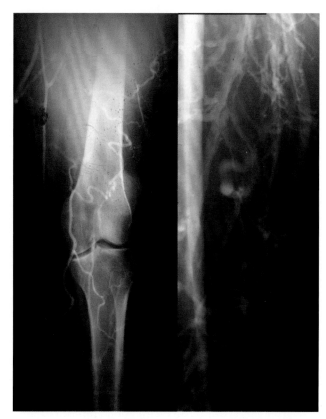

Figure 60.3   Ascending venogram opacifies only superficial network (Left). The deep system appears "wiped out." This is often a technical artifact (see text); ample deep venous elements are demonstrated on descending venography (Right).

clinical symptoms from outflow obstruction. In iliac vein occlusions, collateral flow is mainly through tributaries of the iliac vein itself, requiring reversal of normal flow direction. Collateral flow seems to be less efficient, and residual outflow obstruction is present in nearly half the cases of iliac occlusions.[15] These differential patterns of collateral development and function have clinical import. In patients with symptoms of outflow obstruction, iliac vein pathology is likely to be the culprit,[16] even if associated femoral vein occlusion is more readily seen on ascending venography.

A pattern sometimes seen in severely postthrombotic limbs may arouse concern: the entire outflow appears to occur through the superficial veins with nonvisualization of deep veins, giving the appearance of a "wiped out" deep system.[17] This is invariably an artifact of technique. In most such cases a patent but postthrombotic deep system with numerous collateral elements can be demonstrated on descending venography (Figure 60.3). Presumably, there is a positive gradient across superficial to deep venous connections in these cases so that contrast flow is preferentially restricted to the superficial system. The collateral contribution of the superficial system in such cases is negligible.[13,18] Since the deep system is patent, reconstructive procedures can be planned despite the spurious appearance on ascending venography.

Ascending venography is inadequate for assessment of the iliac vein and the vena cava due to contrast dilution. Transfemoral venography provides better opacification but has a diagnostic sensitivity of only about 50%.[19,20] Exercise femoral venous pressures[20] can be measured concurrently and can be helpful in grading severity of outflow obstruction.

Several authors, beginning with Rokitanski, have documented the development of a dense perivenous sheath in postthrombotic iliac veins. This narrows the venous lumen from restriction. The perivenous sheath also prevents or retards the development of collaterals. Because of these features, venographic appearance can underestimate the severity of stenosis present. Surgical attempts have been made to remove the perivenous sheath in order to improve flow.

INTRAVASCULAR ULTRASOUND (IVUS)

Intravascular ultrasound is superior to venography in the assessment of postthrombotic iliac vein and the inferior vena cava.[19] Perivenous and mural fibrosis, stenoses, and trabeculae are readily seen.

LYMPHANGIOGRAPHY

About 30% of patients with deep venous insufficiency have lymphographic abnormalities such as pooling and delayed or absent lymphatic transport.[21,22] Most are thought to be secondary to venous pathology from lymphatic exhaustion or damage. Some may be reversible with correction of venous pathology.[22] Lymphographic information has prognostic value in resolution of leg swelling, and affected patients may be adequately forewarned before interventions.

AIR PLETHYSMOGRAPHY (APG)

Measurement of ejection fraction and residual volume have been suggested as indirect indices of outflow obstruction. In our own experience and that of others, specificity and sensitivity have been inconsistent. The venous filling index (VFI_{90}) appears to be a useful measure of reflux.[23]

AMBULATORY VENOUS PRESSURE MEASUREMENT

Ambulatory venous pressure measurement provides a global index of venous function in the limb, encompassing multiple components.[24] Postexercise pressure (% drop) has an inconsistent relationship to the severity of outflow obstruction,[15] presumably because of the variability of calf pump efficiency. The recovery time or venous filling time (VFT) has been useful in assessing severity of postthrombotic pathology and reflux.[17] Postthrombotic alterations in venous compliance degrades VFT independent of any reflux present.[25] A postoperative VFT of >5 s bodes well for a good surgical outcome; a VFT of <5 s indicates the opposite. The mean improvement in VFT after successful repairs with good clinical outcome is generally on the order of about 6 ± 4 (SD) seconds. After successful valve repair, postoperative VFT does not reach normal levels in many patients, presumably because of persistent compliance and other abnormalities that influence VFT.[24]

MEASUREMENT OF OUTFLOW OBSTRUCTION

Reduced or absent phasicity on duplex examination is often indicative of outflow obstruction at the iliac vein level,[15] the information being qualitative. The diagnostic sensitivity of this modality is only about 50%.[26] There are no reliable methods of functionally quantifying and grading outflow obstruction at the present time. Plethysmographic outflow fraction measurement, such as with strain gauge technique and APG, yield unacceptably high false positives[13,27] due to compliance changes in the postthrombotic calf; a reduced outflow fraction (<50%) results from subpar emptying of the venous pool from poor compliance as often as from outflow obstruction per se. Poor compliance may also be present without obstruction. Pressure-based tests to detect and grade severity of obstruction, such as the arm/foot venous pressure differential with reactive hyperemia, exercise femoral venous pressures measurement, and intraoperative femoral vein pressure measurement with papavarine, are positive in only about a third of cases.[19] Assessment of iliac vein outflow obstruction currently rests entirely on morphologic methodology (IVUS).

TREATMENT

COMPRESSION THERAPY

Compression therapy remains the initial approach in chronic venous disease including PTS. It has been reported anecdotally to be less effective in PTS than in primary disease, but no systematic study has been undertaken. Some patients fail compression therapy despite faithful compliance. Noncompliance, however, is the major cause of compression failure and recurrent symptoms.[28–30] Noncompliance is high even while under supervision by health care workers.[28,31] The reasons for noncompliance are varied—physical factors related to application, wear comfort, and quality-of-life issues related to daily use. Demands for compliance are unlikely to succeed after previous entreaties have failed and may not be appropriate when therapeutic alternatives have become available.

SAPHENOUS VEIN ABLATION

There has been traditional advice against saphenous ablation in the presence of deep venous obstruction (secondary varices) to preserve its collateral contribution. The collateral contribution of saphenous vein in the presence of deep venous obstruction is insignificant.[13,18] Ablation of a refluxive saphenous vein in PTS cases is safe[32] and can provide significant symptom benefit without jeopardizing the limb.[18] The newer minimally invasive saphenous ablation techniques are easily combined with iliac vein stent placement when indicated.[33]

ILIAC VEIN STENT PLACEMENT IN PTS

Iliac vein stent placement has recently emerged as effective therapy in PTS.[34] Excellent relief of symptoms including healing of stasis ulceration (58% cumulative) appears to be sustained in the long term (>5 years) with stent placement *alone*, even when the associated reflux remained *uncorrected*.[26] This has important implications for the management of PTS, as the majority of patients have combined obstruction/reflux.[8,13,16,35] Most patients should benefit from stent placement alone, a minimally invasive outpatient procedure. Most total occlusions of the IVC-iliac-femoral segments can be recanalized percutaneously.[36] Open veno-venous bypass or valve reconstruction procedures will be required only in recalcitrant cases that have failed initial stent placement and are not precluded. Currently, the need for open surgery in our practice has declined to <5% of PTS patients after stent placement.

VALVULOPLASTY

In PTS patients, direct femoral or popliteal valve repair can be performed if the basic valve architecture is preserved.

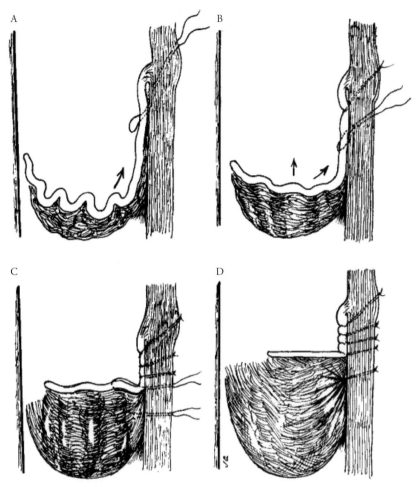

Figure 60.4A Transcommissural valvuloplasty. (A) The initial through-and-through oblique transluminal suture placed at commissural apex catches sagging leaflets and resuspends them. (B and C) Transluminal sutures with each successive suture biting deeper and less oblique than suture above to pull up and tighten cusp edge, deepen sinus, and appose valve attachment lines. (D) Each suture is tied before the next is placed. One or two of the most caudally placed sutures may actually pass through body of leaflet rather than edge, with no subsequent ill effects.

Eriksson stressed the importance of profunda valve repair in postthrombotic cases due to the frequent presence of collateral reflux.[37] We prefer an external or transmural technique[38] without a venotomy (Figure 60.4) in these cases, as these measures are faster and hence multiple repairs (i.e., femoral and profunda) can be performed in a single sitting; and repairs can be carried out even in constricted or small valve stations. The internal technique is disadvantaged in comparison.

The first step in valve reconstruction irrespective of the specific technique is to carry out an adventitial dissection to peel away the fibrous sheath surrounding the valve station.[39] Valve attachment lines should become visible after the dissection. Absent or interrupted valve attachment lines invariably indicate cusp dissolution or damage beyond direct repair. In such cases one should proceed forthwith with alternative repair techniques without wasting time on the performance of a venotomy in a futile search for repairable valve cusps.

Recurrence-free ulcer healing in PTS cases after valve reconstruction at 5 years was ±60%, not different from "primary" valve repairs.[40,41] There was also no difference between the various specific techniques to reconstruct the valve.

Perrin reported clinical results in a large group of postthrombotic cases followed over 5 years.[42] He also noted a postoperative thrombosis rate of 32% in PTS cases using intense surveillance with postoperative venography. Many were localized partial thrombi, and most had recanalized later. He did notice a significant difference between PTS and "primary" cases in ulcer healing (60% and 75% respectively at 5 years) and attributed the difference to the postoperative thromboses. Masuda and Kistner reported long-term results of valve reconstruction in "primary" disease as well as a subset of proximal "primary" reflux with distal thrombosis, presumed secondary to proximal reflux.[43] Internal valvuloplasty or vein segment transfer (end-to-side anastamosis of the femoral vein to the profunda femoris below the profunda valve) was largely used in the PTS subset. PTS results were inferior (43% cumulative) to valve repairs in "primary" cases (73% cumulative) at 10 years. It is not clear whether

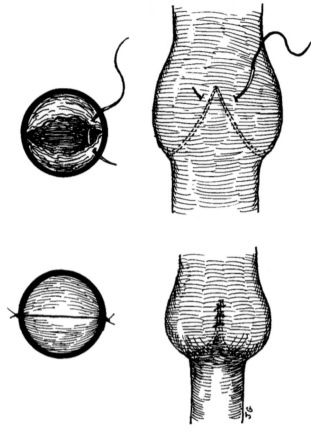

Figure 60.4B Correct suture placement narrows the angle between valve attachment lines and tightens cusps, resulting in good apposition. (By permission, *J Vasc Surg*)

these different results are due to choice of technique (i.e., segment transfer) or other specifics of the PTS subset.

AXILLARY VEIN TRANSFER

Axillary vein transfer[39] is a technically demanding procedure despite its "simple" appearance on the surface. The transferred valve should match the size of the native valve station being reconstructed. In most cases, the axillary vein is the preferred donor site to obtain a good size match. A transverse incision in the armpit along the skin crease is used; exposure of 5 to 6 cm length of axillary vein segment will require ligation and division of three or more tributaries in the area. One or more valves will then come into view. The valve with a good size match is chosen for transfer. A valve high up in the axilla at or near the first rib is consistently present and is the largest. The chosen valve is then tested for competence by negative (emptying the infravalvular segment) and positive (squeezing the supravalvular segment) strip tests. About 40% of axillary valves will fail the strip tests, in which case they should be repaired in situ or on the "bench" before transfer. A 4-cm vein segment housing the valve is excised, and the ends of the remaining vein ligated. A lesser length will interfere with later anastomoses as the excised segment shrinks, placing the valve cusps at risk of

being caught up in the suture lines. Reconstruction of the donor vein is not required; outflow obstructive symptoms in the donor limb are extremely rare. A 1-cm segment of the recipient vein is excised, resulting in retraction of the cut ends and leaving a longer gap. The axillary valve is then transferred to the recipient site in proper orientation. The proximal anastamosis is performed first. Interrupted 6-0 monofilament permanent sutures should be used throughout. Continuous sutures, however expertly applied, will result in postoperative suture line stenosis as the native and transferred vein segments dilate to their normal caliber when freed of intraoperative spasm. Once the upper anastamosis is completed, the valve should be retested for competence by the strip tests. Some axillary valve sinuses are shallow and are prone to de novo reflux with minor distortions of architecture that may occur during the transfer procedure. A rapid external or transcommissural technique is preferred for this and for in situ or bench repairs. Before starting the distal anastamosis, the distal end of the recipient vein should be trimmed to match the length of the donor segment put on a mild stretch. A slack or overstretched donor segment will result in reflux. Proper rotational orientation of the transferred segment is crucial. There should be no hesitancy to take down and redo the distal suture line if imperfections or reflux is discovered after completion. Final positive and negative strip tests are performed to assure competence. The axillary vein has a thinner muscle layer than the native recipient vein. This may result in gradual dilatation of the transferred axillary vein segment with onset of reflux. This problem encountered in early experience was addressed by placing a prosthetic sleeve around the transferred vein segment. Currently an 8- to 10-mm polytetrafluoroethylene (PTFE) sleeve, 3 cm long, is split open and sutured back as a loose-fitting sleeve around the transferred axillary valve with one or two anchoring sutures to the adventitia to prevent migration. Slipping an unopened sleeve over the lower end of the transferred segment before beginning the distal suture line may obscure rotational orientation of the transferred valve, resulting in reflux after completion of the suture line, and is to be avoided. Others have used autogenous tissue as wraps. The incision is closed with a closed drainage system. To avoid compression of the repair by fluid collection in a tight space, only the superficial fascia is closed with interrupted sutures and the deep fascia is left open.

In trabeculated postthrombotic veins, modifications of the basic technique are necessary. The trabeculae at the site of proximal and distal suture lines are excised (Figure 60.5) to create a single lumen at the site for anastamoses.

In a subset of PTS patients, both the femoral and profunda femoral veins are severely postthrombotic with destroyed valve structures. The femoral confluence can be repaired with individual axillary vein transfers or by en bloc transfer of basilic-brachial confluence, provided valves are present and size match requirements are satisfied (Figure 60.6).

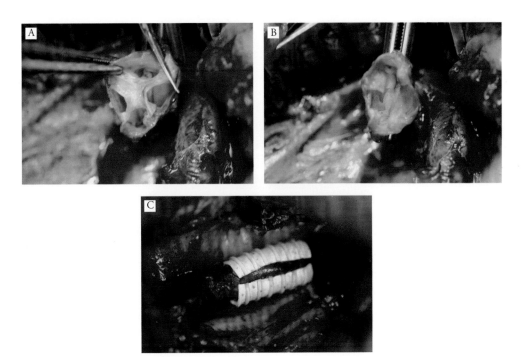

Figure 60.5   Technique in trabeculated veins. Trabeculae are excised (A) to create a single lumen (B) for axillary vein transfer (C).

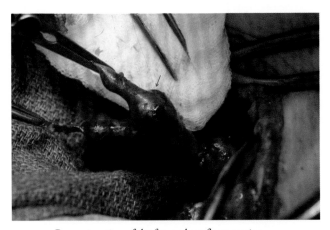

Figure 60.6   Reconstruction of the femoral confluence using Axillary-Brachial-Basilic complex. Proximal clamp is off after completion of the proximal suture line. The brachial valve is competent. Refluxive (de novo) basilic valve is being repaired by transcommissural technique (arrow).

Results of axillary vein transfer in over one hundred trabeculated veins were particularly surprising.[17] Cumulative long-term patency and recurrence-free ulcer healing at 10 years were 83% and >60%, respectively, not different from axillary vein transfer results in a matched group of PTS limbs without trabeculated veins.

MALETI NEOVALVE RECONSTRUCTION

There have been numerous prior attempts at constructing a functional valve where none exists. All have failed or have not advanced beyond trial stage. Creation of a valve

that functions has obvious attractions, especially in postthrombotic cases in which there are limited or no other available repair options. Maleti and Lugli appear to have successfully developed a technique of *neovalve* creation.[44] Through a longitudinal venotomy, mono or bicuspid valve cusps are created by sharp dissection from the intimal and subintimal layers of the vein at the target site (Figure 60.7). A recent report[44] outlined results of the technique in eighteen limbs with venous ulceration. Mean follow-up was 22 months (range 1–42). Ulcer healing occurred in sixteen limbs (89%) within 4 to 25 weeks (median, 12 weeks) afterward, and there were no recurrences. Patency (median, 22 months) and repair competence were confirmed in seventeen cases (95%). A late occlusion occurred in one patient (6%) 8 months after surgery. Minor postoperative complications occurred in three patients (17%).

ENDOPHLEBECTOMY

Surgical disobiliteration of the occluded or stenosed femoral confluence where the profunda femoris joins the femoral vein can be of benefit in selected cases. It can improve limb venous outflow if the iliac veins above the lesion are patent and can facilitate iliac vein stenting if the iliac vein segment is compromised by disease. Endophlebectomy can be combined with valve reconstruction in selected cases. The Straub Clinic group[45] performed endovenectomy in twenty-three deep venous segments combined with fourteen deep venous reconstructions in thirteen patients to treat advanced postthrombotic chronic venous insufficiency. The synechiae and masses attached to the intimal layer were carefully excised under direct vision through a longitudinal venotomy of

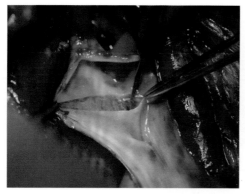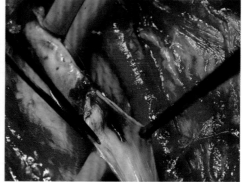

Figure 60.7   Maleti neovalve reconstruction. Single or double valve cusps are developed by sharp dissection from the interior of the target vein (left). The neovalve is shown to be functional and competent with the proximal clamp off (right).   Operative photographs generously provided by Prof. Oscar Maleti, Medona. Italy.

variable length. In ten patients (77%) the treated segments remained primarily patent per duplex at median follow-up of 8 months (range, 1–28 months). Early thrombosis of the repair occurred in three patients, with successful restoration of flow by secondary intervention in two patients. Overall secondary patency rate was 93%. No pulmonary embolism occurred.

POSTOPERATIVE CARE AFTER VALVE RECONSTRUCTION

Hematomas and seromas occur in about 10–15% of cases because of anticoagulation. They should be promptly evacuated to avoid compression and thrombosis of the repair.

Low molecular weight heparins are used at prophylactic dosage starting before surgery and continuing until warfarin anticoagulation started on the first postoperative day achieves therapeutic range. Intraoperative and postoperative pneumatic compression is routine. Warfarin anticoagulation is maintained at therapeutic levels for at least 6 weeks by which time operative endothelial injury is fully healed.[46] Long-term anticoagulation is determined on an individual basis. Thrombophilia, prior thrombotic events without cause or severe diffuse postthrombotic damages with little functional reserve (ambulatory venous pressure) are indications for chronic anticoagulation.

SUMMARY

Postthrombotic disease accounts for 30 to 50% of patients with advanced manifestations of chronic venous disease. Treatment has hitherto mainly centered on compression. Compression is not an option[47] or ineffective[48] in >50% of patients. Patients not controlled by compression suffer a lifetime of morbidity to varying degree with a reduced quality of life. Since many are still at productive age, the socioeconomic costs are substantial. Valve reconstruction techniques were shown to offer benefit to selected patients nearly two decades ago but were not widely adopted. There

is reluctance to undertake open or closed venous interventions in general, and particularly in postthrombotic cases, for fear of thromboembolic complications. Certainly the venographic appearance can be daunting in many PTS cases with trabeculated veins. However, thromboembolic complications have been surprisingly infrequent. The advent of minimally invasive stent technology is a hopeful development. Reported results are excellent with minimal morbidity, and the technique is expected to become widely available. Iliac vein stent placement is the initial procedure of choice in PTS cases, even those with combined obstruction/reflux. Valve reconstruction or veno-venous bypass will be required in only a very small subset that fail initial stent placement. A full range of therapeutic options now exist to address this underserved disease population.

REFERENCES

1. Prandoni P, Lensing AW, Prins MR. Long-term outcomes after deep venous thrombosis of the lower extremities, *Vasc Med.* 1998. *3:* 57–60.
2. Strandness DEJ, Langlois Y, Cramer M, Randlett A, Thiele BL. Long-term sequelae of acute venous thrombosis, *JAMA.* 1983. *250:* 1289–1292.
3. Scott J, Huskisson EC. Graphic representation of pain, *Pain.* 1976. *2:* 175–184.
4. Beebe HG, Bergan JJ, Bergqvist D, et al. Classification and grading of chronic venous disease in the lower limbs: A consensus statement, *Eur J Vasc Endovasc Surg.* 1996. *12:* 487–491; discussion 491–492.
5. Rutherford RB, Padberg FTJ, Comerota AJ, Kistner RL, Meissner MH, Moneta GL. Venous severity scoring: An adjunct to venous outcome assessment, *J Vasc Surg.* 2000. *31:* 1307–1312.
6. Launois R, Rebpi-Marty J, Henry B. Construction and validation of a quality of life questionnaire in chronic lower limb venous insufficiency (CIVIQ), *Qual Life Res.* 1996. *5:* 539–554.
7. Caps MT, Manzo RA, Bergelin RO, Meissner MH, Strandness DEJ. Venous valvular reflux in veins not involved at the time of acute deep vein thrombosis, *J Vasc Surg.* 1995. *22:* 524–531.
8. Johnson BF, Manzo RA, Bergelin RO, Strandness DEJ. Relationship between changes in the deep venous system and the development of the postthrombotic syndrome after an acute episode of lower limb deep vein thrombosis: A one- to six-year follow-up, *J Vasc Surg.* 1995. *21:* 307–312; discussion 13.

9. Killewich LA, Bedford GR, Beach KW, Strandness DEJ. Spontaneous lysis of deep venous thrombi: Rate and outcome, *J Vasc Surg.* 1989. *9*: 89–97.

10. Markel A, Manzo RA, Bergelin RO, Strandness DEJ. Valvular reflux after deep vein thrombosis: Incidence and time of occurrence, *J Vasc Surg.* 1992. *15*: 377–382; discussion 383–384.

11. Raju S, Fredericks RK, Hudson CA, Fountain T, Neglen PN, Devidas M. Venous valve station changes in "primary" and postthrombotic reflux: An analysis of 149 cases, *Ann Vasc Surg.* 2000. *14*: 193–199.

12. Neglen P, Egger JF 3rd, Olivier J, Raju S. Hemodynamic and clinical impact of ultrasound-derived venous reflux parameters, *J Vasc Surg.* 2004. *40*: 303–310.

13. Labropoulos N, Volteas N, Leon M, et al. The role of venous outflow obstruction in patients with chronic venous dysfunction, *Arch Surg.* 1997. *132*: 46–51.

14. Raju S, Fountain T, Neglen P, Devidas M. Axial transformation of the profunda femoris vein, *J Vasc Surg.* 1998. *27*: 651–659.

15. Raju S, Fredericks R. Venous obstruction: An analysis of one hundred thirty-seven cases with hemodynamic, venographic, and clinical correlations, *J Vasc Surg.* 1991. *14*: 305–313.

16. Neglen P, Thrasher TL, Raju S. Venous outflow obstruction: An underestimated contributor to chronic venous disease, *J Vasc Surg.* 2003. *38*: 879–885.

17. Raju S, Neglen P, Doolittle J, Meydrech EF. Axillary vein transfer in trabeculated postthrombotic veins, *J Vasc Surg.* 1999. *29*: 1050–1062; discussion 1062–1064.

18. Raju S, Easterwood L, Fountain T, Fredericks RK, Neglen PN, Devidas M. Saphenectomy in the presence of chronic venous obstruction, *Surgery.* 1998. *123*: 637–644.

19. Neglen P, Raju S. Intravascular ultrasound scan evaluation of the obstructed vein, *J Vasc Surg.* 2002. *35*: 694–700.

20. Negus D, Cockett FB. Femoral vein pressures in post-phlebitic iliac vein obstruction, *Br J Surg.* 1967. *54*: 522–525.

21. Partsch H, Mostbeck A. [Involvement of the lymphatic system in post-thrombotic syndrome], *Wien Med Wochenschr.* 1994. *144*: 210–213.

22. Raju S, Owen SJ, Neglen P. Reversal of abnormal lymphoscintigraphy after placement of venous stents for correction of associated venous obstruction, *J Vasc Surg.* 2001. *34*: 779–784.

23. Criado E, Farber MA, Marston WA, Daniel PF, Burnham CB, Keagy BA. The role of air plethysmography in the diagnosis of chronic venous insufficiency, *J Vasc Surg.* 1998. *27*: 660–670.

24. Raju S, Neglén P, Carr-White P, Fredericks R, Devidas M. Ambulatory venous hypertension: Component analysis in 373 limbs, *Vascular.* 1999. *33*: 257–267.

25. Raju S, Hudson CA, Fredericks R, Neglen P, Greene AB, Meydrech EF. Studies in calf venous pump function utilizing a two-valve experimental model, *Eur J Vasc Endovasc Surg.* 1999. *17*: 521–532.

26. Raju S, Darcey R, Neglén P. Unexpected major role for venous stenting in deep reflux disease, *J Vasc Surg. 51*(2): 401–408; discussion 408.

27. Neglen P, Raju S. Compliance of the normal and post-thrombotic calf, *J Cardiovasc Surg.* 1995. *36*: 225–231.

28. Mayberry JC, Moneta GL, Taylor LMJ, Porter JM. Fifteen-year results of ambulatory compression therapy for chronic venous ulcers, *Surgery.* 1991. *109*: 575–581.

29. Moffatt CJ. Perspectives on concordance in leg ulcer management, *J Wound Care.* 2004. *13*: 243–248.

30. Moffatt CJ, Oldroyd MI. A pioneering service to the community: The Riverside Community Leg Ulcer Project, *Prof Nurse.* 1994. *9*: 486, 8, 90 passim.

31. Erickson CA, Lanza DJ, Karp DL, et al. Healing of venous ulcers in an ambulatory care program: The roles of chronic venous insufficiency and patient compliance, *J Vasc Surg.* 1995. *22*: 629–636.

32. Puggioni A, Marks N, Hingorani A, Shiferson A, Alhalbouni S, Ascher E. The safety of radiofrequency ablation of the great saphenous vein in patients with previous venous thrombosis, *J Vasc Surg.* 2009. *49*: 1248–1255.

33. Neglen P, Hollis KC, Raju S. Combined saphenous ablation and iliac stent placement for complex severe chronic venous disease, *J Vasc Surg.* 2006. *44*: 828–833.

34. Neglen P, Hollis KC, Olivier J, Raju S. Stenting of the venous outflow in chronic venous disease: Long-term stent-related outcome, clinical, and hemodynamic result, *J Vasc Surg.* 2007. *46*: 979–990.

35. Raju S. Endovenous treatment of patients with iliac-caval venous obstruction. *J Cardiovasc Surg.* 2008. *49*: 27–33.

36. Raju S, McAllister S, Neglen P. Recanalization of totally occluded iliac and adjacent venous segments, *J Vasc Surg. 36*: 903–911.

37. Eriksson I, Almgren B. Influence of the profunda femoris vein on venous hemodynamics of the limb: Experience from thirty-one deep vein valve reconstructions, *J Vasc Surg.* 1986. *4*: 390–395.

38. Raju S, Berry MA, Neglen P. Transcommissural valvuloplasty: Technique and results, *J Vasc Surg.* 2000. *32*: 969–976.

39. Raju S, Hardy JD. Technical options in venous valve reconstruction, *Am J Surg.* 1997. *173*: 301–307.

40. Raju S, Fredericks R. Valve reconstruction procedures for nonobstructive venous insufficiency: Rationale, techniques, and results in 107 procedures with two- to eight-year follow-up, *J Vasc Surg.* 1988. *7*: 301–310.

41. Raju S, Fredericks RK, Neglen PN, Bass JD. Durability of venous valve reconstruction techniques for "primary" and postthrombotic reflux, *J Vasc Surg.* 1996. *23*: 357–366; discussion 366–367.

42. Perrin M. Reconstructive surgery for deep venous reflux: A report on 144 cases, *Cardiovasc Surg.* 2000. *8*: 246–255.

43. Masuda EM, Kistner RL. Long-term results of venous valve reconstruction: A four- to twenty-one- year follow-up, *J Vasc Surg.* 1994. *19*: 391–403.

44. Lugli M, Guerzoni S, Garofalo M, Smedile G, Maleti O. Neovalve construction in deep venous incompetence, *J Vasc Surg.* 2009. *49*: 156–162, 62 e1–e2; discussion 62.

45. Puggioni A, Kistner RL, Eklof B, Lurie F. Surgical disobliteration of postthrombotic deep veins—endophlebectomy—is feasible, *J Vasc Surg.* 2004. *39*: 1048–1052; discussion 1052.

46. Raju S, Perry JT. The response of venous valvular endothelium to autotransplantation and in vitro preservation, *Surgery.* 1983. *94*: 770–775.

47. Franks PJ, Oldroyd MI, Dickson D, Sharp EJ, Moffatt CJ. Risk factors for leg ulcer recurrence: A randomized trial of two types of compression stocking, *Age Ageing.* 1995. *24*: 490–494.

48. Raju S, Hollis K, Neglen P. Use of compression stockings in chronic venous disease: Patient compliance and efficacy, *Ann Vasc Surg.* 2007. *21*: 790–795.

61.

EFFICACY OF VENO-ACTIVE DRUGS IN PRIMARY CHRONIC VENOUS DISEASE SURVEY OF EVIDENCE, SYNTHESIS, AND TENTATIVE RECOMMENDATIONS

Michel Perrin and Albert-Adrien Ramelet

INTRODUCTION

Chronic venous disease (CVD) of the lower limb is associated with a range of clinical signs that are quite diverse and include telangiectases, varicose veins, edema, and a spectrum of skin changes including venous eczema, hyperpigmentation, atrophie blanche, lipodermatosclerosis, and venous ulcer.[1,2] Clinical presentations of CVD can be described according to the clinical, etiological, anatomical, and pathophysiological (CEAP) classification.[3-7] The clinical signs in the affected legs are categorized into seven clinical classes designated C_0 to C_6. Symptoms of CVD are also diverse and include tingling, aching or pain, burning, night-time muscle cramps, swelling/throbbing sensation, heaviness, itching, restless legs, and leg tiredness, but none are pathognomic for the condition. In many cases, symptoms vary throughout the day, commonly being exacerbated as the day progresses and by heat, and relieved with rest or elevation of the leg.[8-10] Limbs categorized in any clinical class may be symptomatic (S) or asymptomatic (A). The term "chronic venous disorders" encompasses the full spectrum of signs and symptoms associated with classes C_{0s} to C_6, while the term "chronic venous insufficiency" (CVI) must be reserved to clinical classes C_3 to C_6.[10]

EPIDEMIOLOGY

There seems little doubt that CVD is extremely common in most countries for which data are available. In some studies, the majority of the adult population showed some degree of CVD. For example, in the Edinburgh Vein Study, more than 80% of an age-stratified random sample (aged 18 to 64 years) had mild hyphenweb or reticular varices,[11] while in a sample of Brazilian women aged >48 years only approximately 5% were free of signs and symptoms of CVD.[12] Similarly, in a study in twenty-four Italian cities, only 23% of subjects examined were free of visible signs of CVD,[13] and in the San Diego Population Study visible disease was present in 84% of women and 57% of men.[9] In the twenty countries of the Vein Consult Program spread over Western and Eastern Europe, Latin America, and the Far and Middle East, the worldwide prevalence of CVD was 83.6%: 63.9% of the subjects ranging C_1 to C_6, and 19.7% being C_{0s} subjects.[14] C_1–C_3 appeared to be more frequent among women whatever the country but the rate of severe stages (C_4–C_6) did not differ between men and women. However, reported prevalence of the clinical manifestations of CVD have varied extremely widely. In recent reviews of published literature, prevalence estimates for varicose veins ranged from <1 to 73% in women and from 2 to 56% in men.[15,16] Although some of this variation may be due to differences in the distribution of risk factors in different populations, much of it is likely to be the result of a lack of consistency in diagnostic criteria and terminology, particularly among earlier studies.

Data are scarce regarding venous symptoms in the general population. In some European studies a large proportion of adults (30 to 55%) complain of symptoms, with a substantially higher proportion for women than for men.[8,17-19] In the Vein Consult Program, patients might report one or several symptoms. The most frequently reported symptoms were heavy legs (72.4%), pain (67.7%), swelling sensation (52.7%), and night cramps (44.3%); other symptoms were reported by 24–37% of the population.[14] In the San Diego population study,[9] the prevalence of subjects with pain and without signs was 18%, and that of subjects with pain and without anomaly at duplex scan examination was also 18 %. These patients could be described as C_{0s}, E_n, A_n, P_n patients according to the advanced CEAP classification.[3]

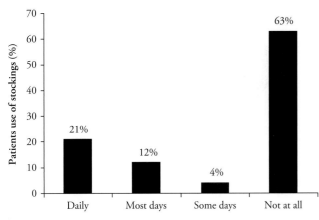

Figure 61.1 Compliance with compression therapy among 3,144 patients with CVD. (Data from Reference 32)

The prevalence of C_{0s} patients was estimated to be 16% in the Acireale project,[20] 13% in a recent subanalysis of the Edinburgh Vein Study,[21] and 19.7% in the Vein Consult Program.[14] In this last survey C0s patients were more frequently men than women whatever the age and the geographical zone.

NONINVASIVE TREATMENTS EMPLOYED IN CVD

A wide range invasive and noninvasive treatments are employed in CVD.[1,22] Invasive therapies include endovenous ablation thermal or chemical, open surgery including surgical removal and ligation of incompetent venous segments, venous reconstructive surgery for deep reflux, and endovascular stent placement to relieve venous outflow obstruction. The main noninvasive treatments are compression therapy and veno-active drug therapy.

Compression Therapy

Compression therapy involving various compressive lower limb garments, particularly stockings, is the mainstay of noninvasive treatment.[23] and has been evaluated in numerous studies over many years.[24–28] Compression stockings improve venous hemodynamics,[29] and reduce edema.[25] The efficacy of compression therapy is widely accepted, but compliance with the treatment protocol is an important factor in treatment success, as has been demonstrated for both ulcer healing and prevention of recurrence.[24,30] Noncompliance with compression therapy is likely to be more common in clinical practice than in trials, and can be a major cause of treatment failure. Noncompliance is a complex and multidimensional problem,[31] for which currently there is no clear, evidence-based solution. In a large study in 3,144 patients referred to a tertiary venous practice in the United States,[32] nearly two-thirds of patients (63%) did not use compression stockings at all, and only 21% used them on a daily

basis (Figure 61.1). If compliance rates are similar in other countries, the inescapable conclusion is that compression therapy is ineffective in the majority of patients with CVD.

Veno-Active Drugs

Veno-active drugs (VADs) constitute a diverse group of medications, most of which are of plant origin. Recent reviewers[22,33–35] have identified five main types, listed below. The first four categories are drugs of plant origin.

1. Alpha-benzopyrones, notably coumarin.

2. Gamma-benzopyrones, also known as flavonoids, which include diosmin, micronized purified flavonoid fraction (MPFF), and the rutosides, including rutin, troxerutin, and hydroxyethylrutosides (HR).

3. Saponins, including horse chestnut seed extract (HCSE) and Ruscus aculateus extract.

4. Other plant extracts, including anthocyans, proanthocyanidins (grape seed extract, red-vine-leaf extract), *Ginko biloba* extract, and *Centella asiatica* extract.

5. Synthetic products (chemical family of quinons) which include naftazone and calcium dobesilate.

Pharmacotherapy is commonly used as part of a repertoire of venous treatments in many parts of Europe, and most VADs are classified as medicines and thus require a marketing authorization and medical prescription. In the UK, however, many of these drugs are not licensed or available. In the United States, VADs such as horse chestnut seed extract, *Gingko biloba*, and maritime pine tree extract are available. Some of these drugs are promoted as "dietary supplements" and can be used without medical advice, while others are "medical food" and are taken under medical supervision.

As expected from the diversity of VADs, they may have multiple actions on the venous system.[22,35] Most VADs enhance venous tone, preventing excessive distension that may damage the vein wall and compromise venous valve function. Recently, attention has focused on the roles of oxidative stress and inflammation in causing adverse changes in the vein wall and venous valves, and subsequent skin changes.[2] At least some VADs have free-radical scavenging actions and can interfere with inflammatory cascades, notably by inhibiting leukocyte-endothelial interactions in the case of MPFF.[2,36] Animal studies suggest that these actions of VADs can protect the vein wall and valves from deleterious changes, with the potential for slowing or preventing the progression of primary CVD.[37] A number of studies have shown that VADs increase capillary resistance and reduce capillary filtration, explaining their anti-edema effect.[22,35] This is seen for MPFF, rutosides, escin, ruscus extracts, proanthocyanidines, and calcium dobesilate. The capillary protective effect of MPFF may be related to inhibition of leukocyte adhesion to capillaries. This is enhanced by micronization.[38]

The positive effect of calcium dobesilate and coumarin on lymphatic circulation has been described by Casley-Smith.[39,40] MPFF improves lymphatic flow and increases the number of lymphatic vessels.[41]

Reduction of blood viscosity and improvement in blood flow have been evidenced for calcium dobesilate[42] and MPFF,[43] while gingko biloba limits red cell aggregation.[44] This may aid reducing the hypoxia that occurs in capillaries and vein wall.

The mechanisms at work in the appearance of venous symptoms are still under investigation. Early work suggested that both hypoxia and venous wall distension (which is increased in varicose veins by 10 to 50%),[45] could produce pain.[46] Edema formation may play a role in pain intensity by the pressure it exerts on nerve endings. Current hypotheses on venous pain mechanisms favor a local inflammatory origin. It has been postulated that proinflammatory mediators released locally by leukocytes can activate C nociceptors and produce venous pain. Unmyelinated C fibers that form these nociceptors were identified in the wall of varicose veins, between endothelial cells and smooth muscle cells of the media.[47] Danziger hypothesized that such nociceptors would be also located in the connective tissue that forms the perivenous space, in close contact with the microcirculation and that their activation would explain the early occurrence of pain.[48] Such nerve fibers may play a key role in symptom onset. The description by Vincent et al. of microvalves in the very small veins in the skin, which incompetence may relate to appearances of reticular veins, corona phlebectatica, and venous flares without reflux in saphenous veins and their major tributaries opens a new avenue to research.[49] The concept might also explain how some people complain of venous symptoms without presenting any visible or detectable sign of venous disease both at physical examination and conventional ultrasound examination. One can hypothesize that such clinical presentation (i.e., the so-called C_{0s} patient) is the result of refluxes in the only microvalves in the small veins that lead to capillary stasis and subsequent inflammatory reaction which in turn activates the nociceptors in the microcirculation and produces pain. Such a postulate remains to be verified.

VADs are prescribed first-line for the relief of CVD-related symptoms, and for prevention of lower limb edema. Some may be efficient in the healing of venous ulcers.[50,51] They are generally regarded as more acceptable to patients than compression therapy, so noncompliance is less of a problem. However, the use of VADs varies widely among different countries, largely related to uncertainty over their efficacy. The efficacy and safety of VADs have been evaluated in numerous clinical studies, but these have generally been small and they have varied in their design,

diagnosis, and selection of patients, and the outcome measures used. There have been a number of international initiatives intended to increase consistency and standardization to the field of CVD in general, and to the conduct of clinical studies in particular.

INITIATIVES TO PROMOTE STANDARDIZATION

DIAGNOSIS AND CLASSIFICATION

There have been several initiatives aimed at standardizing the classification of CVD and improving communication and reporting in the field. Perhaps the most important has been the CEAP (Clinical, Etiologic, Anatomical, and Pathophysiological) classification system.[4] This system has received wide international endorsement and is subject to ongoing appraisal and refinement.[3,5–7] The original CEAP classification of the clinical manifestations involved seven classes (C_0 to C_6), one of which (C_4) has now been split into two subclasses (C_{4a}, pigmentation or venous eczema or both, and C_{4b}, lipodermatosclerosis or atrophie blanche or both).[3] Each clinical class is further characterized for the presence (s, symptomatic) or absence (a, asymptomatic) of CVD-related symptoms. In 2004, a revision of the classification further refined the definitions of CVD, important amendments being the introduction of subclasses in skin changes (C_{4a} and C_{4b}) and the addition of a new descriptor, n, for E, A, and P items when no venous abnormality is identified.[3] This made it possible to classify the often encountered C_{0s}, En, An, Pn subject, which describes a patient with so-called venous symptoms but without any visible or detectable sign of CVD (usually termed "C0s patient"). A second initiative has been the introduction of a common anatomical nomenclature for the veins of the lower limbs,[52,53] and a third has been the proposal of more precise definitions of important terms used in CVD.[3,10] Diagnosis, treatment, research and communication in CVD are thus being placed on an increasingly secure and rigorous foundation, which improved comparability between studies. The association of a clinical examination with a duplex scan investigation, as performed in the Edinburgh Vein Study,[11] may also lead to greater consistency of results.

OUTCOME

CEAP class has been shown to correlate with generic and disease-specific quality of life (QoL)[54] and the presence of venous reflux.[55] Nonetheless, the CEAP system is not ideal for assessing outcome after treatment in practice or in clinical trials. CEAP is not graded or quantitative and, with the exception of the designations for active (C_6) and healed (C_5) venous ulcer, it is not sensitive to improvements in disease severity with treatment. Several severity grading scores have been proposed to overcome this limitation, perhaps most notably the Venous Clinical Severity Score (VCSS) from the American Venous Forum.[56,57] The VCSS has recently undergone a revision to increase its sensitivity to treatments.[57] The VCSS has been characterized and validated in several studies in different clinical settings.[58–61] The VCSS has also been used as an outcome measure in a number of recent clinical studies, notably those evaluating different venous ablation procedures.[62–69] and has been shown to be responsive to the effects of such treatments. For example, the VCSS score decreased progressively with time in patients following saphenous vein radiofrequency ablation.[65] However, the items of the VCSS cover the full spectrum of stages and severity of CVD. For patients with less severe CVD, for example in CEAP classes C_{0S} to C_{2S}, some items will not apply, and the responsiveness of the VCSS to the effects of therapy will be reduced in such patients. Indeed, VCSS scores are often low even for patients in CEAP classes C_4 to C_6.[70] Since VADs are widely used to treat symptoms associated with early stage CVD (CEAP classes C_{0S} to C_{2S}), VCSS score may not be an ideal outcome measure in trials evaluating the efficacy of these drugs.

The 20 question-Chronic Venous Insufficiency Questionnaire (CIVIQ-20) was developed using an iterative process based on features identified by CVD patients as important to their QoL.[71] It has been translated and validated in seventeen languages,[72,73] and shown to be sensitive to change in a large sample of patients including those in CEAP clinical classes C_{0S} to C_4.[71–74] More recently, the CIVIQ-14,[75] VEINES-QoL,[76] and the SQOR-V[77] questionnaires have also been introduced.

The lack of a single, widely accepted instrument for outcome evaluation is an important obstacle to attempts to standardize methodology in clinical studies in CVD, making systematic reviews and meta-analyses more complex and their results more difficult to interpret.

THE GRADE SYSTEM FOR RECOMMENDATIONS

Historically, guideline developers have used a variety of systems to rate the strength of their recommendations. The GRADE (Grading of Recommendations, Assessment, Development and Evaluation) system represents an attempt to produce an explicit, transparent, pragmatic, and comprehensive framework for formulating and grading clinical recommendations. The rationale for the GRADE system was described in a recent series of articles,[78–80] and is being adopted by an increasing number of organizations worldwide. At the heart of the GRADE system is the distinction between the strength of a recommendation and the quality of the evidence on which it is based, although in practice the separation is not absolute and quality of evidence is an important determinant of the strength of a GRADE recommendation.

For simplicity, the GRADE system involves only two grades of recommendation, "strong" and "weak," often represented as "1" and "2," respectively, and four levels of evidence quality—high, moderate, low and very low, often represented as "A" to "D," respectively.[80] Some organizations have combined the low and very low categories.[78] The GRADE system acknowledges that judgments will always be required at each step, and that observational studies can constitute worthwhile evidence, especially if the treatment effect is large.[81] In these respects, GRADE recommendations are fundamentally different from the results of purely statistical meta-analyses of data from randomized trials.

EFFICACY OF VENO-ACTIVE DRUGS

There have been several recent attempts to summarize the available evidence on the efficacy and safety of VADs, and some of these are described below.

THE COCHRANE REVIEW OF PHLEBOTONIC DRUGS, 2005

Clinical trials of a range of different VADs were subjected to a Cochrane review published in 2005.[82] Studies of HCSE were excluded because they were covered in separate Cochrane reviews.[83] All trials of French maritime bark extract were further reviewed in another Cochrane separate document.[84] The main aim of the review was to assess the overall efficacy of VADs as a group; subgroup analyses of the major individual VADs were also performed.

The authors identified 110 randomized, placebo-controlled trials, of which 44 were finally included in the analysis. Studies were excluded for a variety of reasons, including not being double-blinded, having physiological rather than clinical end points, or providing mean data without standard deviation or error. The length of treatment and patient follow-up was 4 to 12 weeks except for one study of 6 months' duration. Only 23% of studies reported the diagnostic classification used; the most frequently used classifications were that of Widmer (five studies) and the CEAP classification (four studies). Most studies included patients with moderately severe CVD, although some included patients with advanced disease including venous ulcers. Of the studies included, twenty-three were of rutosides, ten of MPFF, six of calcium dobesilate, two of *Centella asiatica*, and one each of French maritime pine bark extract, aminaftone, and grape seed extract. Overall, 2,417 patients included in the analysis received a VAD and 1,996 received placebo.

A wide range of outcome variables, including objective signs and subjective symptoms, were analyzed using a random effects statistical model. The effect of treatment was estimated by relative risk (RR) for dichotomous variables

Table 61.1 GLOBAL RESULTS OF COMBINED ANALYSES FOR ALL VENO-ACTIVE DRUGS, FOR ALL OUTCOMES ANALYZED AS DICHOTOMOUS OR CONTINUOUS VARIABLES, FROM THE COCHRANE REVIEW OF PHLEBOTONICS FOR VENOUS INSUFFICIENCY

OUTCOME VARIABLE	DICHOTOMOUS			CONTINUOUS		
	N PTS	RR [95% CI]	HETERO[a]	N PTS	SMD [95% CI]	HETERO[a]
Edema	1,245	0.72 [0.65; 0.81]	No	–	–	–
Ankle circumference	–	–	–	1,390	−0.24 [−0.44; −0.04]	Yes
Lower leg volume	–	–	–	775	−0.73 [−1.45; 0.00]	Yes
Venous ulcer	160	NS	Yes	–	–	–
Trophic disorders[b]	705	0.88 [0.83; 0.94]	No	–	–	–
Pain	2,247	0.63 [0.52; 0.76]	Yes	475	−0.59 [−1.01; −0.17]	Yes
Cramps	1,793	0.72 [0.58; 0.89]	Yes	314	−0.70 [−1.15; −0.24]	Yes
Restless legs	652	0.84 [0.74; 0.95]	No	–	–	–
Itching	405	NS	Yes	60	−0.58 [−1.10; −0.06]	1 study
Heaviness	2,166	0.59 [0.49; 0.72]	Yes	697	−0.94 [−1.47; −0.42]	Yes
Swelling	1,072	0.63 [0.50; 0.80]	Yes	454	−1.49 [−2.42; −0.56]	Yes
Paresthesias[c]	1,456	0.67 [0.50; 0.88]	Yes	188	NS	No
Global assessment by patient	2,213	0.60 [0.46; 0.78]	Yes	402	−0.97 [−1.59; −0.34]	Yes

[a] evidence of significant heterogeneity among studies analyzed
[b] skin changes including telangiectasia, reticular veins, varicose veins, and lipodermatosclerosis
[c] abnormal sensations such as prickling, burning, and tingling
n pts: number of patients included in the analysis; NS: not significant
(From Reference 82)

and by standardized mean difference (SMD) for continuous variables. Dichotomous variables were analyzed on an intention-to-treat basis. However, only seven studies provided an intention-to-treat efficacy analysis; for the other studies, the original data were reanalyzed and an intention-to-treat analysis performed with all missing values imputed as treatment failures. Continuous variables were analyzed either per-protocol or by intention-to-treat, as in the original publication. A chi-squared test of homogeneity was used to establish the presence of significant heterogeneity among studies analyzed together.

The results of the global analyses for all VADs are summarized in Table 61.1. For every outcome variable except venous ulcer, the analyses showed significant treatment benefits for the VADs compared with placebo when analyzed as either a dichotomous or a continuous variable, or both in

some cases. The only nonsignificant effects were for venous ulcer, itching assessed as a continuous variable, and paresthesias assessed as a continuous variable. For edema (RR 0.72, 95% CI 0.65; 0.81), trophic disorders (RR 0.88, 95% CI 0.83; 0.94), and restless legs (RR 0.84, 95% CI 0.74; 0.95), the analyses showed significant benefit of VAD treatment with no evidence of heterogeneity among studies. However, for most analyses there was evidence of heterogeneity.

Adverse events were analyzed using two different hypotheses to take account of patients withdrawn or lost to follow-up, and by both methods the incidence of patients experiencing adverse events was the same with VADs as with placebo (Table 61.2). The authors drew attention to the fact that, given the relatively short duration of most studies, there was a lack of long-term safety data for VADs.

Table 61.2 RELATIVE RISK (RR) OF PATIENTS EXPERIENCING ADVERSE EVENTS IN COMBINED ANALYSES FOR ALL VENO-ACTIVE DRUGS FROM THE COCHRANE REVIEW OF PHLEBOTONICS FOR VENOUS INSUFFICIENCY

	N STUDIES	N PATIENTS	RR [95% CI]	SIGNIFICANCE	HETEROGENEITY
Hypothesis A	38	4,216	0.89 [0.69; 1.14]	NS	Yes
Hypothesis B	31	3,068	1.04 [0.87; 1.24]	NS	No

Hypothesis A: incidence of adverse events calculated assuming that all lost patients experienced an adverse event.
Hypothesis B: incidence of adverse events calculated assuming that lost patients presented the adverse event in the same proportion as those in the observed control group.
NS: not significant
(From Reference 82)

In the subgroup analyses of individual VADs, calcium dobesilate, MPFF, and rutosides all showed significant benefit, relative to placebo and based on multiple studies, for several dichotomous and continuous outcome variables, albeit with evidence of heterogeneity in most of cases (Table 61.3). The VADs differed in the variables for which they showed significant efficacy.

The presence of heterogeneity among studies within a meta-analysis implies that the result should be interpreted carefully. However, in these analyses, data from studies of different VADs were combined. Unless all the different VADs show similar efficacy profiles across the various outcome variables, a degree of heterogeneity is inherent in such an analyses, and the subgroup analyses indicated that the VADs did indeed vary in their efficacy profiles. Other potential sources of heterogeneity include the use of different diagnostic and outcome criteria, and different assessment and measurement methods. Inclusion of one or more studies using different methodology could introduce heterogeneity into an otherwise homogeneous set of data. Given that the publication dates of the studies included ranged from 1971 to 2004, heterogeneity in study methodology was inevitable as scientific and clinical advances were made over time. Between-study heterogeneity was therefore to be expected in these analyses.

In view of the design and scope of the analyses, this Cochrane review, while less than definitive, provided evidence of the efficacy and safety of VADs as a group, and for some of the more intensively studied drugs individually, that was as compelling as could reasonably have been expected.

Table 61.3 SUBGROUP ANALYSES OF SELECTED INDIVIDUAL VENO-ACTIVE DRUGS, SHOWING DICHOTOMOUS AND CONTINUOUS VARIABLES FOR WHICH A SIGNIFICANT BENEFIT WAS SHOWN, RELATIVE TO PLACEBO, FROM THE COCHRANE REVIEW OF PHLEBOTONICS FOR VENOUS INSUFFICIENCY

VENO-ACTIVE DRUG	SIGNIFICANT BENEFIT OF DRUG VERSUS PLACEBO			
	Dichotomous variables		*Continuous variables*	
	Variable	Hetero[a]	Variable	Hetero[a]
Calcium dobesilate	Pain	Yes	Leg volume	No
	Cramps	No		
	Restless legs	No		
	Swelling	No		
MPFF	Trophic disorders	No	Ankle circumference	Yes
	Cramps	Yes	Cramps	1 study
	Swelling	No	Heaviness	1 study
			Swelling	1 study
			Global assessment	1 study
Rutosides	Edema	No	Pain	Yes
	Pain	Yes	Cramps	Yes
	Heaviness	Yes	Itching	1 study
	Swelling	Yes	Heaviness	Yes
	Paresthesias	Yes	Global assessment	Yes
	Global assessment	Yes		
Centella asiatica	Global assessment	1 study		
French maritime pine bark extract	Pain	1 study	Pain	1 study
			Heaviness	1 study
			Swelling	1 study

[a] evidence of significant heterogeneity among studies analyzed
(From Reference 82)

THE COCHRANE REVIEW OF HORSE CHESTNUT SEED EXTRACT AND OF FRENCH MARITIME PINE BARK EXTRACT

Randomized clinical trials of HCSE, whose main active component is the triterpenic saponin escin, were the subjects of Cochrane reviews and meta-analyses, the most recent of which was published in 2006.[83] A total of twenty-nine studies were identified. Of these, seventeen (some unpublished) were of HCSE given as monotherapy, and met the selection criteria for inclusion in the review. Ten studies compared HCSE against placebo, two against compression therapy, and five against other VADs. The included studies were of 2 to 16 weeks' duration; the majority (twelve studies) lasted between 3 and 8 weeks. In fourteen included studies, patients were diagnosed according to the classification of Widmer.[85] Outcome measures included CVD-related symptoms (leg pain, itching) and signs (edema, lower leg volume, calf and ankle circumference).

Assessment and reporting methods varied among studies. For placebo-controlled studies, meta-analysis could only be performed for reduction in lower leg volume (6 studies, 502 patients), and reduction in circumference at the ankle and at the calf (3 studies, 80 patients for both outcome measures). In each meta-analysis, HCSE was significantly superior to placebo. Most individual studies also reported significant benefits for most outcome measures with HCSE compared with placebo (Table 61.4).

Results of testing for heterogeneity among studies were not reported.

The authors concluded that HCSE was efficacious relative to placebo and of similar efficacy to compression therapy in the short-term treatment of CVD. Adverse effects

Table 61.4 OUTCOME VARIABLES FOR WHICH A SIGNIFICANT BENEFIT OF TREATMENT
WAS SHOWN, RELATIVE TO PLACEBO, IN THE COCHRANE REVIEW OF HORSE
CHESTNUT SEED EXTRACT FOR CHRONIC VENOUS INSUFFICIENCY

OUTCOME VARIABLE	N STUDIES	N PATIENTS	EFFECT SIZE
Leg pain, responder ratio (D)	1	418	OR 2.22 [1.50; 3.29]
Leg pain, VAS (C)	1	30	WMD 42.4 [34.9; 49.9]
Edema, responder ratio (D)	1	346	OR 2.78 [1.79; 4.30]
Edema, VAS (C)	1	30	WMD 40.1 [31.6;48.6]
Lower leg volume (C)	6	502	WMD 32.1 [13.5; 50.7]
Ankle circumference (C)	3	80	WMD 4.71 [1.13; 8.28]
Calf circumference (C)	3	80	WMD 3.51 [0.58; 6.45]
Itching, responder ratio (D)	1	196	OR 1.98 [1.11; 3.53]

C: continuous variable; D: dichotomous variable; OR: odds ratio; VAS: visual analogue scale; WMD: weighted mean difference.
(From Reference 83)

were generally mild and infrequent, so the overall risk/benefit ratio for HCSE was favorable.

The Cochrane review of French maritime pine bark extract included fifteen trials with a total of 791 participants for the treatment of seven different chronic disorders.[84] These included asthma (two studies; N = 86), attention deficit hyperactivity disorder (one study; N = 61), chronic venous insufficiency (two studies; N = 60), diabetes mellitus (four studies; N = 201), erectile dysfunction (one study; N = 21), hypertension (two studies; N = 69) and osteoarthritis (three studies; N = 293). Two of the studies were conducted exclusively in children; the others involved adults. The authors concluded that due to small sample size, limited numbers of trials per condition, variation in outcomes evaluated, and outcome measures used, evidence was insufficient to support use of French maritime pine bark extract for the treatment of any chronic disorder comprising chronic venous disorders.[84]

THE INTERNATIONAL CONSENSUS STATEMENT, 2005

A group of fourteen experts, representing the fields of angiology, dermatology, and vascular surgery, from countries in which VADs were available and who had experience of their clinical use, attended a consensus symposium in Siena, Italy in 2005. Attendees evaluated published clinical studies and meta-analyses devoted to the medical treatment of symptomatic CVD of any severity, and a consensus statement was prepared.[34]

Randomized, double-blind, placebo-controlled trials and meta-analyses were included in the analysis, but studies with a crossover design were excluded. No statistical meta-analysis was performed; the experts individually drew on their own clinical experience as well as the trial results, and their conclusions were combined using a secret ballot. In each case, the final classification was based on a large

majority or unanimity of votes cast. Three grades of recommendation were considered, based on the following levels of evidence: Grade A (large randomized controlled trials, meta-analysis of homogeneous results); Grade B (smaller randomized controlled trials, or a single randomized controlled trial); Grade C (nonrandomized controlled trials, observational studies).

A total of eighty-three studies were analyzed, and the experts drew up a list of VADs that had been shown to be safe and efficacious on venous symptoms according to at least one randomized trial, and assigned final grades of recommendation for each (Table 61.5). Calcium dobesilate, MPFF, and HR-oxerutins were all assigned to the highest level (Grade A) of recommendation, while HCSE and *Ruscus* extracts were assigned to Grade B.

The experts also commented on the place of VAD therapy in the management of venous symptoms. They agreed that VADs were indicated to relieve venous symptoms in all classes of CVD, from C0s through to C6s, and were an alternative to compression therapy especially in case of contraindication or poor compliance. VADs are also known to enhance the effects of compression therapy. They also pointed out that VAD therapy can be effective against venous pain when aspirin, paracetamol and other nonsteroidal anti-inflammatory drugs (NSAIDs) are not.

META-ANALYSIS OF MPFF AS ADJUNCTIVE THERAPY IN VENOUS LEG ULCER

The main Cochrane review of phlebotonics[82] included two studies of VADs in the treatment of venous ulcer, neither of which showed significant evidence of benefit relative to placebo. A meta-analysis[50] of trials of MPFF as adjunctive therapy (on top of conventional therapy of compression and appropriate local care) identified five randomized controlled trials (2 placebo-controlled) that met the methodological

Table 61.5 GRADES OF RECOMMENDATION OF THE INTERNATIONAL CONSENSUS STATEMENT

COMPOUND	RECOMMENDATION	NUMBER OF INFLUENTIAL STUDIES	
		RCTS	META-ANALYSES
Calcium dobesilate	Grade A	3	2
MPFF	Grade A	4	1
HR-oxerutins	Grade A	5	1
HCSE (escin)	Grade B	1	2
Ruscus extracts	Grade B	2	1
Diosmin (synthetic)	Grade C	1	
Troxerutin	Grade C	2	
Gingko biloba	Grade C	2	
Proanthocyanidines	Grade C	2	
Troxerutin + coumarin	Grade C	1	
Centella asiatica	Grade C	1	
Naftazone	Grade C	1	

RCTs: randomized clinical trials
(From Reference 34)

characteristics required by the Cochrane Wounds Group. The main end point of the meta-analysis was complete ulcer healing, and the analysis was by intention-to-treat.

At 6 months of treatment (4 trials, 616 patients), 61.3% of patients in the MPFF group were completely healed, compared with 47.7% in the control group, with RR for ulcer persistence of 32% (95% CI 3; 70%) in favor of MPFF (p = 0.03), although there was evidence of heterogeneity among trials. When the analysis was restricted to patients with ulcers ≥5 cm^2 in area at baseline (n = 319), the RR for persistence of ulceration was 53% (95% CI 15; 103%, p = 0.0035) in favor of MPFF, with no evidence of heterogeneity. At 2 months of treatment (5 trials, 723 patients), the reduction in risk of ulcer persistence was 44% (95% CI 7; 94%, p = 0.015) in favor of MPFF, with no evidence of heterogeneity.

The median time to ulcer healing was significantly shorter with MPFF (16.1 weeks) than in the control group (21.3 weeks). Subgroup analyses indicated that MPFF produced no significant additional benefit for ulcers <5 cm^2 in area or of <6 months' duration, possibly because compression treatment alone is sufficient for treating small ulcers or these of short duration.

This analysis indicates that MPFF, when given as an adjunct to conventional therapy, assists in the healing of large and long-standing venous ulcers. Largely on the basis of these results, the recent American College of Chest Physicians evidence-based guidelines[51] recommended that MPFF be added to local care and compression in patients with persistent ulcer as a complication of postthrombotic syndrome. Similarly, MPFF was given a strong recommendation (1B) for use in combination with compression for long-standing or large venous ulcers in the recent edition of the *Handbook of Venous Disorders: Guidelines of the American Venous Forum*.[86]

CONSENSUS STATEMENT ON THE MANAGEMENT OF CHRONIC VENOUS DISORDERS OF THE LOWER LIMBS, 2008

This set of guidelines, prepared under the auspices of several learned societies, including the American Venous Forum, the American College of Phlebology, and the European Venous Forum, covers most aspects of the management of CVD, including investigations, treatment, and management strategy.[22]

When considering VADs, the guidelines largely summarized and endorsed the positive findings of the last Cochrane reviews[82,83] and the grades of recommendation of the International Consensus Statement.[34] The guidelines highlighted the evidence of efficacy of several VADs (calcium dobesilate, MPFF, rutosides, HCSE, proanthocyanidines, and coumarin + rutin) in CVD-related edema, and the efficacy of MPFF as an adjunct to standard treatment in the healing of venous ulcers.

These guidelines also provided recommendations on the indications for VADs, which may be summarized as follows. VADs may be indicated as a first-line treatment for C_{0s} patients and be adjunctive treatment of C_{1s} to C_{6s} patients. In these last patients, VADs may be used in conjunction with sclerotherapy, surgery, endovenous thermal treatment, and/or compression therapy. VADs may accentuate the effects of compression. These guidelines also reiterated the French

Table 61.6 CHANGES IN SYMPTOMS AND SIGNS IN PATIENTS IN THE RELIEF PROSPECTIVE OBSERVATIONAL STUDY

	PATIENTS WITH SYMPTOMS, %			ANKLE CIRCUMFERENCE (CM)	PAIN BY VAS (CM)
	SWELLING	HEAVINESS	CRAMPS		
Baseline	80.2	95.1	71.7	27.3	3.75
6 months	38.0	48.2	19.1	25.3	1.27
p-value	<0.001	<0.001	<0.001	0.007	0.0001

VAS: visual analogue scale
(From Reference 72)

recommended prescribing practices, stating that VADs should not be prescribed in the absence of CVD-related symptoms. It is not appropriate to combine several VADs in the same prescription.

TOWARD A TENTATIVE "GRADE" RECOMMENDATION

Building on recent reviews and meta-analyses, and taking account of additional evidence that was either not available or not included in them, we propose tentative recommendations for the use of VADs, based on the principles of the GRADE system. We stress that these recommendations reflect the opinions and judgments of the authors, and have not been endorsed by learned societies or other organizations.

RECENT AND ADDITIONAL EVIDENCE

Several results that were not available or were not included in the Cochrane meta-analyses[82–84] and previous reviews[34,35,86] are relevant to recommendations based on the GRADE system.

Important evidence was provided by the RELIEF observational study.[72] RELIEF was a large, prospective cohort study in 5,052 symptomatic CVD patients in CEAP clinical classes C_{0s} to C_{4s}. The presence of venous reflux was screened by pocket-Doppler, and its location (superficial or deep) identified by photoplethysmography using tourniquet. All patients were treated with MPFF for a period of 6 months. Study outcomes were changes in CVD-related symptoms (sensations of leg swelling, heaviness and leg cramps), edema assessed by ankle circumference, and pain assessed by 10-cm visual analogue scale. Changes in CEAP clinical class and in quality of life, assessed using the CIVIQ questionnaire,[71] were also evaluated. All study outcomes showed significant improvements, in the study population as a whole and in the subgroups of patients with and without venous reflux knowing that only saphenous veins, their first rank tributaries, and nonsaphenous veins were investigated using pocket-Doppler. Improvements in the

prevalence of CVD-related symptoms were particularly dramatic (Table 61.6). For example, the proportion of patients reporting leg cramps decreased from 71.7% at baseline to 19.1% at 6 months in patients, ($P < 0.001$). Ratings of pain by visual analogue scale decreased from 3.75 cm to 1.27 cm ($P = 0.0001$) while leg circumference decreased from 27.3 cm to 25.3 cm in the same population ($P = 0.007$). These changes took place progressively throughout the study. There was also a progressive improvement in QoL during the study, in patients with and without reflux. Changes between baseline and 6 months achieved significance in all QoL dimensions as well as in the global index (p values equal to 0.0001). This 6-month study also provided evidence of the longer-term safety of MPFF treatment.

In a randomized, double-blind, placebo-controlled trial of twenty patients[87] with chronic pelvic pain diagnosed at laparoscopy with pelvic congestion syndrome with no other severe disease, pelvic pain was significantly reduced after 6 months in the MPFF group.

The benefits of MPFF as part of the pharmacological preoperative care and postoperative recovery for patients with varicose veins who undergo phlebectomy have been evaluated in two randomized controlled trials.[88,89] In both studies, MPFF helped to attenuate pain, decrease postoperative hematomas and accelerate their resorption, and to increase exercise tolerance in the early postoperative period.

In a meta-analysis of ten publications dated between 1975 and 2009 including a total of 1,010 patients, of the benefits of MPFF, hydroxyethylrutoside, *Ruscus* extracts, and diosmin on edema reduction, the mean reduction in ankle circumference was -0.80 ± 0.53 cm with MPFF, -0.58 ± 0.47 cm with *Ruscus* extract, -0.58 ± 0.31 cm with hydroxyethylrutoside, -0.20 ± 0.5 cm with single diosmin, and -0.11 ± 0.42 cm with placebo. The reduction in ankle circumference was significantly superior to that of placebo whatever the drug concerned (P < 0.0001). The comparison between MPFF, *Ruscus* extract and hydroxyethylrutoside on the reduction of ankle edema was in favor of MPFF.[90] This was significant (P < 0.0001).

In patients with edema, ultrasonographic reflux time was significantly reduced in the MPFF group compared with the placebo group (P = 0.03), although no significant changes were seen regarding symptoms in the whole C_1 to C_6 study population (N = 101).[91]

The recent review by Gohel concluded that MPFF evidenced the greatest clinical benefits in patients with venous disease.[92]

Observational study in 1,036 Argentinean patients with symptomatic ankle swelling[93] showed a significant decrease in ankle circumference, together with improvement in the patients' QoL, after 2 months of treatment with *Ruscus* extracts (-21 ± 61.9 mm, P < 0.001). Although symptoms were affirmed to have improved after treatment, no definition of "improvement of symptoms" could be found in the article.

In an open-label clinical trial in sixty-five women CEAP C_{2s} and C_{3s}, improvement in venous pain intensity assessed on VAS was significantly correlated (P = 0.04) with plethysmographic parameter improvement after 28 treatment days with *Ruscus* extracts.[94]

In a randomized controlled study of efficacy of the association coumarin/troxerutin in adjunction to compression therapy on venous edema, 226 patients randomly assigned medical compression stockings with adjunctive coumarin/troxerutin (treatment group) or medical compression stockings plus placebo (control group) for 4 weeks and adjunctive pharmacological therapy or placebo for the consecutive 12 weeks of the study. Lower leg volume was measured by water displacement. After ceasing compression stockings, leg volume increased again by 6.5 ± 12.1 ml in the treatment group and by 36.7 ± 12.1 ml in the control group (p = 0.0402), implying that adjunctive coumarin/troxerutin treatment is edema protective.[95]

Four randomized clinical trials of calcium dobesilate have been published recently.[96-99] One was a double-blind, parallel groups, placebo-controlled, study in 256 adult patients with symptomatic C_3 to C_6 disease and pitting edema.[96] Patients received 1,500 mg of calcium dobesilate per day or placebo during 8 weeks, and their leg volume before and after treatment was assessed based on a truncated cone model. Wearing of compression stockings Class II was admitted during the time of trial and the proportion of patients wearing compression was slightly higher in the treatment group compared with the control one (28% versus 25.8% respectively). At the end of study, the volume of the lower calf diminished in the treatment group by 264.72 + 111.93 cm^3, while it increased by + 0.8 + 152.98 cm^3 in the placebo group (P < 0.0002). The symptoms of pain, discomfort, heavy legs, tired legs, tingling, itching, and cramps, as well as the global assessments by investigators and patients, also improved significantly in favor of calcium dobesilate (P < 0.05). The second was a large study in 509 patients in CEAP classes C_1 to C_6.[97] At the end of the 3-month treatment period, there were no significant differences between the calcium dobesilate and placebo groups in QoL, edema, or CVD-related symptom severity. However, there was a significant difference in favor of calcium dobesilate in

QoL after a further 9 months of follow-up off-treatment. In the third, smaller, study in forty-nine patients,[98] 7 weeks' treatment with calcium dobesilate produced significant reductions, relative to baseline, in leg, calf, and ankle circumference, while there was no change in the placebo group. There were also reductions in pain severity with calcium dobesilate that were significant compared with placebo. In a fourth trial, 253 consecutive outpatients in CEAP classes C_3 to C_4 were treated for 4 weeks.[99] The difference in leg volume was statistically significant (P = 0.0109) in favor of active treatment, but there was no difference between the groups in symptom improvement.

Calcium dobesilate has been associated with possible increased risk of agranulocytosis, a rare but serious condition; in three anecdotal reports[100-102] Including two cases of positive rechallenge.[100-101] A case-control and case-population study confirmed the presence of a significant association (121 cases per million per year).[103] while the prevalence was estimated lower by others, at 0.32 cases per million per year.[104] The incidence of agranulocytosis attributable to calcium dobesilate has been challenged, and no death was reported with such treatment until now.[105]

A total of twenty publications, all authored by Belcaro's team, came out on O-beta-hydroxyrutosides between 2002 and 2011.[106-108] Most of the results drawn from such interesting studies would deserve confirmation from other teams.

A randomized, double-blind and placebo controlled study was carried out with red-vine-leaf extract, 720 mg per day over 12 weeks in 248 patients, CEAP C_3 to C_{4a} and complaining of moderate-to-severe clinical symptoms. Efficacy end points were changes in limb volume determined by water displacement volumetry, symptom improvement assessed on a 10-cm visual analogue scale, and global efficacy evaluation. At the end of the 12-week treatment, lower limb volume was significantly reduced in favor of the treatment group (p < 0.0268), and also for the symptom of "pain in the legs" (p < 0.047). Other symptoms showed no significant improvement over placebo.[109]

TENTATIVE RECOMMENDATIONS

To our knowledge, no VAD has been evaluated in a very large randomized clinical trial of the type that could provide high quality evidence supporting their use in any indication related to CVD. For MPFF and rutosides, there is substantial evidence from smaller trials, supported by meta-analyses and, in the case of MPFF, a large observational study, three recent randomized trials and one meta-analysis, for their efficacy in relieving CVD-related symptoms such as pain, heaviness, and cramps, and in reducing CVD-related lower limb edema. There are insufficient data to specify those CEAP clinical classes as well as anatomical and pathophysiological anomalies for which the benefits will be greatest, but it is reasonable to assume that patients at all stages of the disease may benefit from VADs. There appear to be no

Table 61.7 SUMMARY OF TENTATIVE RECOMMENDATIONS, ACCORDING TO THE PRINCIPLES OF THE GRADE SYSTEM

INDICATION	VENO-ACTIVE DRUG	RECOMMENDATION FOR USE	QUALITY OF EVIDENCE	CODE
Relief of symptoms associated with CVD in patients C0s to C6s and with CVD-related edema	Micronized purified flavonoid fraction (MPFF)	Strong	Moderate	1B
	Nonmicronized diosmins or synthetic diosmins	Weak	Poor	2C
	Rutosides (O-betahydroxyethyl)	Weak	Moderate	2B
	Calcium dobesilate	Weak	Moderate	2B
	HCSE	Weak	Moderate	2B
	Ruscus extracts	Weak	Moderate	2B
	Gingko biloba	Weak	Poor	2C
	Other VADs	Weak	Poor	2C
Healing of large or long-standing venous ulcer, as an adjunct to compressive and local therapy (Reference 86)	Micronized purified flavonoid fraction (MPFF)	Strong	Moderate	1B

HCSE: horse chestnut seed extract; VADs, venoactive drugs
(From Reference 80)

important safety concerns with the use of these drugs, so it is possible to propose a strong recommendation, based on evidence of moderate quality, for their use in these indications. HCSE and *Ruscus* extracts have also shown efficacy against CVD-related symptoms and lower limb edema, and an early trial comparing the efficacy on edema reduction and safety of compression stockings class II and HCSE, 50 mg escin, twice daily was published in the *Lancet*.[110] Significant edema reductions were achieved by HCSE ($p = 0.005$) and compression ($p = 0.002$) compared to placebo, and the two therapies were shown to be equivalent ($p = 0.001$), but diuretic treatment was administered to both groups in the run-in period. Since then, the volume and quality of evidence has been less for HCSE and *Ruscus* extracts than for the previous two drugs. In the apparent absence of important safety concerns, these drugs may be given a weak recommendation based on middle quality evidence.

Calcium dobesilate has shown evidence of efficacy against CVD-related symptoms and edema, but a recent randomized trial in over 500 patients found it to be not superior to placebo in its efficacy on symptoms, edema and QoL.[97] Calcium dobesilate has been associated with a potential safety concern relating to rare cases of agranulocytosis. We consider that it is only possible to give a weak recommendation for its use, given the uncertainty over the balance between benefits and harms with a middle quality evidence. A definitive, favorable resolution of the agranulocytosis issue in future would be grounds for reconsideration.

O-beta-hydroxyrutosides has also shown evidence of efficacy against CVD-related symptoms and edema, but it would deserve additional trials to confirm its efficacy.

There is evidence from meta-analysis of randomized controlled trials that MPFF shows efficacy in the healing of venous ulcers (CEAP class C_6) when used as an adjunct to compression therapy and appropriate local therapy, particularly for ulcers that are large (>5 cm² in area) and/or persistent (>6 months' duration). In the absence of important safety concerns, its use in this indication can be given a strong recommendation based on evidence of moderate quality. These tentative recommendations are summarized in Table 61.7.

CONCLUDING REMARKS

The evidence base for the efficacy and safety of VADs has accrued over a long period of time from studies of variable size, quality, and methodology. In future, it is to be hoped that the various initiatives to increase standardization will bear fruit and lead to improved quality and comparability of studies, and that the pharmaceutical industry will invest the necessary resources to perform large and definitive clinical trials. However, at this time we consider it possible to make strong recommendations, based on evidence of moderate quality, for the use of MPFF for the relief of symptoms associated with CVD and CVD-related edema. Weaker recommendations can be made for the use of rutosides HCSE, *Ruscus* extracts, and calcium dobesilate in these indications. We also consider it possible to make a strong recommendation based on evidence of moderate quality for the use of MPFF as an adjunct to compressive and local therapy in the healing of venous ulcers, with greatest benefit in ulcers

>5 cm² in area and >6 months in duration. We hope that our recommendations will be useful to clinicians and organizations involved in decision-making in this important and undervalued field.

REFERENCES

1. Eberhardt RT, Raffetto, JD. Chronic venous insufficiency, *Circulation.* 2005. *111*: 2398–2409.
2. Bergan JJ, Schmid-Schönbein GW, Coleridge Smith PD, Nicolaides AN, Boisseau MR, Eklöf B. Chronic venous disease, *N Engl J Med.* 2006. *355*: 488–498.
3. Eklöf B, Rutherford RB, Bergan JJ, et al. Revision of the CEAP classification for chronic venous disorders: Consensus statement, *J Vasc Surg.* 2004. *40*: 1248–1252.
4. Porter JM, Moneta GL. Reporting standards in venous disease: An update: International Consensus Committee on Chronic Venous Disease, *J Vasc Surg.* 1995. *21*: 635–645.
5. Allegra C, Antignani PL, Bergan JJ, et al. The "C" of CEAP: Suggested definitions and refinements: An International Union of Phlebology conference of experts, *J Vasc Surg.* 2003. *37*: 129–131.
6. Carpentier PH, Cornu-Thénard A, Uhl JF, et al. Appraisal of the information content of the C classes of CEAP clinical classification of chronic venous disorders: A multicenter evaluation of 872 patients, *J Vasc Surg.* 2003. *37*: 827–833.
7. Antignani PL, Cornu-Thénard A, Allegra C, et al. Results of a questionnaire regarding improvement of "C" in the CEAP classification, *Eur J Vasc Endovasc Surg.* 2004. *28*: 177–181.
8. Carpentier PH, Maricq HR, Biro C, Ponçot-Makinen CO, Franco A. Prevalence, risk factors, and clinical patterns of chronic venous disorders of lower limbs: A population-based study in France, *J Vasc Surg.* 2004. *40*: 650–659.
9. Langer RD, Ho E, Denenberg JO, Fronek A, Allison M, Criqui MH. Relationships between symptoms and venous disease, *Arch Intern Med.* 2005. *165*: 1420–1424.
10. Eklöf B, Perrin M, Delis KT, Rutherford RB, Gloviczki P. Updated terminology of chronic venous disorders: The VEIN-TERM transatlantic interdisciplinary consensus document, *J Vasc Surg.* 2009. *49*: 498–501.
11. Evans CJ, Fowkes FGR, Ruckley CV, Lee AJ. Prevalence of varicose veins and chronic venous insufficiency in men and women in the general population: Edinburgh Vein Study, *J Epidemiol Community Health.* 1999. *53*: 149–153.
12. Scuderi A, Raskin B, Al Assal F, et al. The incidence of venous disease in Brazil based on the CEAP classification, *Int Angiol.* 2002. *21*: 316–321.
13. Chiesa R, Marone EM, Limoni C, Volonté M, Schaefer E, Petrini O. Chronic venous insufficiency in Italy: The 24-cities cohort study, *Eur J Vasc Endovasc Surg.* 2005. *30*: 422–429.
14. Rabe E, Guex JJ, Puskas A, Scuderi A, Fernandez Quesada F, VCP coordinators. Epidemiology of chronic venous disorders in geographically diverse populations: Results from the Vein Consult Program, *Int Angiol.* 2012. *31*: 105–115.
15. Beebe-Dimmer JL, Pfeifer JR, Engle JS, Schottenfeld D. The epidemiology of chronic venous insufficiency and varicose veins, *Ann Epidemiol.* 2005. *15*: 175–184.
16. Robertson L, Evans C, Fowkes FG. Epidemiology of chronic venous disease, *Phlebology.* 2008. *23*: 103–111.
17. Bradbury A, Evans C, Allan P, Lee A, Ruckley CV, Fowkes FG. What are the symptoms of varicose veins? Edinburgh vein study cross sectional population survey, *Br Med J.* 1999. *318*: 353–356.
18. Preziosi P, Galan P, Aissa M, Hercberg S, Boccalon H. Prevalence of venous insufficiency in French adults of the SUVIMAX cohort, *Int Angiol.* 1999. *18*: 171–175.
19. Pannier-Fischer F, Rabe E. Epidemiologie der chronischen Venenerkrankungen, *Hautarzt.* 2003. *54*: 1037–1044.
20. Andreozzi GM, Signorelli S, Di Pino L, et al. Varicose symptoms without varicose veins: The hypotonic phlebopathy, epidemiology, and pathophysiology: The Acireale project. *Minerva Cardioangiol.* 2000. *48*: 277–285.
21. Ruckley CV, Evans CJ, Allan PL, Lee AJ, Fowkes FG. Telangiectasia in the Edinburgh Vein Study: Epidemiology and association with trunk varices and symptoms, *Eur J Vasc Endovasc Surg.* 2008. *36*: 719–724.
22. Nicolaides AN, Allegra C, Bergan J, et al. Management of chronic venous disorders of the lower limbs: Guidelines according to scientific evidence, *Int Angiol.* 2008. *27*: 1–59.
23. Shingler S, Robertson L, Boghossian S, Stewart M. Compression stockings for the initial treatment of varicose veins in patients without venous ulceration, *Cochrane Database Syst Rev.* 2011. *11*: CD008819.
24. Mayberry JC, Moneta GL, Taylor LM Jr, Porter JM. Fifteen-year results of ambulatory compression therapy for chronic venous ulcers, *Surgery.* 1991. *109*: 575–581.
25. Motykie GD, Caprini JA, Arcelus JI, Reyna JJ, Overom E, Mokhtee D. Evaluation of therapeutic compression stockings in the treatment of chronic venous insufficiency, *Dermatol Surg.* 1999. *25*: 116–120.
26. Iglesias C, Nelson EA, Cullum NA, Torgerson DJ, VenUS Team. VenUS I: A randomised controlled trial of two types of bandage for treating venous leg ulcers, *Health Technol Assess.* 2004. *8*: 1–105.
27. Blecken SR, Villavicencio JL, Kao TC. Comparison of elastic versus nonelastic compression in bilateral venous ulcers: A randomized trial, *J Vasc Surg.* 2005. *42*: 1150–1155.
28. O'Meara S, Cullum NA, Nelson EA. Compression for venous leg ulcers, *Cochrane Database Syst Rev.* 2009. *1*: CD000265.
29. Ibegbuna V, Delis KT, Nicolaides AN, Aina O. Effect of elastic compression stockings on venous hemodynamics during walking, *J Vasc Surg.* 2003. *37*: 420–425.
30. Erickson CA, Lanza DJ, Karp DL, et al. Healing of venous ulcers in an ambulatory care program: The roles of chronic venous insufficiency and patient compliance, *J Vasc Surg.* 1995. *22*: 629–636.
31. Van Hecke A, Grypdonck M, Defloor T. A review of why patients with leg ulcers do not adhere to treatment, *J Clin Nurs.* 2009. *18*: 337–349.
32. Raju S, Hollis K, Neglen P. Use of compression stockings in chronic venous disease: Patient compliance and efficacy, *Ann Vasc Surg.* 2007. *21*: 790–795.
33. Ramelet AA, Perrin M, Kern P, Bounameaux H. *Phlebology*, 5e. Paris, France: Elsevier Masson. 2008.
34. Ramelet AA, Boisseau MR, Allegra C, et al. Veno-active drugs in the management of chronic venous disease: An international consensus statement: Current medical position, prospective views, and final resolution, *Clin Hemorheol Microcirc.* 2005. *33*: 309–319.
35. Perrin M, Ramelet AA. Pharmacological treatment of primary chronic venous disease: Rationale, results, and unanswered questions, *Eur J Vasc Endovasc Surg.* 2011. *41*(1): 117–125.
36. Bergan J. Molecular mechanisms in chronic venous insufficiency, *Ann Vasc Surg.* 2007. *21*: 260–266.
37. Bergan JJ, Pascarella L, Schmid-Schönbein GW. Pathogenesis of primary chronic venous disease: Insights from animal models of venous hypertension, *J Vasc Surg.* 2008. *47*: 183–192.
38. Korthuis RJ, Gute DC. Anti-inflammatory actions of a micronized, purified flavonoid fraction in ischemia/reperfusion. *Adv Exp Med Biol.* 2002. *505*: 181–190.
39. Casley-Smith JR. The influence of tissue hydrostatic pressure and protein concentration on fluid and protein uptake by diaphragmatic initial lymphatics- effect of calcium dobesilate, *Microcirc Endothelium Lymphatics.* 1985. *2*: 385–415.
40. Casley-Smith JR, Morgan RG, Piller NB. Treatment of lymphedema of the arms and legs with 5,6-benzo-alpha-pyrone, *N Engl J Med.* 1993. *329*: 1158–1163.
41. Mc Hale NG, Hollywood MA. Control of lymphatic pumping: Interest of Daflon 500 mg, *Phlebology.* 1994. *9*(Suppl 1): 23–25.

42. Tejerina T, Ruiz E. Calcium dobesilate: Pharmacology and future approaches. *Gen Pharmacol.* 1998. *31*(3): 357–360. Review.

43. Le Devehat C, Khodabandehlou T, Vimeux M, Kempf C. Evaluation of haemorheological and microcirculatory disturbances in chronic venous insufficiency: Activity of Daflon 500 mg, *Int J Microcirc Clin Exp.* 1997. *17*(Suppl 1): 27–33.

44. Boisseau MR. Pharmacology of venotonic drugs: Current data on the mode of action, *Angeiologie.* 2000. *52*: 71–77.

45. Nicolaides AN. Investigation of chronic venous insufficiency: A consensus statement, *Circulation.* 2000. *102*: e126–e163.

46. Nicolaides AN. From symptoms to leg edema, *Angiology.* 2003. *54*(Suppl 1): S33–S44.

47. Vital A, Carles D, Conde da Silva Fraga E, Boisseau MR. Unmyelinated C fibers and inflammatory cells are present in the wall of human varicose veins: A clinico-pathological study, *Int Angiol.* 2009. *28*(Suppl 1): 49.

48. Danziger N. Pathophysiology of pain in venous disease, *J Mal Vasc.* 2007. *32*: 1–7. [In French]

49. Vincent JR, Jones GT, Hill GB, van Rij AM. Failure of microvenous valves in small superficial veins is a key to the skin changes of venous insufficiency, *J Vasc Surg.* 2011. *54*(Suppl 6): 62S–69S.

50. Coleridge Smith P, Lok C, Ramelet AA. Venous leg ulcer: A meta-analysis of adjunctive therapy with micronized purified flavonoid fraction, *Eur J Vasc Endovasc Surg.* 2005. *30*: 198–208.

51. Kearon C, Kahn SR, Agnelli G, et al. Anthithrombotic therapy for venous thromboembolic disease: American College of Chest Physicians Evidence-Based Clinical Practice Guidelines (8th Edition), *Chest.* 2008. *133*(Suppl 6): 454S–545S.

52. Caggiati A, Bergan JJ, Gloviczki P, et al. Nomenclature of the veins of the lower limbs: an international interdisciplinary consensus statement. *J Vasc Surg.* 2002. *36*: 416–422.

53. Caggiati A, Bergan JJ, Gloviczki P, et al. Nomenclature of the veins of the lower limbs. *J Vasc Surg.* 2005. *41*: 719–724.

54. Kahn SR, M'lan CE, Lamping DL, et al. Relationship between clinical classification of chronic venous disease and patient-reported quality of life: Results from an international cohort study, *J Vasc Surg.* 2004. *39*: 823–828.

55. Chiesa R, Marone EM, Limoni C, Volonté M, Petrini O. Chronic venous disorders: Correlation between visible signs, symptoms, and presence of functional disease, *J Vasc Surg.* 2007. *46*: 322–330.

56. Vasquez MA, Rabe E, McLafferty RB, et al. Revision of the venous clinical severity score: Venous outcomes consensus statement: Special communication of the American Venous Forum Ad Hoc Outcomes Working Group, *J Vasc Surg.* 2010. *52*(5): 1387–1396.

57. Vasquez MA, Munschauer CE. Revised VCSS: A facile measurement of outcomes in venous disease, *Phlebology.* 2012. *27*(Suppl 1): 119–129.

58. Passman MA, McLafferty RB, Lentz MF, et al. Validation of Venous Clinical Severity Score (VCSS) with other venous severity assessment tools from the American Venous Forum, National Venous Screening Program, *J Vasc Surg.* 2011. *54*(Suppl 6): 2S–9S.

59. Kakkos SK, Rivera MA, Matsagas MI, et al. Validation of the new venous severity scoring system in varicose vein surgery, *J Vasc Surg.* 2003. *38*: 224–228.

60. Ricci MA, Emmerich J, Callas PW, et al. Evaluating chronic venous disease with a new venous severity scoring system, *J Vasc Surg.* 2003. *38*: 909–915.

61. Gillet JL, Perrin MR, Allaert FA. Clinical presentation and venous severity scoring of patients with extended deep axial venous reflux, *J Vasc Surg.* 2006. *44*: 588–594.

62. Hartung O, Otero A, Boufi M, et al. Mid-term results of endovascular treatment for symptomatic chronic nonmalignant venous occlusive disease, *J Vasc Surg.* 2005. *42*: 1138–1144.

63. Masuda EM, Kessler DM, Lurie F, Puggioni A, Kistner RL, Eklöf B. The effect of ultrasound-guided sclerotherapy of incompetent perforator veins on venous clinical severity and disability scores, *J Vasc Surg.* 2006. *43*: 551–556.

64. Rasmussen LH, Bjoern L, Lawaetz M, Blemings A, Lawaetz B, Eklöf B. Randomized trial comparing endovenous laser ablation of the great saphenous vein with high ligation and stripping in patients with varicose veins: Short-term results, *J Vasc Surg.* 2007. *46*: 308–315.

65. Vasquez MA, Wang J, Mahathanaruk M, Boczkowski G, Sprehe E, Dosluoglu HH. The utility of the Venous Clinical Severity Score in 682 limbs treated by radiofrequency saphenous vein ablation, *J Vasc Surg.* 2007. *45*: 1008–1014.

66. Disselhoff BC, der Kinderen DJ, Kelder JC, Moll FL. Randomized clinical trial comparing endovenous laser with cryostripping for great saphenous vein varicose veins, *Br J Surg.* 2008. *95*: 1232–1238.

67. Disselhoff BC, der Kinderen DJ, Kelder JC, Moll FL. Randomized clinical trial comparing endovenous laser ablation of the great saphenous vein with and without ligation of the sapheno-femoral junction: 2-year results, *Eur J Vasc Endovasc Surg.* 2008. *36*: 713–718.

68. Gonzalez-Zeh R, Armisen R, Barahona S. Endovenous laser and echo-guided foam ablation in great saphenous vein reflux: One-year follow-up results, *J Vasc Surg.* 2008. *48*: 940–946.

69. Marston WA, Brabham VW, Mendes R, Berndt D, Weiner M, Keagy B. The importance of deep venous reflux velocity as a determinant of outcome in patients with combined superficial and deep venous reflux treated with endovenous saphenous ablation, *J Vasc Surg.* 2008. *48*: 400–405.

70. Perrin M, Dedieu F, Jessent V, Blanc M-P. Evaluation of the new severity scoring system in chronic venous disease of the lower limbs: An observational study conducted by French angiologists, *Phlebolymphology.* 2006. *13*: 6–16.

71. Launois R, Mansilha A, Jantet G. International psychometric validation of the chronic venous disease quality of life questionnaire CIVIQ-20, *Eur J Vasc Endovasc Surg.* 2010. *40*: 783–789.

72. Jantet G. Chronic venous insufficiency: Worldwide results from the RELIEF study: Reflux assEssment and quaLity of lIfe improvEment with micronized Flavonoids. *Angiology.* 2002. *53*: 245–256.

73. Launois R, Mansilha A, Lozano F. Linguistic validation of the 20 item-chronic venous disease quality of life questionnaire (CIVIQ-20). *Phlebology.* Published online 3 May 2013. DOI: 10.1177/0268355513479582.

74. Erevnidou K, Launois R, Katsamouris A, Lionis C. Translation and validation of a quality of life questionnaire for chronic lower limb venous insufficiency into Greek, *Int Angiol.* 2004. *23*: 394–399.

75. Launois R, Le Moine JG, Lozano FS, Mansilha A. Construction and international validation of CIVIQ-14 (a short form of CIVIQ-20), a new questionnaire with a stable factorial structure, *Qual Life Res.*2012; *21*(6): 1051–1058.

76. Lamping DL, Schroter S, Kurz X, Kahn SR, Abenhaim L. Evaluation of outcomes in chronic venous disorders of the leg: Development of a scientifically rigorous, patient-reported measure of symptoms and quality of life, *J Vasc Surg.* 2003. *37*: 410–419.

77. Guex JJ, Zimmet SE, Boussetta S, Nguyen C, Taieb C. Construction and validation of a patient-reported outcome dedicated to chronic venous disorders: SQOR-V (specific quality of life and outcome response—venous), *J Mal Vasc.* 2007. *32*: 135–147.

78. Guyatt GH, Oxman AD, Vist GE, et al. GRADE: An emerging consensus on rating quality of evidence and strength of recommendations, *Br Med J.* 2008. *336*: 924–926.

79. Guyatt GH, Oxman AD, Kunz R, et al. GRADE: What is "quality of evidence" and why is it important to clinicians, *Br Med J.* 2008. *336*: 995–998.

80. Guyatt GH, Oxman AD, Kunz R, et al. GRADE: Going from evidence to recommendations, *Br Med J.* 2008. *336*: 1049–1051.

81. Glasziou P, Chalmers I, Rawlins M, McCulloch P. When are randomised trials unnecessary? Picking signal from noise, *Br Med J.* 2007. *334*: 349–351.

82. Martinez MJ, Bonfill X, Moreno RM, Vargas E, Capellà D. Phlebotonics for venous insufficiency, *Cochrane Database Syst Rev.* 2005. *3*: CD003229.

83. Pittler MH, Ernst E. Horse chestnut seed extract for chronic venous insufficiency, *Cochrane Database Syst Rev.* 2006. *9*(1): CD003230.

84. Schoonees A, Visser J, Musekiwa A, Volmink J. Pycnogenol® (extract of French maritime pine bark) for the treatment of chronic disorders, *Cochrane Database Syst Rev.* 2012. *18*(4): CD008294.

85. Widmer LK, Stähelin HB. *Peripheral venous disorders: Prevalence and sociomedical importance: Basle Study III.* Bern, Switzerland: Hans Huber. 1978.

86. Coleridge Smith PD. Drug treatment of varicose veins, venous edema, and ulcers. In: Gloviczki P, ed. *Handbook of venous disorders: Guidelines of the American Venous Forum,* 3e. London. Hodder Arnold. 2009. 359–365.

87. Simsek M, Burak F, Taskin O. Effects of micronized purified flavonoid fraction (Daflon) on pelvic pain in women with laparoscopically diagnosed pelvic congestion syndrome: A randomized crossover trial, *Clin Exp Obstet Gynecol.* 2007. *34:* 96–98.

88. Pokrovsky AV, Saveljev VS, Kirienko AI, et al. Surgical correction of varicose vein disease under micronized diosmin protection (results of the Russian multicenter controlled trial DEFANS), *Angiol Sosud Khir.* 2007. *13*(2): 47–55.

89. Veverkova L, Kalac J, Jedlicka V, et al. Analysis of surgical procedures on the vena saphena magna in the Czech Republic and an effect of Detralex during its stripping, *Rozhl Chir.* 2005. *84:* 410–412.

90. Allaert FA. Meta-analysis of the impact of the principal venoactive drugs agents on malleolar venous edema, *Int Angiol.* 2012. *31*(4): 310–315.

91. Danielsson G, Jungbeck C, Peterson K, Norgren L. A randomised controlled trial of micronised purified flavonoid fraction vs placebo in patients with chronic venous disease, *Eur J Vasc Endovasc Surg.* 2002. *23:* 73–76.

92. Gohel MS, Davies AH. Pharmacological agents in the treatment of venous disease: An update of the available evidence, *Curr Vasc Pharmacol.* 2009. *7*(3): 303–308. Review.

93. Guex JJ, Enrici E, Boussetta S, Avril L, Lis C, Taieb C. Correlations between ankle circumference, symptoms, and quality of life demonstrate the clinical relevance of minimal leg swelling reduction: Results of a study in 1,036 Argentinean patients, *Dermatol Surg.* 2008. *34:* 1666–1675.

94. Allaert FA, Hugue C, Cazaubon M, Renaudin JM, Clavel T, Escourrou P. Correlation between improvement in functional signs and plethysmographic parameters during venoactive treatment (Cyclo 3 Fort), *Int Angiol.* 2011. *30*(3): 272–277.

95. Vanscheidt W, Rabe E, Naser-Hijazi B, et al. The efficacy and safety of a coumarin-/troxerutin-combination (SB-LOT) in patients with chronic venous insufficiency: A double blind placebo-controlled randomised study, *Vasa.* 2002. *31*(3): 185–190.

96. Rabe E, Jaeger KA, Bulitta M, Pannier F. Calcium dobesilate in patients suffering from chronic venous insufficiency: A double-blind, placebo-controlled, clinical trial, *Phlebology.* 2011. *26:* 162–168.

97. Martinez-Zapata MJ, Moreno RM, Gich I, Urrútia G, Bonfill X, Chronic Venous Insufficiency Study Group. A randomized, double-blind multicentre clinical trial comparing the efficacy of calcium dobesilate with placebo in the treatment of chronic venous disease, *Eur J Vasc Endovasc Surg.* 2008. *35:* 358–365.

98. Flota-Cervera F, Flota-Ruiz C, Treviño C, Berber A. Randomised, double-blind, placebo-controlled clinical trial to evaluate the lymphagogue effect and clinical efficacy of calcium dobesilate in chronic venous disease, *Angiology.* 2008. *59:* 352–356.

99. Labs KH, Degisher S, Gamba G, Jaeger KA. Effectiveness and safety of calcium dobesilate in treating chronic venous insufficiency: Randomized, double-blind, placebo-controlled trial, *Phlebology.* 2004. *19:* 123–130.

100. Kulessa W, Becker EW, Berg PA. Recurrent agranulocytosis after taking calcium dobesilate, *Dtsch Med Wschr.* 1992. *117:* 372–374. [Article in German]

101. Cladera Serra A, Blasco Mascaro I, Oliva Berini E, Ramos diaz F. Agranulocytosis induced by dobesilate calcium, *Med Clin-Barcelona.* 1995. *105:* 558–559.

102. García Benayas E, Garcia Diaz B, Perez G. Calcium dobesilate-induced agranulocytosis, *Pharm World Sci.* 1997. *5:* 251–252.

103. Ibáñez L, Ballarin E, Vidal X, Laporte JR. Agranulocytosis associated with calcium dobesilate: Clinical course and risk estimation with the case-control and case-population approaches, *Eur J Clin Pharmacol.* 2000. *56:* 763–767.

104. Zapater P, Horga JF, Garcia A. Risk of drug-induced agranulocytosis: The case of calcium dobesilate, *Eur J Clin Pharmacol.* 2003. *58:* 767–772.

105. Allain H, Ramelet AA, Polard E, Bentué-Ferrer D. Safety of calcium dobesilate in chronic venous disease, diabetic retinopathy, and haemorrhoids, *Drug Saf.* 2004. *27:* 649–660.

106. Belcaro G, Cesarone MR, Ledda A, et al. 5-Year control and treatment of edema and increased capillary filtration in venous hypertension and diabetic microangiopathy using O-(beta-hydroxyethyl)-rutosides: A prospective comparative clinical registry, *Angiology.* 2008. *59*(Suppl 1): 14S–20S.

107. Belcaro G, Rosaria Cesarone M, Ledda A, et al. O-(beta-hydroxyethyl)-rutosides systemic and local treatment in chronic venous disease and microangiopathy: An independent prospective comparative study, *Angiology.* 2008. *59*(Suppl 1): 7S–13S.

108. Cesarone MR, Belcaro G, Pellegrini L, et al. HR Venoruton O-(beta-hydroxyethyl)-rutosides in comparison with diosmin + hesperidine in chronic venous insufficiency and venous microangiopathy: An independent, prospective, comparative registry study, *Angiology.* 2005. *56:* 1–8.

109. Rabe E, Stucker M, Esperester A, Schäfer E, Ottillinger B. Efficacy and tolerability of a red-vine-leaf extract in patients suffering from chronic venous insufficiency: Results of a double-blind placebo-controlled study, *Eur J Vasc Endovasc Surg.* 2011. *41:* 540–547.

110. Diehm C, Trampisch HJ, Lange S, Schmidt C. Comparison of leg compression stocking and oral horse-chestnut seed extract therapy in patients with chronic venous insufficiency, *Lancet.* 1996. *347:* 292–294.

62.

MEDICAL MANAGEMENT OF THE VENOUS LEG ULCER

WOUND DRESSINGS AND ADJUVANT AGENTS

Nisha Bunke-Paquette, Teresa Russell, Kevin Broder, and Andrew Li

INTRODUCTION

Leg ulceration of venous origin accounts for over 70% of patients with chronic leg wounds.[1] It is the most severe manifestation of chronic venous insufficiency (CVI) owing to long standing venous hypertension. Venous hypertension is most commonly caused by reflux through incompetent valves, but other causes include venous outflow obstruction and failure of the calf-muscle pump. The majority of venous leg ulcers (VLU) will have a superficial component of venous reflux.[2] Therefore, treatment of the underlying source of venous hypertension should be sought for therapeutic intervention, when patient selection is appropriate. However, treatment of the VLU is often inadequate and poorly addressed, leading to disappointing healing rates and chronicity of the ulcer.

When properly diagnosed, effective treatment of the VLU is available. External compression is the mainstay of treatment of the venous leg ulcer. When used in conjunction with corrective procedures for superficial venous reflux, ulcer recurrence is significantly reduced coupled with an extended ulcer-free time.[3] Various adjunctive wound care therapies and procedures are available that can be utilized as part of a comprehensive approach to healing venous stasis ulcers. These include wound disinfection and debridement using autolytic, chemical, and mechanical methods; pneumatic devices; negative pressure wound therapy; ultrasonic wound bed stimulation; pulsed electromagnetic field therapy; platelet leukocyte gel application; skin substitute grafts; auto skin grafts; tissue flap reconstruction; and use of systemic therapy with agents such as daflon and pentoxifylline. Various topical agents and techniques of applying wound dressings are available, but there is no evidence that one is better than another.

This chapter will discuss adjunctive treatments for wound healing of the venous leg ulcer.

APPROACH TO THE VENOUS LEG ULCER

Effective treatment depends on an accurate diagnosis. The patient's history often includes a prior history of venous ulceration, symptoms of venous insufficiency, and in cases of secondary venous insufficiency, a history of thrombotic events. The clinical appearance is often distinct. The venous ulcer commonly is an exudative wound covered with granulation tissue and a fibrinous layer. The borders tend to be irregular with a sloping edge. The location of the ulcer is usually in the gaiter region, characteristically around the malleoli. Ulcers occurring above the mid calf or on the toes and foot are unlikely to be venous origin. Edema may be present and the surrounding skin may manifest signs of chronic venous insufficiency including skin hyperpigmentation, stasis dermatitis, and lipodermatosclerosis with or without varicose veins (Figure 62.1). The wound may or may not be painful.

The duplex ultrasound examination will support the clinical diagnosis, and vein mapping will help identify targets for therapeutic intervention. Concomitant arterial insufficiency may exist in 20% of venous ulcer patients and should be evaluated when suspected and in all cases of delayed wound healing.[1] An ankle brachial index (ABI) of less than 0.80 may impair wound healing.[4] The differential diagnosis should minimally include small vessel disease, pyoderma gangrenosum, infection, neoplasia, drug reaction, exogenous origin, and calciphylaxis. The approach to the VLU is summarized in Table 62.1.

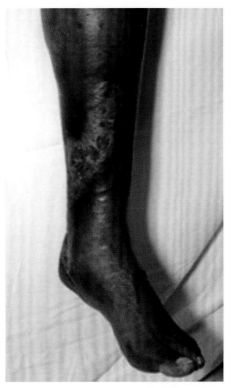

Figure 62.1 Venous leg ulcer. The location of the ulcer in the gaiter region, irregular borders, and surrounding skin hyperpigmentation suggest venous origin.

COMPRESSION

Treatment of venous ulcers has primarily focused on two main targets, normalizing venous hypertension and treatment of the ulcer bed.[5] Compression reduces venous hypertension and edema, and improves the function of the calf muscle while enhancing arterial flow, microcirculation, and lymphatic drainage. Types of compression can be broken down into four areas, inelastic, elastic, multilayer dressings, and pneumatic compression. Compression physiology and types are described in Chapter 9. However, in the context of the venous leg ulcer, compression should be used to increase ulcer healing rates compared with no compression (Grade 1A recommendation)[6]. Other conclusions from the Cochrane database by O'Meara et al.[6] include the following: Multicomponent systems are more effective than single-component systems. Multicomponent systems containing an elastic bandage appear to be more effective than those composed mainly of inelastic constituents. Two-component bandage systems appear to perform as well as the four-layer bandage. Patients receiving the four-layer bandage heal faster than those allocated the short-stretch bandage. Lowest recurrence rates of ulcerations were seen in people who wore the highest compression. Therefore, patients should wear the highest level of compression tolerable. When edema is present, short-stretch compression is most effective as it promotes a lower resting pressure than

elastic dressings and offers a high working pressure that decreases edema and improves venous flow.[5]

For patients with concomitant peripheral arterial disease, compression must be used cautiously, and bandaging is generally contraindicated if the ABI is less than 0.5.

TARGET THE SOURCE OF VENOUS REFLUX

Hemodynamic abnormalities in patients with venous leg ulcers may involve the superficial, perforating, or deep veins. The pathology may be isolated or a combination of the three venous systems. However, superficial venous insufficiency, with or without perforating vein reflux, was the commonest pattern in limbs with primary CVI, whereas deep venous insufficiency was present in most of the limbs with post-thrombotic CVI.[7,8]

These data have significant clinical implications, since reflux in the superficial system can be easily corrected. Superficial venous surgery in addition to compression therapy for chronic venous leg ulceration reduced ulcer recurrence and improved ulcer free time when compared with compression alone.[2]

Treatments to abolish superficial venous reflux include traditional vein-stripping surgery, subfascial perforating vein surgery, phlebectomy, endovenous ablation, and foam sclerotherapy. These procedures are described elsewhere in this text. However, foam sclerotherapy deserves additional attention for its increasing role in the treatment of stasis ulcers. Ultrasound-guided foam sclerotherapy can be used to target the cluster of superficial veins beneath the wound bed (Figure 62.2). The injection is nearly painless, is safe and minimally invasive with little morbidity. Although large randomized controlled studies that demonstrate accelerated wound healing are lacking, it is our experience, and that of others, that superficial venous insufficiency treatment by ultrasound-guided foam sclerotherapy leads to more complete wound healing (Figure 62.3).[9,10]

WOUND INFECTION AND ANTIBIOTICS

At present, there is no evidence to support the routine use of systemic antibiotics to promote healing in venous leg ulcers. Current prescribing guidelines recommend that antibacterial preparations should only be used in cases of clinical infection and not for bacterial colonization.[11] The most common organisms found in the VLU are *Staphylococcus aureus*, *Pseudomonas aeruginosa* (*P. aeurginosa*), *β-haemolytic streptococci*, and *Enterococcus faecalis*.[12] Ulcers with *P. aeruginosa* have been correlated to significantly larger wounds, suggesting that the presence of *P. aeruginosa* in venous leg ulcers can cause wound enlargement and/or delayed healing.

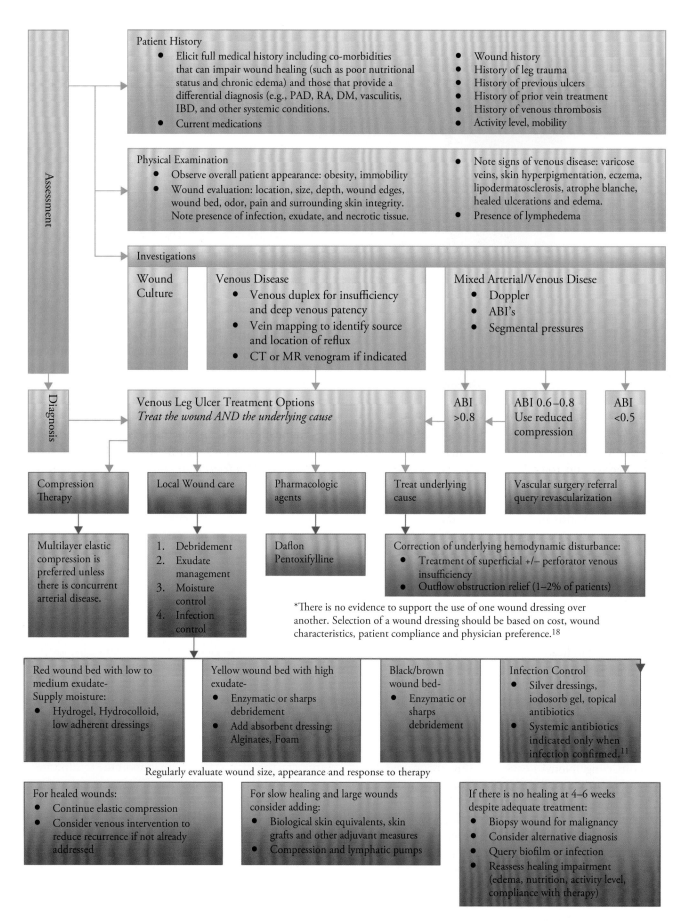

Patient History
- Elicit full medical history including co-morbidities that can impair wound healing (such as poor nutritional status and chronic edema) and those that provide a differential diagnosis (e.g., PAD, RA, DM, vasculitis, IBD, and other systemic conditions.
- Current medications

- Wound history
- History of leg trauma
- History of previous ulcers
- History of prior vein treatment
- History of venous thrombosis
- Activity level, mobility

Physical Examination
- Observe overall patient appearance: obesity, immobility
- Wound evaluation: location, size, depth, wound edges, wound bed, odor, pain and surrounding skin integrity. Note presence of infection, exudate, and necrotic tissue.

- Note signs of venous disease: varicose veins, skin hyperpigmentation, eczema, lipodermatosclerosis, atrophe blanche, healed ulcerations and edema.
- Presence of lymphedema

Investigations

Wound Culture

Venous Disease
- Venous duplex for insufficiency and deep venous patency
- Vein mapping to identify source and location of reflux
- CT or MR venogram if indicated

Mixed Arterial/Venous Disese
- Doppler
- ABI's
- Segmental pressures

Assessment

Diagnosis

Venous Leg Ulcer Treatment Options
Treat the wound AND the underlying cause

ABI >0.8

ABI 0.6–0.8 Use reduced compression

ABI <0.5

Compression Therapy

Local Wound care

Pharmacologic agents

Treat underlying cause

Vascular surgery referral query revascularization

Multilayer elastic compression is preferred unless there is concurrent arterial disease.

1. Debridement
2. Exudate management
3. Moisture control
4. Infection control

Daflon
Pentoxifylline

Correction of underlying hemodynamic disturbance:
- Treatment of superficial +/− perforator venous insufficiency
- Outflow obstruction relief (1–2% of patients)

*There is no evidence to support the use of one wound dressing over another. Selection of a wound dressing should be based on cost, wound characteristics, patient compliance and physician preference.[18]

Red wound bed with low to medium exudate-Supply moisture:
- Hydrogel, Hydrocolloid, low adherent dressings

Yellow wound bed with high exudate-
- Enzymatic or sharps debridement
- Add absorbent dressing: Alginates, Foam

Black/brown wound bed-
- Enzymatic or sharps debridement

Infection Control
- Silver dressings, iodosorb gel, topical antibiotics
- Systemic antibiotics indicated only when infection confirmed.[11]

Regularly evaluate wound size, appearance and response to therapy

For healed wounds:
- Continue elastic compression
- Consider venous intervention to reduce recurrence if not already addressed

For slow healing and large wounds consider adding:
- Biological skin equivalents, skin grafts and other adjuvant measures
- Compression and lymphatic pumps

If there is no healing at 4–6 weeks despite adequate treatment:
- Biopsy wound for malignancy
- Consider alternative diagnosis
- Query biofilm or infection
- Reassess healing impairment (edema, nutrition, activity level, compliance with therapy)

Table 62.1 **APPROACH TO THE VENOUS LEG ULCER**

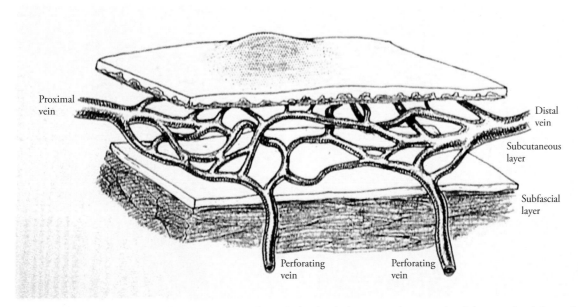

Figure 62.2   The ulcer bed. Note the tangle of incompetent veins beneath the ulcer bed. These can be targeted and eliminated with foam sclerotherapy.

In addition to bacterial colonization, there is increasing evidence that chronic, nonhealing venous leg ulcers are more likely to have biofilm formation, which inhibits wound healing.[13] The biofilm is a polysaccharide substance secreted by surface bacteria. This biofilm increases resistance to antibiotics and topical agents. No prospective studies have reported a benefit for routine use of topical antibiotics. The use of topical antibiotics are discouraged due to the risk of contact dermatitis and bacterial resistance.

DEBRIDEMENT

Healthy granulation tissue is pink in color and is an indicator of healing, whereas unhealthy granulation appears dark red and may bleed on contact. Dark red and excess granulation may be an indicator of infection, in which debridement of the chronic wound should be used to facilitate wound healing.[14] Failure to remove necrotic tissue from the wound bed results in the delayed wound healing and[15] exposes the patient to increased risk for infection due to the high levels of bacteria found in nonviable tissue. Fibrin on more than 50% of the wound bed has also been associated with delayed wound healing.[4] Nonviable tissue may be classified as slough or eschar. Both slough and eschar can harbor pathogenic organisms and should be eliminated by debridement to enhance the formation of new granulation and epithelial tissue and to encourage revascularization of the wound bed.

Debridement can be performed by sharps, surgical, mechanical, autolytic, and enzymatic debridement.

Sharps debridement. This is the quickest and most effective way to remove debris and necrotic tissue from the wound bed and can be performed at the bedside. This type of debridement is used when there is a large surface area, or when there is infected bone and tissue that must be removed.

Surgical debridement. This is usually done in the operating room under sterile conditions, and accommodations are made to control pain during this procedure.

Autolytic debridement. This is the use of appropriate dressings to facilitate the body's own mechanisms to debride itself. Some occlusive wound dressings (hydrocolloids) promote autolytic debridement by providing an oxygen-free environment allowing nonviable tissue to begin the process of breaking down and separating from healthy viable tissue.

Mechanical debridement. There are several types of mechanical debridement. These include saline wet to dry dressings, hydrotherapy, and irrigation. The major disadvantage of mechanical debridement is its nondiscriminatory removal of viable tissue along with necrotic material. It is commonly known that mechanical debridement is less used in the clinical setting in recent years.

Enzymatic debridement. Debriding agents such as Santyl or collaganese ointment provide enzymatic debridement. The most commonly used enzymatic debriding agent is collangese ointment, which has shown to be safe and effective.[16] This enzyme is derived from clostridium histolyticum.[17] This enzyme digests denatured collagen, which is the principal constituent of necrotic tissue, and destroys the stands of endogenous collagen, which tend to anchor necrotic residues to the bed the of the wound.

TOPICAL DRESSINGS

In a systematic review of randomized controlled trials of hydrocolloids, foams, alginates, hydrogels, and other dressings for venous ulcers, it was concluded that the specific

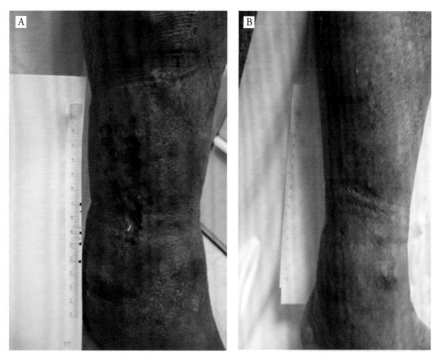

Figure 62.3 A, Chronic leg ulcer before sclerotherapy. This patient presented to our facility with a nonhealing leg ulcer of 10 years duration despite compression therapy. Venous reflux was identified in the greater saphenous vein and tributaries leading to the wound bed. B, Chronic leg ulcer after sclerotherapy. Cannulation of a varicose vein superior to the ulcer allowed for sclerofoam to be manually guided into the superficial varicose vein network beneath the wound bed. Abolition of the distal superficial venous reflux in addition to compression, healed the wound in approximately 6 weeks.

type of dressing applied beneath compression does not affect ulcer healing.[18] However, the role of topical dressings in the venous leg ulcer is to help control infection and maintain an optimal wound-healing environment. Venous wounds may drain moderate to copious amounts of serous and serosanguinous drainage. Because of constant exposure to moisture and types of wound fluid, the periwound skin has the potential to break down as a result of this constant moisture exposure. Therefore, care must be taken to choose the appropriate dressing and the following should be kept in mind while a dressing is being selected; size of the ulcer, amount and type of exudate, granulation or fibrinous debris, and the presence of necrotic tissue or infection. Wound dressings are divided into nine major categories; transparent films, absorptive dressings, foams, alginates, hydrocolloids, collagen based, hydrogels, antimicrobial dressings, and woven gauze dressings. Most occlusive dressings are contraindicated with infected wounds. The classes of wound dressings frequently used in the management of the venous ulcer are described below and are summarized in Table 62.2.

Hydrofibers are a form of absorptive dressings for wounds that are highly exudative. This product combined with wound drainage turns into a wound gel, keeping the wound bed moist. Some of these products have impregnated silver (antimicrobial coverage) to decrease the bioburden within the wound bed. Examples of hydrofibers are Aquacel, Versiva, and Aquacel Silver.

Foams are used to control drainage from highly exudative wounds. Foams are manufactured as either a polyurethane or silicone foam. They provide insulation and protection to the wound bed from large amounts of moisture. Some of the more commonly used foams are Allevyn, Lyofoam, and Coloplast.

Alginates are produced from the naturally occurring calcium and sodium salts of alginic acid found in brown seaweed (*Phaeophyceae*). These dressings have the capacity to absorb large amounts of wound drainage protecting the periwound skin from excessive moisture and eventual maceration. These dressings work well under Unna boots or multilayer compression dressings. Alginates are used as a secondary dressings, such as Kaltostat or Restore.

Hydrocolloid dressings include sodium carboxymethylcellulose, gelatin, pectin, elastomers, and adhesives that are bonded to a carrier of semipermeable film to produce an occlusive, adhesive dressing that forms a gel on the wound surface. This gel promote moisture in clean, low- to medium-exudate wounds. These dressings will break down necrotic tissue and begin the process of debridement but are not recommended to be used under compression dressings. They may be changed only every 3–5 days for best results. Examples are Comfeel, Duoderm, and Restore.

Hydrogels involve the topical application of moisture to a wound bed to keep the wound moist and hydrated. They occur in the form of matrix sheets or amorphous gels that have 20–90% water. They have mild autolytic debridement capabilities and are commonly used for sloughy or necrotic

Table 62.2 WOUND DRESSINGS DESCRIPTIONS AND INDICATIONS

CLASSIFICATION	DESCRIPTION	INDICATIONS	CONTRAINDICATIONS	PRODUCT EXAMPLES
Foams	Foams are used to control drainage from highly exudative wounds.	- Moderate to high exudate wounds - Granular or necrotic wounds - Infected wounds if changed regularly	- Dry wounds - Fragile surrounding skin (adhesive foams)	- Allevyn - Coloplast - CarraSmart Foam - Curafoam - Lyofoam - Mepilex - Mitraflex
Alginates	Seaweed derived dressings that have the capacity to absorb large amounts of wound drainage	- Moderate to heavy exudate wounds. - granular or necrotic wounds	- dry or low exudate wounds	- Carrasorb H - Comfeel Seasorb - Curasorb - Melgisorb - Tegagen - Kaltostat
Hydrocolloids	Dressing that forms a moist gel on the wound bed	- Low exudate wounds - Partial or full-thickness - Granular or necrotic wounds - May be used over absorptive wound fillers, alginates, or hydrogels depending on amount of drainage	- Infected wounds - Wounds with heavy exudate - Fragile surrounding skin	- CarraSmart - Duoderm - Exuderm - Hydrocol - Procol - Restore - Tegasorb - Ultec
Hydrogels	Topical application of moisture to a wound bed to keep the wound moist and hydrated	sloughy or necrotic wounds. Dry to minimally exudating wounds	- high exudate wounds where the wounds should be kept dry to reduce the risk of infection	- Curafil - Intrasite - Tegasorb
Antimicrobial Dressings	Sheets, pastes, foams, films or gauze dressings with antimicrobial properties	- infected wounds - for prevention of infection and bacterial colonization of wounds	- allergies to ingredients	Silver Based - Acticoat - Actisorb - Arglaes Cadexomer Iodine - iodosorb gel

wounds. They are not indicated for wounds producing high exudate, where the wounds should be kept dry to reduce the risk of infection. Common examples are Intrasite, Curafil, and Tegasorb.

Antimicrobial dressings are used for locally infected or colonized wounds. Silver in ionic form, has been used an antimicrobial agent for years in silver sulfadiazine cream. A disadvantage is that it can cause hypersensitivity reactions and should be avoided in patients who have known sulfonamide allergies. Impregnated silver dressings such as Acticoat and Aquacel Silver combine a silver dressing with foam for exudative wounds. Iodine dressings can also be used to reduce the bacterial load in chronic wounds. Iodosorb is a cadexomer iodine which has absorptive properties for wound debrid.

The use of inappropriate wound dressings may result in hypersensitivity reactions, maceration or worsening of the wound and cause infection.

PHARMACOLOGIC TREATMENT

DAFLON

Daflon is a potent venotropic during used in the treatment of CVI. It is a micronized purified flavonoid fraction (MPFF) containing Diosmin and Flavonoids expressed as Hesperidin. MPFFs are described in Chapter 61. Guidelines of the American College of Chest Physicians recommend Daflon to be added to compression (Grade 2B) in the treatment of venous leg ulcers in patients with venous thromboembolic disease.[19]

PENTOXIFYLLINE

Pentoxifylline is a xanthine derivative used in the treatment of peripheral vascular disease. Although it is often classified as a vasodilator, pentoxifylline's primary action reduces blood viscosity, probably due to its effect on erythrocyte deformability, platelet adhesion, and aggregation. Pentoxifylline also inhibits production of cytokine tumor necrosis factor alpha (TNF-a). Studies suggest that pentoxifylline may be effective in increasing the healing rate of chronic venous ulcers with or without compression therapy but at a higher dose than is used for treating claudication (400 mg, three times daily).[20]

OTHER THERAPIES

Negative pressure wound therapy (NPWT)[21] has been shown to increase the rate of granulation tissue formation,[22] significantly decrease wound surface area compared with non-vacuum-treated wounds,[23] and reduce the duration of therapy as compared with standard gauze dressing application.[24] There is no strong evidence to support the physiology behind NPWT, which lies in its ability to remove excess interstitial fluid and reduce interstitial pressure to values below capillary pressure. This improves the microcirculation of periwound tissue.[1]

The viscoelastic nature of skin allows for slow deformation over time with applied mechanical forces, resulting in an increased mitotic rate of stretched tissues with subsequent new tissue production.[1,25,26] Furthermore, applied mechanical forces have been shown to activate the vascular endothelial cell growth factor pathway.[1] The vacuum-assisted device was initially directed toward chronic and difficult-to-treat wounds.[27]

MIST ultrasound therapy (MIST Therapy System; Celleration, Inc., Eden Prairie, MN) is a noncontact delivery of ultrasound frequency energy to treatment sites.[28] It transmits a low-intensity (0.1–0.8 W/cm²) low-frequency ultrasound (40 kHz) via a saline mist and has been reported to improve healing in chronic lower extremity wounds[29,30] associated with neuropathic disease, limb ischemia, chronic renal insufficiency, inflammatory connective tissue disease, diabetic foot disease,[31] and venous stasis disease.[32] Other beneficial effects have been observed in the healing of bony and ligamentous injuries[33–37] as well as partial and full thickness burn wounds.[38]

There are two general mechanisms thought to be responsible for the efficacy of MIST therapy on wound healing.[39] *Cavitation* occurs when the ultrasound energy generates micron-sized bubbles within the mist and fluids within the tissues being treated. Bubbles of the appropriate size will resonate with the ultrasound frequency and deliver the ultrasonic energy to the tissue and cellular level. *Microstreaming* occurs when fluid is moved by the ultrasound energy around and along cell membranes and other acoustic boundaries.[10,40,41] It is thought that the combination of microstreaming and cavitation can effect changes on cell membrane activation.[42]

MIST therapy has been demonstrated to affect leukocyte adhesion, macrophage activity, growth factor production,

collagen production, angiogenesis, fibrinolysis, nitric oxide production, and fibroblast extracellular regulated kinase/jun-N-terminal kinase (ERK/JNK) activation.[43–50] Other reported effects of MIST therapy include statistically significant reduction in bacterial bioburden within 2 weeks of treatment, notably in staphylococcal and beta hemolytic streptococcal species.[51]

Limited evidence suggests that MIST therapy promotes wound healing when used in conjunction with standard wound therapy.[52] A variety of wounds have been treated adjunctively with MIST therapy including those associated with neuropathic disease, limb ischemia, venous insufficiency, and trauma, as well as poorly healing surgical wounds.[32]

Pulsed electromagnetic field therapy (PEMF therapy) involves exposure of a wound to a pulsed electromagnetic field. The application of this field induces a field effect in the treated area,[53] creating currents within the tissue, leading to various downstream biochemical effects.

There exist a few theories explaining the mechanism of action of how PEMF works to augment wound healing. Rohde et al.[54] analyzed wound exudates for levels of TNF-α, vascular endothelial growth factor (VEGF), fibroblast growth factor 2 (FGF-2), and interleukin 1-β (IL-1β) in patients who had undergone breast reduction for symptomatic macromastia and found a much lower concentration of IL-1β in patients treated with PEMF. This reduction was likely responsible for reducing postoperative pain through an improved wound-healing mechanism. An earlier study found that genetic disruption of IL-1 signaling diminished wound fibrosis and collagen deposition, which improved both the architecture of skin as well as tensile strength.[55,56]

PEMF also promotes nitric oxide (NO) production. Fitzsimmons et al.[57] exposed chondrocytes to PEMF, and within 30 minutes of exposure, the chondrocyte culture medium was measured to have significantly higher levels of NO and cyclic guanosine monophosphate (cGMP). Furthermore, increasing calcium in the culture medium produced the same effects, and introducing a calcium/calmodulin inhibitor to the medium obliterated the effect of PEMF on NO. The effects of NO include microvascular dilatation independent of any thermal effects.[58]

Aside from microvascular dilatation, PEMF has also been shown to increase FGF-2 production, augmenting angiogenesis[59] as well as improving wound-healing rates.[60] Other studies have demonstrated reduced wound contracture,[61] increased epithelialization in the early stages of wound repair,[40] increased tensile strength of wounds,[62] and histological demonstration of accelerated wound healing.[63]

PEMF's applications include adjunctive therapy in pressure ulcers,[33] reduction of postoperative pain,[34] and orthopedic nonunions/delayed fractures. Currently, human subject studies on the efficacy of PEMF therapy for soft-tissue injuries demonstrate promising effects on both bony- and soft-tissue healing.[64]

Strong evidence to support the use of NPWT, PEMF, and MIST in the treatment of venous leg ulcers is lacking, but worth mentioning as it may be beneficial for a specific patient.

GROWTH FACTORS

Platelet leukocyte gel (PLG) is produced from whole blood by point-of-care devices that fractionate a patient's blood into various components, including platelet-leukocyte rich plasma (P-LRP).[65,66] The P-LRP can be extracted in various settings whether intraoperatively or in an outpatient clinic. When mixed with thrombin, P-LRP becomes activated, yielding a viscous mixture called PLG,[67] which can be applied to soft tissue wounds in the form of a spray or gel.[46] PLG functions by creating an optimal wound healing environment rich in growth factors that are released from α granules when platelets are activated.[68] PLG has been shown to have a variety of effects, from triggering peripheral blood mononuclear cells to release proinflammatory and proangiogenic cytokines,[69] to stimulating the proliferation of human fibroblasts in a dose-dependent fashion.[70]

Various studies have been performed showing the efficacy of platelet gel on wound healing. Surgical wound healing in horses treated with PLG demonstrated faster epithelial differentiation and increased organization of dermal collagen compared to controls.[71] Used on chronic venous stasis ulcers, PLG has been noted to increase granulation tissue formation and promote complete epithelialization of these ulcers.[72] A randomized controlled trial found that diabetic foot ulcers were statistically significantly more likely to heal with PLG application than ulcers treated with a control (saline) gel.[73] PLG has been used in conjunction with fibrin glue and skin grafting,[74] fat grafting,[75] and negative pressure wound therapy[76] to heal chronic ulcers.

SURGICAL STRATEGIES FOR MANAGEMENT OF CHRONIC WOUNDS

Direct closure of wounds involves coaptation of the various tissue layers including muscle, fascia, subcutaneous tissue, and skin. Direct closure is typically not a viable option for venous stasis ulcers, as the tissues surrounding the ulcer are often stiff and friable and lack the elasticity to obtain a tension-free repair, which is essential to avoid secondary wound breakdown due to dehiscence.

A *xenograft* is a biomaterial taken from another animal species for use as a human tissue substitute. OASIS® wound dressing, made from porcine small-intestine submucosa (SIS), is an example of a xenograft, which contains natural extracellular matrix[77] as well as biologically active ECM components including glycosaminoglycans,[78] proteoglycans, fibronectin,[79] and certain growth factors such

as basic fibroblast growth factor (bFGF)[80,81] and transforming growth factor-beta (TGF-β).[82] These active components promote the proliferation and differentiation of various cell types,[83–87] as well as aid in the sequestration of matrix degrading enzymes (i.e., proteoglycans)[88] thereby preventing them from degrading the developing matrix during the wound-healing process.[56]

In a randomized trial, Mostow et al. found that a statistically significantly greater proportion of venous stasis ulcers healed when SIS was applied to the wounds each week in conjunction with compression therapy. They compared the study group to standard compression therapy alone and studied the effects of the wounds over a 12-week period.[56]

Skin grafts can be used to cover open wounds by healing into the wound bed through three phases. Plasmatic imbibition occurs during the first 24–48 hours and involves passive fluid and nutrient absorption into the graft by diffusion. Inosculation occurs during days 2–3 as connections form between the vasculature of the wound bed and the cut blood vessels in the dermis of the graft. During capillary ingrowth on days 2–5, new blood vessels grow into the graft.[89]

Skin grafting can involve split thickness skin grafts (STSG), which contain epidermis and a variable thickness of dermis. These grafts have a better chance of "take" to the recipient site under less favorable conditions such as a poorly vascularized and edematous wound bed. The disadvantages include contraction, abnormal pigmentation, and easy susceptibility to trauma.

Full thickness skin grafts (FTSG) contain epidermis and all of the underlying dermis. To obtain wound closure, the donor site requires direct closure or additional skin grafting. The main disadvantage is that FTSGs require a well-vascularized wound bed. Advantages include minimal skin graft contraction, better resistance to trauma due to increased thickness, and a more natural aesthetic result.[90]

There are a variety of sources of skin grafts. These include autografts, which are taken from one part of an individual's body and transferred to a different part of that same individual. Allografts are taken from a different individual of the same species. Cadaveric grafts are taken from deceased human subjects. Physician clinical experience has attested to the efficacy of autografting for coverage of venous ulcers, especially when used concomitantly with compression stockings.[91–93]

Artifical skin substitutes have been shown effective in covering venous stasis ulcers. *Apligraf* (Organogenesis, Canton, MA) is a bilayered skin substitute with an epidermal layer consisting of human keratinocytes and a dermal layer composed of human fibroblasts in a bovine Type I collagen matrix. Indications for its use include noninfected partial and full thickness venous ulcers that have been present for greater than 1 year. When applied in conjunction with compression therapy as compared with compression therapy alone (Unna's boot), patients achieved wound closure at a significantly faster rate (181 days versus not attained; p <

0.005).[94] *Dermagraft* (Advanced BioHealing, Westport, CT) is a human fibroblast-derived dermal replacement consisting of a bioresorbable three-dimensional scaffold containing growth factors, matrix proteins, and glycosaminoglycans, on which fibroblasts derived from human newborn foreskin are cultured to produce metabolically active tissue. Hydrolytic degradation takes place, leaving biologically active cellular and extracellular components in the wound bed encouraging epithelialization.[95] Dermagraft has been shown to be associated with improved healing of venous ulceration.[96] High rates of recurrence are anticipated when not used in conjunction with compressive bandage therapy.

Flap reconstruction, although beyond the scope of this chapter, is a further level of surgical reconstruction available for wound coverage. Flaps may incorporate skin, fascia, muscle, or combinations of these various tissue types. The various local, regional, and free tissue flaps, which include their own native blood supply, are typically reserved to reconstruct recalcitrant venous ulcers.[97]

RECALCITRANT ULCERS THAT PERSIST DESPITE OPTIMIZATION

Malignant skin changes are common in chronic leg ulcers. A biopsy should be taken from all suspicious ulcers or ulcers that fail to improve with local care over a 4-week period of time.[98–99]

REFERENCES

1. Korber A, Klode J, Al-Benna S, et al. Etiology of chronic leg ulcers in 31,619 patients in Germany analyzed by an expert survey, *J Dtsch Dermatol Ges*. 2011. *9*(2): 116–121.
2. Obermayer A, Garzon K. Identifying the source of superficial reflux in venous leg ulcers using duplex ultrasound, *J Vasc Surg*. 2010. *52*(5): 1255–1261.
3. Gohel MS, Barwell JR, Taylor M, et al. Long term results of compression therapy alone versus compression plus surgery in chronic venous ulceration (ESCHAR): Randomised controlled trial, *Br Med J*. 2007. *335*(7610): 83.
4. Margolis DJ, Berlin JA, Strom BL. Risk factors associated with the failure of a venous leg ulcer to heal, *Arch Dermatol*. 1999. *135*(8): 920–926.
5. Sackheim K, Dearaujo T, et al. Compression modalities and dressings: Their use in venous ulcers, *Dermatol Ther*. 2006. *19*: 338–347.
6. O'Meara S, Cullum N, Nelson EA, Dumville JC. Compression for venous leg ulcers. *Cochrane Database Syst Rev*. 2012. *11*: CD000265.
7. Tassiopoulos AK, Golts E, Oh DS, Labropoulos N. Current concepts in chronic venous ulceration, *Eur J Vasc Endovasc Surg*. 2000. *20*(3): 227–232.
8. Ioannou CV, Giannoukas AD, Kostas T, et al. Patterns of venous reflux in limbs with venous ulcers. Implications for treatment, *Int Angiol*. 2003. *22*(2): 182–187.
9. Bunke N, Brown K, Bergan J. Foam sclerotherapy: Techniques and uses, *Perspect Vasc Surg Endovasc Ther*. 2009. *21*(2): 91–93.
10. Alden PB, Lips EM, Zimmerman KP, et al. Chronic venous ulcer: Minimally invasive treatment of superficial axial and perforator vein reflux speeds healing and reduces recurrence, *Ann Vasc Surg*. 2013. *27*(1): 75–83.
11. O'Meara S, Al-Kurdi D, Ologun Y, Ovington LG. Antibiotics and antiseptics for venous leg ulcers, *Cochrane Database Syst Rev*. 2010. *1*: CD003557. doi:10.1002/14651858.CD003557.pub3. Review. PubMed PMID: 20091548.
12. Gjodsbol K, Christensen JJ, Karlsmark T, Jorgensen B, Klein BM, Krogfelt KA. Multiple bacterial species reside in chronic wounds: A longitudinal study, *Int Wound J*. 2006. *3*(3): 225–231.
13. Bjarnsholt T, Kirketerp-Moller K, Jensen PØ, et al. Why chronic wounds will not heal: A novel hypothesis, *Wound Rep Reg*. 2008. *16*(1): 2–10. doi: 10.1111/j.
14. Robson MC, Cooper DM, Aslam R, et al. Guidelines for the treatment of venous ulcers, *Wound Rep Reg*. 2006. *14*: 649–662.
15. Ayello EA, Dowsett C, Schultz GS, et al. TIME heals all wounds, *Nursing*. 2004. *34*(4): 36–41; quiz, 41–42.
16. Ramundo J, Gray M. Collagenase for enzymatic debridement: A systematic review, *J Wound Ostomy Continence Nurs*. 2009. *36*(Suppl 6): S4–S11.
17. Marazzi M, Stefani A, et al. Effect of enzymatic debridement with collagenase on acute and chronic hard to heal wounds, *J Wound Care*. 2006. *15*(5): 222–227.
18. O'Donnell TF Jr, Lau J. A systematic review of randomized controlled trials of wound dressings for chronic venous ulcer, *J Vasc Surg*. 2006. *44*(5): 1118–1125. Review.
19. Whitlock RP, Sun JC, Fremes SE, Rubens FD, Teoh KH, American College of Chest Physicians. Antithrombotic and thrombolytic therapy for valvular disease: Antithrombotic Therapy and Prevention of Thrombosis, 9th ed: American College of Chest Physicians Evidence-Based Clinical Practice Guidelines. *Chest*. 2012. *141*(Suppl 2): e576S–600S.
20. Jull AB, Arroll B, Parag V, Waters J. Pentoxifylline for treating venous leg ulcers, *Cochrane Database Syst Rev*. 2012. *12*: CD001733.
21. Morykwas MJ, Simpson J, Punger K, et al. Vacuum-assisted closure: State of basic research and physiologic foundation, *Plast Reconstr Surg*. 2006. *117*: 121S–126S.
22. Morykwas MJ, Faler BJ, Pearce DJ, et al. Effects of varying levels of subatmospheric pressure on the rate of granulation tissue formation in experimental wounds in swine, *Ann Plast Surg*. 2001. *47*: 547–551.
23. Moues CM, Vos MC, van den Bemd GJ, et al. Bacterial load in relation to vacuum-assisted closure wound therapy: A prospective randomized trial, *Wound Repair Regen*. 2004. *12*: 11–17.
24. Moues CM, van den Bemd GJ, Heule F, et al. Comparing conventional gauze therapy to vacuum-assisted closure wound therapy: A prospective randomised trial. *J Plast Reconstr Aesthet Surg*. 2007. *60*: 672–681.
25. Austad ED, Thomas SB, Pasyk K. Tissue expansion: Dividend or loan? *Plast Reconstr Surg*. 1986. *78*: 63–67.
26. Olenius M, Dalsgaard CJ, Wickman M. Mitotic activity in expanded human skin, *Plast Reconstr Surg*. 1993. *91*: 213–216.
27. Argenta LC, Morykwas MJ. Vacuum-assisted closure: A new method for wound control and treatment: Clinical experience. *Ann Plast Surg*. 1997. *38*: 563–576; discussion 577.
28. Kavros SJ, Miller JL, Hanna SW. Treatment of ischemic wounds with noncontact, low-frequency ultrasound: The Mayo Clinic experience, 2004–2006, *Adv Skin Wound Care*. 2007. *20*: 221–226.
29. Ennis WJ, Valdes W, Gainer M, Meneses P. Evaluation of clinical effectiveness of MIST ultrasound therapy for the healing of chronic wounds, *Adv Skin Wound Care*. 2006. *19*: 437–446.
30. Kavros SJ, Schenck EC. The use of noncontact low frequency ultrasound in the treatment of chronic foot and leg ulcerations: A 51 patient analysis, *J Am Podiatr Med Assoc*. 2007. *97*(2): 95–101.
31. Ennis WJ, Foremann P, Mozen N, Massey J, Conner-Kerr T, Meneses P. Ultrasound therapy for recalcitrant diabetic foot ulcers: Results of a randomized, double-blind, controlled, multicenter study, *Ostomy Wound Manage*. 2005. *51*(8): 24–39.

32. Al-Kurdi D, Bell-Syer SEM, Flemming K. Therapeutic ultrasound for venous leg ulcers. *Cochrane Database Syst Rev.* 2008. *1*: CD001180.

33. Warden SJ, Fuchs RK, Kessler CK, Avin KG, Cardinal RE, Stewart RL. Ultrasound produced by a conventional therapeutic ultrasound unit accelerates fracture repair, *Phys Ther.* 2006. *86*: 1118–1127.

34. Warden SJ, Avin KG, Beck EM, DeWolf ME, Hagemeier MA, Martin KM. Low-intensity pulsed ultrasound accelerates and a non-steroidal anti-inflammatory drug delays knee ligament healing, *Am J Sports Med.* 2006. *34*: 1094–1102.

35. Jingushi S, Mizuno K, Matsushita T, Itoman M. Low-intensity pulsed ultrasound treatment for postoperative delayed union or nonunion of long bone fractures, *J Orthop Sci.* 2007. *12*(1): 35–41.

36. Stein H, Lerner A. How does pulsed low-intensity ultrasound enhance fracture healing?, *Orthopedics.* 2005. *28*: 1161–1163.

37. [[Please provide the 37th endnote text]]

38. Samies J, Gehling M. Acoustic pressure wound therapy for management of mixed partial and full thickness burns in a rural wound center, *Ostomy Wound Management.* 2008. *54*(3): 56–59.

39. Webster DF, Pond JB, Dyson M, Harvey W. The role of cavitation in the in vitro stimulation of protein synthesis in human fibroblasts by ultrasound, *Ultrasound Med Biol.* 1978. *4*: 343–351.

40. Sussman C, Dyson M. Therapeutic and diagnostic ultrasound. In: Sussman C, Bates-Jensen B, eds. *Wound care: A collaborative practice manual for physical therapists and nurses,* 2e. Gaithersburg, MD: Aspen. 2001. 596–616.

41. Dijkmans PA, Juffermans LJ, Musters RJ, et al. Microbubbles and ultrasound: From diagnosis to therapy. *Eur J Echocardiogr.* 2004. *5*: 245–256.

42. Dinno MA, Dyson M, Young SR, Mortimer AJ, Hart J, Crum LA. The significance of membrane changes in the safe and effective use of therapeutic and diagnostic ultrasound, *Phys Med Biol.* 1989. *34*: 1543–1552.

43. Maxwell L, Collecutt T, Gledhill M, Sharma S, Edgar S, Gavin JB. The augmentation of leucocyte adhesion to endothelium by therapeutic ultrasound, *Ultrasound Med Biol.* 1994. *20*: 383–390.

44. Ito M, Azuma Y, Ohta T, Komoriya K. Effects of ultrasound and 1,25-dihydroxyvitamin D3 on growth factor secretion in co-cultures of osteoblasts and endothelial cells, *Ultrasound Med Biol.* 2000. *26*: 161–166.

45. Doan N, Reher P, Meghji S, Harris M. In vitro effects of therapeutic ultrasound on cell proliferation, protein synthesis, and cytokine production by human fibroblasts, osteoblasts, and monocytes, *J Oral Maxillofac Surg.* 1999. *57*: 409–419; discussion 420.

46. Young SR, Dyson M. The effect of therapeutic ultrasound on angiogenesis, *Ultrasound Med Biol.* 1990. *16*: 261–269.

47. Young SR, Dyson M. Macrophage responsiveness to therapeutic ultrasound, *Ultrasound Med Biol.* 1990. *16*: 809–816.

48. Francis CW, Onundarson PT, Carstensen EL, et al. Enhancement of fibrinolysis in vitro by ultrasound, *J Clin Invest.* 1992. *90*: 2063–2068.

49. Reher P, Harris M, Whiteman M, Hai HK, Meghji S. Ultrasound stimulates nitric oxide and prostaglandin E2 production by human osteoblasts, *Bone.* 2002. *31*: 236–241.

50. Lai J, Pittelkow MR. Physiological effects of ultrasound mist on fibroblasts, *Int J Dermatol.* 2007. *46*: 587–593.

51. Serena T, Lee KS, Lam K, et al. The impact of non contact, non thermal, low frequency ultrasound on bacterial counts in experimental and chronic wounds, *Ostomy Wound Management.* 2009. *55*(1): 22–30.

52. Ramundo J, Gray M. Is ultrasonic mist therapy effective for debriding chronic wounds?, *J Wound Ostomy Continence Nurs.* 2008. *35*(6): 579–583.

53. Gupta A, Taly AB, Srivastava A, et al. Efficacy of pulsed electromagnetic field therapy in healing of pressure ulcers: A randomized controlled trial, *Neurology India.* 2009. *57*(5).

54. Rohde C, Chiang A, Adipoju O, Casper D, Pilla AA. Effects of pulsed electromagnetic fields on il-1β and post operative pain: A double-blind, placebo-controlled pilot study in breast reduction patients. *Plast Reconstr Surg.* 2010. *125*(6): 1620–1629. doi:10.1097/PRS.0b013e3181c9f6d3

55. Gharaee-Kermani M, Phan SH. Role of cytokines and cytokine therapy in wound healing and fibrotic diseases, *Curr Pharm Des.* 2001. *7*: 1083–1103.

56. Thomay AA, Daley JM, Sabo E, et al. Disruption of interleukin-1 signaling improves the quality of wound healing, *Am J Pathol.* 2009. *174*(6): 2129–2136.

57. Fitzsimmons RJ, Gordon SL, Kronberg J, Ganey T, Pilla AA. A pulsing electric field (PEF) increases human chondrocyte proliferation through a transduction pathway involving nitric oxide signaling, *J Orthop Res.* 2008. *26*: 854–859.

58. Smith TL, Wong-Gibbons D, Maultsby J. Microcirculatory effects of pulsed electromagnetic fields, *J Orthop Res.* 2004. *22*: 80–84.

59. Tepper OM, Callaghan MJ, Chang EI, et al. Electromagnetic fields increase in vitro and in vivo angiogenesis through endothelial release of FGF-2, *FASEB J.* 2004. *18*(11): 1231–1233.

60. Callaghan MJ, Chang EI, Seiser N, et al. Pulsed electromagnetic fields accelerate normal and diabetic wound healing by increasing endogenous FGF-2 release, *Plast Reconstr Surg.* 2007. *121*(1): 130–141.

61. Milgram J, Shahar R, Levin-Harrus T, et al. The effect of short, high intensity magnetic field pulses on the healing of skin wounds in rats, *Bioelectromagnetics.* 2004. *25*: 271–277.

62. Strauch B, Patel MK, Navarro JA, Berdichevsky M, Yu HL, Pilla AA. Pulsed magnetic fields accelerate cutaneous wound healing in rats, *Plast Reconstr Surg.* 2007. *120*(2): 425–430.

63. Athanasiou A, Karkambounas S, Batistatou A, et al. The effect of pulsed electromagnetic fields on secondary skin wound healing: An experimental study, *Bioelectromagnetics.* 2007. *28*: 362–368.

64. Akai A, Hayashi K. Effect of electrical stimulation on musculoskeletal systems: A meta-analysis of controlled clinical trials, *Bioelectromagnetics.* 2002. *23*(2): 132–143.

65. Landesberger R, Moses M, Karpatkin M. Risks of using platelet rich plasma, *J Oral Maxillofac Surg.* 1998. *56*: 1116–1117.

66. Weibrich G, Kleis WKG, Hafner G. Growth factor levels in the platelet-rich plasma produced by 2 different methods: Curasan-type PRP kit versus PCCS PRP system, *Int J Oral Maxillofac Imp.* 2002. *17*: 184–190.

67. Everts PA, Overdevest EP, Jakimowicz JJ, et al. The use of autologous platelet–leukocyte gels to enhance the healing process in surgery: A review, *Surg Endosc.* 2007. *21*: 2063–2068.

68. Zucker-Franklin C. The relationship of alpha granules to the membrane system of platelets and megakaryocytes, *Blood Cells.* 1989. *15*: 73–79.

69. Naldini A, Morena E, Fimiani M, et al. The effects of autologous platelet gel on inflammatory cytokine response in human peripheral blood mononuclear cells, *Platelets.* 2008. *19*(4): 268–274.

70. Krasna M, Domanović D, Tomsic A, et al. Platelet gel stimulates proliferation of human dermal fibroblasts in vitro, *Acta Dermatovenerol Alp Panonica Adriat.* 2007. *16*(3): 105–110.

71. DeRossi R, Coelho AC, de Mello GS. Effects of platelet-rich plasma gel on skin healing in surgical wound in horses. *Acta Cir Bras.* 2009. *24*(4): 276–281.

72. Ficarelli E, Bernuzzi G, Tognetti E, et al. Treatment of chronic venous leg ulcers by platelet gel, *Dermatol Ther.* 2008. *21*(Suppl 1): S13–S17.

73. Driver VR, Hanft J, Fylling CP, Beriou JM, AutoloGel™ Diabetic Foot Ulcer Study Group. A prospective, randomized, controlled trial of autologous platelet-rich plasma gel for the treatment of diabetic foot ulcers, *Ostomy/Wound Manag.* 2006. *52*(6): 68–87.

74. Chen TM, Tsai JC, Burnouf T. A novel technique combining platelet gel, skin graft, and fibrin glue for healing recalcitrant lower extremity ulcers, *Dermatol Surg.* 2010. *36*(4): 453–460.

75. Cervelli V, Gentile P, Grimaldi M. Regenerative surgery: Use of fat grafting combined with platelet-rich plasma for chronic lower-extremity ulcers, *Aesthetic Plast Surg.* 2009. *33*(3): 340–345.

76. Gurvich L. Synergism in using negative pressure wound therapy with alternated applications of autologous platelet-derived growth factors, *Wounds.* 2009. *21*(5): 134–140.

77. Mostow EN, Haraway DG, Dalsing M, et al. Effectiveness of an extracellular matrix graft (OASIS Wound Matrix) in the treatment of chronic leg ulcers: A randomized clinical trial, *J Vasc Surg.* 2005. *41*: 837–843.

78. Hodde JP, Badylak SF, Brightman AO, Voytik-Harbin SL. Glycosaminoglycan content of small intestinal submucosa: A bioscaffold for tissue replacement, *Tissue Eng.* 1996. *2*: 209–217.

79. McPherson TB, Badylak SF. Characterization of fibronectin derived from porcine small intestinal submucosa, *Tissue Eng.* 1998. *4*: 75–83.

80. Hodde JP, Hiles MC. Bioactive FGF-2 in sterilized extracellular matrix, *Wounds.* 2001. *13*: 195–201.

81. Hodde JP, Ernst DMJ, Hiles MC. Bioactivity of FGF-2 in Oasis wound matrix after prolonged storage, *J Wound Care.* 2005. *14*: 23–25.

82. McDevitt CA, Wildey GM, Cutrone RM. Transforming growth factor-β1 in a sterilized tissue derived from the pig small intestine submucosa, *J Biomed Mater Res.* 2003. *67A*: 637–640.

83. Hodde JP, Badylak SF, Brightman AO, Voytik-Harbin SL. Glycosaminoglycan content of small intestinal submucosa: A bioscaffold for tissue replacement, *Tissue Eng.* 1996. *2*: 209–217.

84. McPherson TB, Badylak SF. Characterization of fibronectin derived from porcine small intestinal submucosa, *Tissue Eng.* 1998. *4*: 75–83.

85. Hodde JP, Hiles MC. Bioactive FGF-2 in sterilized extracellular matrix, *Wounds.* 2001. *13*: 195–201.

86. Hodde JP, Ernst DMJ, Hiles MC. Bioactivity of FGF-2 in Oasis wound matrix after prolonged storage, *J Wound Care.* 2005. *14*: 23–25.

87. McDevitt CA, Wildey GM, Cutrone RM. Transforming growth factor-β1 in a sterilized tissue derived from the pig small intestine submucosa, *J Biomed Mater Res.* 2003. *67A*: 637–640.

88. Yu WH, Woessner JF. Heparan sulfate proteoglycans as extracellular docking molecules for matrilysin (matrix metalloproteinase 7), *J Biol Chem.* 2000. *275*: 4183–4191.

89. Song DH, Henry G, Reid RR, et al. *Plastic and reconstructive surgery essentials for students*, 14e. Arlington Heights, IL: Plastic Surgery Educational Foundation. 2007. 11.

90. Rudolph R, Klein L. Healing processes in skin grafts, *Surg Gynecol Obstet.* 1973. *136*: 641–654.

91. Kirsner RS, Eaglstein WH, Kerdel FA. Split thickness skin grafting for lower extremity ulceration, *Dermatol Surg.* 1997. *23*: 85–91.

92. Reffieux PH, Hommel I, Saurat JH. Long-term assessment of chronic leg ulcer treatment by autologous skin grafts, *Dermatology.* *195*: 77–80.

93. Kirsner RS, Mata SM, Falanga V, Kerdel FA. Split thickness skin grafting of leg ulcers, *Dermatol Surg.* 1995. *21*:701–703.

94. Falanga V, Sabolinski M. A bilayered living skin construct (APLIGRAF) accelerates complete closure of hard-to-heal venous ulcers, *Wound Repair Regen.* 1999. *7*: 201–207.

95. Naughton G, Mansbridge J, Gentzkow G. A metabolically active human dermal replacement for the treatment of diabetic foot ulcers, *Artif Organs.* 1997. *21*: 1203–1210.

96. Omar AA, Mavor AI, Jones AM, et al. Treatment of venous leg ulcers with Dermagraft, *Eur J Vasc Endovasc Surg.* 2004. *27*: 666–672.

97. Kumins NH, Weinzweig N, Schuler JJ. Free tissue transfer provides durable treatment for large nonhealing venous ulcers, *J Vasc Surg.* 2000. *32*: 848–854.

98. Mulder GD, Reis TM. Venous ulcers: Pathophysiology and medical therapy, *Am Fam Physician.* 1990. *42*: 1323–1330.

99. Senet P, Combemale P, Debure C, et al. Malignancy and chronic leg ulcers: The value of systematic wound biopsies: A prospective, multicenter, cross-sectional study, *Arch Dermatol.* 2012. *148*(6): 704–708.

PART V

CONGENITAL VENOUS ABNORMALITIES

63.

VENOUS MALFORMATIONS AND TUMORS

ETIOLOGY, DIAGNOSIS, AND MANAGEMENT

B. B. Lee and James Laredo

INTRODUCTION

Since the early 1900s, there have been numerous documentations of vascular malformations, usually describing only the general/natural appearance of this inborn error,[1] mostly based on anecdotal experiences. Its complicated nature was never properly explained, and it was instead often described under the heading of an eponymous "syndrome" (e.g., Klippel-Trenaunay syndrome), which made it seem more enigmatic.[2,3]

Many clinicians attempted to define the nature of these birth defects. But it was difficult to study this multifaceted condition, which involves various locations of the vascular system in various conditions, extents, and severities. This extreme variety of clinical appearance and unpredictable behavior in general, with the stigma of recurrence, made this entire group of vascular malformations an enigma in modern medicine.

Once condemned and abandoned[4] this disease is now known as congenital vascular malformation (CVM). Many confusing terms (e.g., angiodysplasia, cavernous hemangioma, cystic hygroma/lymphangioma) and eponyms (Klippel-Trenaunay syndrome [KTS], Parkes-Weber syndrome [PWS], and so forth), have been replaced by new terminology and new classification.[5,6] This terminology clears up much of confusion surrounding this unique vascular disorder.

The eponymous syndromes in particular made a tremendous contribution to the understanding of CVM when limited information/knowledge meant that diagnoses were made based solely on the clinical evaluation. But with the current technology available to study and characterize individual vascular malformations, the descriptive role of the eponyms became obsolete, and they now act as a source of confusion for clinicians.[7]

A NEW CONCEPT WITH A NEW CLASSIFICATION

Through the last half of the twentieth century, advanced technology made it possible to more accurately investigate CVMs and develop better understanding; and many newly developed diagnostic and therapeutic modalities corrected previous misunderstandings about CVMs.

The Hamburg classification,[6,7] formulated based on the Hamburg consensus in 1988, has been further modified and now well accepted as the foundation for research on CVMs and clinical practice, providing solid ground on which to gather new information on the etiology and anatomopathophysiology of the CVMs and build a precise definition, evaluation, and therapeutic implementation (Table 63.1).[6-10]

For example, in the new classification, the vascular malformation component of KTS is now properly defined as hemolymphatic malformation (HLM)[6,7] which comprises venous malformation (VM), lymphatic malformation (LM), and capillary malformation (CM). The vascular malformation components of PWS are VM, LM, CM, and arteriovenous malformation (AVM).[8-10]

"Cystic/cavernous hemangioma," once a popular name for the CVMs, is now correctly defined as VM, to prevent unnecessary confusion with a true "hemangioma." Genuine hemangioma represents only "infantile/neonatal" hemangioma, which is not a vascular malformation but a vascular tumor.[11,12] The difference between cystic/cavernous hemangioma and true (infantile/neonatal) hemangioma is so crucial for their clinical management that its importance cannot be overemphasized. True hemangioma is a vascular tumor and can be categorized as a vascular anomaly along with the vascular malformation, but hemangioma generally appears in the early neonatal period as a rapidly growing tumor. Hemangioma also has a distinctive pattern of self-limited growth, with an initial proliferate phase followed by slow regression in an involution phase, and it is generally resolved spontaneously with minimum morbidity before the age of 7 to 9 years[13] (Figure 63.1).

In contrast, VM is generally distinctive on birth as an inborn error and steadily grows commensurably in proportion to the general/systemic growth; it never disappears nor

Table 63.1 **THE MODIFIED HAMBURG CLASSIFICATION OF CONGENITAL VASCULAR MALFORMATIONS**

Primary classification*
- Arterial malformations
- Venous malformations
- Arteriovenous malformations
- Lymphatic malformations
- Capillary malformations
- Combined vascular malformations: Hemolymphatic malformation

Anatomical/Embryological subclassification**
- **Extratruncular forms**
  - Diffuse, infiltrating
  - Limited, localized
- **Truncular forms**
  - Obstruction or narrowing
  - Aplasia; Hypoplasia; Hyperplasia
    - Obstruction due to atresia or membranous occlusion
    - Stenosis due to coarctation, spur, or membrane
  - Dilatation
    - Localized (aneurysm)
    - Diffuse (ectasia)

* Based on the predominant vascular structure in the malformation.

** Based on anatomy and developmental arrest at the different stages of embryonal life:

extratruncular form from earlier stages; truncular form from late stage.

regresses. Therefore, its management is naturally quite different from that of hemangioma.

The original Hamburg classification was further modified to accommodate the entire group of CVMs; it grouped various CVMs based on their predominant component: VM, LM, arterial malformation (AM), AVM, and their combined form named as HLM, in addition to CM. Each malformation was further subgrouped into "extratruncular" and "truncular" subtypes, based on the embryologic stage when the developmental arrest/defect occurred. This is crucial for clinicians to formulate appropriate treatment strategies.[14–17]

ETIOLOGY

VM is the most common CVM together with LM. It is neither a hemangioma nor a vascular tumor; VM is one of the birth defects developed along the venous system as a CVM. The majority of VMs exist as a single, independent malformations, but some exist together with other CVMs (e.g., LM). These combined conditions are separately classified as HLM, often known as Klippel-Trenaunay syndrome (KTS).[2,3]

The "extratruncular" VM lesion is an embryonic tissue remnant derived from an early stage of vascular tissue development (the reticular stage). Developmental arrest occurs before the main vascular trunks are formed (pretruncal embryonic lesions).[14–17] These lesions maintain the unique embryonic characteristics of the mesenchymal cells and the ability to proliferate when stimulated externally (e.g., trauma, surgery, and hormone) or internally (e.g., menarche, pregnancy). This embryologic characteristic has never been properly understood until recently, and poor treatment strategy without appropriate consideration of this critical factor only provoked the dormant/silent lesion to grow rapidly. All extratruncular VM lesions carry this risk of recurrence following ill-planned treatment strategy.

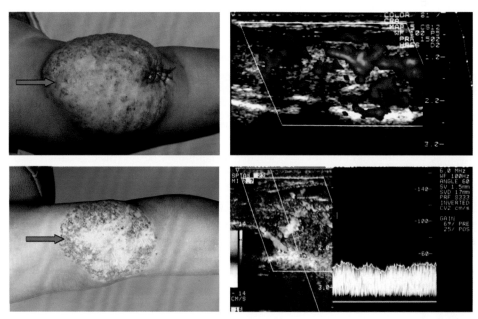

Figure 63.1   Left Column: Top photo depicts a clinical appearance of neonatal hemangioma in its proliferative stage. Due to the alarming rate of the growth, the neonatologist included a tissue biopsy to confirm the clinical diagnosis. The bottom photo shows the outcome of a spontaneous regression of the lesion a year later leaving minimal residual skin change. Right Column: Two photos represent typical duplex ultrasonographic findings of the hemangioma in its proliferative stage.

Extratruncular lesions are further subdivided into diffuse, infiltrating, and localized, limited lesions. Diffuse, infiltrating extratruncular lesions may cause symptoms due to compression of surrounding structures (muscles, nerves). They may also produce significant hemodynamic impact on the involved venous system that is dependent on lesion size and location. Growth is usually slow and proportionate to the person's growth throughout the rest of the person's life. Furthermore, there is no spontaneous regression (cf. hemangioma; Figure 63.2).

In contrast, the "truncular" VM lesion is the result of a developmental arrest that occurs during the "later" stages of vascular trunk formation during fetal development. This arrest occurs long after the embryonic (reticular) stage of vascular development is over.[14–17] These lesions are also known as "posttruncal fetal lesions."

Truncular lesions, therefore, do not have the embryonic characteristic of the mesenchymal cells (angioblasts) as observed in the extratruncular lesions. These lesions do not possess the critical evolutional ability to proliferate. The risk of recurrence after treatment is minimal to none. These lesions have hemodynamic consequences due to congenital valvular incompetence, obstruction (atresia, hypoplasia) or dilatation/aneurysm formation with associated risk of thromboembolism.

Truncular lesions are subdivided into obstruction; aplasia, hypoplasia, or hyperplasia;[18,19] and dilation or aneurysms.[20,21] Immature, incomplete, or abnormal development of the main axial veins results in aplasia, hypoplasia, or hyperplasia of the vessel trunk (e.g., absence of iliac vein, agenesis/rudimentary femoral vein) or in a defective vessel: obstruction (e.g., vein web, spur, annulus, or septum) or dilatation (e.g., popliteal or iliac vein ectasia/aneurysm).

These lesions also manifest as persistent, large, embryonic veins such as the marginal vein or the sciatic vein when a fetal (truncal) vessel fails to undergo normal involution to give complicated hemodynamic impact to the deep vein system.[22,23]

Truncular lesions of an obstructive nature (webs, hypoplasia) may have different hemodynamic impacts on their relevant vascular systems depending on their location, extent/severity, and natural compensation through collaterals. Stenosing truncular lesions may produce venous obstruction leading to a reduction in venous drainage resulting in chronic venous insufficiency in the territory drained by the stenotic vein.

Membranous obstruction of the inferior vena cava in primary Budd-Chiari syndrome is an example of a primary obstructive VM affecting a major hepatic vein outflow to cause portal hypertension. And stenosing lesions of the extracranial jugular veins, superior vena cava, and azygos vein system are also known to cause chronic cerebrospinal venous insufficiency, precipitating multiple sclerosis.[24,25]

Avalvulosis, or absence of valves, is another form of hypoplasia that produces venous reflux. Avalvulosis, atresia of the venous trunks, and venous aneurysms are relatively common. The incidence of aneurysm has been reported to be 4% in nearly 490 cases of congenital anomalies of the venous system.[26]

DIAGNOSIS IN GENERAL

The new concept of the CVM mandated a precise diagnosis to provide accurate information on its histologic, pathologic, hemodynamic, and embryologic characteristics; this new information in turn allowed a new perspective on VM

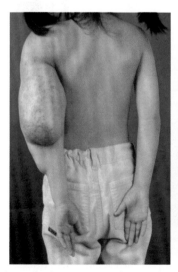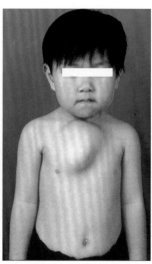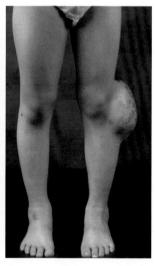

Figure 63.2   Three photos display "extratruncular" VM lesions in various locations; they are an embryonic tissue remnant, so they maintain unique embryological characteristics of the mesenchymal cell and proliferate or grow when stimulated. But the growth is usually slow and proportionate to the person's growth throughout the rest of the person's life. And, there is no spontaneous regression like a hemangioma.

management. Now we know there are many different vascular malformations with different clinical significances other than the VM, but we are able to precisely define the type (e.g., VM, LM, HLM, AVM) and nature (e.g., truncular or extratruncular lesion) of each CVM involved because we have enough knowledge to verify many different aspects of each CVM lesion either existing alone or as combined with other CVMs.[27,28]

Proper clinical evaluation should be based on a thorough history and careful physical examination. Detailed assessment of the VM lesion regarding its extent, severity, and its secondary impact on the related systems/organs should follow, which is also now possible with non- to less-invasive tests alone.[29] Many newly developed tests, mostly noninvasive, can now provide precise diagnosis of VMs and other CVMs to confirm the clinical impression[30] in the majority of VMs: duplex ultrasonography,[31,32] magnetic resonance imaging (MRI),[33,34] whole body blood pool scintigraphy (WBBPS),[35,36] transarterial lung perfusion scintigraphy (TLPS),[37,38] and radionuclide lymphoscintigraphy,[39,40] among others (Table 63.2).

Detailed information on each test has been fully documented in previous publications.[31–40] In most cases the invasive tests (e.g., phlebography) may be reserved for use when needed as a road map for treatment. They may, however, be required for the differential diagnosis of hemangioma or AVM.

The IUP Consensus panel on VMs[41] recommends duplex scanning as the first diagnostic test for all patients with VMs involving the limbs to assess the deep and superficial veins; to identify any aberrant vein, obstruction, dilation, or valvular incompetence; and to define the feeding or draining veins of the VM. This duplex test is safe, noninvasive, cost-effective, and reliable (Grade of recommendation: 1 [strong], level of evidence A [high quality]).[42,43]

Computed tomography (CT) is also recommended by the panel for evaluation of obstructed veins and other truncular anomalies of large veins in the chest, abdomen, or pelvis. CT venography accurately identifies the underlying pathology, confirms venous obstruction or extrinsic compression, and delineates anatomic variations and the extent of venous thrombosis (Grade of Recommendation: 1 [strong], Level of Evidence: B [moderate quality]).[42,43]

MRI and MRV (for magnetic resonance venography) is recommended for evaluation of VMs. The test is reliable, it confirms the extent and type of the VM, delineates feeding and draining vessels, and distinguishes between different soft tissues (muscle, fat) and the vascular structures. This imaging modality is highly accurate in the diagnosis of deep vein thrombosis. MRI and MRV is recommended before performing interventions on VMs, except some small localized VMs (Grade of Recommendation: 1 [strong], Level of Evidence: A [high quality]).[42,43]

Radionuclide lymphoscintigraphy (LSG)[39,40] is essential to rule out lymphatic dysfunction, especially due to the presence of a truncular LM known as primary lymphedema, which often occurs with the VM lesion.

Whole body blood pool scintigraphy (WBBPS), a transvenous angioscan using radioisotope-tagged red blood cells,[35,36] is an optional test to screen for multiple VM lesions scattered throughout the body. It allows qualitative and quantitative evaluation of the VM lesion especially during the course of multisession sclerotherapy as a cost-effective measure. It is an excellent tool for routine follow-up and to assess the progress of treatment and the natural course of the VM lesion

MANAGEMENT

PRINCIPLE

Not all CVMs are equal in terms of clinical management. They should not be treated equally, because they behave differently with different natural course/progress and prognosis.[44] For example, AVM in general is a potentially limb, and/or life threatening condition, but VM is not. Hence, the treatment principles for these two CVMs are inherently different; an AVM requires aggressive treatment regardless of its extent or severity,[45,46] but a VM does not.

The VM, which represents the majority of CVMs, is not a life-threatening condition in general. There are a few unique conditions in which the location of a VM may interfere with or threaten a vital function—seeing, breathing, eating, hearing—or when the proximity of a VM to the active joints presents the risk of injury or trauma (e.g., hemarthrosis).[47] Therefore, the strategy for VM management

Table 63.2 **DIAGNOSTIC TESTS FOR THE VENOUS MALFORMATION**

- **Noninvasive tests**
  - **B-mode to differentiate tumors vs. malformations**
  - **Doppler mode to assess flow characteristics**
- **Minimally invasive tests**
  - **Computed tomography with intravenous contrast**
  - **Magnetic resonance (MR) imaging and MR angiography.**
  - **Whole body blood pool scintigraphy (WBBPS): transvenous angioscan utilizing radioisotope-tagged red blood cells**
  - **Transarterial lung perfusion scintigraphy (TLPS): transarterial angioscan utilizing radioisotope-tagged microsphere albumin**
  - **Radionuclide Lymphoscintigraphy (LSG)**
  - **Microscopic fluorescent lymphangiography**
  - **MR lymphangiography**
  - **Ultrasound lymphangiography-investigational**
  - **Endoscopy/colonoscopy for lesions involving the GI tract.**
- **Invasive diagnostic tests**
  - **Ascending, descending, and/or segmental venography/ phlebography**
  - **Standard and/or selective arteriography**
  - **Percutaneous direct puncture angiography: arteriography, phlebography, varicography, lymphography**

should be different from that for AVM management. Not all the VM lesions require immediate treatment, and the traditional conservative approach is still recommended for the vast majority of VM lesions.[48,49]

A typical VM lesion without abnormal bone growth involvement can be monitored until the age of 2 or more years, when the child is matured enough to tolerate various diagnosis and treatment procedures. But earlier intervention is required when the VM lesion produces the vascular bone syndrome, resulting in discrepancy of long bone growth, or when the lesion is located at a life- or limb-threatening anatomic area, as mentioned above.[50,51]

However, the clinical management of HLM, defined as the coexistence of four different CVMs: AVM, VM, and LM in various combinations,[52,53] is much more complicated because of the interlocking hemodynamic conditions. Additional precaution is mandated when treatment of the VM is required, because it often affects other coexisting CVM negatively, worsening the condition.

MULTIDISCIPLINARY APPROACH

For many decades clinicians challenged this relatively rare vascular condition by surgical means alone. The outcome of a surgical excision based on limited knowledge and experiences was often disastrous; the search for a "cure" as an ultimate and ideal solution often led to surgical excess, resulting in prohibitively high morbidity and complications. Furthermore, following incomplete excision, the extratruncular VMs all recurred, because of their unique embryological characteristics. This led surgeons to mistakenly associate recurrence with all vascular malformations.

Now, based on much improved ability to assess the extent and severity of a VM, including its relationship with surrounding tissues/systems, the decision for treatment and the selection of the treatment modality can be made quite accurately, and a "multidisciplinary team approach" allows a new strategy of combining traditional open surgical therapy with endovascular therapy as a new treatment modality.[54] The traditional surgical treatment[55–57] is now fully integrated with various endovascular therapies[58–60] utilizing modern interventional technology[61] (Table 63.3).

Endovascular therapy with various combinations of emboloscleroagents is now the treatment of choice for "surgically inaccessible" lesions, and open surgical therapy can also be delivered to "surgically accessible" lesions more effectively with much reduced risk of complication and morbidity by perioperative embolosclerotherapy as an adjunct supplemental therapy. Endovascular treatment with sclerotherapy is therefore excellent as an "independent therapy" when surgery is to be avoided, in particular with the diffuse infiltrating type of extratruncular lesion. It is the treatment of choice for extensive lesions beyond deep fascia with involvement of muscle, tendon, and bone (Figure 63.3).

Table 63.3 TREATMENT MODALITIES FOR THE VENOUS MALFORMATION

- Observation and conservative management
- Drug therapy
- Endovascular therapy
  - Ethanol sclerotherapy
  - Sclerotherapy with other liquid sclerosants
  - Ultrasound-guided sclerotherapy with foam sclerosants
  - Fluoroscopic and ultrasound-guided sclerotherapy (FUGS)
  - Embolotherapy with coils, glue, and/or particles embolization
  - Endovenous thermal ablations (laser, radiofrequency, cryoablation)
  - Angioplasty and stent
- Open surgical therapy
- Combined approach: excisional surgery combined with preoperative embolosclerotherapy

But various surgical treatments remain essential for the proper management of the VM. The operation to correct hemodynamic derangement often requires various reconstructive (e.g., venous bypass, venous aneurysmorrhaphy) and/or ablative (excisional) surgery (e.g., removal of marginal vein, excision of the VM lesions; Figure 63.4).

Various orthopedic as well as many plastic and reconstructive surgeries are actively used to correct/improve the consequence of secondary impact of the VM (e.g., Achilles tendon lengthening). But the treatment, either surgical or endovascular, should be undertaken only with appropriate indications, to avoid unnecessary complication and morbidity[62] (Table 63.4); the decision should be made on the basis of the consensus of a multidisciplinary team.

Among various emboloscleroagents available, ethanol is the most powerful scleroagent with excellent long-term

Table 63.4 TREATMENT INDICATIONS FOR THE VENOUS MALFORMATION

- Bleeding
- Signs and symptoms of chronic venous insufficiency (painful varicosity, edema, skin changes, ulcers, recurrent superficial thrombophlebitis)
- Lesions located at a life-threatening region involving or close to vital structures (e.g., proximity to the airway), or located in an area threatening vital functions (e.g., sight, eating, hearing, or breathing)
- Disabling pain
- Functional impairment (e.g., genital region)
- Cosmetically severe deformity
- Lesions located at regions with high risk of complications (e.g., hemarthrosis, thromboembolism)
- Lesions combined producing the vascular-bone syndrome (length discrepancy of the lower extremities, affecting the bone itself) or the destructive angiodysplastic arthritis (Hauert disease)
- Lesions obstructing the outflow and drainage of vital organ (i.e., liver, brain)
- Persistent lymph leak due to a combined lymphatic malformation lesion with/without infection
- Recurrent sepsis, local and/or general, due to a combined lymphatic malformation lesion

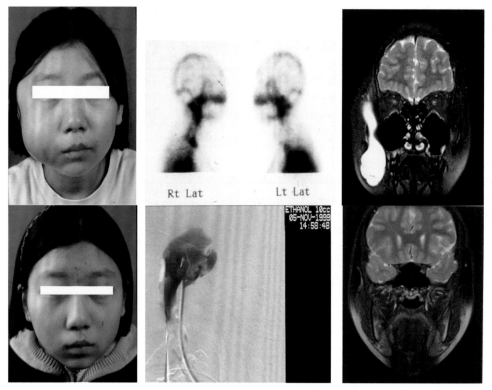

Figure 63.3   Left Column: Two photos present the clinical appearance of the extratruncular VM lesion affecting the right cheek before treatment (top photo) with massive swelling and also after treatment (bottom photo) with satisfactory relief. Middle column: Top photo displays WBBPS (whole body blood pool scintigraphy) findings of the abnormal blood pooling of the VM lesion, and bottom photo shows angiographic findings of the lesion treated with the ethanol sclerotherapy. Right Column: Top photo presents the MRI finding of the lesion before treatment, showing typical intraluminal bleeding, and bottom photo shows the MRI finding of the outcome of the successful therapy 2 years later with complete disappearance of the lesion and no evidence of recurrence.

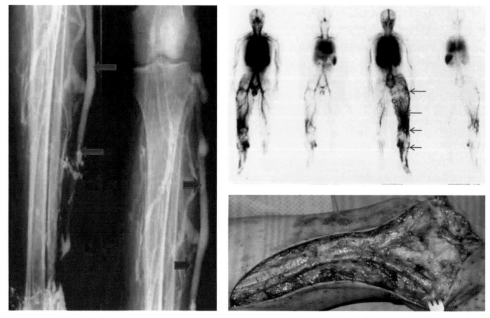

Figure 63.4   Left Column: Two photos, side by side, show the angiographic findings of the marginal vein as a truncular VM along the lateral aspect of the lower leg as the cause of chronic venous insufficiency (CVI). Right Column: Top photo presents the WBBPS (whole body blood pool scintigraphy) findings of same marginal vein running whole lateral aspect of entire right lower extremity up to the gluteal region. Bottom photo depicts surgically exposed marginal vein before the excision to relieve a clinical condition of the CVI.

results/outcome. But it also presents the highest risk of complication/morbidity among the agents; indiscriminating use of ethanol should be discouraged. Not only local (e.g., skin/soft tissue necrosis) and/or regional (e.g., nerve palsy, venous thrombosis) complications, but also systemic complications (e.g., pulmonary spasm) should be anticipated with appropriate preparation.

Recently foam sclerotherapy has gained a momentum over traditional liquid sclerotherapy in the management of VM lesions with excellent interim treatment outcomes and minimum complication/morbidity.[63–65] Although recurrence is high, as expected, it is particularly recommendable for the VM lesion with proximity to the skin or oral mucosa, with or without transdermal extension, to avoid the risk of tissue or skin necrosis: that is, lesions involving finger, palm, toe, sole, oral mucosa, lip and tongue.[66] Repeating therapy to control the recurring lesion makes it possible to maintain favorable results.[66]

CONCLUSION

The VM can be easily diagnosed with proper combination of basic non- to less-invasive tests alone and can also be treated safely following the indications. A Multidisciplinary team approach with fully integrated traditional open surgical therapy with endovascular therapy can improve long-term treatment results with a reduced morbidity and recurrence over the conventional approach.

REFERENCES

1. Malan E. History and nosography. In: Malan E, ed. *Vascular malformations (angiodysplasias)*. Milan, Italy: Carlo Erba Foundation. 1974. 15–19.
2. Klippel M, Trenaunay J. Du noevus variqueux et osteohypertrophique, *Arch Gén Méd*. 1900. 3: 641–672.
3. Servelle M. Klippel and Trenaunay's syndrome: 768 operated cases, *Ann Surg*. 1985. 201(3): 365–373.
4. Szilagyi DE, Smith RF, Elliott JP, Hageman JH. Congenital arteriovenous anomalies of the limbs, *Arch Surg*. 1976. 111: 423–429.
5. Malan E, Puglionisi A. Congenital angiodysplasias of the extremities, note II: Arterial, arterial and venous, and hemolymphatic dysplasias, *J Cardiovasc Surg*. 1965. 6: 255–345.
6. Belov S. Classification, terminology, and nosology of congenital vascular defects. In: Belov S, Loose DA, Weber J, eds. *Vascular malformations*. Reinbek, Germany: Einhorn-Presse. 1989. 25–30.
7. Lee BB, Laredo J, Lee TS, Huh S, Neville R. Terminology and classification of congenital vascular malformations: Special issue, *Phlebology*. 2007. 22(6): 249–252.
8. Belov St. Anatomopathological classification of congenital vascular defects, *Semin Vasc Surg*. 1993. 6: 219–224.
9. Rutherford RB. Classification of peripheral congenital vascular malformations. In: Ernst C, Stanley J, eds. *Current therapy in vascular surgery*, 3e. St. Louis, MO: Mosby. 1995. 834–838.
10. Belov S. Classification of congenital vascular defects, *Int Angiol*. 1990. 9: 141–146.
11. Mulliken JB. Cutaneous vascular anomalies, *Semin Vasc Surg*. 1993. 6: 204–218.

12. Mulliken JB, Glowacki J. Hemangiomas and vascular malformations in infants and children: A classification based on endothelial characteristics, *Plast Reconstr Surg*. 1982. 69: 412–420.
13. Mulliken JB, Zetter BR, Folkman J. In vivo characteristics of endothelium from hemangiomas and vascular malformations, *Surgery*. 1982. 92: 348–353.
14. Van Der Stricht J. Classification of vascular malformations. In: Belov S, Loose DA, Weber J, eds. *Vascular malformations*. Reinbek, Germany: Einhorn-Presse Verlag. 1989. 23.
15. Bastide G, Lefebvre D. Anatomy and organogenesis and vascular malformations. In: Belov S, Loose DA, Weber J, eds. *Vascular malformations*. Reinbek, Germany: Einhorn-Presse Verlag. 1989. 20–22.
16. Woolard HH. The development of the principal arterial stems in the forelimb of the pig, *Contrib Embryol*. 1922. 14: 139–154.
17. Leu HJ. Pathoanatomy of congenital vascular malformations. In: Belov S, Loose DA, Weber J, eds. *Vascular malformations*. Reinbek, Germany: Einhorn-Presse Verlag. 1989. Vol 16, 37–46.
18. Belov S. Congenital agenesis of the deep veins of the lower extremity: Surgical treatment, *J Cardiovasc Surg*. 1972. 13: 594.
19. Lee BB, Villavicencio L, Kim YW, et al. Primary Budd-Chiari syndrome: Outcome of endovascular management for suprahepatic venous obstruction, *J Vasc Surg*. 2006. 43: 101–110.
20. Gillespie DL, Villavicencio JL, Gallagher C, et al. Presentation and management of venous aneurysms, *J Vasc Surg*. 1997. 26: 845–852.
21. Zamboni P, Cossu A, Carpanese L, Simonetti G, Massarelli G, Liboni A. The so-called venous aneurysms, *Phlebology*. 1990. 5: 45–50.
22. Mattassi R. Approach to marginal vein: Current issue, *Phlebology*. 2007. 22(6): 283–286.
23. Kim YW, Lee BB, Cho JH, Do YS, Kim DI, Kim ES. Haemodynamic and clinical assessment of lateral marginal vein excision in patients with a predominantly venous malformation of the lower extremity, *Eur J Vasc Endovasc Surg*. 2007. 33(1): 122–127.
24. San Millan Ruiz D, Gailloud P, Rufenacht DA, Delavelle J, Henry F, Fasel JH. The craniocervical venous system in relation to cerebral venous drainage, *Am J Neuroradiol*. 2002. 23(9): 1500–1508.
25. Zamboni P, Galeotti R, Menegatti E, et al. Chronic cerebrospinal venous insufficiency in patients with multiple sclerosis, *J Neurol Neurosur Ps*. 2009. 80(4): 392–399.
26. Eifert S, Villavicencio JL, Kao TC, Taute BM, Rich NM. Prevalence of deep venous anomalies in congenital vascular malformations of venous predominance, *J Vasc Surg*. 2000. 31: 462–471.
27. Lee BB. Critical issues on the management of congenital vascular malformation, *Annals Vasc Surg*. 2004. 18(3): 380–392.
28. Lee BB, Laredo J, Lee SJ, Huh SH, Joe JH, Neville R. Congenital vascular malformations: General diagnostic principles, *Phlebology*. 2007. 22(6): 253–257.
29. Lee BB. Advanced management of congenital vascular malformation (CVM), *Int Angiol*. 2002. 21(3): 209–213.
30. Lee BB. Statues of new approaches to the treatment of congenital vascular malformations (CVMs): Single center experiences (editorial review), *Eur. J Vasc Endovasc Surg*. 2005. 30(2): 184–197.
31. Lee BB, Mattassi R, Choe YH, et al. Critical role of duplex ultrasonography for the advanced management of a venous malformation (VM), *Phlebology*. 2005. 20: 28–37.
32. Dubois J, Patriquin HB, Garel L, et al. Soft-tissue hemangiomas in infants and children: Diagnosis using Doppler sonography, *Am J Roentgenol*. 1998. 171(1): 247–252.
33. Lee BB, Choe YH, Ahn JM, et al. The new role of MRI (Magnetic Resonance Imaging) in the contemporary diagnosis of venous malformation: Can it replace angiography?, *J Am Coll Surg*. 2004. 198(4): 549–558.
34. Rak KM, Yakes WF, Ray RL, et al. MR imaging of symptomatic peripheral vascular malformations, *Am J Roentgenol*. 1992. 159: 107–112.
35. Lee BB, Mattassi R, Kim BT, Kim DI, Ahn JM, Choi JY. Contemporary diagnosis and management of venous and AV

shunting malformation by whole body blood pool scintigraphy (WBBPS), *Int. Angiol.* 2004. *23*(4): 355–367.

36. Inoue Y, Wakita S, Ohtake T, et al. Use of whole-body imaging using Tc-99m RBC in patients with soft-tissue vascular lesions, *Clin Nucl Med.* 1996. *21*(12): 958–959.

37. Lee BB, Mattassi R, Kim BT, Park JM. Advanced management of arteriovenous shunting malformation with Transarterial Lung Perfusion Scintigraphy (TLPS) for follow up assessment, *Int Angiol.* 2005. *24*(2): 173–184.

38. Lee BB. Mastery of vascular and endovascular surgery. In: Zelenock GB, Huber TS, Messina LM, Lumsden AB, Moneta GL, eds. *Arteriovenous malformation.* Philadelphia, PA: Lippincott, Williams, and Wilkins. 2006. Ch 76, 597–607.

39. Lee BB, Bergan, JJ. New clinical and laboratory staging systems to improve management of chronic lymphedema, *Lymphology.* 2005. *38*(3): 122–129.

40. Choi JY, Hwang JH, Park JM, et al. Risk assessment of dermato-lymphangioadenitis by lymphoscintigraphy in patients with lower extremity lymphedema, *Kor J Nucl Med.* 1999. *33*(2): 143–151.

41. Lee BB, Bergan J, Gloviczki P, et al. Diagnosis and treatment of venous malformations: Consensus document of the International Union of Phlebology (IUP)-2009, *Int Angiol.* 2009. *28*(6): 434–451.

42. Summary of guideline of American venous forum. In: Gloviczki P, ed. *Handbook of venous disorders,* 3e. London: Hodder Arnold. 2008. 706–722.

43. Guyatt GH, Oxman AD, Vist GE, et al. GRADE: An emerging consensus on rating quality of evidence and strength of recommendations, *Br Med J.* 2008. *336*: 924–926.

44. Lee BB. Congenital vascular malformation. In: Geroulakos G, van Urk H, Hobson R, eds. 2nd Ed. *Vascular surgery: Cases, questions, and commentaries.* London: Springer-Verlag. 2006. Ch 41, 377–392.

45. Lee BB, Do YS, Yakes W, et al. Management of arterial-venous shunting malformations (AVM) by surgery and embolosclerotherapy: A multidisciplinary approach, *J Vasc Surg.* 2004. *39*(3): 590–600.

46. Lee BB, Lardeo J, Neville R. Arterio-venous malformation: How much do we know?, *Phlebology.* 2009. *24*: 193–200.

47. Lee BB. Current concept of venous malformation (VM), *Phlebolymphology.* 2003. *43*: 197–203.

48. Lee BB, Do YS, Byun HS, Choo IW, Kim DI, Huh SH. Advanced management of venous malformation with ethanol sclerotherapy: Mid-term results, *J Vasc Surg.* 2003. *37*(3): 533–538.

49. Lee BB, Kim DI, Huh S, et al. New experiences with absolute ethanol sclerotherapy in the management of a complex form of congenital venous malformation, *J Vasc Surg.* 2001. *33*: 764–772.

50. Lee BB, Mattassi R, Loose D, Yakes W, Tasnadi G, Kim HH. Consensus on controversial issues in contemporary diagnosis and management of congenital vascular malformation: Seoul communication, *Int J Angiol.* 2004. *13*(4): 182–192.

51. Lee BB, Kim HH, Mattassi R, Yakes W, Loose D, Tasnadi G. A new approach to the congenital vascular malformation with new concept: Seoul consensus. *Int J Angiol.* 2003. *12*: 248–251.

52. Lee BB, Kim YW, Seo JM, et al. Current concepts in lymphatic malformation (LM), *J Vasc Endovasc Surg.* 2005. *39*(1): 67–81.

53. Lee BB. Lymphedema-angiodysplasia syndrome: A prodigal form of lymphatic malformation (LM), *Phlebolymphology.* 2005. *47*: 324–332.

54. Lee BB, Bergan JJ. Advanced management of congenital vascular malformations: A multidisciplinary approach, *Cardiovasc Surg.* 2002. *10*(6): 523–533.

55. Mattassi R. Surgical treatment of congenital arteriovenous defects, *Int Angiol.* 1990. *9*: 196–202.

56. Loose DA, Weber J. Indications and tactics for a combined treatment of congenital vascular malformations. In: Balas P, ed. *Progress in angiology.* Turin, Italy: Minerva Medica. 1992. 373–378.

57. Loose DA, Weber J. *Indications and tactics for a combined treatment of congenital vascular malformations: Angiology.* Turin, Italy: Minerva Medica. 1991. 373–378.

58. Park JH, Kim DI, Huh S, Lee SJ, Do YS, Lee BB. Absolute ethanol sclerotherapy on cystic lymphangioma in neck and shoulder region, *J Korean Vasc Surg Soc.* 1998. *14*(2): 300–303.

59. Yakes WF, Haas DK, Parker SH, et al. Symptomatic vascular malformations: Ethanol embolotherapy, *Radiology.* 1989. *170*: 1059–1066.

60. Weber J. Embolizing materials and catheter techniques for angiotherapeutic management of the AVM. In: Belov S, Loose DA, Weber J, eds. *Vascular malformations.* Reinbek, Germany: Einhorn-Presse Verlag. 1989. Vol 16, 252–260.

61. Lee BB. Current concept of venous malformation (VM), *Phlebolymphology.* 2003. *43*: 197–203.

62. Lee BB, Kim DI, Do YS, Choo IW. Congenital vascular malformation. In: Geroulakos G, van Urk H, Hobson R, eds. *Vascular surgery: Cases, questions, and commentaries.* London: Springer-Verlag. 2003. Ch 40, 315–323.

63. Yamaki T, Nozaki M, Fujiwara O, Yoshida E. Duplex-guided foam sclerotherapy for the treatment of the symptomatic venous malformations of the face, *Dermatol Surg.* 2002. *28*(7): 619–622.

64. Pascarella L, Mekenas L, Bergan J. Venous disorders: Treatment with sclerosant foam, *J Cardiovasc Surg.* 2006. *47*(1): 9–18.

65. Cabrera J, Cabrera J Jr, Garcia-Olmedo MA, Redondo P. Treatment of venous malformations with sclerosant in microfoam form, *Arch Dermatol.* 2003. *139*(11): 1409–1416.

66. Lee BB, Bergan J. Transition from alcohol to foam sclerotherapy for localized venous malformation with high risk. In: Bergan J, Cheng VL, eds. *A textbook: Foam sclerotherapy.* London: Royal Society of Medicine Press. Ch 12, 129–139.

INDEX

ultrasound therapy, MIST, 534
unfractionated heparin (UFH), 297. *See also* heparin
  for venous thromboembolism prophylaxis after surgery, 308, 311–15
unfractionated heparin (UFH) therapy for deep vein thrombosis, 319–20
  complications of, 320–21
upper extremity superficial veins, anatomy of, 21f
upper extremity veins, anatomy of, 20–21
ureteric vein reflux, 256

V

valve reconstruction, postoperative care after, 512
valve remodeling, 96–97
  produces distal venous hypertension, 463
valve repair. *See also* valvuloplasty
  internal vs. external, 492
  original technique of external, 496f
  results of internal, 492t
valves. *See also* valvuloplasty
  distribution of primary incompetent, 490–91
  failure in chronic venous insufficiency, 40–41
  historical perspective on, 14, 486
  physiology, 39–40
  prosthetic, 499
    animal studies, 499–501
    autogenous valve studies, 501–2
    clinical trials, 500–502
    endovascular surgery, 502–3
    prospects, 502–3
    rationale, 499
valve substitution techniques, 488f
valve surgery, history of, 14, 486–87
valvular hypothesis vs. parietal hypothesis, 203, 204
valvular incompetence. *See* venous reflux
valvular insufficiency. *See* venous reflux
valvular regurgitation. *See* venous reflux
valvuloplasty. *See also* valves
  clinical contributions to the experience of deep vein valve repair, 491–92
  complications, 496
  historical perspective on, 14, 486–87
  influence on the management of CVD, 492–93
  influence on the study of venous disease, 488–90
  outcomes, 492, 492t, 495
  perspective on the value of surgical repair in deep vein valves, 496
  postthrombotic syndrome management, 508–10
  preoperative evaluation, 493–95
  for reflux, 436, 436t

surgical considerations arising from deep vein reflux patterns, 491
surgical considerations in repair of deep vein reflux disease, 493–95
transcommissural, 509, 509f
varicose ulcers. *See* ulcers
varicose veins (VV), 27, 31. *See also* saphenous stripping; sclerotherapy
  defined, 88
  genetics, 67–68
  history of study of, 5–6
  management of postsurgical recurrent, 157
  pathophysiology
    animal models of venous hypertension and, 60
    apoptosis alterations, 59–60
    macroscopic alterations, 67–69
    matrix metalloproteinases, 58–59
    smooth muscle cell, dermal fibroblast, and collagen alterations, 59
    vein wall anatomy, histopathology, and functional alterations, 68–69
  phlebectomy. *See* ambulatory phlebectomy; TriVex
  recurrence. *See* neovascularization; recurrent varicose veins
  risk factors, 96t
  surgery, 183–84
  symptoms, 98t
  treatment indications, 186t, 186–87
  treatment principles, 183–84
vasa vasorum, dilation of small advential vessels in, 195–96
vascular endothelial growth factor (VEGF), 75
VEGF. *See* vascular endothelial growth factor
VEINES. *See* Venous Insufficiency Epidemiological and Economic Study
vein of Giacomini, 228
  bidirectional flow in, 229
vein sizes, limb position and, 103t
vein wall remodeling, thrombus resolution and, 273–74
Velpeau, Louis Marie, 10–11
vena cava filter. *See* inferior vena cava filter
Vena Tech (VT) filters, 360, 373f
Vena Tech low profile filter, 360
veno-active drugs (VADs), 515–16
  efficacy, 517–22, 518t, 519t
venography. *See also* popliteal vein entrapment
  axillosubclavian venous thrombosis and, 410, 410f
  first contrastless venography by multislice CT, 7f
  postthrombotic syndrome and, 506–7
venous anatomy, first systematic description of, 3–4, 4f

Venous Clinical Severity Score (VCSS), 243t, 244, 248t
venous disease, signs of, 141t
venous disorders
  physiologic testing in, 45–49
  proposals for evaluation of, 8t
venous filling time (VFT), 508
venous incompetence. *See* venous reflux
venous insufficiency, 136. *See also* venous reflux; *specific topics*
  treatment, 136
    nonsurgical, 137
    surgical, 136–37
Venous Insufficiency Epidemiological and Economic Study (VEINES), 249
venous leg ulcer (VLU), 435, 528. *See also* wounds
  approach to, 528, 530t
  growth factors and, 535
  meta-analysis of micronized purified flavonoid fraction as adjunctive therapy in, 520–21
  recalcitrant ulcers that persist despite optimization, 536
  treatment, 528, 530t, 534–35
    compression, 529
    debridement, 531
    pharmacologic, 533–34
    targeting the source of venous reflux, 529
    topical dressings, 531–33, 533t
    wound infection and antibiotics, 529, 531
venous malformations (VMs), 541
  diagnosis, 543–44, 544t
  etiology, 542–43
  management
    multidiscliplinary approach, 545, 547
    principle of, 544–45
    treatment indications, 545t
    treatment modalities, 545t
  a new concept with new classification, 541–42
venous obliteration, techniques for, 10f
venous physiology, 39–40
venous pump, compression therapy and, 82–83
venous refilling time (VRT), measurement and diagnostics, 45
venous reflux
  compression therapy and, 82–83
  interrogation points for examination of, 147t
  isolated primary deep vein reflux, 437
  ultrasound examination of, 141–42, 175–76
venous stasis
  as an inappropriate term, 463–64
  defined, 463–64
venous stasis theory, 69

venous stasis ulcer. *See* venous leg ulcer
venous surgery. *See* surgery
venous system, histology of, 18–19
venous thrombectomy. *See* thrombectomy
venous thromboembolism (VTE). *See also* deep vein thrombosis; hypercoagulable states; pulmonary embolism
  clinical signs, symptoms, and events associated with, 297t
  prevention/prophylaxis, 284–87
    after surgery, 306–15
venous thrombosis. *See* thrombosis, venous
venous ulceration. *See* ulcers
venous volume (VV)
  compression therapy and, 82
  measurement, 45
Venturi effect, 402f
Vesalius, André
  omissions, 4–5
  on venous anatomy, 3–4, 4f
  venous system according to, 4f
vitamin K
  biology, 321–23
  interruption, 323
  warfarin reversal, 323
vitamin K antagonists, 321
  long-term treatment of VTE using, 321–22
VNUS Closure. *See* radiofrequency ablation
VRT. *See* venous refilling time
VTE. *See* venous thromboembolism
vulval varicosities, 256
VV. *See* varicose veins; venous volume

W

warfarin
  duration of therapy
    first episode venous thromboembolism, 322
    recurrent VTE and, 322–23
  heparin-induced thrombocytopenia and, 336–37
  laboratory monitoring and therapeutic range, 321
  overanticoagulation
    bleeding risks, 323
    management, 323
  as vitamin K antagonist, 321
warfarin-induced skin necrosis, 280
Weibel-Palade bodies (WPBs), 269–70, 270f
white atrophy, defined, 89
wounds. *See also* venous leg ulcer
  surgical strategies for management of chronic, 535–36

X

xenograft, 535
X-Sizer, and percutaneous mechanical thrombectomy, 404